The GALE ENCYCLOPEDIA of CANCER

A GUIDE TO CANCER AND ITS TREATMENTS

THIRD EDITION

The GALE ENCYCLOPEDIA of CANCER

A GUIDE TO CANCER AND ITS TREATMENTS

THIRD EDITION

VOLUME

1

A–K

JACQUELINE L. LONGE, EDITOR

GALE
CENGAGE Learning™

Detroit • New York • San Francisco • New Haven, Conn • Waterville, Maine • London

Gale Encyclopedia of Cancer: A Guide To Cancer And Its Treatments

Project Editors: Jacqueline L. Longe

Editorial: Kristin Key

Product Manager: Kate Hanley

Editorial Support Services: Andrea Lopeman

Indexing Services: Factiva, a Dow Jones Company

Rights Acquisition and Management: Margaret Abendroth, Dean Dauphinais, and Savannah Gignac

Composition: Evi Abou-El-Seoud

Manufacturing: Wendy Blurton

Imaging: John Watkins

Product Design: Pam Galbreath

For product information and technology assistance, contact us at **Gale Customer Support, 1-800-877-4253.** For permission to use material from this text or product, submit all requests online at **www.cengage.com/permissions.** Further permissions questions can be emailed to **permissionrequest@cengage.com**

While every effort has been made to ensure the reliability of the information presented in this publication, Gale, a part of Cengage Learning, does not guarantee the accuracy of the data contained herein. Gale accepts no payment for listing; and inclusion in the publication of any organization, agency, institution, publication, service, or individual does not imply endorsement of the editors or publisher. Errors brought to the attention of the publisher and verified to the satisfaction of the publisher will be corrected in future editions.

Library of Congress Cataloging-in-Publication Data

The Gale encyclopedia of cancer : a guide to cancer and its treatments. -- 3rd ed. / Jacqueline L. Longe, editor.
   p. ; cm.
   Other title: Encyclopedia of cancer
   Includes bibliographical references and index.
   ISBN-13: 978-1-4144-7598-1 (set)
   ISBN-13: 978-1-4144-7599-8 (vol. 1)
   ISBN-13: 978-1-4144-7600-1 (vol. 2)
   ISBN-10: 1-4144-7598-5 (set)
   [etc.]
   1. Cancer--Encyclopedias. 2. Oncology--Encyclopedias. I. Longe, Jacqueline L. II. Title: Encyclopedia of cancer.
   [DNLM: 1. Neoplasms--Encyclopedias--English. 2. Medical Oncology--Encyclopedias--English. QZ 13 G151 2010]

   RC254.5.G353 2010
   616.99'4003--dc22
                      2010002075

Gale
27500 Drake Rd.
Farmington Hills, MI, 48331-3535

ISBN-13: 978-1-4144-7598-1 (set)   ISBN-10: 1-4144-7598-5 (set)
ISBN-13: 978-1-4144-7599-8 (vol. 1)   ISBN-10: 1-4144-7599-3 (vol. 1)
ISBN-13: 978-1-4144-7600-1 (vol. 2)   ISBN-10: 1-4144-7600-0 (vol. 2)

This title is also available as an e-book.
ISBN-13: 978-1-4144-7601-8 ISBN-10: 1-4144-7601-9
Contact your Gale, a part of Cengage Learning sales representative for ordering information.

Printed in China by China Translation & Printing Services Limited
1 2 3 4 5 6 7 11 10

CONTENTS

LIST OF ENTRIES

R

Radiation dermatitis
Radiation therapy
Radical neck dissection
Radiofrequency ablation
Radiopharmaceuticals
Raloxifene
Receptor analysis
Reconstructive surgery
Rectal cancer
Rectal resection
Renal pelvis tumors
Retinoblastoma
Revtositumomab
Rhabdomyosarcoma
Richter's syndrome
Rituximab

S

Salivary gland tumors
Sarcoma
Sargramostim
Saw palmetto
Scopolamine
Screening test
Second cancers
Second-look surgery
Segmentectomy
Semustine
Sentinel lymph node biopsy
Sentinel lymph node mapping
Sexual dysfunction in cancer patients
Sexuality
Sezary syndrome
Sigmoidoscopy
Sirolimus
Sjogren's syndrome
Skin cancer
Skin cancer, non-melanoma
Small intestine cancer
Smoking cessation
Soft tissue sarcoma
Sorafenib

Spinal axis tumors
Spinal cord compression
Splenectomy
Squamous cell carcinoma of the skin
Stenting
Stereotactic needle biopsy
Stereotactic surgery
Stomach cancer
Stomatitis
Streptozocin
Substance abuse
Sunitinib
Sun's soup
Superior vena cava syndrome
Supratentorial primitive
  neuroectodermal tumors
Suramin
Syndrome of inappropriate
  antidiuretic hormone

T

Tacrolimus
Tamoxifen
Taste alteration
Temozolomide
Temsirolimus
Teniposide
Testicular cancer
Testicular self-exam
Testolactone
Testosterone
Tetrahydrocannabinol
Thalidomide
Thioguanine
Thiotepa
Thoracentesis
Thoracic surgery
Thoracoscopy
Thoracotomy
Thrombocytopenia
Thrombopoietin
Thrush
Thymic cancer
Thymoma
Thyroid cancer
Thyroid nuclear medicine scan

Topotecan
Toremifene
Tositumomab
Tracheostomy
Transfusion therapy
Transitional care
Transitional cell carcinoma
Transurethral bladder resection
Transvaginal ultrasound
Transverse myelitis
Trastuzumab
Tretinoin
Trichilemmal carcinoma
Trimetrexate
Triple negative breast cancer
Triptorelin pamoate
Tube enterostomy
Tumor grading
Tumor lysis syndrome
Tumor markers
Tumor necrosis factor
Tumor staging

U

Ultrasonography
Upper gastrointestinal endoscopy
Upper GI series
Ureterosigmoidoscopy
Ureterostomy, cutaneous
Urethral cancer
Urostomy

V

Vaccines
Vaginal cancer
Valrubicin
Vascular access
Vinblastine
Vincristine
Vindesine
Vinorelbine
Vitamins
Von Hippel-Lindau disease

PLEASE READ—IMPORTANT INFORMATION

The *Gale Encyclopedia of Cancer: A Guide To Cancer And Its Treatments* is a health reference product designed to inform and educate readers about a wide variety of cancers, diseases and conditions related to cancers, nutrition and dietary practices beneficial to cancer patients, and various cancer treatments including drug treatments. Cengage Learning believes the product to be comprehensive, but not necessarily definitive. It is intended to supplement, not replace, consultation with a physician or other healthcare practitioners. While Cengage Learning has made substantial efforts to provide information that is accurate, comprehensive, and up-to-date, Cengage Learning makes no representations or warranties of any kind, including without limitation, warranties of merchantability or fitness for a particular purpose, nor does it guarantee the accuracy, comprehensiveness, or timeliness of the information contained in this product. Readers should be aware that the universe of medical knowledge is constantly growing and changing, and that differences of opinion exist among authorities. Readers are also advised to seek professional diagnosis and treatment for any medical condition, and to discuss information obtained from this book with their healthcare provider.

INTRODUCTION

The *Gale Encyclopedia of Cancer: A Guide to Cancer and Its Treatments* is a unique and invaluable source of information for anyone touched by cancer. This collection of over 450 entries provides in-depth coverage of specific cancer types, diagnostic procedures, treatments, cancer side effects, and cancer drugs. In addition, entries have been included to facilitate understanding of common cancer-related concepts, such as cancer biology, carcinogenesis, and cancer genetics, as well as cancer issues such as clinical trials, home health care, fertility issues, and cancer prevention. This encyclopedia minimizes medical jargon and uses language that laypersons can understand, while still providing thorough coverage that will benefit health science students as well.

Scope

Entries follow a standardized format that provides information at a glance. Rubrics include:

Cancer types
- Definition
- Description
- Demographics
- Causes and symptoms
- Diagnosis
- Treatment team
- Clincial staging, treatments, and prognosis
- Coping with cancer treatment
- Clinical trials
- Prevention
- Special concerns
- Resources
- Key terms

Cancer drugs
- Definition
- Purpose

- Description
- Recommended dosage
- Precautions
- Side effects
- Interactions
    Drugs, herbs, vitamins
- Definition
- Description
- Recommended dosage
- Precautions
- Side effects
- Interactions
- Caregiver concerns
- "Questions to ask the doctor"
- Resources
- Key Terms

Inclusion criteria

A preliminary list of cancers and related topics was compiled from a wide variety of sources, including professional medical guides and textbooks, as well as consumer guides and encyclopedias. The advisory board, made up of medical doctors and oncology pharmacists, evaluated the topics and made suggestions for inclusion. Final selection of topics to include was made by the advisory board in conjunction with the Gale editor.

About the contributors

The essays were compiled by experienced medical writers, including physicians, pharmacists, nurses, and other health care professionals. The advisors reviewed the completed essays to ensure that they are appropriate, up-to-date, and medically accurate.

How to use this book

The *Gale Encyclopedia of Cancer* has been designed with ready reference in mind.

- Straight **alphabetical arrangement** of topics allows users to locate information quickly.

- **Bold-faced terms** within entries direct the reader to related articles.

- **Cross-references** placed throughout the encyclopedia direct readers from alternate names and related topics to entries.

- A list of **key terms** is provided where appropriate to define unfamiliar terms or concepts.

- A list of **questions to ask the doctor** is provided whenever appropriate to help facilitate discussion with the patient's physician.

- The **Resources** section for non-drug entries directs readers to additional sources of medical information on a topic.

- Valuable **contact information** for organizations and support groups is included with each cancer type entry. Appendix II at the back of Volume 2 contains an extensive list of organizations arranged in alphabetical order.

- A comprehensive **general index** guides readers to all topics mentioned in the text.

- A note about **drug entries**: Drug entries are listed in alphabetical order by common **generic names**. However, because many oncology drugs have more than one common generic name, and because in many cases, the brand name is also often used interchangeably with a generic name, drugs can be located in one of three ways. The reader can: find the generic drug name in alphabetical order, be directed to the entry from an alternate name cross-reference, or the reader can use the **index** to look up a **brand name**, which will direct the reader to the equivalent generic name entry. If the reader would like more information about oncology drugs than these entries provide, the reader is encouraged to consult with a physician, pharmacist, or the reader may find helpful any one of a number of books about cancer drugs. Two that may be helpful are: D. Solimando's *Drug Information Handbook for Oncology*, or R. Ellerby's *Quick Reference Handbook of Oncology Drugs*.

Graphics

The *Gale Encyclopedia of Cancer* is also enhanced by color photographs, illustrations, and tables.

FOREWORD

Unfortunately, humans must suffer disease. Some diseases are totally reversible and can be effectively treated. Moreover, some diseases with proper treatment have been virtually annihilated, such as polio, rheumatic fever, smallpox, and, to some extent, tuberculosis. Other diseases seem to target one organ, such as the heart, and there has been great progress in either fixing defects, adding blood flow, or giving medications to strengthen the diseased pump. Cancer, however, continues to frustrate even the cleverest of doctors or the most fastidious of health conscious individuals. Why?

By its very nature, cancer is a survivor. It has only one purpose: to proliferate. After all, that is the definition of cancer: unregulated growth of cells that fail to heed the message to stop growing. Normal cells go through a cycle of division, aging, and then selection for death. Cancer cells are able to circumvent this normal cycle, and escape recognition to be eliminated.

There are many mechanisms that can contribute to this unregulated cell growth. One of these mechanisms is inheritance. Unfortunately, some individuals can be programmed for cancer due to inherited disorders in their genetic makeup. In its simplest terms, one can inherit a faulty gene or a missing gene whose role is to eliminate damaged cells or to prevent imperfect cells from growing. Without this natural braking system, the damaged cells can divide and lead to more damaged cells with the same abnormal genetic makeup as the parent cells. Given enough time, and our inability to detect them, these groups of cells can grow to a size that will cause discomfort or other symptoms.

Inherited genetics are obviously not the only source of abnormalities in cells. Humans do not live in a sterile world devoid of environmental attacks or pathogens. Humans must work, and working environments can be dangerous. Danger can come in the form of radiation, chemicals, or fibers to which we may be chronically exposed with or without our knowledge. Moreover, man must eat, and if our food is contaminated with these environmental hazards, or if we prepare our food in a way that may change the chemical nature of the food to hazardous molecules, then chronic exposure to these toxins could damage cells. Finally, man is social. He has found certain habits which are pleasing to him because they either relax him or release his inhibitions. Such habits, including smoking and alcohol consumption, can have a myriad of influences on the genetic makeup of cells.

Why the emphasis on genes in the new century? Because they are potentially the reason as well as the answer for cancer. Genes regulate our micro- and macrosopic events by eventually coding for proteins that control our structure and function. If the above-mentioned environmental events cause errors in those genes that control growth, then imperfect cells can start to take root. For the majority of cases, a whole cascade of genetic events must occur before a cell is able to outlive its normal predecessors. This cascade of events could take years to occur, in a silent, undetected manner until the telltale signs and symptoms of advanced cancer are seen, including pain, lack of appetite, cough, loss of blood, or the detection of a lump. How did these cells get to this state where they are now dictating the everyday physical, psychological, and economic events for the person afflicted?

At this time, the sequence of genetic catastrophes is much too complex to comprehend or summarize because, it is only in the past year that we have even been able to map what genes we have and where they are located in our chromosomes. We have learned, however, that cancer cells are equipped with a series of self-protection mechanisms. Some of the altered genes are actually able to express themselves more than in the normal situation. These genes could then code for more growth factors for the transforming cell, or they could make proteins that could keep our own immune system from eliminating these interlopers. Finally, these cells are chameleons: if we treat them with drugs to try to kill them, they can "change their colors" by mutation, and then be resistant to the drugs that may have harmed them before.

Then what do we do for treatment? Man has always had a fascination with grooming, and grooming involves removal—dirt, hair, waste. The ultimate removal involves cutting away the spoiled or imperfect portion. An abnormal growth? Remove it by surgery . . . make sure the edges are clean. Unfortunately, the painful reality of cancer surgery is that it is highly effective when performed in the early stages of the disease. "Early stages of the disease" implies that there is no spread, or, hopefully, before there are symptoms. In the majority of cases, however, surgery cannot eradicate all the disease because the cancer is not only at the primary site of the lump, but has spread to other organs. Cancer is not just a process of growth, but also a metastasizing process that allows for invasion and spread. The growing cells need nourishment so they secrete proteins that allow for the growth of blood vessels (angiogenesis); once the blood vessels are established from other blood vessels, the tumor cells can make proteins that will dissolve the imprisoning matrix surrounding them. Once this matrix is dissolved, it is only a matter of time before thecancer cells will migrate to other places making the use of surgery fruitless.

Since cancer cells have a propensity to leave home and pay a visit to other organs, therapies must be geared to treat the whole body and not just the site of origin. The problem with these chemotherapies is that they are not selective and wreak havoc on tissues that are not affected by the cancer. These therapies are not natural to the human host, and result in nausea, loss of appetite, fatigue, as well as a depletion in our cells that protect us from infection and those that carry oxygen. Doctors who prescribe such medications walk a fine line between helping the patient (causing a "response" in the cancer by making it smaller) or causing "toxicity" which, due to effects on normal organs, causes the patient problems. Although these drugs are far from perfect, we are fortunate to have them because when they work, their results can be remarkable.

But that's the problem—"when they work." We cannot predict who is going to benefit from our therapies, and doctors must inform the patient and his/her family about countless studies that have been done to validate the use of these potentially beneficial/potentially harmful agents. Patients must suffer the frustration that oncologists have because each individual afflicted with cancer is different, and indeed, each cancer is different. This makes it virtually impossible to personalize an individual's treatment expectations and life expectancy. Cancer, after all, is a very impersonal disease, and does not respect sex, race, wealth, age, or any other "human" characteristics.

Cancer treatment is in search of "smart" options. Like modern-day instruments of war, successful cancer treatment will necessitate the construction of therapies which can do three basic tasks: search out the enemy, recognize the enemy, and kill the enemy without causing "friendly fire." The successful therapies of the future will involve the use of "living components," "manufactured components," or a combination of both. Living components, white blood cells, will be educated to recognize where the cancer is, and help our own immune system fight the foreign cells. These lymphocytes can be educated to recognize signals on the cancer cell which make them unique. Therapies in the future will be able to manufacture molecules with these signature, unique signals which are linked to other molecules specifically for killing the cells. Only the cancer cells are eliminated in this way, hopefully sparing the individual from toxicity.

Why use these unique signals as delivery mechanisms? If they are unique and are important for growth of the cancer cell, why not target them directly? This describes the ambitious mission of gene therapy, whose goal is to supplement a deficient, necessary genetic pool or diminish the number of abnormally expressed genes fortifying the cancer cells. If a protein is not being made that slows the growth of cells, gene therapy would theoretically supply the gene for this protein to replenish it and cause the cells to slow down. If the cells can make their own growth factors that sustain them selectively over normal cells, then the goal is to block the production of this growth factor. There is no doubt that gene therapy is the wave of the future and is under intense investigation and scrutiny at present. The problem, however, is that there is no way to tell when this future promise will be fulfilled.

No book can describe the medical, psychological, social, and economic burden of cancer, and if this is your first confrontation with the enemy, you may find yourself overwhelmed with its magnitude. Books are only part of the solution. Newly enlisted recruits in this war must seek proper counsel from educated physicians who will inform the family and the patient of the risks and benefits of a treatment course in a way that can be understood. Advocacy groups of dedicated volunteers, many of whom are cancer survivors, can guide and advise. The most important component, however, is an intensely personal one. The afflicted individual must realize that he/she is responsible for charting the course of his/her disease, and this requires the above described knowledge as well as great personal intuition. Cancer comes as a series of shocks: the symptoms, the diagnosis, and the treatment. These shocks can be followed by cautious optimism or profound disappointment. Each one of these shocks either reinforces or chips away at one's resolve, and how an individual reacts to these issues is as unique as the cancer that is being dealt with.

While cancer is still life-threatening, strides have been made in the fight against the disease. Thirty years ago, a young adult diagnosed with testicular cancer had few options for treatment that could result in cure. Now, chemotherapy for good risk Stage II and III testicular cancer can result in a complete response of the tumor in 98% of the cases and a durable response in 92%. Sixty years ago, there were no regimens that could cause a complete remission for a child diagnosed with leukemia; but now, using combination chemotherapy, complete remissions are possible in 96% of these cases. Progress has been made, but more progress is needed. The first real triumph in cancer care will be when cancer is no longer thought of as a life-ending disease, but as a chronic disease whose symptoms can be managed. Anyone who has been touched by cancer or who has been involved in the fight against it lives in hope that that day will arrive.

Helen A. Pass, M.D., F.A.C.S.
Director, Breast Care Center
William Beaumont Hospital
Royal Oak, Michigan

ADVISORS

A number of experts in the medical community provided invaluable assistance in the formulation of this encyclopedia. Our advisory board performed a myriad of duties, from defining the scope of coverage to reviewing individual entries for accuracy and accessibility. The editor would like to express her appreciation to them.

Melinda Granger Oberleitner, R.N., D.N.S.
*Acting Department Head
    and Associate Professor*
Department of Nursing
University of Louisiana
    at Lafayette
Lafayette, Louisiana

Helen A. Pass, M.D., F.A.C.S.
Director, Breast Care Center

William Beaumont Hospital
Royal Oak, Michigan

Marianne Vahey, M.D.
Clinical Instructor in Medicine
Yale University School
    of Medicine
New Haven, Connecticut

James E. Waun, M.D., M.A., R. Ph..
Associate Clinical Professor

Department of Family Practice
Faculty
Center for Ethics and the
    Humanities
Michigan State University
*Adjunct Assistant Professor
    of Clinical Pharmacy*
Ferris State University
East Lansing, Michigan

CONTRIBUTORS

Margaret Alic, Ph.D.
Science Writer
Eastsound, Washington

Lisa Andres, M.S., C.G.C.
*Certified Genetic Counselor
    and Medical Writer*
San Jose, California

Racquel Baert, M.Sc.
Medical Writer
Winnipeg, Canada

Julia R. Barrett
Science Writer
Madison, Wisconsin

Maria Basile, PhD
Neuropharmacologist
Neward, New Jersey

Nancy J. Beaulieu, RPh., B.C.O.P.
Oncology Pharmacist
New Haven, Connecticut

Linda K. Bennington, C.N.S., M.S.N.
Clinical Nurse Specialist
Department of Nursing
Old Dominion University
Norfolk, Virginia

Kenneth J. Berniker, M.D.
Attending Physician
Emergency Department
Kaiser Permanente Medical Center
Vallejo, California

Olga Bessmertny, Pharm.D.
Clinical Pharmacy Manager
Pediatric Hematology/Oncology/
    Bone Marrow Transplant
Children's Hospital of New York
Columbia Presbyterian Medical
    Center
New York, New York

Patricia L. Bounds, Ph.D.
Science Writer
Zürich, Switzerland

Cheryl Branche, M.D.
Retired General Practitioner
Jackson, Mississippi

Tamara Brown, R.N.
Medical Writer
Boston, Massachusetts

Diane M. Calabrese
*Medical Sciences and
    Technology Writer*
Silver Spring, Maryland

Rosalyn Carson-DeWitt, M.D.
Durham, North Carolina

Lata Cherath, Ph.D.
Science Writer
Franklin Park, New York

Lisa Christenson, Ph.D.
Science Writer
Hamden, Connecticut

Rhonda Cloos, R.N.
Medical Writer
Austin, Texas

David Cramer, M.D.
Medical Writer
Chicago, Illinois

Tish Davidson, A.M.
Medical Writer
Fremont, California

Dominic DeBellis, Ph.D.
Medical Writer and Editor
Mahopac, New York

Tiffani A. DeMarco, M.S.
Genetic Counselor
Cancer Control

Georgetown University
Washington, DC

Lori DeMilto
Medical Writer
Sicklerville, New York

Stefanie B. N. Dugan, M.S.
Genetic Counselor
Milwaukee, Wisconsin

Janis O. Flores
Medical Writer
Sebastopol, California

Paula Ford-Martin
Medical Writer
Chaplin, Minnesota

Rebecca J. Frey, Ph.D.
Research and Administrative Associate
East Rock Institute
New Haven, Connecticut

Jason Fryer
Medical Writer
Lubbock, Texas

Jill Granger, M.S.
Senior Research Associate
University of Michigan
Ann Arbor, Michigan

David E. Greenberg, M.D.
Medicine Resident
Baylor College of Medicine
Houston, Texas

Maureen Haggerty
Medical Writer
Ambler, Pennsylvania

Kevin Hwang, M.D.
Medical Writer
Morristown, New Jersey

Michelle L. Johnson, M.S., J.D.
Patent Attorney and Medical Writer
Portland, Oregon

Paul A. Johnson, Ed.M.
Medical Writer
San Diego, California

Cindy L. A. Jones, Ph.D.
Biomedical Writer
Sagescript Communications
Lakewood, Colorado

Crystal H. Kaczkowski, M.Sc.
Medical Writer
Montreal, Canada

David S. Kaminstein, M.D.
Medical Writer
Westchester, Pennsylvania

Beth Kapes
Medical Writer
Bay Village, Ohio

Bob Kirsch
Medical Writer
Ossining, New York

Melissa Knopper
Medical Writer
Chicago, Illinois

Monique Laberge, Ph.D.
Research Associate
Department of Biochemistry
    and Biophysics
University of Pennsylvania
Philadelphia, Pennsylvania

Jill S. Lasker
Medical Writer
Midlothian, Virginia

G. Victor Leipzig, Ph.D.
Biological Consultant
Huntington Beach,
    California

Lorraine Lica, Ph.D.
Medical Writer
San Diego, California

John T. Lohr, Ph.D.
Utah State University
Logan, Utah

Warren Maltzman, Ph.D.
Consultant, Molecular Pathology
Demarest, New Jersey

Richard A. McCartney M.D.
*Fellow, American College
    of Surgeons
Diplomat, American Board
    of Surgery*
Richland, Washington

Sally C. McFarlane-Parrott
Medical Writer
Mason, Michigan

Monica McGee, M.S.
Science Writer
Wilmington, North Carolina

Alison McTavish, M.Sc.
Medical Writer and Editor
Montreal, Quebec

Molly Metzler, R.N., B.S.N.
*Registered Nurse and
    Medical Writer*
Seaford, Delaware

Beverly G. Miller
MT(ASCP), Technical Writer
Charlotte, North Carolina

Mark A. Mitchell, M.D.
Medical Writer
Seattle, Washington

Laura J. Ninger
Medical Writer
Weehawken, New Jersey

Nancy J. Nordenson
Medical Writer
Minneapolis, Minnesota

Teresa G. Odle
Medical Writer
Albuquerque, New Mexico

Melinda Granger Oberleitner
*Acting Department Head and
    Associate Professor*
Department of Nursing
University of Louisiana
    at Lafayette
Lafayette, Louisiana

Lee Ann Paradise
Science Writer
Lubbock, Texas

J. Ricker Polsdorfer, M.D.
Medical Writer
Phoenix, Arizona

Elizabeth J. Pulcini, M.S.
Medical Writer
Phoenix, Arizona

Kulbir Rangi, D.O.
Medical Doctor and Writer
New York, New York

**Esther Csapo Rastegari, Ed.M.,
    R.N., B.S.N.**
Registered Nurse, Medical Writer
Holbrook, Masachusetts

Toni Rizzo
Medical Writer
Salt Lake City, Utah

Martha Floberg Robbins
Medical Writer
Evanston, Illinois

Richard Robinson
Medical Writer
Tucson, Arizona

**Edward R. Rosick, D.O.,
    M.P.H., M.S.**
*University Physician, Clinical
    Assistant Professor*
Student Health Services
The Pennsylvania State
    University
University Park, Pennsylvania

Nancy Ross-Flanigan
Science Writer
Belleville, Michigan

Belinda Rowland, Ph.D.
Medical Writer
Voorheesville, New York

Andrea Ruskin, M.D.
Whittingham Cancer Center
Norwalk, Connecticut

Laura Ruth, Ph.D.
*Medical, Science, & Technology
    Writer*
Los Angeles, California

Kausalya Santhanam, Ph.D.
Technical Writer
Branford, Connecticut

Marc Scanio
Doctoral Candidate in Chemistry
Stanford University
Stanford, California

Joan Schonbeck, R.N.
Medical Writer
Nursing
Massachusetts Department
   of Mental Health
Marlborough, Massachusetts

Kristen Mahoney Shannon, M.S.,
   C.G.C.
Genetic Counselor
Center for Cancer Risk Analysis
Massachusetts General Hospital
Boston, Massachusetts

Judith Sims, MS
Science Writer
Logan, Utah

Genevieve Slomski, Ph.D.
Medical Writer
New Britain, Connecticut

Anna Rovid Spickler, D.V.M., Ph.D.
Medical Writer
Salisbury, Maryland

Laura L. Stein, M.S.
Certified Genetic Counselor
Familial Cancer Program-
   Department of Hematology/
   Oncology
Dartmouth Hitchcock Medical
   Center
Lebanon, New Hampshire

Phyllis M. Stein, B.S., C.C.R.P.
Affiliate Coordinator

Grand Rapids Clinical Oncology
   Program
Grand Rapids, Michigan

Kurt Sternlof
Science Writer
New Rochelle, New York

Deanna M. Swartout-Corbeil
Registered Nurse, Freelance Writer
Thompsons Station, Tennessee

Jane M. Taylor-Jones, M.S.
Research Associate
Donald W. Reynolds Department
   of Geriatrics
University of Arkansas for
   Medical Sciences
Little Rock, Arkansas

Carol Turkington
Medical Writer
Lancaster, Pennsylvania

Samuel Uretsky, PharmD
Medical Writer
Wantagh, New York

Marianne Vahey, M.D.
Clinical Instructor
Medicine
Yale University School of Medicine
New Haven, Connecticut

Malini Vashishtha, Ph.D.
Medical Writer
Irvine, California

Ellen S. Weber, M.S.N.
Medical Writer
Fort Wayne, Indiana

Ken R. Wells
Freelance Writer
Laguna Hills, California

Barbara Wexler, M.P.H.
Medical Writer
Chatsworth, California

Wendy Wippel, M.Sc.
*Medical Writer and Adjunct
   Professor of Biology*
Northwest Community College
Hernando, Mississippi

Debra Wood, R.N.
Medical Writer
Orlando, Florida

Kathleen D. Wright, R.N.
Medical Writer
Delmar, Delaware

Jon Zonderman
Medical Writer
Orange, California

Michael V. Zuck, Ph.D.
Writer
Boulder, Colorado

ILLUSTRATIONS OF BODY SYSTEMS

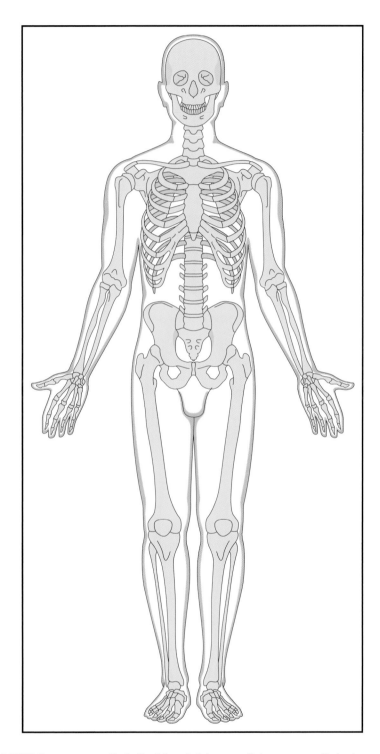

HUMAN SKELETON and SKIN. Some cancers that affect the skeleton are: Osteosarcoma; Ewing's sarcoma; Fibrosarcoma (can also be found in soft tissues like muscle, fat, connective tissues, etc.). Some cancers that affect tissue near bones: **Chondrosarcoma** (affects joints near bones); **Rhabdomyosarcoma** (formed from cells of muscles attached to bones); **Malignant fibrous histiocytoma** (common in soft tissues, rare in bones). SKIN CANCERS: **Basal cell carcinoma**; **Melanoma**; **Merkel cell carcinoma**; **Squamous cell carcinoma of the skin**; and **Trichilemmal carcinoma**. Precancerous skin condition: **Bowen's disease**. Lymphomas that affect the skin: **Mycosis fungoides**; **Sézary syndrome**. *(Illustration by Argosy Publishing Argosy Publishing. Cengage Learning, Gale.)*

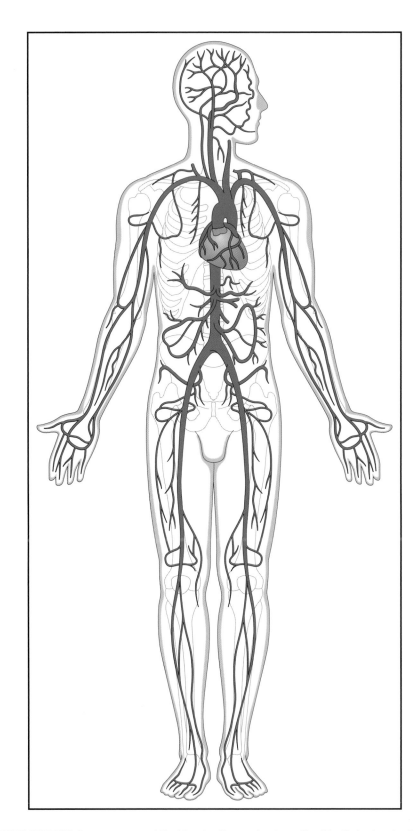

HUMAN CIRCULATORY SYSTEM. Some cancers of the blood cells are: Acute erythroblastic leukemia; Acute lymphocytic leukemia; **Acute myelocytic leukemia**; Chronic lymphocytic leukemia; Chronic myelocytic leukemia; **Hairy cell leukemia**; and **Multiple myeloma**. One condition associated with various cancers that affects blood is called **Myelofibrosis**. *(Illustration by Argosy Publishing Argosy Publishing. Cengage Learning, Gale.)*

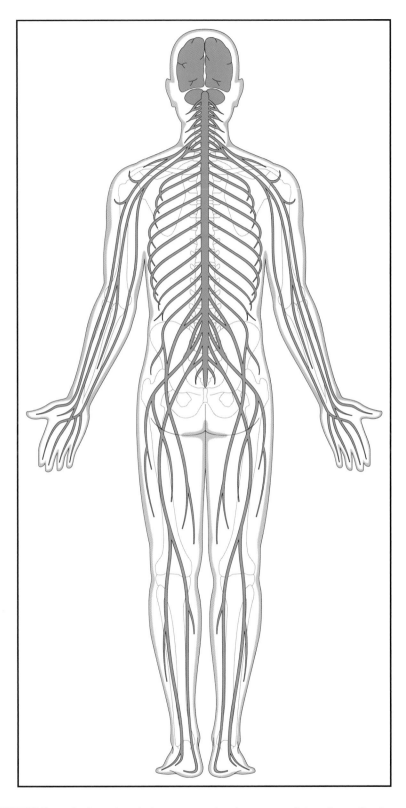

HUMAN NERVOUS SYSTEM. Some brain and central nervous system tumors are: **Astrocytoma; Carcinomatous meningitis; Central nervous system carcinoma; Central nervous system lymphoma; Chordoma; Choroid plexus tumors; Craniopharyngioma; Ependymoma; Medulloblastoma; Meningioma; Oligodendroglioma;** and **Spinal axis tumors**. One kind of noncancerous growth in the brain: **Acoustic neuroma**. *(Illustration by Argosy Publishing Argosy Publishing. Cengage Learning, Gale.)*

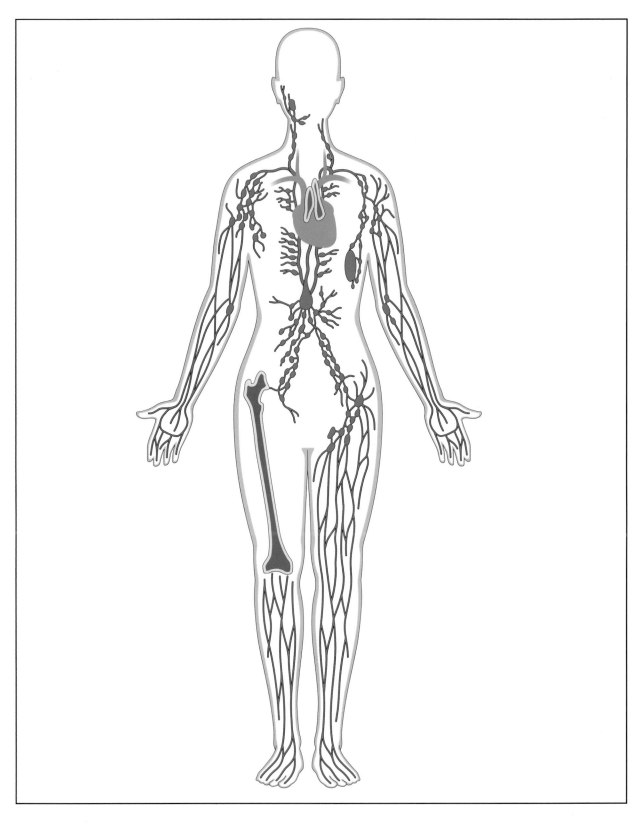

HUMAN LYMPHATIC SYSTEM. The lymphatic system and lymph nodes are shown here in pale green, the thymus in deep blue, and one of the bones rich in bone marrow (the femur) is shown here in purple. Some cancers of the lymphatic system are: Burkitt's lymphoma; Cutaneous T-cell lymphoma; Hodgkin's disease; MALT lymphoma; Mantle cell lymphoma; Sézary syndrome; and **Waldenström's macroglobulinemia**. *(Illustration by Argosy Publishing. Cengage Learning, Gale.)*

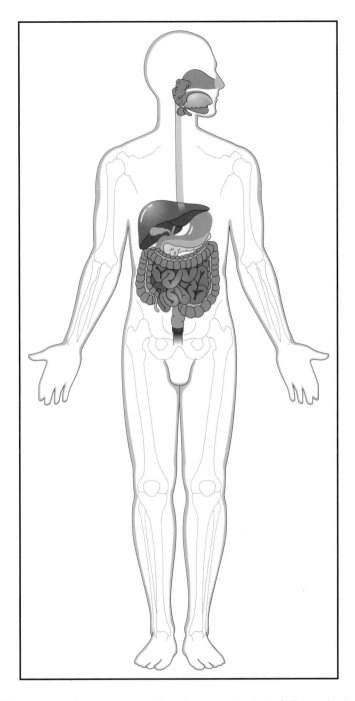

HUMAN DIGESTIVE SYSTEM. Organs and cancers of the digestive system include: Salivary glands (shown in turquoise): Salivary gland tumors. Esophagus (shown in bright yellow): **Esophageal cancer**. Liver (shown in bright red): **Bile duct cancer**; **Liver cancer**. Stomach (pale gray-blue): **Stomach cancer**. Gallbladder (bright orange against the red liver): **Gallbladder cancer**. Colon (green): **Colon cancer**. Small intestine (purple): **Small intestinal cancer**; can have malignant tumors associated with **Zollinger-Ellison syndrome**. Rectum (shown in pink, continuing the colon): **Rectal cancer**. Anus (dark blue): **Anal cancer**. *(Illustration by Argosy Publishing. Cengage Learning, Gale.)*

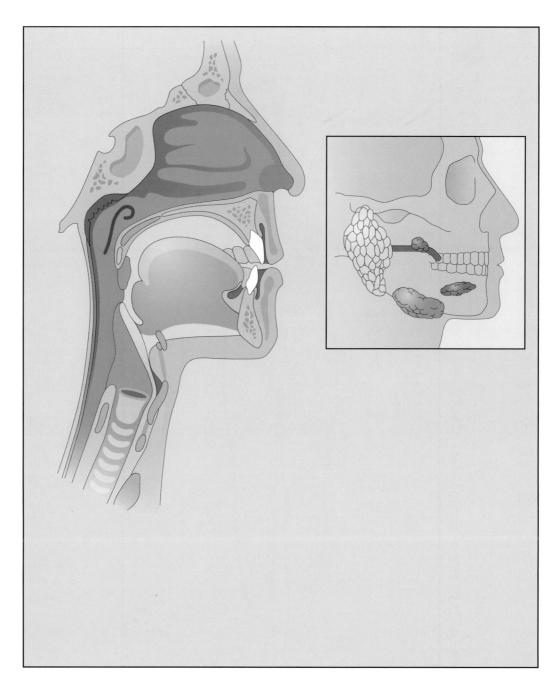

HEAD AND NECK. The pharynx, the passage that leads from the nostrils down through the neck is shown in orange. This passage is broken into several divisions. The area posterior to (behind) the nose is the nasopharynx. The area posterior to the mouth is the oropharynx. The oropharynx leads into the laryngopharynx, which opens into the esophagus (still in orange) and the larynx (shown in the large image in medium blue). Each of these regions may be affected by cancer, and the cancers include: **Nasopharyngeal cancer**; **Oropharyngeal cancer**; **Esophageal cancer**; and **Laryngeal cancer**. **Oral cancers** can affect the lips, gums, and tongue (pink). Referring to the smaller, inset picture of the salivary glands, **salivary gland tumors** can affect the parotid glands (shown here in yellow), the submandibular glands (inset picture, turquoise), and the sublingual glands (purple). *(Illustration by Argosy Publishing. Cengage Learning, Gale.)*

HUMAN ENDOCRINE SYSTEM. The glands and cancers of the endocrine system include: In the brain: the pituitary gland shown in blue (pituitary tumors), the hypothalamus in pale green, and the pineal gland in bright yellow. Throughout the rest of the body: Thyroid (shown in dark blue): **Thyroid cancer**. Parathyroid glands, four of them adjacent to the thyroid: **Parathyroid cancer**. Thymus (green): **Thymic cancer; Thymoma**. Pancreas (turquoise): **Pancreatic cancer, endocrine; Pancreatic cancer, exocrine; Zollinger-Ellison syndrome** tumors can be malignant and can be found in the pancreas. Adrenal glands (shown in apricot, above the kidneys): **Neuroblastoma** often originates in these glands; **Pheochromocytoma** tumors are often found in adrenal glands. Testes (in males, shown in yellow): **Testicular cancer**. Ovaries (in females, shown in dark blue in inset image): **Ovarian cancer**. *(Illustration by Argosy Publishing. Cengage Learning, Gale.)*

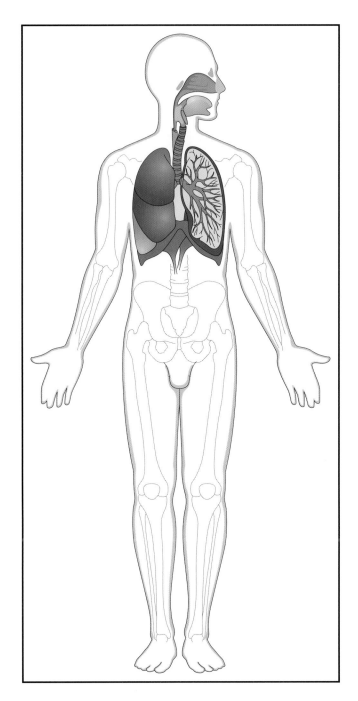

HUMAN RESPIRATORY SYSTEM. Air is breathed in through nose or mouth, enters the pharynx, shown here in orange, and passes through the larynx, shown here as a green tube with a ridged texture. (The smooth green tube shown is the esophagus, which is posterior to the larynx and which is involved in digestion instead of breathing.) The air then passes into the trachea (purple), a tube that divides into two tubes called bronchi. One bronchus passes into each lung, and continues to branch within the lung. These branches are called bronchioles and each bronchiole leads to a tiny cluster of air sacs called alveoli, where the exchange of gases occurs, so that the air and gases breathed in get diffused to the blood. The lungs (deep blue) are spongy and have lobes and can be affected by Lung cancer, both the non-small cell and small-cell types. *(Illustration by Argosy Publishing. Cengage Learning, Gale.)*

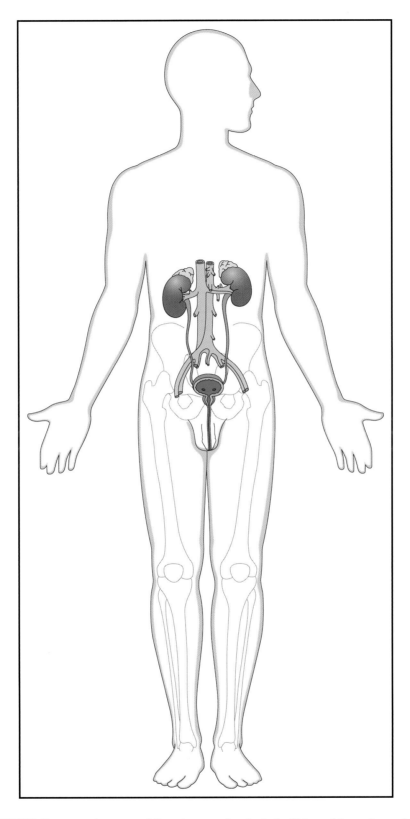

HUMAN URINARY SYSTEM. Organs and cancers of the urinary system include: Kidneys (shown in purple): Kidney cancer; **Renal pelvis tumors**; **Wilms' tumor.** Ureters are shown in green. Bladder (blue-green): **Bladder cancer**. The kidneys, bladder, or ureters can be affected by a cancer type called **Transitional cell carcinoma**. *(Illustration by Argosy Publishing. Cengage Learning, Gale.)*

FEMALE REPRODUCTIVE SYSTEM. Organs and cancers of the female reproductive system include: Uterus, shown in red with the uterine or Fallopian tubes: Endometrial cancer. Ovaries (blue): **Ovarian cancer**. Vagina (shown in pink with a yellow interior or lining): **Vaginal cancer**. Breasts: **Breast cancer**; **Paget's disease of the breast**. Shown in detailed inset only in turquoise, Cervix: **Cervical cancer**. *(Illustration by Argosy Publishing. Cengage Learning, Gale.)*

MALE REPRODCTIVE SYSTEM. Organs, glands, and cancers of the male reproductive system include: Penis (shown in pink): Penile cancer. Testes (shown in yellow): **Testicular cancer**. Prostate gland (shown in full-body illustration in a peach/ apricot color, and in the inset as the dark blue gland between the bladder and the penis): **Prostate cancer**. *(Illustration by Argosy Publishing. Cengage Learning, Gale.)*

A

2-CdA *see* **Cladribine**

5-Azacitidine *see* **Azacitidine**

5-Fluorouracil *see* **Fluorouracil**

6-Mercaptopurine *see* **Mercaptopurine**

6-Thioguanine *see* **Thioguanine**

Abarelix

Definition

Abarelix is an injectable gonadotrophin-releasing hormone (GnRH) antagonist that is used to decrease the production of the male hormone **testosterone**.

Purpose

Abarelix is used in men to treat advanced **prostate cancer** that has not responded to other treatments or when other treatments have been refused. The prostate gland lies under the bladder and surrounds the urethra. Its main function is to produce seminal fluid that mixes with sperm prior to ejaculation. Prostate **cancer** is the most common cancer in men over the age of 50.

Other treatments for prostate cancer should be tried before treatment with abarelix is prescribed. Early stage prostate cancer is often treated with surgery or **radiation therapy** and less often with **cryoablation**. Advanced stage prostate cancer may be treated with other drugs that decrease the production of testosterone. Another approach to treating advanced prostate cancer is surgical removal of the testicles (castration). Some men reject this surgery, making them candidates for treatment with abarelix.

Because abarelix can cause serious side effects, this drug is considered appropriate for use only in the following situations:

- The cancer has spread (metastasized) and is close to the spinal column, so that there is a risk that pressure will cause damage to the spinal nerves.

- The urethra or bladder is blocked because of malignant tissue growth making urination difficult or impossible.

- Prostate cancer causes severe pain in the bones that narcotic pain medication cannot control.

Description

Abarelix works by blocking gonadotropin-releasing hormone (GRH) a hormone released from the anterior pituitary gland that stimulates the production of testosterone. When this messenger hormone from the pituitary is blocked, the level of testosterone in the blood decreases. Prostate cancer cells grow best in the presence of testosterone, so by decreasing the amount available, growth of the tumor is slowed or stopped. Other drugs (**leuprolide acetate** [Lupron], **goserelin acetate** [Zoladex]) are available that also decrease testosterone production. One advantage of abarelix over these other drugs is that the other drugs used to decrease testosterone levels first stimulate the production of testosterone then decrease it. With abarelix, there is no initial increase in testosterone production and decline in production of the hormone begins immediately. However, abarelix may stop working in some men after an initial period of effectiveness. The drug does not cure prostate cancer but can relieve symptoms.

Abarelix is manufactured in the United States by Praecis Pharmaceuticals and sold under the brand name Plenaxis. Generic substitutes are not available, and there is only one American manufacturer. Abarelix was approved for use by the United States Food and Drug Administration (FDA) in December 2003 with restrictions. The drug can only be administered by doctors who are registered in the Plenaxis PLUS Program

(Plenaxis User Safety Program) because of its potentially life-threatening side effects.

Recommended dosage

Abarelix is an injectable liquid. It is supplied as powder in single dose vial to which the physician adds a small amount of saline (saltwater) before use. The resulting liquid is injected into the buttocks muscle. The treatment cycle calls for an initial injection on days 1, 15, and 29 followed by an injection every 28 days. The testosterone level of the blood should be checked after the first month and then about every eight weeks to assure that the drug is continuing to work. Liver function tests should also be done regularly, as abarelix may cause changes in the liver function. These changes are usually not permanent and go away once the drug is stopped.

Precautions

Certain individuals should not use abarelix. These include women, children under age 18, and men with a rare heart condition called prolongation of the QTc interval. Men with osteoporosis, liver disease, and blood clotting disorders should identify these existing problems to their doctor before beginning treatment. Abarelix may stop working in some men and is more likely to stop working in men weighing over 225 lb (102 kg). There are no special dietary restriction when receiving abarelix therapy.

Side effects

Abarelix can cause serious or life-threatening allergic reactions either during or after administration. Therefore, the drug can only be administered by a physician registered in the Plenaxis PLUS safety program. The likelihood of life-threatening reactions increases with each injection of abarelix. For this reason, men receiving an injection of abarelix must remain under observation in the doctor's office for at least 30 minutes following each treatment.

Symptoms of rare but life-threatening reactions include:

- low blood pressure, fainting, shock
- swelling of the face, eyelids, tongue, or throat
- wheezing, asthma, tightness in the chest, difficulty breathing

More common but less serious side effects include:

- hot flashes
- rapid heart beat (tachycardia)
- rash, hives, itching, skin redness
- vomiting
- jaundice (yellowing of the whites of the eyes or skin)
- stomach pain
- breast enlargement
- problems sleeping
- breast, back or other pain
- constipation
- changes in the electrical profile of the heart

Interactions

It is important for patients to discuss with their physician all prescription medications, over-the-counter medications, and herbal or alternative remedies that the patients are taking before treatment with abarelix is begun. Although as of 2005 formal drug interaction studies have not been completed, a number of drugs may interact with abarelix. These include:

- arsenic trioxide
- astemizole (Hismanal)
- bepridil (Vascor)
- certain antibiotics
- cisapride (Propulsid)
- cyclobenzaprine (Flexeril)
- DHEA (dietary supplement)
- dolasetron (Anzemet)
- droperidol
- halofantrine (Halfan)

- estrogen or other female hormones
- levomethadyl (Orlaam)
- medications that regulate heart rhythm
- medications that treat depression
- palonosetron (Aloxi)
- pentamidine (Pentam)
- phenothiazines (found in antihistamines)
- pimozide (Orap)
- probucol (Lorelco)

Tish Davidson, A. M.

Accelerated partial breast irradiation

Definition

Accelerated partial breast irradiation (APBI), also referred to as high dose rate breast brachytherapy, is a shortened course of high dose **radiation therapy** that is given to **breast cancer** patients. It targets the area of the breast where the **cancer** is most likely to recur.

Purpose

One of the purposes of APBI is to reduce the radiation treatment time from seven or eight weeks, which is generally required with conventional whole breast irradiation, to four or five days. Planning for seven or eight weeks of radiation treatment is difficult for many women, especially women who work outside the home, are single parents, and/or live in rural areas. Reducing the treatment time to one week is not only more convenient for many patients, but it also helps them with emotional closure. In other words, the sooner they are done with the treatments, the sooner they can put the cancer behind them.

Another purpose of APBI is to save the breast while still preventing a recurrence of the cancer. Many women are good candidates for breast conserving therapy, in which the lump is surgically removed (**lumpectomy**), and then radiation or **chemotherapy** is used to destroy any remaining cancer cells. Although this treatment leaves the breast intact, many women still choose to have a full removal of the breast (**mastectomy**). There are many reasons women may make this choice, including the long treatment regimen being too difficult or costly to arrange and concerns about exposing surrounding tissue and organs to radiation. Arranging for seven or eight weeks of treatment can be especially burdensome for individuals living far from their treatment center, or who have to juggle multiple obligations family and work. Because APBI is of shorter duration than traditional breast saving treatment, it may be a more viable option for many women. It also targets a smaller area for treatment, meaning that fewer healthy tissues and organs are exposed to the radiation.

In 2009 the American Society for Radiation Oncology issued a consensus statement on accelerated partial breast irradiation. In it, they made recommendations based on a wide range of clinical trial outcomes. They established guidelines for which women are good candidates for APBI instead of the traditional whole breast irradiation.

Demographics

Patients over 60 years of age are considered "suitable" candidates for APBI. Patients from 50 to 59 years of age are considered "cautionary", meaning in some cases the treatment may be appropriate, and patients under age 50 are considered "unsuitable". Guidelines also consider which women are suitable candidates along a variety of other factors, including tumor size (less than or equal to 2 cm), cancer stage (T1) and other factors.

Precautions

Accelerated partial breast irradiation is a relatively new treatment method. Long-term studies of its effectiveness and safety are, as of 2009, still being carried out. For many women it may not be as effective as traditional whole breast irradiation. **Clinical trials** are underway to determine its long-term effectiveness and which patient populations it is most appropriate for. Until more is known about this treatment, the American Society for Radiation Oncology recommend conservative guidelines be used.

Description

High Dose Rate Breast Brachytherapy

There are two ways to accomplish the administration of APBI, both of which can be done on an outpatient basis. One way, called high does rate breast brachytherapy, involves inserting multiple plastic tubes (catheters) in the breast area surrounding the lumpectomy cavity. A tiny radioactive seed, which delivers the correct amount of radiation, is inserted in the catheters. Generally, the treatment is given twice a day for five days, although some treatment regimes vary according to the individual needs of the patient. Treatment sessions usually take no longer than

20 minutes. At the end of the five-day treatment, the catheters are removed.

Mammosite Breast Brachytherapy

Another way to administer APBI is called mammosite breast brachytherapy, which is also known as balloon catheter brachytherapy. In this case, a small balloon is attached to a single catheter, which is inserted into the lumpectomy cavity. Then the balloon is inflated and a computer-controlled machine places the high dose radioactive seed inside the balloon. This therapy requires a fairly narrow range of cavity location and size, so it is not an appropriate treatment for all women.

Preparation

Preparation requirements are different depending on the type of procedure being performed, and the specifics of the patient's breast and previous history. Making plans in advance with family and friends to help in providing transportation, caring for children, preparing meals, or doing housework can provide much needed support during treatment.

Aftercare

Good nutrition, regular light exercise, and plenty of rest are important after any radiation therapy. Additional aftercare information is provided by treatment staff on a case-by-case basis.

Risks

Possible side effects include discomfort due to the insertion and removal of the catheters and pain or soreness around the insertion sited. Other possible side effects include swelling around the irradiated area, soreness, changes in skin coloration, and **fatigue**.

Results

Preliminary evidence suggests that for many women APBI is as effective as traditional whole breast irradiation. However, as of 2009, clinical trials were still underway to determine the long-term effectiveness of the treatment. Patients should ask their physician for the most up-to-date information on recommendations for treatment and outcome statistics.

Resources

BOOKS

Kneece, Judy C. *Breast Cancer Treatment Handbook: Understanding the Disease, Treatments, Emotions, and Recovery from Breast Cancer,* 7th ed. North Charleston, SC: EduCare, 2009.

Miller, Kenneth, D. *Choices in Breast Cancer Treatment: Medical Specialists and Cancer Survivors Tell You What You Need to Know.* Baltimore: Johns Hopkins University Press, 2008.
Wazer, David E. *Accelerated Partial Breast Irradiation.* New York: Springer, 2009.

PERIODICALS
Dirbas, Frederick M. "Accelerated Partial Breast Irradiation: Where Do We Stand? *Journal of the National Comprehensive Cancer Network,* (February 2009), 215-225.
Smith, Benjamin D., et al. "Accelerated Partial Breast Irradiation Consensus Statement from the American Society for Radiation Oncology. *Journal of the American College of Surgeons,* (August 2009), 269-277.

ORGANIZATIONS
American Cancer Society, (800) ACS-2345, www.cancer.org.
National Cancer Institute, 6116 Executive Boulevard Room 3036A, Bethesda, MD, 20892-8322, (800) 4-CANCER (800-422-6237), www.cancer.gov.
Susan G. Komen Foundation, 5005 LBJ Freeway, Suite 250, Dallas, TX, 75244, (877) GO-KOMEN, www.komen.org.

Lee Ann Paradise
Tish Davidson, A.M.

Acoustic neuroma

Definition

An acoustic neuroma is a benign tumor involving cells of the myelin sheath that surrounds the vestibulocochlear nerve (eighth cranial nerve).

False-color magnetic resonance image (MRI) scan of a coronal section of the head & brain of someone suffering from an acoustic neuroma (green circular area). *(Photograph by Mehau Kulyk, Photo Researchers, Inc. Reproduced by permission.)*

Description

The vestibulocochlear nerve extends from the inner ear to the brain and is made up of a vestibular branch, often called the vestibular nerve, and a cochlear branch, called the cochlear nerve. The vestibular and cochlear nerves lie next to one another. They also run along side other cranial nerves. People possess two of each type of vestibulocochlear nerve, one that extends from the left ear and one that extends from the right ear.

The vestibular nerve transmits information concerning balance from the inner ear to the brain and the cochlear nerve transmits information about hearing. The vestibular nerve, like many nerves, is surrounded by a cover called a myelin sheath. A tumor called a schwannoma can sometimes develop from the cells of the myelin sheath. A tumor is an abnormal growth of tissue that results from the uncontrolled growth of cells. Acoustic neuromas are often called vestibular schwannomas because they are tumors that arise from the myelin sheath that surrounds the vestibular nerve. Acoustic neuromas are considered benign (non-

cancerous) tumors since they do not spread to other parts of the body. They can occur anywhere along the vestibular nerve but are most likely to occur where the vestibulocochlear nerve passes through the tiny bony canal that connects the brain and the inner ear.

An acoustic neuroma can arise from the left vestibular nerve or the right vestibular nerve. A unilateral tumor is a tumor arising from one nerve and a bilateral tumor arises from both vestibular nerves. Unilateral acoustic neuromas usually occur spontaneously (by chance). Bilateral acoustic neuromas occur as part of a hereditary condition called Neurofibromatosis Type 2 (NF2). A person with NF2 has inherited a predisposition for developing acoustic neuromas and other tumors of the nerve cells.

Acoustic neuromas usually grow slowly and can take years to develop. Some acoustic neuromas remain so small that they do not cause any symptoms. As the acoustic neuroma grows, it can interfere with the functioning of the vestibular nerve and can cause vertigo and balance difficulties. If the acoustic nerve grows large enough to press against the cochlear nerve, then hearing loss and a ringing (tinnitus) in the affected ear will usually occur. If untreated and the acoustic neuroma continues to grow, it can press against other nerves in the region and cause other symptoms. This tumor can be life threatening if it becomes large enough to press against and interfere with the functioning of the brain.

Causes and symptoms

Causes

An acoustic neuroma is caused by a change or absence of both of the NF2 tumor suppressor genes in a nerve cell. Every person possesses a pair of NF2 genes in every cell of their body including their nerve cells. One NF2 gene is inherited from the egg cell of the mother and one NF2 gene is inherited from the sperm cell of the father. The NF2 gene is responsible for helping to prevent the formation of tumors in the nerve cells. In particular the NF2 gene helps to prevent acoustic neuromas.

Only one unchanged and functioning NF2 gene is necessary to prevent the formation of an acoustic neuroma. If both NF2 genes become changed or missing in one of the myelin sheath cells of the vestibular nerve, then an acoustic neuroma will usually develop. Most unilateral acoustic neuromas result when the NF2 genes become spontaneously changed or missing. Someone with a unilateral acoustic neuroma that has developed spontaneously is not at increased risk for having children with an acoustic neuroma. Some

KEY TERMS

Benign tumor—A localized overgrowth of cells that does not spread to other parts of the body.

Chromosome—A microscopic structure, made of a complex of proteins and DNA, that is found within each cell of the body.

Cranial nerves—The set of twelve nerves found on each side of the head and neck that control the sensory and muscle functions of a number of organs such as the eyes, nose, tongue face and throat.

Computed tomography (CT)—An examination that uses a computer to compile and analyze the images produced by x rays projected at a particular part of the body.

DNA testing—Testing for a change or changes in a gene or genes.

Gene— A building block of inheritance, made up of a compound called DNA (deoxyribonucleic acid) and containing the instructions for the production of a particular protein. Each gene is found on a specific location on a chromosome.

Magnetic resonance imaging (MRI)—A test which uses an external magnetic field instead of x rays to visualize different tissues of the body.

Myelin sheath—The cover that surrounds many nerve cells and helps to increase the speed by which information travels along the nerve.

Neurofibromatosis type 2 (NF2)—A hereditary condition associated with an increased risk of bilateral acoustic neuromas, other nerve cell tumors and cataracts.

Protein—A substance produced by a gene that is involved in creating the traits of the human body such as hair and eye color or is involved in controlling the basic functions of the human body.

Schwannoma—A tumor derived from the cells of the myelin sheath that surrounds many nerve cells.

Tinnitus—A ringing sound or other noise in the ear.

Vertigo—A feeling of spinning or whirling.

Vestibulocochlear nerve (Eighth cranial nerve)— Nerve that transmits information, about hearing and balance from the ear to the brain.

---

unilateral acoustic neuromas result from the hereditary condition NF2. It is also possible that some unilateral acoustic neuromas may be caused by changes in other genes responsible for preventing the formation of tumors.

Bilateral acoustic neuromas result when someone is affected with the hereditary condition NF2. A person with NF2 is typically born with one unchanged and one changed or missing NF2 gene in every cell of their body. Sometimes they inherit this change from their mother or father. Sometimes the change occurs spontaneously when the egg and sperm come together to form the first cell of the baby. The children of a person with NF2 have a 50% chance of inheriting the changed or missing NF2 gene.

A person with NF2 will develop an acoustic neuroma if the remaining unchanged NF2 gene becomes spontaneously changed or missing in one of the myelin sheath cells of their vestibular nerve. People with NF2 often develop acoustic neuromas at a younger age. The mean age of onset of acoustic neuroma in NF2 is 31 years of age versus 50 years of age for sporadic acoustic neuromas. Not all people with NF2, however, develop acoustic neuromas. People with NF2 are at increased risk for developing cataracts and tumors in other nerve cells.

Most people with a unilateral acoustic neuroma are not affected with NF2. Some people with NF2, however, only develop a tumor in one of the vestibulocochlear nerves. Others may initially be diagnosed with a unilateral tumor but may develop a tumor in the other nerve a number of years later. NF2 should be considered in someone under the age of 40 who has a unilateral acoustic neuroma. Someone with a unilateral acoustic neuroma and other family members diagnosed with NF2 probably is affected with NF2. Someone with a unilateral acoustic neuroma and other symptoms of NF2 such as cataracts and other tumors may also be affected with NF2. On the other hand, someone over the age of 50 with a unilateral acoustic neuroma, no other tumors and no family history of NF2 is very unlikely to be affected with NF2.

Recent studies in Europe have suggested a possible connection between the widespread use of mobile phones and an increased risk of developing acoustic neuromas. Some observers, however, question whether mobile phones have been in use long enough to be an identifiable risk factor.

Symptoms

Small acoustic neuromas usually only interfere with the functioning of the vestibulocochlear nerve. The most common first symptom of an acoustic neuroma is hearing loss, which is often accompanied by a ringing sound (tinnitis). People with acoustic neuromas sometimes report difficulties in using the phone and difficulties in perceiving the tone of a musical instrument or sound even when their hearing appears to be otherwise normal. In most cases the hearing loss is initially subtle and worsens gradually over time until deafness occurs in the affected ear. In approximately 10% of cases the hearing loss is sudden and severe.

Acoustic neuromas can also affect the functioning of the vestibular branch of the vestibulocochlear nerve and van cause vertigo and dysequilibrium. Twenty percent of small tumors are associated with periodic vertigo, which is characterized by dizziness or a whirling sensation. Larger acoustic neuromas are less likely to cause vertigo but more likely to cause dysequilibrium. Dysequilibrium, which is characterized by minor clumsiness and a general feeling of instability, occurs in nearly 50% of people with an acoustic neuroma.

As the tumor grows larger, it can press on the surrounding cranial nerves. Compression of the fifth cranial nerve can result in facial pain and or numbness. Compression of the seventh cranial nerve can cause spasms, weakness or paralysis of the facial muscles. Double vision is a rare symptom but can result when the sixth cranial nerve is affected. Swallowing and/or speaking difficulties can occur if the tumor presses against the ninth, tenth, or twelfth cranial nerves.

If left untreated, the tumor can become large enough to press against and affect the functioning of the brain stem. The brain stem is the stalk-like portion of the brain that joins the spinal cord to the cerebrum, the thinking and reasoning part of the brain. Different parts of the brainstem have different functions such as the control of breathing and muscle coordination. Large tumors that impact the brain stem can result in headaches, walking difficulties (gait ataxia) and involuntary shaking movements of the muscles (tremors). In rare cases when an acoustic neuroma remains undiagnosed and untreated it can cause **nausea**, **vomiting**, lethargy and eventually coma, respiratory difficulties and death. In the vast majority of cases, however, the tumor is discovered and treated long before it is large enough to cause such serious manifestations.

Diagnosis

Anyone with symptoms of hearing loss should undergo hearing evaluations. Pure tone and speech audiometry are two screening tests that are often used to evaluate hearing. Pure tone audiometry tests to see how well someone can hear tones of different volume and pitch and speech audiometry tests to see how well someone can hear and recognize speech. An acoustic neuroma is suspected in someone with unilateral hearing loss or hearing loss that is less severe in one ear than the other ear(asymmetrical).

Sometimes an auditory brainstem response (ABR, BAER) test is performed to help establish whether someone is likely to have an acoustic neuroma. During the ABR examination, a harmless electrical impulse is passed from the inner ear to the brainstem. An acoustic neuroma can interfere with the passage of this electrical impulse and this interference can, sometimes be identified through the ABR evaluation. A normal ABR examination does not rule out the possibility of an acoustic neuroma. An abnormal ABR examination increases the likelihood that an acoustic neuroma is present but other tests are necessary to confirm the presence of a tumor.

If an acoustic neuroma is strongly suspected then **magnetic resonance imaging** (MRI) is usually performed. The MRI is a very accurate evaluation that is able to detect nearly 100% of acoustic neuromas. **Computed tomography** (CT scan, CAT scan) is unable to identify smaller tumors; but it can be used when an acoustic neuroma is suspected and an MRI evaluation cannot be performed.

Once an acoustic neuroma is diagnosed, an evaluation by genetic specialists such as a geneticist and genetic counselor may be recommended. The purpose of this evaluation is to obtain a detailed family history and check for signs of NF2. If NF2 is strongly suspected then DNA testing may be recommended. DNA testing involves checking the blood cells obtained from a routine blood draw for the common gene changes associated with NF2.

Treatment

The three treatment options for acoustic neuroma are surgery, radiation, and observation. The physician and patient should discuss the pros and cons of the different options prior to making a decision about treatment. The patient's physical health, age, symptoms, tumor size, and tumor location should be considered.

Microsurgery

The surgical removal of the tumor or tumors is the most common treatment for acoustic neuroma. In most cases the entire tumor is removed during the surgery. If the tumor is large and causing significant symptoms, yet there is a need to preserve hearing in that ear, then only part of the tumor may be removed. During the procedure the tumor is removed under microscopic guidance and general anesthetic. Monitoring of the neighboring cranial nerves is done during the procedure so that damage to these nerves can be prevented. If preservation of hearing is a possibility, then monitoring of hearing will also take place during the surgery.

Most people stay in the hospital four to seven days following the surgery. Total recovery usually takes four to six weeks. Most people experience **fatigue** and head discomfort following the surgery. Problems with balance and head and neck stiffness are also common. The mortality rate of this type of surgery is less than 2% at most major centers. Approximately 20% of patients experience some degree of post-surgical complications. In most cases these complications can be managed successfully and do not result in long term medical problems. Surgery brings with it a risk of stroke, damage to the brain stem, **infection**, leakage of spinal fluid and damage to the cranial nerves. Hearing loss and/or tinnitus often result from the surgery. A follow-up MRI is recommended one to five years following the surgery because of possible regrowth of the tumor.

Stereotactic radiation therapy

During stereotactic **radiation therapy**, also called radiosurgery or radiotherapy, many small beams of radiation are aimed directly at the acoustic neuroma. The radiation is administered in a single large dose, under local anesthetic and is performed on an outpatient basis. This results in a high dose of radiation to the tumor but little radiation exposure to the surrounding area. This treatment approach is limited to small or medium tumors. The goal of the therapy is to cause tumor shrinkage or at least limit the growth of the tumor. The long-term efficacy and risks of this treatment approach are not known; however, as of the early 2000s, more and more patients with acoustic neuromas are choosing this approach over conventional surgery. Periodic MRI monitoring throughout the life of the patient is therefore recommended.

Radiation therapy can cause hearing loss which can sometimes occurs even years later. Radiation therapy can also cause damage to neighboring cranial nerves, which can result in symptoms such as numbness, pain or paralysis of the facial muscles. In many cases these symptoms are temporary. Radiation treatment can also induce the formation of other benign or malignant schwannomas. This type of treatment may therefore be contraindicated in the treatment of acoustic neuromas in those with NF2 who are predisposed to developing schwannomas and other tumors.

Observation

Acoustic neuromas are usually slow-growing; in some cases they will stop growing and even become smaller or disappear entirely. It may therefore be appropriate in some cases to hold off on treatment and to periodically monitor the tumor through MRI evaluations. Long-term observation may be appropriate for example in an elderly person with a small acoustic neuroma and few symptoms. Periodic observation may also be indicated for someone with a small and asymptomatic acoustic neuroma that was detected through an evaluation for another medical problem. Observation may also be suggested for someone with an acoustic neuroma in the only hearing ear or in the ear that has better hearing. The danger of an observational approach is that as the tumor grows larger it can become more difficult to treat.

Prognosis

The prognosis for someone with a unilateral acoustic neuroma is usually quite good provided the tumor is diagnosed early and appropriate treatment is instituted. Long-term hearing loss and tinnitus in the affected ear are common, even if appropriate treatment is provided. Many patients also experience facial weakness, balance problems, and headaches. Regrowth of the tumor is also a possibility following surgery or radiation therapy and repeat treatment may be necessary. The prognosis can be poorer for those with NF2 who have an increased risk of bilateral acoustic neuromas and other tumors.

Resources

BOOKS

Beers, Mark H., MD, and Robert Berkow, MD, editors. "Acoustic Neuroma." in *The Merck Manual of Diagnosis and Therapy*. Whitehouse Station, NJ: Merck Research Laboratories, 2007.

PERIODICALS

Broad, R. W. "Management of Acoustic Neuroma." *New England Journal of Medicine* 340, no. 14 (April 8, 1999): 1119.

Kondziolka, D., L. D. Lundsford, and J. C. Flickinger. "Acoustic Neuroma Radiosurgery. Origins, Contemporary Use and Future Expectations." *Neurochirurgie* 50 (June 2004): 427–435.

Kundi, M., K. Mild, L. Hardell, and M. O. Mattsson. "Mobile Telephones and Cancer—A Review of Epidemiological Evidence." *Journal of Toxicology and Environmental Health, Part B, Critical Reviews* 7 (September-October 2004): 351–384.

Lederman, G., E. Arbit, and J. Lowry. "Management of Acoustic Neuroma." *New England Journal of Medicine.* 340, no. 14 (April 8, 1999): 1119–1120.

O'Donoghue, G.M., T. Nikolopoulos, and J. Thomsen. "Management of Acoustic Neuroma." *New England Journal of Medicine* 340, no.14 (April 8, 1999): 1120–1121.

Ryzenman, J. M., M. L. Pensak, and J. M. Tew, Jr. "Patient Perception of Comorbid Conditions After Acoustic Neuroma Management: Survey Results from the Acoustic Neuroma Association." *Laryngoscope* 114 (May 2004): 814–820.

OTHER

National Institute of Health Consensus Statement Online *Acoustic Neuroma* 9(4)(11-13 December 1991). [cited June 28, 2001]. <http://text.nlm.nih.gov/nih/cdc/www/87txt.html>.

University of California at San Francisco (UCSF) *Information on Acoustic Neuromas.* [cited June 28, 2001]. (18 March 1998).

ORGANIZATIONS

Acoustic Neuroma Association. 600 Peachtree Pkwy, Suite 108, Cumming, GA 30041-6899. Phone:(770) 205-8211. Fax: (770) 205-0239. ANAusa@aol.com. [cited June 28, 2001]. <http://anausa.org>.

Acoustic Neuroma Association of Canada Box 369, Edmonton, AB T5J 2J6. 1-800-561-ANAC(2622). (780)428-3384. anac@compusmart.ab.ca. [cited June 28, 2001]. http://www.anac.ca.

British Acoustic Neuroma Association. Oak House, Ransom Wood Business Park, Southwell Road West, Mansfield, Nottingham, NG21 0HJ. Tel: 01623 632143. Fax: 01623 635313. bana@btclick.com. [cited June 28, 2001].http://www.bana-uk.com/.

Seattle Acoustic Neuroma Group. Emcityland@aol.com. [cited June 28, 2001]. <http://acousticneuromaseattle.org/entryenglish.html>.

Lisa Andres, M.S., CGC
Rebecca J. Frey, PhD

Acquired Immune Deficiency syndrome *see* **AIDS-related cancers**

Actinomycin D *see* **Dactinomycin**

Acute erythroblastic leukemia

Definition

Acute erythroblastic leukemia, a subtype (M6) of acute myelogenous leukemia (AML), is also called erythroid leukemia, DiGuglielmo syndrome, or erythroleukemia, results from uncontrolled proliferation of immature erythrocytes (red blood cells).

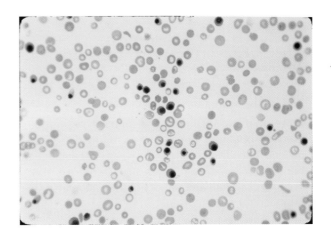

Erythroblastic leukemia cells. *(Copyright Richard Green, Science Source/Photo Researchers, Inc. Reproduced by permission.)*

Description

Acute erythroblastic leukemia, a variant of AML, originates in the blood and in the bone marrow. In this form of leukemia, a large number of abnormal, immature red blood cells are produced. The World Health Organization (WHO) classifies acute erythroid leukemia into two subtypes, erythroleukemia, which includes erythroblastic and myeloblastic components (blast cells are immature cells), and pure erythroid leukemia in which the erythroid component constitutes 80% or more of the bone marrow.

Demographics

According to the American **Cancer** Society, approximately 12,810 people (6,920 males and 5,890 females) will be diagnosed with AML in 2009 with about 9,000 deaths predicted to occur from AML during that same time period. Acute erythroid leukemia accounts for about 3–5% of all cases of AML and constitutes 20–30% of cases of secondary leukemia.

Erythroid leukemia has been reported from the newborn period through age 7, however, this subtype of AML is rare in children. Males are affected slightly more often than females. A small spike in incidence of erythroid leukemia appears in the fourth decade but the disease is more common after age 50. A larger peak in incidence occurs in the seventh decade.

Causes and symptoms

The causes of acute erythroblastic leukemia are largely unknown. However, acute erythroblastic leukemia constitutes 10–20% of leukemias that develop secondary to previous exposures to ionizing radiation,

KEY TERMS

Anemia—A condition in which the number of red blood cells is below normal

Blast cells—Immature cancer cells.

Bone marrow aspiration—Common technique used to obtain a bone marrow sample from a patient. A needle is inserted into a marrow-containing bone, such as the hip (iliac crest) or sternum (breast bone) and a small amount of liquid bone marrow is removed for examination.

Bone marrow biopsy—Another common technique used to obtain a bone marrow sample from a patient. Like bone marrow aspiration, it is performed with a needle, but a larger one is used and a small piece of bone is removed as well as bone marrow.

Chemotherapy—The treatment of disease by means of chemicals. In cancer, the chemicals selectively destroy cancerous tissue. When cancer remission occurs, a course of maintenance chemotherapy is often prescribed so as to prevent recurrence.

Erythrocyte—Red blood cell.

Leukemia—Cancer of the blood-forming tissues.

Myeloid blast cell—Type of cancer cell originating in the bone marrow.

Platelet—A type of blood cell responsible for blood coagulation and for the repair of damaged blood vessels.

Proliferation—Rapid reproduction of tissue.

Remission—Complete or partial disappearance of the symptoms of cancer following treatment.

previous treatment with **chemotherapy** agents known as alkylating agents which may have been used to treat Hodgkin disease, **multiple myeloma**, **ovarian cancer**, **breast cancer** and some other non-cancerous diseases and disorders, or as a result of overexposure to benzene.

Inheritance

There is type of inherited erythroid leukemia which is known as familial erythroleukemia. This familial disorder is rare and most typically occurs in the sixth decade of life.

Patients diagnosed with erythroid leukemia have less than the normal amount of healthy red blood cells

and platelets, which results in insufficient amounts of oxygen being carried through the body. This condition is called **anemia**, and causes patients to experience severe weakness and tiredness. Patients may have less than the normal number of white blood cells as well. Other symptoms include **fever**, chills, loss of appetite and weight, easy bleeding or bruising (due to lower than normal platelet levels), bone or joint pain, headaches, **vomiting**, and confusion. In addition, patients with leukemia may have hepatosplenomegaly, an enlargement of the liver and spleen. Enlargement of these organs is noticed as a fullness or swelling in the abdomen, and can be felt by a doctor during a physical examination. The occurrence of Sweet's syndrome, a rare skin disorder accompanied by fever, inflammation of the joints (arthritis), and the sudden onset of a rash, has also been associated with acute erythroblastic leukemia.

Diagnosis

Patients seeking treatment usually report a vague history of chronic general **fatigue**. Blood tests are used to establish the diagnosis. A sample of blood is examined under a microscope to identify abnormal red cells—which are larger than healthy cells—and to count the number of mature cells and blasts present. Cancer red cell precursors predominate, myeloid blasts may also be seen, and multinucleated red cell precursors are common. However, blasts may not be present at diagnosis in as many as half of the cases.

Other laboratory studies which may be done include:

- blood chemistry profile, liver function tests and serum electrolytes
- blood and urine cultures will be obtained in patients with fever or other signs of infection
- vitamin B_{12} and folate levels should be measured to rule out severe pernicious anemia whose signs and symptoms mimic erythroleukemia
- flow cytometry to determine myeloid markers for the disease
- cytogenetics studies which assess for chromosomal abnormalities. Cytogenetics studies are important in diagnosis and prognosis of the disease. However, no specific chromosomal abnormalities have yet been identified for M6 subtype of AML.

Imaging studies will also be performed at the time of diagnosis. These studies include:

- echocardiogram or multiple-gated acquisition(MU-GA)scan – used to evaluate the status of the cardiac system prior to chemotherapy administration. Some of the chemotherapy medications used to treat this subtype of AML may be toxic to the cardiac system.

- chest x ray is done to evaluate for pulumonary infections, enlargement of the heart, and other heart and lung problems.
- CT scan or MRI will be performed if there is suspicion of neurologic involvement.

Bone marrow examinations are also performed, either by aspiration or **biopsy** to examine the cell types further. These results of these examinations are critical to the accurate diagnosis of erythroleukemia.

A **lumbar puncture** may be performed if neurologic involvement is suspected or is present and is also recommended in patients whose circulating leukemic cell counts are very elevated (higher than $50,000/mm^3$) and for those patients with elevated liver enzyme (LDH) levels.

Treatment

Treatment for acute erythroblastic leukemia depends on the features of the cancer cells present and on the extent of the disease, as well as on the age of the patient, his symptoms, and general health condition. The treatment strategy is based on chemotherapy and in some patients, bone marrow or hemotopoietic stem cell transplantations are indicated as well. Chemotherapy is usually administered in combinations of two or more drugs. **Cytarabine** (Ara-C) is currently the most active chemotherapy agent used in the management of AML and in the erythroid subtype. Various regimens have been designed around the use of Ara-C. Post-remission therapy includes maintenance chemotherapy for most patients.

Prognosis

Acute erythroblastic leukemia is a usually a very aggressive form of leukemia and typically does not respond well to the types of therapy used to treat acute myelocytic leukemia. The prognosis compared to the average for AML is worse for patients with this M6 subtype of AML.

Coping with cancer treatment

Like all types of leukemias, patients with acute erythroblastic leukemia usually experience a number of specific complications and side effects resulting from treatment, as well as emotional concerns. They require supportive care to cope with these issues and to maintain their comfort and quality of life during treatment. As with every serious disease, psychological stress is increased and it is important for patients to

> ### QUESTIONS TO ASK THE DOCTOR
> - How can I obtain information on a rare cancer such as acute erythroblastic leukemia?
> - How are my chances of recovery affected by the fact that this cancer is so rare?
> - Are there current clinical trials in which I may enroll?

be able to discuss their needs and concerns about tests, treatments, hospital stays, and financial consequences of the illness. Family, friends, doctors, nurses, and other members of the health care team are the best sources of support, as well as social workers, counselors, and members of the clergy.

Clinical trials

As of June 2009, one clinical trial to determine if standard chemotherapy given with **idarubicin** and Ara-C can help to control AML is available for patients ages 15 to 75 diagnosed with the M6 subtype of AML and who have less than 20% blasts. Other eligibility (inclusion) criteria apply as well. This clinical trial is sponsored by M.D. Anderson Cancer Center in Houston, Texas.

Prevention

Since this form of cancer is very rare and its causes are largely unknown, no specific preventive measures can be recommended.

Special concerns

Patients diagnosed with acute erythroblastic leukemia require special support in that they must deal with having a rare form of cancer about which there is very little specific information available. This creates additional anxiety and special care must be taken to explain to the patient that an uncommon cancer is not an untreatable one.

See also Bone marrow aspiration and biopsy; Chronic myelocytic leukemia; Myeloproliferative diseases.

Resources

OTHER
Holkova, B., and K. Takeshita. "Erythroleukemia." *eMedicine Hematology* July 18, 2006. http://emedicine.medscape.com/article/199965-print.

ORGANIZATIONS

The Leukemia and Lymphoma Society of America. 1-800-955-4572. http://www.leukemia-lymphoma.org/.

National Cancer Information Center. 1-800-ACS-2345.

National Cancer Institute. Public Inquiries Office, Building 31, Room 10A31, 31 Center Drive, MSC 2580, Bethesda, MD 20892-2580. (301)435-2848. http://www.cancer.gov.

Monique Laberge, PhD
Melinda Granger Oberleitner, R.N., D.N.S.,
A.P.R.N., C.N.S.

Acute lymphocytic leukemia

Definition

Acute lymphocytic leukemia is a **cancer** of the white blood cells known as lymphocytes.

Description

Leukemia is a cancer of white blood cells. In acute leukemia, the cancerous cells are immature forms called blasts that cannot properly fight **infection**; patients become ill in rapid fashion.

The cells that make up blood are produced in the bone marrow and the lymph system. The bone marrow is the spongy tissue found in the large bones of the

False-color scanning electron micrograph (SEM) of white blood cells from a patient with acute lymphocytic leukemia. In this disease, certain types of white blood cells are overproduced, and these abnormal cells suppress the normal function of white and red cells, increasing the susceptibility to infections. *(Copyright Aaron Polliack, Science Source/Photo Researchers, Inc. Reproduced by permission.)*

body. The lymph system includes the spleen (an organ in the upper abdomen), the thymus (a small organ beneath the breastbone), and the tonsils (an organ in the throat). In addition, the lymph vessels (tiny tubes that branch like blood vessels into all parts of the body) and lymph nodes (pea-shaped organs that are found along the network of lymph vessels) are also part of the lymph system. The lymph is a milky fluid that contains cells. Clusters of lymph nodes are found in the neck, underarm, pelvis, abdomen, and chest.

The main types of cells found in the blood are the red blood cells (RBCs), which carry oxygen and other materials to all tissues of the body; white blood cells (WBCs), which fight infection; and the platelets, which play a part in the clotting of the blood. The white blood cells can be further subdivided into three main types: granulocytes, monocytes, and lymphocytes.

The granulocytes, as their name suggests, have particles (granules) inside them. These granules contain special proteins (enzymes) and several other substances that can break down chemicals and destroy microorganisms such as bacteria. Monocytes are the second type of white blood cell. They are also important in defending the body against pathogens. The lymphocytes form the third type of white blood cell. The two types of lymphocytes are B cells, which make antibodies, and T cells, which make other infection-fighting substances. Lymphocytic leukemia can arise in either B or T cells.

B-cell leukemia occurs more frequently than T-cell leukemia. It is the most common form of leukemia in children, but also occurs in adults. At diagnosis, leukemic cells can be found throughout the body, in the bloodstream, the lymph nodes, spleen, liver, occasionally in the central nervous system, and in T-cell ALL, the thymus gland.

Cancerous lymphoblasts take over the bone marrow, reducing both the number and the effectiveness of all types of blood cells. The cancerous cells reduce the ability of healthy white cells to fight infection. Fewer red cells are produced, causing **anemia**, and fewer platelets increases the risk of bleeding and bruising. The presence of the cancerous white cells in the central nervous system can produce headaches, confusion and seizures.

Demographics

ALL is the most common of the four major types of leukemia in children, representing one-third of all pediatric cancers. Peak incidence in children occurs between the ages of two and five years. Conversely, ALL is the least common type of the four major types of leukemia affecting adults.

In 2009, the American Cancer Society estimates about 45,000 Americans will be diagnosed with leukemia. Of those cases, 5,760 of ALL will be diagnosed with 1 in 3 cases or about 1,900 new cases diagnosed in adults. Approximately 3,800 new cases of ALL will be diagnosed in children in the U.S. in 2009. About 1400 deaths from ALL will occur in the U.S. in 2009 with three-fourths of the deaths, about 1,000, occurring in adults. The death rate for children with ALL has dropped nearly 60% in the last 30 years. The overall five-year survival rate for children with ALL is now 80%. The average life-time risk of developing ALL is about 1 in 1000. ALL incidence in adults increases with age.

In the United States, ALL is highest among Caucasians and lowest among Asian-Americans. The incidence of ALL is about 50% higher for men than for women. Death rates in leukemia patients are highest in African-Americans and Caucasians and lowest in Asians.

In children, the highest leukemia rates in the US occur among those of Filipino descent; next highest are white Hispanics, then non-Hispanic whites, and the lowest incidence in children is in African-Americans. Survival is higher for Caucasians than African-Americans. The survival rate for girls is slightly higher, in part due to the risk of relapse occurring in the testicles and in part because boys appear to have a slightly higher risk of bone marrow relapse.

Causes and symptoms

Causes

While specific causes for ALL are not known, there are some known risk factors, including ionizing radiation. Exposure to certain chemicals, particularly benzene (used in the manufacture of plastics, rubber, and some medicines), has also been associated with an increased risk of developing ALL.

Infection with a rare virus, HTLV-1 (rare in the United States), can cause a rare type of ALL. The **Epstein Barr virus** (EBV), which causes mononucleosis, has also been linked to a form of ALL.

The causes of ALL in children are also unknown. Certain inherited genetic abnormalities, such as Down syndrome, increase the risk. Some studies have shown prenatal exposure to ionizing radiation increases a child's risk of ALL. Some contaminants of tap water, such as trihalomethanes, chloroform, zinc, cadmium, and arsenic are associated with an increased risk. A number of reports suggested an increased risk of ALL among children who lived in proximity to high voltage power lines, but several later analyses suggested that was not true. Studies continue in efforts to disprove or confirm this possible connection. ALL is more common in children who are not firstborn and among those whose mothers took **antibiotics** during their pregnancies. Breastfeeding has been found to be protective.

Symptoms

ADULTS. ALL in adults can cause any or all of the following symptoms:

- fevers, chills, sweats
- weakness, fatigue, shortness of breath

- frequent infections
- depressed appetite, weight loss
- enlarged lymph nodes
- easy bleeding or bruising
- rash of small, flat red spots (petechiae)
- bone and joint pain

Symptoms of central nervous system involvement include:

- headache
- nausea and vomiting
- confusion
- seizures

CHILDREN. Symptoms in children are similar, but young children may be unable to communicate them. They include:

- fevers
- frequent infections
- fatigue, irritability, decreased activity levels
- easy bruising or bleeding
- bone or joint pain
- a limp
- swollen belly
- enlarged lymph nodes

T-cell ALL can invade the thymus gland in the upper chest, which can cause compression of the windpipe, cough or shortness of breath, and **superior vena cava syndrome** (compression of a large vein that causes swelling of the head, neck, and arms).

Central nervous system involvement in children produces:

- headache
- nausea and vomiting
- blurred vision
- decline in school performance
- seizures

Spread to the testicles can cause painless swelling in them.

Diagnosis

There are no screening tests for leukemia. The patient's history and physical examination raise the physician's suspicions, triggering orders for appropriate tests. Pallor, swollen lymph nodes, bleeding, bruising, pinpoint red rashes, and in children, a swollen abdomen, will suggest the diagnosis. Testing is similar for adults and children.

The first test is a complete blood count (CBC), examining red cells, platelets and white cells. In early leukemia, the total white blood cell count might be normal, but there will usually be circulating lymphoblasts, which is always abnormal. The red cell and platelet counts may be low.

The abnormal CBC results trigger a referral to a hematologist/oncologist who will perform a **bone marrow aspiration and biopsy**, in which a small sample of marrow is removed with a hollow needle inserted in the hipbone. Although topical anesthetic will numb the skin and bone, most patients experience brief pain during this procedure. The sample will be examined microscopically for evidence of lymphoblasts. The marrow will be further studied to determine whether the lymphoblasts are of T-cell or B-cell origin and the cells tested for chromosomal abnormalities. A pathologist can examine the marrow and make the diagnosis immediately. The chromosome studies require several days to complete. The bone marrow aspirate will be repeated occasionally during treatment to confirm remission and to look for possible relapse.

A **lumbar puncture**, or spinal tap, will be performed to rule out spread of ALL to the central nervous system. A thin needle is inserted between two vertebrae in the lower back, and spinal fluid removed. This fluid is examined microscopically for the presence of lymphoblasts. Topical anesthetics eliminate most of the discomfort of a spinal tap, although many patients experience headaches afterwards. Remaining flat for 30 minutes after a spinal tap decreases the likelihood of headache.

A chest x ray will show enlargement of internal lymph nodes or the thymus gland.

No preparation is necessary for most of the testing done to diagnose ALL. Younger children will often receive mild sedatives before procedures like spinal taps and bone marrow studies. Topical anesthetic cream can be applied an hour in advance of either a bone marrow test or a spinal tap.

When treatment is complete, tests for minimal residual disease can be performed. These new tests detect the presence of lingering leukemic cells that would have been missed by standard testing. The presence of a certain amount of residual disease probably has an impact on prognosis and the likelihood of relapse.

Treatment team

The treatment team consists of a hematologist/oncologist who directs care, oncology nurses familiar with administering **chemotherapy**, and often social workers, who can address both insurance issues and psychological support. The patient's regular physician should be kept informed of all cancer-related care. Because treatment is so prolonged, most patients have long-term intravenous catheters placed by a surgeon.

In many hospitals, a Child Life specialist will participate in the care of children with ALL. They ensure that children with cancer are seen, first and foremost, as children, organizing play times, providing distraction during scary procedures and giving parents some much-needed respite.

Clinical staging, treatments, and prognosis

Classification of ALL based on immunophenotyping has replaced the French American British (FAB) system of classifying ALL in adults. Results of cytogenetic testing, **flow cytometry**, and molecular genetic studies provide detailed information regarding specific subtypes of ALL provide clues to prognosis, and help to determine the best treatment options. ALL in adults is classified by the type of lymphocyte affected, either B cell or T cell, and by the level of differentiation or maturity of the leukemic cell.

The two major subtypes of ALL are B-cell ALL and T-cell ALL. B-cell ALL can be further subdivided or classified into the following categories:

- early pre-B cell ALL – about 10% of cases; this type may also be referred to as pro-B ALL
- common ALL – comprises about 50% of cases
- pre B ALL – approximately 10% of cases
- mature B-cell ALL; also known as Burkitt leukemia; comprises about 4% of cases

T-cell ALL can be further subdivided or classified into the following categories:

- pre-T ALL – about 5–10% of cases
- mature T cell ALL – about 15–20% of cases

Conventional treatment for ALL consists of chemotherapy for disease in the bone marrow and treatment aimed at preventing central nervous system disease.

The type of treatment a person receives for ALL depends on the presence of risk factors for relapse. Children are at standard risk if they are between ages 1 and 9, have a total white cell count of less than 50,000 per microliter of blood, and have B-precursor cell leukemia. Children are at high risk if they are younger than 1 or older than 9, if their white blood cell count exceeds 50,000 per microliter, or if they have T-cell leukemia. Compared to children, adults are all at

higher risk of relapse at the time of diagnosis, but younger adults (less than 50 years old) have a better prognosis. Adults whose initial white blood cell is higher than 50,000/mm3 at the time of diagnosis have a poorer prognosis. In addition, adults who achieve complete remission within 4 to 5 weeks of starting therapy, tend to have a more favorable prognosis.

Generally, T-cell ALL has a more favorable prognosis than B-cell Burkett leukemia. The presence of an antigen called CD20 indicates a more favorable prognosis.

ALL is also classified by karyotype, which is the number and composition of a cell's chromosomes. Normal human cells contain 46 chromosomes. One chromosomal abnormality often seen in ALL is a translocation, in which a piece of one chromosome becomes attached to a different chromosome. Different translocations carry different prognoses. One translocation, labeled t(9;22) is also called the Philadelphia chromosome and is found in 5% of childhood ALL and 20% of adult ALL cases. The Philadelphia chromosome carries a somewhat less favorable prognosis.

The number of chromosomes found in the leukemic cells, particularly in children, also impacts prognosis. The occurrence of more than 50 chromosomes in leukemic cells has a very favorable prognosis. Even the presence of one extra chromosome can be favorable. Children whose leukemic cells have fewer than 45 chromosomes are at highest risk of treatment failure.

ADULTS. The first phase of treatment is remission induction. Combinations of various chemotherapeutic drugs are typically used. Drugs used to treat adult ALL include:

- prednisone
- vincristine
- cytarabine
- cyclophosphamide
- asparaginase
- daunorubicin
- doxorubicin
- etoposide
- teniposide
- 6-mercaptopurine
- methotrexate
- dexamethasone

Most are given intravenously and a few are given orally. Depending on the disease, these drugs can achieve a complete remission in 60–90% of adults. The relapse rate is higher in adults than in children. A 50% 3-year survival has been noted in some research series, and very aggressive treatment with multiple drugs has produced up to a 70% survival rate.

Adverse effects of these drugs include:

- bone marrow suppression
- anemia, pallor, fatigue, shortness of breath, and angina in older patients
- bleeding, bruising
- increased risk of infection
- hair loss (alopecia)
- mouth sores
- nausea and vomiting
- menopausal symptoms
- lower sperm counts
- tumor lysis syndrome, in which the dead cancer cells can harm healthy organs

Treatment that is directed at preventing central nervous system spread is called prophylactic. Because of the blood brain barrier, a physical and chemical barrier that prevents toxins from reaching the brain and spinal cord, chemotherapeutic drugs do not easily reach the central nervous system. Thus, chemotherapeutic drugs are administered directly into spinal fluid, which circulates around the brain and spinal cord. This is called **intrathecal chemotherapy**. The drugs are given by spinal tap or through an **Ommaya reservoir**, which is surgically inserted under the scalp. This reservoir empties into the spinal fluid around the brain.

Some patients receive prophylactic **radiation therapy** to the brain, in addition to or instead of intrathecal chemotherapy.

Some patients with Philadelphia chromosome positive ALL may receive the targeted therapy agents imatinib (Gleevec) or **dasatinib** (Sprycel) to treat their leukemia.

The monoclonal antibody, **rituximab** (Rituxan), may be used to treat adult ALL in patients whose leukemic cells are positive for the CD20 antigen.

CHILDREN. The treatment of ALL in children represents one of the great success stories of modern oncology. In contrast to adults, most children with cancer enter into research protocols, strict treatment regimens with careful follow-up that are built on the most successful aspects of earlier treatments. Childhood ALL now has an 80% long-term survival rate, due in large part to the extensive and widely disseminated research on the disease. Within the United States, research on ALL was conducted for many years under the auspices of either the Children's Cancer Group or the Pediatric Oncology Group. In 1998,

recognizing the benefits of cooperation and collaboration, these two groups joined forces with the National **Wilms' Tumor** Study Group and the Intergroup **Rhabdomyosarcoma** Study Group to form the Children's Oncology Group.

Excluding the treatment of B-cell ALL, the treatment of other types of childhood ALL includes 5 components or phases: induction, consolidation, interim maintenance, delayed intensification, and maintenance.

The goal of the induction phase is to achieve remission or evidence of less than 5% blasts (immature cells) in the bone marrow. Drugs in the induction phase may include a glucocorticoid, **vincristine**, **asparaginase** and sometimes an anthracycline drug. Most patients, over 98%, achieve complete remission as a result of this therapy.

The adverse effects of these drugs include bone marrow suppression, risk of infection, **nausea**, **vomiting**, hair loss, and mouth sores. Although these drugs can reduce sperm counts, most survivors of childhood ALL grow up to have normal fertility.

Treatment may be intensified for some patients based on evidence of minimal residual disease.

Drugs given in the consolidation phase are given in higher doses than those during induction or the patient may be given a different combination of drugs. Drugs which may be used in this phase include high-dose **methotrexate**, 6-mercaptopurine, **etoposide**, **cytarabine** or a combination of drugs.

The goal during the interim maintenance phase is to maintain remission while allowing the bone marrow to recover. This phase, which lasts about 4 weeks, is followed by delayed intensification. Drugs given during the interim maintenance phase are administered orally.

Treatment given during the delayed intensification component is given to eradicate any remaining leukemic cells which may have been resistant to the drugs administered in the other phases of therapy.

The final phase, maintenance, consists of the administration of intrathecal methotrexate every three months in addition to monthly administration of vincristine, weekly methotrexate and daily 6-mercaptopurine.

Like adults, children also receive prophylaxis against central nervous system spread. They receive multiple doses of intrathecal chemotherapy, with the drugs delivered directly to the spinal fluid through a lumbar puncture or spinal tap. Cranial radiation as central nervous system prophylaxis for children is infrequently used. Though once standard, brain radiation produced a high incidence of cognitive and learning disabilities, especially among those younger than five years old. Cranial radiation is reserved for those children felt to be at high risk of central nervous system disease, including those older than ten at the time of diagnosis, those with initial white blood cell counts of more than 50,000 per microliter, and those with T-cell leukemia. Some high-risk children who enter remission rapidly with induction chemotherapy receive intrathecal chemotherapy alone, without radiation therapy.

Alternative and complementary therapies

ADULTS. Individuals with leukemia often employ alternative or complementary therapies. Some of these provide pain relief and improve psychological well being. No controlled studies have yet shown that alternative treatments offer cures for ALL, although some may hold promise of benefit.

Patients with ALL sometimes use acupuncture, which offers relief from generalized pain, nausea, and vomiting. Other methods that may help with the physical and often emotional side effects of treatment include hypnosis, guided imagery, and yoga.

Nutritional supplements and herbs are sometimes utilized by persons with leukemia. **Coenzyme Q10** is an antioxidant, a substance that protects cells from toxic byproducts of metabolism. Early studies suggest, although it is not proven, that coenzyme Q10 can improve immune function and counteract some of the harmful effects of chemotherapy and radiation on healthy cells. Adverse effects of coenzyme Q10 include headache, rash, heartburn and **diarrhea**. Another supplement with potential benefit is polysaccharide K (PSK). A few studies have shown PSK to have some benefit in improving immunity.

Supplements that have not been proven to be of value or are potentially dangerous to those with leukemia include camphor, sometimes called 714-X. Green tea has received much press for its reported abilities to enhance the immune system and fight cancer, but studies have had conflicting results. Some show that green tea has preventive benefits and others show no effect. A few animal studies suggest that growth of tumors might be slowed by green tea, but this has not been shown in humans yet.

Hoxsey is another supplement touted as a cancer treatment, but no studies have confirmed any benefit. Some of its ingredients have serious adverse effects. Vitamin megadoses have long been advocated as beneficial in cancer, but no conclusive studies show

benefit, and they have significant potential for adverse effects, such as diarrhea, kidney stones, iron overload, nerve damage and liver disease.

Laetrile, or amygdalin, was once touted as a cure for cancer and leukemia. No human or animal studies conducted in the decades since have shown any benefit other than relief of some pain. Laetrile can, however, cause cyanide poisoning.

CHILDREN. Complementary and alternative treatments are recommended less frequently for children. Real caution must be used in administering herbal remedies to children, whose metabolisms are very different from those of adults. For example, jin bu hua, a traditional Chinese medicine, can cause heart or breathing problems. Life root and comfrey can both cause fatal liver damage in children.

While many children are too young for formal guided imagery, they can be distracted from the fears and pain associated with some treatments by toys and videotapes. Reading favorite books during scary procedures can relieve some of their fears.

ALL in remission

ADULTS. Remission is achieved in many people within days of beginning treatment. Treatment does not end at that point, but rather enters into the next phases, called consolidation and maintenance. Several different approaches can be used in these. Some patients receive long term chemotherapy with drugs that might include Ara-C (cytarabine), **cyclophosphamide**, methotrexate, **mercaptopurine**, vincristine, prednisone, or **doxorubicin**. Other patients undergo high-dose chemotherapy or combination chemotherapy and radiation therapy to ablate or wipe out their own bone marrow, and then have bone marrow or stem cell transplants. Adverse effects of bone marrow transplant include significant risk of serious infection and **graft-vs.-host disease** (GVHD), in which the transplanted cells fail to "recognize" the host's cells as self and attack the host cells. Medications to decrease this risk include those that suppress the immune system and steroids.

Central nervous system prophylaxis, as either intrathecal chemotherapy or radiation therapy or both, typically continues through at least a portion of the post-remission therapy.

Adults who receive intensive chemotherapy have a 40% likelihood of long-term survival.

Recurrent ALL

ADULTS. Adults who relapse after initial remission and maintenance therapy often undergo reinduction chemotherapy and are then referred for bone marrow or stem cell transplant. Some receive transplants of umbilical cord blood. Such transplants carry the risk of graft versus host disease, but also carry the possibility of graft versus leukemia, in which the transplanted cells attack the residual leukemic cells. Unlike graft versus host disease, graft versus leukemia is useful.

New treatments for relapsed ALL include immunotherapies or **biological response modifiers**. Some reduce adverse effects of treatment and others are used to fight the leukemia. Some of these include cytokines, substances that stimulate the production of blood cells after treatment has suppressed the bone marrow, and colony-stimulating factors, which have the same effect. Other patients may be offered options of bone marrow or peripheral blood stem cell transplantation.

CHILDREN. The treatment and prognosis of children who relapse depends on the timing of that relapse. Relapse that occurs within six months is often treated with **bone marrow transplantation**. Early relapse carries the least favorable prognosis, with only 10–20% chance of long term survival. Relapse that occurs more than a year after initial treatment is finished can be treated with another full round of chemotherapy, and bone marrow transplant or stem cell transplant reserved for those children who relapse a second time. Those with such late relapses have a 30–40% chance of long term survival.

Recurrent disease may occur in a sanctuary site, or a part of the body difficult to penetrate with chemotherapeutic drugs. The central nervous system is the most common site of such recurrences. Children who have an isolated central nervous system relapse during the first 18 months of treatment have a 45% likelihood of long-term survival. Children with central nervous system relapse after the first 18 months of treatment have up to an 80% chance of long-term survival. Treatment for relapse in the central nervous system includes intrathecal chemotherapy, and for most children, the use of radiation therapy to the brain and spinal cord.

The testicles are the second most common site of relapse. Early testicular relapse (within the first 18 months of treatment) carries a 40% chance of long-term survival, and late testicular relapse carries an 85% chance of long-term survival. Another sanctuary site is the eye, but isolated relapse here is unusual.

Coping with cancer treatment

The treatment of ALL can be particularly draining, not only due to adverse effects but due to its prolonged time course. Although much of the treatment can be given on an outpatient basis, many protocols utilize lengthy intravenous infusions of chemotherapy and require hospitalization.

ADULTS. To prevent **nausea and vomiting**, adults can take oral anti-nausea medication an hour or so before scheduled treatments, including intrathecal treatments. To avoid headache, they should remain flat for at least 30 to 60 minutes after intrathecal chemotherapy. Nurses can give instructions in mouth care if mouth sores occur and skin care if rashes occur after radiation treatment. Books, music, and television can provide distraction and reduce anxiety during chemotherapy infusions.

Patients scheduled for inpatient stays can bring their own pillows, pajamas and even food, with their doctor's approval. Temporary issuance of handicapped parking stickers are often helpful.

CHILDREN. The presence of parents during treatment is critical. While some hospitals exclude parents during treatments, others invite them to be present. Blood can be drawn and intravenous catheters placed while children sit in their parents' laps. If at all possible, a parent should spend the night during any hospitalizations.

Like adults, children can take anti-nausea drugs an hour or so before scheduled treatments. Children, and some adults, can apply topical anesthetic creams to sites of bone marrow aspirates or spinal taps. Favorite stuffed animals or blankets can be present for most procedures.

Play and fun are as important to children with cancer as to healthy children. Items such as board games, modeling clay, video games, dolls, and toy cars can be enjoyed even with intravenous lines in place. Play dates with friends should be encouraged, with proper screening to limit exposure to contagious illnesses.

School districts are required to accommodate the special needs of children. Children with ALL might require shorter school days or the provision of a tutor at home. Children who develop learning disabilities due to treatment might require the intervention of a special education team.

Clinical trials

There are numerous **clinical trials** looking at novel strategies for the treatment of ALL in adults and children. Most oncologists consider bone marrow transplants to be state-of-the-art in specific circumstances, and some insurance companies agree. Many

QUESTIONS TO ASK THE DOCTOR

- What type of leukemia do I or does my child have?
- What characteristics of my or my child's illness are favorable? Which are unfavorable?
- What course of therapy do you recommend?
- What medications will you use and what side effects are anticipated?
- Will I or my child need to be hospitalized for those treatments?
- Should I or my child be enrolled in a clinical trial?
- Can I continue to work or can my child go to school?
- Can I stay with my child for procedures? For hospitalizations?
- How and what should we tell our child about this illness?
- What should we tell our other children?

still require extensive reviews before approving coverage for transplant.

A variety of biological agents are currently under study. These include antibodies that react specifically against leukemic cells, causing their death, and chemicals that interfere with the leukemic cells' normal DNA function or their ability to make proteins.

Researchers are developing second and third generation versions of established chemotherapeutic drugs, isolating the molecular components of those drugs that seem to be most useful in ALL and amplifying them.

Locating and enrolling in clinical trials has been made easier by listings on the Internet. A general search under "clinical trials and leukemia" will yield several listings. University-affiliated hospitals and oncologists participate in many trials and can refer patients to other sites if necessary.

Prevention

There are few preventive measures to take against ALL. Those who work with chemicals should be cautious, particularly around benzene. Pregnant women should avoid exposure to ionizing radiation to reduce the risk to their unborn children.

Special concerns

Parents of children with ALL have specific concerns regarding the long-term consequences of treatment for ALL, such as learning disabilities. Organizations devoted to childhood cancer, hospital social workers, pediatric oncologists and other parents can be important resources when advocating for the educational needs of the child with ALL.

When cranial radiation must be used, children have a risk of developing secondary cancers in the central nervous system years later. Some children are left infertile by the treatment. Chicken pox can be lethal in children with ALL. The introduction of the chicken pox vaccine has reduced this risk, but parents must still be vigilant.

Resources

BOOKS

Margolin, J.F., Steuber, C.P., Poplack, D.G. *Acute Lymphoblastic Leukemia in Principles and Practice of Pediatric Oncology, 15th ed.* 2006.

PERIODICALS

de Labarthe, A., et al. "Imatinib Combined with Induction or Consolidation Chemotherapy with de novo Philadelphia Chromosome Positive Acute Lymphoblastic Leukemia: Results of the GRAAPH-2003 Study." *Blood* 109, no. 4 (February 15, 2007):1408–1413.

Pui, C.H. & Evans, W.E. "Treatment of Acute Lymphoblastic Leukemia." *New England Journal of Medicine.* 353, no.2 (January 12, 2006):166–78.

Pui, C.H., Robinson, L.L., & Look, A.T. "Acute Lymphoblastic Leukemia." *Lancet* 371 no. 9617 (March 22, 2008):1030–1043.

ORGANIZATIONS

American Cancer Society. 1599 Clifton Rd., Atlanta, GA, 30329. (800) ACS-2345. http://www.cancer.org.

Cancer Care, Inc. 275 Seventh Ave, Floor 22 New York, NY 10001. (212) 712-8400 or (800) 813-4673. http://www.cancercare.org.

Candlelighters Childhood Cancer Foundation. National Office P.O. Box 498 Kensington, MD 20895-0498. (800) 366-CCCF. http://www.candlelighters.org.

The Leukemia and Lymphoma Society of America (formerly The Leukemia Society of America). 1311 Mamaroneck Ave., White Plains, NY 10605. (800) 955-4572. http://www.leukemia-lymphoma.org.

The National Cancer Institute. Cancer Information Service. Building 31, Room 10A31, 31 Center Dr., MSC 2580, Bethesda, MD 20892-2580. (301) 435-3848. http://www.cancer.gov/.

National Childhood Cancer Foundation. 440 E. Huntington Dr., Suite 400, Arcadia, CA 91066-3776. (800) 458-6223. http://www.curesearch.org.

National Marrow Donor Program. Suite 100, 3001 Broadway St. NE, Minneapolis, MN 55413-1753. (800) MARROW-2. http://www.marrow.org/.

Marianne Vahey, M.D.
Melinda Granger Oberleitner, R.N., D.N.S.,
A.P.R.N., C.N.S.

Acute myelocytic leukemia

Definition

Acute myelocytic leukemia (AML) is an acute **cancer** that affects white blood cells, primarily those of the granulocyte or monocyte types.

Description

Acute myelogenous leukemia and acute nonlymphocytic leukemia (ANLL) are other names for AML and refer to the identical disease.

The cells that make up blood are produced in the bone marrow and the lymph system. The bone marrow is the spongy tissue found in the large bones of the body. The lymph system includes the spleen (an organ in the upper abdomen), the thymus (a small organ beneath the breastbone), and the tonsils (an organ in the throat). In addition, the lymph vessels (tiny tubes that branch like blood vessels into all parts of the body) and lymph nodes (pea-shaped organs that are found along the network of lymph vessels) are also part of the lymph system. The lymph is a milky fluid

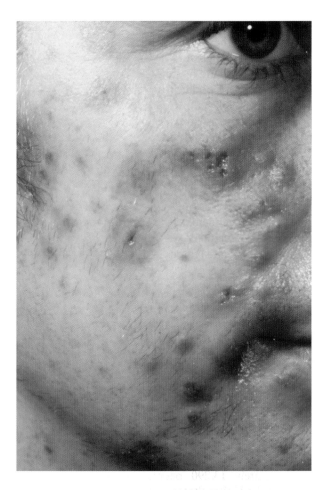

An acute myelocytic leukemia patient with a rash, one of the symptoms of the disease. *(Custom Medical Stock Photo. Reproduced by permission.)*

An enhanced scanning electron microscopy (SEM) image of acute myelocytic leukemia cells. *(Photograph by Robert Becker, Ph.D., Custom Medical Stock Photo. Reproduced by permission.)*

that contains cells. Clusters of lymph nodes are found in the neck, underarm, pelvis, abdomen, and chest.

The main types of cells found in the blood are the red blood cells (RBCs), which carry oxygen and other materials to all tissues of the body; white blood cells (WBCs), which fight **infection**; and the platelets, which play a part in the clotting of the blood. The white blood cells can be further subdivided into three main types: granulocytes, monocytes, and lymphocytes.

The granulocytes, as their name suggests, have particles (granules) inside them. These granules contain special proteins (enzymes) and several other substances that can break down chemicals and destroy microorganisms such as bacteria. Monocytes are the second type of white blood cell. They are also important in defending the body against pathogens. The lymphocytes form the third type of white blood cell.

The bone marrow makes stem cells, which are the precursors of the different blood cells. These stem cells mature through stages into either RBCs, WBCs, or platelets. In **acute leukemias**, the maturation process of the white blood cells is interrupted. The immature cells (or "blasts") proliferate rapidly and begin to accumulate in various organs and tissues, thereby affecting their normal function. This uncontrolled proliferation of the immature cells in the bone marrow affects the production of the normal red blood cells and platelets as well.

Acute leukemias are of two types: **acute lymphocytic leukemia** and acute myelogenous leukemia. Different types of white blood cells are involved in the two leukemias. In acute lymphocytic leukemia (ALL), it is the lymphocytes that become cancerous. AML is a cancer of the monocytes and/or granulocytes.

The reason certain leukemias are now called acute is because of names received decades ago. Before the discovery of modern methods of cancer treatment, these were illnesses that progressed rapidly. In contrast, **chronic leukemias** were, in this period before newer methods had been invented, illnesses that progressed more slowly.

Demographics

According to the American Cancer Society, approximately 13,290 people were diagnosed with AML in the Unites States in 2008. An estimated 8,820 people died of the disease during that same time period. Older persons are considerably more likely to develop AML. As the general population continues to age, it is anticipated that the number of cases of AML will continue to rise as well.

AML sometimes affects children. About 500 children develop AML in the United States every year. Approximately one in five of all children who develop leukemia develop AML. The disease affects boys and girls in roughly equal numbers. Children in all ethnic groups may develop the disease. If one of two identical twins develop AML, the chances are considerable that the other twin will develop the disease as well.

Causes and symptoms

AML is neither contagious nor inherited. However, people who suffer from certain genetic disorders, such as **Fanconi anemia**, Klinefelter syndrome, Patau syndrome, Bloom syndrome, and Down syndrome, are at greater risk of developing AML than the general population. A child with Down syndrome is roughly 14 times as likely as the average child to develop leukemia.

Any person who has been exposed to radiation at high doses is at heightened risk of developing AML, as are people exposed to benzene, a chemical used in the manufacture of plastics, rubber, medicines, and certain other chemicals including petrochemicals. Another group of people at increased risk for developing AML are those who have been treated for cancer previously. The number of treatment-related cases of AML is increasing particularly in survivors of childhood and adolescent cancers such as Hodgkin's disease, **lymphoma**, **sarcoma**, **testicular cancer** and **breast cancer**.

The symptoms of AML are generally vague and non-specific. A patient may experience all or some of the following symptoms:

- weakness or chronic fatigue
- fever of unknown origin
- shortness of breath
- weight loss that is not due to dieting or exercise
- frequent bacterial or viral infections
- headaches
- skin rash
- non-specific bone pain
- easy bruising
- bleeding from gums or nose
- blood in urine or stools
- enlarged lymph nodes and/or spleen
- abdominal fullness

A small minority of patients with AML have a tumor of leukemic cells at diagnosis. Such a tumor may appear in the lung, breast, brain, uterus, ovary, stomach, prostate, or certain other places in the body.

Some children with AML present to their doctor with very few symptoms, while other children present with severe symptoms. **Anemia** is usually present. The symptoms of the anemia may include **fatigue**, dizziness, headache, paleness of the skin, or, infrequently, congestive heart failure. Easy bruising, bleeding gums, and nosebleeds may be present, as may **fever**. There may be swollen gums, **bone pain** or joint pain, or, rarely, an actual tumor. Some infants with AML have skin disorders.

Diagnosis

Like all cancers, acute leukemias are best treated when found early. There are no screening tests available.

A thorough diagnostic evaluation should be conducted. This is important because the doctor must determine more than whether or not AML is present.

If it is suspected, has it affected the general health of the patient? Is the patient capable of undergoing rigorous treatment?

A doctor who suspects leukemia may start by obtaining a thorough medical history. The doctor may then conduct a very thorough physical examination to look for enlarged lymph nodes in the neck, underarm, and pelvic region. Swollen gums, enlarged liver or spleen, bruises, or pinpoint red rashes all over the body are among the signs of the disease. In addition, the physician may examine the teeth and look for dental abscesses, and may explore whether back pain is present.

Urine and blood tests may be ordered to check for microscopic amounts of blood in the urine and to obtain a complete differential blood count. This count will give the numbers and percentages of the different cells found in the blood. An abnormal blood test might suggest leukemia. Patients suffering from AML may have high leukocyte counts and typically have low counts of both red blood cells and platelets. Many patients with AML have low counts of all of the major components of the blood. A microscopic exploration of the blood will usually show that leukemic blast cells are present. However, the diagnosis has to be confirmed by more specific tests.

The doctor may perform a **bone marrow aspiration and biopsy** to confirm the diagnosis of leukemia. Aspiration involves the withdrawal of a liquid sample of marrow. During the **biopsy**, a cylindrical piece of bone and marrow is removed. The tissue is generally taken out of the hipbone. These samples are sent to the laboratory for examination. In addition to diagnosis, the aspiration and biopsy may be repeated during the treatment phase of the disease to see if the leukemia is responding to therapy.

A chest x ray is taken. Cardiac tests, including an electrocardiogram, are conducted. The patient is examined for possible infection. These diagnostic procedures often disclose bleeding in the stomach or intestines, and there may be bleeding in the lungs, brain, or eyes. Anemia is often present and may be severe.

Sophisticated cytogenetic studies, which examine the number and shape of the chromosomes in the DNA of individual blast cells, should be conducted in addition to the immunophenotyping of cells of the bone marrow. This procedure involves applying various stains to the marrow cells. These stains help doctors identify some of the proteins lying on the surface of the cells.

A spinal tap (**lumbar puncture**) is another procedure the doctor may order to diagnose leukemia. In this procedure, a small needle is inserted into the spinal cavity in the lower back to withdraw some cerebrospinal fluid and to look for leukemic cells. Routine screening with lumbar puncture is not warranted in AML patients at the time of diagnosis, however.

Standard imaging tests such as **x rays** may be used to check whether the leukemic cells have invaded other areas of the body, such as the bones, chest, kidneys, abdomen, or brain. Other tests, such as **computed tomography** scans (CT scans), **magnetic resonance imaging** (MRI), or gallium scans, are not typical for AML but may also be performed.

Children with AML undergo most of the same studies used for adults.

Clinical staging, treatments, and prognosis

Unlike several other cancers, AML is not staged. However, a classification system is used to separate different forms of AML. One of the most important classification systems, devised by a team of physicians, is known as the French-American-British (FAB) Classification System. A newer staging system for AML is the World Health Organization (WHO) Staging System which takes into account newer prognostic factors and the results of cytogenetic analyses such as molecular markers and chromosomal translocations. The WHO classification includes a minimum of 17 subclassifications of AML. In general, AML is distinguished from other highly myelodysplastic diseases when the percentage of blast (immature) cells in the bone marrow or in the blood exceeds 30%.

The goal of AML treatment is to achieve a complete remission (CR). What is a complete remission? It is a measure that indicates that the patient's disease has gotten markedly better in several ways. In general, it might be said that CR is achieved once the body has regained its ability to produce blood cells normally. At this point, the number of blood cells of various types should return to normal ranges, while none of the immature cells called leukemic blast cells should be present in the blood or the marrow.

Chemotherapy is the use of drugs to kill cancer cells. It is usually the treatment of choice in AML and is used to relieve symptoms and achieve long-term remission of the disease. Generally, combination chemotherapy, in which multiple drugs are used, is more efficient than using a single drug for the treatment. Some drugs may be administered intravenously through a vein in the arm; others may be given by mouth in the form of pills. If the cancer cells have invaded the brain, then chemotherapeutic drugs may be put into the fluid that surrounds the brain and spinal cord. This is known as intrathecal chemotherapy. Chemotherapy should start soon after diagnosis.

Patients who are anemic or who have low platelet counts should receive transfusions. These transfusions should be sufficient to restore counts of various components of the blood to adequate levels.

There are two general phases of treatment of acute leukemia in adults, the induction phase and the consolidation (post-induction or post-remission) phase. The first phase is called induction therapy. During this phase, the main aim of treatment is to reduce the number of leukemic cells as much as possible and induce a remission in the patient.

Patient characteristics such as age and presence of co-morbidities, play a role significant role in determining the treatment strategies offered during the induction phase. For example, older patients (greater than age 60) may not be able to tolerate the intensity of the induction chemotherapy regimens and may be treated with supportive care or with therapy that is of a lower intensity.

A variety of chemotherapy agents may be used during the induction therapy portion of AML treatment. For patients ages 60 and younger the chemotherapy agent Ara-C (**cytarabine**) is often used in combination with either **daunorubicin** or **idarubicin** (Idamycin). This standard regimen for AML induction therapy has not changed in 25 years. Participation in a clinical trial may be an option for older individuals with a poor cytogentic prognosis. For older AML patients with a better cytogenetic prognosis, enrollment in a clinical trial may also be an option. These individuals may also be treated with standard chemotherapy for AML. Two newer agents, decitabine and clofarabine, are being studied in large scale **clinical trials** at this time as options for induction therapy for older individuals diagnosed with AML.

A second phase of treatment is initiated once CR is achieved. This is called post-remission or consolidation therapy. The goal of therapy now becomes killing any remaining cells and maintaining the remission for as long as possible.

For patients under the age of 60, post-induction or consolidation therapy is determined by the effectiveness of the induction therapy. A bone marrow aspirate and biopsy are conducted one week to 10 days after completion of induction therapy to evaluate the effectiveness of the therapy. If the induction therapy failed to bring the patient into remission, allogeneic stem cell transplant with an HLA-matched donor may be an option. If no matched donor is available, the patient may be enrolled in a clinical trial. For younger patients who are in remission post-induction, 3-4 cycles of high dose cytarabine therapy has been the standard regimen since 1994. Other options may include 1 or more cycles of high dose cytarabine followed by autologous stem cell transplant or allogeneic stem cell transplant from a sibling or unrelated donor.

Transplantation therapy has been studied very thoroughly. It involves taking blood-making cells, whether from the patient or from another person, and infusing them into the patient following removal of the diseased marrow, with either high doses of chemotherapy or total body irradiation. These procedures are potentially very effective because of the remarkable ability of these cells to create a sustained replacement of the patient's blood cells.

Other treatment strategies may also be implemented. Approaches used for patients younger than 60 years of age may differ from those used for patients of older ages. Post-induction therapy for those over the age of 60 also includes an evaluation of the bone marrow 10 to 14 days after the completion of induction therapy. Patients with significant responses to induction therapy will receive standard dose cytarabine plus an anthracycline or anthracenedione agent. Some older patients may be candidates for reduced intensity stem cell transplantation as consolidation therapy.

Post-remission follow-up for older patients includes undergoing a complete blood count and platelet count every one to three months for two years after the completion of consolidation therapy. After two years the CBC and platelet count will be done very 3 to 6 months for five years. Growth factor support may be considered for patients older than 60 after the conclusion of therapy. Patients over the age of 60 whose disease relapses may be treated with the drug, **gemtuzumab** ozogamicin.

Because leukemia cells can spread to all the organs via the blood stream and the lymph vessels, surgery is not considered an option for treating leukemias.

Most children diagnosed with AML undergo treatment in two phases: induction and intensification (consolidation). Often two or three medicines are used in conjunction with one another. After remission is achieved in a young patient, typically after 2 or 3 treatments, postremission therapy is started. The type of postremission therapy depends largely on the type of AML the patient has. It may involve additional chemotherapy or stem cell transplantation. Chemotherapy to the central nervous system (CNS) is given to most children, since without it, roughly one in five will develop CNS relapse. The CNS includes the brain and spinal cord.

The prognosis of patients with AML varies, however, outcomes for AML, particularly for older patients, have not changed appreciably in 30 years. A number of different matters should be examined before the prognosis of any individual patient is assessed. The most important of these is whether or not the patient attains a complete remission (CR). The most important consideration in terms of whether a patient is likely to achieve CR is the patient's age. However, it may be that chronological age is not what really matters. Rather, to a large extent, what is truly significant is the patient's ability to survive the difficulties associated with induction therapy. For example, the patient who has some other disease in addition to AML may have a more difficult time with the rigors of the therapy. Yet, it is also true that older patients are more likely to have AML that expresses certain characteristics associated with poorer outcomes.

Other factors also affect the patient's prognosis. For example, in the tests performed during diagnosis, the chromosomes of cells are examined. Some chromosomal findings are associated with a good prognosis. Others are only mildly good, while still others indicate the patient is less likely to achieve CR.

Other factors that may provide physicians with hints as to the patient's prognosis include: how long symptoms were present before the illness was diagnosed, and how quickly immature blast cells disappear after treatment is started.

Coping with cancer treatment

One of the most important aspects of treatment is guaranteeing that the patient will have the supportive care needed to come through the treatment period with physical and emotional strength intact. Part of what this means is that AML should be treated in major cancer centers, because only these centers have the medical and nursing expertise necessary to provide not only the right medicine but also the intensive supportive care reqired during treatment for AML.

One way physicians help AML patients cope with treatment is to guarantee that adequate blood bank support is available. Many patients require platelet transfusions.

One of the great dangers to patients during induction treatment and other steps of treatment is the threat of serious infectious disease. These patients have deficient blood components and are therefore more susceptible to infectious illness than the average person is. The leading cause of death for patients

receiving induction treatment and chemotherapy following remission is infectious illness.

To help build the patient's white cell count, doctors may prescribe growth factors. These encourage the body to produce certain types of blood cells. The types of growth factors prescribed most frequently are granulocyte-colony stimulating factor (G-CSF) and granulocyte-macrophage colony stimulating factor (GM-CSF).

The psychological aspects of cancer treatment are a major concern. Patients should ask their physician about local support groups and survivor networks that can help with the stresses associated with this disease.

Prevention

High doses of radiation and exposure to the chemical benzene (used in the manufacture of plastics, rubber, and medicines) are strong risk factors. With the exception of people with such rare genetic conditions as Fanconi anemia, Klinefelter syndrome, Patau syndrome, Bloom syndrome, and Down syndrome, there is no known genetic predisposition to AML.

Resources

PERIODICALS

Applebaum, F.R., Gundacker, H, Head, D.R. "Age and Acute Myeloid Leukemia." *Blood* 107 (2006): 3481–3485.

Kantarjian, H., O'Brien, S., Cortes, Jl, et al. "Results of Intensive Chemotherapy in 998 Patients Age 65 Years and Older with Actue Myeloid Leukemia or High

Risk Myelodysplastic Syndrome" *Cancer* 106 (2006): 1090–1098.

Smith, M., Barnett, M., Bassen, R., et al."Adult Acute Myeloid Leukemia." *Critical Reviews in Onc/Hem.* 50 (2004): 197–222.

Storb, R. "Can Reduced-Intensity Allogeneic Transplantation Cure Older Adults with AML." *Best Prac Res Clin Haematol.* 20 (2007): 85–90.

OTHER

"Acute Myeloid Leukemia." National Comprehensive Cancer Network (NCCN) Practice Guidelines in Oncology, v.1.2009. http://www.nccn.org.

"Acute Myelogenous Leukemia (AML). Emotional Aspects of Childhood Leukemia. Making Intelligent Choices About Therapy. Understanding Blood Counts." Patient Aid Program. Family Support Group. Information Resource Center. The Leukemia and Lymphoma Society. (800) 955-4572. http://www.leukemia-lymphoma.org.

"Acute Myeloid Leukemia Treatment, Childhood. Acute Myeloid Leukemia Treatment, Adult." National Cancer Institute. (800) 4-CANCER. http://www.nci.cancer.gov.

"Adult Acute Leukemia." American Cancer Society. (800) ACS-2345. http://www.cancer.org.

"How Is Childhood Leukemia Treated." American Cancer Society. (800) ACS-2345. http://www.cancer.org.

Lata Cherath, Ph.D.
Bob Kirsch
Melinda Granger Oberleitner, R.N., D.N.S., A.P.R.N., C.N.S.

Acute myelogenous leukemia *see* **Acute myelocytic leukemia**

Acute promyelocytic leukemia *see* **Acute myelocytic leukemia**

Acyclovir *see* **Antiviral therapy**

Adenocarcinoma

Definition

Cancer that begins in the epithelial cells that line certain internal organs and have glandular (secretory) properties. Some types of adenocarcinomas include cancers of the breast, thyroid, colon, stomach, pancreas, and prostate, cervix, as well as certain types of lung cancer.

Description

There are many different types of cancers. One way of classifying cancers is to group them based on the specific cell type which produced the cancer. The four major categories for classifying cancers using this methodology include: carcinomas (which includes adenocarcinoma), sarcomas, lymphomas, and leukemias. Most cancers arise from one of these major cell types.

Carcinomas are cancers which develop in the cells that line the inside of organs. These cells are called epithelial cells. Epithelial cells form the outer layers of skin and are found in the tissues lining the digestive tract, the bladder, the uterus, and all of the tubes and ducts which are found in virtually every body organ.

Sarcomas develop from cells in the body's connective tissues such as bone, muscle, cartilage, and fibrous tissues.

Lymphomas arise from cells in the lymph system, which is a component of the immune system. Organs in the lymph system include lymph nodes, the spleen, bone marrow, and the thymus gland.

Leukemias, which can be classified as acute or chronic, develop from the white blood cells circulating in the body. Leukemias also affect the bone marrow and the spleen.

Carcinomas are the most common of the four major cell types that produce cancer, constituting about 85% of all cancers.

Carcinomas can be further divided into sub-groups depending on which specific type of epithelial cell is responsible for originating the cancer and in which specific part of the body the cancer originated. The four major types of epithelial cells are: squamous cells, adeno cells, transitional cells, and basal cells. Squamous cells are found in the skin, the lining of the mouth and digestive tract, the trachea, and the bronchi in the lungs as well as in other parts of the body. Adeno cells line all of the glands in the body including the breasts, kidneys and in the digestive organs such as the stomach, bowel and pancreas and many other organs. Transitional cells are found only in the lining of the bladder and other parts of the urinary tract and basal cells form one of the layers of the skin.

Therefore, when a cancer starts in the transitional cells in the lining of the bladder that tumor is called a **transitional cell carcinoma** of the bladder. If an individual develops **skin cancer** in the basal cells of the skin that cancer is called a **basal cell carcinoma** of the skin. A woman who develops a cancer of the glands in the breast would be diagnosed with adenocarcinoma of the breast.

As stated earlier, adenocarcinomas can originate in many different body organs including the colon and rectum, the breast, the lung, the pancreas, the stomach, the ovary and in several other organs.

Adenocarcinomas are malignant tumors that have the ability to metastasize to other parts of the body. Determining the type of cell in which the cancer originated plays an important role in determining the best treatment options for the patient.

Kate Kretschmann
Melinda Granger R.N.,D.N.S., A.P.R.N., C.N.S.

Adenoma

Definition

An adenoma is a benign (noncancerous) tumor that forms from the cells lining the inside or the surface of an organ.

Demographics

Certain types of adenomas are more common in women than in men (e.g., **pituitary tumors** and liver adenoma), and some are more common in older adults (e.g., adenomas of the colon, pituitary). Specific demographics depend on the specific type of adenoma. Adrenal adenomas are found in less than 1% of individuals younger than 30 years, but are found in 7% of individuals 70 years or older. Adenomas of the colon are found in are found in 30–40% of individuals 60 years or older.

Description

Adenomas arise from epithelial cells that are specialized for secretion. This type of epithelial cell is found in glands. Glands produce sweat, saliva, mucus, milk, digestive juices, hormones, and an array of other substances. Hormone-secreting (endocrine) glands include the thyroid, pituitary, parathyroids, adrenals, ovaries, and testes. Adenomas can arise from most gland cells in the body.

Adenomas arise from excessive growth of normal epithelial cells in much the same way as malignant (cancerous) tumors. In healthy cells, cell division and growth is controlled so that new cells are created in an orderly way only when the body needs them. When cells continue to divide uncontrollably and grow beyond what the body needs, a mass or tumor is formed. Unlike malignant tumors, adenomas are not cancerous and do not spread (metastasize) to nearby tissue or other parts of the body. Some adenomas have specialized names, depending on where they are located. A gastrinoma is found in the small intestine or pancreas; a bronchial adenoma is found in the lungs; and a villous adenoma is found in the intestines.

The two major medical concerns related to all tumors found in glands are whether they are malignant and whether they are secreting hormones. Many adenomas affect the normal functioning of the gland in which they arise, most often by secreting a hormone. Elevated hormone levels in the blood and can cause uncomfortable symptoms and sometimes life-threatening conditions.

Tumors found in some glands are more likely to be adenomas than malignant. For example, 80% of **adrenal tumors** are both benign and nonfunctioning, meaning that they are not cancerous and produce no hormones. Hormone-secreting adenomas of the adrenal are associated with Cushing syndrome, a disorder caused by excess levels of the hormone cortisol. Adenomas also form in the gastrointestinal system. About half of tumors that secrete the hormone gastrin (gastrinomas) that are associated with **Zollinger-Ellison syndrome** are benign. Other glands that tend to have a high level of adenomas include the pituitary gland and the salivary glands.

In most cases, the occurrence of an adenoma does not indicate an increased risk for the later development of a **carcinoma**. The exceptions, however, are **colon cancer** and **rectal cancer**, which are thought to develop from adenomas. Also, one type of lung adenoma called a bronchial adenoma can potentially develop into lung **cancer**.

Risk factors

Advanced age appears the be the most common risk factor for the development of an adenoma.

Causes and symptoms

The cause of most adenomas is unknown (idiopathic). Liver adenomas in women have been linked to the use of oral contraceptives, and some conditions, such as a type of adrenal adenoma know as a **pheochromocytoma**, and colon adenomas, can be inherited.

No single set of symptoms can be applied to all adenomas. Some disorders have similar or identical symptoms whether due to an adenoma or carcinoma. Ultimately, the signs and symptoms depend on the location of the adenoma:

- Adrenal glands: an adrenocortical adenoma often shows the same symptoms of an adrenocortical carcinoma, including abdominal pain and loss of weight. A benign and malignant pheochromocytoma also has the same symptoms, including headaches, sweating, and chest pains.
- Breast: a marble-like benign fibroadenoma causes no symptoms and can be either too small to detect by touch or several inches across and easily detected.

- Colon or rectum: persistent diarrhea can indicate villous adenomas of the rectum. Blood in stool samples can indicate adenomas in the colon or rectum. Many other conditions can cause similar symptoms.
- Liver: a hepatic adenoma causes pain and a mass that is detectable by touch.
- Lung: a chronic or bloody cough, fever, chills, and shortness of breath can indicate a bronchial adenoma.
- Pancreas: pain in the abdomen, diarrhea, stomach pain, persistent fatigue, fainting, and weight gain can indicate one of the various types of pancreatic adenomas or pancreatic cancer.
- Parathyroid: weakness, fatigue, constipation, kidney stones, loss of appetite, and bone pain are signs of a condition known as hyperparathyroidism, in which excess parathyroid hormone is secreted. This condition can occur in individuals with either parathyroid adenomas or parathyroid cancer.
- Salivary gland: adenomas are small and usually painless but can cause swelling around the chin or jawbone, numbness of the face, and pain in the face, chin, or neck.
- Stomach and intestine: a gastrinoma causes a peptic ulcer in the intestines or stomach. The occurrence of many ulcers in the stomach, intestine, and pancreas that do not respond well to treatment can indicate Zollinger-Ellison syndrome.
- Sweat gland: adenomas may appear as many small, smooth, and firm bumps on the lower eyelids and upper parts of the cheek (syringomas), or as small bumps with bluish or dark-brown coloration on the head and neck area (hidrocystoma). Solitary adenomas (poromas) occur on the sole of the foot or palm of the hand.
- Thyroid: a lump in the neck region accompanied by a cough and difficulty swallowing or breathing often indicates a benign thyroid nodule; however, these are the same symptoms for thyroid cancer.

Diagnosis

Most adenomas are found incidentally during an imaging procedure related to another condition or in the process of diagnosing confusing symptoms. Once found, a variety of techniques are used to determine whether the mass is an adenomas or a malignant tumor.

Tests

Blood and urine samples are taken to detect elevated levels of hormones or other substances associated with a specific adenoma. Tumors are located using a combination of **ultrasonography**, **computed tomography** scan (CT scan), **magnetic resonance**

imaging (MRI), and possibly radionuclide imaging. A **biopsy** may be performed to determine whether a tumor is benign or malignant.

Treatment

Treatment depends on the location of the adenoma, whether it is secreting a hormone, and the symptoms it is causing, and whether it is related to an underlying condition. Surgical removal is the recommended treatment for many adenomas, especially colon and rectal adenomas, as they are associated with an increased risk for cancer. In some cases, surgery may be impractical, and symptoms of some adenomas, such as some occurring in the pituitary, can be treated with medication.

Prognosis

Outcome depends on the location of the adenoma, whether it is active and is producing symptoms, the symptoms it is causing, the presence of an underlying disease, the type of treatment (surgical or drug therapy) and the response to treatment.

Prevention

Adenomas cannot be prevented because their cause is unknown.

ORGANIZATIONS

National Endocrine and Metabolic Diseases Information Service, 6 Information Way, Bethesda, MD, 20892-3569, (888) 828-0904; TTY (866) 569-1162, (703) 738-4929, endoandmeta@info.niddk.nih.gov, http://www.endocrine.niddk.nih.gov/pubs/cushings/cushings.htm.

Monica NcGee, M.S.
Tish Davidson, A.M.

Adjuvant chemotherapy

Definition

Adjuvant **chemotherapy** is **cancer** treatment that is administered after the primary therapy. For example, when the primary therapy to treat a cancerous tumor is surgery, chemotherapy would be an adjuvant therapy.

Purpose

Even if there is no clear sign that the cancer has spread, adjuvant chemotherapy is administered to prevent the chance of a recurrence by killing any cancer cells that *may have* spread. The rationale behind adjuvant chemotherapy is that the chemotherapy drugs are more effective when they are given immediately after the tumor has been removed and any remaining cancer is in small amounts.

For some cancers, especially breast and colorectal cancers, adjuvant chemotherapy has been shown to decrease the chance the cancer will return. In addition, cancer patients who received adjuvant chemotherapy tend to live longer than those who do not receive the treatment.

Description

Patient selection

Patients selected for adjuvant chemotherapy are usually considered to have a high risk of recurrence. In order to determine the chance of recurrence, physicians look at the prognostic factors, which means they study the characteristics of the tumor. Tumor size, histology, and the proliferation rates are three prognostic factors that help determine the necessity for adjuvant chemotherapy. For example, patients with small tumors (2 centimeters or less) have a better prognosis, in general, than patients with large tumors (5 centimeters or more). Histology (or histologic grade) refers tow hat the tumor cells look like under a microscope. In other words, are the cells close to normal or are they far from normal. The term used to describe them is *differentiated.* When a tumor is well differentiated, the prognosis is better, because the cells closely resemble normal cells. When a tumor is poorly differentiated, the prognosis is considered to be not as good because the cells look very little like normal cells. A high proliferation rate refers to the rate in which cancer cells divide to make more cells. When the cancer cells are multiplying quickly, the cancer is described as aggressive, which often means adjuvant chemotherapy is needed.

Other prognostic factors may need to be considered, depending on the cancer type. For example, the degree of lymph node involvement is an important consideration when the patient has **breast cancer**. During the tumor surgery, physicians often remove some of the underarm lymph nodes to see if they contain any cancerous cells. Positive lymph nodes indicate a higher risk of recurrence, because research shows if the cancer has spread to the lymph nodes, it may have spread to other parts of the body. Hormone receptor status (high levels of estrogen or progesterone that affect cell growth) may also impact the decision whether or not to treat a patient with adjuvant chemotherapy. It should be noted, however, that a panel of experts at a conference sponsored by the National Institutes of Science concluded that "adjuvant chemotherapy improves survival [of breast cancer patients] and should be offered to most women with primary breast cancers (larger than 1 centimeter in diameter) regardless of tumor involvement in the lymph nodes under the arm, menopausal status, or hormone receptor status." Despite the value of analyzing prognostic factors, physicians cannot predict with 100% certainty what the outcome of adjuvant chemotherapy will be. Treatment decisions must be made on an individual basis, taking into account the patient's general health, as well as his or her preferences.

Treatment specifics

In general, adjuvant chemotherapy is started as soon as possible after surgery. In the case of colorectal cancer patients, for example, physicians don't like to wait more than six weeks after surgery to begin adjuvant chemotherapy. Chemotherapy regimes generally include more than one drug, but not always. The drug combinations are selected based on the kind of cancer being treated and individual patient considerations.

Adjuvant chemotherapy treatments are usually given over a period of months in cycles, meaning a treatment is followed by a recovery period. The treatments can be administered orally, intravenously (through a vein), by injection, or by a patch on the skin. Most patients receive adjuvant chemotherapy as an outpatient in a hospital or clinic, but, in some cases, the treatments can be given at home.

Preparation

Each patient should talk with his or her doctor regarding any preparations that need to be made prior to treatment. Patients who work outside the home might want to plan, if possible, to take the entire day off from work on the day the chemotherapy is given. Depending on how a patient responds to treatment, the patient may need the next day off as well. The laws vary from state to state regarding employee rights, but many states have specific laws that address what the obligations of an employer are to an employee who is seriously ill. Patients concerned that they might be treated unfairly should consult an attorney.

Many patients prefer to have someone with them when they receive chemotherapy treatments, especially with regard to driving them home. Some cancer treatment centers insist that a patient have someone provide transportation. Patients who do not have friends or family available to help them can call the American Cancer Society. They manage a volunteer program that provides cancer patients with rides to and from the hospital or clinical where they will receive their treatments. For patients that live over 30 miles away from the nearest treatment center or hospital, the American Cancer Society also tries to arrange free-of-charge hotel rooms for cancer patients.

Patients with children may want to arrange to have someone stay with them while they are having chemotherapy, especially the day of or the day after the treatments. Patients should ask their physicians what local support groups exist in their area that specialize in this type of assistance. Church groups often have volunteers who will be willing to lend a hand as well. In addition, the hospital or cancer treatment center is likely to have a list of available services from a variety of sources.

Aftercare

Patients can expect to have some side effects associated with chemotherapy, although the particular side effects will vary depending on the patient and the drug combinations. Most patients lose their hair during chemotherapy treatment. Patients can also expect to be more prone to **infection** and feel fatigued,

even for a period of time after the therapy is all done. For example, patients whose gums tend to bleed when they brush their teeth may be advised to brush their teeth gently and use a soft brush. Other cautions may be to avoid crowds and people who patients know are sick. Other common side effects are **nausea**, **vomiting**, **diarrhea**, and mouth sores.

Chemotherapy doses can be adjusted and medication can be prescribed to help the patient overcome nausea. Patients should refrain from taking any medications (over-the-counter or prescription) without first talking to their oncologist (a physician who specializes in cancer treatment). In general, it is a good idea for patients to talk with all their treatment team regarding the toxic effects associated with adjuvant chemotherapy.

Risks

There is some concern that woman over 70 years of age, for example, are more likely to develop severe side effects than younger women. However, in a large randomized clinical trial conducted by Muss and colleagues, which was published in the *Journal of the American Medical Association*, it was concluded that age alone was not a significant enough reason to avoid treating elderly women with adjuvant chemotherapy. In the study, the researchers tracked 6,487 breast cancer patients, all of whom had a high risk of recurrence, to see how they responded to high doses of chemotherapy. The study included 542 patients who were 65 years of age or older and 159 of them were 70 years of age and older. Although the researchers found that older patients did have a slightly higher risk of bad reactions to the chemotherapy, the researchers concluded that the risks did not outweigh the benefits of treatment.

Results

Treatment results vary from patient to patient, depending on a variety of factors. However, research shows that the benefits of adjuvant chemotherapy often outweigh the risks, especially for patients with breast or colorectal cancers. A patient's physician will perform various tests to determine if the treatment is working, such as blood tests and physical examinations. Some patients think that the side effects provide some indication as to how the treatment is working. The truth is, however, that the severity or lack of severity of the side effects has nothing to do with the effectiveness of the treatment.

Resources

PERIODICALS

Muss, H. B., Woolf, S., Berry, D., et al. "Adjuvant chemotherapy in older and younger women with lymph node-positive breast cancer." *Journal of the American Medical Association* 293 (2005): 1118–1120.

OTHER

American Cancer Society. "Older Women Less Likely To Be Offered Adjuvant Chemotherapy." *American Cancer Society* 9 May 2003 American Cancer Society. 24 Feb 2005 http://www.cancer.org/.

National Cancer Institute "Adjuvant Therapy for Breast Cancer: Questions and Answers. *National Cancer Institute* 13 May 2002 National Cancer Institute. 24 Feb. 2005 http://www.cancer.gov/.

Susan G. Komen Breast Cancer Foundation. "Recommendations for Adjuvant Therapy for Breast Cancer Updated by the National Institute of Health Consensus Panel." *Susan G. Komen Breast Cancer Foundation* 2 Jan 2001 Susan G. Komen Breast Cancer Foundation. 19 March 2005 http://www.cancer.org/.

Susan G. Komen Breast Cancer Foundation. "Adjuvant Therapy Improves Survival for Women with Fast Growing Localized Breast Cancer." *Susan G. Komen Breast Cancer Foundation* 2 Feb 2002 Susan G. Komen Breast Cancer Foundation. 19 March 2005 http://www.cancer.org/.

Lee Ann Paradise

Adrenal fatigue

Definition

Adrenal **fatigue** refers to suboptimal functioning of the adrenal glands, particularly the inadequate secretion of the hormone cortisol. The syndrome is characterized by a collection of generalized symptoms, especially lack of energy, fatigue, and anxiety. Adrenal fatigue is an accepted diagnosis among practitioners of alternative medicine, but is not widely recognized in conventional medicine. Adrenal fatigue is also referred to as:

- adrenal apathy
- adrenal neurasthenia
- hypoadrenalism
- neurasthenia
- non-Addison's hypoadrenia
- sub-clinical hypoadrenia

Demographics

Because adrenal fatigue is not widely recognized as a medical condition, there are no reliable statistics about its incidence. Some proponents assert that at some point in their lives an estimated 80% of people in industrialized nations are affected by adrenal fatigue. The condition is believed to be stress-related and, by some estimations, 75–90% of visits to primary care physicians in the United States are stress-related.

Description

The adrenal glands, also called the suprarenal glands, are walnut-sized organs located near the top of each kidney. The adrenals, along with the hypothalamus and pituitary gland, constitute the master control network of the endocrine system. The adrenal glands produce a large number of essential hormones including epinephrine, norepinephrine, sex hormones, and cortisol. Among its many other functions, cortisol is an important component of the body's stress response. It is the major "fight or flight" hormone that helps the human body respond to danger and other stressful situations.

Cortisol affects virtually every system of the body. It is responsible, in part, for regulating:

- blood sugar (glucose) levels through its control of fat, protein, and carbohydrate metabolism
- blood pressure and heart and blood vessel tone and contraction
- central nervous system activation
- immune system responses
- anti-inflammatory activity

Stress is believed to play a role in many diseases, particularly cardiovascular and gastrointestinal disorders. It also causes generalized anxiety and sleep disorders. The contribution of stress to disease is thought to be due, in part, to increased production of cortisol and other stress hormones and the resulting decrease in immune system functioning.

In addition to its secretion in response to stress, cortisol is secreted in response to 24-hour circadian rhythms. Cortisol secretion by the adrenals is at its lowest level at about 4 A.M. and peaks at about 8 A.M.

Adrenal insufficiency or Addison's disease is a serious condition in which an underlying disease or disorder results in inadequate production of cortisol and possibly other adrenal hormones. Adrenal fatigue is usually defined as a mild form of adrenal insufficiency. It can occur when the adrenal glands do not respond adequately to the demands of stress or when they do not function at an adequate level even when the body is at rest. This diminished adrenal function—the inability to secrete the hormones necessary for maintaining the body's homeostasis—is said to result from over-stimulation of the adrenal glands.

Proponents claim that adrenal fatigue can contribute to a broad spectrum of conditions including:

- frequent infections
- allergies
- chemical sensitivities
- premenstrual syndrome (PMS) and menopausal symptoms
- imbalances in thyroid hormones
- chronic anxiety
- mild depression
- chronic fatigue syndrome
- autoimmune diseases such as fibromyalgia and rheumatoid arthritis
- obesity

Risk factors

Some practitioners believe that adrenal fatigue appears to run in families and may be inherited. Other commonly cited risk factors include:

- chronic illness
- recurrent infections
- a life crisis
- chronic stress caused by financial or other pressures
- poor diet
- sleep deprivation
- smoking
- substance abuse
- pregnancy

Causes and symptoms

Adrenal insufficiency has a variety of causes including:

- genetic disorders such as congenital adrenal hyperplasia, in which the adrenals do not make sufficient cortisol and in which other hormones may be out of balance
- pituitary tumors, since the activity of the adrenal glands is controlled by the pituitary gland
- bleeding
- infections

In contrast, it is usually argued that adrenal fatigue is caused by physical, mental, and/or emotional stress that is frequent, persistent, or severe. Stress activates the "fight or flight" response, resulting in increased secretion of cortisol, epinephrine, and norepinephrine by the adrenal glands. These hormones increase heart rate, blood pressure, and blood sugar levels and shunt blood away from the digestive system. Proponents of adrenal fatigue argue that the adrenal glands cannot produce hormones in sufficient quantities to meet the demands of a body that is often in a "fight or flight" state of arousal. They further argue that chronic, frequent, or persistent stress—and the demands that it puts on the adrenals—disrupts the normal circadian release of cortisol and perhaps other hormones. These disruptive effects on the adrenal glands can continue long after the stress has passed.

A wide range of stresses can stimulate the release cortisol and the catecholamine stress hormones epinephrine and norepinephrine and lead to suboptimal adrenal function. These stresses include:

- caloric restriction
- poor diet
- sleep deprivation
- excessive exercise
- extreme weather (too hot or too cold)
- life-changing events
- various mental states
- injury
- surgery
- metal toxicity, such as exposure to lead, mercury, cadmium, or aluminum
- acute or chronic infections, especially respiratory infections such as flu, bronchitis, or pneumonia

The primary symptom of adrenal fatigue is tiredness that is not relieved by sleep and a general malaise. Patients with adrenal fatigue usually:

- wake in the morning feeling tired
- do not feel completely awake until after their noon meal
- feel low between 2 P.M. and 4 P.M.
- feel better after 6 P.M.
- are usually tired again by 9 P.M. In the most severe cases, patients may have difficulty spending more than a few hours a day out of bed.

Other symptoms of adrenal fatigue may include:

- lack of energy
- sleep disturbances
- insomnia
- muscle weakness
- body aches
- nervousness, anxiety, or stress

- inability to relax or exercise
- depression
- cravings for sweet or salty snacks
- decreased sex drive
- increased PMS or perimenopausal or menopausal symptoms
- absentmindedness, forgetfulness
- digestive problems
- mild constipation alternating with diarrhea
- low blood pressure
- weight loss
- lightheadedness, dizziness, fainting
- loss of body hair
- memory loss

Diagnosis

Examination

A complete medical history and physical examination is conducted. The symptoms of adrenal fatigue are similar to those of Addison's disease. The healthcare provider also must rule out conditions such as **depression** and fibromyalgia that can cause similar symptoms

Tests

Adrenal insufficiency is typically diagnosed by blood tests to measure the levels of adrenal hormones. However it is claimed that these tests are not sensitive enough to reveal the smaller hormonal deficiencies of adrenal fatigue:

- The most accurate measure of adrenal function may be an ACTH stimulation test, in which the adrenal steroids are measured in urine collected over a 24-hour period and then compared with a second 24-hour urine collection following an injection of ACTH to stimulate the adrenals.
- Commercially available saliva tests measure cortisol in the saliva at four times during the day: 8 A.M., noon, 4 P.M., and between 11 P.M. and midnight, although sometimes only the morning cortisol level is determined. These tests can also measure sex hormone levels.
- Postural hypotension, also called orthostatic hypotension—lowered blood pressure that occurs when rising from a seated or prone posture—can be determined by repeatedly measuring blood pressure as the patient is moved between horizontal and upright positions on a tilt table.
- Thyroid tests are usually performed to rule out hypothyroidism.

Treatment

Traditional

Pituitary tumors that cause cortisol deficiency can be treated with surgery or microsurgery, **radiation therapy**, **chemotherapy**, or a combination of these therapies.

Drugs

Adrenal hormone insufficiencies are treated with replacement hormone. Hydrocortisone (Cortef) is administered if the adrenals are not producing cortisol. Some people take these every day and others only when they are ill.

Alternative

Adrenal fatigue is most often treated by an alternative medical practitioner. A wide variety of botanicals, nutritional supplements, and combinations are commercially available for treating adrenal fatigue.

Adaptogens are botanicals that improve the general response to stress and promote recovery from stress. The term was coined in the 1940s by the Russian physician I. I. Brekhman who defined the properties of adaptogens as follows:

- They are harmless.
- Their effects are generally nonspecific.
- They increase resistance to physical, chemical, or biological stressors.
- They act as general stabilizers or normalizers.

Adaptogens that are thought to act primarily on the adrenal glands include:

- *Panax ginseng*—Korean ginseng or its active ingredients, particularly in combination with multivitamins and minerals
- *Eleutherococcus senticosus*, also known as *Acanthopanax senticosus*, Ciwujia, or Siberian ginseng
- *Withania somnifera*, also called ashwagandha or Indian ginseng, which is used in Ayurvedic medicine to counteract the effects of extreme stress including changes in blood sugar, adrenal weight, and cortisol levels

Glycyrrhiza glabra (licorice) and *Glycyrrhiza uralensis* have been postulated to act synergistically with cortisol. Glycyrrhizin, a component of licorice which is structurally similar to cortisol, can bind to corticoid receptors, weakly mimicking the role of cortisol. Therefore it may increase the effective half-life of endogenous cortisol and reduce the demand on the adrenals for cortisol secretion. Licorice may elevate blood pressure and should not be used by patients with a history of hypertension or renal failure or who are using digitalis preparations such as digoxin. *G. uralensis* has been used in China, in combination with **corticosteroids**, to treat early-stage Addison's disease.

The reported effects of *Rhodiola rosea* include:

- prevention of stress-induced depletion of adrenal catecholamines
- decreased salivary cortisol
- improved concentration and mental performance
- decreased stress-related fatigue
- improved physical fitness and coordination
- improved sleep
- improved motivation
- greater mood stability
- improved general well-being
- improvement of general anxiety disorder symptoms

Various substances have been suggested to modulate the effects of cortisol and counteract stress-induced activation of the hypothalamus-pituitary-adrenal axis:

- Phosphatidylcholine may reduce the levels of cortisol and ACTH released in response to physical stress and relieve soreness and depression.
- Fish oil may reduce stress-induced cortisol and epinephrine levels.
- Plant sterols/sterolins may reduce the levels of physical-stress-induced cortisol.
- Gamma-aminobutyric acid (GABA), the major inhibitory neurotransmitter in the brain, may reduce levels of cortisol and the adrenal stress marker chromogranin A.
- Thiamine (vitamin B_1) may protect against surgery-induced adrenal fatigue, reducing cortisol levels before and during surgery and preventing post-surgical reduction in blood cortisol levels.
- Pantetheine/pantothenic acid (vitamin B_5) may enhance adrenal cortex activity and down-regulate cortisol over-secretion in response to stress.
- Methylcobalamin (vitamin B_{12}) may normalize cortisol peaks, resetting the cortisol peak to the circadian rhythm.
- Ascorbic acid (vitamin C) can reduce high cortisol levels.
- A combination of ascorbic acid and vitamins B_1 and B_6 may improve adrenal glucocorticoid function and normalize the rhythmic activities of glucocorticoid hormones.

Home remedies

Many practitioners believe that adrenal fatigue can be effectively treated at home with lifestyle and dietary changes, nutritional supplements, stress-reducing techniques, and possibly detoxification. Other recommendations include frequent rest periods during the day, sleeping in late whenever possible, and an early bedtime.

Dietary recommendations for treating adrenal fatigue include:

- breakfast before 10 A.M., lunch before noon, a nutritious snack between 2 P.M. and 3 P.M., an evening meal between 5 P.M. and 6 P.M., and a small nutritious snack before bed
- slow, deliberate eating
- a combination of protein, fat, and complex carbohydrates such as whole grains at every snack and meal
- whole grains as the primary source of carbohydrates
- combinations of grains and legumes or legumes and seeds or nuts for complete protein
- lightly cooked or raw protein and avoidance of processed proteins
- 6–8 daily servings of a wide variety of vegetables variously prepared, especially brightly colored vegetables
- 1–2 tablespoons daily of essential oils (olive, grape seed, safflower, flax, etc.) in grains, vegetables, or meat
- moderate salt, except in the rare cases where adrenal fatigue is accompanied by high blood pressure

Foods to avoid include:

- fruit in the mornings
- sugar and white flour products
- hydrogenated and partially hydrogenated oils such as vegetable shortening, margarine, and oils added to commercial peanut butters
- caffeine, chocolate, soft drinks, and alcohol
- deep-fried foods
- fast and junk foods

Nutritional supplements for treating adrenal fatigue include:

- vitamin C, 2,000–4,000 mg/day of sustained-release tablets
- vitamin E with mixed tocopherols, 800 IU/day
- vitamin B complex
- niacin, 125–150 mg/day as inositol hexaniacinate
- vitamin B_6, 150 mg/day
- ...id, 1,200–1,500 mg/day

- magnesium citrate, 400–1,200 mg/day
- liquid trace minerals (zinc, manganese, selenium, chromium, molybdenum, copper, iodine) for their calming effects
- S-adenosylmethionine (SAMe; 200 mg twice a day) and D,L-phenylalanine (DLPA; 500 mg twice a day) if depression is present

Prognosis

Alternative practitioners generally believe that adrenal fatigue can be overcome with a good diet, physical and mental rest and relaxation, and possibly nutritional and/or botanical supplementation.

Prevention

Stress is usually unavoidable in daily life and can be associated with disease and mortality. However a healthy diet, adequate exercise, and stress-reducing techniques such as meditation can help prevent adrenal fatigue.

Resources

BOOKS

Bharadvaj, Daivati. *Natural Treatments for Chronic Fatigue Syndrome*. Westport, CT: Praeger, 2008.
Null, Gary, and Amy McDonald. *Be a Healthy Woman*. New York: Seven Stories Press, 2009.
Watson, James L. *Adrenal Fatigue: The 21st Century Stress Syndrome*. Petaluma, CA: Smart Publications, 2007.

PERIODICALS

Head, Kathleen A., and Gregory S. Kelly. "Nutrients and Botanicals for Treatment of Stress: Adrenal Fatigue, Neurotransmitter Imbalance, Anxiety, and Restless Sleep." *Alternative Medicine Review* 14, no. 2 (June 1, 2009): 114-140.
Singh, Karta Purkh. "Avert Adrenal Fatigue." *Better Nutrition* 70, no. 10 (October 2008): 28.
"SOS for Adrenal Fatigue." *Better Nutrition* 70, no. 10 (October 2008): 30-31.

OTHER

"Adrenal Gland Disorders." *National Institute of Child Health and Human Development*.http://www.nichd.nih.gov/health/topics/Adrenal_Gland_Disorders.cfm
Dr. James Wilson's www.AdrenalFatigue.org.http://www.adrenalfatigue.org.
Grimes, Melanie. "A Stressful Lifestyle Can Cause Adrenal Fatigue." *HealthNews*.http://www.healthnews.com/blogs/melanie-grimes/disease-illness/a-stressful-lifestyle-can-cause-adrenal-fatigue-3572.html.
Nippoldt, Todd B. "Is There Such a Thing as Adrenal Fatigue?" *MayoClinic.com*.http://www.mayoclinic.com/print/adrenal-fatigue/AN01583/METHOD=print.
Wade, Vicki. "Adrenal Fatigue." *Project AWARE*.http://www.project-aware.org/Resource/articlearchives/adrenalfatigue.shtml.

ORGANIZATIONS

The American Institute of Stress, 124 Park Avenue, Yonkers, NY, 10703, (914) 963-1200, (914) 965-6267, Stress125@optonline.net, http://www.stress.org.
National Institute of Child Health and Human Development (NICHD) Information Resource Center, PO Box 3006, Rockville, MD, 20847, (800) 370-2943, (866) 760-5947, NICHDInformationResourceCenter@mail.nih.gov, http://www.nichd.nih.gov.

Margaret Alic, PhD

Adrenal tumors

Definition

Tumors that occur on one or both of the adrenal glands. Adrenal tumors are rare tumors that are characterized by overproduction of hormones produced by the adrenal glands.

Description

The two small adrenal glands, one located just above each kidney, are among the many endocrine (hormone-secreting) glands in the body. All endocrine glands make and store hormones. Hormones are chemical messages that are sent from an endocrine gland and are received by an organ or a cell to trigger a specific reaction. When the body requires hormone levels to rise, endocrine glands secrete them into the bloodstream. Adrenal gland tumors often cause overproduction of one or a combination of the adrenal hormones.

An adrenal tumor is shown at lower left. The gallbladder is white, and the nearby liver is deep red. *(Custom Medical Stock Photo. Reproduced by permission.)*

Adrenal glands are comprised of two parts. The outer portion of the gland is called the cortex. The inner portion of the gland is called the medulla. Nervous system hormones are produced by the adrenal medulla.

Most tumors that arise from the adrenal cortex are benign and are termed benign adenomas. Benign adenomas are usually small tumor and typically produce no symptoms. Should symptoms arise the tumors can be removed by surgically removing the adrenal gland that houses the benign tumor. Some benign adenomas can be treated with medications while others require no treatment.

A malignant adrenal tumor (**cancer**) that arises in the adrenal cortex is called an adrenal cortical **carcinoma** and can produce high blood pressure, weight gain, excess body hair, weakening of the bones and diabetes.

A malignant adrenal tumor (cancer) in the adrenal medulla is called a **pheochromocytoma** and can cause high blood pressure, headache, palpitations, and excessive perspiration.

An adrenal gland has two parts, each of which secretes different hormones. The inner part is called the adrenal medulla, and the outer part is the adrenal cortex.

The adrenal medulla secretes the nervous system hormones epinephrine and norepinephrine. These hormones help maintain normal blood pressure. In high-stress situations, they help prepare the body for quick action by increasing heartbeat and breathing rate, increasing the flow of blood to the heart and lungs, and increasing blood pressure.

The adrenal cortex secretes aldosterone and cortisol. They also make small amounts of androgens, which affect the expression of female and male sex characteristics. Aldosterone helps maintain normal salt levels in the blood and the normal functioning of the kidneys. Cortisol (also called hydrocortisone) is the major adrenal hormone.

Cortisol is a steroid, an organic compound that affects metabolism. Many hormones and drugs used to relieve swelling and inflammation are steroids. Cortisol helps maintain blood pressure and is crucial in the breakdown of proteins, carbohydrates, and fats. It also raises blood sugar (glucose) when levels are too low, thus providing needed energy for the body's activities. Cortisol also prevents inflammation and is important for the normal response to stress.

The level of cortisol in the blood is carefully controlled. When the body needs cortisol, a small area of the brain called the hypothalamus releases coricotripoin-releasing hormone (CRH). The pituitary gland, located at the base of the brain, receives the message from the hypothalamus and begins secreting adrenocorticotropic hormone (ACTH). ACTH is received by the cortex of the adrenal glands, which responds by producing cortisol. When the level of cortisol meets the body's need, the pituitary stops producing ACTH, which then stops the adrenal cortex from secreting cortisol.

Demographics

About 8% of people worldwide develop benign (noncancerous) adrenal tumors. Malignant (cancerous) tumors are very rare, occurring in two out of every one million people worldwide. The exact incidence of adrenal cancers in the United States is unknown but is thought to be about 300–500 new adrenal cancers per year. This cancer is more common in women than in men. Although adrenal cancers can happen at any age, most are diagnosed in adults ages 45 to 50.

Causes and symptoms

It is not known what causes adrenal gland cancer, but some cases are associated with hereditary diseases. Symptoms of adrenal cancer are related to the specific hormones produced by that tumor. An **adrenocortical carcinoma** typically secretes high amounts of cortisol, producing Cushing's syndrome. This syndrome produces progressive weight gain, rounding of the face, and increased blood pressure. Women can experience menstrual cycle alterations and men can experience feminization. The symptoms for pheochromocytoma include hypertension, acidosis, unexplained **fever** and **weight loss**. Because of the hormones produced by this type of tumor, anxiety is often a feature also.

Diagnosis

It is often difficult for a pathologist to distinguish between a benign and a malignant adrenal tumor. Several criteria are used to make a diagnosis, including the size and weight of the tumor, whether hormones are produced, and what hormones are produced. A benign tumor (**adenoma**) is usually less than 4–6 centimeters (1.57–2.3 inches) in diameter and likely causes changes in the blood level of only one hormone or may cause no changes at all. A malignant tumor is larger and may alter the level of several adrenal hormones. One reliable indicator for a malignant tumor is evidence that the cancer has spread (**metastasis**).

Tests which may be used in the diagnosis of adrenal cancers include:

- chest x ray
- computed tomography (CT)
- positron emission tomography (PET scan)
- magnetic resonance imaging (MRI)
- biopsy
- laparoscopy
- blood and urine tests

Types of cancers

Adrenal cortex

A disorder caused by an adrenal cortex tumor can occur alone, but often two or more conditions occur simultaneously. These disorders include

- Cushing's syndrome: a disorder resulting from prolonged exposure to high levels of cortisol. Most cases are the result of a pituitary gland dysfunction that causes excessive secretion of ACTH, but 20–25% are caused by a benign adrenal tumor, of which about 50% are malignant. Symptoms include obesity, moon-shaped face, increased fat in neck region, skin that bruises easily, severe fatigue, weak muscles, and high blood pressure. The common treatment is surgical removal of the affected gland. The outcome for a Cushing's syndrome patient with a benign adrenal adenoma is very good. Surgery usually results in a cure. The outcome is variable for malignant tumors.

- Aldosteronism: a condition resulting from an abnormally high level of the hormone aldosterone. It is usually caused by an adenoma and rarely is the result of a malignant adrenal tumor. Symptoms include headaches, weakness, fatigue, high blood salt levels, frequent urination, high blood pressure, and an irregular heartbeat. An adenoma is usually removed surgically, although medication that controls the secretion of aldosterone is an effective treatment in many cases.

- Virilization syndrome (also called adrenal virilism or adrenogenital syndrome): a disorder caused by an excessive secretion of androgen hormones, leading to high levels of the male hormone testosterone. Adenomas that cause virilization are rare. When the condition accompanies Cushing's syndrome it may indicate an adrenocortical carcinoma. In males, the symptom is early onset of puberty, whereas in females symptoms include deepening of voice, a masculine build, and abnormal hairiness. The recommended treatment depends on the cause. If the condition is caused by an adenoma, use of medications that surpress ACTH secretion by the pituitary is the preferred treatment.

- Adrenocortical carcinoma: a rare cancer that is often not detected until it has spread to the liver or lung. The symptoms can include that of Cushing's syndrome, aldosteronism, virilization, or a combination of each of these conditions. The preferred treatment depends on the stage of the cancer, but usually involves surgery to remove the tumor, chemotherapy, and radiation therapy. If the cancer is caught at an early stage, the long-term survival can be good. If found at a later stage, about 30% of patients will survive five years after the initial diagnosis.

Adrenal medulla

Only one type of tumor is associated with the adrenal medulla:

- Pheochromocytoma: a tumor that produces and secretes epinephrine and norepinephrine. Excessive secretion of these hormones can cause life-threatening hypertension and an irregular heartbeat. About 90% of these tumors are benign. Five percent of those diagnosed with this tumor have either Von Hippel-Lindau syndrome, type 2 of the multiple endocrine neoplasia syndromes (MEN), Von Recklinghausen's neurofibromatosis, or another inherited disorder. Symptoms include headaches, sweating, and chest pains. Treatment involves medication to control hypertension and the surgical removal of the affected gland. Long-term survival depends on early detection of the tumor and whether the tumor is benign or malignant.

Treatment

Treatment is aimed at removing the tumor by surgery. In some cases, this can be done by **laparoscopy**. Surgery is sometimes followed by **chemotherapy** and/or **radiation therapy**. Because the surgery removes the source of many important hormones, hormones must be supplemented following surgery. If adrenocortical cancer recurs or has spread to other parts of the body (metastasized), additional surgery may be done followed by chemotherapy.

Prognosis

The prognosis for adrenal gland cancer is variable. For localized pheochromocytomas the 5-year survival rate is 95%. This rate decreases with aggressive tumors that have metastasized. The prognosis for adrenal cortical cancer is dependent upon stage at diagnosis. Tumors diagnosed in stages I and II have a 50–60% five year survival rate while tumors diagnosed in more advanced stages (Stages III and IV) have more dismal survival rates of 20% and less than 10% respectively.

Prevention

Since so little is known about the cause of adrenal gland cancer, it is not known if it can be prevented.

See also Endocrine system tumors.

Resources

PERIODICALS

Cook, L.K. "Pheochromocytoma." *American Journal of Nursing* 109 (2009):50–53.

Kissane, N.A. & Cendran, J.C. "Patients with Cushing's Syndrome Are Care-Intensive Even in the Era of Laproscopic Adrenalectomy." *American Surgery* 75(2009):279–83.

Miller, J.C., Blake, M.A., Boland, G.W., Copeland, P.M., Thrall, J.H., Lee, S.I. "Adrenal Masses." *Journal of the American College of Radiology* 6(2009):206–11.

ORGANIZATIONS

American Association of Clinical Endocrinologists. 1000 Riverside Avenue Suite 205, Jacksonville, FL 32204. 904-353-7878. http://www.aace.com.

National Adrenal Diseases Foundation. 505 Northern Boulevard, Great Neck, NY 11021. 516-487-4992. http://www.medhelp.org/nadf.

Monica McGee, M.S.
Cindy L.A. Jones, PhD
Melinda Granger Oberleitner, R.N., D.N.S., A.P.R.N., C.N.S.

Adrenocortical carcinoma

Definition

Adrenocortical **carcinoma** is a malignant growth that originates in the cortex, or the outer portion, of one of the two adrenal glands.

Description

There are two adrenal glands in the body. Each one is paired with a kidney. The adrenal gland rests atop the kidney, on the side of the kidney that is nearest to the head.

An adrenal gland has two parts. The inner part (medulla) produces hormones such as epinephrine (adrenaline) that increases the heart rate. The cortex, or outer part, is made up of layers of epithelial cells, the cells that form coverings for the surfaces of the body. The cortex produces cortical hormones that are essential to well-being, or homeostasis.

The hormones produced by the cortex include glucocorticoids, mineralocorticoids, and sex hormones. Among the many hormones the cortex makes, three—aldosterone, cortisol and adrenal sex hormones—are very important. Aldosterone helps regulate salt and water content in the body. Cortisol helps keep sugars, fats and proteins in balance. Adrenal sex hormones influence sex organ development and sex drive (libido).

Adrenocortical carcinoma is a **cancer** that originates in the cortex of the adrenal gland. When a tumor grows in the adrenal cortex, it interferes with the production of hormones. Consequently, the effects of adrenocortical carcinoma can be severe and are almost always a threat to life.

There are two types of adrenocortical carcinoma. In one type, a tumor functions—that is, it makes hormones. In the other type, the tumor does not function. If the tumor functions, it acts like the cells in the cortex from which it grew and thus, produces hormones. But since it grows large, it produces extra

KEY TERMS

Biopsy—Tissue sample is taken from body for examination.

Carcinoma—A cancer that originates in cells that developed from epithelial tissue, a tissue found on skin and mucosal surfaces.

Computed tomography (CT)—X rays are aimed at slices of the body (by rotating equipment) and results are assembled with a computer to give a three-dimensional picture of a structure.

Homeostasis—Self-regulating mechanisms are working, body is in equilibrium, no uncontrolled cell growth.

Hormone—A chemical released by one organ of the body that affects the activity of another organ.

Inferior vena cava—The large vein that returns blood from the lower body to the heart.

Lymph nodes—Part of the lymphatic system, these clusters of tissue help to protect the body from foreign substances, organisms, and cancer cells.

Magnetic resonance imaging (MRI)—Magnetic fields used to provide images of the internal organs of the body.

Pituitary—A gland at the base of the brain that produces hormones.

Venography—Technique used for examining veins for blockage, using a dye to make the vein visible with scans similar to x ray.

QUESTIONS TO ASK THE DOCTOR

- In which stage is the carcinoma?
- With this type of carcinoma, what is the five-year survival rate for a person of my age and gender? What is the one-year survival rate?
- Is there a center that specializes in treating this type of cancer?
- Are there any clinical trials in which I might be eligible to participate?
- Does this health care institution have a support group for individuals with my type of carcinoma?
- What is your approach to relieving pain?

amounts of hormones and the body is thrown far out of balance in any one of a number of ways.

When a tumor functions

How excess hormones cause the symptoms they produce is complex because more than one hormone from the adrenal cortex can be involved in producing a single symptom. For example, both aldosterone and cortisol, when present in extra quantities, may contribute to the increase in blood pressure (hypertension) many patients experience. Extra amounts of adrenal sex hormones can cause children to begin to display the sexual characteristics (hair growth, genital maturation) of adults. And adults with extra amounts of sex hormones often begin to display the sexual characteristics of the opposite sex. A woman may grow excess facial hair. A man may begin to develop fatty tissue in his breasts. Large quantities of adrenal sex hormones coursing through the body disrupt what would be a normal loop of feedback from the pituitary area of the brain. The pituitary is geared to send information, via a stimulating hormone, to the adrenal cortex, to prompt the tissue to manufacture adrenal sex hormone. When there is an extra amount of adrenal sex hormone in the body, the pituitary stops sending instructions to the adrenal cortex, as well as to other organs that produce the hormones responsible for male features. Thus, a man can begin to look like a woman because he does not have enough male hormones. A woman can begin to look like a man because she has too much adrenal sex hormone.

When a tumor does not function

If the tumor does not function, it just grows large, and may go unnoticed for a long time. Sometimes a tumor that does not function is called dormant. Often, the tumor that does not function first gets attention when it grows large enough to push against the body wall or an organ and cause pain; or when it has spread (metastasized) to another organ.

The adrenocortical carcinoma that does not function has a high likelihood of metastasizing before it is discovered. The two most common sites for metastases are the lungs and liver. Thus, even a non-functioning tumor may cause serious complications.

Demographics

Adrenocortical carcinoma is rare. Fewer than two in one million people, and perhaps as few as one in four million people, are diagnosed in a year. Two age groups are most likely to be diagnosed: those between zero and ten years of age, and those between 40 and 50 years.

Causes and symptoms

Causes

The cause of adrenocortical carcinoma is not known. **Infection** with bacteria or parasites is linked to other conditions of the adrenal glands, and there could be a connection with adrenocortical carcinoma. There is also evidence that adrenocortical carcinoma in children is caused by some chemical to which they were exposed as fetuses— possibly a chemical that the women carrying the children were exposed to in food, drink, or in the air.

Many tumors of the adrenal cortex have cells with extra copies of chromosomes, the beads of genetic material or DNA. Chemicals in the environment that are known to affect cells and cause mutations are being investigated as possible causes for adrenocortical carcinoma.

Symptoms

Depending on whether or not the tumor interferes with the production of hormones, the tumor may or may not be linked to symptoms during its early growth. A group of Japanese surgeons led by K. Kunieda reported the case of a 52-year-old man who had a tumor weighing more than two pounds at the time it was discovered. The tumor had not been producing extra hormones, and was not producing symptoms.

An adrenocortical tumor that functions produces many symptoms. Some of them are similar to those linked to other conditions, and many of these conditions have names that are based on a collection of symptoms and not on the cause. A combination of the following symptoms, known as **Cushing's syndrome**, could be caused by a tumor in the pituitary area of the brain, as well as by adrenocortical carcinoma:

- an abnormal accumulation of fatty pads in the face (creating the distinctive "moon face" of Cushing's syndrome); in the trunk (termed "truncal obesity"); and over the upper back and the back of the neck (giving the individual what has been called a "buffalo hump")
- purple and pink stretch marks across the abdomen and flanks
- high blood pressure
- weak, thinning bones (osteoporosis)
- muscle atrophy (due to protein loss)
- low energy

- thin, fragile skin, with a tendency toward both bruising and slow healing
- abnormalities in the processing of sugars (glucose), with occasional development of actual diabetes
- increased risk of infections
- irregular menstrual periods in women
- decreased sex drive in men and difficulty maintaining an erection
- abormal hair growth in women (in a male pattern, such as in the beard and mustache area), as well as loss of hair from the head (receding hair line)

Similarly, virilization syndrome, or the tendency of a child to exhibit adult sexual features, or a female adult to exhibit male features, can be caused by other conditions, such as tumors in the pituitary, or by adrenocortical carcinoma. So, too, with feminization, or the tendency of a male individual to exhibit female characteristics, such as enlarged breasts and fat deposits on the hips.

Diagnosis

Symptoms usually cause a patient to talk with a physician. Blood and urine samples are examined to learn whether hormones are out of balance. Venography, a way of getting a picture of the inside of veins, is a technique that is still used to examine the adrenal glands prior to any decision about surgery. But the **magnetic resonance imaging** (MRI) scan has replaced venography in many facilities. **Computed tomography** (CT) scan is also used to examine the adrenal cortex.

Treatment team

Depending on symptoms, the first specialized physician an individual consults may either be an endocrinologist (a physician who focuses on hormones) or a urologist (a physician who focuses on the study of the kidneys and nearby structures). Either one of them, or a medical oncologist (a physician who focuses on treating patients with cancer) will lead the treatment team. A surgeon will be on the team too because in almost all cases removal of the adrenocortical carcinoma to the fullest extent possible is standard procedure.

Nurses will be on the team to help with administering drugs and monitoring the status of the patient. And if the patient is given **chemotherapy**, technicians skilled in the treatment will be part of the team.

Clinical staging, treatments, and prognosis

Adrenocortical tumors are assigned to one of four stages.

- Stage I tumors have not spread beyond the cortex of the adrenal gland and are less than two in (5 cm) in their greatest dimension.
- Stage II tumors have not spread beyond the cortex of the adrenal gland and are more than two inches.
- Stage III tumors have either spread into tissues around the adrenal cortex or they have spread into lymph nodes near the adrenal glands, or both.
- Stage IV tumors have spread to lymph nodes and other organs near the adrenal cortex or to other organs of the body.

A plan for treatment is based on the size and extent of the tumor. Surgical removal of the tumor, radiation and chemotherapy are all used. Method of treatment depends on how large the carcinoma is and whether it has spread to other organs. In some cases the treatment is strictly palliative (provides comfort) and is not expected to halt the course of the cancer. Palliative treatment can include surgery to reduce the size of the tumor, as well the pain a large tumor causes by pushing against other organs.

Because adrenocortical carcinoma that metastasizes often moves into the renal (kidney) vein and then, the inferior vena cava, venography or MRI scan prior to surgical removal of all or part of the tumor is important. If the tumor has grown into a vein, a piece of it can be dislodged and become a dangerous object. The piece of tumor begins to move in the blood flow and it is capable of getting stuck in a small blood vessel in the heart or the brain, and causing a stroke.

The drug **mitotane** gives some good results is slowing tumor growth in certain patients. But the only therapy that provides relief in most patients is the removal of the tumor.

The outlook for individuals with adrenocortical carcinoma depends on the stage of the cancer. Because seven in ten individuals are diagnosed only after the cancer has reached stage III or stage IV the five-year survival rate for all stages is 40%. And for individuals with stage IV carcinoma it is much less, with most patients dying within nine months of diagnosis.

Alternative and complementary therapies

Yoga, biofeedback, or other relaxation techniques may help manage pain.

Coping with cancer treatment

Being an active member of the treatment team is important. Premier cancer centers encourage patients to play such a role. A support group can also help.

Clinical trials

The Cancer Information Service at the National Institutes of Health, Bethesda, Md., offers information about **clinical trials** that are looking for volunteers. The Service offers a toll-free number at 1-800-422-6237.

Prevention

No prevention is known.

Special concerns

The excess production of hormones that indicate functioning tumors in adrenocortical carcinoma can also be symptoms of other conditions. A tumor in the pituitary gland can cause the pituitary to produce too much of the hormone that stimulates the adrenal cortex to make cortical hormones. The symptoms are identical to those for the adrenocortical tumor. A pituitary tumor must sometimes be ruled out when an adrenocortical carcinoma is suspected. Brain scans may be necessary.

Resources

PERIODICALS

Kunieda, K., et al. "Recurrence of giant adrenocortical carcinoma in the contralateral adrenal gland 6 years after surgery." *Surgery Today* 30 (March 2000): 294-7.

Wajchenber, B. L., et al. "Adrenocortical carcinoma: clinical and laboratory observations." *Cancer* 88 (February 15, 2000):711-36.

Diane M. Calabrese

Adult cancer pain

Definition

Most adult **cancer** pain is caused by the cancer itself, although treatment and other cancer-related conditions also can cause pain. Not all cancer patients have pain and the pain varies greatly from day to day and patient to patient. Controlling cancer pain is an integral part of cancer treatment.

Demographics

Many—but not all—cancer patients have pain. About 70% of cancer patients experience pain at some point during their illness. Between 30% and 40% of patients undergoing cancer treatment report pain and 70–90% of those with advanced cancer have pain. However fewer than 50% receive adequate treatment for their pain.

According to the World Health Organization (WHO), in most parts of the world the majority of cancer patients are not presented for treatment until their cancers are advanced and pain relief is the only treatment possible. However in many countries cancer pain relief is limited by national drug laws. In developing countries cancer pain relief also may be limited by geographical barriers, medical infrastructure, and financial resources.

Description

There are two categories of pain. Nociceptive pain is pain caused during the normal process of an outside agent (or disease) acts upon the body's tissues and causes damage. Neuropathic pain is caused by the peripheral or central nervous system (CNS) incorrectly processing sensory input.

Not all cancers cause pain and the pain can almost always be controlled and managed. The existence of cancer pain and its severity depends on:

- the location of the cancer
- the type of cancer
- the type of damage that the cancer is causing
- the stage or extent of the cancer
- treatments
- the patient's pain threshold or tolerance for pain and how the patient experiences pain

There are different types of adult cancer pain:

- Acute pain is mild to severe, comes on quickly, and lasts only a short time.
- Chronic pain is mild to severe and lasts longer than three months or recurs often.
- Breakthrough pain occurs in patients with chronic pain that is controlled by round-the-clock medication. Breakthrough pain is an intense sudden increase in pain that may occur several times in a day, but usually lasts less than one hour. It may occur as the last dose of medication begins to wear off. However it often is unpredictable.

Risk factors

The risk of cancer pain depends on a variety of factors. The major risk for pain is advanced cancer.

Causes and symptoms

There are various causes of cancer pain. Most cancer pain is caused by the cancer itself; however cancer treatments can also cause pain. More advanced cancer is likely to cause more pain:

- A tumor that is growing or spreading and pressing on surrounding tissues such as organs, bones, nerves, or the spinal cord can cause pain.
- Spinal cord compression occurs when a tumor spreads to the spine and presses on the spinal cord. It often begins with back and/or neck pain that is made worse by coughing, sneezing, or other movements.
- Cancer that has spread to the bones can cause bone pain.
- Medical tests and procedures that are performed to diagnose and stage cancer or to measure the effectiveness of treatment can cause pain. These include biopsies, spinal taps, and bone marrow tests.
- Chemotherapy and radiation can cause painful sores in the mouth and throat that make it difficult to eat and drink.
- Radiation therapy can also cause painful skin burns, scarring, or injury to the throat, intestines, or bladder.
- Surgical pain usually lasts from a few days to a few weeks.
- Other conditions related to cancer—such as stiffness from inactivity, muscle spasms, bedsores, and constipation—can cause pain.

There are three major types of cancer treatment pain:

- Neuropathic pain may occur when certain types of chemotherapy or the cancer itself damages nerves. It is often a burning, shooting, or sharp pain.
- Peripheral neuropathy is pain in the arms, legs, hands, or feet.
- Phantom pain comes from a body part that has been surgically removed. It is not well understood; however it lasts longer than pain from the surgery.

Cancer pain that is not treated may cause patients to become fatigued, worried, stressed, angry, lonely, and depressed. The pain may interfere with daily activities and make it difficult to eat and sleep.

Diagnosis

Examination

The physician will take a medical history and perform physical and neurological examinations. However diagnosis of adult cancer pain usually depends on the patient's self-report, possibly with the help of a family member or friend. The physician must have the following information from the patient:

- the location of the pain
- whether the pain is constant or intermittent, sharp or dull, throbbing, burning, or shooting

- the pain intensity
- the pain duration
- the time of day or activities during which the pain occurs
- factors that ease and worsen the pain
- whether the pain interferes with daily activities

Openly sharing details about their cancer pain helps the pain control team determine how the cancer and treatments are affecting the body and how to best control the pain. Patients may be asked to keep a pain control record that lists:

- the name and dose of all pain medications
- when the medications are administered
- when more or less than the prescribed dose is administered
- any side effects
- the duration of a single dose's effectiveness
- any over-the-counter (OTC) drugs, alternative, herbal, or home remedies used
- other pain relief methods
- activities that ease or worsen the pain
- activities that the pain interferes with
- any medications taken for other health problems
- allergies to any drugs

Procedures

There are several procedures for determining a patient's pain threshold and measuring the effectiveness of the pain treatment plan:

- The most common procedure is a numeric pain intensity scale: patients rate their pain on a scale of zero to ten, with 0 as no pain and 10 as the worst possible pain.
- With a simple descriptive pain intensity scale, patients use words to describe their pain.
- With a visual analog scale (VAS), patients are shown pictures of faces with a range of expressions and choose the face that best describes how they feel.

Treatment

Traditional

Controlling cancer pain is an integral component of overall cancer treatment. Pain is much easier to treat and control when it first begins than after it has become more severe. Cancer pain is sometimes treated by a pain specialist, who may also be an oncologist, anesthesiologist, neurologist, surgeon, other physician, nurse, or pharmacist. Some patients have a pain control team that may include a psychologist or social worker. Pain control plans are always individualized for the patient.

Although cancer pain is most often treated with drugs, other treatments also may be used:

- Radiation therapy can shrink the tumor and reduce pain.
- Surgery can remove part or all of a tumor that is pressing on nerves or other parts of the body.
- Neurosurgery can cut the nerves, usually those near the spinal cord, that transmit pain messages to the brain.
- Nerve blocks are local anesthetics, possibly combined with a steroid, that an anesthesiologist injects into or around a nerve or into the spine. Sometimes phenol or alcohol is injected for longer-lasting pain relief.
- Transcutaneous electric nerve stimulation (TENS) counteracts pain by transmitting a gentle electric current from a small power pack that patients hold or attach to themselves.
- Occasionally radiofrequency ablation may be used to destroy tumors in certain areas of the body to relieve pain.

Drugs

There are a wide variety of medications for treating cancer pain and each patient is medicated differently, depending, in part, on the type of pain and its severity. Different pain medications are more effective for some people than for others and there is no correct dose for cancer pain. The goal is to control the pain, whatever it takes. It is important that the medications always be taken as prescribed to prevent pain from starting or becoming worse. It is harder to control pain that has already started and it is much easier to control pain when it is mild.

Cancer patients who take their pain medications as prescribed rarely become addicted to them; nor do their bodies become immune to pain medication, so there is no reason to avoid or put off taking stronger medications. However tolerance to pain medication is a common problem with cancer patients and may require increasing the dose, changing medications, or adding a medication.

Cancer pain is most often treated with analgesics:

- Nonopioids are used for mild to moderate pain—one to four on a scale of zero to ten—as well as for pain from fever and swelling. OTC drugs often are all that is needed. These include acetaminophen (Tylenol) and nonsteroidal anti-inflammatory drugs (NSAIDs) such as aspirin, naproxen (Aleve), and ibuprofen (Advil,

Motrin). Acetaminophen only treats pain. NSAIDs also treat inflammation. There are prescription-strength as well as OTC nonopioids.

- Opioids or narcotics are used to treat moderate to severe pain, often in combination with acetaminophen, aspirin, or ibuprofen. Common opioids include codeine, fentanyl, hydromorphone, levorphanol, meperidine, methadone, morphine, oxycodone, and oxymorphone. Drugs to treat chronic or persistent cancer pain are long-acting or sustained-release and are taken on a regular schedule, usually every 8–12 hours or via a skin patch.

- Rapid-onset opioids are used to treat breakthrough pain. Sometimes called rescue medicines, they act quickly for a short period of time. They are taken as needed immediately upon experiencing breakthrough pain or as a preventative if the breakthrough is predictable. They include fast-acting oral morphine and fentanyl in a lozenge that is sucked and absorbed through the mouth.

Pain medications are most often pills or liquids taken by mouth. However they also can be:

- placed inside the cheek or under the tongue
- rectal suppositories as capsules or pills
- skin patches that slowly release medication over two to three days
- injections under the skin (subcutaneous) or into a vein (intravenous, IV)
- epidural injections into the space around the spinal cord
- intrathecal injections into the fluid around the spinal cord, often with a patient-controlled analgesia (PCA) pump that enables patients to dose themselves as needed
- a surgical implant that injects medication directly into the spinal fluid or the space around the spine

Other types of drugs used to treat cancer pain include:

- Antidepressants such as amitriptyline, nortriptyline, and desipramine—alone or in combination with nonopioids and opioids—can relieve tingling and burning pain from nerve damage caused by cancer treatments.
- Anti-seizure drugs, also called anticonvulsants—such as carbamazepine, gabapentin, and phenytoin—also help control tingling and burning from nerve damage.
- Steroids, such as prednisone or dexamethasone, are prescribed for pain caused by swelling.
- Stimulants and amphetamines, such as caffeine or dextroamphetamine, can increase the pain-relieving

effects of opioids and reduce the drowsiness they cause.

- Chemotherapy drugs can shrink a tumor, which may relieve pain.
- Hormone therapy can be used to shrink prostate tumors to reduce pain.
- Radioactive materials that settle in diseased bone and bisphosphonates that strengthen bones may be used to treat bone pain.
- Antibiotic therapy can relieve pain caused by infections.

Alternative

Alternative and complementary therapies for relieving pain, as well as stress and anxiety, and for helping patients cope with cancer include:

- acupuncture
- hypnosis
- biofeedback
- massage
- therapeutic touch
- physical therapy
- reiki
- tai chi
- yoga
- psychological therapies to influence pain perception

Home remedies

Home remedies for controlling cancer pain include:

- cold packs to numb pain or heat to relieve muscle soreness, for no more than ten minutes at a time
- guided imagery
- meditation
- distraction to move the focus away from the pain, such as watching television, listening to music, singing, praying, talking, or engaging in other activities
- exercise therapy
- relaxation techniques such as visual concentration, rhythmic massage, slow rhythmic breathing, breathing and muscle tensing, progressive relaxation of body parts, relaxation CDs, music or art therapy
- skin stimulation such as massage, pressure, vibration, heat, cold, or menthol
- social and spiritual support to influence pain perception

Prognosis

All pain can be treated and most cancer pain can be relieved or controlled. Cancer pain can be reduced to the point where it is possible to pursue normal activities, work, eat and sleep well, enjoy family and friends, have sexual intimacy, avoid **depression**, and enjoy life. However if pain medication is avoided or delayed, the pain may become worse, may take longer to control, or may require higher doses of the medication.

Prevention

The best means of preventing cancer pain is to treat it before it starts or becomes worse. Communicating openly about pain with the healthcare team is the best way to ensure that the pain is properly treated.

Resources

BOOKS

Fisch, Michael J., and Allen W. Burton. *Cancer Pain Management*. New York: McGraw-Hill, 2007.

Patt, Richard B., and Susan S. Lang. *The Complete Guide to Relieving Cancer Pain and Suffering*. New York: Oxford University Press, 2007.

Shannon, Joyce Brennfleck. *Pain Sourcebook*, 3rd ed. Detroit: Omnigraphics, 2008.

PERIODICALS

Brawley, Otis W., Daniel E. Smith, and Rebecca A. Kirch. "Taking Action to Ease Suffering: Advancing Cancer Pain Control as a Health Care Priority." *Ca: A Cancer Journal for Clinicians* 59, no. 5 (September/October 2009): 285.

McMains, Vanessa. "Study Tries to Put Pain in Perspective." *Chicago Tribune* (August 16, 2009): 13.

Savage, Liz. "Chemotherapy-Induced Pain Puzzles Scientists." *Journal of the National Cancer Institute* 99, no. 14 (July 18, 2007): 1070-1071.

OTHER

"Global Cancer Facts & Figures 2007.' *American Cancer Society*.http://www.cancer.org/downloads/STT/Global_Facts_and_Figures_2007_rev2.pdf.

"Pain." *StopPain.org*.http://www.stoppain.org/palliative_care/content/symptom/pain.asp.

"Pain Control: A Guide for People with Cancer and Their Families." *American Cancer Society*.http://www.cancer.org/docroot/MIT/content/MIT_7_2x_Pain_Control_A_Guide_for_People_with_Cancer_ *Chest x ray of patient with Hodgkin's disease*.Chest x ray of patient with Hodgkin's disease.Custom Medical Stock Photo. Reproduced by permission.and_Their_Families.asp

"Pain Control: Support for People with Cancer." *National Cancer Institute*.http://www.cancer.gov/cancertopics/paincontrol.

ORGANIZATIONS

American Cancer Society, 1599 Clifton Road NE, Atlanta, GA, 30329-4251, (800) ACS-2345, http://www.cancer.org.

American Pain Foundation, 201 North Charles Street, Suite 710, Baltimore, MD, 21201-4111, (888) 615-PAIN (7246), info@painfoundation.org, http://www.painfoundation.org.

National Cancer Institute, NCI Public Inquiries Office, 6116 Executive Boulevard, Room 3036A, Bethesda, MD, 20006, (800) 4-CANCER, http://www.cancer.gov.

The Wellness Community, 919 18th St. NW, Washington, DC, 20006, (202) 659-9709, (888) 793-well, (202) 659-9703, help@thewellnesscommunity.org, www.thewellnesscommunity.org.

Margaret Alic, PhD

Advance directives

Definition

An advance directive is a written document in which people clearly specify how medical decisions affecting them are to be made if they are unable to make them, or to authorize a specific person to make such decisions for them.

Description

Advance directives are recognized in most industrialized countries of the world. In the United States, by law, the creation of an advance directive is the right of

KEY TERMS

Competent—Duly qualified; having sufficient ability or authority; possessing all the requirements of law.

Dialysis—A technique used to remove waste products from the blood and excess fluid from the body as a treatment for kidney failure.

Hyperalimentation—The administration of a nutrient solution into a large, central vein near the heart. It is often used supplementary to eating, but can provide complete nourishment.

Tube feeding—Administration of nourishment, in nutritionally complete solutions, via tube into the stomach or intestines. Tubes can be either nasogastric, or inserted through the nose into the stomach via the esophagus, or surgically implanted directly into the stomach. These are usually used to sustain life when a person is unable to eat or take fluids by mouth.

all competent adults. The goal of this legislation is to empower all health care consumers to make their own judgments regarding medical decision-making, to approve of potential treatment they believe they would want, and to refuse care they do not perceive as being in their best interest. These directives are generally divided into living wills or durable powers of attorney.

Federal law requires that all health care providers (health maintenance organizations, or HMOs, skilled nursing care facilities, hospices, home health care providers, and hospitals) make information regarding advance directives available to all people in their care. Many states require that two people witness such advance directives.

Living wills

Living wills go into effect while the individual is still living, but is unable to communicate his/her wishes regarding care. Traditionally, a living will has specified the individual's wishes concerning procedures that would sustain life if he/she were terminally ill. Newer advance directives do not limit such preferences to terminal illness but instead go into effect whenever the individual is unable to speak for him/herself.

There are several ways of preparing a living will. Sometimes a preprinted form is provided, or people may create their own form, or may simply write down their wishes. Though all 50 states and the District of Columbia recognize the validity of advance directives,

each state's laws have differences as to whether one or all of these types of preparation of the document are legal and binding in that state. It is recommended that people speak to their attorney or physician to ensure that their wishes are carried out.

Durable power of attorney for health care

A durable power of attorney for health care is the second type of advance directive. This is a signed, dated, and witnessed document that authorizes a designated person (usually a family member or close friend) to act as an agent, or proxy. This empowers the proxy to make medical decisions for a person when the person is deemed unable to make these decisions him/herself. Such a power of attorney frequently includes the person's stated preferences in regard to treatment. Several states do not allow any of the following people to act as a person's proxy:

- the person's physician, or other health care provider
- the staff of health care facilities that is providing the person's care
- guardians (often called conservators) of the person's financial affairs
- employees of federal agencies financially responsible for a person's care
- any person that serves as agent or proxy for 10 people or more

As in the case of living wills, regulations regarding such powers of attorney vary from state to state. Some states provide printed forms, and require witnesses, while other states do not.

Causes

As medical advances provide greater than ever means of extending life, it becomes increasingly important for people to evaluate which of the available means they would wish used. If this is not done, people run the risk of having health care providers make critical decisions regarding their care. The absence of advance directive information can also create dilemmas and increased stress for loved ones. Some of the terms describing now-routine medical interventions that can maintain life under dire circumstances include:

- cardiopulmonary resuscitation (CPR), the use of chest compressions and/or mouth-to-mouth resuscitation to restart heart beat and/or respirations

- ventilators or respirators that physically deliver oxygen via a tube into the windpipe when the lungs are unable to work on their own

- Life-sustaining care encompasses the use of machinery or equipment that prolongs life by keeping the body functioning. Examples of life-sustaining care include hyperalimentation, tube feedings, and kidney dialysis.

In contrast, life-enhancing care, sometimes referred to as Care and Comfort Only, involves the provision of high quality, but non-heroic medical care until death occurs naturally. Important examples of life-enhancing care include administration and monitoring of medications, carrying out other measures to control pain, comfort measures such as bathing and massage, and offering food and fluids.

Special concerns

Though specifics vary, all states have laws allowing people to spell out their health care wishes for a time when they might be unable to speak for themselves. But, as noted, there is a potential for disparity in how advance directives are interpreted. In most hospitals, an ethics committee is available to assist and support both patients and families faced with decisions regarding medical care. In 1995, the American Association of Retired Persons (AARP), with the help of the American Bar Association (ABA) and the American Medical Association (AMA), produced a combined living will and power of attorney for health care document that provides very specific and detailed statements of a person's wishes. Further information regarding the laws in individual states can be obtained from the AARP, ABA, or AMA.

The AARP recommends that those individuals considering making an advance directive address the following issues:

- What the person's goals for medical treatment are: Should treatment be used to sustain life, regardless of the quality of that life?

- Who should act as the person's proxy or agent? It is important for the person making an advance directive to actually speak with this designated person and make his/her wishes known.

- Though there is no formula for specificity, the AARP recommends that instructions be made as clear and specific as possible, but should not restrict the proxy from making informed decisions at the time that cannot be anticipated in advance.

- To ensure that an advance directive is carried out, copies of it should be given to a person's physician, proxy, family, or any other interested party.

Resources

ORGANIZATIONS

American Association of Retired Persons Legal Counsel for the Elderly., P.O. Box 96474, Washington, DC, 20090-6474.

American Bar Association. http://www.abanet.org.

American Medical Association. http://www.ama-assn.org.

Center for Healthy Aging. http://www.careproject.net.

Choices In Dying, Inc., 200 Varick Street, New York, New York 10014-4810. (800) 989-WILL.

Joan Schonbeck, R.N.

AIDS-related cancers

Definition

The AIDS-related cancers are a group of cancers that occur more frequently in persons with human immunodeficiency virus (HIV) **infection** than in the general population. Individuals with HIV/AIDS are at high risk for developing certain cancers, particularly Kaposi's **sarcoma** (KS), non-Hodgkin **lymphoma** (NHL), and **cervical cancer**. Because these cancers occur so frequently in patients diagnosed with HIV/AIDS they are known as AIDS-defining conditions. The most common form of AIDS-related **cancer**, **Kaposi's sarcoma** (KS), was one of the first indications of the AIDS epidemic in the early 1980s.

Other types of cancers which may develop in patients diagnosed with HIV/AIDS include **anal cancer**, **liver cancer**, several different types of **skin cancer**, Hodgkin lymphoma, angiosarcoma, **testicular cancer** and colorectal cancer.

Demographics

The demographic distribution of AIDS-related cancers varies somewhat depending on the type of cancer. KS has reached epidemic proportions in areas such as southern Africa due to the large numbers of people infected with AIDS in that area of the world. In Africa, KS is most likely to occur in men although incidence is increasing among African women and children. In the United States, incidence of KS is decreasing. HIV/AIDS-related KS is most commonly diagnosed in gay men and is over 20,000 times more common in individuals with AIDS than it is in individuals without AIDS.

Numbers of cases of HIV/AIDS-related NHL, the second most commonly occurring AIDS-related cancer, continue to increase slightly. Approximately 4 – 10% of people with HIV/AIDS develop NHL. HIV/AIDS-related NHL is observed in all high risk groups for the development of HIV/AIDS including intravenous drug users and in children of HIV-positive individuals

Women diagnosed with HIV/AIDS are at higher risk for developing the pre-cancerous condition cervical intraepithelial neoplasia (CIN). CIN occurs in as much as 30% of women with HIV/AIDS. Women with HIV/AIDS are more likely to be diagnosed with a more aggressive form of CIN which can eventually develop into invasive cervical cancer.

Description

In order to understand the causes and treatment of AIDS-related cancers, it is useful to begin with a basic description of HIV infection. AIDS, or acquired immunodeficiency syndrome, is a disease of the immune system that is caused by HIV. HIV is a retrovirus, a single-stranded virus containing ribonucleic acid (RNA) and an enzyme called reverse transcriptase. This enzyme enables the retrovirus to make its genetic material part of the DNA in the cells that it invades. HIV selectively infects and destroys certain subtypes of white blood cells called CD4 cells, which are an important part of the body's immune system. As an infected person's number of CD4 cells drops, he or she is at risk of developing opportunistic infections, disorders of the nervous system, or an AIDS-related cancer. HIV is transmitted through blood or blood products that enter the bloodstream—most commonly through sexual contact or contaminated hypodermic needles.

Kaposi's sarcoma

Kaposi's sarcoma is the most common type of cancer related to HIV infection. There are two other major subtypes of KS—so-called classic KS and African KS—with different causes that are not yet well understood. AIDS-related KS (also called epidemic KS) is characterized by purplish or brownish lesions (areas of diseased or injured tissue) on the skin, in the mouth, or in the internal organs. The lesions may take the form of small patches or lumps (nodular lesions), large patches that grow downward under the skin (infiltrating lesions), or lumpy swellings in the lymph nodes. Unlike other cancers that typically develop in one organ or area of the body, KS often appears simultaneously in many different parts of the body. It may be the first indication that the patient has AIDS.

Non-Hodgkin's lymphoma

Lymphomas are cancers of the immune system that develop when white blood cells called lymphocytes begin to grow and multiply abnormally. The increased numbers of lymphocytes cause the lymph nodes, the organs that produce these white blood cells, to swell and form large lumps that can be felt. Lymphomas are divided into two major categories: **Hodgkin's disease** (HD), and **non-Hodgkin's lymphoma** (NHL). HD can be differentiated from NHL by the presence of Reed-Sternberg cells in the lymphatic tissue; these cells are not found in any other type of cancer.

NHL occurs more often than Hodgkin's disease. NHL can involve the spleen, liver, bone marrow, or digestive tract as well as the lymph nodes. Most AIDS related lymphomas are categorized as aggressive B cell type tumors. Three important types AIDS-related lymphomas are:

- Primary central nervous system lymphomas (PCNSL). This type accounts for about 20% of NHL cancers found in AIDS patients, but only 1% to 2% of NHL cancers in patients not infected by HIV. Lymphomas of this type start in the brain or the spinal cord. Symptoms include headaches, paralysis, seizures, and changes in the patient's mental condition. Patients diagnosed with PCNSL are more likely to suffer from advanced HIV infection than patients with other types of NHL.
- Systemic lymphomas. These also are called peripheral lymphomas. They begin in the lymph nodes or other parts of the lymphatic system and may spread throughout the body. Burkitt's lymphoma (BL) is a type of systemic lymphoma that is 1,000 times more common in AIDS patients than in the general population.
- Primary effusion lymphomas, also called body cavity-based lymphomas (BCBL). This type of NHL is relatively rare, but seems to be related to infection by human herpesvirus 8 (HHV-8) in addition to HIV.

Many cases of this type of HIV/AIDS-related NHL are also associated with the Epstein-Barr virus.

Cervical cancer

In women, cancer of the cervix (the lower end of the uterus or womb) is more likely to occur in HIV-infected individuals than in the general female population. About 60% of women with HIV infection are found to have some kind of abnormal tissue growth or cell formation in the cervix when a Pap test is performed. The **human papilloma virus** (HPV) is thought to be a co-factor in the development of cervical cancers. Papilloma viruses are a group of tumor-causing viruses that also cause genital warts. Cervical cancers develop more rapidly in HIV-positive than in HIV-negative women, are harder to cure, and are more likely to recur.

Risk factors

Risk factors associated with the development of HIV/AIDS-related cancers include:

- Infection with the human papillomavirus (HPV) – infection with this virus is a risk factor for the development of cervical cancer.
- Infection with the human herpesvirus 8(HHV-8)-associated with the development of KS and with primary effusion lymphoma
- Infection with the **Epstein-Barr Virus** (EBV) – EBV is a herpes-related virus implicated in the development of several types of lymphomas

Causes and symptoms

The most common types of AIDS-related cancers have been linked to oncogenic (tumor-causing) viruses:

- Human herpesvirus 8 (HHV-8) is associated with KS and some of the less common types of AIDS-related lymphomas (ie. cancers of the lymphatic system).
- Epstein-Barr virus (EBV) is associated with the more common types of AIDS-related lymphomas, particularly PCNSL and Burkitt's lymphoma.
- Human papillomavirus (HPV) is associated with anal cancer and with cervical cancer in women.

Oncogenic viruses cause cancer by changing the genetic material inside tissue cells. When this genetic material is changed, the cells begin to grow and multiply uncontrollably. The abnormal tissue formed by this uncontrolled growth is called a tumor. A healthy human immune system has a greater ability to protect the body against oncogenic viruses and to stop or slow down tumor formation. Since the retrovirus that causes AIDS weakens the immune system, persons with AIDS are at greater risk of developing cancers caused by oncogenic viruses.

Some types of AIDS-related cancers, such as **Burkitt's lymphoma**, have been linked to changes in human chromosomes (translocations). In a translocation, a gene or group of genes moves from one chromosome to another. Burkitt's lymphoma is associated with exchanges of genetic material between chromosomes 8 and 14 or between chromosomes 2 and 22.

Symptoms associated with AIDS-related KS include the presence of purplish or brownish lesions (areas of diseased or injured tissue) on the skin, in the mouth, or in the internal organs. The lesions may take the form of small patches or lumps (nodular lesions), large patches that grow downward under the skin (infiltrating lesions), or lumpy swellings in the lymph nodes. Unlike other cancers that typically develop in one organ or area of the body, KS often appears simultaneously in many different parts of the body. It may be the first indication that the patient has AIDS.

Other symptoms of KS include lymphedema or swelling in an arm or leg, a cough that is unexplained, chest pain, pain in the stomach or intestines, bleeding from the mouth and/or rectum, as well as **diarrhea** and/or symptoms resulting from the gastrointestinal system being blocked by KS lesions.

Symptoms of AIDS-related NHL are dependent upon the location of the cancer and can include enlarged lymph nodes, enlarged liver and spleen, unexplained **fever**, **weight loss**, and sweating and chills.

Unusual periods, bleeding between periods or after menopause, pain during intercourse and increased vaginal discharge are symptoms of cervical cancer.

Diagnosis

The diagnosis of an AIDS-defining condition such as KS, NHL, or cervical cancer may indicate that a person infected with the HIV virus has progressed to the development of AIDS.

Procedures and tests which may be used to diagnose HIV/AIDS-related malignancies include tissue **biopsy** and imaging scans in addition to a variety of other tests depending on the specific type of cancer and on the location of the cancer in the body.

Treatments

AIDS-related Kaposi's sarcoma treatment

KS differs from other solid tumors in that it lacks a stage or site of origin in which it can be cured. In addition, there is no relationship between the stage of KS and its response to treatment. Currently, there is no indication that treatment of KS improves survival. Small localized lesions may be treated by surgical excision, electrode dessication, and/or by curettage **cryotherapy**. KS tumors typically respond well to treatment with **radiation therapy** which is generally reserved to treat localized lesions on the skin and in the oral cavity. Localized lesions also respond to treatment using injections of the **chemotherapy** drug **vinblastine** directly into the lesion. The topical treatment alitretinoin (Panretin) 0.1% gel may also be used to treat KS skin lesions.

The use of systemic chemotherapy to treat AIDS-related KS is limited. Drugs which have been used as single agent therapy or as combination therapy include **bleomycin**, **docetaxel**, **doxorubicin**, **etoposide**, paclitaxel, vinblastine, and **vincristine**.

AIDS-related Non-Hodgkin's lymphoma

AIDS-related NHL is typically treated using chemotherapy and/or radiation therapy. The primary treatment choice is treatment with chemotherapy. The monoclonal antibody, **rituximab** (Rituxan), is used in combination with chemotherapy in most cases.

Cervical cancers

Treatment of CIN in women diagnosed with HIV/AIDS is more difficult than in women without HIV/AIDS. Recurrence of CIN is high HIV/AIDS affected women after treatment. Women infected with HIV/AIDS who progress to cervical cancer are treated with surgery initially. Disease progression after surgery may be treated with chemotherapy. HIV/AIDS infected women are also treated with anti-retroviral therapy to improve the treatment outcomes for the cervical cancer.

Prognosis

Treatment with anti-retroviral drugs has proven to be very effective in treating HIV/AIDS. As a result, incidence of AIDS-related cancers is decreasing overall. However, as individuals affected by HIV/AIDS live longer they are increasingly being diagnosed with cancers not typically associated with HIV/AIDS. Results of recent research reported in 2009 that analyzed data from more than 100,000 patients treated in the Veterans Administration System between 1997 and 2004, indicated HIV patients were 60% more likely to develop anal cancer, lung cancer, Hodgkin lymphoma, **melanoma**, or liver cancer as compared to patients without HIV infection. The researchers offer several theories to explain this increase: use of

antiretroviral therapy may increase the risk for developing non-AIDS related cancers, HIV-infected patients are more affected by risk factors for those cancers than other people and/or infection with the HIV virus or another undetected virus may increase a person's risk for developing one of these cancers.

Prevention

AIDS-related cancers develop as a result of infection with the HIV virus. Incorporating strategies to maintain a healthy immune system, including adherence to treatment with anti-retroviral drugs, is critical for patients diagnosed with HIV/AIDS to minimize the potential for development of AIDS-related cancers.

See also Immunologic therapies.

Resources

PERIODICALS

Bedimo, R.J., McGinnis, K.A., Dunlap, M., Rodriguez-Barradas, M.C., & Justice, A.C. "Incidence of Non-AIDS-Defining Malignancies in HIV-Infected Versus Non-Infected Patients." *Journal of Acquired Immune Deficiency Syndromes* 52(Oct. 2009):203–8.

Di Lorenzo, G., Konstantinopoulos, P.A., Pantanowitz, L., et al. "Management of AIDS-related Kaposi's Sarcoma." *Lancet Oncology* 8(2007):167–76.

Graber, S., Abraham, B., Mahamat, A., et al. "Differential Impact of Combination Antiretroviral Therapy in Preventing Kaposi's Sarcoma With and Without Visceral Involvement." *J Clin Oncol* 24(2006):3408–14.

ORGANIZATIONS

AIDS Clinical Trials Group (ACTG). c/o William Duncan, PhD, National Institutes of Health. 6003 Executive Boulevard, Room 2A07, Bethesda, MD 20892.

American Cancer Society (ACS). 1599 Clifton Road, NE, Atlanta, GA 30329. (404) 320-3333 or (800) ACS-2345. Fax: (404) 329-7530. http://www.cancer.org.

National Cancer Institute, Office of Cancer Communications. 31 Center Drive, MSC 2580, Bethesda, MD 20892-2580. (800) 4-CANCER. TTY: (800) 332-8615. http://www.cancer.gov.

San Francisco AIDS Foundation (SFAF). 995 Market Street, #200, San Francisco, CA 94103. (415) 487-3000 or (800) 367-AIDS. Fax: (415) 487-3009. http://www.sfaf.org.

Rebecca J. Frey, Ph.D.
Melinda Granger Oberleitner, R.N., D.N.S., A.P.R.N.,C.N.S

AJCC *see* **American Joint Commission on Cancer**

Alcohol consumption

Definition

Alcohol consumption is the ingestion of substances containing ethyl alcohol (ethanol), including beer, wine, and distilled spirits such as gin, whiskey, or vodka.

Purpose

In earlier times in subsistence agricultural societies, alcoholic beverages, usually beer or mead (fermented honey and water), provided a substantial proportion of dietary calories. Today people drink alcohol to relax and socialize, to get high, or because they are physically addicted to it.

Alcohol has an effect on almost every system of the body and it can be a dangerous substance of abuse. However a large number of studies have found some health benefits from the consumption of moderate amounts of alcohol by middle-aged and older adults. Moderate alcohol consumption can reduce the risk of heart attack, sudden cardiac death, peripheral vascular disease, and stroke caused by blood clots (ischemic stroke) by 25–40%. This risk reduction occurs in both men and women and in people who have no apparent heart disease, as well as those who are at high risk of heart disease because of type 2 diabetes, high blood pressure (hypertension), angina (chest pain), or a previous heart attack. Researchers suggest that this protective effect occurs because alcohol increases the amount of high-density lipoprotein (HDL; "good" cholesterol) and also because alcohol affects various proteins in ways that reduce the risk of blood clots. However, although moderate alcohol consumption may be recommended for reducing the risk of heart disease, other lifestyle factors, such as a healthy diet and exercise, reduce the risk of both heart disease and **cancer**.

Studies have also found that moderate alcohol consumption appears to decrease the risk of developing type 2 diabetes and gallstones. Gallstones are hard masses of cholesterol and calcium that form in the gallbladder. Although the risks of alcohol consumption outweigh its potential health benefits, moderate social drinking can also provide psychological benefits. Heavy alcohol consumption has no health benefits and poses many health risks.

Description

Ethanol is produced by yeast fermentation of the natural sugars in plants, such as grapes (wine), hops (beer), sugar cane (rum), agave (tequila), and rice (saki). The process of fermenting plants to produce alcohol is at least 10,000 years old and developed independently in many cultures. Although alcohol sales and consumption are prohibited in some countries and by some religions, the production of alcoholic beverages is a huge industry worldwide.

Recommended dosage

The federal government's *Dietary Guidelines for Americans* defines moderate alcohol consumption as one drink per day for women and two drinks for men. This gender difference is because women tend to be smaller than men and their bodies contain a lower percentage of water. Therefore equivalent amounts of alcohol consumption result in a higher blood alcohol concentration in women than in men. A drink, as defined by these guidelines, contains about 14 grams of alcohol and is equivalent to approximately:

- 12 fluid ounces of regular beer
- 5 fluid ounces of wine
- 1.5 fluid ounces of 80-proof distilled spirits

Heavy alcohol consumption is defined as 15 or more alcoholic drinks per week for men and 8 or more drinks per week for women. Between moderate and heavy alcohol consumption is a gray area of potentially problem drinking that includes binge drinking—heavy alcohol consumption that occurs intermittently. Bingeing is defined as 5 or more drinks in a period of about two hours for men and 4 or more drinks in the same period for women. About 60% of American men ages 18–25 binge drink.

Some people should never drink any alcohol:

- children and adolescents under age 21
- women who are pregnant, breastfeeding, or who could become pregnant

- people who cannot control their drinking and keep it at the level of moderate consumption
- people who plan to drive a car, fly a plane, operate dangerous equipment, act as a lifeguard, or perform any activity that requires quick reactions, good judgment, and coordination
- people who are unable to control their aggression when they drink
- people taking certain medications
- people with liver or kidney damage
- recovering alcoholics

Precautions

By far the greatest risk of frequent moderate alcohol consumption is that it can lead to heavy alcohol consumption, alcohol abuse, and alcohol dependency. Twin and family studies indicate that there is an inherited tendency for some individuals to develop alcohol abuse disorders.

In women even moderate alcohol consumption is associated with a modest increase in the risk of developing **breast cancer**. Research has shown that women who consume only one alcoholic drink per day have a 30% higher risk of dying from breast cancer than abstainers. However, some researchers suggest that taking at least 600 micrograms (mcg) of **folic acid** daily will counteract this increased risk.

Pediatric

Alcohol interferes with brain development in fetuses, children, and adolescents. Recent research indicates that the human brain continues to undergo development until people are in their early 20s. In addition, alcohol consumption by adolescents substantially increases their risk for:

- fatal and nonfatal motor-vehicle accidents
- risky sexual behavior
- school failure
- suicide
- death by homicide

Furthermore, adolescents are particularly susceptible to alcohol poisoning, a potentially fatal condition. Children who begin drinking before age 15 are five times more likely to develop alcoholism than those who begin drinking at age 21.

Geriatric

It is generally recommended that older men and women limit their alcohol consumption to one drink per day:

- Older adults have a lower tolerance for the effects of alcohol.
- Age-associated reductions in lean body mass can cause decreases in total body water, leading to higher blood alcohol concentrations in older adults than in younger people who consume the same amount of alcohol.
- Older adults are more likely to have medical conditions that are adversely affected by alcohol consumption.
- Older adults are more likely to be taking medications that interact with alcohol.
- Some research suggests that even moderate alcohol consumption in postmenopausal women increases their risk of breast cancer.

Pregnant or breastfeeding

There is no known safe level of alcohol consumption during pregnancy. Any level of alcohol consumption by a pregnant woman has the potential to damage the developing fetus, resulting in fetal alcohol syndrome disorders, including mental retardation or other conditions. Breastfeeding women should also abstain from alcohol, as it can pass through the breast milk to the infant.

Other conditions or allergies

Although approximately 34% of Americans never consume alcohol, about 7%, or more than 17 million people, are alcohol dependent or have alcoholism. Alcohol abuse is more common in men than in women and alcoholic men started drinking at an earlier age than women alcoholics. Costs related to alcohol disorders are estimated to be more than $185 billion annually. Alcohol disorders are related to increased rates of motor-vehicle deaths, homicides, suicides, and domestic violence.

Heavy alcohol consumption leads to two alcohol abuse disorders that are recognized in the *Diagnostic and Statistical Manual for Mental Disorders* (*DSM-IV-TR*) published by the American Psychiatric Association.

Alcohol dependence is diagnosed when one or more of the following occur within a 12-month period:

- Repeated alcohol use causes failure to fulfill obligations at work, home, or school.
- Driving or hazardous activities such as operating machinery occurs while under the influence of alcohol.
- Alcohol use results in legal problems.
- Alcohol use continues despite causing problems in relationships.

Alcohol abuse, or alcoholism, is diagnosed when three or more of the following occur within a 12-month period:

- Tolerance develops to the effects of alcohol.
- Abstaining causes, or would cause, physical symptoms of withdrawal.
- More alcohol is regularly consumed than is intended.
- Efforts to reduce alcohol consumption are unsuccessful.
- Obtaining alcohol, consuming it, and recovering from its consumption takes up a great deal of time.
- Work, social, and recreational activities are replaced by drinking or recovering from drinking.
- Alcohol use continues despite obvious physical and/ or psychological problems resulting from it.

Alcoholism is a chronic progressive disease that is often fatal. It is a primary disorder, although it can also be a symptom of another disease or emotional disorder. Factors such as psychology, culture, genetics, and response to physical pain influence the severity of alcoholism.

The best-known treatment for alcohol abuse disorders is the 12-step program of Alcoholics Anonymous. This program uses social support, rewards, and mentoring to change behavior. For it to succeed, the alcoholic must want to recover and must be willing to work at achieving sobriety. Relapses are common. Families of alcoholics may be helped by Al-Anon and Alateen for adolescents, regardless of whether their alcoholic family member participates in Alcoholics Anonymous.

Two other common forms of treatment for alcoholism are cognitive-behavioral therapy and interactional group psychotherapy based on a 12-step program. People with mild to moderate withdrawal symptoms are usually treated in outpatient programs through counseling and/or support groups. Alcoholics may be treated in a general or psychiatric hospital or substance-abuse rehabilitation facility if they:

- have not responded to more conservative treatments
- have coexisting medical or psychiatric disorders
- have a difficult home environment
- are a danger to themselves or others Inpatient programs may include detoxification, physical activities, psychotherapy or cognitive-behavioral therapy, and a 12-step program.

The U.S. Food and Drug Administration (FDA) has approved three medications for the treatment of alcoholism:

- Disulfiram (Antabuse) causes illness with alcohol consumption.
- Naltrexone (Depade, ReVia) acts on the brain to reduce the craving for alcohol.
- Acamprosate (Canpral) reduces withdrawal symptoms.

Side effects

The effect of alcohol consumption on the body depends on the alcohol content of the drinks, how much is consumed, and how often it is consumed. One of the most common side effects of alcohol consumption is the altering of sleep patterns. Alcohol consumption can cause a wide range of disorders, from poisoning to malnutrition to liver disease to cancer. There is also a broad spectrum of physical and mental disorders that result from fetal alcohol exposure.

Alcohol poisoning occurs when an overdose of alcohol shuts down the control of breathing and the gag reflex. Alcohol poisoning can cause a person to stop breathing and can cause irreversible brain damage. Binge drinking can result in a person continuing to drink beyond a fatal dose before losing consciousness. Signs of alcohol overdose include:

- mental confusion
- vomiting
- breathing that is slow (less than eight breaths per minute) or irregular (10 seconds or more between breaths)
- hypothermia (low body temperature, bluish skin color, paleness)
- seizures
- unconsciousness

Alcoholics generally do not eat healthy balanced diets and they may replace food with alcohol. Alcohol can decrease eating by interfering with the body's mechanisms for regulating food intake. Like food, alcohol contains energy in the form of calories. Alcohol contains approximately 7 calories per gram, whereas carbohydrates and protein contain about 4 calories per gram:

- One regular beer contains about 144 calories; light beer averages 108.
- One glass of wine averages about 100 calories.
- One shot of distilled spirits has about 96 calories plus the calories in any mixer.

Alcoholism is a major cause of malnutrition because serious nutritional deficiencies develop when at least 30% of total calories come from alcohol, which does not contain many of the nutrients required by the body. Alcohol also decreases the absorption, metabolism, and storage of nutrients from food. Alcoholics may have deficiencies in:

- protein
- essential amino acids
- carbohydrates
- fats
- B-complex vitamins, especially vitamins B_1 (thiamine), B_2, B_6, folate, and B_{12}
- fat-soluble vitamins (A, E, and K)
- vitamin C
- minerals such as calcium and magnesium Alcoholics may have either a deficiency or an excess of vitamin A.

Alcohol can further compromise nutritional status via:

- inducing early satiation
- immune system suppression
- respiratory disorders
- liver, gastrointestinal, and pancreatic damage

One of the most common side effects of chronic alcohol consumption is liver disease: steatosis (fatty liver), alcoholic hepatitis, and cirrhosis—liver damage that leads to scarring and dysfunction. Alcohol abuse is responsible for 60–75% of cirrhoses and worldwide about 32% of alcoholics die of cirrhosis. Cirrhosis is also a major risk factor for the development of primary **liver cancer**.

Alcohol consumption is an important risk factor for many types of cancer including cancer of the pharynx, larynx, mouth, breast, liver, lung, esophagus, stomach, pancreas, urinary tract, prostate, and brain. It also increases the risk for ovarian and colorectal cancer, **lymphoma**, and leukemia. The risk of breast and other cancers rises with increased alcohol consumption. Approximately 75% of esophageal cancers and 50% of cancers of the mouth, throat, and larynx are due to alcoholism, although wine appears to pose less of a danger than beer or hard liquor. People who consume 40–100 grams of alcohol per day have a 3–8-fold increased risk for **esophageal cancer**. A 2004 study reported that although moderate wine consumption might help protect against the formation of precancerous polyps in the colon, heavy alcohol consumption greatly increases the risk of developing colorectal cancer. Even moderate alcohol consumption can have detrimental effects on the health of cancer patients.

Other possible side effects of alcoholism include:

- immune system suppression resulting in infections, especially pneumonia

- gastrointestinal problems, especially diarrhea and hemorrhoids
- mental and neurological disorders, including depression, confusion, and destruction of gray matter in the brain, leading to mental disturbances and psychosis
- male impotence
- osteoporosis

Heavy drinking and alcoholism are also risk factors for:

- loss of judgment
- loss of motor skills
- loss of memory
- damage to the endocrine, immune, and hematopoietic systems
- stroke and cardiovascular disease
- brain damage
- violent death

Alcoholism takes an emotional and psychological toll on relationships and families, especially children.

Interactions

Alcohol is a central nervous system depressant that can interact with more than 150 different drugs. Some of these interactions can be fatal, especially those involving narcotic drugs that also depress the central nervous system. Categories of drugs that interact with alcohol include:

- narcotics
- sleeping pills
- antidepressants
- antianxiety medications
- antihistamines

Alcohol consumption can also:

- cause hypoglycemia (a drop in blood sugar), which is particularly dangerous for diabetics taking insulin
- interfere with the effectiveness of anticancer therapy and possibly cause the patient to become even sicker

- when combined with smoking, significantly increase the risk of developing mouth, throat, pharynx, larynx, and esophageal cancers

Resources

BOOKS

American Psychiatric Association. *Diagnostic and Statistical Manual of Mental Disorders (DSM-IV-TR)*, 4th ed., text rev. Arlington, VA: American Psychiatric Association, 2007.

Califano, Joseph A., Jr. *High Society: How Substance Abuse Ravages America and What to Do About It*. New York: Public Affairs Press, 2007.

National Center on Addiction and Substance Abuse (CASA) at Columbia University. *Women under the Influence*. Baltimore: Johns Hopkins University Press, 2006.

Sher, Leo. *Research on the Neurobiology of Alcohol Use Disorders*. New York: Nova Science Publishers, 2008.

PERIODICALS

Butler, Katy. "The Grim Neurology of Teenage Drinking." *New York Times* (July 4, 2006): F1.

"Heavy Alcohol Consumption Linked to CRC." *Patient Care* (January 2004): 8–10.

Miller, J. W., et al. "Binge Drinking and Associated Health Risk Behaviors Among High School Students." *Pediatrics* 119 (2007): 76–85.

Young, Emma. "Inside the Brain of an Alcoholic." *New Scientist* 189 (February 4—10, 2006): 18.

OTHER

"Alcohol: Frequently Asked Questons." *Centers for Disease Control and Prevention*. http://www.cdc.gov/alcohol/faqs.htm.

"FAQ for the General Public." *National Institute on Alcohol Abuse and Alcoholism*. http://www.niaaa.nih.gov/FAQs/General-English/default.htm.

"Fetal Alcohol Spectrum Disorders." *National Institutes of Health*. http://www.nih.gov/about/researchresultsfor thepublic/FetalAlcohol.pdf.

Harvard School of Public Health. "Alcohol: Balancing Risks and Benefits." *The Nutrition Source*. http://www.hsph.harvard.edu/nutritionsource/what-should-you-eat/alcohol-full-story/index.html.

Higdon, Jane. "Alcoholic Beverages." *Micronutrient Information Center*. http://lpi.oregonstate.edu/infocenter/foods/alcohol.

National Institute on Alcohol Abuse and Alcoholism. "Alcohol Calorie Counter." *College Drinking—Changing the Culture*. http://www.collegedrinkingprevention.gov/CollegeStudents/calculator/alcoholcalc.aspx.

National Institutes of Health. "Discussing Drinking: A Back-to-School Conversation You Need to Have." *NIH News in Health*. http://newsinhealth.nih.gov/2006/September/docs/01features_01.htm.

Rosenbloom, Margaret J., and Adolf Pfefferbaum. "Magnetic Resonance Imaging of the Living Brain: Evidence for Brain Degeneration Among Alcoholics and Recovery With Abstinence." *National Institute on Alcohol Abuse and Alcoholism*. http://pubs.niaaa.nih.gov/publications/arh314/362-376.htm.

U.S. Department of Agriculture and Department of Health and Human Services. "Alcoholic Beverages." *Dietary Guidelines for Americans*. http://www.health.gov/DIETARYGUIDELINES/dga2005/document/html/chapter9.htm.

ORGANIZATIONS

Al-Anon/Alateen, 1600 Corporate Landing Parkway, Virginia Beach, VA, 23454-5617, (757) 563-1600, (757) 563-1655, wso@al-anon.org, http://www.al-anon.alateen.org.

Alcoholics Anonymous, PO Box 459, New York, NY, 10163, (212) 870-3400, http://www.aa.org.

National Clearinghouse for Alcohol and Drug Information, P.O. Box 2345, Rockville, MD, 20847-2345, (877) SAMHSA7, (240) 221-4292, http://ncadi.samhsa.gov/default.aspx.

National Council on Alcoholism and Drug Dependence, 244 East 58th Street, 4th Floor, New York, NY, 10022, (212) 269-7797, (800) NCA-CALL, (212) 269-7510, national@ncaad.org, http://www.ncadd.org.

National Institute on Alcohol Abuse and Alcoholism (NIAAA), 5635 Fishers Lane, MSC 9304, Bethesda, MD, 20892-9304, (301) 443-3860, http://www.niaaa.nih.gov/.

Tish Davidson, AM
Crystal Heather Kaczkowski, MS
Margaret Alic, PhD

▌ Aldesleukin

Definition

Aldesleukin is interleukin-2 (IL-2), or specific kind of biological response modifier, that is used to treat metastatic renal cell **carcinoma** (a form of **kidney cancer**) and metastatic malignant **melanoma**.

U.S. brand names

Aldesleukin is also known as interleukin-2, IL-2 and the trademarked brand name Proleukin.

Purpose

When patients diagnosed with renal cell carcinoma and metastatic melanoma (**cancer** of the skin that arises in the pigmented cells of the skin or eyes) do not respond to other therapies, they may be candidates for treatment with aldesleukin.

Description

Aldesleukin is a biological response modifier (BMR). It promotes the development of T cells, or the cells in the lymphatic system that can fight cancer cells in cell-to-cell interaction. The human body produces aldesleukin naturally.

For use in therapy, aldesleukin is manufactured in a laboratory setting, using biotechnology methods, or methods that combine biological mechanisms and tools from technology. In the instance of aldesleukin, the compound is made in large quantities by using recombinant DNA technology. The DNA, or hereditary material, that provides instructions for making aldesleukin, is put in bacterial cells under laboratory confinement. The cells then produce large quantities of the human compound that are harvested, purified, and used for treatment.

Treatment with aldesleukin may control the growth of tumors, but this treatment does not produce a cure. In some cases, aldesleukin is used together with an anticancer drug.

Recommended dosage

Standard treatment with aldesleukin is via an intravenous line. The standard dose is 0.037 milligrams per kilogram (600,000 IU/kg) of body weight every eight hours to a maximum of 14 doses. The patient then remains off of the drug for 9 days. Following the 9 day rest period, the schedule is repeated for another 14 doses (the total is a maximum of 28 doses per course of treatment) as tolerated. Treatment with aldesleukin may result in severe side effects, therefore, lowering doses, withholding doses, and interrupting doses during treatment with this drug are not uncommon occurrences.

Each treatment course should be separated by a rest period of at least 7 weeks from the date of hospital discharge prior to initiation of the next course of treatment. Additional treatment is warranted only if there is evidence of decrease in tumor size since the last course and/or if there are no other contraindications to treating the patient again with aldesleukin.

Precautions

Side effects from aldesleukin are generally very severe. Therefore, the drug should only be administered in a hospital setting under the supervision of clinicians (oncology nurses, oncologists, and pharmacists) who are experienced in the administration of cancer therapies. Access to an intensive care unit is required when administering this drug.

Aldesleukin should only be given to patients with normal cardiac and pulmonary function as validated by thallium stress testing and pulmonary function testing. Patients with normal thallium stress test and pulmonary function test results but who have a history of prior cardiac or pulmonary disease and who are to be treated with aldesleukin should be treated with extreme caution.

Patients treated with aldesleukin may develop capillary leak syndrome (CLS) which results in hypotension and reduced perfusion of organs which may result in death. CLS is also associated with many other serious conditions including heart attack, breathing difficulties, renal problems and mental status changes.

Patients with bacterial infections or those prone to developing **infection** should be free of any infection prior to the start of therapy with aldesleukin.

Continued administration of aldesleukin to patients who develop lethargy may result in coma.

Pediatric

Aldesleukin in not approved for use in children.

Geriatric

As stated earlier, patients who may be candidates for aldesleukin therapy must have normal cardiac and pulmonary functioning. This drug is contraindicated in patients with significant renal, hepatic, and/or central nervous system impairment.

Pregnant or breastfeeding

At this time in 2009, there have been no studies which have determined whether aldesleukin is safe for use in pregnant woman. The drug should be given in pregnancy only if potential benefit to the mother justifies the potential risk to the fetus. It is not yet known whether aldesleukin is excreted in human breast milk. However, there is potential for serious adverse reactions in infants of breastfeeding mothers. Therefore, women who have been prescribed aldesleukin while breastfeeding should make the decision to discontinue breastfeeding or to discontinue the drug.

Other conditions and allergies

The effect of aldesleukin on fertility has not been studied. The manufacturer recommends this drug not be administered to fertile persons of either gender who are not using effective contraceptive methods and practices.

Side effects

Aldesleukin causes changes in the ways body fluids accumulate in the body that can lead to **ascites** and pleural effusions. Changes in personality are common due to the influence the drug has on the central nervous system. Among the most severe side effects is the possibility a patient will slip into a coma, or unconscious state. Other side effects may include alterations in liver function, skin reactions, such as rash, and infections may be severe and life threatening. Less serious, and almost always transient side effects, include flu-like symptoms, such as **nausea and vomiting**.

Interactions

Aldesleukin interacts with drugs that affect the central nervous system and it should not be taken with drugs that are used to modify moods or disposition (psychotropic agents). Many drugs, including those used to control blood pressure, heart beat and kidney function, increase the toxicity of aldesleukin and should not be taken in combination with it. **Corticosteroids** also interfere with the action of aldesleukin.

Physicians must be informed about every drug a patient is taking so interactions can be avoided.

Other drugs used to treat cancer which may interact with aldesleukin include **dacarbazine**, cisplatinum, **tamoxifen** and interferon-alfa.

Some patients (approximately 11–28% of patients in one study) previously treated with IL-2 containing regimens who then underwent radiological procedures which required use of iodinated contrast media, experienced adverse reactions including **fever**, chills, **nausea** and **vomiting**, rash, **diarrhea**, hypotension and other adverse effects.

Diane M. Calabrese
Melinda Granger Oberleitner, R.N., D.N.S.,
A.P.R.N., C.N.S.

Alemtuzumab

Definition

Alemtuzumab is an anti-cancer chemotherapeutic drug used to treat a type of **cancer** of the blood and bone marrow called leukemia.

Purpose

Alemtuzumab is used to treat a type of leukemia called B-cell **chronic lymphocytic leukemia**, also known as chronic lymphoid leukemia (CLL). Alemtuzumab is considered a first line agent for treatment of CLL, meaning that it may be a part of the first group of medicines used once a patient is diagnosed with CLL. Alemtuzumab is also used to treat CLL that has not responded to other drugs. Chronic lymphoid leukemia is cancer of a white blood cell called a lymphocyte. Lymphocytes are part of the immune defense of the body useful in fighting infections. The type of lymphocyte that creates antibodies against foreign invaders is the B cell. B cells are formed in the bone marrow, mature in lymph nodes, and travel via the blood and lymphatic system to fight **infection**. In CLL, the B cells are abnormal and do not fight infection. Instead the B cells present in CLL grow at an abnormally high rate, fill up the bone marrow and blood with abnormal B cells, and keep other normal immune system cells from growing. Most patients with CLL are greater than 50 years of age and male, but CLL can occur in either gender and at any age. Reports of patients with CLL less than 35 years of age are rare. Alemtuzumab is currently being investigated for possible use in other types of cancer in addition to CLL.

Description

Alemtuzumab is a type of monoclonal antibody used in the treatment of leukemia. **Monoclonal antibodies** are produced in the laboratory as substances that can locate and bind to cancer cells to destroy them. Alemtuzumab is marketed as the drug Campath by Bayer and Berlex Labs.

Studies have shown that use of alemtuzumab increases median survival time and progression-free survival compared to placebo. Median survival time is a term used to describe the time from either diagnosis or treatment at which half of the patients with a given disease are expected to still be alive. The term progression-free survival describes the length of time during and after treatment in which a patient is living with a disease that does not get worse. In a clinical trial

KEY TERMS

Anaphylactic shock—Acute systemic allergic reaction that can be life threatening.

Aplastic anemia—Type of anemia in which the bone marrow does not produce enough new cells to replenish the blood.

Autoimmune hemolytic anemia—Type of anemia in which the immune system of the body attacks its own red blood cells and destroys them in a process known as hemolysis.

Autoimmune thrombocytopenia—Condition in which the immune system of the body attacks its own blood system, resulting in decreased number of platelets necessary for normal blood clotting.

B cell—Type of white blood cell that creates antibodies to fight infection.

Bone marrow suppression—Disorder often caused by anti-cancer drugs in which the bone marrow no longer produces enough of the blood cells necessary for oxygen transport and the immune system often causing anemia and life-threatening infections.

Gout—Disease caused by elevated levels of uric acid in the bloodstream that deposit as crystals in

joints, tendons, and the big toe causing painful arthritic attacks.

Leukemia—Group of cancers of the blood or bone marrow characterized by an abnormal multiplication of white blood cells.

Lymphocyte—White blood cells of the immune system.

Monoclonal antibody—Antibodies produced by one type of B cell that are all clones of the parent cell and so are identical.

Multiple sclerosis—Autoimmune disease where the immune system is attacking the nervous system causing scars in the brain and spinal cord and physical and cognitive difficulty.

Oral mucositis— Painful inflammation and ulceration of the lining of the mouth, usually as a side effect of chemotherapy in the treatment of cancer.

Pancytopenia—Disorder in which all blood elements are deficient, red blood cells, white blood cells, and platelets.

Psoriasis—Chronic autoimmune disease that affecting skin and joints that causes red scaly patches of inflammation on the skin.

designed to test out a cancer drug in humans, both median survival time and progression-free survival are ways to measure how effective a treatment is.

Recommended dosage

Alemtuzumab therapy is dependent on a maintenance dose, the dose required to maintain a therapeutic level or range of alemtuzumab present in the bloodstream. However, the maintenance dose is often too high for patients to tolerate without working up to it gradually. Alemtuzumab therapy is begun at low doses and increased on a daily basis over a period of days or up to several weeks, to gradually bring the patient to the maintenance dose necessary for therapeutic effect. Alemtuzumab is given as an intravenous infusion over 2 hours three times per week, at a dose of 30 mg per infusion. Infusions are given on alternate days. The total duration of therapy, including initial dosage and dosage escalation, is up to 12 weeks. Single doses exceeding 30 mg or cumulative weekly doses exceeding 90 mg increase the incidence of toxicity and treatment related blood disorders.

Alemtuzumab intravenous therapy is associated with severe infusion reactions, ranging from skin

inflammation and **itching**, to life-threatening drop in blood pressure, difficulty breathing, heart attack, collapse of the blood vessels, and shock. To help prevent infusion reactions both diphenhydramine (Benadryl) and acetaminophen (Tylenol) are given 30 minutes prior to the alemtuzumab infusion during dose escalation. The doses used are 50 mg of diphenhydramine and 500 mg to 1 g acetaminophen.

Alemtuzumab depresses the immune system and makes a patient more susceptible to infections. Opportunistic infections are infections that may not normally occur in a healthy individual whose immune system is strong enough to fight them off. However, in individuals with depressed immune systems these infectious organisms are often able to get a foothold. To minimize this risk, several medications are given prophylactically when starting alemtuzumab therapy and continued for a time after therapy. The antibiotic sulfamethoxazole/trimethoprim is given in a dose of 800mg/160mg twice a day three times in a week. This antibiotic protects against an opportunistic **pneumonia** called Pneumocystis jiroveci. The antiviral drug famciclovir may be given in a dose of 250 mg twice a day to prevent herpes infection. These therapies are continued for 2 months after alemtuzumab treatment or when the immune system has healthy levels of immune cells again (whichever is later).

Precautions

Alemtuzumab is a pregnancy category C drug, and is used during pregnancy only when medically necessary. A pregnancy category C drug is one for which studies done in animals have shown potential harm to a fetus but there is not sufficient data in humans. If the potential benefits for the patient outweigh the potential risks to the fetus, the drug may be used during pregnancy. However, alemtuzumab may cause harm to a fetus. Alemtuzumab is contraindicated for use during breastfeeding and cannot be used within 3 months of beginning breastfeeding. The safety and effectiveness of alemtuzumab has not been established in patients less than 18 years of age. Clinical studies done on alemtuzumab did not include sufficient numbers of patients greater than 65 years of age to determine any differences in response in this age group, however no differences in geriatric patients have been reported. Patients should not have any vaccinations while taking alemtuzumab without the consent of their treating physician, and live **vaccines** should not be given. Patients taking alemtuzumab should also avoid being around people who have recently had the oral polio vaccine or the inhaled flu vaccine, as these are both live vaccines.

Some serious and even fatal side effects have been observed with alemtuzumab therapy. Alemtuzumab may cause fatal blood cell toxicities, including autoimmune **hemolytic anemia**, autoimmune **thrombocytopenia**, and pancytopenia. Alemtuzumab therapy has caused serious bone marrow suppression and immune system suppression resulting in increased risk for dangerous opportunistic infections. Serious and fatal reactions to the infusion have occurred including respiratory arrest, heart attack, cardiac arrhythmias, loss of consciousness, severe **fever**, chills, **nausea**, and **vomiting**, dangerously low blood pressure, and anaphylactoid shock. Most infusion reactions occur within the first week of therapy.

Several different types of monitoring tests are done during alemtuzumab therapy. Blood is monitored weekly in most patients, more frequently if initial signs of blood abnormality occur. Blood monitoring checks for disorders such as developing **anemia**, deficiency in any blood cells, and to check immune system cells are present in appropriate amounts.

QUESTIONS TO ASK YOUR PHARMACIST OR DOCTOR

- How long will I need to take this drug before you can tell if it helps for me?
- Is this drug safe to take with the other drugs that I am currently taking?
- What side effects should I watch for? When should I call the doctor about them?

Alemtuzumab may not be suitable for patients who have a form of anemia called autoimmune hemolytic anemia or aplastic anemia, thrombocytopenia, bacterial infections, bone marrow depression, fungal Infections, HIV infection, heart disorders, depressed immune system, or viral Infections. Monitoring is done for any sign of an infusion reaction, especially in the first several weeks of therapy. Because the immune system is depressed by alemtuzumab therapy, patients are monitored for opportunistic cytomegalovirus (CMV) infection throughout therapy and for 2 months after completion of treatment. During therapy CMV testing may be done weekly, then biweekly after therapy.

Side Effects

Alemtuzumab is used when the medical benefit is judged to be greater than the risk of side effects. Potential side effects include anemia, mouth sores, infusion reactions, rash, dizziness, **fatigue**, cough, nausea, vomiting, fever, chills, muscle stiffness, heart disorders, heart attack, difficulty breathing, sweating, headache, itchiness, wheezing, abdominal pain and cramping, **diarrhea**, constipation, loss of appetite, increased bacterial, viral, and fungal infections, sudden low blood pressure, high blood pressure, increased bleeding and bruising, racing heartbeat, anxiety, insomnia, and shock. Side effects involving infusion reactions are most likely to appear within the first week of treatment.

Interactions

Alemtuzumab may cause multiple different potentially serious adverse effects. Use of alemtuzumab in the same time period as other drugs that cause similar medical problems may cause an additive effect. Use of alemtuzumab with the psoriasis drug alefacept, the immunosuppressant drugs **azathioprine** or **corticosteroids**, the antipsychotic drug clozapine, the antiviral drug ganciclovir, or the gout drug **allopurinol** may cause toxicity in the form of immunosuppression. There are many drugs with which alemtuzumab may cause additive immunosupression, and the treating physician should be made aware of all medications the patient is taking before starting therapy with alemtuzumab. Use of alemtuzumab with the multiple sclerosis drug natalizumab may increase risk of infection. Use of alemtuzumab within 24 hours before, during, or 24 hours after the oral **mucositis** drug palifermin may increase the severity of mouth sores.

Resources

BOOKS

Goodman and Gilman's The Pharmacological Basis of Therapeutics, Eleventh Edition. McGraw Hill Medical Publishing Division, 2006.
Tarascon Pharmacopoeia Library Edition. Jones and Bartlett Publishers, 2009.

OTHER

Medscape*Alemtuzumab.*<http://www.medscape.com.>
RxList*Alemtuzumab.*<http://www.rxlist.com.>

ORGANIZATIONS

National Cancer Institute. 6116 Executive Boulevard, Room 3036A, Bethesda, MD 20892-8322. (800)4-CANCER. http://www.cancer.gov.
FDA U.S. Food and Drug Administration. 10903 New Hampshire Ave, Silver Spring, MD 20993. (888)INFO-FDA. http://www.fda.gov.

Maria Basile, Ph.D.

Allopurinol

Definition

This medication, also known as (Zyloprim), is used for the treatment and prevention of gout attacks and certain types of kidney stones. It is also used to treat elevated uric acid levels in the blood and urine, which can occur in patients receiving **chemotherapy** for the treatment of leukemia, **lymphoma** and other types of **cancer**. If left untreated, high uric acid levels in patients receiving cancer chemotherapy can cause kidney stones and kidney failure.

Description

Allopurinol decreases uric acid levels in the blood and urine by inhibiting a certain enzyme responsible for production of uric acid. It has been used for over three decades for prevention of gouty arthritis, kidney stones, and **tumor lysis syndrome** in cancer patients.

KEY TERMS

ACE inhibitors—A group of drugs used to treat high blood pressure. These drugs work by decreasing production of a certain chemical in the kidneys that causes constriction of blood vessels.

Gout—A disease, especially common in men, in which patients may have high uric acid levels in the blood and sudden attacks of severe joint pain and swelling caused by the deposits of uric acid crystals in those joints. These gout attacks most commonly affect the big toe.

Kidney stone—A concretion in the kidney made of various materials, such as uric acid crystals, calcium, or lipids. These concretions, or stones, cause severe pain when they are transported from the kidney into the bladder and out of the body.

Tumor lysis syndrome—A potentially life-threatening condition caused by cancer chemotherapy associated with very high blood levels uric acid, phosphate, and potassium, low calcium, and acute kidney failure.

Uric acid—White, poorly soluble crystals found in the urine. Sometimes uric acid forms small solid stones or crystals that are deposited in different organs in the body, such as the kidney. High levels of uric acid can be seen in patients with gout or cancer.

Recommended dosage

Adults

GOUT. 200–300 mg per day for mild gout and 400–600 mg per day for severe gout. Patients greater than 65 years of age should be started at 100 mg per day. Their dose can be increased until desired uric acid levels in the blood are reached.

Children over 10 years of age and adults

PREVENTION OF URIC ACID KIDNEY STONES IN CANCER PATIENTS. 600–800 mg per day divided into several doses, usually starting 1-2 days before cancer chemotherapy and stopped two to three days after the chemotherapy is completed for that cycle.

Total daily dose greater than 300 mg should be given in divided doses.

Children less than 10 years of age

PREVENTION OF URIC ACID KIDNEY STONES IN CANCER PATIENTS. 10 mg per kg per day of allopurinol in two to three divided doses up to a maximum dose of 800 mg per day. Another alternative is to give 150 mg per day in three divided doses for children 6 years of age and 300 mg per day in two to three divided doses for children 6-10 years of age.

Administration

Allopurinol should be taken after meals to avoid stomach upset. Patients should drink plenty of fluids (at least eight glasses of water per day) while taking this medicine unless otherwise directed by a physician. Drinking a lot of water can prevent formation of kidney stones.

Precautions

The use of allopurinol in pregnant women should be avoided whenever possible because its effects on the human fetus are not known.

Allopurinol should be used with caution by the following populations:

- Patients who have had an allergic reaction to allopurinol in the past.
- Patients who are taking certain medicines for high blood pressure such as diuretics (water pills) or angiotensin converting enzyme (ACE) inhibitors (captopril, lisinopril, enalapril). These people may be at higher risk of hypersensitivity with allopurinol.
- Breast-feeding mothers.
- Children (except those who have high uric acid levels caused by cancer, chemotherapy, or genetic diseases).

Patients should call a doctor immediately if any of these symptoms develop:

- rash, itching, swelling of lips or mouth, trouble breathing (also known as hypersensitivity reaction)
- yellowing of the skin or eyes
- pain when urinating or blood in the urine
- unusual bleeding or bruising

Patients with kidney problems may need to use lower doses of allopurinol.

Patients taking allopurinol will need to see a physician before starting therapy and occasionally during therapy to do blood tests for monitoring of kidney and liver function and complete blood count.

Side effects

Allopurinol is usually well tolerated by most patients. The most common side effect is skin rash, hives and **itching**. Loss of hair, **fever**, and feelings of discomfort or uneasiness can happen alone or in

combination with a rash. The risk of rash is higher in people with kidney disease or people taking amoxicillin or ampicillin. The use of allopurinol should be discontinued at first sign of a rash. Other side effects include **nausea**, **vomiting**, decreased kidney function and drowsiness (especially during the first few days of therapy). Because allopurinol can cause drowsiness, caution should be taken when performing tasks requiring alertness, such as cooking or driving.

Interactions

Patients should consult their doctor before drinking alcoholic beverages; alcohol can decrease the effectiveness of allopurinol. People consuming large amounts of vitamin C can be at an increased risk for kidney stones.

Allopurinol can prolong the effects of blood thinners such as **warfarin** (Coumadin) and put patients at risk for bleeding. It can also increase chances of low blood sugar with chlorpropamide (Diabinese) and nerve toxicity with vidarabine. Allopurinol can decrease breakdown of **azathioprine** (Imuran), **mercaptopurine** (6-MP), **cyclosporine** (Neoral, Sandimmune) and theophylline (Theo-Dur, Theolair, Theo-24) by the liver, increasing blood levels and side effects. Doses of azathioprine and mercaptopurine need to be reduced when they are used together with allopurinol. Mercaptopurine can be substituted for **thioguanine** (6-TG) to avoid this interaction altogether.

The use of amoxicillin and ampicillin should be avoided if possible in patients taking allopurinol because of increased risk of rash. Water pills such as hydrochlorthiazide (Diuril) can increase the risk of toxicity and allergic reaction when used with allopurinol.

Olga Bessmertny, Pharm.D.

Alopecia

Definition

Alopecia is the loss of hair for any reason. It can refer to thinning hair, patchy bald spots, partial or complete baldness, or hair loss confined to specific parts of the body. Androgenetic alopecia—also called adrogenic alopecia or pattern baldness or hair loss—is the thinning of scalp hair in response to androgens or male hormones, which is a natural part of aging in both men and women.

Demographics

Up to 70% of all men and approximately one-third of women are affected by alopecia at some point in their lives. In males androgenetic alopecia begins anytime after puberty. It usually becomes noticeable during the third decade of life and almost always by the fourth decade. Androgenetic alopecia affects about 50% of Caucasian men over age 40, but is less common and often less severe in Asian, Native American, and African-American men. It has been estimated that about 13% of premenopausal and about 37% of postmenopausal women have some degree of androgenetic alopecia.

Description

Alopecia can be a natural process, a symptom of an underlying physical or mental health condition, or the result of **cancerchemotherapy** or other drug treatments. Alopecia may affect only the hair and or the underlying skin as well. For example, some systemic diseases selectively affect hair growth, whereas others cause alopecia by altering the scalp skin.

- Alopecia areata is the loss of patches of hair due to an unknown cause.
- Alopecia totalis is complete baldness.
- Alopecia universalis is loss of hair all over the body.

The average person has 5 million hairs growing all over the body except the lips, palms, and soles of the feet. The scalp usually has about 100,000 hairs. Each hair grows out of a microscopic **depression** in the skin called a hair follicle. No new follicles are formed after birth. Each hair normally grows to its maximum length, stops growing, and is shed and replaced:

- About 88% of hairs are in the growing or anagen stage, which lasts for two to six years. Hair generally grows about one inch every four months.
- When a hair stops growing, it enters the catagen or transitional stage that lasts two to four weeks.
- It then enters the telogen or resting stage, which lasts for two to five months.
- In the exogen stage the hair falls out and a new hair begins to grow, beginning the cycle anew. Most people lose about 50–100 hairs each day. Alopecia of the scalp becomes noticeable only after about half of the hair has fallen out.

Hair follicles contain receptors for androgens circulating in the blood. Androgens binding to these receptors affect the hair-growth cycle in both makes and females. Although scalp hair grows in the absence of androgens, body hair is dependent on androgens.

Although alopecia itself is a harmless, painless condition, it can significantly affect **body image**, self-esteem, and **sexuality**. It can cause people to limit their social activities and bring on depression.

Risk factors

Androgenetic alopecia has a genetic basis. A family history of androgenetic alopecia increases one's risk of inheriting the condition. It is also associated with coronary heart disease, prostate enlargement in men, and polycystic ovary syndrome in women.

Other risk factors for alopecia include:

- a family history of alopecia areata
- various diseases including diabetes, thyroid disease, lupus erythematosus, or infection
- chemotherapy or other drug treatments

Causes and symptoms

- Androgenetic alopecia or pattern baldness is caused by a shortened anagen stage and the regrowth of thinner more fragile hair. With each growth cycle the hair is less firmly rooted and more easily shed. Androgenetic alopecia occurs in response to circulating androgens in the blood and is the most common cause of alopecia in both men and women.
- Male-pattern hair loss or hereditary baldness is considered normal in adult males. It is easily recognized by hair loss over the top and front of the head, with a receding hairline at the temples and balding on top, eventually leading to partial or complete baldness. The scalp remains healthy.
- Female pattern hair loss is also hereditary androgenetic alopecia, although the pattern is somewhat different than in men. It is characterized by a reduction in hair density over the crown and frontal scalp—thinning at the front, sides, or crown—but without a receding hairline. Hair loss in women is more common with advancing age and tends to be very gradual, although it accelerates during pregnancy and menopause.
- Hormonal changes or imbalances can cause temporary hair loss. These include pregnancy, giving birth, discontinuing birth control pills, entering menopause, or an underactive or overactive thyroid gland.
- Poor nutrition resulting from lack of protein or iron in the diet, fad or crash diets, or eating disorders can cause alopecia.
- Alopecia areata ranges from patchy hair loss to complete baldness. Most often it is characterized by a few small round smooth patches on the scalp, about the size of quarters. However it can occur anywhere on

the body, including the eyelashes or beard. Rarely, alopecia areata extends to the loss of all body hair. Soreness and itching may precede the hair loss. Although the hair regrows, the condition is often cyclical with hair repeatedly falling out and regrowing. Although the cause is unknown, it is believed to be an autoimmune condition. Most people with alopecia areata are otherwise healthy and there is little or no inflammation of the scalp.

- Several systemic autoimmune diseases—conditions in which the body's immune system attacks its own cells—cause alopecia by affecting the skin and/or hair. Lupus erythematosus causes alopecia by affecting the skin. Hyperthyroidism—excess thyroid hormone—causes the hair to become thin and fine. Hypothyroidism—thyroid hormone deficiency—thickens both the hair and skin, causing alopecia. Diabetes can also cause alopecia.

- Tinea capitis, or ringworm of the scalp, is a common contagious infection caused by mold-like fungi similar to those that cause athlete's foot. It usually causes patchy hair loss. Other scalp infections can also cause alopecia

- Cicatricial (scarring) hair loss is a rare condition in which inflammation permanently damages and scars the hair follicle, preventing new hair from growing. It may be accompanied by itching or pain. Although the precise cause of the inflammation is unknown, it is associated with several conditions including lupus erythematosus and a skin disease called lichen planus.

- Telogen effluvium is the sudden loss of clumps of hair that occurs when washing, combing, or simply gently tugging on the hair. Telogen effluvium usually results in thinning rather than bald patches. It occurs when the hair-growth cycle is prematurely forced into the telogen stage, often as the result of physical or emotional trauma.

- Trichotillomania is a mental disorder in which people compulsively pull out their own hair, resulting in bald spots.

- Traction apolecia results from hairstyles—such as tight pigtails, braids, cornrows, or tight curlers—that pull on the scalp. Hair loss usually occurs at the spots where the hair is pulled. Over-styling and excessive brushing can also cause hair loss from damage and breakage.

- Harsh hair treatments, including tinting, dyeing, bleaching, straightening, or permanents, can cause alopecia. African-American women often suffer from alopecia as a result of harsh chemical treatments that damage the hair shaft and follicles.

- Complete hair loss is a common side effect of the toxic drugs used in cancer chemotherapy.

- Occasionally drugs for treating gout, arthritis, depression, heart problems, or high blood pressure or birth control pills can cause alopecia.

- Radiation therapy causes hair loss only in the area of skin being treated.

- In children, alopecia is usually caused by drug treatments, radiation therapy, a skin disorder, or a hormone imbalance.

In addition to killing rapidly growing cancer cells, chemotherapy drugs also kill normal body cells that are growing rapidly. These include the cells of the hair bulb at the base of each hair. The hair falls out when these cells are killed. Some drugs affect the hair bulb, causing the hair to narrow and weaken and leading to breakage during normal brushing or shampooing.

Most patients undergoing chemotherapy, especially those who are being treated with more than one drug, will suffer from hair loss. Alopecia usually occurs between two and three weeks after the first cancer treatment. Hair loss is usually gradual, occurring over a three-to-four-week period. However the chemotherapy drug paclitaxel can cause all of the hair of the body to fall out within a 24-hour period. Other cancer treatments also can cause hair loss on the face, including the eyelashes and eyebrows, as well as the hair of the genitals, underarms, and other body areas. Loss of head hair usually begins on the top (crown) and sides of the head, presumably due to friction caused by pillows, bed linens, and hats.

Although many chemotherapy drugs can cause alopecia, certain drugs are more likely to cause hair loss than others. The likelihood of alopecia is also affected by the way in which the drug is administered, the dose, and the treatment schedule. The rapid administration of large doses, called bolus-dosing, is more toxic to the hair bulb than the slow administration of lower doses. Chemotherapy drugs with very high potential for causing alopecia include:

- cyclophosphamide
- daunorubicin
- doxorubicin (at doses higher than 50 milligrams)
- etoposide
- ifosamide
- paclitaxel
- docetaxel (Taxotere)

Radiation treatments also kill rapidly dividing cells. However hair loss occurs only at the site receiving the radiation. A high dose of radiation (greater than 6,000 cGy) usually permanently damages the hair follicles, preventing the hair from regrowing. If hair regrowth does occur, the hairs may be finer than before the treatment. Hair usually regrows following low doses of radiation (less than 6,000 cGy).

Genetic profile

Genetic factors determine the degree to which circulating androgens affect hair follicles in men. Androgens can activate genes that shorten the anagen cycle, causing the hair follicles to shrink. As the follicles shrink, the hair becomes shorter and finer and loses its pigment. Androgenic alopecia in women also appears to have a genetic component, but is not well-understood and may result from a combination of androgen-dependent and androgen-independent mechanisms. Genetic factors also influence the age at which alopecia begins, the speed that it progresses, and the pattern and extent of hair loss.

Diagnosis

Examination

Dermatologists can often diagnosis the cause of alopecia by its appearance. Androgenetic alopecia is easily recognized by the pattern of hair loss on the top and front of the head and by the healthy condition of the scalp. Dermatologists use the Norwood scale to evaluate the extent of androgenetic alopecia in men. Female pattern hair loss is less easily recognizable. Dermatologists use the Ludwig scale or the Savin scale to evaluate female androgenetic alopecia. For other types of alopecia, a complete patient and family medical history, physical examination, and possibly a psychological evaluation may be required.

Tests

If the cause of the alopecia is not apparent tests may include:

- Pull testing, in which several dozen hairs are gently tugged to observe how many are removed, is used to determine the stage of shedding and diagnose or rule out telogen effluvium.

- Skin scrapings remove small samples of skin and a few hairs to be examined for infection.

- The fungus causing tinea capitis usually glows under ultraviolet light.

- Systemic diseases underlying alopecia, such as diabetes, lupus, or thyroid disease, usually require a battery of specialized tests for diagnosis.

Procedures

Diagnosis of more unusual diseases or conditions underlying alopecia may require a skin punch **biopsy**. Using a local anesthetic, a circular tool removes a tiny bit of the deeper layers of skin for microscopic examination. Skin biopsies are often used to diagnose alopecia areata or cicatricial (scarring) apolecia.

Treatment

Traditional

Temporary alopecia requires successful treatment of the underlying cause. This may require an effective cure of the scalp fungus, control of a systemic disease, or completion of chemotherapy.

There are various surgical treatments for androgenetic alopecia or other permanent hair loss:

- Hair transplantation involves the surgical transplantation of thousands of individual hair follicles. Tiny plugs of skin, each containing one to several hairs, are removed from the back side of the scalp and implanted into the bald sections.

- Hair grafting, in which micrografts of one or two hairs are transplanted per follicle, tends to give the best results with the fewest complications.

- Scalp reduction involves reducing the bald area by stretching the skin, removing the hairless area of scalp, and closing the space with hair-covered scalp.

- Rotation flaps involve folding skin with hair over an area of bald skin.

Drugs

Minoxidil (Rogaine) and finasteride (Propecia) are the only approved drugs for promoting hair growth. They are effective in a significant minority of patients, especially those with male pattern baldness or alopecia areata and they are both considered to be safe when used as directed. However any new hair growth ceases as soon as the treatment is discontinued.

Minoxidil is an over-the-counter 2% liquid or foam that is rubbed into the scalp twice a day. When used continuously for long periods of time, minoxidil produces satisfactory results—regrowth and/or a slower rate of loss—in about 25% of patients with androgenic alopecia and as many as half of patients with alopecia areata, although the new hair may be shorter and is often thinner and lighter in color. It can take 12 weeks of treatment to regrow any hair. If there is no regrowth within six months, further treatment is unlikely to be effective. Minoxidil appears to increase the length of the anagen phase, enlarge the hair follicles, and rouse the follicles from catagen. Minoxidil can be effective for both men and women, but an over-the-counter extra-strength (5%) form of minoxidil is approved for use by men only. Minoxidil may cause scalp irritation.

Finasteride is a prescription drug that is taken orally. It prevents the conversion of the male hormone **testosterone** to dihydrotestosterone (DHT), the hormone that shrinks hair follicles. Many men experience slowed hair loss with finasteride and occasionally some regrowth, although results may take several months. Finasteride should not be used by women of childbearing age because it adversely affects male fetuses. Pregnant women should not even handle the drug. Finasteride has not been shown to be effective in women with postmenopausal androgenetic alopecia.

Other drugs that are sometimes used to treat alopecia include:

- hormones, which can sometimes reverse hair loss due to hormonal changes or imbalances
- monthly corticosteroid injections into the scalp for alopecia areata
- oral corticosteroids for extensive hair loss
- corticosteroid ointments and lotions, although these are less effective
- anthralin (Dritho-Scalp) cream or ointment, a psoriasis drug, which may stimulate new hair growth in alopecia areata when applied to the scalp
- topical or oral antifungal medications for tinea capitis

Alternative

Patients suffering from alopecia may benefit from certain **vitamins**, minerals, and supplements that promote healthy hair:

- zinc
- selenium
- magnesium
- iron
- vitamins A, B-complex, and C
- vitamin E massaged into the scalp
- evening primrose oil and flaxseed oil, which are rich sources of omega-3 and omega-6 fatty acids that are important for healthy hair

Herbalists recommend rinsing hair with sage tea or massaging the scalp with essential oil of rosemary to improve blood circulation and stimulate hair follicles. Chinese medicinal herbs that promote hair growth include

- cornus
- Chinese foxglove root
- Chinese yam
- lycium fruit
- polygonum

Cancer patients should check with their oncologist before taking any vitamin, mineral, or herbal supplements because of the possibility that they could interfere with the effectiveness of chemotherapy.

Home remedies

There are a variety of hair-replacement methods, including weaving remaining hair together with hair from another person. Spray-on scalp dye treatments can help disguise hair loss by making the remaining hair appear thicker.

Cancer patients are encouraged to buy a wig before they lose their hair, so it will be available when needed and match the color and texture of their normal hair. Patients with long hair can have a wig made with their own hair. A doctor's prescription is required if the wig is covered by insurance. Some patients prefer to shave their head once hair loss begins.

Prognosis

The prognosis for alopecia depends on the cause of the hair loss. It is generally much easier to lose one's hair than to regrow it and regrown hair is often thinner and less attractive.

Androgenetic alopecia is almost always permanent and there are no truly effective treatments. Generally the more extensive the hair loss, the less effective medications will be. However female androgenetic alopecia rarely results in complete baldness. Cicatricial alopecia is also permanent.

Hair loss due to hormonal changes, alopecia areata, tinea capitis, and telogen effluvium is usually temporary. However with telogen effluvium it may take months for the hair to regrow. If the pulling that causes traction alopecia is discontinued before the roots are permanently damaged or the scalp is scarred, the hair usually grows back normally.

Chemotherapy-induced alopecia is usually temporary. Hair typically regrows in about three to five months, although it may be of a different color or type than before treatment. Radiation-induced alopecia may be permanent.

QUESTIONS TO ASK YOUR DOCTOR

- What is causing my hair loss?
- Will it grow back?
- What are my treatment options?
- What are the side effects of treatment?

Prevention

Steps for maintaining healthy hair and minimizing alopecia include:

- a nutritionally balanced diet
- handling hair gently
- avoiding tight hairstyles such as buns, pigtails, and braids
- avoiding twisting, rubbing, or pulling hair
- using a mild shampoo
- using hair brushes with soft bristles
- avoiding the use of hair dryers, hot curlers, and curling irons
- using the lowest setting on a hair dryer
- avoiding hair dyes
- avoiding permanent-wave solutions
- wearing sunscreen or a hat outdoors
- using satin pillowcases

Alopecia resulting from cancer treatment is unavoidable. The safety and effectiveness of various methods for preventing chemotherapy-induced alopecia are somewhat controversial. Certain medications are sometimes used. A scalp tourniquet, which puts pressure on the scalp to block blood flow, may prevent the drugs from damaging hair follicles. Scalp hypothermia uses ice or a cooling device to reduce the amount of drug taken up by the hair bulb cells.

Resources

BOOKS

Haber, Robert S., and Dow B. Stough. *Hair Transplantation*. Philadelphia: Elsevier Saunders, 2006.

Hoffman, Candace. *Breaking the Silence on Women's Hair Loss*. Orem, UT: Woodland Publishing, 2006.

Levy, Janey. *Alopecia Areata*. New York: Rosen Publishing Group, 2007.

National Cancer Institute. *Hair Loss (Alopecia)*. Bethesda, MD: U.S. Department of Health and Human Services, National Institutes of Health, 2008.

Sherrow, Victoria. *Encyclopedia of Hair: A Cultural History*. Westport, CT: Greenwood Press, 2006.

PERIODICALS

Harrison, S., and W. Bergfeld. "Diffuse Hair Loss: Its Triggers and Management." *Cleveland Clinic Journal of Medicine* 76, no. 6 (June 2009): 361–367.

Rogers, N. E., and M. R. Avram. "Medical Treatments for Male and Female Pattern Hair Loss." *Journal of the American Academy of Dermatology* 59 (2008): 547–566.

Rulon, E., et al. "Clinical Inquiries: What is the Best Diagnostic Approach to Alopecia in Women?" *Journal of Family Practice* 58, no. 7 (July 2009): 378–380.

"Treating Female Pattern Hair Loss. Noticeable Hair Loss Can Be Deeply Distressing. Here Are Some Medical Treatments that May Help." *Harvard Women's Health Watch* 16, no. 10 (June 2009): 1–3.

OTHER

"Alopecia Areata." *National Institute of Arthritis and Musculoskeletal and Skin Diseases*. http://www.niams.nih.gov/Health_Info/Alopecia_Areata/alopecia_areata_ff.asp.

"Best Rx Options for Hair Loss in Women: Dermatologists Say First Find the Cause." *American Academy of Dermatology*. http://www.skincarephysicians.com/agingskinnet/hair_loss_options.html.

"Hair Diseases and Hair Loss." *MedlinePlus*. http://www.nlm.nih.gov/medlineplus/hairdiseasesandhairloss.html.

"Hair Loss." *American Cancer Society*. http://www.cancer.org/docroot/MIT/content/MIT_7_2X_Hair_Loss.asp.

"Is Your Hair Taking a Break? Dermatologists Can Help Women Get to the Root of Hair Loss." *American Academy of Dermatology*. http://www.aad.org/media/background/news/Releases/Is_Your_Hair_Taking_a_Break_Dermatologists_Can_Hel/

"Male and Female Pattern Hair Loss Information." *Androgenetic Alopecia.com*. http://www.androgeneticalopecia.com

Mayo Clinic Staff. "Hair Loss." *MayoClinic.com*. http://www.mayoclinic.com/health/hair-loss/DS00278

ORGANIZATIONS

American Academy of Dermatology, PO Box 4014, Schaumburg, IL, 60168, (847) 240-1280, (866) 503-SKIN (7546), (847) 240-1859, http://www.aad.org.

American Cancer Society, 1599 Clifton Road NE, Atlanta, GA, 30329-4251, (800) ACS-2345, http://www.cancer.org.

National Institute of Arthritis and Musculoskeletal and Skin Diseases (NIAMS), Information Clearinghouse, National Institutes of Health, 1 AMS Circle, Bethesda, MD, 20892-3675, (301) 495-4484, (877) 22-NIAMS (226-4267), (301) 718-6366, NIAMSinfo@mail.nih.gov, http://www.niams.nih.gov.

Belinda Rowland, PhD
Beth A. Kapes
Margaret Alic, PhD

Alternative therapies *see* **Complementary cancer therapies**

Altretamine

Definition

Altretamine, also known by the brand name Hexalen, is an anticancer agent used to treat **ovarian cancer**.

Purpose

Altretamine is used to treat persistent or recurrent ovarian **cancer**, usually after treatment of the cancer with **cisplatin** and/or an alkylating agent fails to effectively treat the tumor.

Description

The mechanism of action of altretamine is not known. However, it is thought that it may inhibit DNA and RNA synthesis.

Recommended dosage

Alretamine is administered orally. Doses for the drug may be different depending on the protocol that is used by the physician. Some example dosing regimens are: 4 to 12 mg per kg in three to four divided doses for 21 to 90 days; 240 to 320 mg per square meter of body surface area in three to four divided doses for 21 days, repeated every six weeks; 260 mg per square meter of body surface area per day for 14 to 21 days of a 28 days cycle in four divided doses; or 150 mg per square meter of body surface area in three to four divided doses for 14 days of a 28 day cycle. The dose of altretamine may be decreased if the patient has intolerable stomach side effects, low blood count of cells that fight **infection** (white blood cells) or cells that prevent bleeding (platelets), or if the patient has progressive toxicity affecting the nerves of the brain and body.

Precautions

Caution is usually taken in prescribing altretamine to patients with decreased kidney or liver function or damage to nerves due to previous **chemotherapy**. Careful monitoring of nerve, kidney, and liver function is required for these patients.

Pregnant women should be warned before taking this drug, as it may cause permanent harm to the fetus. Women who are of childbearing age should apply contraceptive methods to avoid pregnancy until they have discontinued drug use. Altretamine may also affect fertility. Additionally, although it is

KEY TERMS

Antiemetic—Agents used to alleviate nausea and vomiting, used during and sometimes following treatment with chemotherapy or radiotherapy.

Peripheral neuropathy—Symptoms resulting from damage to the peripheral nerves, that is, nerves not found in the spinal cord or brain.

not known whether this drug is excreted in the breast milk, nursing mothers are cautioned not to breast feed while being treated with altretamine.

Side effects

Nausea and vomiting may gradually occur as patients receive continuous high dose of altretamine. In most instances, **antiemetics** can help control these side effects. However, some patients may experience severe **nausea** and **vomiting** that requires either reducing the dose or stopping treatment with altretamine. Other common side effects include loss of appetite (**anorexia**) and **diarrhea**. Patients may also experience nerve toxicity, which is described as numbness, tingling, and burning sensations in the fingers and toes. Patients can also have difficulty walking because of these sensation changes. Patients may also commonly experience: **thrombocytopenia**, a decrease of the platelet cells responsible for blood clotting; **anemia**, a decrease of the red blood cells responsible for oxygen transport to tissues and organs; and leukopenia, a decrease of the white blood cells responsible for fighting infections. Less common side effects include seizures, **depression**, dizziness, stomach cramps, liver toxicity, rash, and hair loss (**alopecia**).

Interactions

Persons taking altretamine and monoamine oxidase inhibitors (MAO inhibitors) may experience severe hypotension (low blood pressure) when standing up. Additionally, the drug cimetidine may increase the toxicity of altretamine. Prior to starting any over-the-counter medications, herbal medications, or new medications, patients should consult with their physician, nurse, or pharmacist to ensure that there are no potential drug interactions.

Michael Zuck, Ph.D.

Amantadine

Definition

Amantadine is a synthetic antiviral drug, similar to rimantadine, in a class known as M2 inhibitors or M2-channel blockers. It is also considered to be an anticholinergic drug and a central nervous system stimulant and has strong anti-parkinsonian properties.

Purpose

Amantadine is used to prevent and treat viral infections caused by some strains of influenza A. It inhibits the replication of influenza A subtypes H1N1, H2N2, and H3N2. It is not active against influenza B. Amantadine may be used to prevent influenza A symptoms when a flu vaccine is unavailable or contra-indicated or in the period after a flu vaccination before the vaccine becomes effective. It is also used to treat early-stage uncomplicated respiratory tract infections caused by influenza A viruses. However flu viruses can develop resistance to amantadine quite rapidly, so it is not usually the drug of choice during flu season.

Amantadine is also used to treat Parkinson's disease and parkinsonism or parkinsonian symptoms that occur as side effects of antipsychotic medications for mental disorders such as schizophrenia. These side effects, called drug-induced extrapyramidal reactions, are similar to symptoms of Parkinson's disease and include tremors, difficulties with voluntary movements such as walking, and poor muscle tone. Amantadine is also used to treat parkinsonism caused by encephalitis, nervous system damage from carbon monoxide poisoning, and cerebral arteriosclerosis. However it is less effective in treating Parkinson's disease than other drugs such as L-dopa. Amantadine increases the level of dopamine—a central nervous system stimulant and neurotransmitter—and helps restore the chemical balance between dopamine and acetylcholine in the brain.

Amantadine is sometimes used off-label to treat other conditions including Creutzfeldt-Jakob disease.

Description

For flu prevention amantadine is administered in anticipation of an influenza outbreak, before or after contact with infected persons, or for two to four weeks after a flu vaccination until the vaccine can take effect. It is continued for at least 10 days following exposure to the flu. For treating influenza A the drug should be started within 24–48 hours of the appearance of signs and symptoms and continued for 24–48 hours after their disappearance.

Amantadine is available in 100-milligram (mg) tablets and capsules and as a syrup containing 50 mg per teaspoon (5 milliliters).

U.S. brand names

Amantadine is available under the brand name Symmetrel and as a generic drug, amantadine hydrochloride.

Canadian brand names

- Symmetrel
- Endantadine
- PMS-Amantadine

International brand names

- Symmetrel
- Amantadin
- Mantadix
- PK-Merz
- Viregyt-K

Recommended dosage

The usual dose of amantadine for adults and children over age nine is 200 mg once a day or 100 mg twice a day. Splitting the dose may reduce central nervous system side effects. Some patients may need a total daily dose as high as 300 mg, especially patients with Parkinson's disease who find the drug's effectiveness decreasing after a few months of use. Patients who are taking other anti-parkinsonian drugs concomitantly may take a lower dose, such as 100 mg daily. Elderly patients and those with kidney disease or on hemodialysis must take lower doses, ranging from 100 mg daily to as little as 200 mg every seven days. The dosage for children aged one through nine is 2–4 mg per lb of body weight daily (4.4–8.8 mg/kg/day), not to exceed 150 mg per day.

Precautions

Amantadine can cause visual disturbances and affect mental alertness and coordination. Patients should not operate motor vehicles or dangerous machinery while taking amantadine if they have central nervous system effects or blurred vision from the drug. Suicide attempts and completed suicides have been reported in patients taking amantadine, often for flu prevention or treatment.

Pediatric

The safety and effectiveness of amantadine in infants under one year-of-age have not been established.

Geriatric

Elderly patients should take lower doses of amantadine and be carefully monitored.

Pregnant or breastfeeding

Adequate human studies on amantadine during pregnancy have not been performed; however the drug should not be taken during pregnancy unless the potential benefits outweigh the risk to the fetus. Amantadine enters breast milk and should not be used by nursing mothers.

Other conditions and allergies

- Because amantadine increases the levels of dopamine in the brain, patients with a history of epilepsy or other seizure disorders should be carefully monitored while taking this drug.
- Patients with kidney or liver disease or a history of congestive heart failure or peripheral edema should also be closely monitored while taking amantadine. Kidney insufficiency significantly reduces clearance of the drug from the body.
- Amantadine can exacerbate mental disturbance in patients with histories of psychiatric disorders or substance abuse.
- Amantadine should not be discontinued abruptly in patients with Parkinson's disease because of the risk of a severe symptomatic episode.
- All patients should be carefully observed if the dose of amantadine is abruptly reduced or the drug is discontinued.
- It should not be given to patients who have a hypersensitivity to amantadine or to any of the inactive ingredients in the medication.

Side effects

About 5–10% of patients taking amantadine experience some or all of the following nervous system side effects:

- dizziness or lightheadedness
- insomnia
- nervousness or anxiety
- impaired concentration

About 1–5% of patients taking amantadine experience some or all of the following nervous system side effects:

- irritability or agitation
- depression
- confusion
- lack of coordination
- nightmares
- fatigue
- headache

Up to 1% of patients may experience:

- hallucinations
- euphoria (excitement)
- extreme forgetfulness
- aggressive behavior
- personality changes
- seizures Seizures are the most serious side effects associated with amantadine.

Amantadine can also cause gastrointestinal side effects. About 5–10% of patients experience **nausea**. Up to 5% of patients experience dry mouth, loss of appetite, constipation, and **vomiting**. In most cases these side effects can be treated symptomatically.

About 1–5% of patients taking amantadine report a bluish tinge to their skin, usually on the legs, which is associated with enlargement of the blood vessels (livedo reticularis). This side effect usually appears from one month to one year after starting the drug and subsides within weeks or months after the drug is discontinued. Patients experiencing this or other side effects from any medication should consult their physician.

Overdoses of amantadine can result in cardiac dysfunction or respiratory, renal, or nervous system toxicity. As little as 1,000 mg of amantadine can be fatal.

Interactions

Taking amantadine together with other drugs used to treat parkinsonism or parkinsonian side effects may cause increased confusion or even hallucinations. The combination of amantadine and other central nervous system stimulants, such as amphetamines or decongestants, may increase central nervous system side effects and the likelihood of seizures. Alcohol can also increase the central nervous system side effects of amantadine and should be avoided.

Resources

BOOKS

Factor, Stewart A., and William J. Weiner. *Parkinson's Disease: Diagnosis and Clinical Management*, 2nd ed. New York: Demos, 2008.

PERIODICALS

Cady, Sarah D., and Mei Hong. "Amantadine-Induced Conformational and Dynamical Changes of the Influenza M2 Transmembrane Proton Channel." *Proceedings of the National Academy of Sciences USA* 105, no. 5 (February 5, 2008): 1483.

Donfrancesco, Renato, et al. "Open-Label Amantadine in Children with Attention-Deficit/Hyperactivity Disorder." *Journal of Child and Adolescent Psychopharmacology* 17, no. 5 (2007): 657–663.

Stouffer, Amanda L., et al. "Amantadine-Structural Basis for the Function and Inhibition of an Influenza Virus Proton Channel." *Nature* 451 (January 31, 2008): 596–600.

OTHER

"Amantadine." *University of Maryland Medical Center.* http://www.umm.edu/altmed/drugs/amantadine-003900.htm.

American Society of Health-System Pharmacists. "Amantadine." *MedlinePlus.* http://www.nlm.nih.gov/medlineplus/druginfo/meds/a682064.html.

Di Minno, Mariann, and Michael J. Aminoff. "Treatment Options." *National Parkinson Foundation.* http://www.parkinson.org/Page.aspx?&pid = 227&srcid = 244.

National Institute of Neurological Disorders and Stroke. "Parkinson's Disease: Hope Through Research." *NIH Publication No. 06-139.* http://www.ninds.nih.gov/disorders/parkinsons_disease/detail_parkinsons_disease.htm

"Symmetrel (Amantadine Hydrochloride, USP) Tablets and Syrup: Package Insert." *Endo Pharmaceuticals.* http://www.endo.com/PDF/symmetrel_pack_insert.pdf.

ORGANIZATIONS

Centers for Disease Control and Prevention, 1600 Clifton Road, Atlanta, GA, 30333, (888) 232-6348, (301) 563-6595, cdcinfor@cdc.gov, http://www.cdc.gov.

National Institute of Neurological Disorders and Stroke (NINDS), NIH Neurological Institute, PO Box 5801, Bethesda, MD, 20824, (301) 496-5751, (800) 352-9424, http://www.ninds.nih.gov/index.htm.

National Parkinson Foundation, Inc., 1501 N.W. 9th Avenue/Bob Hope Road, Miami, FL, 33136-1494, (305) 243-6666, (800) 327-4545, (305) 243-6073, contact@ parkinson.org, http://www.parkinson.org.

U.S. Food and Drug Administration, 10903 New Hampshire Ave., Silver Spring, MD, 20993-0002, (888) INFO-FDA, http://www.fda.gov.

Jack Raber, PharmD
Ruth A. Wienclaw, PhD
Margaret Alic, PhD

Amenorrhea

Definition

Amenorrhea is the absence of menstruation and is a symptom, not a diagnosis.

Primary amenorrhea refers to the absence of the onset of menstruation by age 16 whether or not normal growth and secondary sexual characteristics are present, or the absence of menses after age 14 when normal growth and signs of secondary sexual characteristics are present. Secondary amenorrhea is the absence of menses for three cycles or six months in women who have previously menstruated.

In terms of the relationship of amenorrhea to **cancer**, amenorrhea may be a symptom of a gynecologic tumor, or the pause or cessation in menstruation may develop as a side effect of cancer treatment.

Demographics

The prevalence of primary amenorrhea is 0.3% and secondary amenorrhea occurs in approximately 1–3% of women. However, among college students and athletes the incidence can range from 3–5% and 5–60%, respectively.

For cancer-related amenorrhea, one clinician noted that nine out of ten women under his care reported secondary amenorrhea following bone marrow transplants. **Chemotherapy** and abdominal-pelvic **radiation therapy** likewise produce similar outcomes.

Causes

Normal menstrual bleeding occurs between menarche and menopause and has an average length of 28 days but varies from woman to woman. The normal menstrual cycle depends on cyclic changes in estrogen and progesterone levels, as well as the integrity of the clotting system and the ability of the spiral arterioles in the uterus to constrict. Abnormalities in any of these components may cause bleeding to stop or increase.

Primary amenorrhea

There are multiple causes for primary amenorrhea once pregnancy, lactation and missed abortion are ruled out. These include:

- anorexia nervosa/bulimia/malnutrition
- extreme obesity
- hyperthyroidism/hypoglycemia
- congenital heart disease
- cystic fibrosis/Crohn's disease
- genetic abnormalities
- obstructions: imperforate hymen/vaginal or cervical absence
- ovarian, pituitary (craniopharyngioma) or adrenal tumors
- polycystic ovarian disease
- testicular feminization

It is rare for primary amenorrhea to be caused by tumors but it can be a cause and should always be a consideration if other factors are ruled out.

Gonadal failure (a nonfunctioning sex gland) is the most common cause of primary amenorrhea, accounting for almost half the patients with this syndrome. The second most common cause is uterovaginal agenesis (absence of a uterus and/or vagina) with an incidence of about 15% of individuals with this syndrome. One of the most important, and probably most common, causes of amenorrhea in adolescent girls is **anorexia** nervosa, which occurs in about 1 in 1,000 white women. It is uncommon in women older than 25 and rare in women of both African and Asian descent. When women lose weight 15% below ideal body weight, amenorrhea can occur due to central nervous system-hypothalamic dysfunction. When **weight loss** drops below 25% ideal body weight, pituitary gonadotrophin function (follicle stimulating hormone and luteinizing hormone) can also become abnormal.

Each year of athletic training before menarche (the beginning of menstrual function) delays menarche about four to five months. Amenorrhea associated with strenuous exercise is related to stress, not weight loss, and is most probably caused by an increase in central nervous system endorphins and other compounds which interfere with gonadotrophin-releasing hormone release.

Secondary amenorrhea

Once pregnancy, lactation and menopause are ruled out, the causes for secondary amenorrhea include:

- extreme obesity
- prolonged or extreme exercise
- anxiety or emotional distress
- non-oral contraceptives (Norplant/Depo-Provera)
- D & C (dilatation and curettage)(Asherman's syndrome)
- early menopause
- autoimmune dysfunction
- pituitary tumors and central nervous system lesions

Cancer and secondary amenorrhea

As mentioned, not only does amenorrhea occur as a symptom of a tumor and/or lesion, but it often develops in women undergoing treatment for cancer.

RADIATION. Radiation therapy is used in conjunction with chemotherapy in a number of clinical situations, including **Hodgkin's disease** and childhood leukemia and lymphomas. Ovarian damage occurs under these circumstances to varying degrees, depending upon the total dosage of radiation as well as the age of the patient at the time of exposure.

CHEMOTHERAPY. Premenopausal women receiving single or multi-agent chemotherapy are at risk for short-term amenorrhea, as well as ovarian damage. Even young women who resume menstruation following chemotherapy are at risk for early menopause; therefore, those treated in childhood and adolescence should be counseled regarding the chance of early menopause in order to plan ahead for childbearing.

WEIGHT LOSS. Side effects of cancer as well as treatments can cause a decrease in appetite and **nausea and vomiting**, which, in turn, can cause severe weight loss as associated with malnutrition. Thus, menstruation may cease for the same reasons as it does in young adolescents with anorexia nervosa—hypothalamic dysfunction.

STRESS. Stress has always been noted to play a large role in the cause of amenorrhea, so the actual stress of having cancer and undergoing treatments may also cause amenorrhea to occur.

RETURN OF NORMAL OVARIAN FUNCTION FOLLOWING TREATMENT. Research on the recovery of normal ovarian function with young girls and/or young women has not revealed any reliable data. There are individual success stories especially with new advances in assisted reproductive technologies (ARTs), but overall, the return of normal ovarian function seems to be age-dependent. One researcher recently reported on ovarian function in 65 women who underwent high-dose chemotherapy and bone marrow transplants for aplastic **anemia**. All women younger than 26 years at the time of chemotherapy recovered ovarian function, while 7 of the 18 women aged 26 to 38 years did not recover ovarian function. Thus, the risk of ovarian dysfunction appears to increase with advancing age when ovarian reserve decreases. Additionally, the risk of dysfunction increases with the dose of alkylating agents, notably **cyclophosphamide**.

Treatments

Even with the possibility of ovarian compromise, women previously treated for cancer have successfully achieved pregnancy via ART's. Advances in the area of ART's include the use of donor eggs, the possibility of freezing embryos, and eventual oocyte (immature ovum) pretreatment offer more options to young women facing cancer chemotherapy.

Special concerns

The need for effective contraception during and after cancer treatment is imperative. Normal menstrual cycles do not imply normal fertility and likewise, irregular menses or even amenorrhea does not imply a lack of fertility. Women with dysfunctional bleeding or amenorrhea are still capable of spontaneous ovulation and conception.

The most reliable form of birth control for any population of women is injectable progestins, which suppress luteinizing hormone secretion. Depo-Provera, 150 mg injected intramuscularly, will effectively block ovulation for four months. Norplant (six rubber capsules placed under anesthesia in the upper arm) will effectively block ovulation for five years. If the treatment or the specific cancer diagnosis contraindicates the use of either of these contraceptives, other options should be considered, i.e., sterilization for the woman or her partner, an intrauterine device (IUD), or barrier methods (condoms, diaphragm or spermicides).

See also Fertility and cancer.

Resources

BOOKS

Jarvis, Carolyn. *Physical Examination and Health Assessment.* Philadelphia: W. B. Saunders Company, 2000.
Trimble, E. *Cancer Obstetrics and Gynecology.* Philadelphia: Lippincott William & Wilkins, 1999.

Linda K. Bennington, C.N.S., M.S.N.

American Joint Commission on Cancer

Definition

The American Joint Commission on Cancer (AJCC) is an organization dedicated to creating and promoting a universal system of classifying tumors according to their location in the body and involvement with surrounding tissues.

Description

Created in 1959, the AJCC works with the International Union Against Cancer (UICC), its European counterpart, and other organizations to standardize cancer-related information and data collection. The AJCC bases its classification on the TNM staging system, a universally accepted method of describing the extent of cancer, and other clinical information. The result is a standardized method of categorizing tumors that helps physicians to predict patient prognosis and develop treatment guidelines. The AJCC periodically publishes its *Cancer Staging Manual*, which is used widely by health care professionals in the diagnosis and treatment of cancer patients.

See also Tumor staging.

Tamara Brown, R.N.

Amifostine

Definition

Amifostine, also known as the brand name Ethyol and as ethiofos or WR2721, is a medicine that helps protect certain tissues of the body from damage caused by **chemotherapy** or **radiation therapy**.

Purpose

Amifostine is a protectant agent that is used in combination with the chemotherapy drug **cisplatin** or in combination with radiation therapy. Amifostine is approved by the Food and Drug Administration (FDA) to prevent kidney damage caused by repeat doses of the chemotherapy agent cisplatin in patients who have a diagnosis of **ovarian cancer** or **non-small cell lung cancer**. It is also FDA approved for patients with head and neck **cancer** who are receiving radiation therapy after surgery. In this group of patients, amifostine helps decrease radiation damage to the salivary glands, which can cause dry mouth.

Description

Amifostine has been on the market since the mid-1990s. A clear colorless solution, it is administered into a vein before chemotherapy and has been shown to decrease kidney damage by greater than 50% in advanced ovarian cancer patients who have received multiple cycles of cisplatin. It is also used before radiation therapy to prevent damage to the salivary gland known as the parotid gland.

When cisplatin is given to patients, it becomes broken down into toxic substances that destroy cancer cells and normal cells. When amifostine is administered into the body, it is broken down by an enzyme that occurs in large quantities in normal cells but not in cancerous cells. It then is converted into a substance called free thiol, which combines with the poisonous cisplatin by-products in the normal cells and makes them nontoxic.

In patients who receive radiation to the mouth area, including the salivary glands, the radiation causes the release of substances called free oxygen species, which damage cells of the mouth. An enzyme in cells of the mouth breaks down amifostine into a substance called free thiol. The free thiol blocks the free oxygen substances from damaging the salivary cells and decreases the amount of dry mouth patients suffer from when they receive radiation to the head and neck area.

Recommended dosage

Before dosing amifostine in chemotherapy or radiation therapy patients, intravenous fluids need to be given to keep the body well flushed with fluid and to maintain a normal blood pressure. All patients will receive amifostine lying down, sometimes with the head of the body lower than the feet. Patients should also receive medication to help prevent the **nausea and vomiting** that occurs due to amifostine.

Amifostine dosages can be determined using a mathematical calculation that measures a person's body surface area (BSA). This number is dependent upon a patient's height and weight. The larger the person, the greater the body surface area. Body surface area is measured in units known as square meter (m^2). To determine the actual dose a patient is to receive, the body surface area is calculated and then multiplied by the drug dosage in milligrams per squared meter (mg/m^2).

The recommended dosage of amifostine for protection of the kidney is $910 mg/m^2$ administered as a 15-minute infusion into a vein. This is to begin 30 minutes before chemotherapy administration. If a patient has difficulty with this dose, the dosage can be lowered to $740 mg/m^2$.

The recommended dosage of amifostine for radiation therapy patients is $200 mg/m^2$ administered once a day into a vein over a three-minute time period 15 to 30 minutes before the patient receives radiation treatment.

Precautions

Amifostine can cause a decrease in blood pressure when it is administered. During the 24 hours before receiving amifostine, patients need to drink a lot of liquids. When amifostine is being administered, medical personnel will be monitoring the patient's blood pressure. If the blood pressure drops significantly, the infusion of amifostine will be stopped until blood pressure returns to normal. The doctor will decide if the patient should receive any additional amifostine. Patients who have low blood pressure to begin with or patients who are not drinking a lot of fluids—referred to as being dehydrated—should not receive amifostine.

Patients with a known previous allergic reaction to aminothiol drugs should not receive amifostine.

Patients who may be pregnant, thinking of becoming pregnant, or who have a history of heart problems or strokes should tell their doctor before receiving amifostine.

Side effects

The most common side effect from receiving amifostine is a lowering of blood pressure, which occurs in approximately 62% of patients treated at a dose of $910mg/m^2$. This lowering of blood pressure occurs within the first 15 minutes of administering the drug. Blood pressure is monitored throughout the infusion of amifostine. If the blood pressure drops to certain level then the drug is stopped and restarted only when blood pressure returns to normal.

Nausea and **vomiting** are common side effects. They occur rapidly and can be severe. Usually, patients are given medicines before receiving amifostine that can help prevent or decrease these side effects. Other side effects include sneezing, hiccups, a warm feeling and redness of the face, sleepiness and dizziness, metallic taste, **fever**, rash, and chills.

Rare side effects of amifostine are: a lowering of calcium levels in the blood, seizures, allergic reactions which include symptoms of fever, shaking chills, **itching**, low blood pressure, shortness of breath, and rashes. There have been rare reports of throat swelling, chest tightness, and heart stopping.

All side effects a patient experiences should be reported to their doctor.

Interactions

Amifostine causes a decrease in blood pressure and should be used with caution in patients who take blood pressure lowering medicines or other medications that may lower blood pressure. If patients are taking blood pressure medications, they may be asked to stop taking these medications for 24 hours before receiving amifostine.

Patients should tell their doctors if they have a known allergic reaction to amifostine or any other medications or substances, such as foods and preservatives. Before taking any new medications, including nonprescription medications, **vitamins**, and herbal medications, patients should notify their doctors.

Nancy J. Beaulieu, RPh., BCOP

Aminoglutethimide

Definition

Aminoglutethimide, also known by the brand name Cytadren, is a **cancer** drug which inhibits the formation of hormones like adrenal glucocorticoids, mineralocorticoids, estrogen, androgens, and aldosterone.

Purpose

Aminoglutethimide is used to treat Cushing's disease, **breast cancer**, or **prostate cancer**. It blocks the conversion of cholesterol to delta-5-pregnenolone, a precursor for the formation of the **corticosteroids**.

Description

Aminoglutethimide is used clinically to reduce the amount of the hormones that can sometimes cause tumors to grow more quickly or are necessary for the survival of the tumor. For example, estrogen is important for the growth of some breast tumors. Lowering estrogen production by the administration of aminoglutethimide might reduce tumor growth or contribute to the destruction of the tumor.

Recommended dosage

Aminoglutethimide is given orally and dosages vary from patient to patient based on a number of factors, including the underlying disease process.

Precautions

Because some corticosteroid is necessary for normal function, patients should receive steroid replacement in addition to aminoglutethimide. Patients may require more corticosteroid when undergoing surgery, illness, or other conditions that cause stress. Hormones that affect the balance of sodium in the body may also be affected by aminoglutethimide and might have to be replaced as a result. If they are not replaced, patients may experience constant low blood pressure or low blood pressure upon standing.

Pregnant women should be warned that aminoglutethimide administration could cause fetal abnormalities. Pregnant patients should consult their physician about the current state of knowledge regarding risks and alternatives before beginning administration of aminoglutethimide. Female patients of childbearing age should attempt to avoid pregnancy while taking this drug. Mothers who are nursing should discontinue nursing while taking this drug.

Side effects

Common side effects from the administration of aminoglutethimide is rash (possibly associated with **fever**) which usually occurs in the first two weeks of therapy. It is usually self-limiting and gets better in a about a week. If the rash continues after one week patient should contact his/her physician or nurse. **Fatigue** is another common side effect of the drug and usually occurs in the first week of therapy. It may take about a month before it gets better. It can be very severe in some patients and if this is the case the patient's physician or nurse should be notified. Female patients may experience masculinization: new and excessive hair growth, a deeper voice, and irregular, abnormal, or absent menstrual periods. Thyroid function may be decreased after several weeks of therapy and the patient's thyroid should be monitored by the physician. Mild **nausea and vomiting** may also occur, as well as dizziness, **depression**, shaking, difficulty speaking, and increased heart rate. Any of these effects, or other unusual symptoms, should be reported to the patient's physician.

Interactions

Dexamethasone, blood-thinning medications, theophylline, and digoxin doses for patients taking aminoglutethimide may need to be increased by the physician. Patients should tell their doctors if they have a known allergic reaction to aminoglutethimide medications or substances, such as foods and preservatives. Before taking any new medications, including nonprescription medications, **vitamins**, and herbal medications, patients should notify their doctors.

Michael Zuck, Ph.D.

Amitriptyline

Definition

Amitriptyline is a member of a class of drugs known as tricyclic antidepressants. It is prescribed to treat **depression** and pain and to prevent migraine headaches.

Purpose

Amitriptyline helps relieve various forms of depression and pain. However amitriptyline and other tricyclic antidepressants are increasingly being replaced by a newer and more effective group of antidepressant drugs called selective serotonin reuptake inhibitors (SSRIs). Amitriptyline is prescribed to treat and manage pain associated with the nerves (neuropathic pain), particularly post-herpetic neuralgia—the burning and stabbing nerve pains or aches that may last for months or years after an attack of shingles—and the tingling or burning sensation that results from **cancer** treatment. It is sometimes prescribed to treat various types of chronic pain, as well as eating disorders, and to prevent migraine headaches. Amitriptyline is usually taken at bedtime to help patients sleep better.

Description

Amitriptyline increases the levels of neurotransmitters in the brain—the chemicals that transmit nerve messages—by blocking their reabsorption by neurons.

U.S. brand names

Amitriptyline is available in the United States as a generic drug in the form of 10-, 25-, 50-, 70-, and 150-milligram (mg) tablets that are taken by mouth. It is also available in an injectable form. It was previously available under the brand names Endep and Elavil. Amitriptyline is also available in combination with chlordiazepoxide, an antianxiety drug, as Limbitrol and Limbitrol DS, and in combination with perphenazine, an antipsychotic, as Duo-Vil 2-10 and Duo-Vil 2-25.

Canadian brand names

- Apo-Amitriptyline
- Levate
- Novo-Triptyn
- PMS-Amitriptyline

International brand names

- Adepril
- Amicen
- Amilent
- Amilit
- Amineurin
- Amiplin
- Amiprin

- Amitrip
- Amyline
- Amyzol
- Anapsique
- Domical
- Elatrol
- Elatrolet
- Enafon
- Etravil
- Lantron
- Laroxyl
- Larozyl
- Lentizol
- Miketorin
- Novoprotect
- Novotriptyn
- Pinsanu
- Pinsaun
- Quietal
- Redomex
- Saroten Retard
- Saroten
- Sarotena
- Sarotex
- Syneudon
- Teperin
- Trepiline
- Tridep
- Tripta
- Triptizol
- Trynol
- Tryptal
- Tryptanol
- Tryptine
- Tryptizol
- Trytomer
- Uxen
- Vanatripp

Recommended dosage

The usual adult dose of amitriptyline for **pain management** is 10–150 mg taken at bedtime to help the patient sleep. Patients are generally started on a low dose that is increased as needed. However side effects may make it difficult to increase the dosage in older adults.

For treating depression the dosage of amitriptyline is usually 75–150 mg, less for teens and older adults. It is taken at bedtime or in up to four divided doses during the day. It should be taken at the same time every day. If the nightly dose is missed, an extra dose should not be taken the next morning. Patients should check with their doctors if the daily dose is skipped. However those taking amitriptyline more than once per day should take a missed dose as soon as it is noted, unless it is almost time for the next dose, in which case the missed one should be skipped. Patients should not take two doses at one time.

Precautions

Patients should not stop taking amitriptyline abruptly; rather the dose should be gradually decreased before discontinuing. Stopping the drug abruptly may cause experience headache, **nausea**, lack of energy, discomfort throughout the body, and a worsening of the original symptoms. Amitriptyline's effects last for three to seven days after the medication has been discontinued.

Other precautions include:

- Taking amitriptyline during waking hours can result in noticeable side effects.
- Patients should not drive or operate machinery or appliances while taking amitriptyline.
- Injectable amitriptyline should not be used long-term; patients should switch to tablets as soon as possible.
- Patients may need to stop this medication before surgery.
- It is possible that a patient's mental health may change in unexpected ways—including becoming suicidal—with amitriptyline or another antidepressant, especially when the medication is first started or the dose is changed.

Pediatric

This medication should not be given to children under 12. It is generally not given to children under age 18. Children, adolescents, and young adults up to 24 years-of-age who take amitriptyline or other antidepressants for depression or mental illness may be somewhat more likely to have suicidal thoughts or to become suicidal, compared with those who do not take antidepressants as treatment for these conditions.

Geriatric

Older adults usually are more prone to some side effects of amitriptyline. Taking a lower dose may help resolve these. Amitriptyline can also increase the risk of falls in older adults.

Pregnant or breastfeeding

Taking amitriptyline during pregnancy has been associated with fetal deformities. Therefore pregnant women should carefully discuss the risks and benefits of this medication with their doctor. Women should not breastfeed while taking amitriptyline because it is secreted into the milk and could affect the baby.

Other conditions and allergies

Amitriptyline:

- should not be taken by anyone with allergies to the drug
- should not be taken by patients recovering from a heart attack
- may increase or decrease blood sugar levels in diabetics
- may increase psychiatric symptoms in patients with schizophrenia

Amitriptyline should be administered with caution to patients with:

- glaucoma
- seizures
- urinary retention
- overactive thyroid
- poor liver or kidney function
- alcoholism
- asthma
- digestive disorders
- enlarged prostate
- heart disease

Side effects

Common side effects associated with amitriptyline include:

- dry mouth
- drowsiness
- constipation
- dizziness or lightheadedness when standing

Sucking on ice cubes or sugarless hard candy can combat dry mouth. Increased fiber in the diet and additional fluids may help with constipation. Dizziness is usually caused by a drop in blood pressure when changing position. Patients should rise slowly from a sitting or lying position if they experience dizziness.

Other side effects of amitriptyline may include:

- blurred vision
- increased appetite
- weight gain

- weakness or fatigue
- unpleasant taste in the mouth
- nausea
- diarrhea
- vomiting
- heartburn
- nightmares
- headaches
- pain, burning, or tingling in the hands or feet
- irregular or fast heartbeat or palpitations
- raising or lowering of blood pressure
- skin that is more sun-sensitive

Taking this medication with food may decrease digestive side effects. Patients should avoid direct sunlight, wear protective clothing, and apply sunscreen with a protective factor of 15 or higher.

Less common side effects of amitriptyline include:

- muscle tremors
- nervousness
- impaired sexual drive or function
- sweating
- rash
- itching
- hair loss
- ringing in the ears
- changes in blood composition

Symptoms of amitriptyline overdose may include:

- irregular heartbeat
- drowsiness
- difficulty concentrating
- agitation
- confusion
- hallucinations
- muscle rigidity
- vomiting
- fever
- lowered body temperature
- seizures
- coma

Geriatric

Older adults are usually more prone to some side effects of amitriptyline, especially:

- drowsiness
- blurred vision
- dry mouth

QUESTIONS TO ASK YOUR PHARMACIST

- Will amitriptyline interact with any of my other prescription or over-the-counter medications?
- What time of day should I take amitriptyline?
- Should I take it with food?
- What if I miss a dose?
- Can I stop amitriptyline whenever I choose?

- difficulty urinating
- constipation
- dizziness
- mental confusion

Interactions

Patients should always tell all of their doctors and dentists that they are taking this and all other medications. Patients should always tell their doctor and pharmacist about any and all prescription and nonprescription medications, **vitamins**, nutritional supplements, or herbal preparations that they are taking. They should not start any dietary supplements while taking amitriptyline without first consulting their physician.

Amitriptyline should not be taken in combination with any other antidepressant. It should not be taken within 14 days of taking any monoamine oxidase inhibitor (MAOI) such as isocarboxazid (Marplan), phenelzine (Nardil), selegiline (Eldepryl, Emsam, Zelapar), or tranylcypromine (Parnate). High **fever**, convulsions, and death can occur if amitriptyline is taken in combination with an MAOI. It is important to inform the doctor if the patient has stopped taking the antidepressant fluoxetine (Prozac, Sarafem) within the past 5 weeks.

Amitriptyline should not be taken in combination with:

- epinephrine and other adrenaline-type drugs, as this can cause severe high blood pressure
- methylphenidate, a central nervous system stimulant
- cisapride (Propulsid; not available in the United States)
- Tagamet (cimetidine) or Neo-Synephrine, a nasal spray, because these can increase the blood levels and side effects of amitriptyline
- St. John's wort (*Hypericum perforatum*)
- belladonna (*Atropa belladonna*)

- henbane (*Hyoscyamus niger*)
- scopolia (*Scopolia carniolica*)

Amitriptyline has other interactions:

- Alcohol and other central nervous system depressants can increase drowsiness induced by amitriptyline.
- Alcohol blocks the antidepressive action of amitriptyline.
- Amitriptyline may decrease the effectiveness of some drugs used to treat high blood pressure.
- Amitriptyline may interact with valproate, which is used to treat the manic phase of bipolar disorder and seizures and to prevent migraines.
- Black tea may decrease the absorption of amitriptyline. There should be at least two hours between ingesting tea and the drug.

Resources

BOOKS

Hales, Robert E., Stuart C. Yudofsky, and Robert H. Chew. *What Your Patients Need to Know about Psychiatric Medications.* Washington, DC: American Psychiatric Publishing, 2007.

Stahl, S. M. *Essential Psychopharmocology: The Prescriber's Guide: Antidepressants.* New York: Cambridge University Press, 2006.

PERIODICALS

Berger, A., S. Mercadante, and G. Oster. "Use of Antiepileptics and Tricyclic Antidepressants in Cancer Patients with Neuropathic Pain." *European Journal of Cancer Care* 15, no. 2 (May 2006): 138–145.

Frese, A., and S. Evers. "Pharmacologic Treatment of Central Post-Stroke Pain." *Clinical Journal of Pain* 22, no. 3 (March 2006): 252–260.

Miyasaki, J. M., et al. "Practice Parameter: Evaluation and Treatment of Depression, Psychosis, and Dementia in Parkinson Disease (an Evidence-Based Review): Report of the Quality Standards Subcommittee of the American Academy of Neurology." *Neurology* 66, no. 7 (April 2006): 96–1002.

Sterr, Andrea, et al. "Electroencephalographic Abnormalities Associated with Antidepressant Treatment: A Comparison of Mirtazapine, Venlafaxine, Citalopram, Reboxetine, and Amitriptyline." *Journal of Clinical Psychiatry* 67, no. 2 (February 2006): 325–326.

Veldhuijzen, D. S., et al. "Acute and Subchronic Effects of Amitriptyline on Processing Capacity in Neuropathic Pain Patients Using Visual Event-Related Potentials: Preliminary Findings." *Psychopharmacology* 183, no. 4 (2006): 462–470.

Weber-Hamann, B., et al. "Resistin and Adiponectin in Major Depression: The Association with Free Cortisol and Effects of Antidepressant Treatment." *Journal of Psychiatric Research* 41, nos. 3–4 (April–June 2007): 344–350.

OTHER

American Society of Health-System Pharmacists. "Amitriptyline." *MedlinePlus Drug Information*. http://www.nlm.nih.gov/medlineplus/druginfo/meds/a682388.html

ORGANIZATIONS

American Academy of Family Physicians, 11400 Tomahawk Creek Parkway, Leawood, KS, 66211-2680, (913) 906-6000, (800) 274-6000, (913) 906-6075, http://www.aafp.org/online/en/home.html.

National Alliance on Mental Health, 2107 Wilson Blvd., Suite 300, Arlington, VA, 22201-3042, (703) 524-7600, (800) 950-NAMI, (703) 524-9094, http://www.nami.org.

National Institute of Mental Health, 6001 Executive Boulevard, Room 8184, MSC 9663, Bethesda, MD, 20892-9663, (301) 443-4513, (866) 615-6464, (301) 443-4279, nimhinfo@nih.gov, http://www.nimh.nih.gov.

National Mental Health Information Center, PO Box 2345, Rockville, MD, 20847, (240) 221-4021, (800) 789-2647, (240) 221-4295, http://mentalhealth.samhsa.gov.

U.S. Food and Drug Administration, 10903 New Hampshire Ave., Silver Spring, MD, 20993-0002, (888) INFO-FDA, http://www.fda.gov.

Mark Mitchell, MD
Ruth A. Wienclaw, PhD
Margaret Alic, PhD

Amphotericin B *see* **Antifungal therapy**

Amphotericin B liposomal *see* **Antifungal therapy**

Amputation

Definition

Amputation is the intentional surgical removal of a limb or body part. Traumatic amputation is the accidental severing of some or all of a body part. Congenital amputations are birth defects in which the child is born without a limb or missing part of a limb.

Purpose

Amputation is performed for the following reasons:

- to remove tissue that no longer has an adequate blood supply
- to remove malignant tumors
- because of severe trauma to the body part

Demographics

Arms, legs, hands, feet, fingers, toes, and ears can be amputated. Many amputations involve small body parts such as a finger, rather than an entire limb. According to the National Limb Loss Information center, about surgical 134,000 limb amputations are performed in the United States each year. About 90% of these are due to problems associated with blood supply to the body part, and almost blood-supply-related amputations are of the lower limb. This category of amputations is increasing because of the increase in diabetes in the United States.

Trauma is the second leading cause of amputation in the United States. About 30,000 traumatic amputations occur in United States each year. Of these, about 69% are amputations of an upper limb. Four of every five traumatic amputees are male, and most of them are between the ages of 15 and 30. The rate of traumatic amputations has been decreasing since the 1970s.

Amputations due to **cancer** also have been decreased since the 1980s. A little over one-third of cancer-related amputations are either above or below the knee limb amputations.

Congenital amputations, which are not surgical procedures but are birth defects, have remained steady since the 1970s at about 26 per 100,000 live births. Upper limb defects accounted for about 58% of all congenital amputations.

Precautions

Amputations cannot be performed on patients with uncontrolled diabetes mellitus, heart failure, or **infection**. Patients with blood clotting disorders also are not good candidates for amputation.

Description

The blood supply to an extremity can be cut off because of injury to the blood vessel, hardening of the arteries, arterial embolism, impaired circulation as a complication of diabetes mellitus, repeated severe infection that leads to gangrene (tissue death), severe frostbite, Raynaud's disease, or Buerger's disease. Most amputations in the United States, occur because of complications of diabetes and involve the lower limbs and feet. When the blood supply is cut off, the body part must be surgically removed in order to prevent more extensive tissue death and infection.

Traumatic amputation most often affects limbs and appendages such as the arms, ears, feet, fingers, hands, legs, and nose. Amputations may be partial (some tissue connects the amputated part to the

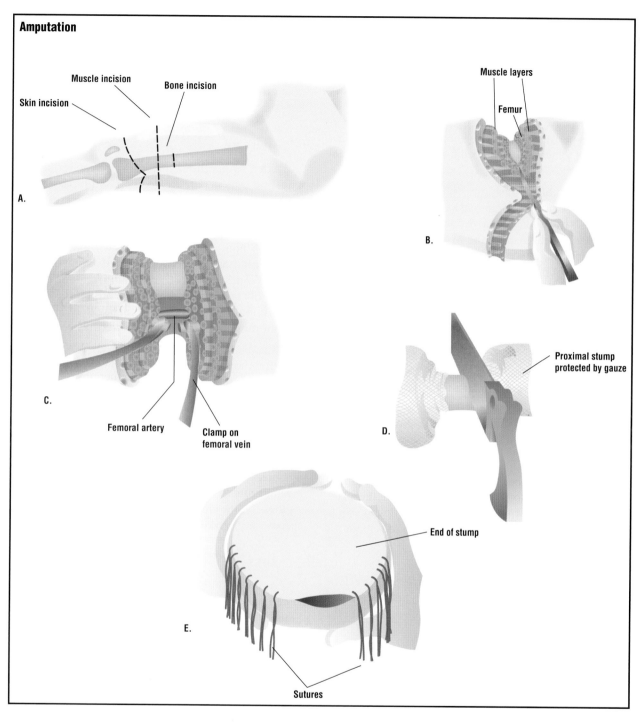

Amputation of leg. A: The muscle is cut and the main artery exposed. B: The surgeon severs the main artery and veins. C: The surgeon saws through the femur bone. D: The muscles are sutured over the bone. *(Illustration by Electronic Illustrators Group. Cengage Learning, Gale.)*

body) or complete (the amputated part is completely severed from the body). Traumatic amputation begins with an accidental severing of the body part. Surgical amputation may follow when repair of the body part is not possible.

Some of the more common causes of traumatic amputations are accidents with lawnmowers, automobiles, motorcycles, power tools, and farm equipment. Amputations may be caused by sharp objects such as knives or blades ("guillotine" amputation) or by heavy objects or mechanisms (crushing amputation). Crushing injuries are the more common cause of traumatic amputations. Traumatic amputations are a common injury to warfighters.

Amputations can be either planned or emergency procedures. Injury and arterial embolisms are the main reasons for emergency amputations. The operation is performed under regional or general anesthesia by a general or orthopedic surgeon in a hospital operating room.

Details of the operation vary slightly depending on what part is to be removed. The goal of all amputations is twofold: to remove diseased tissue so that the wound will heal cleanly, and to construct a stump that will allow the attachment of a prosthesis or artificial replacement part.

The surgeon makes an incision around the part to be amputated. The body part is removed, and the bone is smoothed. A flap is constructed of muscle, connective tissue, and skin to cover the raw end of the bone. The flap is closed over the bone with sutures (surgical stitches) that remain in place for about one month. Often, a rigid dressing or cast is applied that stays in place for about two weeks.

Preparation

Before an amputation is performed, extensive testing is done to determine the proper level of amputation. The goal of the surgeon is to find the place where healing is most likely to be complete, while allowing the maximum amount of limb to remain for effective rehabilitation.

The greater the blood flow through an area, the more likely healing is to occur. Multiple tests are done that measure blood flow through the limb. Several or all of the following tests are done to help choose the proper level of amputation.

- measurement of blood pressure in different parts of the limb
- xenon 133 studies, which use a radiopharmaceutical to measure blood flow
- oxygen tension measurements in which an oxygen electrode is used to measure oxygen pressure under the skin. If the pressure is 0, the healing will not occur. If the pressure reads higher than 40mm Hg (40 milliliters of mercury), healing of the area is likely to be satisfactory.
- laser Doppler measurements of the microcirculation of the skin
- skin fluorescent studies that also measure skin microcirculation
- skin perfusion measurements using a blood pressure cuff and photoelectric detector
- infrared measurements of skin temperature

No single test is highly predictive of healing, but taken together, the results give the surgeon an excellent idea of the best place to amputate.

Aftercare

After amputation, medication is prescribed for pain, and patients are treated with **antibiotics** to discourage infection. The stump is moved often to encourage good circulation. Physical therapy and rehabilitation are started as soon as possible, usually within 48 hours. Studies have shown that there is a positive relationship between early rehabilitation and effective functioning of the stump and prosthesis. Length of stay in the hospital depends on the severity of the amputation and the general health of the amputee, but ranges from several days to two weeks.

Rehabilitation is a long, arduous process, especially for above the knee amputees. Twice daily physical therapy is common. In addition, psychological counseling is an important part of rehabilitation. Many people feel a sense of loss and grief when they lose a body part. Others are bothered by phantom limb syndrome, where they feel as if the amputated part is still in place. They may even feel pain in the limb that does not exist. Many amputees benefit from joining self-help groups and meeting others who are also living with amputation. Addressing the emotional aspects of amputation often speeds the physical rehabilitation process.

Risks

Amputation is major surgery. All the risks associated with the administration of anesthesia exist, along with the possibility of heavy blood loss and the development of blood clots. Infection is of special concern to amputees. Infection rates in amputations average 15%. If the stump becomes infected, it is necessary to remove the prosthesis and sometimes to amputate a second time at a higher level.

Failure of the stump to heal is another major complication. Nonhealing usually is due to an inadequate blood supply. The rate of nonhealing varies from 5–30% depending on the facility and the site of amputation. Centers that specialize in amputation usually have the lowest rates of complication.

Most amputees experience some degree of persistent pain in the stump or phantom limb syndrome. About 80% of all amputees over age four experience tingling, **itching**, numbness, or pain in the place where the amputated part used to be. About 30% of amputees experience a sensation of the amputated part "telescoping" or shrinking into the viable part of the limb. Phantom sensations may begin immediately after the amputation, or they may develop months or years later. They often occur after an injury to the site of the amputation. Treatment of phantom limb pain is difficult.

Finally, many amputees give up on the rehabilitation process and discard their prosthesis. Better fitting prosthetics and earlier rehabilitation have decreased the incidence of this problem. Researchers and prosthetic manufacturers continue to refine the materials and methods used to try to improve the comfort and function of prosthetic devices for amputees.

Results

The five-year survival rate for all lower extremity amputees is less than 50%. For diabetic amputees, the rate is less than 40%. Up to 50% of people who have one leg amputated because of diabetes will lose the other leg within five years. Amputees who walk using a prosthesis have a less stable gait. Three to five percent of these people fall and break bones because of this instability. Although the fractures can be treated, about one-half of amputees who experience them then remain wheelchair-bound.

Resources

BOOKS

Cristian, Adrian *Lower Limb Amputation: A Guide to Living a Quality Life* New York: Demos Medical Pub., 2006.

OTHER

"Amputees." Medline Plus August 12, 2009 [September 14, 2009]. http://www.nlm.nih.gov/medlineplus/amputees.html.

"Amputation, Traumatic." MedlinePlus July 29, 2008 [September 14, 2009]. http://www.nlm.nih.gov/medlineplus/ency/article/000006.htm.

ORGANIZATIONS

American Diabetes Association, 1701 North Beauregard Street, Alexandria, VA, 22311, (800) DIABETES (342-2383), http://www.diabetes.org.

Amputee Coalition of America, 900 East Hill Avenue, Suite 205, Knoxville, TN, 37915-2566, (865) 524-8772; TTY: (865) 525-4512, (888) AMP-KNOW (888) 267-5669) , (865) 525-7917, http://www.amputee-coalition.org.

National Amputation Foundation, 40 Church Street, Malverne, NY, 11565, (516) 887-3600, (516) 887-3667, amps76@aol.com, http://www.nationalamputation.org.

Tish Davidson, A.M.

Amsacrine

Definition

Amsacrine is an antitumor agent used to treat adult acute leukemia. It is no longer commercially available in the United States, although it is available in Canada.

Purpose

Amsacrine is an investigational drug used to treat refractory acute lymphocytic and nonlymphocytic leukemias, **Hodgkin's disease**, and **non-Hodgkin's lymphoma**. It may also have some activity against **head and neck cancers**.

Description

Amsacrine inhibits the synthesis of DNA. It also inhibits the enzyme responsible for cutting the strands of DNA, and untwists DNA so that replication of DNA cannot occur.

Recommended dosage

The dose for amsacrine may be different depending on the protocol used by the physician. The drug is given through the vein as a 30- to 90- minute infusion or as a 24-hour continuous infusion. Example doses for adults are: 60–160 mg per square meter of body surface area every three to four weeks, or 40–120 mg per square meter of body surface area for five to seven days every three to four weeks. The dose for children is 120–150 mg per square meter of body surface area per day for five days. The dose of amsacrine is usually decreased in patients with decreased kidney or liver function.

Precautions

Amsacrine is usually given with caution to patients with underlying heart disease, severe kidney or liver disease, or to patients who have received high doses of anthracycline **chemotherapy** drugs, such as **doxorubicin**.

Although the effects of amsacrine treatment on children are currently unknown, caution is still indicated. Women of childbearing age should take precautions to prevent pregnancy while on this drug. Women should not breastfeed while taking this medication.

Side effects

Toxicity to the heart is a common side effect of amsacrine, and patients receiving this drug are usually very closely monitored by their physician. Other common side effects of amsacrine include **nausea and vomiting**, **diarrhea**, ulcerations of the mouth and the gastrointestinal tract, decreased white blood cells and platelets, and decreased liver function. Patients may notice orange-red discoloration of the urine, but should not be alarmed as this is normal. The urine will clear again once all the drugs have been eliminated from the body. Other common side effects include headache, dizziness, confusion, seizures, abnormal touch sensation such as burning and prickling, and blurred vision. As with any side effects that occur while taking any medications, patients should notify their doctor or nurse immediately.

Interactions

To prevent any drug interactions, patients should consult their physician, nurse, or pharmacist prior to taking any over-the-counter medications, herbal medications, or new medications. Many physicians recommend bringing the containers with the names of the drugs to an appointment.

Michael Zuck, Ph.D.

Anagrelide

Definition

Anagrelide, also known by the brand name Agrylin, is used to treat patients with thrombocytosis, a condition in which patients have too many platelet cells in their blood. Platelets are a cell type formed in the bone marrow that are involved in the blood clotting process.

Purpose and description

Anagrelide reduces the platelet count in patients with blood disorders.

Recommended dosage

Adult patients taking anagrelide should receive 0.5 mg of the drug four times daily or one mg twice daily. Based on the response to therapy, the dose of anagrelide can be increased by 0.5 mg per day every seven to 14 days if necessary. The goal is to maintain platelets at a count of less than 600,000 at the lowest dose of the drug possible to keep side effects at a minimum.

Precautions

Patients with heart disease should be given anagrelide with caution. Anagrelide should be given with caution, if at all, in patients taking drugs that affect platelet aggregations such as aspirin, clopidrogel, ticlopodine, or non-steroidal agents.

Pregnant mothers should be warned that anagrelide administration may cause fetal abnormalities. Pregnant patients should consult their physician about the current state of knowledge regarding risks and alternatives before beginning administration of anagrelide. Female patients of childbearing age should attempt to avoid pregnancy while taking this drug. Mothers who are nursing should discontinue nursing while taking this drug.

Side effects

The most common side effects of anagrelide are palpitations, fluid gain resulting in swelling, headaches, dizziness, **diarrhea**, stomach discomfort, mild to moderate **nausea**, passing gas, weakness, shortness of breath, and decreased platelets. Less common side effects of anagrelide include increased heart rate and chest pain, malaise, rash, **vomiting**, and decreased appetite. As with all medications, patients should contact their physician or nurse if any of these side effects occur.

Interactions

There are no proven interactions between anagrelide and other drugs. The drug sucralfate may interfere with the absorption of anagrelide. Prior to starting any over-the-counter medications, herbal medications, or new medications, patients should consult their physician, nurse, or pharmacist to prevent drug interactions.

Michael Zuck, Ph.D.

Anal cancer

Definition

Anal **cancer** is an uncommon cancer occurring in the tissues that make up the opening through which stool passes out of the body.

Description

The anus is the opening at the end of the large intestine (rectum) through which solid waste passes out of the body. The anus is a junction between two types of tissues: mucosa, which lines the intestines, and skin. Cancer located at the junction between the rectum and anus is called "anal canal cancer" (also known as transitional cell, squamous, epidermoid, or basal cell cancer). Cancer located near the external skin is called "anal margin cancer." Anal canal cancer is more common in women, and anal margin cancer is more common in men.

Demographics

Approximately 5,070 new cases of anal cancer were diagnosed in the United States in 2008. Less than 700 Americans died as a result of anal cancers in 2008. Anal cancer accounts for about 2% of the cancers of the digestive system. Although anal cancer is considered to be a rare type of cancer, incidence rates of anal cancer are rising in the United States. The average age at diagnosis is in individuals over 50 years old. Most anal cancers are squamous cell carcinomas.

Women are much more likely than men to develop anal cancer. Anal cancer is more prevalent in Caucasians than other races.

Causes and symptoms

Risk factors

Risk factors associated with anal cancer include:

- Human papilloma virus (HPV) infection (presence of anal-genital warts,
- history of receptive anal intercourse or presence of sexually transmitted disease (STD),
- history or cervical, vulvar, or vaginal cancer,
- immunosuppression as a result of organ transplantation or human immunodeficiency virus (HIV) infection,
- current smoker or history of smoking

Currently, in 2009, it is believed that the association between anal cancer and persistent **infection** with the HPV-16 virus is the strongest association.

Symptoms of anal cancer may include:

- bleeding from the anus (most common presenting symptom)
- pain around the anus
- the sensation of anal pressure or a mass
- anal itching
- anal discharge
- straining to pass stool (rectal tenesmus)
- change in diameter of stool
- swollen lymph nodes in the anal and/or groin areas
- About 30% of patients complain of pain or the sensation of a rectal mass at the time of diagnosis.

Diagnosis

Examination

According to the 2009 National Comprehensive Cancer Network Clinical Practice Guidelines for Anal Cancer, the clinical evaluation of patients with suspected anal canal or anal margin cancer are the same except that a positron emission scan (PET scan) is not included in the workup for anal margin cancers.

To diagnose anal cancer, the physician will first examine the skin of the anus and then will perform a **digital rectal examination** by inserting a greased, gloved finger into the rectum to feel for lumps. He or she will look for blood on the glove. If a lump is felt, a small sample of the lump will be removed (**biopsy**) through a small endoscope (flexible viewing instrument) to examine the tissue under a microscope.

Procedures

The biopsy may be performed using local anesthesia in the physician's office. The physician will also carefully palpate the lymph nodes in the groin area. If inguinal lymph node involvement is suspected, a biopsy by fine needle aspiration (FNA) may be performed. Another alternative procedure which may be performed is an excisional biopsy of enlarged or suspicious lymph nodes.

Although the diagnosis of anal cancer can be made by the examination alone, the cancer may be further evaluated by conducting other procedures. Endoscopic examinations of the anus (**anoscopy**) may be performed to see the tumor. **Endorectal ultrasound**, in which a wand-like ultrasound probe is inserted into the anus, enables the physician to determine how deep the tumor lies and whether or not nearby organs have been affected.

Tests

Other possible diagnostic procedures include x ray and/or **computed tomography** (CT scan) to detect tumor spread (**metastasis**). A PET scan may be ordered even if lymph nodes appear normal-sized on the CT scan.

HIV testing and measurement of CD4 levels are also recommended at the time of diagnosis. It is also recommended that women undergo a gynecologic examination at the time of diagnosis to include **cervical cancer** screening due to the strong association of anal cancer and HPV infection.

Treatment team

The treatment team for anal cancer may include a colorectal surgeon, gastroenterologist, oncologist, radiation oncologist, nurse oncologist, psychiatrist, psychological counselor, and social worker.

Clinical staging, treatments, and prognosis

Clinical staging

Most anal tumors are staged based on the size of the primary tumor as noted on direct examination and then confirmed microscopically. The American Joint Committee on Cancer (AJCC) Staging System is used to stage anal cancers. Anal canal cancer is categorized into five stages (0, I, II, III, and IV) which may be further subdivided (A and B) based on the depth or spread of cancerous tissue. This staging system does not apply to anal melanomas or sarcomas. Seventy-five percent of anal cancer patients have stage I or stage II disease. The stages of anal cancer are:

- Stage 0. Cancer has not spread below the limiting membrane of the first layer of anal tissue.
- Stage I. Cancer is 2 cm (approximately 0.75 in) or less in greatest dimension and has not spread anywhere else.
- Stage II. Cancer is between 2 and 5 cm in diameter and has spread beyond the topmost layer of tissue. There is no evidence of regional lymph node metastasis or distant metastasis.
- Stage IIIA. Cancer has spread to adjacent organs (e.g. vagina, bladder) or to the perirectal lymph nodes. Tumor may be of any size.
- Stage IIIB. Cancer has spread to nearby lymph nodes in the abdomen or groin or has spread to both adjacent organs and perirectal lymph nodes. Tumor may be of any size.
- Stage IV. Cancer has spread to distant abdominal lymph nodes or to distant organs in the body.

The AJCC Staging System for **skin cancer** is used to stage anal margin cancers as anal margin cancers are biologically comparable to other skin cancers.

Treatments

The specific treatment depends on the stage of cancer, type of cancer, and the age and overall health of the patient. Anal cancer is most frequently treated with a combination of **radiation therapy** and **chemotherapy**. Current recommendations for the primary treatment of anal cancers do not involve surgical excision.

Radiation therapy uses high-energy radiation from **x rays** and gamma rays to kill the cancer cells. Radiation given from a machine that is outside the body is called external radiation therapy. Radiation given internally is called internal radiation therapy or brachytherapy. Sometimes applicators containing radioactive compounds are placed directly into the cancerous lesion (interstitial radiation). The skin in the treated area may become red and dry and may take as long as a year to return to normal. **Fatigue**, upset stomach, **diarrhea**, and **nausea** are also common complaints of patients having radiation therapy. Women may develop vaginal narrowing (stenosis) caused by radiation therapy in the pelvic area, which makes intercourse painful. Radiation may injure the anal sphincter and may cause anal ulcers and anal stenosis.

Chemotherapy uses **anticancer drugs** to kill the cancer cells. The drugs are given by mouth (orally) or intravenously. They enter the bloodstream and can travel to all parts of the body to kill cancer cells. Generally, a combination of drugs is given because it is more effective than a single drug in treating cancer. The side effects of chemotherapy are significant and include stomach upset, **vomiting**, appetite loss (**anorexia**), hair loss (**alopecia**), mouth sores, and fatigue. Women may experience vaginal sores, menstrual cycle changes, and premature menopause. There is also an increased chance of infections.

In the past, patients with invasive anal cancers were treated surgically with abdominoperineal resection. This procedure is typically no longer recommended as a primary treatment for anal cancer because local recurrence rates were high, five year survival rates were limited and because of the physical and psychological complications associated with a permanent **colostomy**.

Concurrent chemoradiation (chemoRT) alone is the recommended primary treatment for patients with anal canal cancer. Anal canal cancer is treated with the chemotherapy drugs 5-FU and mitomycin administered concurrently with radiation therapy. Anal margin tumors can be treated with either local surgical excision or chemoRT depending on the clinical stage of the tumor. Inclusion of bilateral inguinal/pelvic lymph nodes in the radiation field is recommended in the treatment of cancers that are more advanced.

Prognosis

Prognosis of anal cancer is related to the size of the primary tumor and the presence of lymph node involvement. For most people, anal cancer is considered a curable disease. Most (60-70%) of anal tumors are in the early stages (stage 1 or II) at the time of diagnosis. Tumors that are located in the anal canal, are less than 2 cm in diameter, and are well-differentiated have a favorable prognosis with a five year survival rate of approximately 80% after treatment with chemoRT. The five year survival rate for patients with tumors larger than 5cm at the time of diagnosis is less than 50% currently. Patients with lymph node involvement of the tumor at the time of diagnosis have a five year survival rate of 10-40%.

Anal cancer can spread locally and invade other pelvic organs such as the vagina, prostate gland, and bladder. Anal cancer that spreads through the bloodstream (hematogenous spread) most often metastasizes to the liver and lungs.

Alternative and complementary therapies

Although alternative and complementary therapies are used by many cancer patients, very few controlled studies on the effectiveness of such therapies exist. Mind-body techniques such as prayer, biofeedback, visualization, meditation, and yoga have not demonstrated any effect in reducing cancer but can reduce stress and have been shown to lessen some of the side effects of cancer treatments.

Coping with cancer treatment

The patient should consult their treatment team regarding any side effects or complications of treatment. Many of the side effects of chemotherapy can be relieved by medications. Vaginal stenosis can be prevented and treated by vaginal dilators, gentle douching, and sexual intercourse. A water-soluble lubricant may be used to make sexual intercourse more comfortable. Patients should consult a psychotherapist and/or join a support group to deal with the emotional consequences of cancer and its treatment.

Clinical trials

As of 2009, there are about ten active **clinical trials** that are specifically studying anal cancer. There are other trials underway that include all types of **gastrointestinal cancers**, which may include anal cancer. Patients should consult with their treatment team to determine if they are candidates for any ongoing studies. The National Cancer Institute also provides information on clinical trials, and can be reached at (800) 4-CANCER or at http://www.cancer.gov/clinicaltrials/search.

Prevention

There is moderately strong evidence linking anal cancer with human immunodeficiency virus (AIDS) infection, cigarette smoking, or long term use of **corticosteroids**. Other factors that are strongly associated with the development of anal cancer include:

- Anogenital warts. Warts in and around the genitals and anus are found in 20% of women and heterosexual men and in 50% of homosexual men with anal cancer.
- Sexual activity. Having more than 10 sexual partners or being the recipient of anal intercourse increases the risk of developing anal cancer.
- Infections. Infection by sexually transmitted microbes, such as human papilloma virus HPV, herpesvirus, *Neisseria gonorrhoeae*, or *Chlamydia trachomatis*, places one at a higher risk of developing anal cancer.
- Gynecologic cancer. Women with a history of vaginal, vulvar, or cervical cancer are at risk of developing anal cancer. This risk is not due to therapeutic radiation exposure for gynecologic cancer.
- Chronic immunosuppression. The long-term use of drugs by organ transplant recipients to suppress the immune system increases the chance of developing a squamous carcinoma, such as anal cancer.

Because anal cancer is believed to be caused by HPV, like cervical cancer, it may be a preventable disease. Practicing safe-sex methods should help to prevent anal cancer. Persons who are at a high risk of developing anal cancer may benefit from routine screening by a physician.

Special concerns

The effect of pelvic radiation therapy on fertility can be a concern for both men and women. The need for a colostomy raises many issues, including those related to **body image** and self esteem.

See also Fertility issues.

QUESTIONS TO ASK THE DOCTOR

- What type of cancer do I have?
- What stage of cancer do I have?
- What is the 5 year survival rate for persons with this type and stage of cancer?
- Has the cancer spread?
- What are my treatment options?
- What are the risks and side effects of these treatments?
- What medications can I take to relieve treatment side effects?
- Are there any clinical studies underway that would be appropriate for me?
- What effective alternative or complementary treatments are available for this type of cancer?
- How debilitating is the treatment? Will I be able to continue working?
- Are there any local support groups for anal cancer patients?
- What is the chance that the cancer will recur?
- Is there anything I can do to prevent recurrence?
- How often will I have follow-up examinations?

Resources

BOOKS

Cummings, B.J., Ajani, J.A., & Swallow, C.J. "Cancer of the Anal Region." In *Cancer: Principles & Practice of Oncology 8th edition*, edited by DeVita, V.T., Lawrence, T.S., and Rosenberg,S.A. Philadelphia: Lippincott Williams & Wilkins, 2008.

PERIODICALS

Daling, J.R., Madeleine, M.M., Godefroy, J.L, et al. "Human Papilloma Virus, Smoking, and Sexual Practices in the Etiology of Anal Cancer." *Cancer* 101 (2004):270–289.

Dezube,B.J. "HIV-associated Anal Squamous Cell Cancer: An Otherwise Preventable Disease." *J Clin Oncol* 24(2006):4516–4517.

Uronis, H.E., Bendell, J.C. "Anal Cancer: An Overview." *Oncologist* 12(2007):534–534.

ORGANIZATIONS

American Cancer Society. 1599 Clifton Rd. NE, Atlanta, GA 30329. (800) ACS-2345. http://www.cancer.org.

Cancer Research Institute, National Headquarters. One Exchange Plaza, 55 Broadway, Suite 1802 New York, NY 10006. (800) 992-2623. http://www.cancer research.org.

National Institutes of Health. National Cancer Institute. 9000 Rockville Pike, Bethesda, MD 20982. (800) 4-CANCER. http://www.cancer.gov.

OTHER

"Anal Cancer." *National Comprehensive Cancer Network Clinical Practice Guidelines in Oncology* 2009[cited June 19, 2009]. http://www.nccn.org.

Belinda Rowland, Ph.D.
Melinda Granger Oberleitner, R.N., D.N.S., A.P.R.N., C.N.S.

Anastrozole *see* **Aromatase inhibitors**

Anemia

Description

Anemia is characterized by an abnormally low number of red blood cells in the circulating blood. It frequently affects patients with **cancer**. In fact, in many cancer diagnoses such as **multiple myeloma** and acute leukemia, the presence of anemia may be what initially prompts a doctor to suspect an underlying tumor (neoplasm). Whether or not anemia develops depends on the type of cancer found, the treatment used, and the presence or absence of other underlying medical disorders.

Symptoms of malignancy-associated anemia may range from weakness, paleness, and **fatigue** to shortness of breath and increased heart rate. Symptoms of anemia can compromise a patient's ability to tolerate treatment, and may severely interfere with activities of daily living. Anemia may be particularly problematic in older individuals with cancer. The incidence and severity of anemia tends to increase as the cancer progresses.

Blood is comprised of three major cell types: white blood cells, which help the body fight **infection**; platelets, which help the blood to clot when necessary; and red blood cells, which transport oxygen from the lungs to the tissues in the body, and then transport carbon dioxide from those tissues back to the lungs. This exchange is enabled by the most important component of red blood cells—the protein called hemoglobin that binds easily to oxygen and carbon dioxide.

Red blood cells are produced in the bone marrow through a process called erythropoiesis. When the bone marrow functions normally, it continuously replaces red blood cells to maintain a normal level that allows for adequate oxygenation of the tissues.

The hormone **erythropoietin** stimulates red blood cell production and sends a message to the bone marrow to increase production when oxygen levels in the body are low. This mechanism is often impaired in patients with cancer.

Causes

The causes of anemia are multiple, and often the factors act in conjunction with one another. Generally, anemia may result from a direct effect of a cancerous tumor, or from an indirect effect of the tumor. The cancer process may directly cause anemia through two main mechanisms: blood loss or bone marrow replacement. However, most cases of anemia in cancer patients result from the indirect effects of the cancer.

Direct effects of the tumor

Anemia is a frequent complication of cancers due to bleeding. Cancers of the head and neck, the gastrointestinal and genitourinary system, and the cervix are frequently associated with endogenous bleeding, or bleeding that occurs within the body. Bleeding occasionally develops within the tumor itself, particularly in sarcomas, melanomas, and ovarian and liver carcinomas.

A second direct cause of anemia in cancer is bone marrow replacement, which inhibits the body's ability to appropriately produce red blood cells. Certain cancers, such as acute leukemia, **lymphoma** and **myeloma**, directly suppress bone marrow function, thereby causing anemia. Other types of cancer, such as prostate or **breast cancer**, often spread to the bone marrow, inhibiting red blood cell production by actually replacing the bone marrow itself.

Indirect effects of the tumor

Anemia of chronic disease, also called anemia of malignancy, is the most common type of anemia seen in individuals with cancer. It is a diagnosis made only after other possible causes are ruled out and if very specific conditions are met. The presence of low levels of iron coupled with normal levels of storage iron helps distinguish anemia of chronic disease from iron deficiency anemia. Factors that cause anemia of chronic disease are not entirely clear. However, it is believed that cytokines (non-antibody proteins) produced by the tumor reduce production of and impair responsiveness to erythropoietin. Typically, this type of anemia develops slowly. Rapid development of anemia may indicate another cause.

Treatments used to manage cancer have been implicated in the development of anemia in cancer patients. **Radiation therapy** to large areas of bone marrow, as in the hip area, may suppress bone marrow function and lead to anemia. **Chemotherapy** can also cause bone marrow suppression, and some drugs specifically target red blood cell production. Studies have shown that 10% to 40% of patients taking **cisplatin** develop significant anemia. Cisplatin, a chemotherapy drug with potentially toxic effects to the kidneys, is believed to reduce the production of the hormone erythropoietin in the kidneys. Although most treatment-induced bone marrow suppression is short term, there is some evidence to support the possibility of long-term problems with blood cell production.

Treatment can increase the risk of anemia in other ways. Chemotherapy, for example, causes bone marrow suppression that may reduce the immune system's ability to fight off opportunistic infection. The resulting infections can impact the bone marrow's functioning, possibly leading to the development of anemia.

Hemolytic anemia is a type of anemia in which the red blood cell has a shortened life span (normal life span is 90-120 days). Because the bone marrow is not able to compensate by producing more red blood cells, anemia results. Abnormalities in the red blood cells may originate in the body (intrinsic) or may be caused by environmental factors such as auto-antibodies to red blood cells or damage from chemotherapy.

Although one factor may have a greater influence, it is important to realize that several factors may be causing anemia. For example, approximately 70% of patients with multiple myeloma are anemic at the time of diagnosis. Anemia in these cases is caused by a combination of mechanisms including bone marrow replacement with cancer cells, bone marrow suppression from chemotherapy, and impaired production of erythropoietin.

Treatments

Treatment of the anemia is directed at the underlying cause. In many cases, treating or removing the cancer corrects the red blood cell deficit. Management of autoimmune hemolytic anemia, which can be associated with **chronic lymphocytic leukemia**, may range from the administration of **corticosteroids** to the surgical removal of the spleen. More commonly, cancer-related anemias are treated with blood transfusions and/or a drug called epoetin alfa.

Blood transfusions

Blood transfusions have been the principle treatment for anemia for many years. Until the 1960s, only whole blood was given. Then, methods of separating whole blood were devised, allowing only particular components, such as platelets, red blood cells, or plasma, to be transfused.

Blood transfusions are not without risk, and must be used carefully. Many patients react to the white blood cell antigens by developing a **fever**. This is so common that patients are routinely premedicated to prevent fever from developing. Individuals with long-term transfusion needs, such as patients with leukemia, may be given blood products with a reduced number of white blood cells to reduce the risk of sensitization to transfused blood.

Cytomegalovirus (CMV) is a virus that may be present in blood products. Although it has no effect on individuals with normally functioning immune systems, cancer patients often have a diminished ability to fight infection. These patients may be at risk for CMV if they are CMV negative and receive CMV-positive blood.

Transfusion-associated graft-versus-host disease (TA-GvHD) is another risk factor associated with blood transfusions in cancer patients. Although it is very rare, it is often fatal. With TA-GvHD, the patient's immune system does not recognize the white blood cells in the donor blood as "nonself." The donor white blood cells, however, recognize the patient as "nonself," and an immune-mediated reaction ensues. To prevent this reaction in at-risk patients, blood may be irradiated prior to transfusion.

Epoetin alfa

As mentioned previously, erythropoietin is a protein produced in the kidneys that stimulates red blood cell production. Using DNA technology, this hormone has been replicated to create the drug epoetin alfa for the treatment of anemia in select cancer patients. (The drug is also called erythropoietin.) The use of this drug in the cancer setting has shown great promise, both in the treatment of cancer-related anemia, and in the reduction in the need for blood transfusion.

However, epoetin alfa therapy is not advisable for everyone. This drug is not recommended for use in cancer-related anemia caused by bleeding, hemolysis, or iron deficiencies. Nor is it recommended for patients with hypertension or albumin sensitivity. Because no human studies are available to determine its effect on a fetus, women taking epoetin alfa should take measures to prevent pregnancy.

Cancer patients with anemia who are undergoing chemotherapy may benefit from this drug. Studies have shown an increased hematocrit (the volume percentage of red blood cells in whole blood) level and a decreased need for blood transfusions after the first month of therapy in this population. Epoetin alfa may be injected up to three times a week, and throughout therapy, blood cell counts are monitored closely. In 2004, it was reported that a form of the drug could be injected only once every two weeks in some cancer patients with the same effect, making its use more convenient.

Resources

BOOKS

Abeloff, M., et al., editors. "Hematopoietic Dysfunction by Hematologic Lineage." In *Clinical Oncology*. 2nd ed. New York: Churchill Livingstone Publishers, 2000.

Lee, G., and C. Bennett, editors. "Nonmetastatic Effects of Cancer: Other Systems." In *Cecil Textbook of Medicine*. 21st ed. Philadelphia, PA: W. B. Saunders Co., 2000.

Lee, G., et al., editors. *Wintrobe's Clinical Hematology*. Baltimore, MD: Williams & Wilkins Publishing, 1999.

PERIODICALS

"Studies: Aranesp Dosed Semiweekly Is Comparable to Epoetin Alfa Once a Week." *Obesity, Fitness & Wellness Week* July 10, 2004:59.

Tamara Brown, R.N.
Teresa G. Odle

Angiogenesis inhibitors

Definition

Angiogenesis inhibitors are medicines that stop the formation of new blood vessels in and around cancerous tumors.

Description

Angiogenesis inhibitors are a group of medicines that prevent the formation of tiny new blood vessels to the area of cancerous tumors. Angiogenesis refers to the ability of **cancer** cells to form new blood vessels that invade the tumor and other surrounding areas. Tumors need a blood supply to nourish the cancer cells, and as tumors grow they must constantly form new blood vessels. These blood vessels are also used by the cancer cells to metastasize or spread the cancerous cells from one area to the next. Angiogenesis inhibitors are important because the scientific theory is that if one can remove and/or prevent the formation of new blood vessels in the tumors, the cancer cells will not be able to grow any further. This could cause the tumors to stay the same size or shrink. In addition, it may be possible to prevent the tumors from spreading by cutting off their ability to invade other surrounding areas through these newly formed blood vessels. There are a few drugs today thought to work as angiogenesis inhibitors, such as **thalidomide**. Additional agents being studied in ongoing oncology **clinical trials**.

Nancy J. Beaulieu, RPh., BCOP

Angiography

Definition

Angiography is the x-ray study of the blood vessels. An angiogram uses a radiopaque substance, or dye, to make the blood vessels visible under x ray. Arteriography is a type of angiography that involves the study of the arteries.

Purpose

Angiography is used to detect abnormalities or blockages in the blood vessels (called occlusions) throughout the circulatory system and in some organs. The procedure is commonly used to: identify atherosclerosis; diagnose heart disease; evaluate kidney function and detect kidney cysts or tumors; detect an aneurysm (an abnormal bulge of an artery that can rupture and lead to hemorrhage), tumor, blood clot, or arteriovenous malformations (abnormal tangles of

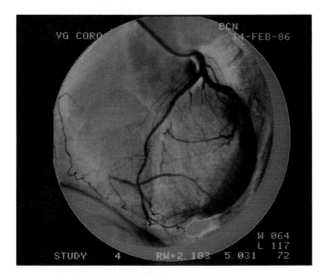

An angiogram of a coronary artery. (Copyright CNRI/Phototake NYC. Reproduced by permission.)

arteries and veins) in the brain; and to diagnose problems with the retina of the eye. It is also used to give surgeons an accurate "map" of the heart prior to open-heart surgery, or of the brain prior to neurosurgery.

Precautions

Patients with kidney disease or injury may suffer further kidney damage from the contrast mediums used for angiography. Patients who have blood clotting problems, have a known allergy to contrast mediums, or are allergic to iodine, a component of some contrast mediums, may also not be suitable candidates for an angiography procedure. Because **x rays** carry risks of ionizing radiation exposure to the fetus, pregnant women are also advised to avoid this procedure.

Description

Angiography is usually performed at a hospital by a trained radiologist and assisting technician or nurse. It takes place in an x-ray or fluoroscopy suite, and for most types of angiograms, the patient's vital signs will be monitored throughout the procedure.

Angiography requires the injection of a contrast dye that makes the blood vessels visible to x ray. Tissues such as bones and blood vessels absorb x rays as they pass through the body. They show up with a clear, white outline when captured on film. The dye is injected through a procedure known as arterial puncture. The puncture is usually made in the groin area, inside elbow, or neck. The site is cleaned with an antiseptic agent and injected with a local anesthetic. First, a small incision is made in the skin to help the needle pass. A needle containing an inner wire called a stylet is inserted through the skin into the artery. When the radiologist has punctured the artery with the needle, the stylet is removed and replaced with another long wire called a guide wire. It is normal for blood to spout out of the needle before the guide wire is inserted.

The guide wire is fed through the outer needle into the artery and to the area that requires angiographic study. A fluoroscopic screen that displays a view of the patient's vascular system is used to pilot the wire to the correct location. Once it is in position, the needle is removed and a catheter is slid over the length of the guide wire until it to reaches the area of study. The guide wire is removed and the catheter is left in place in preparation for the injection of the contrast medium, or dye.

Depending on the type of angiography procedure being performed, the contrast medium is either injected by hand with a syringe or is mechanically

Arteriosclerosis—A chronic condition characterized by thickening and hardening of the arteries and the buildup of plaque on the arterial walls. Arteriosclerosis can slow or impair blood circulation.

Carotid artery—An artery located in the neck.

Catheter—A long, thin, flexible tube used in angiography to inject contrast material into the arteries.

Cirrhosis—A condition characterized by the destruction of healthy liver tissue. A cirrhotic liver is scarred and cannot break down the proteins in the bloodstream. Cirrhosis is associated with portal hypertension.

Computed tomography (CT)—A non-invasive diagnostic tool radiologists may use instead of x-ray angiography.

Embolism—A blood clot, air bubble, or clot of foreign material that travels and blocks the flow of blood in an artery. When blood supply to a tissue or organ is blocked by an embolism, infarction, or death of the tissue the artery feeds, occurs. Without immediate and appropriate treatment, an embolism can be fatal.

Femoral artery—An artery located in the groin area that is the most frequently accessed site for arterial puncture in angiography.

Fluorescein dye—An orange dye used to illuminate the blood vessels of the retina in fluorescein angiography.

Fluoroscopic screen—A fluorescent screen which displays moving x rays of the body. Fluoroscopy allows the radiologist to visualize the guide wire and catheter he is moving through the patient's artery.

Guide wire—A wire that is inserted into an artery to guide a catheter to a certain location in the body.

Ischemia—A lack of normal blood supply to a organ or body part because of blockages or constriction of the blood vessels.

Magnetic resonance imaging (MRI)—A non-invasive diagnostic tool radiologists may use instead of x-ray angiography. MRI scans use magnetic waves to create a picture of structures in the body.

Necrosis—Cellular or tissue death; skin necrosis may be caused by multiple, consecutive doses of radiation from fluoroscopic or x-ray procedures.

Plaque—Fatty material that is deposited on the inside of the arterial wall.

Portal hypertension—A condition caused by cirrhosis of the liver. It is characterized by impaired or reversed blood flow from the portal vein to the liver, an enlarged spleen, and dilated veins in the esophagus and stomach.

Portal vein thrombosis—The development of a blood clot in the vein that brings blood into the liver. Untreated portal vein thrombosis causes portal hypertension.

injected with an automatic injector connected to the catheter. An automatic injector is used frequently because it is able to propel a large volume of dye very quickly to the angiogram site. The patient is warned that the injection will start, and instructed to remain very still. The injection causes some mild to moderate discomfort. Possible side effects or reactions include headache, dizziness, irregular heartbeat, **nausea**, warmth, burning sensation, and chest pain, but they usually last only momentarily. To view the area of study from different angles or perspectives, the patient may be asked to change positions several times, and subsequent dye injections may be administered. During any injection, the patient or the camera may move.

Throughout the dye injection procedure, x-ray pictures and/or fluoroscopic pictures (moving x rays) will be taken. Because of the high pressure of arterial blood flow, the dye will dissipate through the patient's system quickly, so pictures must be taken in rapid succession. An automatic film changer is used because the manual changing of x-ray plates can eat up valuable time.

Once the x rays are complete, the catheter is slowly and carefully removed from the patient. Pressure is applied to the site with a sandbag or other weight for 10 to 20 minutes in order for clotting to take place and the arterial puncture to reseal itself. A pressure bandage is then applied.

Most angiograms follow the general procedures outlined above, but vary slightly depending on the area of the vascular system being studied. In addition to x rays, technological advances have allowed physicians to use other diagnostic tools for angiography, such as **computed tomography** (CT) scans and **magnetic resonance imaging** (MRI). A variety of common angiography procedures are outlined below:

Cerebral angiography

Cerebral angiography is used to detect aneurysms, blood clots, and other vascular irregularities in the brain. The catheter is inserted into the femoral artery (the main artery of the thigh) or the carotid artery in the neck, and the injected contrast medium travels through the blood vessels of the brain. Patients frequently experience headache, warmth, or a burning sensation in the head or neck during the injection portion of the procedure. A cerebral angiogram takes two to four hours to complete.

Coronary angiography

Coronary angiography is administered by a cardiologist with training in radiology or, occasionally, by a radiologist. The arterial puncture is typically given in the femoral artery, and the cardiologist uses a guide wire and catheter to perform a contrast injection and x-ray series on the coronary arteries (arteries that supply the heart with oxygenated blood). The catheter may also be placed in the left ventricle to examine the mitral and aortic valves of the heart. If the cardiologist requires a view of the right ventricle of the heart or of the tricuspid or pulmonic valves, the catheter will be inserted through a large vein and guided into the right ventricle. The catheter also serves the purpose of monitoring blood pressures in these different locations inside the heart. The angiogram procedure takes several hours, depending on the complexity of the procedure. Some cardiologists prefer to use a compbination of CT and x-ray angiography to study the heart.

Pulmonary angiography

Pulmonary, or lung, angiography is performed to evaluate blood circulation to the lungs. It is also considered the most accurate diagnostic test for detecting a pulmonary embolism, although some physicians prefer CT or MRI scans because they are less invasive.

New technology has improved the accuracy of these alternative methods. The procedure differs from cerebral and coronary angiograms in that the guide wire and catheter are inserted into a vein instead of an artery, and are guided up through the chambers of the heart and into the pulmonary artery. Throughout the procedure, the patient's vital signs are monitored to ensure that the catheter does not cause arrhythmias, or irregular heartbeats. The contrast medium is then injected into the pulmonary artery where it circulates through the lung capillaries. The test typically takes up to 90 minutes.

Kidney angiography

Patients with chronic renal disease or injury can suffer further damage to their kidneys from the contrast medium used in a kidney angiogram, yet they often require the test to evaluate kidney function. These patients should be well-hydrated with a intravenous saline drip before the procedure, and may benefit from available medications (e.g., dopamine) that help to protect the kidney from further injury due to contrast agents. During a kidney angiogram, the guide wire and catheter are inserted into the femoral artery in the groin area and advanced through the abdominal aorta, the main artery in the abdomen, and into the renal arteries. The procedure will take approximately one hour.

Fluorescein angiography

Fluorescein angiography is used to diagnose retinal problems and circulatory disorders. It is typically conducted as an outpatient procedure. The patient's pupils are dilated with eye drops and he rests his chin and forehead against a bracing apparatus to keep it still. Sodium fluorescein dye is then injected with a syringe into a vein in the patient's arm. The dye will travel through the patient's body and into the blood vessels of the eye. The procedure does not require x rays. Instead, a rapid series of close-up photographs of the patient's eyes are taken, one set immediately after the dye is injected, and a second set approximately 20 minutes later once the dye has moved through the patient's vascular system. The entire procedure takes up to one hour.

Celiac and mesenteric angiography

Celiac and mesenteric angiography involves x-ray exploration of the celiac and mesenteric arteries, arterial branches of the abdominal aorta that supply blood to the abdomen and digestive system. The test is commonly used to detect aneurysm, thrombosis, and signs of ischemia in the celiac and mesenteric arteries, and to locate the source of gastrointestinal bleeding. It is also used in the diagnosis of a number of conditions, including portal hypertension and cirrhosis. The procedure can take up to three hours, depending on the number of blood vessels studied.

Splenoportography

A splenoportograph is a variation of an angiogram that involves the injection of contrast medium directly into the spleen to view the splenic and portal veins. It is used to diagnose blockages in the splenic vein and portal vein thrombosis and to assess the strength and location of the vascular system prior to liver transplantation.

Most angiography procedures are typically paid for by major medical insurance. Patients should check with their individual insurance plans to determine their coverage.

Preparation

Patients undergoing an angiogram are advised to stop eating and drinking eight hours prior to the procedure. They must remove all jewelry before the procedure and change into a hospital gown. If the arterial puncture is to be made in the armpit or groin area, shaving may be required. A sedative may be administered to relax the patient for the procedure. An IV line will also be inserted into a vein in the patient's arm before the procedure begins in case medication or blood products are required during the angiogram.

Prior to the angiography procedure, patients will be briefed on the details of the test, the benefits and risks, and the possible complications involved, and asked to sign an informed consent form.

Aftercare

Because life-threatening internal bleeding is a possible complication of an arterial puncture, an overnight stay in the hospital is sometimes recommended following an angiography procedure, particularly with cerebral and coronary angiograms. If the procedure is performed on an outpatient basis, the patient is typically kept under close observation for a period of six to twelve hours before being released. If the arterial puncture was performed in the femoral artery, the patient will be instructed to keep his leg straight and relatively immobile during the observation period. The patient's blood pressure and vital signs will be monitored and the puncture site observed closely. Pain medication may be prescribed if the patient is experiencing discomfort from the puncture, and a cold pack is applied to the site to reduce swelling. It

is normal for the puncture site to be sore and bruised for several weeks. The patient may also develop a hematoma, a hard mass created by the blood vessels broken during the procedure. Hematomas should be watched carefully, as they may indicate continued bleeding of the arterial puncture site. Patients may be given intravenous fluids and may experience a frequent need to urinate due to the x-ray dye.

Angiography patients are also advised to enjoy a few days of rest and relaxation after the procedure in order to avoid placing any undue stress on the arterial puncture. Patients who experience continued bleeding or abnormal swelling of the puncture site, sudden dizziness, chest pains, chills, nausea, headaches, or numbness in the days following an angiography procedure should seek medical attention immediately.

Patients undergoing a fluorescein angiography should not drive or expose their eyes to direct sunlight for 12 hours following the procedure.

Risks

Because angiography involves puncturing an artery, internal bleeding or hemorrhage are possible complications of the test. As with any invasive procedure, **infection** of the puncture site or bloodstream is also a risk, but this is rare.

A stroke or heart attack may be triggered by an angiogram if blood clots or plaque on the inside of the arterial wall are dislodged by the catheter and form a blockage in the blood vessels or artery. The heart may also become irritated by the movement of the catheter through its chambers during pulmonary and coronary angiography procedures, and arrhythmias may develop.

Patients who develop an allergic reaction to the contrast medium used in angiography may experience a variety of symptoms, including swelling, difficulty breathing, heart failure, or a sudden drop in blood pressure. If the patient is aware of the allergy before the test is administered, certain medications can be administered at that time to counteract the reaction.

Angiography involves minor exposure to radiation through the x rays and fluoroscopic guidance used in the procedure. Unless the patient is pregnant, or multiple radiological or fluoroscopic studies are required, the small dose of radiation incurred during a single procedure poses little risk. However, multiple studies requiring fluoroscopic exposure that are conducted in a short time period have been known to cause skin necrosis (cell death) in some individuals. This risk can be minimized by careful monitoring and documentation of cumulative radiation doses administered to these patients.

Normal results

The results of an angiogram or arteriogram depend on the artery or organ system being examined. Generally, test results should display a normal and unimpeded flow of blood through the vascular system. Fluorescein angiography should result in no leakage of fluorescein dye through the retinal blood vessels.

Abnormal results

Abnormal results of an angiography may display a restricted blood vessel or arterial blood flow (ischemia) or an irregular placement or location of blood vessels. The results of an angiography vary widely by the type of procedure performed, and should be interpreted and explained to the patient by a trained radiologist.

Resources

BOOKS

Baim, Donald S., and William Grossman, editors. *Grossman's Cardiac Catheterization, Angiography and Intervention.* 6th ed. Philadelphia: Lippincott Williams & Wilkins, 2000.

OTHER

Angiography Fact Sheet. Beth Israel Hospital, 2001. [cited June 22, 2001].
Angiography Overview. Northwestern Memorial Hospital, 2001. [cited June 22, 2001].
Coronary Angiography and angioplasty. Video. Timonium, MD: Milner-Fenwick, 1999.
Coronary Angiography Fact Sheet. American Heart Association, 2001. [cited June 22, 2001].

Paula Anne Ford-Martin

Anorexia

Definition

Anorexia is characterized by a loss of appetite or lack of desire to eat.

Description

Anorexia is common in **cancer** patients with reported incidence between 15% and 40%. Primary anorexia is especially prevalent in patients with advanced malignancy, and is frequently a side effect of cancer treatments. Sometimes, early symptoms may remain undiagnosed, or will be masked by a more generalized wasting of the body from chronic disease, known as cachexia.

KEY TERMS

Anorexia—A condition frequently observed in cancer patients characterized by a loss of appetite or desire to eat.

Cancer—A term for diseases in which abnormal cells divide without control. Cancer cells can invade nearby tissues and can spread through the bloodstream and lymphatic system to other parts of the body.

Candidiasis—A yeast-like fungal infection occurring on the skin or mucous membranes, i.e. mouth.

Chemotherapy—Chemotherapy kills cancer cells using drugs taken orally or by needle in a vein or muscle. It is referred to as a systemic treatment due to fact that it travels through the bloodstream and kills cancer cells outside the small intestine.

Hypercalcemia— A high calcium blood concentration above 10.5 milligrams per deciliter of blood. Increased gastrointestinal tract absorption or increased intake of calcium may lead to hypercalcemia.

Malignant (also malignancy)— Meaning cancerous; a tumor or growth that often destroys surrounding tissue and spreads to other parts of the body.

Radiation therapy—Also called radiotherapy; uses high-energy x-rays to kill cancer cells.

Satiation—A feeling of fullness or satisfaction during or after food intake.

Uremia—An excess of nitrogenous substances in the blood that are toxic and usually excreted by the kidneys.

When patients experience appetite loss, decreased energy consumption will subsequently lead to **weight loss**. When inadequate calories are consumed, the body may become weaker and less able to tolerate cancer therapies. As body weight decreases, cachexia sets in, and a general failure to thrive may make it more difficult to fight off illness and **infection**. A poor response to cancer treatments, reduced quality of life, and death may result from substantial weight loss. The spiraling effect of a patient's reluctance to eat is a source of frequent anxiety for caregivers. Weight loss due to anorexia may be temporary or may continue at a life-threatening pace if the patient continues to consume inadequate energy to sustain bodyweight.

Causes

It is normal for a patient to consume less energy when not as active. It is also natural to lose interest in food when individuals are seriously ill. However, it is essential in anorexic patients to consider whether the loss of appetite is the result of a natural disinterest in eating (primary anorexia), or is due to some reversible cause (secondary anorexia).

Secondary anorexia may be a result of:

- nausea with or without fear of vomiting after food consumption
- fatigue
- constipation
- sores in the mouth or mouth pain
- candidiasis
- unappetizing food or change in food preference due to cancer-related treatments
- depression
- odors in the environment, or heightened sensitivity to odors as a result of cancer-related treatments
- early satiation
- metabolic causes such as hypercalcemia and uremia
- radiation therapy or chemotherapy
- drugs such as antibiotics or drugs that can cause nausea

Special concerns

In order to allow normal tissue repair following aggressive cancer therapies, patients require adequate energy and macronutrients in the form of protein, carbohydrates, and fat. Inadequate consumption of food and/or poor nutrition may impair the ability of a patient to tolerate a specific therapy. If a low tolerance to therapy necessitates a decrease in dose, the therapy's effectiveness could be compromised. Wound healing may also be impaired with poor nutrition and inadequate energy intake.

Individuals who experience pain, **nausea**, or **diarrhea** due to the side effects of radiation and **chemotherapy** may want to discuss treatments options with their doctor to ease these side effects.

Treatments

Dietary tips for managing anorexia

- Serve food when the patient is hungry. A microwave oven often helps.
- Have the patient eat small meals every one to two hours, or time meals corresponding to when the patient feels best (typically early in the day).
- If only a little food is consumed by the patient, it should ideally be high in protein and calories. Avoid empty calories (i.e. foods without protein and nutrients).

- Add extra calories and protein to foods with the use of butter, skim milk powder, commercially prepared protein powder, honey, or brown sugar.
- Try to tempt the patient with tiny portions on small plates.
- Serve food in an attractive manner.
- Food is more likely to be eaten if it is served at frequent intervals unrelated to standard meal times.
- Avoid strong aromas if the patient finds them bothersome.
- Avoid liquids with meals to decrease problems of early satiety.
- A small alcoholic drink of the patient's choice may help unless contraindicated.
- Consider flavors, consistency and quantity of food when preparing meals.
- Encourage eating with friends or family members; a meal in a social setting may help the patient to eat.
- Stimulate appetite with light exercise.
- Treat any underlying cause and, if a particular drug appears to be the cause, modify drug regimen.
- Have the patient take medications with high-calories fluids, i.e. commercial liquid supplements unless medication necessitates an empty stomach.

Often, patients may experience difficulty with eating due to upper gastrointestinal blockage such as problems with swallowing, esophageal narrowing, tumor, stomach weakness, paralysis, or other conditions that preclude normal food intake. In those circumstances, enteral nutrition may be administered through a tube into the gastrointestinal tract via the nose, or through surgically placed tubes into the stomach or intestines. If the gastrointestinal tract is working and will not be affected by the cancer treatments, then enteral support by feeding directly into the gut is preferable. Parenteral nutrition (most often an infusion into a vein) can be used if the gut is not functioning properly or if there are other reasons that prevent enteral feeding.

An appetite stimulant may be given such as **megestrol acetate** or **dexamethasone**. In **clinical trials**, both these medications appear to have similar and effective appetite stimulating effects with megestrol acetate having a slightly better toxicity profile. **Fluoxymesterone** has shown inferior efficacy and an unfavorable toxicity profile.

Alternative and complementary therapies

Depression may affect approximately 15–25% of cancer patients, particularly if the prognosis for recovery is poor. If anorexia is due to depression, there are antidepressant choices available through a physician.

Counseling may be also be sought through a psychologist or psychiatrist to deal with depression.

St. John's Wort has been used as a herbal remedy for treatment of depression, but it and prescription antidepressants is a dangerous combination that may cause symptoms such as nausea, weakness, and may cause one to become incoherent. It is important to check with a dietitian or doctor before taking nutritional supplements or alternative therapies because they may interfere with cancer medications or treatments.

Resources

BOOKS

Quillin, Patrick, and Noreen Quillin. *Beating Cancer With Nutrition-Revised*. Sun Lakes, AZ: Bookworld Services, 2001.

PERIODICALS

Kant, Ashima, et al. "A Prospective Study of Diet Quality and Mortality in Women." *JAMA* 283, no. 16 (2000): 2109-2115.

Loprinzi, C.L., et al. "Randomized comparison of megestrol acetate versus dexamethasone versus fluoxymesterone for the treatment of cancer anorexia/cachexia." *Journal of Clinical Oncology* 17, no. 10 (1999): 3299-306.

Singletary, Keith. "Diet, Natural Products and Cancer Chemoprevention." *Journal of Nutrition* 130 (2000): 465S-466S.

Willett, Walter C. "Diet and cancer." *The Oncologist* 5, no. 5 (2000): 393-404.

ORGANIZATIONS

American Institute for Cancer Research. 1759 R Street N.W., Washington, D.C. 20009. (800) 843-8114 or (202) 328-7744. http://www.aicr.org.

The National Cancer Institute (NCI). For information contact the Public Inquiries Office: Building, 31, Room 10A31, 31 Center Drive, MSC 2580, Betheseda, MD 20892-2580 USA. (301) 435-3848, 1-800-4-CANCER. <http://cancer.gov/publications>, <http://cancernet.nci.nih.gov>.

National Center for Complementary and Alternative Medicine (NCCAM). 31 Center Dr., Room #5B-58, Bethesda, MD 20892-2182. (800) NIH-NCAM, Fax (301) 495-4957. <http://nccam.nih.gov>.

Crystal Heather Kaczkowski, MSc.

Anoscopy

Definition

Anoscopy is a diagnostic procedure that allows a gastroenterologist or other physician to visually examine the rectum, anus, and anal canal.

Purpose

Doctors use anoscopy to diagnose **rectal cancer** and **cancer** of the anus. This procedure can also help the doctor:

- detect any lesions that could not be felt during a digital examination
- determine whether squamous cell carcinomas involving lymph nodes in or near the groin (inguinal lymph nodes) originated in the genital area or in or near the anus or rectum
- confirm the source of malignancies that have spread to the anorectal area from other parts of the body

Doctors also perform anoscopy to determine whether a patient has hemorrhoids or anal:

- growths or nodules (polyps)
- ulcer-like grooves (fissures)
- inflammation
- infection

Description

After removing underwear, the patient bends forward over the examining table or lies on one side with knees drawn up to the chest. The doctor performs a digital examination to make sure no tumor or other abnormality will obstruct the passage of a slender lubricated tube (anoscope). As the doctor gently guides the anoscope a few inches into the rectum, the patient is told to bear down as though having a bowel movement, then relax.

By tensing and relaxing, the patient makes it easier for the doctor to insert the anoscope, and discover growths in the lining of the rectum that could not be detected during the digital examination.

Directing a light into the anoscope gives the doctor a clear view of any tears or other irregularities in the lower anus or rectum. A doctor who suspects that a patient may have cancer will remove tissue for **biopsy** in the course of this procedure.

Slowly withdrawing the anoscope allows the doctor to thoroughly inspect the entire anal canal. As the procedure is being performed, the doctor explains what is happening, and why the patient feels pressure.

Removing tissue samples for biopsy can pinch, but anoscopy does not usually cause pain. Patients do experience the sensation of needing to have a bowel movement.

Preparation

The rectum should be emptied of fecal matter (stool) before the procedure is performed. The doctor may suggest using:

- a laxative
- an enema
- or some other preparationto clear the rectum

Aftercare

As soon as the procedure is completed, the doctor can tell the patient whether the results are normal or abnormal, and the patient can resume normal activities.

Risks

Removing tissue for biopsy may cause a little bleeding and some slight pain, but there are no significant risks associated with anoscopy.

Normal results

A normal anoscopy reveals no evidence of:

- tumor
- tissue irregularities
- polyps
- fissures
- hemorrhoids
- inflammation
- infection or other abnormalities

The size, color, and shape of the anal canal look like they should.

Abnormal results

Abnormal results of anoscopy can indicate the presence of:

- cancer
- abscesses
- polyps
- inflammation
- infection
- fissures
- hemorrhoids

See also Anal cancer; Digital rectal examination.

Resources

OTHER

Anoscopy. [cited May 14, 2001].
Diagnostic tests:anoscopy. [cited May 17, 2001].

Maureen Haggerty

Antiandrogens

Definition

Antiandrogens, including flutamide (brand name Eulexin or Euflex), bicalutamide (brand name Casodex), and nilutamide (brand name Nilandron), are medicines used in the treatment of advanced **prostate cancer**.

Purpose

Antiandrogens are approved by the Food and Drug Administration (FDA) for the treatment of prostate gland **cancer** that has spread to other areas of the body.

Purpose

Antiandrogen therapy stops or blocks the effect androgen presence has on tumor cells of the prostate. Antiandrogens are combined with either surgery or drug therapy that shuts down male hormone production. The common drugs used with antiandrogens are known as luteinizing hormone releasing hormone (LHRH) agonists, referred to by the brand names Lupron or Zoladex. The LHRH agonists produce side effects that the antiandrogens can keep under control; thus the combination of the two types of agents has improved survival in prostate cancer patients.

KEY TERMS

Adrenal gland—Small organ located above the kidneys that produce hormones.

Food and Drug Administration—A government agency that oversees public safety in relation to drugs and medical devices. The FDA gives approval to pharmaceutical companies for commercial marketing of their products.

LHRH agonists—Luteinizing hormone-releasing hormone drugs that initially stimulate the testes to make and release testosterone. With time, as the amount of testosterone in the blood rises, it stops the production of luteinizing hormone, which results in stopping overall production of testosterone.

Monotherapy—Treatment of a disease or disorder with the use of a single drug.

Osteoporosis—A condition in which the loss of minerals from the bone leads to fractures after minor trauma. Osteoporosis can develop in men taking antiandrogen drugs for prostate cancer.

Newer trends in antiandrogen therapy include intermittent treatment with the drugs rather than continuous dosage; and antiandrogen monotherapy for patients whose cancer is still localized. Monotherapy means that the patient is given only the antiandrogen drugs without any LHRH agonists. As of late 2003, however, antiandrogen monotherapy is considered an investigational treatment.

Description

Antiandrogens will not cure prostate cancer, but they will help improve some of the disease's symptoms. They may also increase survival time.

Androgens are made naturally in the body and include the hormone **testosterone** and its related compound, dihydrotestosterone. The testes produce the majority of testosterone. The adrenal glands also produce androgens in smaller amounts. Prostate cancer cells grow due to normal levels of androgens produced by the body. Some patients have prostate tumors that are extra-sensitive to androgens in the blood. The androgens attach to receptors on the tumor cells and send a signal to the tumor cells causing them to grow and multiply. Antiandrogen drugs block the receptors on the prostate cancer cell that are sensitive to the androgen hormones. By blocking these receptors, known as androgen-receptors, the cancer cells cannot

be instructed to grow and multiply. Antiandrogens also cause the body to decrease production of androgens and, as a result, their effects.

Recommended dosage

Flutamide

Flutamide is an oral capsule dosed at 250 mg three times a day in combination with the LHRH agonist or surgical removal of the testis.

Bicalutamide

Bicalutamide is an oral tablet dosed at 50 mg once a day in combination with the LHRH agonist. The dose may need to be decreased in patients with decreased liver function.

Nilutamide

Nilutamide is an oral tablet dosed at 300 mg once a day for 30 days then 150 mg once a day in combination with surgical removal of the testis.

Precautions

Although antiandrogens are primarily given to men, women taking them should avoid pregnancy. Antiandrogens block the male hormone called testosterone and, as a result, can adversely affect the developing fetus. Blood counts will be monitored while on antiandrogen therapy.

Side effects

The most common side effects from all antiandrogens are due to the decreased levels of hormones. These commonly include hot flashes, loss of sex drive, tiredness, and impotence (the inability of males to have sexual intercourse).

Antiandrogens can also cause mild **nausea, vomiting, diarrhea**, loss of appetite, enlarged breasts or breast tenderness, skin reactions, muscle aches, liver problems, blood in the urine and generalized pain and decrease in blood counts. Nilutamide may cause visual disturbances, with patients having difficulty with the dark. Rarely, lung problems have occurred due to nilutamide or bicalutamide, including cough and shortness of breath.

These drugs must be used with caution in patients who are receiving the blood-thinning drug Coumadin (**warfarin**) or the drugs **phenytoin** and theophylline. Combining these drugs with antiandrogen therapy may increase the effects or side effects of these agents.

Another potentially troublesome side effect of antiandrogens is bone loss. Men who are taking these

Antibiotics

drugs are at increased risk of osteoporosis and consequent bone fractures. Doctors are now recommending that male patients taking these drugs should have a baseline assessment of their bone mineral density, and should be given zoledronic acid (Zometa) if there is evidence of serious bone loss.

Interactions

Patients should tell their doctors if they have a known allergic reaction to antiandrogens or any other medications or substances, such as foods and preservatives. Before taking any new medications, including nonprescription medications, **vitamins**, and herbal medications, the patients should notify their doctors.

Resources

PERIODICALS

Cooperberg, M. R., E. J. Small, A. D'Amico, and P. R. Carroll. "The Evolving Role of Androgen Deprivation Therapy in the Management of Prostate Cancer." *Minerva Urologica e Nefrologica* 55 (December 2003): 219–238.

Higano, C. S. "Management of Bone Loss in Men with Prostate Cancer." *Journal of Urology* 170, 6 pt. 2 (December 2003): S59–S63.

Holzbeierlein, J. M., E. P. Castle, and J. B. Thrasher. "Complications of Androgen-Deprivation Therapy for Prostate Cancer." *Clinical Prostate Cancer* 2 (December 2003): 147–152.

Morote, J., E. Martinez, E. Trilla, et al. "Osteoporosis During Continuous Androgen Deprivation: Influence of the Modality and Length of Treatment." *European Urology* 44 (December 2003): 661–665.

ORGANIZATIONS

American Urological Association (AUA). 1000 Corporate Boulevard, Linthicum, MD 21090. (866) RING-AUA or (410) 689-3700. http://www.auanet.org.

United States Food and Drug Administration (FDA). 5600 Fishers Lane, Rockville, MD 20857-0001. (888) INFO-FDA (463-6332). http://www.fda.gov.

Nancy J. Beaulieu, RPh., BCOP
Rebecca J. Frey, PhD

Antibiotics

Definition

Antibiotics are drugs that are used to treat infections caused by bacteria and other organisms, including protozoa, parasites, and fungi.

KEY TERMS

Gram-negative—Types of bacteria that do not retain Gram stain.

Gram-positive—Types of bacteria that retain Gram stain.

Mycobacteria—Rod-shaped bacteria, some of which cause human diseases such as tuberculosis.

***Pneumocystis carinii* pneumonia (PCP)**—Serious type of pneumonia caused by the protozoan *Pneumocystis carinii*.

Protozoa—Single-celled animals.

Toxoplasmosis—Infection caused by the protozoan parasite *Toxoplasma gondii*, affecting animals and humans with suppressed immune systems.

Trichomoniasis—Infection caused by a protozoan of the genus *Trichomonas*; especially vaginitis caused by *Trichomonas vaginalis*.

Purpose

Many treatments for **cancer** destroy disease-fighting white blood cells, thereby reducing the body's ability to fight **infection**. For example, bladder, pulmonary, and urinary tract infections may occur with **chemotherapy**. Single-celled organisms called protozoa are rarely a problem for healthy individuals. However, they can cause serious infections in individuals with low white blood cell counts. Because of the dangers that infections present for cancer patients, antibiotic treatment often is initiated before the exact nature of the infection has been determined; instead, the choice of antibiotic may depend on the site of the infection and the organism that is likely to be the cause. Often, an antibiotic that kills a broad spectrum of bacteria is chosen and several antibiotics may be used together.

Description

The common antibiotics that are used during cancer treatment include:

- Atovaquone (Mapren): antiprotozoal drug used to prevent and treat a very serious type of pneumonia called *Pneumocystis carinii* pneumonia (PCP), in individuals who experience serious side effects with SMZ-TMP (Sulfamethoxazole/Trimethoprim, brand name Bactrim).
- Aztreonam (Azactam): monobactam antibiotic used to treat gram-negative bacterial infections of the

urinary and lower respiratory tracts and the female organs, and infections that are present throughout the body (systemic infections or septicemia).

- Cefepime (Maxipime), ceftazidime (Ceptaz, Fortaz, Tazicef, Tazidime), and ceftriaxone sodium (Rocephin): members of a group of antibiotics called cephalosporins used to treat bacterial infections of the urinary and lower respiratory tracts, and infections of the skin, bones, joints, pelvis, and abdomen.

- Ciprofloxacin (Cipro): fluoroquinolone antibiotic used to treat certain gram-negative and gram-positive bacteria and some mycobacteria.

- Clindamycin phosphate (Cleocin): used to treat gram-positive and gram-negative bacterial infections and, in individuals who are allergic to sulfadiazine, toxoplasmosis caused by a parasitic protozoa.

- Gentamicin (gentamycin) sulfate (generic name product, Garamycin, G-Mycin, Jenamicin): aminoglycoside antibiotic used to treat serious infections by many gram-negative bacteria that cannot be treated with other medicines.

- Metronidazole hydrochloride (Flagyl, Metric 21, Metro I.V., Protostat): used for anaerobic bacteria and protozoa.

- Pentamidine (generic name product, Pentam 300): used to treat PCP if serious side effects develop with SMZ-TMP.

- Pyrimethamine (Daraprim): antiprotozoal medicine used together with sulfadiazine to treat toxoplasmosis; or in combination with other medicines for treating mild to moderate PCP, in individuals who cannot tolerate the standard treatment.

- Sulfadiazine (generic name product): sulfonamide antibiotic used with pyrimethamine to treat toxoplasmosis.

- Sulfamethoxazole-Trimethoprim (SMZ-TMP) (generic name product, Bactrim, Cofatrim Forte, Cotrim, Septra, Sulfatrim): the sulfonamide antibiotic, sulfamethoxazole, used in combination with trimethoprim, to prevent and treat PCP and bacterial infections, such as bronchitis and middle ear and urinary tract infections.

- Trimethoprim (generic name product, Proloprim, Trimpex): primarily used to prevent or treat urinary tract infections.

- Vancomycin hydrochloride (generic name product, Vancocin): glycopeptide antibiotic used to treat a variety of serious gram-positive bacterial infections for which other medicines are ineffective, including strains of *Staphylococcus* that are resistant to most oral antibiotics.

Most of these antibiotics kill bacteria by preventing them from making protein for their cell walls. Ciprofloxacin and metronidazole prevent bacteria from reproducing by interfering with their ability to make new DNA. All of these drugs are approved for prescription by the U.S. Food and Drug Administration.

Recommended dosage

Dosages of antibiotics depend on the individual, the infection that is being treated, and the presence of other medical conditions. For children, the dosage usually is based on body weight and is lower than the adult dosage. To be effective, an entire treatment with antibiotics must be completed, even if the symptoms of infection have disappeared. Furthermore, it is important to keep the level of antibiotic in the body at a constant level during treatment. Therefore, the drug should be taken on a regular schedule. If a dose is missed, it should be taken as soon as possible. If it is almost time for the next dose, the missed dose should be skipped. Doubling up doses is generally not recommended.

Average adult dosages of common antibiotics for cancer patients are as follows:

- Atovaquone: for PCP treatment, 750 mg oral suspension twice a day, or tablets three times per day, for 21 days; for PCP prevention, 1,500 mg oral suspension, once a day; must be taken with balanced meals.

- Aztreonam: 1–2 gm every 6–12 hours, injected into a vein, over a 20–60 minute-period.

- Cefepime: 500 mg to 2 gm, injected into a vein or muscle, every 8–12 hours for 7–10 days.

- Ceftazidime: 250 mg to 2 gm, injected into a vein or muscle, every 8–12 hours.

- Ceftriaxone: 1–2 gm, injected into a vein or muscle, every 24 hours.

- Ciprofloxacin: 500–750 mg of the tablet or suspension, every 12 hours, for 3–28 days, taken two hours after meals with 8 oz of water; bone and joint infections usually are treated for at least 4–6 weeks; 200–400 mg injected every 8–12 hours.

- Clindamycin: 150–300 mg of capsule or solution, every six hours; 300–600 mg every six to eight hours or 900 mg every eight hours, injected into a vein or muscle.

- Gentamicin: dosage determined by body weight, every 8–24 hours for at least 7–10 days, injected into a vein or muscle.

- Metronidazole: for bacterial infections, 7.5 mg per kg (3.4 mg per lb) of body weight up to a maximum of 1 gm, every six hours for at least seven days (capsules or tablets); 15 mg per kg (6.8 mg per lb) for the first dose, followed by half that dosage every six hours for at least seven days (injected into a vein); for protozoal infections caused by amebas, 500–750 mg of oral medicine, three times per day for 5–10 days; for trichomoniasis, 2 gm for one day or 250 mg three times per day for seven days (oral medicine); extended-release tablets for vaginal bacterial infections, 750 mg once a day for seven days.

- Pentamidine: for treating PCP, 4 mg per kg (1.8 mg per lb) of body weight, once per day for 14–21 days, injected into a vein over one to two hours, while lying down.
- Pyrimethamine: for toxoplasmosis, 25–200 mg tablets, taken with other medicine, for several weeks.
- Sulfadiazine: for bacterial and protozoal infections, 2–4 gm for the first dose, followed by 1 gm every four to six hours (tablets).
- SMZ-TMP: 800 mg of sulfamethoxazole and 160 mg of trimethoprim, (tablet or oral suspension), every 12 hours for bacterial infections and every 24 hours for prevention of PCP; dosage based on body weight for PCP treatment; injections based on body weight, every six, eight or 12 hours for bacterial infections and every six hours for PCP treatment.
- Trimethoprim: 100 mg tablet every 12 hours for 10 days; for prevention of urinary tract infections, once a day for a long period.
- Vancomycin: 7.5 mg per kg (3.4 mg per lb) of body weight, or 500 mg–1 gram, injected or taken orally, every 6–12 hours.

Precautions

Stomach or intestinal problems or colitis (inflammation of the colon) may affect the use of:

- Atovaquone
- Cephalosporins
- Clindamycin

Kidney or liver disease may affect the use of:

- Aztreonam
- Cefepime
- Ceftazidime
- Ciprofloxacin
- Clindamycin
- Gentamicin
- Metronidazole
- Pentamidine
- Pyrimethamine
- Sulfadiazine
- SMZ-TMP

- Trimethoprim
- Vancomycin

Central nervous system or seizure disorders may affect the use of:

- Ciprofloxacin
- Metronidazole
- Pyrimethamine

Anemia (low red blood cell count) or other blood disorders may affect the use of:

- Metronidazole
- Pentamidine
- Pyrimethamine
- Sulfadiazine
- SMZ-TMP
- Trimethoprim

Ciprofloxacin may not be suitable for individuals with tendinitis or with skin sensitivities to sunlight. Gentamicin may not be suitable for people with hearing problems, **myasthenia gravis**, or Parkinson's disease. Metronidazole may not be suitable for individuals with heart disease, oral or vaginal yeast infections, or a history of alcoholism. Pentamidine may not be suitable for individuals with heart disease, bleeding disorders, or low blood pressure. Pentamidine may affect blood sugar levels, making control of diabetes mellitus or hypoglycemia (low blood sugar) difficult. Vancomycin may not be appropriate for individuals with hearing problems.

Many antibiotics should not be taken during pregnancy or while breast-feeding. Older individuals may be more susceptible to the side effects of sulfadiazine, SMZ-TMP, or trimethoprim.

Side effects

Some individuals may have allergic reactions to antibiotics. If symptoms of an allergic reaction (such as rash, shortness of breath, swelling of the face and neck), severe **diarrhea**, or abdominal cramping occur, the antibiotic should be stopped and the individual should seek medical advice.

Because antibiotics can affect bacteria that are beneficial, as well as those that are harmful, women may become susceptible to infections by fungi when taking antibiotics. Vaginal **itching** or discharge may be symptoms of such infections. All patients may develop oral fungal infections of the mouth, indicated by white plaques in the mouth.

Injected antibiotics may result in irritation, pain, tenderness, or swelling in the vein used for injection.

Antibiotics used in cancer patients may have numerous side effects, both minor and severe; however, most side effects are uncommon or rare.

The more common side effects of atovaquone, aztreonam, cephalosporins, ciprofloxacin, clindamycin, gentamicin, metronidazole, and SMZ-TMP include:

- nausea and vomiting
- diarrhea
- loss of appetite

Eating active cultured yogurt may help counteract diarrhea, but if a patient has low white blood cells, this remedy is not recommended. For mild diarrhea with cephalosporins, only diarrhea medicines containing kaolin or attapulgite should be taken. With clindamycin, diarrhea medicines containing attapulgite should be taken several hours before or after the oral antibiotic. Diarrhea following antibiotics like clindamycin may indicate a bacterial infection that needs additional therapy, and a physician should be consulted.

Other side effects of atovaquone may include:

- fever
- skin rash
- cough
- headache
- insomnia

Other side effects of ciprofloxacin may include:

- abdominal pain
- increase in blood tests for kidney function
- dizziness or light-headedness
- inflammation or tearing of a tendon
- drowsiness
- insomnia

Other common side effects of clindamycin include abdominal pain and **fever**. Side effects may occur up to several weeks after treatment with this medicine.

Gentamicin and vancomycin may cause serious side effects, particularly in elderly individuals and newborn infants. These include kidney damage and damage to the auditory nerve that controls hearing. Other, more common side effects of gentamicin may include:

- changes in urination
- increased thirst
- muscle twitching or seizures
- headache
- lethargy

When gentamicin is injected into a muscle, vein, or the spinal fluid, the following side effects may occur:

- leg cramps
- skin rash
- fever
- seizures

Side effects from gentamicin may develop up to several weeks after the medicine is stopped.

More common side effects of metronidazole include:

- mouth dryness
- unpleasant or metallic taste
- dizziness or light-headedness
- headache
- stomach pain

Sugarless candy or gum, bits of ice, or a saliva substitute may relieve symptoms of dry mouth.

Pentamidine, pyrimethamine, sulfonamides, SMZ-TMP, and trimethoprim can lower the number of white blood cells, resulting in an increased risk of infection. These drugs also can lower the number of blood platelets that are important for blood clotting. Thus, there is an increased risk of bleeding or bruising while taking these drugs.

Serious side effects of pentamidine may include:

- heart problems
- low blood pressure
- high or low blood sugar
- other blood problems
- decrease in urination
- sore throat and fever
- sharp pain in upper abdomen

Some of these symptoms may not occur until several months after treatment with pentamidine.

Pyrimethamine and trimethoprim may lower the red blood cell count, causing anemia. **Leucovorin** or the vitamin **folic acid** may be prescribed for anemia.

Some individuals become more sensitive to sunlight when taking sulfonamides, SMZ-TMP, or trimethoprim. Other common side effects of sulfonamides and SMZ-TMP include:

- dizziness
- itching
- skin rash
- headache
- mouth sores or swelling of the tongue
- fatigue

If vancomycin is injected into a vein too quickly, it can cause flushing and a rash over the neck, face, and chest, wheezing or difficulty breathing, and a dangerous decrease in blood pressure.

Interactions

Many prescription and non-prescription medicines can interact with these antibiotics. Therefore, it is important to consult a complete list of known drug interactions. Among the more common or dangerous interactions:

- Antibiotics that lower the number of blood platelets, with blood thinners (anticoagulants), such as warfarin
- Aztreonam and metronidazole with alcohol; it is important not to consume alcohol until at least three days after treatment with these antibiotics
- Ciprofloxacin with antacids, iron supplements, or caffeine
- Pentamidine or pyrimethamine with previous treatments with x rays or cancer medicines (increased risk of blood cell damage)
- Trimethoprim with diuretics to remove excess fluid in the elderly

Many medicines can increase the risk of hearing or kidney damage from gentamicin. These include:

- cisplatin
- combination pain medicine with acetaminophen and aspirin or other salicylates (taken regularly in large amounts)
- cyclosporine
- inflammation or pain medicine, except narcotics
- lithium
- methotrexate
- other medicines for infection

The following drugs may increase the risk of liver effects with sulfadiazine or SMZ-TMP:

- acetaminophen, long-term, high-dose (eg Tylenol)
- birth control pills containing estrogens
- disulfiram (Antabuse)
- other medicines for infection

Resources

BOOKS

American Cancer Society. *Consumers Guide to Cancer Drugs*. Atlanta: Jones and Bartlett, 2000.

OTHER

American Cancer Society. *Cancer Drugs*. Cancer Resource Center. 2000. [cited May 27, 2001].

American Cancer Society. *Infections in Individuals with Cancer*. Cancer Resource Center. 30 Sep. 1999. [cited May 27, 2001].

MEDLINEplus Drug Information. U.S. National Library of Medicine. 24 Jan. 2001. [cited May 22, 2001]. http://www.nlm.nih.gov/medlineplus/druginformation.html.

Margaret Alic, Ph.D.

Anticancer drugs

Definition

Anticancer drugs, also called antineoplastic drugs, are chemicals that are used to treat malignancies, or cancerous growths, either alone or in combination with other treatments such as surgery or **radiation therapy**. **Chemotherapy** drugs target rapidly growing cells, including **cancer** cells. Chemotherapy drugs include:

- alkylating agents
- platinium drugs
- antimetabolites
- antitumor antibiotics
- topoisomerase inhibitors
- mitotic inhibitors
- corticosteroids Other, newer classes of anticancer drugs include:
- hormone therapies
- immunotherapies
- targeted therapies
- differentiating agents
- angiogenesis inhibitors

Purpose

Anticancer drugs are used to kill or control the growth of malignant cancer cells. These cells grow uncontrollably, with loss of differentiation, and commonly metastasize or spread the cancer to other tissues and organs. Anticancer drugs may destroy the cancer, prolong life, or relieve cancer symptoms for improved quality of life. The drugs used in cancer treatment depend on the type and stage of the cancer and other factors including the patient's age and health. Two or more anticancer drugs are often used in combination.

The majority of anticancer drugs are chemotherapy drugs that act by interfering with cell growth, since cancer cells grow more rapidly than other cells. Since these drugs target cells that are reproducing, they commonly affect not only cancer cells, but other cells that reproduce quickly, including those of hair follicles, ovaries and testes, and blood-forming organs. There are two classes of chemotherapy drugs: cycle-specific drugs act only at specific points in a cell's duplication cycle, such as anaphase or metaphase; non-cycle-specific drugs may act at any point in the cell cycle.

Alkylating agents directly damage DNA (deoxyribonucleic acid, the genetic material in the nucleus of the cell), thereby preventing cells from reproducing. Alkylating agents are non-cycle-specific and include:

- nitrogen mustards
- nitrosoureas
- alkyl sulfonates
- triazines
- ethylenimines

Other classes of chemotherapy drugs have different mechanisms of action:

- Platinium drugs also damage DNA, but are less likely than alkylating agents to cause leukemia.
- Antimetabolites damage DNA and RNA (ribonucleic acid, used in protein synthesis) by substituting incorrect components into the DNA and RNA as they are produced. Antimetabolites are cycle-specific and are used most often to treat leukemias, breast cancer, ovarian cancer, and intestinal cancer.
- Antitumor antibiotics include anthracyclines, which interfere with the synthesis of enzymes needed to replicate DNA. They work at all stages of the cell cycle and are used to treat many types of cancer, but have the potential to damage the heart in high doses.
- Topoisomerase inhibitors interfere with enzymes that control the replication of DNA.
- Mitotic inhibitors prevent mitosis—the process by which cells divide. They are often derived from natural products.
- Corticosteroids are multipurpose drugs that are related to hormones. In cancer treatment they are used to slow cell growth and prevent nausea and vomiting caused by other anticancer drugs.
- Asparaginase, an enzyme, interferes with the growth of cancer cells. It is used to treat acute lymphocytic leukemia.
- Bortezomib, a proteosome inhibitor, interferes with protein synthesis.

Some new classes of anticancer drugs target characteristics of cancer cells other than their rapid growth. These drugs may have fewer side effects than

chemotherapy drugs and may be used in combination with chemotherapy.

Hormone-therapy drugs counteract the effects of hormones that stimulate the growth of cancer cells. For example breast cancers are often stimulated by estrogens and may be treated with drugs that inactivate these female sex hormones. Similarly, **prostate cancer** may be treated with drugs that inactivate androgens, the male sex hormones. Hormone-therapy drugs include:

- estrogens
- anti-estrogens
- progestins
- luteinizing hormone-releasing hormone (LHRH) agonists
- aromatase inhibitors
- anti-androgens

Immunotherapy drugs enhance or stimulate the body's immune system. They include:

- monoclonal antibodies, a passive imnmunotherapy
- immunostimulating drugs that non-specifically stimulate the body's immune response
- immunomodulating drugs that alter the immune response

Other newer anticancer drugs include:

- targeted therapies that are aimed at cancer cells expressing certain genes
- differentiating agents that cause cancer cells to mature into normal cells
- angiogenesis inhibitors that interfere with the formation of blood vessels that feed tumors and contribute to tumor growth

Description

The majority of anticancer drugs are administered intravenously, either by injection or by continuous infusion. Other drugs are administered orally, as a liquid, tablet, or capsule.

U.S. brand names

Alkylating agents include:

- nitrogen mustards: mechlorethamine (nitrogen mustard, Mustargen), chlorambucil (Leukeran), cyclophosphamide (Cytoxan, Neosar), isofamide (isophosphamide, Ifex), melphalan (Alkeran)
- nitrosoureas: streptozocin (Zanosar), carmustine (BCNU, Gliadel), lomustine (CeeNU)
- the alkyl sulfonate busulfan (Busulfex, Myleran)

- triazines: dacarbazine (DTIC-Dome), temozolomide (Temodar)
- ethylenimines: thiotepa (Thioplex), altretamine or hexamethylmelamine (Hexalen)

Platinium drugs include:

- cisplatin (Platinol)
- carboplatin (Paraplatin, Carboplatin Novaplus)
- oxaliplatin (Eloxatin)

Antimetabolites include:

- 5-fluorouacil (5-FU; Adrucil)
- capecitabine (Xeloda)
- 6-mercaptopurine (6-MP; Purinethol)
- methotrexate (Rheumatrex, Trexall)
- gemcitabine (Gemzar)
- cytarabine (Cytosar, Tarabine, Ara-C)
- fludarabine (Fludara)
- pemetrexed (Alimta)

Anthracyclines include:

- daunorubicin (Cerubidine)
- doxorubicin (Adriamycin, Rubex)
- epirubicin (Ellence)
- idarubicin (Idamycin)

Other antitumor **antibiotics** include:

- actinomycin-D or dactinomycin (Cosmegen)
- bleomycin (Blenoxane)
- mitomycin (Mutamycin)
- mitoxantrone (Novantrone)

Topoisomerase inhibitors include:

- topotecan (Hycamtin)
- irinotecan (Camptosar)
- etoposide or VP-16 (Toposar, VePesid)
- teniposide (Vumon)
- mitoxantrone (Novantrone)

Mitotic inhibitors include:

- taxanes: paclitaxel (Taxol, Onxal), docetaxel (Taxotere)
- epothilones: ixabepilone (Ixempra)
- vinca alkaloids: vinblastine (Velban), vincristine (Vincasar), vinorelbine (Navelbine)
- estramustine (Emcyt)

Anticancer **corticosteroids** include:

- prednisone (Prednisone Intensol, Sterapred)
- methylprednisolone (Medrol)
- dexamethasone (Decadron)

Asparaginase is marketed as Elspar.

Hormone-therapy drugs include:

- anti-estrogens: tamoxifen (Nolvadex), toremifene (Fareston), fulvestrant (Faslodex)
- progestin: megestrol acetate (Megace)
- LHRH agonists: leuprolide (Lupron, Eligard, Viadur), goserelin (Zolodex)
- aromatase inhibitors: anastrozole (Arimidex), exemestane (Aromasin), letrozole (Femara)
- anti-androgens: bicalutamide (Casodex), flutamide (Eulexin), nilutamide (Nilandron)

Immunotherapy drugs include:

- monoclonal antibodies: rituximab (Rituxan), alemtuzumab (Campath)
- immunostimulating drugs: interleukin-2 (Il-2 or aldesleukin, Proleukin); interferon alfa-2 (Intron A, Roferon-A); BCG vaccine (TheraCys, TICE BCG)
- immunomodulating drugs: thalidomide (Thalomid), lenalidomide (Revlimid)

Targeted therapies include:

- bortezomib (Velcade)
- imatinib (Gleevec)
- gefitinib (Iressa)
- erlotinib (Tarceva)

Differentiating agents include:

- retinoids: tretinoin (ATRA, Atralin, Vesanoid), bexarotene (Targretin)
- arsenic trioxide (Trisenox)

Angiogenesis inhibitors include **bevacizumab** (Avastin).

Canadian brand names

Alkylating agents include:

- nitrogen mustards: Mustargen (mechlorethamine); Leukeran (chlorambucil); Cytoxan, Procytox (cyclophosphamide); Alkeran (melphalan)
- nitrosoureas: Zanosar (streptozocin); BiCNU (carmustine); CeeNU (lomustine)
- Busulfex, Myleran (busulfan)
- triazines: DTIC (dacarbazine); Temodal, Temodar (temozolomide)
- Hexalen (altretamine)

Platinium drugs include Paraplatin-AQ (**carboplatin**).

Antimetabolites include:

- Adrucil (5-fluorouacil)
- Xeloda (capecitabine)
- Purinethol (6-mercaptopurine)

- Methotrexate
- Gemzar (gemcitabine)
- Cytosar (cytarabine)
- Fludara (fludarabine)

Anthracyclines include:

- Cerubidine (daunorubicin)
- Adriamycin (doxorubicin)
- Ellence, Pharmorubicin (epirubicin)
- Idamycin (idarubicin)

Other antitumor antibiotics include:

- Cosmegen (dactinomycin)
- Blenoxane (bleomycin)
- Mutamycin (mitomycin)
- Novantrone (mitoxantrone)

Topoisomerase inhibitors include:

- Hycamtin (topotecan)
- Camptosar (irinotecan)
- VePesid (etoposide)
- Vumon (teniposide)
- Novantrone (mitoxantrone)

Mitotic inhibitors include:

- taxanes: Taxol (paclitaxel); Taxotere (docetaxel)
- vinca alkaloids: Vincasar, PFS (vincristine); Navelbine (vinorelbine)
- Emcyt (estramustine)

Anticancer corticosteroids include:

- Apo-Prednisone, Winpred (prednisone)
- Medrol (methylprednisolone)
- Decadron, Dexasone, Diodex, Maxidex (dexamethasone)

Asparaginase is marketed as Elspar and Kidrolase.

Hormone-therapy drugs include:

- anti-estrogens: Apo-Tamox, Gen-Tamoxifen, Nolvadex, Novo-Tamoxifen, PMS-Tamoxifen, Tamofen (tamoxifen); Fareston (toremifene)
- progestin: Megestrol, Megace
- LHRH agonists: Viadur, Lupron (leuprolide); Zoladex (goserelin)
- aromatase inhibitors: Arimidex (anastrozole); Aromasin (exemestane); Femara (letrozole)
- anti-androgens: Casodex (bicalutamide); Flutamide, Euflex, Eulexin (flutamide); Anandron (nilutamide)

Immunotherapy drugs include:

- monoclonal antibodies: rituximab (Rituxan)

- immunostimulating drugs: Proleukin (Il-2); Immu-Cyst, Oncotice, Pacis (BCG)
- immunomodulating drugs: Thalomid (thalidomide)

Targeted therapies include:

- Velcade (bortezomib)
- Gleevec (imatinib)

Differentiating agents include the retinoids Vesanoid (**tretinoin**) and Targretin (**bexarotene**).

Angiogenesis inhibitors include Avastin (bevacizumab).

International brand names

Alkylating agents include:

- nitrogen mustards: Mustargen, Nitromin (mechlorethamine); Leukeran (chlorambucil); Cytoxan, Procytox, Endoxan (cyclophosphamide); Alkeran (melphalan)
- nitrosoureas: Zanosar (streptozocin); Bicnu, Gliadel (carmustine); CeeNU (lomustine)
- Busulfex, Myleran, Busilvex (busulfan)
- triazines: Dacarbazin, Deticene, DTIC-Dome (dacarbazine); Temodal (temozolomide)
- ethylenimines: Thioplex, Thiotepa (thiotepa); Hexalen (altretamine)

Platinium drugs include:

- Platinol, Platidiam, Platinex, Platosin (cisplatin)
- Carboplatin, Carbosin, Paraplatin (carboplatin)
- Eloxatin (oxaliplatin)

Antimetabolites include:

- Xeloda (capecitabine)
- Puri-Nethol, Purinethol (mercaptopurine)
- Methotrexate
- Gemzar (gemcitabine)
- Alexan, Cytosar (cytarabine)
- Fludara (fludarabine)
- Alimta (pemetrexed)

Anthracyclines include:

- Cerubidine, Daunoblastina (daunorubicin)
- Adriamycin, Adriblastina, Caelyx, Doxorubicin, Myocet, Rastocin, Rubex (doxorubicin)
- Farmorubicina, Farmorubicin, Pharmorubicin (epirubicin)
- Zavedos (idarubicin)

Other antitumor antibiotics include:

- Cosmegen (dactinomycin)
- Blenoxane, Bleocin (bleomycin)
- Mitomycin C, Mutamycin (mitomycin)
- Novantrone, Onkotrone (mitoxantrone)

Topoisomerase inhibitors include:

- Hycamtin (topotecan)
- Campto, Camptosar (irinotecan)
- Etopophos, Ebewe, VePesid (etoposide)
- Vumon (teniposide)
- Novantrone, Onkotrone (mitoxantrone)

Mitotic inhibitors include:

- taxanes: Anzatax, Taxol (paclitaxel); Taxotere (docetaxel)
- vinca alkaloids: Velbe (vinblastine); Oncovin, Vincristine (vincristine); Navelbine (vinorelbine)
- Emcyt (estramustine)

Anticancer corticosteroids include:

- Prednisone, Meticorten (prednisone)
- Medrol, Metypred (methylprednisolone)
- Alin, Decadron, Dexalocal, Maxidex (dexamethasone)

Asparaginase may be marketed as Elspar, Leunase, and Kidrolase.

Hormone-therapy drugs include:

- anti-estrogens: Nolvadex, Tamofen, Tamoplex, Tamoxifen, Zitazonium (tamoxifen); Fareston (toremifene); Faslodex (fulvestrant)
- progestin: Megestrol
- LHRH agonists: Zoladex (goserelin); Viadur, Lupron (leuprolide)
- aromatase inhibitors: Arimidex (anastrozole); Aromasin, Aromasil, Aromasine (exemestane); Femara, Femar (letrozole)
- anti-androgens: Casodex (bicalutamide); Eulexin, Flutamid (flutamide); Anandron (nilutamide)

Immunotherapy drugs include:

- monoclonal antibodies: Mabthera (rituximab); Mabcambath (alemtuzumab)
- immunostimulating drugs: Proleukin (Il-2)
- immunomodulating drugs: Thalix (thalidomide)

Targeted therapies include:

- Velcade (bortezomib)
- Gleevec, Glivec (imatinib)
- Iressa (gefitinib)

Differentiating agents include:

- the retinoid Targretin (bexarotene)
- arsenic trioxide (Trisenox)

Recommended dosage

Dosages of anticancer drugs depend on a variety of factors including the specific drug, method of administration, the type of cancer being treated, and the patient's health. Although dosages are often calculated based on body weight, they may also be based on blood cell counts, in order to avoid **anemia** (red cell depletion), **neutropenia** (white cell deficiency), or **thrombocytopenia** (platelet deficiency). Children and the elderly may be dosed differently than others. Because of the frequency and severity of side effects from anticancer drugs, chemotherapy is commonly administered in cycles, allowing time for recovery from the effects before administering the next dose.

Precautions

Individual anticancer drugs all carry their own precautions, including the risk of their causing additional cancers. General precautions include:

- Patients should be well-informed concerning the benefits and risks of their anticancer drugs and be emotionally prepared for the side effects, some of which—including possible sterility—may be permanent.
- When anticancer drugs are self-administered, patients must be familiar with proper use of the drugs, including dose scheduling and interactions with food or other drugs.
- Since many adverse effects do not appear until several days after a dose of an anticancer drug, patients must know which side effects should be reported to their physician.
- Chemotherapy patients are at risk for infections due to reduced white blood cell counts. Prophylactic antibiotics may be necessary and patients should follow good hygiene practices to minimize exposure to infections. Live virus immunizations—and contact with others who have recently received a live virus immunization—are contraindicated until the patient has fully recovered from the effects of chemotherapy.

Geriatric

Some anticancer drugs are only used in elderly patients. Others are generally not used in the elderly, who may be more sensitive to the toxic effects.

Pregnant or breastfeeding

Because most anticancer drugs can harm a fetus, women of childbearing age should use two concurrent effective methods of birth control while they or their males partners are being treated with anticancer drugs. Breastfeeding should be avoided during treatment.

Other conditions and allergies

The existence of any of the following conditions should be taken into consideration before administering anticancer drugs:

- chickenpox or recent exposure to someone with chickenpox
- shingles (Herpes zoster)
- mouth sores
- current or past seizures
- head injury
- nerve or muscle disease
- hearing problems
- infection of any kind
- gout
- colitis
- intestinal blockage
- stomach ulcers
- kidney stones
- kidney disease
- liver disease
- current or past alcohol abuse
- immune system disease
- cataracts or other eye problems
- high cholesterol

Side effects

Because most anticancer drugs do not target specific cell types, they can have numerous side effects. Drugs that target specific cell types may have more specific side effects. **Nausea and vomiting** are among the most common side effects of anticancer drugs and in some cases may be severe enough to cause dose reduction or discontinuation of treatment. Other common side effects include:

- hair loss due to effects on hair follicles
- menstrual cycle changes
- itchy skin
- loss of appetite
- anemia
- immune system impairment
- blood clotting problems due to damage to the blood-forming organs, leading to a reduction in the number of red blood cells, white blood cells, and platelets

Steps to minimize side effects include:

- antinausea medications to reduce nausea and vomiting
- maintaining fluid levels to reduce drug toxicity, particularly to the kidneys
- application of a scalp tourniquet to reduce blood flow to the scalp and minimize hair loss

Other side effects of anticancer drugs can include:

- joint pain
- skin rash
- hearing problems or ringing in the ears
- numbness or tingling in the fingers or toes
- trouble walking or balance problems
- swelling of the feet or lower legs
- unusual tiredness or weakness
- loss of taste
- seizures
- dizziness
- confusion
- agitation
- headache
- dark urine
- yellow eyes or skin
- flushing of the face

Uncommon but serious side effects of anticancer drugs may include:

- black, tarry, or bloody stools
- blood in the urine
- diarrhea
- fever or chills
- cough or hoarseness
- wheezing or shortness of breath
- sores in the mouth or on the lips
- unusual bleeding or bruising
- swelling of the face
- red "pinpoint" spots on the skin
- redness, pain, or swelling at the point of injection
- pain in the side or lower back
- problems urinating or painful urination
- fast or irregular heartbeat

Interactions

Anticancer drugs can interact with numerous other drugs, affecting the actions of one or both or increasing the risk of side effects. The physician should be aware of all prescription and nonprescription (over-the-counter) medicines that a patient is taking, as well as radiation treatments or other anticancer drugs administered in the past.

Resources

BOOKS

Abeloff, M. D., et al. *Abeloff's Clinical Oncology*, 4th ed. Philadelphia: Churchill Livingstone, 2008.

Nathan, David G. *The Cancer Treatment Revolution: How Smart Drugs and Other New Therapies are Renewing Our Hope and Changing the Face of Medicine.* Hoboken, NJ: John Wiley & Sons, 2007.

Thurston, David E. *Chemistry and Pharmacology of Anti-cancer Drugs.* Boca Raton, FL: CRC Press/Taylor & Francis, 2007.

PERIODICALS

Dawood, S., and B. Leyland-Jones. "Pharmacology and Pharmacogenetics of Chemotherapeutic Agents." *Cancer Investigation* 27, no. 5 (June 2009): 482–488.

OTHER

"Anticancer Drugs." *University of Maryland Medical Center*. http://www.umm.edu/altmed/articles/anticancer-drugs-002712.htm

"Cancer Center." *Drugs.com*. http://www.drugs.com/cancer.html

"Cancer Chemotherapy." *MedlinePlus*. http://www.nlm.nih.gov/medlineplus/cancerchemotherapy.html.

"Drug Information Summaries." *National Cancer Institute*. http://www.cancer.gov/cancertopics/druginfo/alphalist

"Guide to Cancer Drugs." *American Cancer Society*. http://www.cancer.org/docroot/CDG/cdg_0.asp

"What Are the Different Types of Chemotherapy Drugs?" *American Cancer Society*. http://www.cancer.org/docroot/ETO/content/ETO_1_4X_What_Are_The_Different_Types_Of_Chemotherapy_Drugs. asp?sitearea=ETO

ORGANIZATIONS

American Cancer Society, 1599 Clifton Road NE, Atlanta, GA, 30329-4251, (800) ACS-2345, http://www.cancer.org.

National Cancer Institute, NCI Public Inquiries Office, 6116 Executive Boulevard, Room 3036A, Bethesda, MD, 20892-8322, (800) 4-CANCER, http://www.cancer.gov.

Samuel D. Uretsky, PharmD
Margaret Alic, PhD

Antidiarrheal agents

Definition

Antidiarrheal agents are prescription and non-prescription medicines that are used to treat **diarrhea**.

Purpose

Some types of **cancer** may cause diarrhea. In addition, diarrhea is a common side effect of **chemotherapy** treatments for cancer. This is because **anticancer drugs** can damage the cells of the intestines. Radiation treatment for cancer directed at the abdominal region also may cause diarrhea. Diarrhea can result in dehydration and the loss of minerals such as potassium. It may prevent the elimination of waste products in the urine, as the body attempts to conserve water.

Description

The common medicines for treating diarrhea that results from cancer and cancer treatments are:

- atropine and diphenoxylate
- loperamide
- octreotide
- opium tincture

Atropine and diphenoxylate are prescribed as a combination medicine with the brand names:

- Lofene
- Logen
- Lomocot
- Lomotil
- Lonox
- Vi-Atro

The generic name product also may be available. Atropine and diphenoxylate, antiperistaltic and anticholinergic agents, relax muscles and slow down the movements of the gastrointestinal tract. Diphenoxylate is similar to some narcotics and may be habit-forming if taken in dosages higher than prescribed. Since higher doses of atropine have unpleasant effects, it is unlikely that the combination medicine will be taken in high enough doses to cause diphenoxylate-dependence.

Loperamide slows down the movements of the intestines. The common brand names for this medicine are:

- Imodium
- Kaopectate II
- Maalox Anti-Diarrheal
- Pepto Diarrhea Control

Octreotide (brand name Sandostatin) is used to treat diarrhea and other symptoms of some types of intestinal cancers. It also is used to treat insulin-producing tumors of the pancreas and diarrhea caused by chemotherapy.

Opium tincture, also known as camphorated opium tincture or laudanum, is a narcotic that is used to treat severe diarrhea.

Except for loperamide liquid or tablets, all of these medicines require a prescription. Dosages vary with the individual.

Recommended dosage

The atropine-diphenoxylate combination is taken by mouth as a solution or a tablet. It may be taken with food to reduce stomach upset. The initial average dosage is 5 mg (2 tsp or two tablets) three to four times daily. Subsequent doses are once daily, as needed.

Loperamide is taken orally, as a liquid, tablet, or capsule. The usual dosage for adults and teenagers is 4 mg (2 capsules or tablets, 4 tsp of liquid) after the first loose bowel movement, followed by 2 mg after each successive loose bowel movement. The maximum dose is 16 mg of the capsules or 8 mg of the tablets or liquid in 24 hours. Loperamide should not be taken for more than two days unless ordered by a physician.

Following therapy with **irinotecan** (Camptosar), loperamide doses of 2 mg every two hours while awake and 4 mg every four hours at night are utilized at the onset of diarrhea to prevent severe dehydration and possible hospitalization.

Octreotide is packaged as a kit, for injection into a vein. For treating severe diarrhea from intestinal tumors, the average initial dosage of the long-acting form, for adults and teenagers, is 20 mg injected into the gluteal muscle of the buttocks, once every four weeks for two months. The dosage may then be adjusted by the physician. For the short-acting form, the average initial dose is 50 micrograms (mcg) injected under the skin, two to three times per day. The dosage may be gradually increased up to 600 mcg per day for the first two weeks. The average dosage after two weeks is 50–1500 mcg per day. For children, the usual dosage is 1–10 mcg per kg (0.45–4.5 mcg per lb) of body weight per day.

Opium tincture is taken orally, as a liquid. It may be taken with food to prevent stomach upset. The average adult dose is 5–16 drops, measured from the dropper in the bottle, four times per day, until diarrhea is controlled. It may be diluted with water. After several weeks of treatment, it may be necessary to lower the dosage gradually before stopping the medicine, to lessen the risk of side effects from opium withdrawal.

Precautions

Antidiarrheal agents may cause allergic reactions in some individuals. Atropine and diphenoxylate should not be given to children. Loperamide should not be given to children under six. Opium may cause breathing problems in children up to two years of age. Older adults are more sensitive to diphenoxylate and opium than younger individuals and these drugs may cause breathing problems. Diphenoxylate and loperamide may mask the symptoms of dehydration caused by diarrhea in older individuals, so it is very important to drink sufficient fluids.

Atropine and diphenoxylate

Other medical conditions may affect the use of atropine and diphenoxylate:

- alcohol or drug abuse may increase the risk of diphenoxylate addiction
- colitis (inflammation of the colon) may become more severe
- Down syndrome may cause more severe side effects
- dysentery may worsen

- emphysema, asthma, bronchitis, or other chronic lung diseases increase the risk of breathing problems
- enlarged prostate or urinary tract blockage may cause severe problems with urination
- gall bladder disease or gallstones may worsen
- glaucoma may result in severe eye pain (rare)
- heart disease may worsen
- hiatal hernia may worsen with atropine (rare)
- high blood pressure may increase (rare)
- intestinal blockage may worsen
- kidney disease may cause atropine to accumulate in the body, resulting in side effects
- liver disease may cause central nervous system side effects, including coma
- myasthenia gravis may become worse
- overactive or underactive thyroid may cause effects on breathing and heart rate
- incontinence may worsen

An overdose of atropine and diphenoxylate can lead to unconsciousness and death. Symptoms of overdose include:

- severe drowsiness
- breathing problems
- fast heartbeat
- warmth, dryness, and flushing of skin
- vision problems
- severe dryness of mouth, nose, and throat
- nervousness or irritability

Loperamide and octreotide

Other medical conditions may affect the use of loperamide:

- colitis (inflammation of the colon) may worsen
- dysentery may worsen
- liver disease may increase the risk of side effects

Loperamide should not be used in the presence of **fever** or blood or mucus in stools.

Medical conditions that may affect the use of octreotide include:

- diabetes mellitus, since octreotide may affect blood sugar levels
- gallbladder disease or gallstones, since octreotide may cause gallstones
- severe kidney disease that may cause octreotide to remain in the body longer

Opium tincture

Side effects of opium tincture may be increased or become dangerous when combined with the following medical conditions:

- alcohol or drug abuse
- colitis (inflammation of the colon)
- heart disease
- kidney disease
- liver disease
- underactive thyroid
- head injury or brain disease
- emphysema, asthma, bronchitis, or other chronic lung disease
- problems with urination or enlarged prostate
- gallbladder disease or gallstones
- seizures

Opium tincture may be habit-forming, causing mental or physical dependence that can lead to side effects of withdrawal when stopping the medicine. The use of opium tincture during pregnancy can cause dependency in the fetus and symptoms of drug withdrawal or breathing problems in the newborn infant.

Symptoms of opium overdose include:

- seizures
- confusion
- severe restlessness or nervousness
- severe dizziness
- severe drowsiness
- slow or irregular breathing
- severe weakness
- cold, clammy skin
- low blood pressure
- slow heartbeat
- contracted eye pupils

Side effects

Atropine and diphenoxylate

At low doses, taken for short periods of time, side effects of atropine and diphenoxylate are rare. However, serious side effects may include:

- bloating
- constipation
- loss of appetite
- stomach pain with nausea and vomiting

Other, less common or rare side effects of atropine and diphenoxylate include:

- dizziness
- drowsiness
- blurred vision
- confusion
- difficult urination
- dry skin or mouth
- fever
- headache
- depression
- numbness in hands or feet
- skin rash or itching
- swelling of gums

Rare side effects that may occur after stopping atropine and diphenoxylate include:

- sweating
- trembling or chills
- muscle cramps
- nausea or vomiting
- stomach cramps

Loperamide

Side effects are rare with low dosages of loperamide, taken for a short time. However, severe side effects may include:

- bloating
- constipation
- loss of appetite
- stomach pain with nausea and vomiting
- skin rash
- dry mouth
- dizziness or drowsiness

Octreotide

More common side effects of octreotide may include:

- irregular or slow heartbeat
- constipation
- diarrhea
- flatulence
- discomfort at the site of injection

Less common or rare side effects of octreotide may include:

- dizziness or light-headedness
- fever
- flushing or redness of the face
- swelling of feet or lower legs
- inflammation of the pancreas with stomach pain, nausea, or vomiting
- hair loss
- seizures
- unconsciousness

Symptoms of high blood sugar (hyperglycemia) from octreotide include:

- blurred vision
- drowsiness and fatigue
- dry mouth
- flushed, dry skin
- fruity breath odor
- increased urination
- ketones in urine
- loss of appetite
- increased thirst
- nausea or vomiting
- stomach ache
- rapid, deep breathing

Symptoms of low blood sugar (hypoglycemia) from octreotide include:

- anxiety and nervousness
- confusion
- blurred vision
- cold sweats
- cool, pale skin
- drowsiness, fatigue, weakness
- hunger
- fast heartbeat
- headache
- nausea
- nightmares and restless sleep
- shakiness
- slurred speech

Opium tincture

Side effects of opium tincture that are more common with higher dosages may include:

- drowsiness
- dizziness, light-headedness, faintness
- nervousness
- weakness or fatigue
- painful or strained urination
- frequent urination
- decreased volume of urine

Lying down and rising slowly from a seated or lying position may help relieve dizziness.

Rare side effects of opium tincture include:

- bloating
- constipation
- loss of appetite
- nausea or vomiting
- stomach cramps
- fast or slow heartbeat
- sweating
- rash, hives, or itching
- redness or flushing of the face
- depression
- troubled breathing
- convulsions (seizures)

The following side effects may occur after stopping treatment with opium tincture:

- runny nose or sneezing
- body aches
- loss of appetite
- diarrhea
- stomach cramps
- nausea or vomiting
- fever
- sweating
- nervousness or irritability
- trembling
- insomnia
- dilated pupils
- severe weakness

Interactions

Atropine and diphenoxylate

Other drugs may interact with atropine and diphenoxylate:

- Antibiotics (cephalosporins, clindamycin, erythromycins, tetracyclines) can counteract the effects of atropine and diphenoxylate and make the diarrhea worse.
- Central nervous system depressants (alcohol, antihistamines, sedatives, pain medicines or narcotics, barbiturates, seizure medicine, muscle relaxants, anesthetics) may increase effects, such as drowsiness, from both the depressant and the antidiarrheal agent.

- Monoamine oxidase inhibitors may cause severe side effects if taken within two weeks of diphenoxylate and atropine.
- Opioid antagonists (naltrexone) may cause withdrawal from diphenoxylate addiction; naltrexone will counteract the antidiarrheal effects of the medicine.
- Other anticholinergics to reduce stomach acid or cramps may increase the effects of atropine.

Loperamide and octreotide

Antibiotics may interact with loperamide and make the diarrhea worse. Narcotic pain medicines in combination with loperamide may cause severe constipation.

Because octreotide may cause high or low blood sugar, it can interact with the following medicines:

- antidiabetic medicines, sulfonylurea
- diazoxide (Proglycem)
- glucagon
- insulin
- growth hormone

Opium tincture

The following medicines may increase side effects from opium tincture:

- anticholinergics for abdominal or stomach cramps
- other antidiarrheal medicines
- tricyclic antidepressants

Naltrexone (Trexan) makes opium less effective for treating diarrhea. Alcohol, narcotics, and other central nervous system depressants, including antihistamines, sedatives, prescription pain medicines, barbiturates, seizure medicines, muscle relaxants, or anesthetics, may lead to unconsciousness or death in combination with opium tincture.

Margaret Alic, Ph.D.

Antiemetics

Definition

Antiemetic drugs are drugs used to combat **nausea and vomiting**.

KEY TERMS

Depersonalization—An alteration in the perception of self.

Tardive dyskinesia—A disorder brought on by antipsychotic medication use, characterized by uncontrollable muscle spasms.

Purpose

Antiemetic drugs are used to prevent **vomiting** (emesis) in **chemotherapy** patients and postoperative patients. Aside from the difficulty of maintaining proper nutrition and a healthy weight, chronic vomiting can result in dehydration, which can be a medical emergency. Following are descriptions of many common antiemetic drugs in use as of 2004.

Description

Promethazine

Promethazine is also known as phenergan and mepergan. It is also used to treat motion sickness, reduce allergic symptoms, and for sedation. It is one of the drugs of the phenothiazine type. In addition to other qualities, it is an antihistamine.

Prochlorperazine

Prochlorperazine is also known as compazine. Like promethazine, it is a member of the class of phenothiazines. Unlike promethazine, however, prochlorperazine also belongs to the class of drugs known as antipsychotics, or neuroleptics. Antipsychotic drugs are used to treat psychoses and other psychiatric disorders. In addition to its use as an antiemetic and anti-psychotic drug, prochlorperazine is also used to treat non-psychotic anxiety.

Serotonin receptor antagonists

The serotonin receptor antagonists include granisetron (kytril), dolasetron (anzemet), and ondansetron (zofran). These drugs are used for postoperative **nausea** and emesis as well as nausea and vomiting associated with chemotherapy, and are often used in combination with a corticosteroid. Ondansetron is approved for nausea and vomiting associated with **radiation therapy**.

Neurokinin receptor antagonists

The Neurokinin receptor antagonists are a new class of antiemetics. Aprepitant (Emend) was approved in 2004 for use in **cancer** patients. It is used in combination with other antiemetics for relief of acute and delayed nausea and vomiting caused by high-dose chemotherapy, most often caused by the chemotherapy drug **cisplatin**.

Dronabinol

Dronabinol (marinol) is used to combat **anorexia** in AIDS patients, and emesis in cancer patients who haven't responded to other antiemetics. Marinol is the synthetic or extracted form of the active ingredient found in marijuana.

Other antipsychotic (neuroleptic) drugs

The other neuroleptic (antipsychotic) drugs used to treat nausea and emesis are droperidol (inapsine), haloperidol (haldol), chlorpromazine (thorazine), and perphenazine (trilafon). One other antipsychotic, triethylperazine (torecan or norzine), was used as an antiemetic, but is no longer widely available. Some of the antipsychotics are also used to treat aggressive or violent behavior or incontrollable hiccups (chlorpromazine). These drugs are similar to prochlorperazine in terms of their actions and potentially severe side effects.

Dosage

Promethazine

Promethazine is given in doses of 12.5 to 25 mg every 4 hours if injected into the muscle or as a suppository. As a syrup, 25 mg should be given every 4 to 6 hours. Doses for children vary by age, weight, and severity of condition.

Prochlorperazine

Generally, the dose is 5 to 10 mg, 3 to 4 times per day. However, the effect of medication varies widely from patient to patient, so the dose should be tailored to each individual. Prochlorperazine is available as a syrup, tablet, 25 mg slow-release capsule, and in injectable form.

Aprepitant

One 125-mg capsule is given by mouth one hour before chemotherapy begins. An 80-mg capsule is taken each morning for two days following the chemotherapy treatment.

Dronabinol

The effective dose of dronabinol varies widely from patient to patient and should be monitored and tested by the physician. The basic dose is $5mg/m^2$ given 4 to 6 times per day.

Precautions

Promethazine

Patients with cardiovascular disease or impaired liver function should either use this drug with caution or not at all. Children should also use this drug cautiously for two reasons. First, some side effects may suggest, or mask, underlying disease, such as Reye's syndrome. Second, large doses of this drug, or any antihistamine, may cause convulsions, hallucinations, or death in children. Patients taking this medication should not drive, operate heavy machinery, or engage in any hazardous activity while under the influence of this drug. This drug has not been established as safe for use during pregnancy, or in nursing mothers.

Prochlorperazine

Persons allergic to any other phenothiazine (such as promethazine) should not take prochlorperazine. Patients who have heart problems, glaucoma, or bone marrow depression should take this drug with caution, or not at all, and inform their physician of their condition. People who will be around high temperatures should also avoid this drug. In addition, those who experience seizures should be aware that administration of this drug makes seizures more likely.

Breast cancer patients may wish to avoid this drug because it increases levels of prolactin in the blood. Increased prolactin may help some types of breast cancer to thrive.

Prochloroperazine, like promethazine, may mask symptoms of Reye's disease in children. It may also mask symptoms of intestinal obstructions or brain disease. In addition, children who are acutely ill, under two years of age, or under 20 pounds should not be given this drug.

This drug has not been established as safe for use during pregnancy and is found in the breast milk of lactating mothers. Therefore, caution should be used when administering this drug to pregnant women and extreme caution should be used when administering to nursing women.

Aprepitant

Patients should not drink grapefruit juice while taking aprepitant. The physician should be told if the patient is pregnant, breast feeding, or becomes pregnant while taking the drug.

Serotonin receptor antagonists

Patients with allergies to any drug in this category should not take any other drug in this category. Also, patients with hypokalemia, hypomagnesia, or certain heart problems should avoid taking these drugs. The effect of these drugs on the children or fetuses of nursing or pregnant mothers is not known, so they should be used with caution.

Dronabinol

Dronabinol is inadvisable for patients with a known allergy to either sesame oil or any part of the cannabis plant. Patients taking this drug should not drive, operate heavy machinery, or engage in hazardous tasks until used to this medication.

This medication also should be used cautiously, if at all, for persons with depression, mania, or schizophrenia, elderly patients, patients with cardiac disorders, and for pregnant and nursing women. It is especially inadvisable for nursing women, since marinol is concentrated in the breast milk.

Side effects

Promethazine

Patients taking promethazine may experience a large number of side effects, including drowsiness, ringing in the ears, a lack of coordination, problems with vision, **fatigue**, euphoria, nervousness, tremors, seizures, a catatonic-like state, and hysteria. These effects are usually reversible. At high doses, patients may also exhibit extrapyramidal reactions. Extrapyramidal reactions can briefly be described as agitation (jitteriness, sometimes insomnia), muscle spasms, and/or pseudo-Parkinson's (a group of symptoms including, but not limited to, drooling, tremors, and a shuffling gait).

Patients may also experience rashes, asthma, jaundice, abnormally low production of white blood cells, and abnormalities in how fast or slow their heart beats. Patients may sometimes experience unusual side effects not known as typical for the medication they are taking. These should be reported to the physician.

Prochlorperazine

Prochlorperazine has many side effects, including low blood pressure, dizziness, blurred vision, skin reactions, and jaundice. Patients also may suffer jaw, neck, and back muscle spasms, slow or difficult speech, and difficulty swallowing, as well as rhythmic face, mouth, or jaw movements. However, the most severe side effects stem from damage to the brain after long-term use. These symptoms may be reversed by treating the patient with drugs effective in treatment of Parkinson's patients (except levodopa). A reduction or elimination in the amount of the antipsychotic medication may also be necessary to eliminate these symptoms.

Two other (rare) disorders, tardive dyskinesia and neuroleptic malignant syndrome (NMS), are also associated with antipsychotic drug use. Patients with NMS have high temperatures, rigid muscles, an altered mental state, and symptoms such as excessive sweating and irregular blood pressure or heart rhythm. Patients with NMS usually respond to treatment. Patients with tardive dyskinesia have involuntary movement of muscles in the chest, arms, and legs, or in the muscles in and around the face (including the tongue). Tardive dyskinesia may be irreversible.

Aprepitant

Side effects of aprepitant include fatigue, dizziness, stomach pain, nausea, hiccups, **diarrhea**, constipation, and loss of appetite. More serious, but less common, side effects have been reported, including hives, skin rash, difficulty breathing or swallowing, hoarseness, and swelling in the face, throat, tongue, lips, eyes, feet, ankles, or lower legs. If any of these more serious side effects occur, the patient should contact the treating physician immediately.

Serotonin receptor antagonists

Side effects include rashes, increased sweating, problems with taste or vision, flushing, agitation, sleep disorder, depersonalization, headache, fatigue, nausea, weakness, abdominal pain, constipation, diarrhea, hypertension, dizziness, chills and shivering, and dry mouth. Patients may also have abnormal liver function tests.

Dronabinol

Possible side effects are fatigue, weakness, abdominal pain, nausea, vomiting, heart palpitations, fast heart rate, facial flushing, amnesia, anxiety, an abnormal mental state, depersonalization, confusion, dizziness, and euphoria.

There are certain additional precautions and side effects associated with each of these drugs. Patients should be sure to notify their physician of any health concerns (including pregnancy) or medications they are taking. Patients should also ask about potential side effects for each individual medication before receiving any of these drugs.

Interactions

Promethazine

Promethazine interacts with central nervous system depressants, like alcohol and barbiturates. Therefore, the physician should be alerted to any medications the patient is taking, and doses of the drugs should be adjusted accordingly. Alcohol should be avoided. It has not been proven, but promethazine may interfere with the action of epinephrine.

Prochlorperazine

Like promethazine, prochlorperazine should be used cautiously, or not at all, with central nervous system depressants like alcohol and barbiturates. Prochlorperazine has also been shown to interact with anticonvulsant medication, guanethidene, propanolol, thiazide diuretics, and oral anticoagulants (like **warfarin** and coumadin).

Aprepitant

A physician can check the long list of possible drug interactions, which include possible effects on the action of certain chemotherapy drugs. Aprepitant also may interact with the blood thinner warfarin (Coumadin) and other popular drugs. The treating physician or pharmacist will need a complete list of other drugs the patient is taking before prescribing this antiemetic.

Serotonin receptor antagonists

These drugs may have very negative effects on the patient when combined with diuretics, anti-arrhythmia drugs, or high doses of anthracycline.

Dronabinol

Dronabinol interacts with the antiemetic prochlorperazine synergistically. Therefore, the use of these two drugs in combination results in a greater antiemetic effect. Patients taking central nervous system depressants, such as barbiturates or alcohol should notify their physician before taking marinol, since marinol may increase their effect. Although no drugs have been shown to interact with marinol, many drugs similar to marinol do interact with a number of other drugs, including central nervous system depressants such as alcohol or barbiturates, or drugs like flouxetine or disulfiram. Again, the physician should be alerted to any medications the patient is taking before beginning a course of dronabinol.

See also Corticosteroids; Lorazepam; Metoclopramide; Scopolamine.

Resources

PERIODICALS

Boothby, Lisa A., and Paul L. Doering. "New Drug Update 2003: Part 1." *Drug Topics* (February 23, 2004): 54.

Michael Zuck, PhD

Antiestrogens

Definition

Antiestrogens are a group of medications that block the effect that estrogen has on the growth of a tumor.

Purpose

For about 20 years, antiestrogens have been used mainly to help prevent and treat **breast cancer**. Since many breast **cancer** tumors use hormones to fuel their growth, blocking the hormones limits their ability to grow.

Description

Antiestrogens refer to a group of drugs. Many breast cancer tumors grow due to normal levels of estrogen, a hormone found in the bloodstream. Some patients have tumors that are extra-sensitive to this normal estrogen level. The estrogen attaches to the area on the outside of the tumor cells and sends a signal to the cell that causes it to grow and multiply. Antiestrogens block the protein on the outside wall of the estrogen-sensitive breast cancer cell. By blocking this protein, known as the estrogen receptor, the free-floating estrogen cannot stimulate the cancer cells to grow and multiply any further.

The drug **tamoxifen** is a common antiestrogen that has proven to have a positive effect in breast cancer patients for both treatment and prevention.

The drug **raloxifene** is a newer antiestrogen. Early research showed that raloxifene worked against breast cancer with fewer side effects than tamoxifene. In 2003, research also showed that raloxifene may be effective in decreasing new fractures among women with low bone mineral density. However, further **clinical trials** on raloxifene are needed.

Precautions

Use of tamoxifen has been associated with a number of side effects, including vaginal bleeding, menstrual irregularities, and **hypercalcemia** (excess calcium in the blood). Most women also experience hot flashes while using the drug. Serious side effects include **endometrial cancer** and thromboembolism (blocking of a blood vessel by a particle of a blood clot at the site the blood clot formed). In late 2003, cancer experts were beginning to recommend a new group of drugs called **aromatase inhibitors** (Arimidex, common name anastrozole or Femara and Novartis, common name letrozole) as an alternative to tamoxifen or following tamoxifen therapy. These drugs fight breast cancer differently, but early research shows they fight it as effectively and with fewer side effects.

Resources

PERIODICALS

Lewis, Jilene. "Breast Cancer Guidelines Suggest Alternative to Standard Therapy." *Drug Topics* August 18, 2003: 22.
Pennachio, Dorothy L. "Letrozole Improves Breast Cancer Outlook." *Patient Care* December 2003: 4.
"Raloxifene Decreases New Fractures in Women with Vertebral Cracks at Baseline." *Women's Health Weekly* December 4, 2003: 84.
"Revised Guidelines Show Changes for Breast Cancer Treatment." *Biotech Week* December 24, 2003: 296.

OTHER

Hormonal Therapy, Breast Cancer Treatment. People Living with Cancer. http://www.peoplelivingwithcancer.org.

Nancy J. Beaulieu, RPh.,BCOP
Teresa G. Odle

Antifungal therapy

Definition

Antifungal drugs are used to treat infections caused by fungi and to prevent the development of fungal infections in patients with weakened immune systems.

Purpose

Fungal infections

A fungus is a living organism that can cause **infection** when it grows in the human body. In healthy people, fungal infections tend to be mild and treatable. For **cancer** patients, however, fungal infections can become severe and must be treated quickly. Cancer patients, particularly those with leukemia or

KEY TERMS

Aspergillosis—A fungal infection that can be life-threatening to patients with a weakened immune system.

Candidiasis—A fungal infection that can be mild or very serious depending on what part of the body it infects.

Cryptococcosis—A fungal infection that can cause meningitis.

Intravenous—A treatment that is given directly into the bloodstream.

Prophylactic—Referring to a drug or other treatment given to prevent disease.

Topical—A treatment that is applied directly to the skin.

lymphoma, tend to have weakened immune systems as a result of **chemotherapy** or the disease. Once they are infected, their weak immune system allows the fungus to grow quickly. Because of this risk, some cancer patients with no obvious fungal infection are given antifungal therapy to help prevent infection from developing. This approach to treatment is called prophylaxis or prophylactic therapy.

Fungal infection can occur in two ways. Some fungi, such as candida, are usually found in the bodies of healthy people and cause little or no harm. When the immune system is weak, however, these fungi begin to grow and cause infection. Other fungi, such as aspergillus and cryptococcus, are found in the air. Infection occurs when the fungus is either inhaled into the lungs or comes into contact with an operative wound. The most common fungal infections found in patients with weakened immune systems are candidiasis, aspergillosis and cryptococcosis.

Diagnostic innovations in antifungal therapy in cancer patients include the increased use of nonculture-based tests to speed up the process of diagnosis.

Treatment

The treatment of a fungal infection depends on the type and location of infection. Superficial infections that affect the skin, hair, and nails can be treated with topical (cream or ointment) or oral antifungal drugs. Systemic infections that affect the internal organs require aggressive treatment with either oral or intravenous drugs.

Description

There are three classes of drugs typically used to treat fungal infections: polyenes, azoles, and echinocandins.

Polyenes

Polyenes are drugs that work by attaching to the sterol component found in the fungal membrane, causing the cells to become porous and die. The two polyenes most commonly used are nystatin (Mycostatin) and amphotericin B (Fungizone). Nystatin is often used as a topical agent to treat superficial infections, or is taken orally to treat such candidal infections as oral or esophageal candidiasis.

Amphotericin B was the first antifungal drug to be approved for use, and it is still the standard therapy for the most severe systemic fungal infections. Recently, several new types of amphotericin B (Abelcet, Amphotec and AmBisome) have been introduced. These drugs, called lipid formulations, cause fewer side effects than traditional amphotericin B but are more expensive.

Azoles

Azoles stop fungal growth by preventing fungi from making an essential part of their cell wall. Three typical azoles are ketoconazole (Nizoral), fluconazole (Diflucan), and itraconazole (Sporanox). Ketoconazole is the oldest of these three drugs, and has been used since the 1970s. It is slightly more toxic than the other azoles and does not work for aspergillosis and many candidiasis infections.

Although fluconazole is effective against both superficial and systemic candidiasis, some strains of this fungus have now become resistant to the drug. Itraconazole, the newest of the azoles, is effective against a range of different fungal infections. Unlike ketoconazole or fluconazole, it can be used to treat aspergillosis.

Newer azole medications include voriconazole (Vfend), approved by the FDA in the fall of 2001, and posaconazole, approved in September 2006.

Echinocandins

Echinocandins are a new class of antifungal drugs that work by disrupting the wall that surrounds fungal cells. Caspofungin (Cancidas) is the first of this new class of drugs to be approved. It is an effective treatment for severe systemic fungal infections, and is given to patients who do not respond to other therapies. Micafungin, another drug in this class, has been used in Japan to treat aspergillosis in leukemia patients but has not been approved by the FDA for use in the United States.

Recommended dosage

Although dosages differ for the various antifungal treatments, most therapies continue even after there is no sign of infection.

Polyenes

Topical nystatin should be liberally applied two to three times daily. Liquid formulations of the drug are usually taken in doses of 400,000 to 600,000 units four times a day for adults and children. The dose for the oral tablets is 500,000 to 1 million units every 8 hours. Both traditional amphotericin B and the new lipid formulations of the drug are given intravenously. Dosages are adjusted according to each patient's tolerance and the severity and location of the infection. Patients receiving amphotericin B treatment are usually hospitalized.

Azoles

Ketoconazole is available as a tablet and as a topical treatment. Both treatments are usually given once daily. Treatment can last for several weeks for superficial infections, or up to a year for more serious infections. Fluconazole and itraconazole are both administered either orally or intravenously. The dose depends on the type of fungal infection, the patient's condition and the response to treatment.

Echinocandins

Caspofungin is given intravenously once daily, and most patients receive the same dose.

Precautions

Patients who are given topical or oral antifungal therapy should make sure they use their medication regularly, and for as long as their doctor thinks is necessary. Infections that are not completely eradicated frequently recur.

Side effects

Antifungal drugs that are applied topically rarely cause side effects unless the patient is allergic to the drug. Side effects are more common when drugs are taken orally or intravenously. The most common reactions from azole drugs are **nausea**, **diarrhea** and other gastrointestinal symptoms. These symptoms usually affect less than 10% of patients. Caspofungin also

produces few side effects. The most common side effect is a rash.

Amphotericin B can be quite toxic and most patients experience side effects. These include **fever**, rigors, and chills. Premedication with acetaminophen, diphenhydramine, hydrocortisone, and sometimes **meperidine** can be given to prevent these side effects. Amphotericin B can also seriously damage the kidneys. However, patients are carefully monitored while taking this drug. If symptoms develop, the liposomal alternative is usually given. Lipid formulations of amphotericin B are far less damaging to the kidneys.

Interactions

Drug interactions are significant with antifungal treatment. Patients taking amphotericin B should not take any other drug that can cause kidney damage. Potentially serious reactions can occur when patients taking azole antifungal therapies also take certain antihistamines such as astemizole (Hismanal) or the statin drug lovastatin (Mevacor). Patients on antifungal therapy who plan to take other prescribed, over the counter, or alternative medicines should always check with their doctor first.

Resources

BOOKS

Beers, Mark H., MD, and Robert Berkow, MD, editors. "Systemic Fungal Diseases (Systemic Mycoses)." In *The Merck Manual of Diagnosis and Therapy*. Whitehouse Station, NJ: Merck Research Laboratories, 2007.

Wilson, Billie Ann, Margaret T. Shannon, and Carolyn L. Stang. *Nurse's Drug Guide 2003*. Upper Saddle River, NJ: Prentice Hall, 2003.

PERIODICALS

Hubel, K., J. Chemnitz, H. G. Brochhagen, and O. A. Cornely. "Successful Treatment of Chronic Disseminated Candidiasis with Caspofungin and Itraconazole in a Patient with Progressive Acute Leukemia and Prolonged Neutropenia." *International Journal of Hematology* 79 (April 2004): 289–292.

Karthaus, M., A. J. Ullmann, and O. A. Cornely. "Current Development in the Diagnostics and Therapy of Systemic Fungal Infections in Cancer Patients." [in German] *Wiener medizinische Wochenschrift* 154 (May 2004): 199–208.

Ostrosky-Zeichner, L. "Novel Approaches to Antifungal Prophylaxis." *Expert Opinion on Investigational Drugs* 13 (June 2004): 665–672.

Ota, S., J. Tanaka, K. Kahata, et al. "Successful Micafungin (FK463) Treatment of Invasive Pulmonary Aspergillosis in a Patient with Acute Lymphoblastic Leukemia in a Phase II Study." *International Journal of Hematology* 79 (May 2004): 390–393.

Rubin, Z. A., and J. Somani. "New Options for the Treatment of Invasive Fungal Infections." *Seminars in Oncology* 31 (April 2004): 91–98.

ORGANIZATIONS

American Society of Health-System Pharmacists (ASHP). 7272 Wisconsin Avenue, Bethesda, MD 20814. (301) 657-3000. www.ashp.org.

United States Food and Drug Administration (FDA). 5600 Fishers Lane, Rockville, MD 20857-0001. (888) INFO-FDA. www.fda.gov.

Alison McTavish, M.Sc.
Rebecca J. Frey, PhD

Antimicrobials

Definition

Antimicrobial drugs are used to fight infections caused by bacteria, fungi, and viruses.

Description

Antimicrobial drugs are drugs designed to kill, or prevent the growth of microorganisms (bacteria, fungi, and viruses). Bacteria, fungi, and viruses are responsible for almost all of the common infectious diseases found in North America from athlete's foot, to AIDS, to ulcers. Interestingly enough, many disorders formerly thought to be caused by other factors, like stress, are now known to be caused by bacteria. For example, it has been shown that many ulcers are caused by the bacteria *Helicobacter pylori*, and not by stress, as many originally thought. Thus, antimicrobials represent an important part of medicine today.

The history of antimicrobials begins with the observations of Pasteur and Joubert, who discovered that one type of bacteria could prevent the growth of another. They did not know at that time that the reason one bacteria failed to grow was that the other bacteria was producing an antibiotic. Technically, **antibiotics** are only those substances that are produced by one microorganism that kill, or prevent the growth, of another microorganism. Of course, in today's common usage, the term antibiotic is used to refer to almost any drug that cures a bacterial **infection**. Antimicrobials include not just antibiotics, but synthetically formed compounds as well.

The discovery of antimicrobials like penicillin and tetracycline paved the way for better health for millions around the world. Before 1941, the year penicillin was discovered, no true cure for gonorrhea, strep throat, or pneumonia existed. Patients with infected wounds often had to have a wounded limb removed, or face death from infection. Now, most of these infections can be easily cured with a short course of antimicrobials.

However, the future effectiveness of antimicrobial therapy is somewhat in doubt. Microorganisms, especially bacteria, are becoming resistant to more and more antimicrobial agents. Bacteria found in hospitals appear to be especially resilient, and are causing increasing difficulty for the sickest patients–those in the hospital. Currently, bacterial resistance is combated by the discovery of new drugs. However, microorganisms are becoming resistant more quickly than new drugs are being found, Thus, future research in antimicrobial therapy may focus on finding how to overcome resistance to antimicrobials, or how to treat infections with alternative means.

Michael Zuck, PhD

Antineoplastic agents

Definition

Antineoplastic agents are a group of specialized drugs used primarily to treat **cancer** (the term "neoplastic" refers to cancer cells). Some patients and clinicians refer to antineoplastic agents as **chemotherapy**.

Description

The first antineoplastic agents, used in the 1940s, were made from either synthetic chemicals or natural plants. Antineoplastic agents are classified by origin and by how they work to destroy cancer cells. As of 2009, there are over one hundred of these agents approved by the Food and Drug Administration (FDA) to be used in the United States. These include: **methotrexate**, 5-fluorouracil (**fluorouracil**), **doxorubicin**, paclitaxel, and **cyclophosphamide** to name a few.

Antineoplastic agents can be administered to patients alone or in combination with other antineoplastic drugs. They can also be given before, during or after a patient receives surgery, **radiation therapy**, biological therapies and/or bone marrow or hematopoietic stem cell transplants. Antineoplastic agents can be given via many different routes including orally, intravenously, intramuscularly, intra-arterially, intra-peritoneally and topically as well as by other routes of administration.

The treatment plan is disease-specific. It is important that patients receive treatment on schedule.

Antineoplastic agents travel the body and destroy cancer cells. Side effects are expected to occur when treated with these agents, and can include **nausea**, mouth sores, hair loss, and lowering of the blood counts. Many of the side effects associated with antineoplastic agents occur because chemotherapy treatment destroys the body's normal cells in addition to cancerous cells. Healthcare providers should be able to assist patients in managing these side effects so that antineoplastic therapy is a tolerable treatment.

Nancy J. Beaulieu, RPh., BCOP
Melinda Granger Oberleitner, R.N., D.N.S.,
A.P.R.N., C.N.S.

Antioxidants

Definition

Antioxidants are chemical compounds that can bind to free oxygen radicals preventing these radicals from damaging healthy cells.

Purpose

Preliminary studies have suggested that antioxidants are useful in a number of ways in regards to **cancer**. For instance, they may improve the effectiveness of **chemotherapy**, decrease side effects of chemotherapy and radiotherapy, and prevent some types of cancer. Sufficient epidemiological studies have shown that ingesting foods high in antioxidants, such as fruits and vegetables, can decrease the risk of many types of cancer. Studies also found that cancer patients have lower levels of antioxidants in their blood.

In early 2004, the National Cancer Institute (NCI) released a new fact sheet concerning **cancer prevention** and antioxidants. Fruits and vegetables are high in antioxidants and evidence continued to support the role of **vitamins** C, E, and A, as well as lycopene and beta-carotene in helping to prevent cancer. However, clinical trial results have not been consistent. The NCI reported that three large **clinical trials** were trying to better answer the role of antioxidants in cancer prevention.

Precautions

Studies of antioxidant supplements to decrease the risk of cancer have not been conclusive. Most antioxidant research has centered around vitamins A (and its provitamin, beta-carotene), C, E (alpha-tocopherol), and the trace element selenium. While some studies have shown positive effects for antioxidants in preventing cancer, they have been conducted mostly in underfed populations or persons otherwise deficient in these antioxidants. The CARET studies in the early 1990s found that if smokers take beta-carotene and vitamin A supplements they actually increase their risk of developing lung cancer. Rather than isolated antioxidants found in supplements, it may be the combination of antioxidants found in foods that are responsible for decreasing the risk of cancer. The American Institute of Cancer Research warns that antioxidant supplements cannot substitute for whole foods. Individuals who may want to consider supplements include those who are underfed, have certain medical conditions, chronic dieters, some vegetarians, some seniors, and newborns.

Concern has developed about potential negative interactions between high doses of antioxidants and chemotherapy. Anthracycline antitumor **antibiotics** used as chemotherapy act by creating free oxygen radicals to kill tumor cells through a process known as apoptosis. Although patients taking antioxidants may improve their tolerance to chemotherapy drugs, they may be decreasing the effectiveness of treatment and risking a recurrence of the tumor in the long run. This viewpoint is theoretical, however, and no clinical studies have as yet addressed it. Patients interested in

KEY TERMS

Apoptosis—A type of cell death. A mechanism by which one cell dies if it becomes severely mutated as a means of protecting the entire organism.

Cisplatin—An anticancer drug.

Doxorubicin—An anticancer antibiotic therapy. Its trade name is Adriamycin

Fluorouracil—An anticancer drug. Its trade names include Adrucil, 5-FU, Efudex, and Fluoroplex.

Mutation—A change in the genetic structure of the cell.

Oxidative stress—A condition where the body is producing an excess of oxygen-free radicals.

using antioxidants during chemotherapy or radiotherapy should discuss this option with their physicians.

High doses of vitamins and minerals can be toxic. The National Academy of Sciences has suggested safe upper intake levels for adults for some antioxidants. These limits are 2,000 milligrams of vitamin C per day from both foods and supplements combined, 1,000 milligrams of vitamin E per day, and 400 micrograms per day of selenium from both supplements and foods. It is not known how higher levels than these will affect healthy persons.

Side effects of vitamin E overdose may include **fatigue**, intestinal cramping, breast soreness, thrombophlebitis, acne, and **diarrhea**, and increase in blood pressure in certain people. Blood clotting time has been shown to increase. Vitamin E is antagonistic to iron at certain levels. Patients with **anemia** who are taking iron supplements should not take the two supplements at the same time. Vitamin E also may interfere with vitamin K. Selenium toxicity is characterized by dermatologic lesions, brittle hair, fragile or black fingernails, metallic taste, dizziness, and **nausea**.

Description

Free radicals are naturally produced in the body through the normal metabolism of amino acids and fats. These free radicals are unstable molecules that can freely react with and destroy healthy cells. They can bind to and alter the structure of DNA thus leading to mutations and eventually to cancer. Besides cancer, this oxidative stress on the cells can lead to heart, eye, and neurological diseases.

Glutathione, lipoic acid, and CoQ10 are antioxidants formed naturally by the body but their levels decline with age. Vitamins C and E are necessary antioxidants but not produced by the body and must be obtained from the diet. The most common antioxidants are the vitamins A, C, and E. Additional antioxidants are natrol, found in grapes and wine; selenium; and melatonin. Flavonoids consist of a large family of antioxidant compounds found in fruits and vegetables. Among the well-studied flavonoids in terms of cancer prevention are catechins from green tea, genistein from soy, curcumin from turmeric, anthocyanosides from blueberries, and quercetin from yellow vegetables. More recent studies have added clack beans to the list of foods high in antioxidants and a 2003 study in Rome reported that women who ate dark chocolate showed some antioxidant benefits.

Although controversy will surround the topic of supplemental antioxidants for some time, there is little if any controversy that dietary levels of antioxidants are useful in preventing cancer. Because of this evidence, the American Cancer Society suggests five servings of fruits and vegetables each day.

Resources

BOOKS

Moss, Ralph W. *Antioxidants Against Cancer*. Brooklyn, NY: Equinox Press, Inc., 2000.

PERIODICALS

"Chocolate's Dark Health Secret." *Muscle & Fitness/Hers* December 2003: 22.

Kelly, Kara M. "The Labriola/Livingston Article Reviewed." *Oncology* 13, no. 7 (1999): 1008-1011.

Labriola, Dan, and Robert Livingston. "Possible Interactions Between Dietary Antioxidants and Chemotherapy." *Oncology* 13, no. 7 (1999): 1003-1008.

Lamson, Davis W, and Matthew S. Brignall. "Antioxidants in Cancer Therapy: Their Actions and Interactions with Oncologic Therapies."*Alternative Medicine Review* 4, no. 5 (1999): 304-329.

"'Musical Fruit' Rich Source of Healthy Antioxidants; Black Beans Highest." *Cancer Weekly* December 23, 2003: 102.

"Update on Antioxidants." *Nutrition Today* January–February 2004: 25–31.

OTHER

http://www.medical.com.hk/english_site/pharmacy_site/vitamins_s/selenium/selenium_m.htm.

ORGANIZATIONS

American Cancer Society. http://www.cancer.org.

American Institute for Cancer Research. 1759 R Street, NW, PO Box 97167, Washington, DC 20090-7167. (800)843-8114. http://www.aicr.org.

National Academy of Science. http://www.nas.edu.

Cindy Jones, Ph.D.

Antiviral therapy

Definition

Antiviral therapy is often used by **cancer** patients to treat viral infections. Commonly used antiviral medications include acyclovir, famciclovir, ganciclovir, valacyclovir, and foscarnet.

Description

Viral infections occur in almost all people at some time in their lives. The common cold is the most easily recognizable example of a virus that can be unpleasant but generally does not cause serious problems. For people with cancer, however, viruses can often cause life-threatening illnesses.

Viral infections in cancer patients can be much more serious and debilitating than in patients without cancer. Cancer patients will often have weakened immune systems from **chemotherapy** or from the cancer itself. Cancer patients who have bone marrow transplants are at especially high risk for life-threatening viral infections. Immediately after the transplant, the patient will have very few, if any, white blood cells, which are the body's main **infection** fighters. Viral infections such as **herpes simplex** virus (HSV), **herpes zoster** virus (HZV), and cytomegalovirus are often seen in cancer patients, and all can cause serious, life-threatening infections.

Until the development of the antiviral drug acyclovir 1974, no relatively safe and effective anti-viral medications for cancer patients were available. By the mid-1980s, acyclovir was being routinely used for cancer patients with herpes infections. Besides treating the infection itself, acyclovir can be taken on a daily basis to prevent infection from occurring. This can be especially important in people with very depressed immune systems, such as cancer patients who have undergone a bone marrow transplant.

Since the introduction of acyclovir, other antiviral medications have been developed that have been very useful in the treatment of viral illnesses. For reasons that are still unknown, certain herpes infections in certain cancer patients do not respond to acyclovir. Fortunately, two other newer medications similar to acyclovir, called famciclovir and valaciclovir, are helpful in treating herpes infections, especially ones that are resistant to acyclovir.

While antiviral drugs such as acyclovir have made a large difference in treating herpes infections in cancer patients, there are other viral infections that do not respond to acyclovir. Cytomegalovirus is a common viral infection among cancer patients, and especially common among cancer patients who have had bone marrow transplants. Some antiviral medications like acyclovir are not effective against cytomegalovirus. Fortunately, two other antiviral medications known as ganciclovir and foscarnet are both effective against cytomegalovirus.

Recommended dosage

The recommended dosage for the various antiviral medications can vary considerably, depending on the health of the patient and how the medication is administered. For the treatment of herpes simplex and herpes zoster, the drugs acyclovir, famciclovir, and valacyclovir can be used. The recommended oral dosage ranges from 500 mg twice a day for valacyclovir, 500 mg three times a day for famciclovir, to 800 mg every four hours for acyclovir. There is also a formulation for the drug to be given administered though the vein. The dose for injection is different than the dose for oral therapy.

For the treatment of Cytomegalovirus, ganciclovir or foscarnet can be used. Both medications are generally given intravenously, although there is an oral formulation available for ganciclovir. The dosage is 5 mg per kg of body weight every 12 hours for 14 to 21 days, followed by maintenance therapy at a dose of 5 mg per kg per day as a single daily dose. The dosage for foscarnet ranges from 40 mg per kg to 90 mg per kg, depending on the diagnosis.

Precautions

The drugs acyclovir, famciclovir, valcyclovir, ganciclovir and foscarnet should all be used with caution by patients with kidney problems. With higher doses of these drugs, patients who do have kidney problems should have their kidney functioning monitored closely on a daily basis. The dosage is usually decreased depending on the degree of decreased kidney function. Kidney failure has been reported in patients taking high doses of foscarnet.

Ganciclovir should be used with extreme caution in women who may be pregnant, since it is teratogenic (causes abnormalities), as well as toxic, to developing embryos. There are no well-controlled studies of the other antiviral agents in pregnant women and it is not known whether these agents are excreted in breast milk. Therefore, it is not recommended that these antiviral agents be given to pregnant or nursing mothers unless the benefit outweighs the risk.

Side effects

Side effects common to all the antiviral medications include **nausea**, **vomiting**, **diarrhea**, headaches, and dizziness, rash, and decreased kidney function. Of the drugs used to treat herpes simplex, acyclovir seems to have more reported side effects than the other medications.

The two drugs that are used to treat cytomegalovirus, ganciclovir and foscarnet, have very different side effect profiles. Ganciclovir's major side effect is the lowering of white blood cells, a condition known as **neutropenia**. Because of this, a patient on ganciclovir should have their white blood cell count monitored closely. Foscarnet, while generally not causing a marked decrease in white blood cells, can cause sudden kidney failure. Patients who are taking foscarnet should make sure they maintain their fluid intake and have their kidney functions monitored closely.

Interactions

The antiviral drugs used to treat herpes simplex and zoster should be used with caution with other drugs that cause kidney problems. Also, they all interact with probenecid, a medication commonly used to treat gout.

Drug interactions with foscarnet and ganciclovir are more numerous and potentially dangerous. Both, especially foscarnet, must be used with caution with other drugs that cause kidney problems. Both must also be used with caution with other medications that lower seizure thresholds. Patients should notify their physician or consult with their pharmacist prior to starting any over the counter or herbal medications due to the numerous drug interactions that can occur with these agents.

Edward R. Rosick, DO, MPH, MS

Aromatase inhibitors

Definition

Aromatase inhibitors are a class of hormone drugs. They inhibit aromatase, an enzyme that regulates the production of estrogen.

Purpose

The aromatase inhibitors decrease blood and tumor levels of estrogen in postmenopausal women. They are used in the treatment of some types of **breast cancer** in post-menopausal women.

Description

Aromatase inhibitors lower a postmenopausal woman's estrogen levels, thereby preventing the **cancer** cells that are dependent on estrogen from growing.

U.S. brand names

Aromatase inhibitors in the United States include Arimidex, Aromasin, and Femara.

Anastrazole (trade name Arimidex)

Anastrazole is a non-steroidal aromatase inhibitor that lowers blood levels of estradiol to prevent the rapid growth of cancerous cells. It is usually used in postmenopausal women as a treatment for advanced breast cancer that has not responded to other therapies, or it can be used as first-line therapy in breast cancer patients. Anastrazole is also indicated in the treatment of post-menopausal breast cancer which is hormone receptor positive early breast cancer. It is also indicated to treat advanced breast cancer in post-menopausal women whose cancer has progressed following treatment with **tamoxifen.**

Exemestane (trade name Aromasin)

Exemestane is an aromatase inhibitor that reduces the concentration of estradiol in the bloodstream. It is also called an aromatase inactivator because it inactivates aromatase irreversibly, potentially providing continued benefits after treatment is stopped. It is used to treat advanced breast cancers in postmenopausal women whose cancers have not responded to other antiestrogen therapies. It is also indicated in the adjuvant treatment of post-menopausal women with estrogen receptor positive (ER positive) early breast cancer who received 2-3 years of tamoxifen therapy and who are switched to exemestane theapy for a total of five consecutive years of adjuvant hormonal therapy.

Letrozole (trade name Femara)

Letrozole is a non-steroidal aromatase inhibitor that lowers blood estrogen levels by hindering the conversion of androgens to estrogens. Letrozole therapy is prescribed as part of adjuvant treatment for post-menopausal women with hormone receptor positive early breast cancer; as extended adjuvant treatment of early breast cancer in post-menopausal women who have received five years of adjuvant therapy with tamoxifen; and for the first-line treatment of post-menopausal women with hormone receptor positive or unknown, locally advanced or metastatic breast cancer. It is used in postmenopausal women with advanced breast cancer that has progressed while on other antiestrogen therapy.

Recommended dosage

- Anastrazole: The adult dose is 1 mg a day by mouth
- Exemestane: The adult dose is 25 mg a day by mouth, after a meal
- Letrozole: The adult dose is 2.5 mg a day by mouth. Reduction in the dose of letrozole is recommended in women with cirrhosis and severe liver dysfunction.

Precautions

Pregnant or breastfeeding

Aromatase inhibitors are not used in pregnant women because of the risk to the fetus. Since these drugs are generally prescribed for postmenopausal women, pregnancy is not usually an issue.

Except in life-threatening conditions, anastrazole, exemestane, and letrozole are not used in pregnancy because of risks to the fetus. These drugs should be avoided by people allergic to them and by nursing mothers.

Side effects

The aromatase inhibitors are generally tolerated well. Side effects are similar to the effects of decreased estrogen, such as hot flashes. People should report any side effects to the doctor.

Anastrazole

Rash is the most common side effect of anastrazole. Less common side effects include:

- hot flashes
- headache, light-headedness, dizziness, confusion
- depression, insomnia, anxiety
- chest pain, high blood pressure, obstruction of blood vessels
- nausea and vomiting, diarrhea, constipation, abdominal pain
- dry mouth, altered taste, appetite loss
- vaginal bleeding, vulvar itching
- hair thinning
- bone pain, tumor pain, weakness, muscle aches
- cough, sinusitis
- abnormally low red blood cell levels (anemia)
- abnormally low white blood cell counts (leukopenia)

Exemestane

Side effects include:

- hot flashes
- headache, fatigue, insomnia
- depression, anxiety
- high blood pressure
- nausea, vomiting
- increase in appetite
- diarrhea, constipation, abdominal pain
- cough, difficulty breathing

Letrozole

Common side effects include:

- headache
- nausea, vomiting
- lethargy

- appetite loss (anorexia)
- rash, itching

Less common side effects include:

- drowsiness, dizziness
- depression, anxiety
- high blood pressure
- constipation, diarrhea, heartburn
- hair loss
- hot flashes, sweating
- cough, difficulty breathing

Interactions

Patients who are taking any kind of prescription drug, over-the-counter drug, or herbal remedy should notify their physician before beginning any treatment with aromatase inhibitors.

See also Megestrol acetate; Tamoxifen.

Resources

PERIODICALS

Deeks, E.D. & Scott, L.J. "Exemestane: A Review of Its Use in Postmenopausal Women with Breast Cancer." *Drugs* 2009:889–918.

Nabholtz, J.M., et al. "Comparative Review of Anastrzole, Letrozole, and Exemestane in the Management of Early Breast Cancer." *Expert Opin Pharmacother.* 2009:1435–47.

Rhonda Cloos, R.N.
Teresa G. Odle
Melinda Granger Oberleitner, R.N., D.N.S.,
A.P.R.N., C.N.S.

▌Arsenic trioxide

Definition

Arsenic trioxide is an antitumor agent used in the treatment of a specific type of leukemia known as acute promyelocytic leukemia (APL).

Purpose

Arsenic trioxide is used to treat acute promyelocytic leukemia in patients who have not responded to standard treatment or who have relapsed following standard treatment. The drug is indicated for those patients whose APL is characterized by the presence of a specific chromosome translocation, t(15;17), or PML/RAR-alpha gene expression as confirmed by cytogenetic testing.

Description

U.S. brand names

The brand name for arsenic trioxide in the United States is Trisenox.

The exact mechanism of action of arsenic trioxide is not completely known at this time. However, the drug appears to cause damage to the fusion protein PML/RAR alpha, which is a protein present in APL. Once the gene which produces this fusion protein is corrected, the body no longer produces immature malignant myelocytic cells and normal white blood cells are again able to be produced by the body. Once this occurs, cytogenetic complete response to therapy has been achieved.

Arsenic trioxide, like many other antineoplastic (antitumor) agents, acts by interfering with the growth of cells. Unfortunately, these drugs affect the growth of normal cells and tumor cells. In some patients the drug may have to be discontinued because normal cell growth is too severely affected. For example, a patient taking a large dose of arsenic trioxide might see tumor growth stop. However, the dosage might be high enough to also stop the body's normal growth of platelet cells. The loss of platelets might cause severe internal bleeding–a consequence more immediately toxic than the tumor.

Recommended dosage

Doses vary from individual to individual and depend on body weight as well as other medications the patient is taking. The dose to induce remission in acute promyelocytic leukemia for adults and children five years of age and older are up to 60 doses of 0.15 mg/kg of body weight per day until bone marrow remission occurs. Three to six weeks after induction therapy is finished, consolidation therapy with arsenic trioxide is started at a dose of 0.15 mg/kg/d for 25 doses within a period of no more than 5 weeks. This medication is administered intravenously.

Precautions

Pregnant or breastfeeding women

Arsenic trioxide has been shown to cause fetal abnormalities and miscarriage in animals. Women who might become pregnant should take precautions to ensure they do not become pregnant while taking this drug. Women who are nursing their infants should discontinue nursing while this medication is in their system.

Pediatric

There is limited data related to the effectiveness of arsenic trioxide in the treatment of patients under the age of 18. Children younger than five years of age should not be administered this drug as safety and effectiveness of arsenic trioxide in this age group have not been studied.

Recommended blood testing for patients undergoing treatment with arsenic trioxide include monitoring of electrolyte values and complete blood count (CBC) with coagulation profile at least twice per week in the induction phase of therapy. Critically ill patients may require more frequent lab testing. During the consolidation phase of treatment lab studies should be monitored at least weekly. EKG testing should also be conducted prior to the initiation of therapy and at least once every week during active phases of treatment with arsenic trioxide. Monitoring of kidney function will also be done during therapy with this drug.

Patients with bone marrow problems, heart problems, kidney problems, or low levels of magnesium or potassium in the blood should notify their physician before taking any of this medicine. Patients should notify their physician of any illnesses they may have before taking arsenic trioxide.

Because persons taking arsenic trioxide may have decreased immunity, it is important for them to avoid **infection**. Caution should be taken to avoid unnecessary exposure to crowds and people with infections.

Patients may experience unusual or excessive bruising and/or bleeding and should avoid situations in which it is likely they could cut or bruise themselves. Patients should consult their physician immediately if they have any indication of excessive bleeding or bruising, including black and tarry stools, blood in the urine or stools, unusual bleeding or bruising, pinpoint red marks on their skin, vomit containing blood or what appears to be coffee grounds (dried blood). Severe symptoms may indicate a medical emergency.

Side effects

Symptoms such as **fever**, difficulty breathing, weight gain and symptoms related to cardiac and pulmonary side effects may be experienced by some patients during treatment. These symptoms may indicate the occurrence of APL differentiation syndrome and can be fatal if not corrected. Treatment with high dose steroids should be started immediately by the physician and should be continued for at least three days.

Patients should always notify their physician about any unusual symptoms they experience while on this medication.

Interactions

Patients should tell their doctors if they have a known allergic reaction to arsenic trioxide or any other medications or substances, such as foods and preservatives. Before taking any new medications, including nonprescription medications, **vitamins**, and herbal medications, the patients should notify their doctors.

This drug should be administered with caution in patients who are concurrently receiving medications which may cause EKG changes such as a prolonged QT interval or electrolyte abnormalities. These medications include certain antiarrhythmic drugs, the drug thioridazine, diuretic drugs and the drug amphotericin B.

Michael Zuck, Ph.D.
Melinda Granger Oberleitner, R.N., D.N.S.,
A.P.R.N., C.N.S.

Arteriography, Angiogram *see* **Angiography**

Ascites

Description

Ascites is defined as an excessive amount of fluid built up within the peritoneal cavity. Both the abdominal organs and the abdomen itself are lined with membranes called the peritoneum. Between these two linings is a space referred to as the peritoneal cavity. In pathological conditions that result in edema, or excessive fluid accumulation in bodily tissues, fluid can build up in the peritoneal cavity.

Smaller abdominal fluid amounts usually do not produce symptoms. However, larger accumulations can cause:

• rapid weight gain

• abdominal discomfort and distention

• shortness of breath and actual dyspnea, or difficulty breathing

• swollen ankles

Severe cases of ascites can result in the retention of literally gallons (each gallon equals nearly four liters) of liquid in the peritoneal cavity. If fluid retention is sufficiently severe, the abdomen becomes swollen and even painful. Breathing can be affected as the fluid-filled peritoneal cavity presses upon the diaphragm, a very necessary component of respiration. The diaphragm is made up of a dome-shaped sheet of muscles that separates the thoracic, or chest, cavity from the abdomen. When the muscle fibers of the diaphragm contract, the space in the chest cavity is enlarged, and air enters the lungs to fill the enlarged space. When pressure on the diaphragm from fluid build-up occurs, it lessens the ability of these diaphragm muscular fibers to expand and contract, and results in impaired breathing.

Ascites, in itself, is not a disease, but rather a symptom of several other pathological conditions. These include:

• Cirrhosis of the liver, which is responsible for 80% of all instances of ascites in the United States.

• Pancreatic ascites develops when a cyst that has thick, fibrous walls (pseudocyst) bursts and permits pancreatic juices to enter the abdominal cavity.

• Chylous ascites, which has a milky appearance caused by lymph that has leaked into the abdominal cavity. Although chylous ascites is sometimes caused by trauma, abdominal surgery, tuberculosis, or another peritoneal infection, it is usually a symptom of lymphoma or some other cancer.

• Cancer causes 10% of all occurrences of ascites in the United States. It is most commonly a consequence of disease that originates in the peritoneum (peritoneal carcinomatosis) or of cancer that spreads (metastasizes) from another part of the body. Tumors especially prone to malignant ascites formation include ovarian cancer and metastatic gastrointestinal tumors.

• Endocrine and renal ascites are rare disorders. Endocrine ascites, sometimes a symptom of an endocrine system disorder, also affects women who are taking fertility drugs. Renal ascites develops when blood levels of albumin dip below normal. Albumin is the major protein in blood plasma. It functions to keep fluid inside the blood vessels.

Causes

The two most important factors in the production of ascites due to chronic liver disease are low levels of albumin in the blood and an increase in the pressure within the branches of the portal vein that run through liver (portal hypertension). Low levels of albumin in the blood cause a change in the pressure necessary to prevent fluid exchange (osmotic pressure). This change in pressure allows fluid to seep out of the blood vessels. The scarring that occurs in cirrhosis causes portal hypertension. Blood that cannot flow through the liver because of the increased pressure leaks into the abdomen and causes ascites.

Other conditions that contribute to ascites development include:

• hepatitis

• heart or kidney failure

• inflammation and fibrous hardening of the sac that contains the heart (constrictive pericarditis)

Persons who have systemic lupus erythematosus but do not have liver disease or portal hypertension occasionally develop ascites. Depressed thyroid activity sometimes causes pronounced ascites, but inflammation of the pancreas (pancreatitis) rarely causes significant accumulations of fluid.

Treatments

Reclining minimizes the amount of salt the kidneys absorb, so treatment generally starts with bed rest and a low-salt diet. Urine-producing drugs (diuretics) may be prescribed if initial treatment is ineffective. The weight and urinary output of patients using diuretics is normally carefully monitored, often on a daily basis. This scrutiny involves watching for signs of:

• Hypovolemia (massive loss of blood or fluid) that can often result in drastic drops in blood pressure.

• Azotemia (abnormally high blood levels of nitrogen-bearing materials).

• Potassium imbalance that can result in cardiac arrhythmia.

• High sodium concentration. Sodium should be restricted from the diet as much as possible.

Because of the discomfort and respiratory difficulty moderate-to-severe accumulations of fluid can produce, fluid removal, or **paracentesis**, is often the treatment of choice. Paracentesis involves the extraction of fluid from the abdominal cavity via a needle that is usually inserted into the peritoneum under local anesthesia. This is a relatively safe and painless method of relieving fluid build-up. It is considered safer than diuretic therapy, resulting in fewer complications and requiring shorter hospital stays.

Large-volume paracentesis is also the preferred treatment for massive ascites. Diuretics are sometimes used to prevent new fluid accumulations, and the procedure may need to be repeated periodically.

In cases of ascites that do not respond appropriately to the treatments described above, a **peritoneovenous shunt** may be inserted. This device is equipped with a one-way valve that allows fluid from the peritoneal cavity to pass into the venous blood circulatory system. From there the fluid is eliminated by the kidneys. In cases of malignant ascites, there is a concern that the use of such a shunt could enhance the spread of the **cancer**. This relatively small risk must be balanced against the positive effect the shunt can have on the individual's quality of life as well as against his or her expected survival period.

Alternative and complementary therapies

Dietary alterations, focused on reducing salt intake, are an important facet of treatment. Potassium-rich foods like low-fat yogurt, mackerel, cantaloupe, and baked potatoes help balance excess sodium intake and help ensure proper heart function. Such complementary therapies should always be considered an adjunct to, not a substitute for, the conventional treatments described above.

Resources

PERIODICALS

Bieligk, S.C., B.F. Calvo, and D.G. Coit. "Peritoneovenous Shunting for Nongynecologic Malignant Ascites." *Cancer* 91, no. 7 (April 2001): 1247–9.

ORGANIZATIONS

National Cancer Institute, National Institute of Health. 31 Center Drive, MSC 2580, Bethesda, MD 20892-2580. (800) 4-CANCER. http://www.nci.nih.gov.

Joan Schonbeck, R.N.

Asparaginase

Definition

Asparaginase is a medicine used to stop growth of **cancer** and formation of new cancer cells.

Purpose

Asparaginase is used primarily as part of an induction regimen for the treatment of **acute lymphocytic leukemia** (ALL) in children. According to the manufacturer, asparaginase is not recommended for use during the maintenance phase of treatment.

Description

U.S. brand names

Asparaginase, also known as L-asparaginase, is sold under the brand name Elspar in the United States.

Asparaginase is an enzyme made from the bacteria *escherichia coli* (E. coli). In this country, two forms of asparaginase are available: one made from E. coli, and a slightly changed version of the E.Coli form linked to polyethylene glycol (PEG) molecule. This PEG-linked asparaginase is called **pegaspargase**. This version was made available in 1994, is more expensive than the other form, and is used in patients who have developed an allergy to E. Coli. Asparaginase kills cancer cells by depleting a certain protein in the blood (L-asparagine) that is necessary for survival and growth of tumor cells in patients with ALL. Fortunately, normal cells are not dependent on L-asparagine for survival.

Asparaginase is mainly given in combination with **vincristine** and steroids (either prednisone or **dexamethasone**) for the first three weeks of therapy.

Recommended dosage

Adults and children

INDUCTION CHEMOTHERAPY FOR ALL. Doses vary between different **chemotherapy** protocols. The usual dose is 6,000-10,000 units per square meter of body surface area given for 10 days. Patients should refer to individual protocol for recommended dose.

Administration

This medicine can be given directly into the muscle (intramuscular) or into the vein (intravenous). Intramuscular injection of asparaginase lowers the risk of severe allergic reactions (also known as hypersensitivity or anaphylaxis). The risk of hypersensitivity reaction is higher with the second and third dose of the drug.

Precautions

Pregnant or breastfeeding

Breastfeeding mothers should use asparaginase with caution. It is not yet known whether this drug crosses into breast milk. Women who are pregnant or may become pregnant should avoid this drug unless the benefits to the mother outweigh the risks to the child.

The use of this medication should be avoided in patients with active pancreatitis (inflammation of the pancreas) or history of pancreatitis, and in patients with serious allergic reaction to asparaginase in the past.

Asparaginase should only be given in a hospital. A patient's blood pressure will need to be monitored every 15 minutes for the first hour. A small test dose may be given to check if patient is allergic to this medicine.

This medication can lower the body's ability to fight infections. Patients should avoid contact with crowds or any individual that may have an **infection**.

Contact a doctor immediately if any of these symptoms develop:

- fever, chills, sore throat
- yellowing of the skin or eyes
- puffy face, skin rash, trouble breathing, joint pain
- drowsiness, confusion, hallucinations, convulsions
- unusual bleeding or bruising
- stomach pain with nausea, vomiting and loss of appetite

A physician will perform blood tests before starting therapy and during therapy to monitor complete blood count, blood sugar, and pancreas, kidney, and liver functions.

Side effects

Asparaginase is a very potent medicine that can cause serious side effects. An allergic reaction with skin rash, **itching**, joint pain, puffy face, and difficulty breathing can occur very quickly after injection with his drug. This side effect is managed by having the drugs epinephrine, diphenhydramine, and steroids available near the bedside to counter the allergic reaction if it occurs. Other common side effects include **nausea**, **vomiting**, **diarrhea**, loss of appetite, stomach cramps, and yellowing of the eyes or skin. Less frequent side effects include high blood sugar, drowsiness, confusion, hallucinations, convulsions, decreased kidney function, increased blood clotting, mouth sores, and decreased ability to fight infections. Usually the side effects of asparaginase are more severe in adults than in children.

Interactions

Asparaginase can decrease effectiveness of **methotrexate** in killing cancer cells when given right before and together with methotrexate. The use of these two medicines together should be avoided.

Asparaginase can decrease breakdown and increase toxicity of **cyclophosphamide**.

Risk of liver disease may be increased in patients receiving both asparaginase and **mercaptopurine**.

This medicine can increase blood sugar especially when given in together with steroids.

Asparaginase should be given after vincristine instead of before or with vincristine because it can increase the risk of numbing, tingling and pain in hands and feet.

Olga Bessmertny, Pharm.D.
Melinda Granger Oberleitner, R.N., D.N.S.,
A.P.R.N., C.N.S.

Astrocytoma

Definition

Astrocytoma is a tumor that arises from astrocytes, star-shaped cells that play a supportive role in the brain.

Demographics

Astrocytoma is the most common type of brain tumor in children. Astrocytoma usually strikes within the first ten years of life, most commonly between ages

Magnetic resonance image (MRI) of the head and neck of a 15-year-old boy showing the recurrence of an astrocytoma of the spinal cord. The tumor appears about halfway down the neck. *(© Simon Fraser, Neuroradiology Dept., Newcastle General Hospital, Science Source/Photo Researchers, Inc. Reproduced by permission.)*

five and nine. This type of tumor occurs slightly more often in males than in females. It is also slightly more common in Caucasians than in those of African or Asian descent. Although it affects both adults and children, children usually develop a less serious form with a better prognosis. The annual incidence of astrocytomas, is approximately 14 newly diagnosed cases out of every million children under the age of 15 years.

Description

The brain acts as a computer that controls all of the functions of the body. It stores information, memories, and with the use of hormones and electrical impulses, regulates and sends instructions to the rest of the body. Because of the brain's importance, cancers in the brain can affect many of the body's functions. The location of a tumor within the brain determines which effects it will have. Astrocytomas may occur in the cerebrum, the site of thought and language, the cerebellum, the area responsible for movement and muscle co-ordination, or the brainstem, the location that regulates critical activities like breathing and heartbeat. Childhood astrocytomas are most commonly located in the cerebellum, while adults usually develop astrocytoma in the cerebrum.

Astrocytomas rarely metastasize (spread) outside the brain to other parts of the body; however, they may grow and spread within the brain. As there is no extra room in the skull, the presence of a brain tumor causes an increase in intracranial (within the skull) pressure, resulting in headaches and possibly affecting normal brain function by compressing delicate brain tissue.

Astrocytomas are a type of glioma, a tumor of glial cells (specialized cells that give physical support and electrical insulation between neurons). They are sometimes called gliomas, anaplastic astrocytomas, or glioblastoma multiforme. Oligoastrocytomas are a type of mixed glioma similar to astrocytomas. They usually contain cells that originate from oligodendrocytes as well as astrocytes, and are usually low grade (grading is an estimate of the tumor's malignancy and aggressiveness; lower-grade tumors require less drastic therapy than high-grade tumors).

Causes and symptoms

The cause of astrocytoma is not known. Brain **cancer** may occasionally be caused by previous radiation treatments; however, **x rays** are not believed to play a role. As of 2001, studies indicated that the moderate use of handheld cellular phones does not cause brain cancer; ongoing research will determine if long-term cellular phone use causes an increase in cancer incidence.

Some studies suggest that **brain tumors** may occur more frequently in people who have occupational exposure to certain chemicals, including some pesticides, formaldehyde, vinyl chloride, phenols, acrylonitrile, N-nitroso compounds, polycyclic aromatic hydrocarbons, lubricating oils, and organic solvents. The greatest risk is associated with exposure before birth or during infancy.

There is a slightly higher incidence of astrocytoma in the siblings and parents of people with this tumor; however, only one type of astrocytoma is known to have a genetic cause. The rare subependymal giant cell astrocytoma occurs in conjunction with tuberous sclerosis, a hereditary disorder.

A wide variety of symptoms develop as a result of astrocytoma including the following:

- headache
- nausea and vomiting
- neck stiffness or pain
- dizziness
- seizures
- unsteadiness in walking or unusual gait
- lack of coordination, decreased muscle control
- visual problems such as blurring, double vision, or loss of peripheral vision
- weakness in arms or legs
- speech impairment

• altered behavior
• loss of appetite

Because there are several different types of astrocytoma, not all patients will show the same symptoms. The location of the tumor within the brain will determine which symptoms a patient will experience. Because the tumor causes an increase in intracranial pressure, most people with astrocytoma will develop headaches and **nausea and vomiting**.

Diagnosis

In the first stage of diagnosis the doctor will take a history of symptoms and perform a basic neurological exam, including an eye exam and tests of vision, balance, coordination and mental status. The doctor will then require a computerized tomography (CT) scan and **magnetic resonance imaging** (MRI) of the patient's brain. During a CT scan, x rays of the patient's brain are taken from many different directions; these are combined by a computer, producing a cross-sectional image of the brain. For an MRI, the patient relaxes in a tunnel-like instrument while the brain is subjected to changes of magnetic field. An image is produced based on the behavior of the brain's water molecules in response to the magnetic fields. A special dye may be injected into a vein before these scans to provide contrast and make tumors easier to identify.

If a tumor is found it will be necessary for a neurosurgeon to perform a **biopsy** on it. This simply involves the removal of a small amount of tumor tissue, which is then sent to a neuropathologist for examination and staging. The biopsy may take place before surgical removal of the tumor or the sample may be taken during surgery. Staging of the tumor sample is a method of classification that helps the doctor to determine the severity of the astrocytoma and to decide on the best treatment options. The neuropathologist stages the tumor by looking for atypical cells, the growth of new blood vessels, and for indicators of cell division called mitotic figures.

Treatment

Treatment team

Treatment of astrocytoma will involve a neurosurgeon to remove the tumor, a neuropathologist to examine the tumor sample, and an oncologist to monitor the patient's health and coordinate **radiation therapy** and **chemotherapy** if necessary. Nurses and radiation therapists will also play a role. After treatment, the patient may be followed up by a neurologist to ensure that the tumor does not grow or recur.

There are several different systems for staging astrocytomas. The World Health Organization (WHO) system is the most common; it has four grades of increasing severity based on the appearance of the astrocytoma cells. Other methods of staging correspond fairly closely to the WHO system. Grades I and II are sometimes grouped together and referred to as low-grade astrocytomas. Over time, tumors may progress from a low-grade form with a relatively good prognosis to a higher-grade form and poorer prognosis. Additionally, tumors may recur at a higher grade.

Grade I Pilocytic Astrocytoma

This is also sometimes referred to as juvenile astrocytoma because it occurs more frequently in children than adults. Under a microscope, the astrocytes are thin and elongated, and known as pilocytes. They are accompanied by Rosenthal fibers. The tumor mass does not invade surrounding tissues and is sometimes enclosed in a cyst. In children, pilocytic astrocytoma often occurs in the cerebellum, but may also occur in the cerebrum.

Treatment of this grade depends on the patient's age and the location of the tumor. Surgery is the preferred treatment for this type of astrocytoma; it is performed by a procedure known as a **craniotomy**. An incision is made in the skin and an opening is made in the skull. After the tumor is removed, the bone is normally replaced and the incision closed. The neurosurgeon may also insert a shunt (drainage system) to relieve intracranial pressure; this involves inserting a catheter into a cavity inside the brain called a ventricle, then threading the other end under the skin to a drainage area where the fluid is absorbed.

If the tumor can be completely surgically removed, the patient may not need further therapy and may be monitored only for recurrence. If the tumor cannot be completely removed, patients may be given chemotherapy as well. If the tumor is not completely resected or if it continues to grow after chemotherapy, radiation therapy may be necessary. Radiation therapy is not normally given to children under the age of three in order to prevent permanent damage to the child's healthy brain tissue. Radiation treatment may cause swelling in the brain; steroids may be prescribed to reduce the swelling.

The best indicator for prognosis is complete removal of the tumor. With complete tumor removal, 80% of patients are alive ten years later. Location of the tumor in the cerebellum also suggests a better prognosis than other locations.

Grade II Low-Grade Diffuse Astrocytoma

These astrocytomas spread out and invade surrounding brain tissues but grow very slowly. Under the microscope, fibrous structures are present. Grade II astrocytomas may occur anywhere in the brain, in the cerebellum and brain stem, or in the cerebrum, including the optic pathways. Genetic studies indicate that mutations of the tumor suppressor gene p53 occur frequently in these tumors.

Surgical removal of the tumor is the first choice for treatment, but it may not be possible due the tumor's location. Surgery is usually followed by radiation. Patients under 35 years of age have a better prognosis than older patients; in older patients, low-grade tumors progress to higher grades more rapidly. Overall median survival is four to five years.

Pleimorphic xanthoastrocytoma, a tumor originating in cells of a mixture of glial and neuronal origin, is often considered a grade II astrocytoma. It is relatively benign and treated only with surgery.

Grade III Anaplastic Astrocytoma

Anaplastic astrocytoma occurs most frequently in people aged 50 to 60. The term anaplastic means that the cells are not differentiated; they have the appearance of immature cells and cannot perform their proper functions. Researchers believe this is due to a gradual accumulation of genetic alterations in these cells. These tumor cells invade surrounding healthy brain tissue.

Anaplastic astrocytomas may be inoperable because of their location and their infiltration into normal tissue; in this case radiation therapy is recommended. Chemotherapy may include various combinations of alkylating agents and other drugs, including **carmustine**, **cisplatin**, **lomustine**, **procarbazine** and **vincristine**. These tumors tend to recur more frequently than grade I and II tumors. Following treatment, median survival is 12 to 18 months. The five-year survival rate for these patients is approximately 10% to 35%.

Grade IV Glioblastoma Multiforme

Glioblastoma Multiforme (GBM) is the most common primary brain tumor in adults. These tumors aggressively invade adjacent tissue and may even spread throughout the central nervous system. They frequently occur in the frontal lobes of the cerebrum. Tumor biopsies may show large areas of necrosis, or dead cells, surrounded by areas of rampant growth. There may also be a mixture of cell types within the biopsy. Genetic studies show that a number of different types of mutations can take place in genes for tumor suppressor p53 and other proteins that play a role in controlling the normal growth of cells.

Often GBM cannot be entirely surgically removed because it affects large areas of the brain. Radiation therapy will be given regardless of whether surgery is possible, except to very young children. Conventional radiation may be performed, but more specialized types, such as stereotactic radiosurgery, which uses imaging and a computer to treat the tumor very precisely, or interstitial radiation, which delivers radiation by placing radioactive material directly on the tumor, may also be used. Chemotherapy will follow radiation; it may include carmustine, lomustine, procarbazine, and vincristine.

GBM is most common in patients over 50 years of age and rarely occurs in patients under 30. Increasing age is associated with a poorer prognosis. Median survival is 9 to 11 months following treatment. Fewer than 5% of patients are alive five years later. Because of the poor prognosis of GBM, it is treated more aggressively than low-grade astrocytomas; many **clinical trials** take place to test new treatments.

Alternative and complementary therapies

While no specific alternative therapies have become popular for this particular type of brain cancer, patients interested in pursuing complementary therapies should discuss the idea with their doctor. A doctor may be able to provide information about the efficacy of certain techniques and whether they may interfere with conventional treatment.

Coping with cancer treatment

Patients may experience unpleasant side effects due to their treatment. Patients should discuss any side effects they experience with their doctors; occasionally an effect may be unexpected or dangerous and dosages may need to be adjusted. Doctors can help alleviate **nausea** with antinausea medications and may prescribe antidepressants to help the patient deal with the cancer on a psychological level. Joining support groups will also help patients deal with the psychological effects of treatment. Cancer survivors can help provide encouragement and offer advice for coping with cancer on a day-to-day basis.

Clinical trials

Clinical trials are an important treatment possibility, especially for patients with tumors that are inoperable or do not respond well to treatment. Participation in clinical trials also gives patients an opportunity to make contributions to the search to find a cure for their cancer. A wide variety of clinical trials are available, particularly for the higher-grade astrocytomas. Trials for higher-grade astrocytomas may test new drugs, new combinations of drugs, drug implants, and higher doses of drugs, possibly in combination with different methods of radiation therapy. Some studies may examine the use of gene therapy or immune therapy, including **vaccines**.

Trials for lower-grade astrocytomas focus on finding chemotherapy that causes fewer side effects. Some studies may also feature new combinations of drugs while others may attempt to treat the tumor by using lower dosages of drugs spread out over a longer period of time.

Prevention

Currently, scientists do not know what causes the majority of brain cancers. There may be a slight genetic predisposition, as family members of astrocytoma patients have a slightly increased incidence of the disease. Clinical studies show that a large number of genetic alterations take place in the higher grade astrocytomas; although this helps to explain what is going wrong in the cells, it does not explain what is causing these genetic mutations to take place.

While it is known that ionizing radiation can cause brain tumors, most people are not exposed to this type of radiation unless they are being treated for cancer. Ongoing studies are examining the long-term risks of other types of radiation, but as of 2001, neither x rays, electromagnetic fields, or cellular phones appear to increase the likelihood of brain cancers.

Although evidence is not yet conclusive, some studies suggest that some brain tumors may be caused by environmental exposure to certain organic chemicals. Exposure is most harmful to the developing fetus and infants, so pregnant women may wish to consider whether they have any occupational exposure to organic chemicals. Parents of infants should be aware of pesticides and any other potentially harmful chemical their child could come into contact with.

Additionally there is some evidence that supplements containing **vitamins** A, C, E, and folate may have a protective effect when taken during pregnancy. The children of women who take these supplements during pregnancy are half as likely to develop brain tumors before age five.

Special concerns

Children who develop astrocytoma should be monitored regularly by their physicians to ensure

---

QUESTIONS TO ASK THE DOCTOR

- Where inside my brain is the cancer located and where will it spread?
- What types of treatment are recommended?
- What are the possible side effects of this treatment?
- How can the side effects be minimized?
- Am I eligible for any clinical trials?
- Are there any alternatives to this treatment?
- What are the chances that the cancer will return?
- Will this cause any disabilities?
- How will this affect my daily life?

---

that the tumor does not recur. A follow-up schedule should be discussed with the doctor; the child may be examined twice a year initially, then tested annually afterwards. In addition to the possibility of recurrence, other health problems due to treatment may arise in the child. The child may have lower levels of growth hormone or thyroid hormone or delayed growth as a result of radiation. There may also be decreased intellectual capacity or learning or physical disabilities that can be detected during follow-up. Parents can then arrange for rehabilitation or special education for their child.

Adults may also experience permanent negative effects as a result of their treatment. Radiation damage to healthy tissue may occasionally cause delayed effects such as decreased intellect, impaired memory, changes in personality, and confusion. These types of side effects should be reported to a health professional; the patient can be referred to rehabilitation specialists who can help with regaining abilities.

See also Brain and central nervous system tumors; Childhood cancers; Tumor grading.

Resources

BOOKS

Abeloff, MD et al. *Clinical Oncology*. 3rd ed. Philadelphia: Elsevier, 2004.

Behrman RE, et al. *Nelson Textbook of Pediatrics*. 17th ed. Philadelphia: Saunders, 2004.

Goetz, CG. *Goetz's Textbook of Clinical Neurology*. 3rd ed. Philadelphia: Saunders, 2007.

ORGANIZATIONS

American Brain Tumor Association. 2720 River Rd., Des Plaines, IL 60018. (800) 886-2282. http://www.abta.org.

The Brain Tumor Society. 124 Watertown St., Suite 3-H, Watertown, MA 02472. (800) 770-8287. http://www.tbts.org.

National Brain Tumor Foundation. 414 13th St., Suite 700, Oakland, CA 94612-2603. (800) 934-2873. http://www.braintumor.org.

OTHER

BRAINTMR T.H.E. Brain Trust. Electronic mailing list. [cited June 22, 2001]. http://www.braintrust.org.

Racquel Baert, M.S.

ATG, anti-thymocyte globulin *see* **Lymphocyte immune globulin**

Atropine *see* **Antidiarrheal agents**

Axillary dissection

Definition

Axillary dissection is a surgical procedure that incises (opens) the armpit (axilla or axillary) to identify, examine, or remove lymph nodes (small glands, part of the lymphatic system, which filters cellular fluids).

Purpose

Axillary dissection is utilized to stage **breast cancer** in order to determine the necessity of further treatment based on **cancer** cell spread. Additionally, axillary dissection includes removal and pathological examination of axillary lymph nodes for persons having operable breast cancer. The anatomy of the axilla is complex and composed of several critical nerves, arteries, and muscles. Because of this complex anatomy and connection with the breast, the axilla is a common route for possible metastatic (cancer cell spread to distant areas within the body) involvement from breast cancer. The absence or presence of cancer cells in axillary lymph nodes is the most power prognostic (outcome) indicator for breast cancer. Axillary dissection is an accurate procedure for axillary node assessment (removal and pathological examination). Clinical examination of the breast (more specifically palpation, or feeling the affected area for lumps) for the axillary region is inaccurate and unreliable. The only method to identify whether or not a lymph node has cancer cells, is to surgically remove the node and perform examination with a microscope to detect abnormal cancer cells.

Demographics

If axillary dissection is not performed, recurrence of cancer in the armpit is common even after breast surgery. Recent evidence suggests that persons who underwent **lumpectomy** alone without axillary dissection had a 10-year average recurrence rate of 28% in the axilla. Generally, recent evidence also suggests that the more nodes and tissues removed in the axilla, the lower the risk of recurrence of cancer. Research also indicates that 10-year axillary cancer recurrence rates are low (10% for node negative and 3% for node positive) for women who have **mastectomy** and axillary node removal. The recurrence rate for breast cancer is approximately 17% for women who did not have axillary node removal.

Description

Lymph nodes (or lymph glands) are filtering centers for the lymphatic system (a system of vessels that collects fluids from cells for filtration and reentry into the blood). Additionally, there is a complex arrangement of muscles, tissues, nerves and blood vessels. Axillary dissection is surgically explained in terms of three levels. Level I axillary dissection is also called lower axillary dissection because it is the removal of all tissue below the axillary vein and extending to the side where the axillary vein crosses the tendon of a muscle called the latissimus dorsi. Level II dissection is continuous—it includes the removal of level tissues and further extensive removal of cancerous tissues. Level II dissection removes diseased tissues deeper in the middle (medial) area of another muscle called the pectoralis minor. Level III dissection is the most aggressive breast cancer axillary surgery, and it entails the removal of all nodal tissue (tissues related to the lymphatic system) from the axilla.

Diagnosis/Preparation

Operable breast cancer is the primary indication for axillary dissection. Persons receiving this surgery have been diagnosed with breast cancer and are undergoing surgical removal of the breast. Diagnosis of breast cancer typically involves palpation of a lump (mass), and other tests such as **mammography** (special type of x ray used to visualize deep into breast tissues) and **biopsy**. The specific diagnosis to estimate the extent of axillary (cancerous) involvement can be made by performing a sentinel node biopsy. The sentinel node is the first lymph node that drains fluid from the primary tumor site. If there is no presence of cancerous cells in the sentinel node, the likelihood that higher echelon lymph nodes have cancer is very small. Conversely, if cancerous cells are detected in the sentinel node, then axillary dissection is recommended.

Preparation for axillary dissection is the same as that for **modified radical mastectomy**. This includes but is not limited to preoperative assessments (special tests and blood analysis), patient education, postoperative care, and follow-up consultations with surgeon and cancer specialist (medical hematologist/oncologist). Psychotherapy and/or community-centered support group meetings may also be beneficial to treatment.

Aftercare

One of the major problems that can result from axillary lymph node removal is lymphedema (fluid accumulation in the arm). Postoperative aftercare should include the use of compression garments, pneumatic compression pumps, and massage to combat fluid retention. Additionally, persons may have pain and should discuss this with the attending surgeon. Other surgical measures for aftercare should be followed similar to persons receiving a modified radical mastectomy. Skin care is important and caution should be exercised to avoid cuts, bites, and skin infections in the affected area. Further measures to control lymphedema can include arm exercises and maintenance of normal weight.

Risks

There are several direct risks associated with axillary surgery. A recent study indicated that approximately 31% of persons may have numbness and tingling of the hand and 10% develop carpal tunnel syndrome. In females who have had a previous breast surgery before the axillary surgery, recurrent wound infections and progression of lymphedema can occur. Additionally, persons may also feel tightness and heaviness in the arm as a result of lymphedema.

Normal results

Normal results can include limited but controlled lymphedema and adequate wound healing. Persons receiving axillary dissection due to breast cancer require several weeks of postoperative recovery to regain full strength.

Morbidity and mortality rates

Sickness and/or death are not necessarily related to axillary surgery per se. Rather, breast cancer outcome is related to breast cancer staging. Staging determined by axillary surgery can yield valuable

WHO PERFORMS THE PROCEDURE AND WHERE IS IT PERFORMED?

The procedure is performed in a hospital equipped to perform major surgery. A general surgeon usually performs the operation with specialized formal training in surgical oncology (the specialty of surgery that provides surgical treatment for operable cancers).

QUESTIONS TO ASK THE DOCTOR

- How do I prepare for the procedure?
- How long does it take to know the results?
- What postoperative care will be needed?
- What are the possible risks involved in this procedure?

information concerning disease progression. Early stage (stage I) breast cancer usually has a better outcome, whereas advance stage cancer (stage 4) is correlated with a 10-year survival rate.

Alternatives

Currently research does not support other therapies. Further study is required but other therapies are currently not recommended. There are no adequate alternatives to axillary surgery in breast cancer persons. The most recent evidence suggests that removal of lymph nodes and tissues in the armpit is correlated with elevated survival rates.

Resources

BOOKS

Hanna, L., Crosby, T., and Macbeth, F. *Practical Clinical Oncology.* 1st ed. Cambridge, UK: Cambridge University Press., 2008.

Noble, J. *Textbook of Primary Care Medicine.* 3rd ed. St. Louis, MO: Mosby, Inc., 2001.

Townsend, C., Beauchamp, D., Evers, B., and Mattox, K. *Sabiston Textbook of Surgery.* 18th ed. St. Louis: W. B. Saunders Company, 2007.

PERIODICALS

Cantin, J., H. Scarth, M. Levine, and M. Hugi. "Clinical practice guidelines for the care and treatment of breast cancer." *Canadian Medical Association Journal* 165 (July 24, 2001).

Fiorica, James. "Prevention and Treatment of Breast Cancer." *Obstetrics and Gynecology Clinics* 28 (December 2001).

Hugi,M. R., I. A. Olivotto, and S. R. Harris. "Clinical practice guidelines for the care and treatment of breast cancer:11.Lymphedema." *Canadian Medical Association Journal* 164 (January 23,2001).

ORGANIZATIONS

American Cancer Society. (800) ACS-2345. http://www.cancer.org.

Y-ME National Breast Cancer Organization. 212 W. Van Buren, Suite 500 Chicago, IL 60607. (312) 986-8338. Fax: (312) 294-8597. (800) 221-2141 (English). (800) 986-9505 (Español). <http://http://www.y-me.org.

OTHER

Cancernews. [cited May 15, 2003]. http://www.cancernews.com.

Laith Farid Gulli, MD, MS
Nicole Mallory, MS, PA-C
Bilal Nasser, MD, MS
Laura Jean Cataldo, RN, EdD

Azacitidine

Definition

Azacitidine, is an antineoplastic (antitumor) agent that acts by interfering with the growth of cells.

Purpose

Azacitidine is a **chemotherapy** drug used primarily to treat adults and children with acute myelocytic leukemia that has not responded to traditional therapy. It is also used to treat **myelodysplastic syndrome**. There is limited data that azacitidine may be useful for chronic myelogenous leukemia, sickle cell **anemia**, and cancers that have spread to other organs in the body. It should also be noted that azacitidine does not appear on the FDA's approved drug list. Currently, azacitidine is prescribed only as an experimental drug.

Description

DNA can be thought of as the blueprint for the cell, and RNA as the messenger to carry out the instructions of the DNA. RNA, or ribonucleic acid, is a close relative of DNA, deoxyribonucleic acid. Both are made up of four different bases, adenine, guanine, cytosine, and thymine. Azacitidine pretends to be cytosine, and is incorporated into the RNA and

DNA of cells, inhibiting them from carrying out their normal functions and causing cell death.

Recommended dosage

The dose of azacitidine depends on the reason it is being administered and whether any other drugs are involved in treatment. The usual dose for azacitidine is 50 to 200 mg per square meter of body surface area per day for five to 10 days. This is repeated at two to three week intervals. Azacitidine is administered either through the vein or injected under the skin. It may be injected under the skin at a dose of 75 mg per square meter of body surface area per day for seven days, to be repeated every 4 weeks.

Precautions

Pregnant women should not take this drug, and should be aware that this drug has been shown to cause death or abnormality in the fetuses of laboratory animals. Women who might become pregnant while taking this medication should take steps to ensure that they do not. Nursing mothers should discontinue nursing while taking this medication. All patients should have this drug administered by a health care professional and their progress regularly monitored.

Side effects

The most common side effect of azacitidine is the decreased production of white blood cells, which are important in fighting infections, and platelets, which are important in preventing bleeding. **Nausea, vomiting**, and **diarrhea** are also very common with this drug.

Other side effects include **fever**, general muscle pain, weakness, and lethargy. Decreased liver function, low blood pressure, and changes in kidney function have also been reported with azacitidine. Also, injections of the drug under the skin can cause redness, swelling, or mild pain.

Interactions

Azacitidine has no known interactions with other drugs. However, prior to initiating any over-the-counter, herbal, or new medications, patients should consult their physician, nurse, or pharmacist to prevent possible drug interactions.

Michael Zuck, Ph.D.

Azathioprine

Definition

Azathioprine is a nonspecific immunosuppressant antimetabolite that can be used as a chemotherapeutic agent to inhibit lymphocyte purine metabolism. In the United States, azathioprine is also known by the brand name Imuran.

Purpose

In 1968 the Food and Drug Administration approved azathioprine for use after organ transplantation to decrease the chance of the body rejecting the transplanted organ. Azathioprine, however, is also an experimental drug that can be used during treatment of such cancers as leukemia and **lymphoma**. In the body, azathioprine is converted to **mercaptopurine** (6-MP) and thus has the same effects as that **chemotherapy** drug. They both are purine analogs that interfere with the metabolism of purine-based nucleotides found in DNA.

The use of azathioprine results in killing cells such as T-lymphocytes. This effect is important in treating such cancers as lymphocytic leukemia. The idea is that if T-lymphocyte reproduction is inhibited by interfering with DNA synthesis, then the cancer cell reproduction will also be inhibited. Certain types of leukemia and lymphoma are treated with radiation and chemotherapy, which destroy dividing cells such as those in the bone marrow. As a result, the patient is no longer able to produce blood cells. To combat the loss of blood cells, a bone marrow transplant may be performed to provide the patient with healthy marrow. The body may react against the foreign bone marrow. Therefore, an additional benefit of azathioprine use as an immunosuppressant could be to produce fewer white blood cells, thus interfering with the body's natural **immune response** to foreign proteins, such as those found on the cell surfaces of bone marrow coming from a bone marrow donor.

Because azathioprine has anti-inflammatory action, it is also used to treat such disorders of the digestive tract as irritable bowel disease (IBD) as well as the vasculitides, which are a group of disorders characterized by inflammation of blood or lymphatic vessels.

Description

Azathioprine is a derivative of mercaptopurine, a purine analog antimetabolite, which interferes with the enzymatic pathways for biosynthesis of nucleic

KEY TERMS

Analog—A chemical compound with a structure similar to another chemical, but differing in a certain way.

Antimetabolite—A drug that resembles a substance that occurs naturally in a metabolic pathway, interfering with metabolism.

Bone marrow—The soft tissue inside of bones that produces blood cells.

Gout—A form of arthritis that involves ureic acid.

Leukopenia—Decrease in the amount of white blood cells.

Lymphocytes—A type of white blood cell and part of the immune system.

Macrocytic anemia—Anemia where blood cells are much larger than normal.

Myelosuppression—Decrease in the proliferation of bone marrow cells.

Pancytopenia—Decrease in all the cellular components of the blood.

Purine—A base found in nucleotides and nucleic acids that are used to make DNA.

Vasculitis (plural, vasculitides)—Inflammation of blood or lymphatic vessels.

acids by substituting for normal metabolites. In this way, it can act as an immunosuppressant by interfering with the production of white blood cells such as lymphocytes.

Recommended dosage

Azathioprine can be taken either orally (50 milligram scored tablets) or through an injection (100 milligram vials for intravenous use). Dosing is based on body weight and size of the patient. Initially, the oral dosage is approximately 3 to 5 milligrams per kilogram of body weight, while the injection dosage is approximately 1 milligram per kilogram of body weight. At time goes on, the physician may decrease the dosage. Patients can take this medicine in a single dose per day. The duration of treatment will continue until the fear of transplant rejection has passed.

Precautions

Since this medication is an immunosuppressant and results in a lower white blood cell count, there is a higher risk of developing **infection**. Therefore, patients using azathioprine should limit their contact with people that have existing infections, they should not have dental work done while on this medication, and they should not touch their eyes or inside of their nose unless they have just washed their hands. Patients should also take care not to cut themselves and should be careful when using a regular toothbrush and dental floss.

Although some early studies performed in animals stated that azathioprine should not be used during pregnancy, two groups of researchers in Italy and Canada respectively reported in 2004 that the drug has a very small potential for harm to the fetus. Moreover, although azathioprine can cross into breast milk, there is no evidence that the small amounts absorbed by a nursing infant are harmful.

Side effects

The most common and less serious side effects include **fatigue**, weakness, loss of appetite (**anorexia**), **nausea and vomiting**, and upset stomach. Upset stomach can be alleviated if azathioprine is taken with food or milk.

Other side effects may occur that require the attention of a medical professional. These include:

- cough or hoarseness
- fever or chills
- lower back or side pain
- extreme fatigue
- black tarry stools
- blood in the urine
- red spots on the skin
- fast heartbeat
- shortness of breath
- liver problems

Since the immune system is depressed when azathioprine is used, the result can be pancytopenia, including leukopenia and **thrombocytopenia** as well as macrocytic **anemia**. The severity of these is dependent on the dose, and the dose may be lowered by the physician as needed.

Azathioprine has been used in children and has not been shown to induce side effects different from those found in adults. However, as with many medications there have not been any specific tests done with the elderly. It is not expected to cause any different side effects from those encountered in younger adults.

Interactions

There are medications and other medical conditions that can interact with azathioprine. A medication called **allopurinol** is used to treat gout and can increase the effects and toxicity of azathioprine because it interferes with the removal of azathioprine from the body.

Both kidney disease and liver disease can increase the effects and toxicity of azathioprine. Both diseases interfere with the removal of azathioprine from the body. If the patient has either of these diseases, the physician may make adjustments in the dosage given.

Resources

BOOKS

Beers, Mark H., MD, and Robert Berkow, MD, editors. "Transplantation." In *The Merck Manual of Diagnosis and Therapy*. Whitehouse Station, NJ: Merck Research Laboratories, 2007.

Wilson, Billie Ann, Margaret T. Shannon, and Carolyn L. Stang. *Nurse's Drug Guide 2003*. Upper Saddle River, NJ: Prentice Hall, 2003.

PERIODICALS

Danesi, R., and M. Del Tacca. "Teratogenesis and Immunosuppressive Treatment." *Transplantation Proceedings* 36 (April 2004): 705–707.

Moskovitz, D. N., C. Bodian, M. L. Chapman, et al. "The Effect on the Fetus of Medications Used to Treat Pregnant Inflammatory Bowel-Disease Patients." *American Journal of Gastroenterology* 99 (April 2004): 656–661.

Russell, J. P., and R. H. Weenig. "Primary Cutaneous Small Vessel Vasculitis." *Current Treatment Options in Cardiovascular Medicine* 6 (April 2004): 139–149.

Su, C., and G. R. Lichtenstein. "Treatment of Inflammatory Bowel Disease with Azathioprine and 6-Mercaptopurine." *Gastroenterology Clinics of North America* 33 (June 2004): 209–234.

Younger, D. S. "Vasculitis of the Nervous System." *Current Opinion in Neurology* 17 (June 2004): 317–336.

ORGANIZATIONS

American Society of Health-System Pharmacists (ASHP). 7272 Wisconsin Avenue, Bethesda, MD 20814. (301) 657-3000. www.ashp.org.

United States Food and Drug Administration (FDA). 5600 Fishers Lane, Rockville, MD 20857-0001. (888) INFO-FDA. www.fda.gov.

Sally C. McFarlane-Parrott
Rebecca J. Frey, PhD

Aztreonam *see* **Antibiotics**

B

Bacillus Calmette Guérin

Definition

Bacillus Calmette Guérin, or BCG, is a genetically engineered bacterium that is used to treat **bladder cancer**. BCG also is known by the brand names ImmuCys, TheraCys and TICE BCG.

Purpose

Excision (cutting out) of bladder tumors can lead to extreme discomfort in patients because of the damage done to the bladder, the organ that collects and holds urine until it can be released from the body. In certain kinds of bladder cancers, treatment with BCG seems to cause cancers to shrink or disappear. Thus, when BCG treatment is effective, it is possible to preserve the bladder.

Description

BCG is made by altering the DNA, or hereditary material, of a bacterium. The bacterium that is altered is one that has been used for decades to vaccinate against tuberculosis. There are several different ways in which BCG has been modified by genetic engineering. In each case, however, the DNA added to the BCG from human cells gives instructions for the production of compounds that stimulate the immune system. The compounds are all proteins and are known by the scientific category name of cytokines.

Even BCG that has not been modified by genetic engineering seems to reduce the growth of superficial tumors in the bladder. But when the BCG introduced to the bladder contains DNA that gives instructions for cytokines, the tumor-fighting ability it confers on the organ is greater.

The live BCG is put inside the bladder where it causes an inflammatory response. This means that the bladder responds as though an **infection** were present

and mounts an attack from the body's immune system. Somehow the response inhibits, or stops, tumor growth, but the way it does so is not understood.

Recommended dosage

BCG is delivered directly to the bladder via a catheter, or a tube that is inserted in the urethra. The method of delivery is called intravesical, which means it is sent directly into the cavity, or holding space, of the bladder.

The patient takes treatment once a week for six weeks and then once a month for six to twelve months. Large quantities of BCG are used. One standard dose of TheraCys calls for 81 milligrams in the first series of treatments.

Precautions

Care providers who have an immune system that is not functioning optimally should not handle BCG. Patients with HIV are at high risk for infection from BCG. All materials from BCG administration are considered biohazards.

Side effects

Most side effects fall into the category of flu-like symptoms and include chills, **fever**, and **nausea and vomiting**. There is also discomfort related to the inflammation of the bladder, particularly the feeling of an urgent need to urinate.

In a very few individuals BCG has spread throughout the body and caused infection and death. A form of **pneumonia** is a rare but possible side effect, and is treatable.

Interactions

Antibiotics, or drugs given to fight infection, can stop the activity of the BCG and should not be given at the same time. Chemicals that suppress the immune system can also interfere with the action of BCG, as can **radiation therapy**.

Resources

PERIODICALS

"Eosiniphilic Pneumonia Is a Risk in Calmette-Guerin Therapy for Bladder Cancer." *Gastroenterology Week* December 15, 2003: 8.

ORGANIZATIONS

American Cancer Society. 1599 Clifton Rd., NE, Atlanta, GA 30329-4251. (800) 227-2345. http://www.cancer.org.
American Foundation for Urologic Disease. 300 W. Pratt St., Suite 401. Baltimore, MD 21201. Phone: (800) 828-7866.

Diane M. Calabrese

Barium enema

Definition

A barium enema, also known as a lower GI (gastrointestinal) exam, is a diagnostic test using x-ray examination to view the large intestine (colon and rectum). There are two types of this test: the single-contrast technique, in which barium sulfate solution is injected into the rectum to gain a profile view of the large intestine; and the double-contrast (or air contrast) technique, in which air and barium sulfate are injected into the rectum.

Purpose

A barium enema may be performed to assist in diagnosing or detecting:

X ray of sigmoid colon after implementation of a barium enema. *(Custom Medical Stock Photo. Reproduced by permission.)*

- colon or rectal cancer (colorectal cancer)
- inflammatory diseases such as ulcerative colitis
- polyps (small benign growths in the tissue lining of the colon and rectum)
- diverticula (pouches pushing out from the colon)
- structural changes in the large intestine

The double-contrast barium enema is more accurate than the single-contrast technique for detecting small polyps or tumors, early inflammatory disease, and bleeding caused by ulcers because it gives a better view of the intestinal walls.

The decision to perform a barium enema is based on the patient's history of altered bowel habits. These alterations may include **diarrhea**, constipation, lower abdominal pain, blood, mucus or pus in the stool. It is also recommended that this exam be used every five to 10 years beginning at age 50 to screen healthy people for **colon cancer**, the second most deadly type of **cancer** in the United States. Those who have a close relative with colon cancer or who have had a precancerous polyp are considered to be at an increased risk for the disease and should be screened more frequently to detect abnormalities.

Precautions

Although the barium enema is an effective screening method and may lead to a timely diagnosis of a variety of gastrointestinal diseases, the test may not detect all abnormalities present in the colon and rectum. In addition, the barium enema visualizes only the large intestine; the small intestine may also require examination with an **upper GI series** to rule out abnormalities in that area of the digestive tract. Another drawback is that intestinal gas may hinder the accuracy of test results.

Numerous studies have shown that a **colonoscopy** performed by an experienced gastroenterologist is a more accurate initial diagnostic tool for detecting early signs of colorectal cancer than a barium enema. Colonoscopy allows a physician to examine the entire colon and rectum for polyps. In addition, if abnormalities such as polyps are observed during the procedure, these often-precancerous growths may be removed during the procedure and later examined (**biopsy**). However, a colonoscopy almost always involves conscious sedation, while the barium enema is an unsedated procedure.

Some physicians use flexible **sigmoidoscopy** (proctosigmoidoscopy) plus a barium enema instead of colonoscopy. However, sigmoidoscopy only visualizes the rectum and the portion of the colon immediately above it (sigmoid colon) and does not allow the physician to remove polyps but only to obtain tissue or stool samples. In 2009, debate continued on the use of virtual colonoscopy to replace colonoscopy and perhaps barium enema for colon and **rectal cancer** screening. Virtual colonoscopy refers to the use of imaging, usually with **computed tomography** (CT) scans or **magnetic resonance imaging** (MRI) to produce images of the colon. Studies showed that virtual colonoscopy was as effective as colonoscopy for screening purposes and

it offered the advantage of being less invasive and less risky. However, many physicians were unwilling to accept it as a replacement for colonoscopy, particularly since some patients might still require the regular colonoscopy as a follow-up to the virtual procedure if a polyp or abnormality is found that requires biopsy. Studies have shown virtual colonoscopy uses less radiation that barium enema and may be more beneficial for use in children in particular. As of late 2009, the American Cancer Society still recommended a barium enema examination every five years as part of regular colon cancer screening for people over age 50.

Description

To begin a barium enema, the patient lies flat on his or her back on a tilting radiographic table in order to have **x rays** of the abdomen taken. After being assisted to a different position, a well-lubricated rectal tube is inserted through the anus. This tube allows the physician or assistant to slowly administer the barium sulfate into the intestine. While this filling process is closely monitored, it is important for the patient to keep the anus tightly contracted against the rectal tube to help maintain its position and prevent the barium from leaking. This step is important because the test may be inaccurate if the barium leaks. A rectal balloon may also be inflated to help retain the barium. The table may be tilted or the patient moved to different positions to aid in the filling process.

As the barium fills the intestine, x rays of the abdomen are taken to distinguish significant findings. There are many ways to perform a barium enema. One way is that shortly after filling, the rectal tube is removed and the patient expels as much of the barium as possible. Upon completing this expulsion, an additional x ray is taken, and a double-contrast enema exam may follow. If this procedure is done immediately, a thin film of barium will remain in the intestine, and air is then slowly injected to expand the bowel lumen (space in the intestine). Sometimes no x rays will be taken until after the air is injected. The entire test takes about 20-30 minutes.

Preparation

In order to conduct the most accurate barium enema test, the large intestine must be empty. Thus, patients must follow a prescribed diet and bowel preparation instructions prior to the test. This preparation commonly includes restricted intake of dairy products and a liquid diet for 24 hours prior to the test, in addition to drinking large amounts of water or clear liquids 12 to 24 hours before the test. Patients may also be given **laxatives** and asked to give themselves a cleansing enema.

In addition to the prescribed diet and bowel preparation prior to the test, the patient can expect the following during a barium enema:

- The patient will be well draped with a gown and secured to a tilting x-ray table.
- As the barium or air is injected into the intestine, the patient may experience cramping pains or the urge to defecate.
- The patient will be instructed to take slow, deep breaths through the mouth to ease any discomfort.

Aftercare

Patients should follow several steps immediately after undergoing a barium enema, including:

- Drinking plenty of fluids to help counteract the dehydrating effects of bowel preparation and the test.
- Taking time to rest because a barium enema and the bowel preparation taken before it can be exhausting.
- Administering a cleansing enema may help to eliminate any remaining barium. The patient may have light-colored stools for 24 to 72 hours following the exam.

Risks

Although a barium enema generally is considered a safe **screening test**, it can cause complications in certain people. For example, patients with a rapid heart rate, severe ulcerative colitis, toxic megacolon (acute dilation of the colon that may progress to rupture), or a presumed perforation in the intestine should not undergo a barium enema. Patients with a known blocked intestine, diverticulitis, or severe bloody diarrhea may be tested with caution on the advice of a physician. Also, administering a barium enema to a pregnant woman is not advisable because of radiation exposure to the fetus.

Although the barium enema may cause minor stomach or abdominal discomfort in some people, more serious complications include:

- severe cramping
- nausea and vomiting
- perforation of the colon
- water intoxication
- barium granulomas (inflamed nodules)
- allergic reactions

These complications, however, are all very rare.

Normal results

When the patient undergoes a single-contrast enema, the intestine is steadily filled with barium to differentiate the colon's markings. A normal result displays uniform filling of the colon. As the barium is expelled, the intestinal walls collapse. A normal result on the x ray after the barium is expelled shows an intestinal lining with a standard, feathery appearance and no abnormalities.

The double-contrast enema expands the intestine, which is already lined with a thin layer of barium; however, the addition of air displays a detailed image of the mucosal pattern. Varying positions taken by the patient allow the barium to collect on the dependent walls of the intestine by way of gravity.

Abnormal results

A barium enema visualizes abnormalities appearing on a series of x rays, thus aiding in the diagnosis of a variety of gastrointestinal disorders and the early signs of cancer. However, most colon cancers occur in the rectosigmoid region, or upper part of the rectum and adjoining portion of the sigmoid colon, and are better detected with flexible sigmoidoscopy or colonoscopy.

Abnormal findings on a barium enema examination may include polyps, lesions or tumors, diverticula, inflammatory disease, such as ulcerative colitis, obstructions, or hernias. Structural changes in the intestine, gastroenteritis, and the size, position, and motility of the appendix may also be apparent.

Resources

BOOKS

Fischbach, Frances Talaska. *A Manual of Laboratory and Diagnostic Tests.* 6th ed. Philadelphia: Lippincott Williams and Wilkins, 2000.

PERIODICALS

Fletcher, Robert H. "The End of Barium Enemas?" *The New England Journal of Medicine* 342 (June 15, 2000): 1823–1824.

Mahoney, Diana. "Virtual Colonoscopy Finds Lesions Fast: High Sensitivity, Specificity." *Pediatric News* January 2004: 39–41.

"Professional Organization Recommends Standard Colonoscopy Over Virtual." *Biotech Week* December 31, 2003: 422.

"Study Shows Virtual Colonoscopy as Effective as Traditional Colonoscopy." *Biotech Week* December 31, 2003.

Winawer, Sidney J., Edward T. Stewart, Ann Zauber, et al. "A Comparison of Colonoscopy and Double-Contrast Barium Enema for Surveillance After Polypectomy." *The New England Journal of Medicine* 342 (June 15, 2000): 1766–1772.

Zoorob, Roger, Russell Anderson, Charles Cefalu, and Modamed Sidari. "Cancer Screening Guidelines." *American Family Physician* 63 (March 15, 2001): 1101–1112.

ORGANIZATIONS

American Cancer Society. 1599 Clifton Road, NE, Atlanta, GA 30329-4251. Phone: 1-800-ACS-2345. http://www.cancer.org.

American College of Gastroenterology. 4900 B South 31st Street, Arlington, VA 22206. Phone: 703-820-7400. Health Hotline: 1-800-978-7666. http://www.acg.gi.org.

American College of Radiology. http://www.acr.org.

Beth Kapes

Barrett's esophagus

Definition

Barrett's esophagus is pre-cancerous condition in which normal cells lining the esophagus are replaced with abnormal cells that, in some people, develop into a type of **cancer** of the esophagus called **adenocarcinoma**.

Endoscopic view of a mid-esophageal stricture in a patient with Barrett's esophagus. *(Custom Medical Stock Photo. Reproduced by permission.)*

Description

The esophagus is a tube 10–13 inches (25–33 cm) long and about 1 inch (2.5 cm) wide that carries food from the mouth to the stomach. Normally, the esophagus is lined with squamous epithelial cells. These cells are similar to skin cells, and look smooth and pinkish-white.

The stomach makes acid to help digest food. A different type of cell that is resistant to acid lines the stomach. These cells look red and velvety. At the place where the esophagus meets the stomach, there is a ring of muscle called the lower esophageal sphincter (LES) muscle that normally keeps acid stomach juices from backflowing into the esophagus. When this sphincter is not working correctly, due to a hiatal hernia, medications, or loss of muscle tone, acid material enters the bottom portion of the esophagus. This backflow is called reflux. When reflux occurs frequently over an extended period of time, it is called gastroesophageal reflux disease (GERD).

Acid and digestive enzymes from the stomach irritate the cells lining the esophagus. The result is inflammation of the esophagus called esophagitis, or heartburn. When the cells lining the lower esophagus are frequently exposed to stomach juices, they erode and are replaced with abnormal cells. These new cells are more resistant to stomach acids and, while they look similar to the cells lining the stomach, they are different. Under the microscope, they appear as a precancerous type of cell not normally found in the body.

These new, pre-malignant cells are called specialized columnar cells. Once specialized columnar cells appear, even if the GERD is controlled and the esophagus heals, the abnormal cells remain and are not

QUESTIONS TO ASK THE DOCTOR

- How would you characterize the changes in the cells in my esophagus?
- What kind of drugs will you prescribe to control my reflux?
- What frequency of endoscopic monitoring do you propose?
- What are the chances of my Barrett's esophagus progressing to adenocarcinoma?
- If high-grade dysplasia is present, where can I get a second opinion?
- If high-grade dysplasia is present, what is involved in a esophagectomy?
- What is daily life like after an esophagectomy?
- Where can I find out more about clinical trials using drugs and light from a laser (called endoscopic laser photablation) to treat adenocarcinoma?
- What changes in my lifestyle can I make to help control my reflux?
- If my GERD cannot be controlled with medication, what is involved in surgery to control reflux?
- Are there any particular signs or symptoms that suggest that I should see a doctor immediately rather than waiting until my next scheduled endoscopy?

replaced with normal cells. The presence of patches of these abnormal red cells in the esophagus is known as Barrett's esophagus. The condition is named after British surgeon Norman Barrett (1903–1979).

Cancer that develops from Barrett's esophagus is called adenocarcinoma. It is one of two types of cancer of the esophagus. This type of cancer cannot occur unless the normal cells lining the esophagus have been damaged and replaced with abnormal cells.

Heartburn is an extremely common complaint. About 10% of people in the United States, or more than 20 million Americans, experience severe or frequent symptoms. Of those people who have frequent heartburn for five years or more, 10–20% develop Barrett's esophagus. From this group, approximately 5–10% go on to develop cancer. Overall, people with Barrett's esophagus have a 30- to 125-fold higher risk of developing adenocarcinoma than the general population.

Demographics

White men over age 45 who experience frequent heartburn for more than 10 years are at highest risk of developing adenocarcinoma arising from Barrett's esophagus. Adenocarcinoma is one of the most rapidly increasing types of cancer in the United States and Western Europe. Often, when the esophagus is damaged by stomach acid, the lining at the entrance to the stomach becomes thick and hard and the opening of the esophagus into the stomach narrows (stricture). People with strictures appear to be at higher risk of developing Barrett's esophagus than other people with GERD. Barrett's esophagus is rare in children.

Causes and symptoms

Barrett's esophagus is caused by gastroesophageal reflux disease that allows the stomach's contents to damage the cells lining the lower esophagus. However, every person who has GERD does not develop Barrett's esophagus. Researchers have thus far been unable to predict which people who have heartburn will develop Barrett's esophagus. While there is no relationship between the severity of heartburn and the development of Barrett's esophagus, there is a relationship between chronic heartburn and the development of Barrett's esophagus. Sometimes people with Barrett's esophagus will have no heartburn symptoms at all. In rare cases, damage to the esophagus may be caused by swallowing a corrosive substance such as lye.

The change from normal to pre-malignant cells that indicates Barrett's esophagus does not cause any particular symptoms. However, warning signs that should not be ignored include:

- frequent and long-standing heartburn
- trouble swallowing (dysphagia)
- vomiting blood
- pain under the breast bone where the esophagus meets the stomach
- unintentional weight loss because eating is painful

Diagnosis

Tissue biopsies and an endoscopy are used to diagnose Barrett's esophagus. An endoscopy is normally done in a clinic under sedation or light anesthesia. A flexible fiber-optic tube is inserted through the mouth and down into the esophagus, which allows a doctor to observe the lining of the esophagus.

Sometimes the line dividing the esophagus from the stomach is not clear. Many people who have trouble with heartburn have a condition called hiatal hernia. A hiatal hernia is a stretching, or dilation, of the hole of the diaphragm that allows a bit of the stomach to bulge up into the esophagus. Because the abnormal cells that develop with Barrett's esophagus look like the cells that normally line the stomach, simply looking at the esophagus during an endoscopy is often not enough to diagnose Barrett's esophagus.

Depending on what is observed, the doctor will use tiny clips at the end of the endoscope to collect samples of tissue. This is a painless procedure. The samples are sent to the laboratory where they are examined under the microscope. Microscopic findings that abnormal cells have replaced normal cells are the only definitive diagnosis of Barrett's esophagus.

Currently, trials are underway to find alternative ways to recognize abnormal esophageal cells. One trial involves the use of laser-induced spectroscopy to visually pinpoint abnormal cells during endoscopy. This has the advantage of requiring no tissue biopsies, and allows the doctor to make an immediate diagnosis rather than wait several days for laboratory results. The technique, however, is still in the experimental stage and is not part of normal clinical practice.

Treatment team

A gastroenterologist (a specialist in diseases of the digestive system) will diagnose and monitor Barrett's esophagus. Should the pre-malignant cells of Barrett's esophagus develop into adenocarcinoma, an oncologist (cancer specialist) or a cancer surgeon will take over treatment of the cancer.

Clinical staging, treatments, and prognosis

The American College of Gastroenterologists (ACG) recognizes five stages of cellular changes in **biopsy** samples obtained from the esophagus. These are (in increasing severity):

- Negative: No abnormal changes in the cells.
- Indefinite: A few cellular changes; often difficult to distinguish from low-grade dysplasia.
- Low-grade dysplasia: Some signs of cellular abnormality are present.
- High-grade dysplasia: Many signs of cellular abnormality are present.
- Carcinoma: Malignant cells are present.

Treatment and monitoring of Barrett's depends on the results of the biopsies. First-line treatment is aimed at stopping stomach acid from entering the esophagus and giving the lining of the esophagus a chance to heal. Two categories of drugs are used to prevent the stomach from producing acid. Histamine$_2$ blockers include cimetidine (Tagamet), ranitidine (Zantac), and nizatidine (Axid). Proton pump inhibitors include omeprazole (Prilosec) and lansoprazole (Prevacid). Lifetime therapy is usually necessary to control GERD, and higher than normal doses of these drugs may be necessary for people with Barrett's esophagus. Surgery to control GERD is recommended only when these drugs are ineffective or if the patient is unwilling or unable to continue taking them.

Monitoring by endoscopy with biopsies has been the standard approach to Barrett's esophagus. However, there is some debate about the effectiveness of the monitoring in detecting adenocarcinomas and about how cost-effective the monitoring is. Research in this area continues, but ACG guidelines suggest the following monitoring program:

- Negative or indefinite biopsies: At least two follow-up endoscopies and biopsies at two- to three-year intervals.
- Low-grade dysplasia: Endoscopies and biopsies every six months for a year, then every year if low-grade dysplasia continues.

Treatment of high-grade dysplasia is controversial. Diagnosis of high-grade dysplasia requires confirmation by at least one expert pathologist, with two experts' opinions recommended. One treatment choice is surgery to remove the esophagus (esophagectomy). About 40–45% of people who have high-grade dysplasia also have previously undetected adenocarcinoma. The advantage of surgically removing the esophagus is that the cancerous cells are also removed. However, in 2004 physicians emphasized that acid suppression is definitely favored over surgery, as is a new form of surgery called duodenal diversion.

The alternative to surgery is to continue to monitor cellular changes with endoscopies and biopsies every three months. The choice of treatment depends both on the health of the patient and on the patient's preference.

Surgical removal of the esophagus is the only effective way known to treat adenocarcinoma. The survival rate for people who progress from Barrett's esophagus to adenocarcinoma is poor, with fewer than 10% surviving five years. However, the earlier the cancer is detected and the esophagus removed, the greater the chances of survival.

Alternative and complementary therapies

Several non-medical ways to prevent GERD can be used effectively along with drug treatments that block the production of stomach acid. These include:

- raising the head of the bed a few inches on bricks to encourage gravity to keep the stomach contents from rising into the esophagus
- eliminating caffeine, acidic foods such as orange juice, and spicy foods from the diet
- eating smaller, more frequent meals, rather than large meals
- not eating within three hours of going to bed None of these methods have any reported adverse side effects.

Clinical trials

Since adenocarcinoma arising from Barrett's esophagus is one of the fastest-growing cancers in the United States and Europe, it has sparked new research activity concerning more sensitive ways to identify high-grade dysplasia, the best methods of monitoring Barrett's esophagus, and the techniques to remove adenocarcinoma without removing the entire esophagus. One of these **clinical trials** involves using drugs to make cancer cells more sensitive to light, and then using a laser to kill these cells in the esophagus. Another clinical trial involves determining if genetic markers can be used to predict which people with Barrett's esophagus are at risk for developing cancer.

The selection of clinical trials underway changes frequently. Current information on clinical trials in process and where they are being held is available by entering the search term "Barrett's esophagus" at the following Websites:

- National Cancer Institute: http://cancertrials.nci.nih.gov or 1-800-4-CANCER
- National Institutes of Health Clinical Trials: http://clinicaltrials.gov
- Center Watch: A Clinical Trials Listing: http://www.centerwatch.com

Prevention

People cannot get esophageal adenocarcinoma unless the cells lining the esophagus are damaged. Prevention, therefore, involves prompt treatment of GERD. Some studies have found that factors that increase the risk of a person with the Barrett's esophagus condition developing into adenocarcinoma include heavy smoking, being overweight, and a family history of gastric cancer. People with chronic gastroesophageal reflux symptoms, particularly those over age 50, should have a screening upper endoscopy.

Special concerns

People who are diagnosed with Barrett's esophagus should expect to eliminate caffeine from their diet as caffeine stimulates the production of stomach acid. Other foods that may need to be eliminated include citrus fruits and juices, tomatoes, and spicy foods.

People with high-grade dysplasia are faced with the stressful decision of whether to undergo surgical removal of the esophagus and endure the lifestyle changes that loss of the esophagus involves, or whether to proceed with intensive monitoring, realizing that monitoring is not totally effective and that cancer may not always be detected early. People faced with this decision should discuss the matter with their physicians, their loved ones, and support group members to get a balanced picture of how their lives may be changed by their choices.

Resources

BOOKS

Sharma, Prateek, Richard E. Sampliner, and Bradley Marino. *Barrett's Esophagus and Esophageal Adenocarcinoma.* 2nd ed. Boston: Blackwell Science, 2001.

PERIODICALS

D'Eprio, Nancy. "Barrett's Esophagus: Put Guidelines Into Practice." *Patient Care* 33 (September 1999): 73.

Jankowski, Janusz, et. al. "Barrett's Metaplasia." *The Lancet* 356 (December 2000): 2079.

McGarrity, Thomas. "Barrett's Oesophagus: The Continuing Conundrum." *British Medical Journal* 321 (November 2000): 1238.

Morales, Thomas G., and Richard E. Sampliner. "Barrett's Esophagus." *Archives of Internal Medicine.* 159 (July 1999): 1411.

"Researchers Describe Guidelines for Barrett Esophagus Screening." *Biotech Week* April 28, 2004: 606.

"Results of Surgical Treatment of Barrett Esophagus 1980—2003 Are Not Optimal." *Biotech Week* May 19, 2004: 582.

OTHER

Cancerlinksusa. http://cancerlinksusa.com.

OncoLink University of Pennsylvania Cancer Center. http://cancer.med.upenn.edu.

ORGANIZATIONS

American Cancer Society. (800) ACS-2345. http://www.cancer.org.

Tish Davidson, A.M.
Teresa G. Odle

Basal cell carcinoma

Definition

A basal cell **carcinoma** is a **skin cancer** that originates from basal keratinocytes in the top layer of the skin, the epidermis. Sometimes these tumors are called "rodent ulcers."

Demographics

Basal cell carcinomas are most common from middle age until old age. They are more frequent in men than women. These cancers seem to be associated with exposure to ultraviolet light; they tend to develop on sun-exposed areas and are more common in people living near the equator. Those who have lighter skin are more susceptible; fair-haired blonds are more likely to develop tumors than people with darker complexions. In the United States, Caucasians have a 23–39% chance of developing a basal cell carcinoma over a lifetime.

Weakened immunity may also play a role. Those who have had an organ transplanted or who have contracted acquired immune deficiency syndrome (AIDS) are more likely to develop one of these cancers.

Basal cell carcinomas are particularly common among individuals with a rare genetic disease called nevoid basal cell carcinoma syndrome (Gorlin's syndrome). Individuals with this disease can be born with basal cell carcinomas or begin to develop them in childhood. Some have few or no cancers; others have more than 250. These tumors seldom grow much before puberty, but during and after adolescence they can spread rapidly. Other symptoms include small pits in the palms and soles, cysts in the jaw, and other abnormalities in the bones.

A basal cell carcinoma tumor. *(Custom Medical Stock Photo. Reproduced by permission.)*

Description

Basal keratinocytes are unpigmented skin cells found deep in the epidermis, hair follicles, and sweat glands. When they become cancerous, these cells invade the dermis (the layer of skin just below the epidermis) and spread out into the normal skin. They become visible as a small growth or area of change in the skin's appearance. These tumors can appear anywhere on the body, but most become evident on the face and neck.

Most basal cell carcinomas are small tumors that can be cured with simple surgeries. They usually grow quite slowly. However, neglected or aggressive tumors can invade vast amounts of skin. These cancers can also spread along bones, cartilage, muscles, and, more rarely, nerves. Some tumors may eventually reach the eye or brain or become large enough to significantly disfigure the face. These serious consequences are more likely if the tumor lies close to bone and cartilage—for instance, at the corner of the eye. Very few basal cell carcinomas spread to more distant organs; the incidence of metastatic basal cell carcinoma is less than 0.1%. Most that do are very large, deep cancers that have been visible for years.

Causes and symptoms

Basal cell carcinomas are caused by genetic damage to a skin cell. Exposure to ultraviolet light and **x rays**, suppression of the immune system, and genetic factors seem to increase the risk that this will happen. Frequent or severe sunburns during childhood, frequent sunbathing or exposure through tanning beds, occupational exposure to sunlight due to outdoor employment (farming, construction, fishing), treatment of acne using x rays, or exposure to arsenic through drinking well water may all increase a person's risk of developing basal cell carcinoma.

Several types of basal cell carcinomas exist. Nodular basal cell carcinomas are the most common form. These tumors begin as a tiny red or clear bump on the skin. Over time, they develop into a growth with clear or white "pearly" raised edges and, often, a depressed area in the middle. A network of tiny blood vessels usually crisscrosses the surface, and the tumor may bleed repeatedly or crust over. Morpheaform (sclerosing, morpheic) basal cell carcinomas are more difficult to detect. These tumors are usually pale, firm, flat growths that can blend into the normal skin around them. Many look just like a scar. Superficial basal cell carcinomas are flat, red, scaly plaques that can look like psoriasis or eczema. Unlike other basal cell carcinomas, they are usually found on the arms, legs, and torso. Pigmented basal cell carcinomas are brown, black, or blue; they are usually of the nodular type and can look like a **melanoma**.

Some general characteristics of skin cancers include:

- irregular or ragged borders
- non-symmetrical shape
- a change in color
- a size greater than 0.2 inches (6 mm)

Diagnosis

Basal cell carcinomas are usually diagnosed with a skin **biopsy** taken in the doctor's office. This is generally a brief and simple procedure. Biopsy may or may not require numbing of the skin with injection of local anesthetic. A shave biopsy removes a tiny bit of superficial tissue; a punch biopsy removes a slightly larger, deeper sample. The skin biopsy must be sent to a trained pathologist to be analyzed. It may take up to a week for the biopsy results to come back. Sometimes the tumor is removed immediately after the biopsy, before the results are known.

Clinical staging, treatments, and prognosis

Basal cell carcinomas rarely spread into the lymph nodes and internal organs. For this reason, doctors tend not to stage them. If staging is needed, the TNM (tumor, lymph node, and metastases) system is usually used. For basal cell carcinomas, this can be simplified into the following five categories:

- Stage 0: The cancer is very small and has not yet spread from the epidermis to the dermis.
- Stage 1: The cancer is less than 0.8 inches (2 cm) in diameter. No cancer cells can be found in lymph nodes or other internal organs.
- Stage 2: The cancer is more than 0.8 inches (2 cm) in diameter. No cancer cells can be found in lymph nodes or other internal organs.
- Stage 3: Cancer cells have been found either in nearby lymph nodes or in the bone, muscle, or cartilage beneath the skin (or in both locations).
- Stage 4: Cancer cells have been discovered in internal organs, most often the lungs or lymph nodes, that are distant from the skin. A stage four cancer can be any size.

Treatment

Treatment options for non-metastatic, non-staged tumors

For most non-metastatic, non-staged cancers, there may be several treatment options. The recommended treatment depends on the size and type of tumor, its location, and cosmetic considerations. The cure rates for most of the following techniques are approximately 85–95%, but vary with tumor size and other factors. Mohs' micrographic surgery has a five-year cure rate of 96%. Success rates for recurrent tumors are approximately 50% with most techniques and 90% with **Mohs' surgery.**

In conventional surgery, the doctor numbs the area with an injection of local anesthetic, then cuts out the tumor and a small margin of normal skin around it. The wound is closed with a few stitches. One advantage to conventional surgery is that the wound usually heals quickly. Another benefit is that the complete **cancer** can be sent to a pathologist for evaluation. If the skin around the tumor is not completely free of cancer cells, the tumor can be treated again immediately.

Mohs' micrographic surgery is a variation of conventional surgery. In this procedure, the surgeon examines each piece of skin under the microscope as it is removed. If any cancer cells remain, another slice is taken from that area and checked. These steps are repeated until the edges of the wound are clear of tumor cells, then the wound is closed. The advantage to this technique is that all of the visible cancer cells are removed but as much normal skin as possible is spared. Mohs' surgery is often used for larger or higher risk tumors and when cosmetic considerations are important. The main disadvantage is that it takes much longer than conventional surgery and requires a specially trained surgeon.

A laser is sometimes used as a cutting instrument instead of a scalpel. Laser light can also destroy some cancer cells directly. A disadvantage to laser surgery is that the wounds from some lasers heal more slowly than cuts from a scalpel. The advantage is that bleeding is minimal.

In electrodessication and curettage, the physician scoops out the cancer cells with a spoon-shaped instrument called a curette. After most of the tumor is gone, the remaining cancerous tissue is destroyed with heat from an electrical current. The wound is left open to heal like an abrasion. It leaks fluid, crusts over, and heals during the next two to six weeks. This is a safe and easy method for removing many basal cell carcinomas. One disadvantage is that there is no skin sample to confirm that the tumor is completely gone. The electrical current used during this surgery can interfere with some pacemakers and larger tumors may heal with a noticeable scar.

In cryosurgery, liquid nitrogen is used to freeze the tumor and destroy it. This treatment is another type of blind destruction; there is no skin sample to make sure the cancer cells have all been killed. Patients report swelling and pain after cryosurgery, and a wound appears a few days later where the cells were destroyed. When the site heals, it has usually lost its normal pigment. There is a risk of nerve damage with this technique.

Radiation therapy is an uncommon treatment for basal cell carcinoma. One disadvantage is the inconvenience: multiple treatments, over a period of weeks, are necessary. Tumors that return after radiation also tend to grow more quickly than the original cancer. In addition, x rays may promote new skin cancers. Radiation therapy may be an option for patients who cannot undergo even minor surgery. It is also used occasionally as an adjunct to surgery. One advantage is that the cosmetic results can be very good.

Occasionally a lotion containing **fluorouracil** is applied to the tumor. This drug cannot penetrate very far and cancer cells in the deeper parts of the tumor may not be destroyed. The main advantage to this treatment is its simplicity.

Treatment options for metastatic cancers

Cancers that have spread to internal organs are treated with a combination of surgery, radiation, and **chemotherapy**.

Special concerns

Because many basal cell carcinomas are found on the face and neck, cosmetic concerns are a priority for many patients. If there is a risk of noticeable scarring or damage, a patient may wish to ask about alternative types of removal or inquire about the services of a plastic surgeon.

After treatment, it is important to return to the doctor periodically to check for regrowth or new skin cancers. Approximately 36% of all patients find a new basal cell or squamous cell carcinoma within the next five years. Having a basal cell carcinoma before the age of 60 may also increase the chance of developing other cancers in internal organs.

Prognosis

The prognosis for small, uncomplicated basal cell carcinomas is very good. The vast majority of these tumors can be successfully removed. However, cancers that were not completely destroyed may regrow. If the edges of the removed skin contain cancer cells, the chance that the tumor will return within the next five years is about 40%. Regrowth is more likely with cancers larger than 0.8 inches (2 cm), those on the face (particularly around the nose, eye, and ear), and higher risk types such as morpheaform tumors. Tumors can redevelop in the scar from the surgery, on the edges of the surgery site, or deep in the skin. These cancers may not look like the original tumor. Patients should be particularly watchful for minor changes in the appearance of the scar or sores that appear nearby.

Cancers that metastasize spread most often to the lymph nodes and lungs. The prognosis for metastatic cancers is poor, even with treatment. Survival after spread of the cancer to internal organs is eight months on the average and seldom more than a year and a half.

Prevention

The risk factors for basal cell carcinoma include:

- ethnic background
- complexion
- geographic location
- increasing age
- exposure to x rays and ultraviolet light (both UVA and UVB)
- a history of premalignant skin lesions or skin cancer
- genetic disorders such as nevoid basal cell carcinoma syndrome, xeroderma pigmentosum, and albinism
- suppression of the immune system by AIDS or an organ transplant

Some important preventive steps include wearing protective clothing and hats in the sun, using a sunscreen, avoiding the sun between 10 A.M. and 4 P.M., and staying away from suntanning booths. Checking the skin for early signs of cancer also is critical.

Drugs related to vitamin A (including beta-carotene, retinol, and isotretinoin), vitamin E, **nonsteroidal anti-inflammatory drugs** (NSAIDS), and selenium have been suggested as possibly preventing basal cell carcinoma. A 2003 study reported that selenium is not effective in preventing basal cell carcinoma and may even increase risk of squamous cell carcinoma.

Resources

BOOKS

Abeloff, MD et al. *Clinical Oncology*. 3rd ed. Philadelphia: Elsevier, 2004.
Habif TP. *Clinical Dermatology*. 4th ed. St. Louis: Mosby, 2004.

OTHER

"Non-Melanoma Staging." *Oncology Channel*. Mar. 2001. [cited June 29, 2009]. http://oncologychannel.com/nonmelanoma/staging.shtml.
"Nonmelanoma Skin Cancer Treatment—Health Professionals." *CancerNet, National Cancer Institute*. Aug. 2000. [cited June 25, 2009].
"Skin Cancer." *CancerLinksUSA*. 1999. [cited June 29, 2009]. http://www.cancerlinksusa.com.

ORGANIZATIONS

Nevoid Basal Cell Carcinoma Syndrome Support Network. 162 Clover Hill Street, Marlboro, MA 01752. (800) 815-4447. souldansur@aol.com.
Skin Cancer Foundation. 245 Fifth Ave., Suite 2402, New York, NY 10016. (212) 725-5176. http://www.skincancer.org.

Anna Rovid Spickler, D.V.M.,Ph.D.
Teresa G. Odle

BCG *see* **Bacillus Calmette Guérin**

BCR-ABL inhibitors

Definition

BCR-ABL inhibitors are a group of **anticancer drugs** that interfere with the actions of a tyrosine kinase protein called BCR-ABL. BCR-ABL inhibitors are also called tyrosine kinase inhibitors (TKIs). The BCR-ABL protein causes hematopoietic stem cells (immature blood cells) to grow and reproduce abnormally so that they are malignant (cancerous). The BCR-ABL protein is active in two types of leukemia.

Purpose

BCR-ABL inhibitors are used to treat chronic myeloid leukemia and Philadelphia positive acute lymphoblastic leukemia (Ph + ALL). Chronic myeloid leukemia (CML), also called chronic myelogenous leukemia, is **cancer** that develops in myeloid cells in the bone marrow and results in the production of abnormal blood cells. These blood cells mature incorrectly or incompletely and live longer than normal so that they slowly build up in the blood, usually over several years, before causing symptoms of CML. Acute lymphoblastic leukemia (ALL), also called **acute lymphocytic leukemia**, is cancer that develops in white blood cells in the bone marrow called lymphocytes. Unlike CML, ALL spreads rapidly through the blood to other organs. BCR-ABL inhibitors are under investigation as a treatment for other cancers as well.

Description

BCR-ABL is not found in normal, healthy cells. It comes into existence because of a non-inherited genetic defect. When cells divide, their chromosomes double and also divide in order for each cell to have a complete set of genetic information. Sometimes during this doubling and division process, material from one chromosome incorrectly gets attached to or exchanged with material from another chromosome. This process is called translocation. CML starts when part of chromosome 9 is exchanged with part of chromosome 22. The resulting abnormal chromosome 22 is known as the Philadelphia chromosome. People who have it are said to be Philadelphia chromosome positive or Ph +. Although it is not clear what factors cause this translocation, almost everyone with CML is Ph + and some people with acute lymphoblastic leukemia are also Ph + (ALL Ph +).

The translocation between chromosomes 9 and 22 forms a new oncogene called bcr-abl on the Philadelphia chromosome. This gene produces a tyrosine kinase protein called BCR-ABL. BCR-ABL causes myeloid cells to become malignant. These malignant cells grow and reproduce abnormally. In people with ALL Ph + lymphocytes a type of white blood cell becomes malignant. BCR-ABL inhibitors interfere with the activities of the BCR-ABL protein and stop the production of cancerous cells while allowing the production of normal blood cells to continue.

Imatinib mesylate (Gleevec) manufactured by Novartis Pharmaceuticals was the first BCR-ABL inhibitor to be developed. The United States Food and Drug Administration approved it for use in treating CML in July 2001. Imatinib rapidly became the standard treatment for CML. The drug works well for most patients, and with it, many patients go into long periods of remission. Imatinib is also approved for treatment of a rare form of cancer called gastrointestinal stromal tumor (GIST).

Although many people respond well to imatinib, some Ph + cancers are resistant to the drug, and some people cannot tolerate the side effects of the drug. Resistance is thought to occur because of variations in the break point where the translocation between chromosome 9 and 22 occurs. This means that all Philadelphia chromosomes are not exactly identical, and some produce a variant of the BCR-ABL protein that is not affected or less affected by imatinib. The search for a TKI drug to that is effective in resistant leukemias has led to the development of the second generation of BCR-ABL inhibitors.

As of October 2009, the FDA has approved two second-generation BCR-ABL inhibitors. **Dasatinib**, manufactured by Bristol-Myers Squibb is sold in the United Sates and the European Union under the brand name of Sprycel. The drug was first given accelerated approval by the United Sates Food and Drug Administration (FDA) on July 28, 2006. After additional data collection and evaluation, it received full FDA approval for treating CML on May 26, 2009.

Nilotinib, manufactured by Novartis Pharmaceuticals is sold in the United Sates and the European Union under the brand name of Tasigna. The United Sates Food and Drug Administration (FDA) first approved nilotinib on October 27. 2007, and the European Union approved it on November 17, 2007. This drug also is approved in the European Union to treat gastrointestinal stromal tumors, a type of digestive system cancer.

Most often an individual with CML or ALL Ph + is treated first with imatinib. If their cancer fails to respond or if they cannot tolerate side effects of imatinib, then they are treated with either dasatinib or nilotinib.

All approved BCR-ABL inhibitors continue to be tested in **clinical trials** for use against other cancers and in combination with other therapies. In addition, several new TKIs are in clinical trials. These include bosutinib (SKI-606) manufactured by Wyeth, INNO-406 manufactured by CtyRx, and saracatnib (AZD 0530) manufactured by AstraZeneca. A list of clinical trials currently enrolling volunteers can be found at http://www.clinicaltrials.gov.

Recommended dosage

Recommended dosage varies with the specific BCR-ABL inhibitor prescribed. Dosage also varies depending on the health status of the patient. Some BCR-ABL inhibitors have requirements about when and how they must be taken. For example, nilotinib is normally taken twice daily at 12-hour intervals and must not be taken with food; nothing may be eaten for at least 2 hours before and one hour after each dose. The safety and effectiveness of all BCR-ABL inhibitors have not been established in children. See individual drug entries and consult a physician or pharmacist for additional information.

Precautions

BCR-ABL drugs have potentially severe and life-threatening side effects. For example, nilotinib carries a black box warning stating that it can prolong a phase of the heart contraction cycle called the QT interval. It should not be used in patients with long QT intervals, and heart monitoring (regular electrocardiograms [ECGs]) must be done while it is being taken.

Precautions and warnings vary somewhat with each drug. See individual drug entries and consult a physician or pharmacist for additional information about specific drugs. Some precautions that generally need to be observed with all BCR-ABL inhibitors are as follows:

- Heart contractions may be altered by prolonging a phase of the heart contraction cycle called the QT interval. Heart monitoring may be necessary. Prolonged QT interval generally requires discontinuation of the drug.
- Severe decrease in the number of normal blood cells (myelosuppression) may occur. Decrease in the number of blood platelets (thrombocytopenia) may reduce the ability of the blood to clot and increase the risk of bleeding episodes. Decrease in the number of neutrophils (neutropenia) may decrease the ability of the body to fight infection. Decrease in the number of red blood cells (anemia) may reduce the ability of the blood to supply oxygen. Blood count should be monitored frequently; dosage may need to be reduced or the drug discontinued.
- Edema (fluid retention) may occur not only in the arms and legs, but also around the heart (pericardial effusion), lungs (pleural effusion), and in the abdomen (ascites). Edema should be monitored and treated as needed.
- The risk of bleeding is increased because of a decrease in platelets. Gastrointestinal bleeding can be severe enough to require transfusion. Bleeding in the brain (intracranial hemorrhage) also may occur.
- The risk of infection is increased because of a decrease in neutrophils. Pneumonia may occur.

- Abnormal blood levels of phosphate, potassium, calcium, and sodium may develop. Electrolytes should be monitored and corrected.

Pregnant or breastfeeding

All BCR-ABL inhibitors described in this entry are pregnancy category D drugs. Woman who are pregnant or who might become pregnant should not use nilotinib. It is not known whether these drugs are excreted in breast milk. Women taking these drug should avoid breastfeeding, as there is the potential for these drugs to cause serious harm to nursing infants.

Side effects

Serious side effects are discussed above in the Precautions section. Common but less serious side effects that may occur include:

- fever
- constipation
- diarrhea
- headache
- skin rash
- fatigue
- nausea

Side effects and their frequency vary somewhat with each drug. See individual drug entries and consult a physician or pharmacist for additional information about specific drugs.

Interactions

BCR-ABL inhibitors interact in a variety of ways with many drugs. A pharmacist or physician must be consulted for information about interactions for the specific drug being taken. All interactions are not known. Patients should provide their doctor and pharmacist with a complete list of all prescription and nonprescription drugs, herbs, and dietary supplements that they are taking.

Resources

PERIODICALS

Weisberg, Ellen, et al. "Second Generation Inhibitors of BCR-ABL for the Treatment of Imatinib-Resistant Chronic Myeloid Leukaemia." *Nature Reviews Cancer* 7 (May 2007) 345–356.

OTHER

Detailed Guide Leukemia, Chronic Myeloid (CML) American Cancer Society. 2009 [October 6, 2009]. http://www.cancer.org/docroot/CRI/CRI_2_3x.asp?rnav = cridg&dt = 83
Leukemia, Adult Chronic. MedlinePlus. September 30, 2009 [October 6, 2009]. http://www.nlm.nih.gov/medlineplus/leukemiaadultchronic.html
Markman, Maurie. Chronic Myeloid Leukemia and BCR-ABL. eMedicine.com. August 20, 2009 [October 7, 2009]. http://emedicine/medscape.com/article/1723784-overview

ORGANIZATIONS

American Cancer Society, 1599 Clifton Rd., NE, Atlanta, GA, 30329, (404) 320-3333, (800) ACS-2345, http://www.cancer.org.
Leukemia & Lymphoma Society, 1311 Mamaroneck Avenue, Suite 310 , White Plains, NY, 10605, (800) 955-4572, http://www.leukemia-lymphoma.org.
National Cancer Institute Public Inquires Office, 6116 Executive Boulevard, Room 3036A, Bethesda, MD, 20892-8322, (800) 4-CANCER. TTY (800) 332-8615, http://www.cancer.gov.

Tish Davidson, A.M.

Bendamustine hydrochloride

Definition

Bendamustine hydrochloride (Treanda) is an alkylating agent used in the treatment of **chronic lymphocytic leukemia** and B-cell non-Hodgkin's **lymphoma**.

Purpose

Bendamustine hydrochloride is used to treat two types of **cancer**: chronic lymphocytic leukemia (CLL) and slow growing (indolent) B-cell non-Hodgkin's lymphoma (NHL). CLL is a cancer of white blood cells called lymphocytes. It develops in the bone marrow and blood. Cancerous (malignant)lymphocytes mature incorrectly or incompletely and live longer than normal so that they build up in the blood, usually over several years, before causing symptoms of CLL. B-cell non-Hodgkin's lymphoma (NHL) is a cancer of B-cells, which are white blood cells that help to fight **infection** by making antibodies. B-cell NHL develops in the lymph nodes and accounts for about 85% of all non-Hodgkin's lymphomas. Bendamustine hydrochloride is used specifically to treat indolent B-cell NHL that has progressed during or within six months of treatment with **rituximab** (Rutixan).

Description

Bendamustine hydrochloride is sold in the United States under the brand name Treanda. Bendamustine is marketed under the brand name Ribomustin in Germany. The United States Food and Drug Administration (FDA) first approved Treanda for the treatment of CLL on March 20, 2008. It was approved for the treatment of B-cell NHL on October 31, 2008. The drug is an alkylating agent that kills cells by binding with and linking deoxyribonucleic acid (DNA) strands. It is effective against both actively dividing and non-dividing (quiescent) cells. The drug is an off-white powder that must be reconstituted with sterile water before use.

Bendamustine hydrochloride continues to be tested in **clinical trials** in the United States for use against other cancers and in combination with other therapies. A list of clinical trials currently enrolling volunteers can be found at http://www.clinicaltrials.gov.

Recommended dosage

Bendamustine hydrochloride is infused intravenously (into a vein). The drug has different dosage regimens for treating CLL and B-cell NHL. For CLL, the standard dosage is 100 mg/m^2 infused over 30 minutes once a day for two consecutive days followed by 26 days when no drug is given. This 28-day cycle is repeated up to six times. For B-cell NHL, the standard dosage is 120 mg/m^2 infused over 60 minutes once a day for two consecutive days followed by 19 days in which no drug is given. This cycle can be repeated up to 8 times.

In both dosage regimens, the dose may be delayed or reduced because of **myelosuppression** and a resulting decrease in red blood cells, platelets, and various types of white blood cells. The dose also may be delayed or reduced if other serious side effects occur. The safety and efficacy of this drug have not been determined in children. Overdosage information is not available.

Precautions

The following precautions should be observed.

- Severe decrease in the number of normal blood cells (myelosuppression) may occur. Decrease in the number of blood platelets (thrombocytopenia) may reduce the ability of the blood to clot and increase the risk of serious bleeding episodes. Decrease in the number of neutrophils (neutropenia) may decrease the ability of the body to fight infection. Decrease in the number of red blood cells (anemia) may reduce the ability of the blood to supply oxygen. Blood count should be monitored frequently. In severe cases, drug administration may need to be delayed or reduced.

- Infection, including pneumonia and systemic infection (sepsis) may occur and be serious enough to require hospitalization. Sepsis has resulted in patient deaths during clinical trials. Patients should immediately report any signs of infection to their physician.

- Infusion reactions are common with bendamustine hydrochloride. Common symptoms include fever, chills, and rash. If a severe infusion reaction occurs, bendamustine hydrochloride should be discontinued. In rare cases anaphylaxis can occur, most often during the second of later cycle. Severe anaphylaxis can result in death. Individuals who are allergic to mannitol (Osmitrol) are at high risk for anaphylaxis and should not be given bendamustine hydrochloride.

- Patients may experience tumor lysis syndrome that results in kidney (renal) failure and, if untreated, death. Blood chemistries should be monitored regularly.

- Serious skin rashes, blistering, itching, and peeling of the skin may occur, especially if bendamustine hydrochloride is given with other drugs.

- Some people using bendamustine hydrochloride in clinical trials have developed other cancers. It is unclear what role, if any, bendamustine hydrochloride played in the development of these malignancies.

Pregnant or breastfeeding

Bendamustine hydrochloride is a pregnancy category D drug. Woman who are pregnant or who might become pregnant should not use bendamustine hydrochloride. It is not known whether the drug is excreted in breast milk. Women taking this drug should not breastfeed, as there is the potential for this drug to cause serious harm to the nursing infant.

Side effects

Bendamustine hydrochloride has many potential side effects, the most serious of which are listed above

QUESTIONS TO ASK YOUR PHARMACIST OR DOCTOR

- How long will I need to take this drug before you can tell if it helps for me?
- How often do I have to have blood work and other laboratory tests done to check the effect the drug is having?
- Is this drug safe to take with the other drugs that I am currently taking?
- What side effects should I watch for? When should I call the doctor about them?
- Are there any clinical trials of this drug combined with other therapies that might benefit me?

in Precautions. In addition, the following side effects may occur:

- chest pain
- difficulty breathing
- difficulty swallowing
- fast heartbeat (tachycardia)
- fatigue
- nausea and vomiting
- diarrhea or constipation
- swelling and fluid retention (edema)
- heartburn
- dry mouth or bad taste in mouth
- decreased ability to taste
- loss of appetite and weight loss
- headache
- anxiety
- depression
- insomnia
- bone or joint pain
- sweating or night sweats

Side effects that require immediate medical attention include signs of infection (e.g., chills, **fever**, cough), or signs of an allergic reaction and anaphylaxis (e.g., difficulty breathing, difficulty swallowing, swelling of the face, tongue, ears, lips). Patients should report other side effects to their doctor promptly.

Interactions

All interactions with bendamustine hydrochloride are not known. Patients should provide their doctor and pharmacist with a complete list of all prescription and nonprescription drugs, herbs, and dietary supplements that they are taking before starting this drug.

Bendamustine hydrochloride is thought to interact with certain drugs, especially a group of drugs called fluoroquinolones (the "oxacin" drugs). Drugs interacting with bendamustine hydrochloride include:

- ciprofloxacin (Cipro)
- gemifloxacin (Factive)
- levofloxacin (Levaquin)
- moxifloxacin (Avelox)
- norfloxacin (Noroxin)
- ofloxacin (Floxin)
- cimetidine (Tagamet)
- omeprazole (Prilosec)
- ticlopidine (Ticid)

Since all drug, herb, and supplement interactions are not yet known, patients should check with their doctor or pharmacist for the most up-to-date information.

Resources

OTHER

Detailed Guided Leukemia, Chronic Lymphocytic (CLL). American Cancer Society. 2009 [October 8, 2009]. http://www.cancer.org/docroot/lrn/lrn_0.asp.

Detailed Guide: Lymphoma, Non-Hodgkin Type. American Cancer Society 2009 [October 8, 2009]. http://www.cancer.org/docroot/CRI/CRI_2_3x.asp?dt = 32.

Leukemia, Adult Chronic. MedlinePlus September 30, 2009 [October 8, 2009]. http://www.nlm.nih.gov/medlineplus/leukemiaadultchronic.html.

Lymphoma. MedlinePlus September 30, 2009 [October 8, 2009]. http://www.nlm.nih.gov/medlineplus/lymphoma.html.

"Oncolink." Abramson Cancer Center of the University of Pennsylvania 2009 [October 8, 2009]. http://www.oncolink.upenn.edu.

ORGANIZATIONS

American Cancer Society, 1599 Clifton Rd., NE, Atlanta, GA, 30329, (404) 320-3333, (800) ACS-2345, http://www.cancer.org.

Leukemia & Lymphoma Society, 1311 Mamaroneck Avenue, Suite 310 , White Plains, NY, 10605, (800) 955-4572, http://www.leukemia-lymphoma.org.

National Cancer Institute Public Inquires Office., 6116 Executive Boulevard, Room 3036A, Bethesda, MD, 20892-8322, (800) 4-CANCER. TTY (800) 332-8615, http://www.cancer.gov.

Tish Davidson, A.M.

Benzodiazepines

Definition

Benzodiazepines are a family of tranquilizers used to treated anxiety and insomnia. In **cancer** patients, it is used primarily to treat **nausea** resulting from **chemotherapy**.

Purpose

Everyone at times feels nervous or anxious. Usually, the feeling is related to something happening in the person's life, such as an upcoming job interview or a speech to a large audience, and it goes away when life returns to normal. This type of anxiety does not need medical treatment. But some people feel anxious almost all the time, or they respond to slightly stressful events with feelings that are out of proportion to the actual situation. The constant anxiety, irrational worries, and sense of impending doom can seriously interfere with their daily lives. For people with such intense or prolonged anxiety, benzodiazepines can help bring their feelings under control and reduce symptoms such as rapid heartbeat, breathing problems, irritability, nausea, and faintness. Benzodiazepines are prescribed for severe general anxiety and for specific anxiety disorders, such as phobias, panic disorder, obsessive-compulsive disorder (OCD), and post-traumatic stress disorder. Physicians may sometimes prescribe these drugs for other conditions, such as sleep disorders, epilepsy, and other seizure disorders. In cancer patients, they are sometimes used to treat people who are overly anxious about their condition, but more commonly, they are prescribed to treat nausea associated with **radiation therapy** and chemotherapy.

Description

Benzodiazepines have a large number of uses, including treatment of panic attacks, treatment of anxiety, short-term treatment of insomnia, control of the symptoms of alcohol withdrawal, including hallucinations, and as skeletal muscle relaxants. In cancer therapy, they are used in combination with other drugs for control of **nausea and vomiting**. In both cancer and surgery, the benzodiazepines may be used to impair memory of unpleasant experiences. This may be particularly useful in some types of cancer therapy where the adverse effects of the treatment may be so severe that patients resist returning for additional courses of therapy. One benzodiazepine (Midazolam) has been useful in induction of anesthesia prior to surgery.

Benzodiazepines, and drugs which are similar to benzodiazepines, have been widely used as sedatives because they are relatively non-toxic. Unlike barbiturates, which were commonly used as sleeping pills, overdoses of the benzodiazepines are almost never fatal.

unfortunately, benzodiazepines are addictive, and so efforts must be made to limit their use whenever possible.

The most common causes of nausea and **vomiting** in cancer patients include treatment with chemotherapy and radiation therapy; tumor spread to the gastrointestinal tract, liver, and brain; constipation; **infection**; and use of some opioid drugs used to treat cancer pain. The mechanisms that control nausea and vomiting are not fully understood, but both are controlled by the central nervous system. The prevention and control of nausea and vomiting are extremely important for patients receiving cancer treatment, particularly chemotherapy (the treatment of cancer with strong chemical agents).

Unrelieved nausea and vomiting may lead to nutritional deficiencies, dehydration, electrolyte imbalances, and a general deterioration of the patient's mental and physical status. The drugs used to treat nausea and vomiting are known as **antiemetics**. Benzodiazepines are valuable tools in the prevention and treatment of nausea and vomiting when given in combination with other antiemetics. They are especially useful in preventing anticipatory nausea and vomiting.

When nausea and vomiting result from chemotherapy administration, the nausea and vomiting can be classified as anticipatory, acute, or delayed. Anticipatory nausea and vomiting occur prior to the actual chemotherapy treatment and is a response primarily to an environmental stimulus, such as a specific odor, which is then associated with the chemotherapy treatment in the future. Acute nausea and vomiting occur within 24 hours of administration of the chemotherapeutic agent.

Delayed nausea and vomiting occur after the acute phase and may last 48 or more hours after chemotherapy administration.

Benzodiazepines may be used in conjunction with antiemetics in the prevention and treatment of anxiety and anticipatory chemotherapy-induced nausea and vomiting. These agents appear to be especially effective in therapy regimens that have a high risk of causing vomiting when given to children. The benzodiazepines have only modest antiemetic properties. Therefore, they are usually used as adjuncts to antiemetic agents.

The family of antianxiety drugs known as benzodiazepines includes alprazolam (Xanax), chlordiazepoxide (Librium), clonazepam (Clonipin), **diazepam** (Valium), and **lorazepam** (Ativan). Benzodiazepines take effect fairly quickly, starting to work within an hour after they are taken. Note that there may be considerable variation between individuals in metabolism of benzodiazepines, so patient response may not be predictable.

As of 2005, there are 13 benzodiazepines in use in the United States, but additional drugs of this type are used in other nations. Although most of these drugs have similar properties, they may be used for different purposes depending on their onset and duration of action.

- Alprazolam (Xanax) is an intermediate acting drug, used both for treatment of anxiety and for panic attacks. Alprazolam has been useful in controlling anxiety that stems from depression.

- Chlordiazepoxide (Librium) is an intermediate acting benzodiazepine which has been used for short-term treatment of anxiety, control of alcohol withdrawal, and control of the anxiety that precedes surgery.

- Clonazepam (Klonopin) has an intermediate onset and relatively long duration of action. It is used to control panic attacks, but most often is used in treatment of seizure disorders. For this purpose, it has been useful in control of some types of seizures that have resisted other types of anti-epileptic medications.

- Clorazepate (Tranxene) is used to treat anxiety disorders, for treatment of alcohol withdrawal, and in combination with other drugs for the treatment of partial seizures.

- Diazepam (Valium) is used to control anxiety, for control of the symptoms of alcohol withdrawal, for relief of the anxiety seen prior to surgical procedures, and as a muscle relaxant. For this purpose it is used to control muscle spasms and as part of the treatment of tetanus. As an anti-convulsant, diazepm is used to treat severe seizures including status epilepticus.

Because diazepam, like other drugs in this class, can impair short-term memory, it is sometimes administered after some medical procedures to blur the effects of an unpleasant experience.

- Estazolam (Pro Som) is used as a sedative in short-term treatment of insomnia.
- Flurazepam (Dalmane) is used as a sedative for short-term treatment of insomnia.
- Lorazepam (Ativan) is used to treat anxiety, including the anxiety associated with depression, for control of resistant seizures, including status epilepticus, and relax surgical patients before administration of anesthesia.
- Midazolam (Versed) is used to relax surgical patients before administration of anesthesia, and, for short surgical or diagnostic procedures, it may be the sole source of anesthesia. The Midazolam package insert has an important warning regarding its use: *Midazolam IV has been associated with respiratory depression and respiratory arrest. In some cases, where this was not recognized promptly and treated effectively, death or hypoxic encephalopathy resulted. Use Midazolam IV only in hospital or ambulatory care settings, including physicians' offices that provide for continuous monitoring of respiratory and cardiac function. Assure immediate availability of resuscitative drugs and equipment and personnel trained in their use.*
- Oxazepam (Serax) is approved for treatment of anxiety disorders and the short-term treatment of anxiety, including anxiety associated with depression. Oxazepam is approved for control of symptoms of alcohol withdrawal and control of anxiety, tension, agitation, and irritability in the elderly.
- Quazepam (Doral) is used for short-term treatment of insomnia.
- Temazepam (Restoril) is used for short-term treatment of insomnia.
- Triazolam (Halcion) is used for the short-term treatment of insomnia.

Although not officially approved for this use, several of the benzodiazepines (chlordiazepoxide, diazepam, clorazepate, lorazepam, oxazepam, and alprazolam) have been used, with some success, in control of irritable bowel syndrome. Alprazolam has been studied for use in treatment of premenstrual syndrome.

Recommended dosage

Benzodiazepine dosage should be individualized to minimize sedation. The normal dose of alprazolam is 0.25–0.5 mg. The usual dose of lorazepam is 2–3 mg. The normal dosage of clonazepam is 0.5–2 mg. The usual dosage range of temazepam (Restoril) is 15–30 mg. Doses may be repeated if necessary.

There can be great differences from person to person in the length of time it takes to remove benzodiazepines from the body. For example, the half-life of diazepam, the length of time it takes to remove half of a single dose of the drug, can range from 20 to 80 hours. In addition, it has an active metabolite, desmethyldiazepam, which has a half-life that ranges from 30 to 200 hours. These differences may be even greater in the elderly. Some benzodiazepines, such as alprazolam, clonazepam, lorazepam, and triazolam, do not have active metabolites, and so their duration of action is easier to predict. Even so, the half lives of these drugs may vary by 100% from one person to the next. Because elderly people normally metabolize drugs at a slower rate than younger patients, careful monitoring and dose adjustments are essential.

Precautions

Prolonged use of benzodiazepines in therapeutic doses can lead to dependence. Withdrawal syndrome has occurred after as little as 4 to 6 weeks treatment. It is more likely if the drug is short acting, taken regularly for over three months and abruptly discontinued. It was once believed that benzodiazepines with a long duration of action, or long lasting metabolites, could not cause withdrawal symptoms because the slow elimination of the drug would act as a form of dose adjustment. This is not true, and all benzodiazepines that have been used for a month or longer should be discontinued by slowly lowering the dose.

Benzodiazepines should not be used in patients with psychosis, acute narrow angle glaucoma, or liver disease. The drugs can act as respiratory depressants and should be avoided in patients with respiratory conditions. Benzodiazepines are potentially addictive and should not be administered to patients with **substance abuse** disorders. Because benzodiazepines are sedatives, they should be avoided in patients who must remain alert. Their use for periods over four months has not been documented. These drugs should not be used during the second and third trimester of pregnancy, although use during the first trimester appears to be safe. They should not be taken by women who are breastfeeding their babies. Parents should consult specialized references for use in children.

Benzodiazepines have long been known to pose serious risks to older people that include impaired thinking, unsteady gait, dizziness, and increased risk of hip fracture. Most of these drugs are cleared from the body more slowly in older adults, thus leading to dangerous accumulation with repeated use.

Patients should never stop taking a benzodiazepine abruptly. Doing so can lead to withdrawal symptoms such as convulsions, tremor, abdominal and muscle cramps, vomiting, and sweating. When it is time to discontinue the medication, the doctor will probably reduce the dosage gradually to avoid withdrawal symptoms. Patients who follow their prescribed medication schedules carefully should have no problems. However, sometimes a patient accidentally takes too much medication, which can result in continuing confusion, severe drowsiness, shakiness, slurred speech, staggering, unusually slow heartbeat, and severe weakness. Anyone experiencing these reactions should seek medical help at once.

When used in patients in whom several different types of seizure disorders coexist, clonazepam may increase the incidence or precipitate the onset of generalized tonic-clonic (grand mal) seizures. This may require the addition of other anticonvulsants or an increase in their dosage.

Side effects

Benzodiazepines are effective in the treatment of anxiety and nausea in cancer patients yet is controversial because of their dependency potential. Benzodiazepines work quickly and have usually few serious side effects. An increased risk of falls and memory impairment, particularly in the elderly, have been noted. Tolerance to their sedative effects develops, but not to their antianxiety properties.

The most common side effects of benzodiazepines include sedation and sleepiness. More rare side effects are:

- depression
- lethargy
- apathy
- fatigue
- hypoactivity
- lightheadedness
- memory impairment
- disorientation
- anterograde amnesia
- restlessness
- confusion
- crying or sobbing
- delirium
- headache
- slurred speech

- aphonia (loss of voice)
- dysarthria
- stupor
- seizures
- coma
- fainting
- rigidity
- tremor
- dystonia
- dizziness
- euphoria
- nervousness
- irritability
- difficulty in concentration
- agitation
- inability to perform complex mental functions
- uncontrollable limb and body movements
- unsteadiness
- lack of coordination
- weakness
- vivid dreams
- psychomotor (bodily movement triggered by mental activity, especially voluntary muscle action)
- retardation
- "glassy-eyed" appearance
- paradoxical reactions such as over-excitability, hallucinations, insomnia, and rage

Other reactions include changes in heart rate and blood pressure, changes in bowel function, severe skin rash and changes affecting the genital and urinary organ functions. Other adverse effects have been reported.

Interactions

The sedating effect of these drugs also can be greatly increased if taken with other drugs that are central nervous system (CNS) depressants, such as antihistamines or other medicines for allergies or colds, sedatives, sleeping medicine, and prescription pain relievers, including narcotics. The metabolism of alprazolam may be increased by: cimetidine, oral contraceptives, disulfiram, fluoxetine, isoniazid, ketoconazole, metoprolol, propoxyphene, propranolol, and valproic acid. The absorption of all benzodiazepines is inhibited by concomitant use of antacids. Benzodiazepines may increase blood levels of digoxin, and reduce the efficacy of levodopa. Other drug interactions have been reported.

It is particularly important to avoid alcohol when taking a benzodiazepine. Alcohol is a powerful central nervous system depressant. Combining large amounts of these two substances can lead to unconsciousness and even death. Use of the ulcer drug cimetidine (Tagamet) along with diazepam or chlordiazepoxide may slow down the metabolism of the anti-anxiety drugs, thus keeping them in the bloodstream longer and prolonging their effects.

Ken R. Wells

Bevacizumab

Definition

Avastin is the trade name for the chemical compound called bevacizumab, an anti-cancer drug. Bevacizumab is in a class of medications known as angiogenesis-inhibitors that block the growth of blood vessels inside tumors, thereby inhibiting their ability to live and grow.

Purpose

Bevacizumab was the first drug of its class used in the United States to treat various types of **cancer**. It is mainly used for metastatic cancer, which is cancer that has traveled from its point of origin to various other parts of the body. The types of metastatic cancer bevacizumab is used to treat include **colon cancer**, some types of lung cancer, and certain breast cancers, all with varying results. Clinical studies are underway to explore possible use for other types of cancer. There are varying opinions and study results in the medical community regarding the effectiveness of bevacizumab in extending survival time of patients treated and in preventing recurrence of the cancer.

Although not approved by the FDA for this purpose, bevacizumab may also be used in diseases of the eye involving abnormal blood vessels. Similar compounds have been developed for this use.

Description

Bevacizumab was the first commercially available drug in its class of anti-cancer drugs, specifically **angiogenesis inhibitors**. It is a humanized monoclonal antibody. The drug was first developed as a genetically engineered version of a mouse antibody that contained components originating from both humans and mice. Bevacizumab binds to and inhibits a growth factor known as vascular endothelial growth factor (VEGF) that is responsible for the formation of tumor blood vessels. It specifically binds to the growth factor target secreted by cancer cells to prevent the process of angiogenesis, tumor blood vessel growth. Once a solid tumor reaches a certain size, it needs blood vessels in order for its cells to remain alive, and to continue to grow. Blood vessels that grow in tumors also contribute to its ability to metastasize to other parts of the body.

Bevacizumab has both cytotoxic and cytostatic effects. Cytotoxic means that the drug is toxic to the cancer cells and hence is able to kill cancer cells. Cytostatic drugs do not kill the cancer cells directly, but rather stop the cancer cells from multiplying and growing further. Bevacizumab has both these functions, resulting in a reduction in tumor growth, increases in median survival time, and increases in time to tumor progression. Median survival time is a term used to describe the time from either diagnosis or treatment at which half of the patients with a given disease are expected to be still alive. In a clinical trial designed to test effects of a cancer drug in humans, median survival time is one way to measure how effective a treatment is. The term time to tumor progression describes a period of time from when disease is diagnosed (or treated) until the disease starts to get worse.

Bevacizumab is produced by Roche/Genentech under the trade name Avastin. It was first approved for use in metastatic colon cancer in 2004, and later for multiple other types of cancer including some types of lung and **breast cancer**. In May 2009, the FDA granted approval for use of bevacizumab as a single chemotherapeutic agent for treatment of a form of brain cancer known as glioblastoma. Glioblastomas are tumors that originate from a type of brain cells known as glial cells, which provide chemical and physical support for the growth of neurons. Bevacizumab is one of multiple drugs that may be used to treat glioblastomas.

Bevacizumab is considered first-line treatment for metastatic colorectal cancer in combination with other chemotherapeutic agents. First-line drug therapy is a term used to describe the drug or combination of drugs that have been evaluated as the most effective treatment for a given disease, and therefore the drug of choice in the absence of factors that would prohibit use of the first-line therapy. There are also preliminary studies that suggest bevacizumab may be a possible treatment for pancreatic, prostate, ovarian, kidney, and liver cancers, as well as for **melanoma** and a form of blood cancer called acute myelogenous leukemia. While bevacizumab is used for colon cancer that has metastasized, a study released in April of 2009 showed that following surgery, bevacizumab is not

KEY TERMS

Acute myelogenous leukemia—Type of cancer of the blood, characterized by the rapid growth of abnormal white blood cells that accumulate in the bone marrow and interfere with the production of normal blood cells.

Angina—Ischemic heart disease that produces chest pain.

Angiogenesis—Physiological process involving the growth of new blood vessels from pre-existing blood vessels, process used by some cancers to create their own blood supply.

Cerebrovascular accident—Terminology that may be used to describe a stroke.

Cytostatic—Inhibiting or suppressing cellular growth and multiplication.

Cytotoxic—Having a toxic effect on cells.

Encephalopathy—Syndrome of global brain disease or injury.

Fistula—Abnormal connection or passageway between two epithelium-lined organs or vessels that normally do not connect.

Glioblastoma—Most aggressive and common type of primary brain tumor.

Humanized monoclonal antibody—Human-like antibodies usually genetically engineered in mice and used in therapeutic manner.

Myocardial infarction—Heart attack.

Pulmonary embolism—Formation in a blood vessel of a clot (thrombus) that breaks loose (embolus) and is carried by the blood stream to plug a vessel in the lungs.

Stroke—Medical condition in which blood flow to a part of the brain is compromised due to blockage of the blood vessel or blood vessel hemorrhage.

Thromboembolic event—Formation in a blood vessel of a clot (thrombus) that breaks loose (embolus) and is carried by the blood stream to plug another vessel, such as in a stroke.

Transient ischemic attack—Changes in the blood supply to a particular area of the brain, resulting in brief neurologic dysfunction that persists less than 24 hours.

VEGF—Vascular endothelial growth factor, chemical compound in the body that contributes to the growth of new blood vessels.

effective at preventing the recurrence of non-metastatic colon cancer.

Bevacizumab is an expensive drug. While it may extend the lifespan of some cancer patients, it does not significantly treat the disease. For this reason, its cost has been criticized by parts of the medical community in light of the perceived value of benefit. Some studies have shown that bevacizumab may increase lifespan by several months at a cost of approximately $40,000 to $50,000, a price that not all cancer patients are able to pay given that it is often not covered by medical insurance companies.

Recommended dosage

Bevacizumab is given intravenously and may be mixed with other chemotherapeutic agents. It may be given to adults for **chemotherapy** in doses of 5–15 mg/kg, usually administered once every 14 days. The dose used varies with the type of cancer, other drugs used in combination with bevacizumab, and the individual's medical history. It may be given in one 90 minute, one 60 minute, and then multiple 30 minute infusions. The dose used does not need to be modified

for patients with mild liver or kidney impairment. While bevacizumab does distribute throughout the body and is cleared from the body differently in male and female patients, studies have shown that doses do not need to be modified based on these factors. Ethnicity does not affect the dose used.

Bevacizumab is not approved for use in children. Patients greater than 65 years of age may experience a higher rate of serious side effects in comparison to younger patients. There are no human studies on the effects of bevacizumab in pregnant women, but animal studies have shown fetal toxicity. In the United States, bevacizumab is listed as a Category C drug. Category C are drugs in which animal reproduction studies have shown an adverse effect on the fetus and there are not adequate studies in humans, however potential benefits to the patient and medical necessity may sometimes warrant use of the drug in pregnant women despite its potential risks.

It is unknown whether or not bevacizumab is excreted in breast milk, but other similar compounds are known to be excreted in this way. The use of bevacizumab in nursing mothers is a clinical decision based on risk and benefits, if the drug is critical enough for the mother a doctor may advise ceasing breastfeeding in order to take bevacizumab.

Precautions

Because bevacizumab interferes with the formation of new blood vessels, it may cause problems for people who have atherosclerosis (blocked blood vessels), coronary artery disease (in blood vessels of the heart), or peripheral artery disease (in blood vessels of the arms or legs). In these disease states, the formation of new blood vessels around the diseased vessels is important for maintenance of blood flow in what is known as collateral circulation. Use of bevacizumab increases the risk of perforation of the nasal septum, the cartilage wall that divides the right and left nostrils of the nose. There have been some cases of bowel perforation, where the wall of the stomach or intestines is broken and its contents leak into the abdominal cavity. Patients who already have a history of bowel perforation may be at risk. Bevacizumab may cause a problem with wound healing after some surgical procedures. The risk of fatal surgical complications is increased in patients taking this drug. For this reason bevacizumab is discontinued for 28 days prior to and after surgical procedures, and until all surgical wounds are healed. Bleeding problems are also reported with this drug and so patients with a history of hemorrhage are at risk. Bevacizumab may not be suitable for use in any of these cases.

In August 2004, the FDA and the Genentech Inc. company issued a drug warning to healthcare providers that there is evidence of an increased risk of serious arterial thromboembolic events. A thromboembolic event is the formation of a clot (thrombus) in a blood vessel, where the clot breaks loose and is carried by the blood to plug another vessel elsewhere in the body. The clot may plug a vessel in the lungs (pulmonary embolism) or in the brain (stroke) causing death. The types of medical complications associated with thromboemboli and use of bevacizumab include cerebrovascular accident, myocardial infarctions, transient ischemic attacks, and angina.

In September 2006, another drug warning was issued stating that there is an increased risk of getting a negative clinical side effect known as reversible posterior **leukoencephalopathy** syndrome (RPLS). RPLS is a rare brain-capillary leaking syndrome associated with high blood pressure, fluid retention, and toxic effects on the lining of blood vessels.

Additionally, in September 2007, a safety labeling update was issued stating that in patients receiving bevacizumab, fistula formation had been reported in parts of the body outside of the gastrointestinal tract,

including the vagina and the bladder. Fistulas are an abnormal connection or passageway that forms between two organs or blood vessels that would not normally be connected. Most of the Bevacizumab-associated fistulas occurred within the first six months of treatment, and made discontinuation of the drug necessary.

Side effects

When used systemically (use to treat cancer as opposed to local use in the eye), bevacizumab is known to cause high blood pressure (hypertension), and increase the risk of bleeding problems. Headache, nosebleeds, alterations of taste, **nausea**, **vomiting**, and dry skin may occur. Infections such as **pneumonia**, catheter infections, and wound infections may occur. There have been some cases of bowel perforation without previous history of such. Other side effects such as myocardial infarction (heart attack), stroke, congestive heart failure, kidney problems, some types of encephalopathy (brain injury) and perforation of the nasal septum have also been reported. When bevacizumab is used directly and applied to the eye it does not significantly enter the rest of the body and most of these side effects are avoided.

Interactions

Patients should make their doctor aware of any and all medications or supplements they are taking before using bevacizumab. Bevacizumab has been combined with multiple other chemotherapeutic agents in **clinical trials** with no clinical problems. However, bevacizumab is known to interact with one other chemotherapy agent called **sunitinib**, causing a severe form of **anemia** known as **hemolytic anemia**.

Resources

BOOKS

Goodman and Gilman's The Pharmacological Basis of Therapeutics, Eleventh Edition. McGraw Hill Medical Publishing Division, 2006.

Tarascon Pharmacopoeia Library Edition. Jones and Bartlett Publishers, 2009.

OTHER

Medscape. "Bevacizumab." <http://www.medscape.com/viewarticle/505771_8.>

RxList. "Bevacizumab." <http://www.rxlist.com.>

ORGANIZATIONS

FDA U.S. Food and Drug Administration. 10903 New Hampshire Ave, Silver Spring, MD 20993. (888)INFO-FDA <http://www.fda.gov/Safety/MedWatch/default.htm.>

National Cancer Institute. 6116 Executive Boulevard, Room 3036A, Bethesda, MD 20892-8322. (800)4-CANCER <http://www.cancer.gov.>

Maria Basile, Ph.D.

Bexarotene

Definition

Bexarotene, also known by the brand name Targretin, is an antitumor agent of the class known as retinoids.

Purpose

Bexarotene is used to treat cutaneous T-cell lymphomas that have not responded to therapy with other drugs commonly used to treat this disease. Cutaneous T-cell lymphomas are characterized by tumors found on the skin and originate from cells of the immune system.

Description

Bexarotene is one of a group of drugs called retinoids, a derivative of vitamin A. Retinoids are involved with the process of stimulating some cells to mature to normal cells, and with inhibiting some cells from growing. It is thought that bexarotene binds to the retinoic acid receptors on cells. This binding ultimately results in the regulation of the growth and maturation of the cells.

Recommended dosage

Doses vary from individual to individual and depend on body weight and other factors. Bexarotene

---

is taken by mouth in capsule form. The initial dose is usually 300 mg per square meter of body surface area per day. The maintenance dose is 300 to 400 mg per square meter of body surface area per day.

Precautions

Pregnant women should not take bexarotene. The risks of fetal abnormality are high, and women should take precautions to ensure they do not become pregnant.

Patients should limit their intake of vitamin A supplements to avoid additive toxic effects with bexarotene, which is a vitamin A derivative. Patients with diabetes and who are receiving insulin or oral medications for their diabetes are usually prescribed bexarotene with caution, and their blood sugar should be frequently monitored. Bexarotene may enhance the effects of the medications for diabetes, and patients may have low blood sugar levels.

Patients taking bexarotene may experience photosensitivity, or increased sensitivity to sunlight. In order to prevent rash, **itching**, or severe sunburn, patients should avoid direct sunlight exposure, avoid sunlamps or tanning beds, use sunblock lotion that is SPF 15 or greater, and wear a lip balm that is SPF 15 or greater. Patients should also wear sunglasses, a hat, and garments covering as much skin as possible when outside.

Side effects

The most common side effects of bexarotene increased levels of triglycerides, cholesterol, and high-density lipoprotein cholesterol. Some patients may require medications to control this rise in lipids. Decreased thyroid function also occurs frequently, and thyroid hormone replacement therapy may be necessary in some patients. Other common side effects include headaches, rash, red and scaly inflammation of the skin, hair loss (**alopecia**), decreased red and white blood cells, and cataracts of the eyes. Patients should have eye examinations if they have any visual difficulties. Patients may be at increased risk of infections due to decreased white blood cells and experience **fatigue** due to decreased red blood cells. Other less common side effects include fluid gain causing swelling of extremities, insomnia, chills, **fever**, **anorexia**, **nausea and vomiting**, abdominal pain, back pain, flu-like symptoms, and dry skin. As with all medications, patients experiencing any of these (or other) side effects should notify their physician.

Interactions

There are an extremely large number of drugs that interact with bexarotene. Patients should consult their physician, nurse, or pharmacist about any medications they are taking before beginning a course of Bexarotene. Many physicians recommend bringing the containers with the names of all the drugs the patient is taking to their appointment with the physician.

Michael Zuck, Ph.D.

Bicalutamide *see* **Antiandrogens**

Bile duct cancer

Definition

Bile duct **cancer**, or cholangiocarcinoma, is a malignant tumor of the bile ducts within the liver (intrahepatic), or leading from the liver to the small intestine (extrahepatic). It is a rare tumor with poor outcome for most patients.

Cancer of the bile duct. (© Biophoto Associates, Science Source/Photo Researchers, Inc. Reproduced by permission.)

Description

Bile is a substance manufactured by the liver that aids in the digestion of food. Bile ducts are channels that carry the bile from the liver to the small intestine. Like the tributaries of a river, the small bile ducts in the liver converge into two large bile ducts called the left and right hepatic ducts. These exit the liver and join to form the common hepatic duct. The gallbladder, which concentrates and stores the bile, empties into the common hepatic duct to form the common bile duct. Finally, this large duct connects to the small intestine where the bile can help digest food. Collectively, this network of bile ducts is called the biliary tract.

Bile duct cancer originates from the cells that line the inner surface of the bile ducts. A tumor may arise anywhere along the biliary tract, either within or outside of the liver. Bile duct tumors are typically slow-growing tumors that spread by local invasion of neighboring structures and by way of lymphatic channels.

Demographics

Bile duct cancer is an uncommon malignancy. In the United States, approximately one case arises per

100,000 people per year, but it is more common in Southeast Asia. It occurs in men only slightly more often than in women. The most common time of diagnosis is during the fifth and sixth decades of life.

Causes and symptoms

A number of risk factors are associated with the development of bile duct cancer:

- Primary sclerosing cholangitis. This disease is characterized by extensive scarring of the biliary tract, sometimes associated with inflammatory bowel disease.
- Choledochal cysts. These are abnormal dilatations of the biliary tract that usually form during fetal development. There is evidence that these cysts may rarely arise during adulthood.
- Hepatolithiasis. This is the condition of stone formation within the liver (not including gallbladder stones).
- Liver flukes. Parasitic infection with certain worms is thought to be at least partially responsible for the higher prevalence of bile duct cancer in Southeast Asia.
- Thorotrast. This is a chemical that was previously injected intravenously during certain types of x rays. It is not in use anymore. Exposure to Thorotrast has been implicated in the development of cancer of the liver as well as the bile ducts.

Symptoms

Jaundice is the first symptom in 90% of patients. This occurs when the bile duct tumor causes an obstruction in the normal flow of bile from the liver to the small intestine. Bilirubin, a component of bile, builds up within the liver and is absorbed into the bloodstream in excess amounts. This can be detected in a blood test, but it can also manifest as yellowish discoloring of the skin and eyes. The bilirubin in the bloodstream also makes the urine appear dark. Additionally, the patient may experience generalized **itching** due to the deposition of bile components in the skin. Normally, a portion of the bile is excreted in stool; bile actually gives stool its brown color. But when the biliary tract is obstructed by tumor, the stools may appear pale.

Abdominal pain, **fatigue**, **weight loss**, and poor appetite are less common symptoms. Occasionally, if obstruction of the biliary tract causes the gallbladder to swell enormously yet without causing pain, the physician may be able to feel the gallbladder during a physical examination. Sometimes the biliary tract can become infected, but this is normally a rare consequence of invasive tests. **Infection** causes **fever**, chills, and pain in the right upper portion of the abdomen.

Diagnosis

Certain laboratory tests of the blood may aid in the diagnosis. The most important one is the test for elevated bilirubin levels in the bloodstream. Levels of alkaline phosphatase and CA 19-9 may also be elevated.

When symptoms, physical signs, and blood tests point toward an abnormality of the biliary tract, then the next step involves radiographic tests. Ultrasound and **computed tomography** (CT scan) are noninvasive and rapid. These tests can often detect the actual tumor as well as dilatation of the obstructed biliary tract. If these tests indicate the presence of a tumor, then cholangiography is required. This procedure involves injecting dye into the biliary tract to obtain anatomic images of the bile ducts and the tumor. The specialist that performs this test can also insert small tubes, or stents, into a partially obstructed portion of the bile duct to prevent further obstruction by growth of the tumor. This is vitally important since it may be the only intervention that is possible in certain patients. Cholangiography is an invasive test that carries a small risk of infection of the biliary tract. The objective of these radiological tests is to determine the size and location of the tumor, as well as the extent of spread to nearby structures.

The treatment of bile duct tumors is usually not affected by the specific type of cancer cells that comprise the tumor. For this reason, some physicians forego **biopsy** of the tumor.

Treatment team

The treatment team may include the patient's primary physician, a surgeon, and a gastroenterologist who specializes in the **stenting** technique described above for palliation of bile duct strictures.

Clinical staging, treatments, and prognosis

Staging

Bile duct tumors are staged according to the tumor-node-metastasis (TNM) system of the **American Joint Commission on Cancer**. This staging scheme assesses the invasiveness of the tumor, the involvement of nearby lymph nodes, and the extent of distant **metastasis**.

- Stage I tumors are confined to the bile duct itself.
- Stage II tumors extend to the immediately adjacent tissues.
- Stage III tumors have spread to associated lymph nodes.
- Stage IV tumors have invaded local structures or have metastasized to distant structures. A higher stage signifies worse prognosis.

Treatment

The only hope for cure lies with surgical resection (removal) of the tumor and all involved structures. Unfortunately, sometimes the cancer has already spread too far when the diagnosis is made. Thus, in the treatment of bile duct cancer, the first question to answer is if the tumor may be safely resected by surgery with reasonable benefit to the patient. If the cancer involves certain blood vessels or has spread widely throughout the liver, then resection may not be possible. Sometimes further invasive testing is required.

Angiography can determine if the blood vessels are involved. **Laparoscopy** is a surgical procedure that allows the surgeon to directly assess the tumor and nearby lymph nodes without making a large incision in the abdomen. Only about 45% of bile duct cancers are ultimately resectable.

If the tumor is resectable, and the patient is healthy enough to tolerate the operation, then the specific type of surgery performed depends on the location of the tumor. For tumors within the liver or high up in the biliary tract, resection of part of the liver may be required. Tumors in the middle portion of the biliary tract can be removed alone. Tumors of the lower end of the biliary tract may require extensive resection of part of the pancreas, small intestine, and stomach to ensure complete resection.

Unfortunately, sometimes the cancer appears resectable by all the radiological and invasive tests, but is found to be unresectable during surgery. In this scenario, a bypass operation can relieve the biliary tract obstruction, but does not remove the tumor itself. This does not produce a cure but it can offer a better quality of life for the patient.

Chemotherapy and **radiation therapy** have not been proven effective in the treatment of bile duct cancer.

Prognosis

Prognosis depends on the stage and resectability of the tumor. If the patient cannot undergo surgical resection, then survival is expected to be less than one year. If the tumor is resected, survival improves but is still dismal. Only 20% of these patients survive past five years.

Clinical trials

Studies of new treatments in patients are known as **clinical trials**. These trials seek to compare the standard method of care with a new method, or the trials may be trying to establish whether one treatment is more beneficial for certain patients than others. Sometimes, a new treatment that is not being offered on a wide scale may be available to patients participating in clinical trials, but participating in the trials may involve some risk. To learn more about clinical trials, patients can call the National Cancer Institute (NCI) at 1-800-4-CANCER or visit the NCI web site for patients at http://www.cancer.gov/clinicaltrials.

Prevention

Other than the avoidance of infections caused by liver flukes, there are no known preventions for this cancer.

Resources

BOOKS

Ahrendt, Steven A. and Henry A. Pitt. "Biliary Tract." In *Sabiston Textbook of Surgery*, edited by Courtney Townsend Jr., 16th ed. Philadelphia: W.B. Saunders Company, 2001, pp. 1076-1111.

"Cholangiocarcinoma." In *Clinical Oncology*, edited by Abeloff, Martin D., second ed. New York: Churchill Livingstone, 2000, pp.1722-1723.

ORGANIZATIONS

The American Cancer Society. Phone: 1-800-ACS 2345. Web site: http://www.cancer.org.

American Liver Foundation. Phone: 1-800-GO-LIVER (1-800-465-4837). Web site: http://www.liverfoundation.org.

National Cancer Institute Cancer Information Service. Phone: 1-800-4-CANCER. Web site: http://www.nci.nih.gov.

Kevin O. Hwang, M.D.

Biliary tract cancers *see* **Bile duct cancer; Gall bladder cancer**

Biological response modifiers

Definition

Biological or biologic response modifiers (BRMs) are a diverse class of drugs that affect immune system responses. Although they occur naturally in the body, BRMs are produced in the laboratory as pharmaceuticals. BRMS include:

- interferons (IFNs)
- interleukins (ILs)
- colony-stimulating factors (CSFs)
- monoclonal antibodies (MOABs or MoABs)
- vaccines
- gene therapies
- nonspecific immunomodulating agents
- factors that target specific immune system components

Purpose

BRMs are used to:

- boost, restore, or redirect the body's immune system to fight cancer, infections, and other diseases
- stimulate immune system cells, such as T cells, natural killer (NK) cells, and macrophages, for destroying cancer cells, infectious agents, and pathogens
- inhibit specific immune system components that promote cancer and other diseases, especially autoimmune diseases

In addition BRMS are used in **cancer** therapies to:

- block or reverse processes by which normal or precancerous cells transform into cancer cells
- directly attack tumors
- alter cancer cells so that they can be recognized and destroyed by the immune system
- alter growth patterns of cancer cells so that they behave more like normal cells
- halt, control, or suppress processes that allow for cancer growth
- prevent the spread or metastasis of cancer cells to other parts of the body
- lessen some side effects from certain cancer treatments
- enhance the body's ability to repair or replace normal cells that have been damaged or destroyed by cancer treatments such as chemotherapy or radiation
- prevent cancer recurrences

Interferons were the first cytokines to be produced for use as BKMs. Various types of interferons:

- boost immune system activity against cancer cells
- stimulate T cells, NK cells, and macrophages

Biological response modifiers

U.S. brand name BRMs	Canadian brand name BRMs	International brand name BRMs
Infergen, Alferon N, Intron A, Pegasys, PEG-Intron, Roferon-A (alfa-INFs)	Infergen, Alferon N, PEG-Intron, Pegasys (alfa-INFs)	Infergen, Inferax, Pegintron, ViraferonPeg (alfa-INFs)
Avonex, Rebif, Betaseron (beta-INFs)	Avonex, Betaseron (beta-INFs)	
Actimmune (gamma-INF)		
Proleukin (IL-2)	Proleukin (IL-2)	Proleukin (IL-2)
Neupogen (G-CSF)	Neupogen (G-CSF)	Granulokine, Neupogen (G-CSF)
Leukine (GM-CSF)	Leukine (GM-CSF)	
Epogen, Procrit (epoetin)	Eprex (epoetin)	Eprex, Hemax (epoetin)
Neumega (IL-11)		Neumega (IL-11)
Rituxan (rituximab)	Rituxan (rituximab)	Mabthera (rituximab)
Herceptin (trastuzumab)	Herceptin (trastuzumab)	Herceptin (trastuzumab)
Remicade (infliximab)	Remicade (infliximab)	Remicade (infliximab)
Humira (adalimumab)		Humira (adalimumab)
Engerix-B, Recombivax HB (HBV vaccine)	Engerix-B, Recombivax HB (HBV vaccine)	Engerix-B, Recombivax HB (HBV vaccine)
Gardasil (HPV vaccine)		Cervarix (HPV vaccine)
TheraCys, TICE BCG (BCG vaccine)	ImmuCyst, Oncotice, Pacis (BCG vaccine)	
Ergamisol (levamisole)		
Enbrel (etanercept)	Enbrel (etanercept)	Enbrel (etanercept)
Kineret (anakinra)	Kineret (anakinra)	Kineret (anakinra)
Orenica (abatacept)		

(Table by GGS Creative Resources. Cengage Learning, Gale.)

- stimulate tumor-specific cytotoxic T cells that destroy tumor cells
- possibly slow the growth of cancer cells or promote their development into more normal cells
- dampen the immune response
- reduce the production of inflammatory cytokines

Alfa-interferons are used to treat various cancers and viral infections including:

- hairy cell leukemia
- malignant melanoma
- chronic myeloid leukemia
- AIDS-related Kaposi's sarcoma
- kidney and bladder cancers
- non-Hodgkin's lymphoma
- ovarian cancer
- prolonging remission of multiple myeloma
- recurring or refractory genital or venereal warts

Beta-interferons are used to prevent multiple sclerosis (MS) and decrease flare-ups and slow the progression of MS. Gamma-interferon is used to treat chronic granulomatous disease, an inherited immune-system disorder.

Of the many different interleukins, IL-2 or **aldesleukin** is the most important for cancer treatment. IL-2 stimulates the growth and activity of various immune system cells including lymphocytes. The U.S. Food and Drug Administration (FDA) has approved IL-2 for the treatment of metastatic **kidney cancer** and metastatic **melanoma**. Interleukins are being studied for the treatment of:

- leukemia
- lymphoma
- brain cancers
- colorectal cancer
- breast, ovarian, and prostate cancers
- multiple myeloma
- HIV infection and AIDS

CSFs, also called hematopoietic growth factors, stimulate bone marrow stem cells to divide and develop into red and white blood cells and platelets that have may been depleted by **chemotherapy**, leaving patients susceptible to **anemia**, infections, and bleeding. CSFs are used in conjunction with high-dose chemotherapy:

- Granulocute colony stimulating factor (G-CSF, filgrastim) and granulocyte-macrophage colony stimulating factor (GM-CSF, sargramostim) increase white blood cells, thereby reducing the risk of infection, and stimulate the production of stem cells for stem cell or bone marrow transplants.
- Epoetin (erythropoietin) increases the production of red blood cells, reducing the need for transfusions. Epoetin also is used to treat anemia caused by a variety of other conditions.
- Interleukin-11 (oprelvekin) stimulates platelet production, reducing the need for platelet transfusions.

CSFs also are being studied as treatments for a wide variety of cancers.

MOABs are antibodies that are produced by a single type of cell and bind to a specific antigen:

- MOABs that are specific for a particular type of immune system cell or cancer cell can stimulate an immune response against those cells.
- MOABs that are specific for a growth factor can interfere with that factor's stimulation of cancer cell growth.
- MOABs that bind specifically to a particular type of cancer cell can be linked to an anticancer drug, a radioisotope, a toxin, or another BRM that will destroy those cancer cells.
- Rituximab blocks the activation of CD20+ B cells and is used to treat non-Hodgkin lymphoma and rheumatoid arthritis.
- Trastuzumab inhibits the HER2 growth factor receptor and is used to treat HER2+ breast cancer.
- Infliximab and adalimumab target tumor necrosis factor (TNF) for the treatment of rheumatoid arthritis.

Vaccines stimulate the immune system to combat **infection** and destroy damaged or abnormal cells. Therapeutic vaccines that recognize cancer cells are being designed to:

- eradicate small tumors
- stop tumor growth
- kill cancer cells that remain after other treatments
- prevent cancer from recurring

Prophylactic or preventative vaccines stimulate the immune system to destroy viruses that can cause cancer. There are two FDA-approved prophylactic cancer vaccines: a vaccine for hepatitis B virus (HBV), which can cause **liver cancer** in chronically infected people; and a vaccine against **human papilloma virus** (HPV) types 6, 11, 16, and 18. HPV 16 and 18 cause 70% of cervical cancers and chronic infection also may be associated with cancers of the anus, penis, and oropharynx. HPV types 6 and 11 cause about 90% of all cases of genital warts. The vaccine also prevents HPV-associated vulvar and vaginal cancers. An HPV vaccine approved for use in Europe protects only against types 16 and 18.

Gene therapies are experimental treatments that inject genetic material into cells to stimulate the immune system or to enable immune system cells to recognize and destroy cancer cells.

Nonspecific immunomodulating agents either directly or indirectly stimulate the immune system. Bacillus Calmette-Guerin (BCG) is a tuberculosis vaccine that is used to treat superficial **bladder cancer** following surgery. BCG may stimulate inflammatory and perhaps immune responses in the bladder. **Levamisole** is used in conjunction with the chemotherapy drug **fluorouracil** (5-FU) to treat stage III **colon cancer**. It appears to restore depressed immune function.

Other BRMS target specific immune system components and are used to treat arthritis:

- Etanercept targets TNF.
- Anakinra targets IL-1.
- Abatacept blocks T cell activation.

Description

BRMs may be used:

- as standard treatment for some cancers and diseases
- alone or in combination with other drugs
- in combination with chemotherapy or radiation therapy
- in clinical trials

BRMs are supplied and administered in various forms:

- IFNs as reconstituted powders, solutions, or pre-filled syringes for infusions or injections
- IL-2 as a reconstituted powder for injection or infusion
- G-CSF as a solution for injection or infusion
- GM-CSF as a reconstituted powder or solution for infusion
- epoetin as a solution for injection
- IL-11 as a reconstituted powder for injection
- rituximab as a solution for injection
- trastuzumab and infliximab as reconstituted powders for infusion
- adalimumab as a solution for injection
- HBV and HPV vaccines as injected suspensions
- BCG as a reconstituted powder for intravesical administration through a tube into the bladder
- etanercept as a reconstituted powder or solution for injection
- anakinra as a solution for injection
- abatacept as a reconstituted powder for infusion

U.S. brand names

- Infergen, Alferon N, Intron A, Pegasys, PEG-Intron, Roferon-A (alfa-INFs)
- Avonex, Rebif, Betaseron (beta-INFs)
- Actimmune (gamma-INF)
- Proleukin (IL-2)
- Neupogen (G-CSF)
- Leukine (GM-CSF)
- Epogen, Procrit (epoetin)
- Neumega (IL-11)
- Rituxan (rituximab)
- Herceptin (trastuzumab)
- Remicade (infliximab)
- Humira (adalimumab)
- Engerix-B, Recombivax HB (HBV vaccine)
- Gardasil (HPV vaccine)
- TheraCys, TICE BCG (BCG vaccine)
- Ergamisol (levamisole)
- Enbrel (etanercept)
- Kineret (anakinra)
- Orenica (abatacept)

Canadian brand names

- Infergen, Alferon N, PEG-Intron, Pegasys (alfa-INFs)
- Avonex, Betaseron (beta-INFs)
- Proleukin (IL-2)
- Neupogen (G-CSF)
- Leukine (GM-CSF)
- Eprex (epoetin)
- Rituxan (rituximab)
- Herceptin (trastuzumab)
- Remicade (infliximab)
- Engerix-B, Recombivax HB (HBV vaccine)
- ImmuCyst, Oncotice, Pacis (BCG vaccine)
- Enbrel (etanercept)
- Kineret (anakinra)

International brand names

- Infergen, Inferax, Pegintron, ViraferonPeg (alfa-INFs)
- Proleukin (IL-2)
- Granulokine, Neupogen (G-CSF)

- Eprex, Hemax (epoetin)
- Neumega (IL-11)
- Mabthera (rituximab)
- Herceptin (trastuzumab)
- Remicade (infliximab)
- Humira (adalimumab)
- Engerix-B, Recombivax HB (HBV vaccine)
- Cervarix (HPV vaccine)
- Enbrel (etanercept)
- Kineret (anakinra)

Recommended dosage

Dosages of BRMs vary greatly depending on factors including:

- the specific drug
- the condition being treated
- the duration of treatment
- the patient's age
- the patient's weight and general health
- the patient's response to the treatment

Precautions

BMFs are powerful drugs and there are specific precautions for the use of each one. INFs and drugs that target immune system components increase susceptibility to infection.

Geriatric

Elderly patients often require lower doses of BRMs.

Pregnant or breastfeeding

Most BMFs are in pregnancy categories B or C, meaning that there have been no adequate human studies on the risks that they may pose to the fetus. It is not known whether most BMFs pass into breast milk, so caution is advised. The following BMFs do enter into breast milk and should not be used while breastfeeding:

- INFs
- IL-2
- rituximab
- trastuzumab
- infliximab
- adalimumab
- etanercept

> ## QUESTIONS TO ASK YOUR PHARMACIST
>
> - How should I store this medication?
> - How do I administer this medication?
> - Will this medication interact with any of my other medications?
> - Can I drink alcohol while taking this medication?
> - What if I miss a dose?
> - What side effects can I expect?
> - When should I contact my doctor about side effects?

Other conditions and allergies

Many conditions can be exacerbated by INFs and other BRMs. Many BRMs cannot be administered to patients who are immunocompromised or otherwise susceptible to infections. Although any BRM can cause an allergic or hypersensitivity reaction, allergic reactions may be more common with MOABs.

Side effects

The side effects of BRMs vary greatly depending on the specific agent and the individual patient. Some side effects may be serious and severe. INFs and ILs, in particular, sometimes cause severe side effects.

Common side effects of BRMs may include:

- redness, pain, heat, itching, swelling, or rash at the injection site
- fatigue
- blood pressure effects, especially low blood pressure
- flu-like symptoms including fever, chills, muscle aches, nausea, vomiting, and loss of appetite
- fluid accumulation
- bone pain with CSFs

Many BRMs can cause side effects through their actions on the central nervous system. Symptoms of central nervous system side effects include:

- nervousness
- numbness or tingling of fingers, toes, and face
- difficulty concentrating
- confusion
- mental depression

Interactions

BRMs can interact with a wide variety of over-the-counter and prescription medications and with alcohol. They should not be taken in combination with any other medication except under a physician's supervision. The treatment team should be made aware of all medications, over-the-counter drugs, and nutritional and alternative supplements used by the patient. Antimicrobial and immunosuppressive drugs may be of particular concern.

Medications that affect the central nervous system may interact with some BRMs. These medications include:

- antihistamines
- sedatives
- tranquilizers
- sleeping medications
- prescription pain medicines
- seizure medications
- muscle relaxants
- narcotics
- barbiturates

Resources

BOOKS

Perry, Michael C. *The Chemotherapy Source Book,* 4th ed. Philadelphia: Wolters Kluwer Health/Lippincott Williams & Wilkins, 2008.

Ruzic, Neil P., and David Neil Ruzic. *Racing to a Cure: A Cancer Victim Refuses Chemotherapy and Finds Tomorrow's Cures in Today's Scientific Laboratories.* Urbana: University of Illinois Press, 2006.

Young, Annie M., Lewis Rowett, and David J. Kerr. *Cancer Biotherapy: An Introductory Guide.* New York: Oxford University Press, 2006.

PERIODICALS

Emens, L. A. "Cancer Vaccines: On the Threshold of Success." *Expert Opinion on Emerging Drugs* 13, no. 2 (2008): 295-308.

Finn, O. J. "Cancer Immunology." *New England Journal of Medicine.* 358, no. 25 (2008): 2704-2715.

Lollini, P. L., et al. "Vaccines for Tumour Prevention." *Nature Reviews Cancer* 6, no. 3 (2006): 204-216.

Waldmann, T. A. "Effective Cancer Therapy Through Immunomodulation." *Annual Review of Medicine* 57 (2006): 65-81.

OTHER

"Biological Therapies for Cancer: Questions and Answers." *National Cancer Institute Fact Sheet.* http://www.cancer.gov/cancertopics/factsheet/Therapy/biological.

"Cancer Vaccines." *National Cancer Institute Fact Sheet.* http://www.cancer.gov/cancertopics/factsheet/cancervaccine.

"Immunotherapy: What It Is and How It Can Help Fight Cancer." *SkinCancerNet.* http://www.skincarephysicians.com/skincancernet/immunotherapy.html.

"Rheumatoid Arthritis—Medications." *University of Maryland Medical Center.* http://www.umm.edu/patiented/articles/what_specific_drugs_used_treating_rheumatoid_arthritis_000048_8.htm.

ORGANIZATIONS

American Academy of Dermatology, PO Box 4014, Schaumburg, IL, 60168, (847) 240-1280, (866) 503-SKIN (7546), (847) 240-1859, http://www.aad.org.

American Cancer Society, 1599 Clifton Road NE, Atlanta, GA, 30329-4251, (800) ACS-2345, http://www.cancer.org.

National Cancer Institute, NCI Public Inquiries Office, 6116 Executive Boulevard, Room 3036A, Bethesda, MD, 20006, (800) 4-CANCER, http://www.cancer.gov.

Margaret Alic, Ph.D.

Biology of cancer *see* **Cancer biology**

Biopsy

Definition

Biopsy is a diagnostic procedure in which a piece of tissue and/or cells are removed to be examined under a microscope by a pathologist.

Purpose

Biopsies are performed to determine the presence of **cancer** cells, establish **tumor grading**, and provide more information for treatment.

Precautions

Most biopsies should not be done on patients with blood clotting problems. If the patient has a low blood platelet count, a platelet transfusion can be given as a temporary relief measure, and a biopsy can then be performed. The physician should be notified of any bleeding problems—as well as any allergies, current medications, or pregnancy—well in advance.

Patients receiving IV sedation for a biopsy procedure will continue to feel drowsy for several hours, and should refrain from cooking, driving, or operating any equipment that requires careful attention. A ride home from the clinic should be arranged in advance.

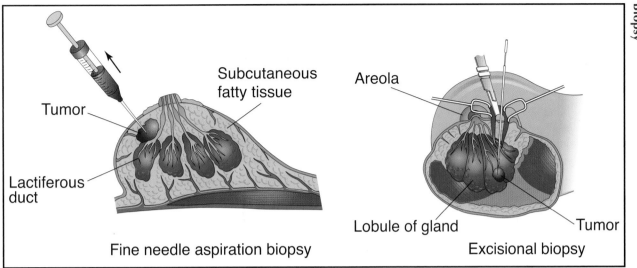

Of the four different types of biopsy discussed, two are shown here: Fine needle aspiration biopsy and Excisional biopsy. A fine needle aspiration biopsy uses a very thin needle to withdraw fluid and cells from the growth to be examined. An excisional biopsy is a surgical procedure in which the entire area of concern and some surrounding tissue is removed for analysis. *(Illustration by Electronic Illustrators Group. Cengage Learning, Gale.)*

Description

There are several different types of biopsies, and the decision on which one is most effective depends on where the tumor is located and the general health of the patient. Four common categories of biopsy are fine needle aspiration, core needle biopsy, excisional biopsy, and incisional biopsy.

Fine needle aspiration biopsy

Fine needle aspiration biopsy, also known as suction biopsy or needle aspiration biopsy, involves applying negative pressure through the use of a syringe and hollow, hypodermic needle. This type of biopsy is often used as a diagnostic procedure on neck and thyroid masses. It results in the removal of tissue that is fragmented into cells, as opposed to one sample of undamaged tissue. Fine needle aspiration biopsy is a frequently performed procedure that results in minimum discomfort and is less costly than many other types of biopsy.

Core needle biopsy

Core needle biopsy, also known as wide-core needle biopsy or cutting core biopsy, involves the use of a large-bore needle and is the simplest method of pathologic diagnosis of cancer. It results in minimal disturbance of surrounding tissues and a solid, intact sample. Tumors located in the liver and breast are commonly biopsied with this technique.

Incisional biopsy

This refers to the removal of part of the tumor from the larger tumor mass. An incisional biopsy is employed for tumors located deep within the body and after an initial needle biopsy has failed to supply enough tissue for diagnosis. Biopsies of this type are the preferred technique for diagnosing soft tissue cancers and osteosarcomas.

Excisional biopsy

Also known as surgical biopsy, the excisional biopsy entails the surgical removal of the entire tumor mass and is a diagnostic technique that simultaneously serves as a treatment. For example, a **lumpectomy** removes the entire primary tumor mass associated with **breast cancer**. Excisional biopsy is also useful for diagnosing and removing surface tumors of the skin, such as those associated with squamous cell **carcinoma**, **basal cell carcinoma**, and malignant **melanoma**.

Preparation

Many biopsies can be performed in the doctor's office or in the hospital on an outpatient basis. Most do not require much special preparation on the part the patient, but patients should ask their physician for special instructions. Prior to the procedure, most require the use of anesthesia. Prior to and during a biopsy, special imaging techniques may be employed to assist in locating the tumor and guidance of biopsy procedures using a needle. Such imaging techniques include **computed tomography** scan (CT guided biopsy), fluoroscopy, **magnetic resonance imaging** (MRI), nuclear medicine scan, and ultrasound (ultrasound guided biopsy). Patients who undergo imaging scans may be injected with or asked to drink a contrast agent (dye) prior to biopsy.

Fine needle aspiration biopsy

Some routine blood work (blood counts, clotting profile) should be completed two weeks prior to biopsy. Patients may be asked not to eat for a specified time before the procedure. Those taking blood thinners (anticoagulants) or aspirin should talk to their physicians about whether they should discontinue using them prior to biopsy.

Core needle biopsy

Women undergoing breast biopsy should not wear talcum powder, deodorant, lotion, or perfume under their arms or on their breasts on the day of the procedure (since these may cause image artifacts or other problems). A comfortable two-piece garment should be worn. Patients may be asked not to eat for a specified time before the procedure. Those taking blood thinners or aspirin should talk to their physicians about whether they should discontinue using them prior to core needle biopsy.

Incisional biopsy

Patients should follow instructions provided by their doctor and give notification of any allergies. Those expecting general anesthesia should not eat or drink for at least 8 hours before an incisional biopsy. Patients should also bathe thoroughly before the procedure and allow time to rest afterward.

Excisional biopsy

Patients may be asked to: sign a consent form allowing the physician to perform this test; refrain from eating or drinking for at least 8 hours prior to surgery; and arrange for a ride home from the hospital (most patients can go home on the same day as the surgery). Those taking insulin, aspirin, non-steroidal anti-inflammatory drugs, or any medicines that affect blood clotting should notify their doctor well before the procedure.

Aftercare

Fine needle aspiration biopsy

After the biopsy, patients should be able to drive home, return to work, or perform any other routine activity. This biopsy does not affect medication schedules.

Core needle biopsy

Most patients can resume normal activities right after the biopsy. If there is excessive redness, pain, or drainage from the puncture site, patients should call their doctor immediately.

Incisional biopsy

After recovering from anesthesia, the patient will be observed for a few hours before returning home. During this time, an analysis may come back from the lab and the doctor may explain the nature of the abnormality. This analysis is the result of only one test and will not be 100% accurate. In about two days, lab testing should be complete. Patients should call their doctor immediately if there is drainage from the wound or a **fever** develops.

Excisional biopsy

Depending on the invasiveness of the procedure, the patient may receive varied instructions for after-care. The incision site should be kept clean, dry, and free of lotion, medication, or ointments. The patient may be required to remain in a certain position until sufficient time has passed to warrant the release of the patient from medical care. For example, patients are required to remain on their right side for approximately four hours to allow for healing to occur after a liver punch biopsy. Some patients, however, may be able to return to normal activities on the same day. Those who develop a fever, or notice bleeding, drainage, strong pain, or redness and warmth at the biopsy site should contact their doctor immediately.

Risks

Although most biopsies end with success, there are a certain number of risks to keep in mind. For example, complications can arise if other organs are nicked during a biopsy using a long needle. As with any procedure, there is a slight risk of allergic reaction to anesthesia. To be well informed, patients should consult with their physician about the risks prior to undergoing the procedure.

Fine needle aspiration biopsy

This biopsy poses no significant risks. Some minor bleeding may occur and some patients report a mild, dull, and throbbing sensation in the area of the biopsy, which usually subsides within 30 to 60 minutes. The risk of **infection** exists any time the skin is penetrated, but is extremely rare with this procedure. The error rate of diagnosis, however, is substantially higher than that of other biopsy procedures; major surgical resections should not be undertaken solely on the basis of the evidence of aspiration biopsy.

Core needle biopsy

A lumpy scar called a keloid may form in the area of puncture. Infection and bleeding may also occur at or under the biopsy site; however, this risk is uncommon. Core needle biopsy, like fine needle aspiration, only removes samples of a mass and not the entire area

of concern. Therefore, it is possible that a more serious diagnosis may be missed by limiting the sampling of an abnormality.

Incisional biopsy

A keloid may form in the incision area. In rare cases, infection and bleeding may occur.

Excisional biopsy

Some patients may experience infection, bleeding, or bruising around the biopsy site. The physician should be consulted about any risks that may be related to a patient's medical history.

Normal results

The tissue sample obtained from the biopsy needs to be prepared for examination by a pathologist, and results usually are reported to the patient within a few days of the procedure. Normal (negative) results indicate that no malignancy is present.

Abnormal results

Abnormal results indicate that a malignancy or other abnormality is present. In some cases, results are indeterminate and patients are subject to further diagnostic procedures.

See also Bone marrow aspiration and biopsy; CT-guided biopsy; Liver biopsy; Pleural biopsy; Stereotactic needle biopsy.

Resources

BOOKS

Bast, Robert C., et al.*Cancer Medicine.* 5th ed. Hamilton, ON: B.C. Decker Inc., 2000.

OTHER

"An Alternative to Excisional Breast Biopsy: Core Needle Breast Biopsy." *Washington Radiology Associates.* [cited June 25, 2009]. http://www.wrapc.com/corenedl.htm.

Harvard Health Online. [cited June 25, 2009]. http://www.health.harvard.edu.

National Cancer Institute. [cited June 25, 2009]. http://www.nci.nih.gov.

Sally C. McFarlane-Parrott

Bisacodyl *see* **Laxatives**

Bisphosphonates

Definition

Bisphosphonates are a class of drugs that lower calcium levels in the blood and can slow down bone loss that results from **cancer** or other causes.

Purpose

Bisphosphonates are used to slow down the loss of bone that results from **multiple myeloma** or from **breast cancer** that has spread, or metastasized, to the bones. These cancers cause bone to dissolve, in a process called resorption. This results in bone weakness and fractures. Bisphosphonates can prevent the holes that form in the bones from multiple **myeloma**. They can ease **bone pain** caused by cancer. They also help to prevent bone fractures and compression of the spinal cord, as well as the high calcium levels in the blood (**hypercalcemia**) caused by bone loss. Hypercalcemia can cause kidney failure and death. Bisphosphonates may help prevent breast cancer from spreading to the bones and other organs. **Clinical trials** are evaluating bisphosphonates for the treatment of bone metastases from other types of cancers.

Description

The most commonly used bisphosphonates are pamidronate disodium (APD; brand name Aredia) and etidronate disodium (EHDP; brand name Didronel). Both drugs are approved by the U.S. Food and Drug Administration. These drugs are classified as antihypercalcemics, meaning that they can lower blood calcium levels. They also are classified as bone resorption inhibitors, meaning that they can prevent bone from dissolving.

Other bisphosphonates include cladronate and alendronate. Cladronate is used less frequently because it is not completely absorbed by the digestive system and can cause stomach upset. **Zoledronate** and ibandronate are new, much more powerful bisphosphonates that are being evaluated, but are not yet available for routine use.

For cancer treatment, bisphosphonates may be used in conjunction with **chemotherapy**. Treatment with bisphosphonates may be accompanied by the injection of fluids into a vein (intravenous) so that large amounts of urine are excreted.

Recommended dosage

Pamidronate and etidronate are solutions that are injected into a vein. For the treatment of hypercalcemia,

KEY TERMS

Antihypercalcemic—Drug that lowers the levels of calcium in the blood.

Hypercalcemia—High levels of calcium in the blood.

Metastasis—Spread of cancer from its point of origin to other parts of the body.

Resorption—Dissolving of bone, as with multiple myeloma or bone metastases from other cancers.

30–90 mg of pamidronate are injected over a period of 2–24 hours. For the treatment of bone metastases from breast cancer, 90 mg are injected over a two-hour period every 3–4 weeks. For multiple myeloma, the 90-mg injection is over a four-hour period once a month. The usual dosage of etidronate is 7.5 mg per kg (3.4 mg per pound) of body weight, injected over two hours, for two or more days. The treatment may be repeated after at least one week off.

Etidronate also may be taken as a tablet, with water, on an empty stomach. The usual dosage for the treatment of hypercalcemia is 20 mg per kg (9.1 mg per pound) of body weight per day for 30 days. The maximum length of treatment usually is 90 days, but the treatment may be repeated after at least 90 days off of the drug. Cladronate is also taken as a pill.

Precautions

The amount of calcium in the diet may be important when taking bisphosphonates. Too much calcium in the diet may prevent absorption of oral etidronate. However, it is important to consume adequate amounts of calcium and vitamin D.

Other medical problems that may affect the use of bisphosphonates include:

- heart problems that may be aggravated by fluid retention
- kidney disease that could result in high levels of bisphosphonate in the blood
- intestinal problems or bowel disease, because etidronate can cause diarrhea
- bone fractures, particularly of the arm or leg, since etidronate can increase the risk of fractures

Bisphosphonates may cause allergic reactions in some individuals. Children may experience temporary changes in bone growth while being treated with etidronate and they should not take pamidronate. Older individuals may suffer from fluid retention if

174

bisphosphonates are given with large amounts of fluid. Bisphosphonates should not be taken during pregnancy. It is not known whether these drugs pass into breast milk.

Side effects

Although bisphosphonates usually are well tolerated, some patients may experience side effects. The most common side effects include:

- fatigue
- fever
- nausea
- vomiting
- abdominal cramps
- low red blood cell levels (anemia)
- bone or joint pain
- muscle stiffness or pain
- pain or swelling at the site of injection or in the vein-However, some of these symptoms may result from the cancer or from other treatments for the cancer. A mild pain reliever can reduce or prevent the muscle and joint pain. Bisphosphonates that are taken by mouth can cause irritation and ulcers in the esophagus (the tube between the mouth and the stomach).

Additional side effects that may occur with pamidronate, particularly at dosages above 60 mg, include:

- chills
- confusion
- muscle spasms
- sore throat
- constipation
- decreased appetite

Additional side effects that may occur with etidronate include:

- decreased levels of magnesium and phosphorus in the blood
- diarrhea
- bone fracture, particularly of the thigh
- increases in test results for kidney function
- hives, skin rash, or itching (rare)
- swelling of the arms, legs, face, lips, tongue, or throat (rare)
- loss or altered sense of taste (with drug injection)

Interactions

Substances that may interact or interfere with bisphosphonates include:

- mineral supplements, antacids, or other substances containing calcium, iron, magnesium, or aluminum, particularly if taken within two hours of taking etidronate
- substances containing vitamin D

Margaret Alic, Ph.D.

Bladder cancer

Definition

Bladder cancer is a disease in which the cells lining the urinary bladder lose the ability to regulate their growth and start dividing uncontrollably. This abnormal growth results in a mass of cells that form a tumor.

Description

The urinary bladder is a hollow muscular organ that stores urine from the kidneys until it is excreted out of the body. Two tubes called the ureters bring the urine from the kidneys to the bladder. The urethra carries the urine from the bladder to the outside of the body.

Bladder cancer has a very high rate of recurrence following treatment. Even after superficial tumors are completely removed, there is a 75% chance that new tumors will develop in other areas of the bladder. Patients need very frequent and thorough follow-up care. When detected at the early stages, the prognosis for bladder cancer is excellent. At least 94% of patients survive five years or more after initial diagnosis. If the disease has spread to the nearby tissues, however, the survival rates drop to 49%. If it has metastasized to distant organs such as the lung or liver, only 6% of patients will survive five years or more.

Demographics

Bladder cancer is the sixth most common cancer in the United States. The American Cancer Society (ACS) estimated that in 2009, approximately 70,980 new cases of bladder cancer would be diagnosed (about 52,810 men and 18,170 women), causing approximately 12,400 deaths.

The highest occurrences of bladder cancer are found in industrialized countries such as the United

Excised specimen of a cancerous human bladder, showing a large tumor mass. *(Copyright Science Photo Library, Science Source/Photo Researchers, Inc. Reproduced by permission.)*

Bladder cancer on the inner lining of the bladder. *(Illustration by Argosy Publishing. Cengage Learning, Gale.)*

An immunofluorescent light micrograph of cells cultured from squamous carcinoma of the bladder. *(Photograph by Nancy Kedersha, Photo Researchers, Inc. Reproduced by permission.)*

States, Canada, France, Denmark, Italy, and Spain. In all countries, the incidence of bladder cancer is higher for men than women. Among men, the highest rates occur in white non-Hispanic males (33.1 per 100,000). The rates for men of African descent and Hispanic men are similar and are approximately one-half of the rate among white non-Hispanic men. The lowest rate of bladder cancer occurs in the Asian population. Among women, the highest rates also occur in

white non-Hispanic females and are approximately twice the rate for Hispanics. Women of African descent have higher rates of bladder cancer than Hispanic women.

Age is also an important factor: bladder cancer is significantly more common in older men and women in all populations. Bladder cancer rates for people aged 70 years and older are two to three times higher than for people in the 55 to 69 age group, and approximately 15 to 20 times higher than for people between the ages of 30 and 54.

Causes and symptoms

Although the exact cause of bladder cancer is not known, smokers are twice as likely to get the disease as are nonsmokers. Smoking is subsequently considered to be the greatest risk factor for bladder cancer. Workers who are exposed to certain chemicals that are used in the dye, rubber, leather, textile, and paint industries are also believed to be at a higher risk for bladder cancer.

Frequent urinary infections, kidney and bladder stones, and other conditions that cause long-term irritation to the bladder may increase the risk of getting bladder cancer. A past history of tumors in the bladder also increases one's risk of developing new tumors.

One of the first warning signals of bladder cancer is blood in the urine. There may be enough blood in the urine to change its color to a yellow-red or dark red. At other times, the color of the urine appears normal but chemical testing of the urine reveals the presence of blood cells. Painful urination, increased frequency, and increased urgency (the sensation of having to urinate immediately but being unable to do so) are other

KEY TERMS

Biopsy—The surgical removal and microscopic examination of living tissue for diagnostic purposes.

Chemotherapy—Treatment with drugs that selectively destroy cancer cells.

Computed tomography (CT) scan—A medical procedure in which a series of x rays are taken and analyzed by a computer in order to form detailed pictures of areas inside the body.

Cystoscopy—A diagnostic procedure in which a hollow lighted tube (cystoscope) is used to look inside the bladder and the urethra.

Electrofulguration—A procedure in which a high-energy laser beam is used to burn the cancerous tissue.

Immunotoxins—Antibodies produced in the laboratory that recognize specific substances that are more abundant in cancer cells than in normal cells; immunotoxins identify cancer cells and deliver a powerful toxin that kills the cells.

Intravenous pyelogram (IVP)—A procedure where an injected dye outlines the urinary system on an x ray to help reveal potential abnormalities.

Magnetic resonance imaging (MRI)—A medical procedure used for diagnostic purposes where pictures of areas inside the body can be created using a magnet linked to a computer.

Partial cystectomy—A surgical procedure where the cancerous tissue is removed by cutting out a small piece of the bladder.

Photodynamic therapy—A combination of special light rays and drugs that are used to destroy the cancerous cells.

Radiation therapy—Treatment using high-energy radiation from x-ray machines, cobalt, radium, or other sources.

Radical cystectomy—A surgical procedure that removes the entire bladder and occasionally other adjoining organs.

Stoma—An artificial opening between two cavities or between a cavity and the surface of the body.

Transurethral resection— A surgical procedure to remove abnormal tissue from the bladder using an instrument called a cystoscope.

Urostomy—A surgical procedure in which the ureters are disconnected from the bladder and connected to an opening (see stoma) on the abdomen, allowing urine to flow into a collection bag.

---

possible signs of bladder cancer. All of these symptoms may also be caused by conditions other than cancer, so it is important to see a doctor to have the symptoms evaluated.

In 2003, studies showed that hormone replacement therapy (HRT), a treatment used by many postmenopausal women, significantly increased the risk of bladder and other cancers.

Diagnosis

If a doctor has any reason to suspect bladder cancer, several tests may be used to find out if the disease is present. A complete medical history will be taken to check for any risk factors. A thorough physical examination will be conducted to assess all the signs and symptoms. Laboratory testing of a urine sample will help to rule out the presence of a bacterial **infection**. In a urine **cytology** test, the urine is examined under a microscope to look for any abnormal or cancerous cells. A catheter (tube) can be advanced into the bladder through the urethra and a salt solution passed through it to wash the bladder. The solution can then be collected and examined under a microscope to check for the presence of any cancerous cells.

A test known as the intravenous pyelogram (IVP) is an x-ray examination performed after a dye is injected into a vein in the arm. The dye travels through the blood stream and reaches the kidneys to be excreted, clearly outlining the kidneys, ureters, bladder, and urethra. Multiple **x rays** are taken to detect any abnormalities in the lining of these organs.

The physician may use a procedure known as a **cystoscopy** to view the inside of the bladder. A thin hollow lighted tube is introduced into the bladder through the urethra. If any suspicious-looking masses are seen, a small piece of the tissue can be painlessly removed using a pair of **biopsy** forceps. The tissue is then examined microscopically to verify if cancer is present, and if so, the type of cancer will be identified.

If cancer is detected and there is evidence showing that it has metastasized to distant sites in the body, imaging tests such as chest x rays, **computed tomography** (CT) scans, and **magnetic resonance imaging** (MRI) may be done to determine which organs are affected. Bladder cancer tends to spread to the lungs, liver, and bone.

Treatment team

Treatment for bladder cancer depends on the stage of the disease and how deeply the cancer has penetrated the bladder wall. It also depends on the grade of the cancer and on the patient's general health status and personal preferences. Most likely, a team of specialists including a urologist, an oncologist, a surgeon, and a radiation oncologist will be responsible for treatment. The treatment team will develop a plan tailored to the individual patient and may recommend one treatment method or a combination of methods.

Clinical staging, treatments, and prognosis

Staging

The following stages are used by health care providers to classify the location, size, and spread of the cancer, according to the TNM (tumor, lymph node, and metastases) staging system:

- Stage 0: Cancer is found only on the inner lining of the bladder (a noninvasive carcinoma).
- Stage I: Cancer has spread to the layer of tissue beyond the inner lining of the bladder but not to the bladder muscles.
- Stage II: Cancer has spread to the muscles in the bladder wall but not to the fatty tissue surrounding the bladder.
- Stage III: Cancer has spread to the fatty tissue surrounding the bladder and potentially to the prostate, vagina, or uterus, but not to the lymph nodes or other organs.
- Stage IV: Cancer has spread to the lymph nodes, pelvic or abdominal wall, and/or other organs.
- Recurrent: Cancer has recurred in the bladder or at another site after having been treated.

Standard treatments

The three standard modes of treatment that are available for bladder cancer are surgery, **radiation therapy**, and **chemotherapy**.

Surgery is considered to be an option only when the disease is in its early stages. If the tumor is localized to a small area and has not spread to the outer layers of the bladder, then the surgery is done without entering the abdomen. A cystoscope is introduced into the bladder through the urethra, and the tumor is removed. This procedure is called a transurethral resection (TUR). Passing a high-energy laser beam through the cystoscope to burn cancer cells, a procedure known as electrofulguration, may treat any remaining cancer.

If the cancer has invaded the wall of the bladder, surgery will be done through an incision in the abdomen. Cancer that is not very large can be removed by partial **cystectomy**, a procedure where a part of the bladder is removed. If the cancer is large or is present in more than one area of the bladder, a radical cystectomy is done. The entire bladder is removed in this procedure; adjoining organs may also be removed. In men, the prostate is removed, while in women, the uterus, ovaries, and fallopian tubes are removed.

If the entire urinary bladder is removed, then an alternate storage place must be created for urine before it is excreted out of the body. To do this, a piece of intestine is converted into a small bag and attached to the ureters. This is connected to an opening (stoma) that is made in the abdominal wall. The procedure is called a **urostomy**. In some urostomy procedures, the urine from the intestinal sac is routed into a bag that is placed over the stoma in the abdominal wall. The bag is hidden by clothing and has to be emptied occasionally by the patient. In a different procedure, the urine is collected in the intestinal sac, but there is no bag on the outside of the abdomen. The intestinal sac has to be emptied by the patient by placing a drainage tube through the stoma.

Radiation therapy that uses high-energy rays to kill cancer cells is generally used after surgery to destroy any remaining cancer cells. If the tumor is in a location that makes surgery difficult or if it is large, radiation may be used before surgery to shrink the tumor. In cases of advanced bladder cancer, radiation therapy is used to ease the symptoms such as pain, bleeding, or blockage. External beam radiation focuses a beam of radiation on the area of the tumor. Alternatively, a small pellet of radioactive material may be placed directly into the cancer. This is known as interstitial radiation therapy.

Chemotherapy uses **anticancer drugs** to destroy the cancer cells that may have migrated to distant sites. The drugs are injected into the patient intravenously or taken orally in pill form. Generally a combination of drugs is more effective than any single drug in treating bladder cancer. Chemotherapy may be given following surgery to kill any remaining cancer cells. Called neoadjuvant chemotherapy, this treatment may allow people with bladder cancer to live up to 31 months longer than previous treatments allowed. Chemotherapy also may be given even when no remaining cancer cells can be seen (**adjuvant chemotherapy**). Anticancer drugs, including **thiotepa, doxorubicin**, and mitomycin, may also be instilled directly into the bladder (intravesicular chemotherapy) to treat superficial tumors. In 2003, the FDA was giving fast track designation to a form of paclitaxel, a common anticancer drug, that was shown effective in treating metastatic or locally advanced bladder cancer.

Immunotherapy or biological therapy uses the body's own immune cells to fight the disease. To treat superficial bladder cancer, bacillus Calmette-Guérin (BCG) may be instilled directly into the bladder. BCG is a weakened (attenuated) strain of the tuberculosis bacillus that stimulates the body's immune system to fight the cancer. This therapy has been shown to be effective in controlling superficial bladder cancer.

A 2003 report stated that giving patients with bladder cancer chemotherapy followed by surgery may improve their outcomes. In the study of 307 patients, those with this combination of therapy lived two years longer than those treated with surgery only.

Photodynamic treatment is a novel mode of treatment that uses special chemicals and light to kill the cancerous cells when the bladder cancer is in its early stages. First, a drug is introduced into the bladder that makes the cancer cells more susceptible to light. A special light is then shone on the bladder in an attempt to destroy the cancerous cells.

Alternative and complementary therapies

Gene therapy is a new method being tested as a complementary therapy for bladder cancer. Research has shown that mutations in tumor suppressor genes can cause abnormal growth of bladder cells. Gene therapy involves infecting bladder cancer cells with specially designed viruses that contain a normal gene in order to restore a normal cell growth process.

Immunotherapy is another area that is expected to contribute new complementary treatment methods. Immunotoxins are antibodies produced in the laboratory that recognize specific substances that are more abundant in cancer cells than in normal cells. Once the immunotoxins identify a cancer cell, they deliver a powerful toxin attached to the antibody that enters and kills the cell.

Coping with cancer treatment

As with any cancer, shock and stress are natural reactions to a confirmed bladder cancer diagnosis. Coping is often made easier with access to helpful information and support services. Many patients want to learn all they can about the disease and their treatment choices so as to be fully involved in the decisions that are being made concerning their medical care. National cancer organizations are an important source of medical information. Many associations have also been organized to allow patients the opportunity to meet others undergoing similar experiences in support groups.

Patients are often uncomfortable during the first few days after bladder surgery. They may also experience **fatigue** and weakness. Those undergoing radiation therapy or chemotherapy may experience side effects such as pain, fatigue, rashes, or bleeding. Pain can be controlled with medication and patients should feel free to discuss aspects of pain relief with their physician or nurse.

Clinical trials

The National Cancer Institute (NCI) supports bladder cancer **clinical trials** to evaluate a variety of anticancer drugs. Some trials study new treatments involving radiation therapy, chemotherapy, biological therapies, and new combinations of various therapies. Other trials study ways to lower the side effects of treatment. Patients who take part in these studies often have the chance to benefit from promising new drugs and developments. Those interested in taking part in a trial should discuss the possibility with their physician and consult an NCI booklet entitled, "Taking Part in Clinical Trials: What Cancer Patients Need To Know" (NIH Publication #97-4250).

Prevention

Since it is not known what exactly causes bladder cancer, there is no certain way to prevent its occurrence. Avoiding risk factors whenever possible is the best alternative. Since smoking doubles one's risk of getting bladder cancer, avoiding tobacco may prevent at least half the deaths that result from bladder cancer. Taking appropriate safety precautions when working with organic cancer-causing chemicals is another way of reducing one's risk.

Those with a history of bladder cancer, kidney stones, urinary tract infections, and other conditions that cause long-term irritation to the bladder are advised to undergo regular screening tests such as urine cytology, cystoscopy, and x rays of the urinary tract, so that cancer may be detected at an early stage and treated appropriately.

Special concerns

Special concerns may arise for those who have undergone partial or radical cystectomy. For example, if the bladder has to be removed, the patient will need to learn a new way to store and pass urine. Women who have had a radical cystectomy are not able to have children because their uterus has also been removed. Men who have had a radical cystectomy will become impotent (unable to sustain an erection) if their prostate and seminal vesicles have also been removed.

See also Metastasis; Intravenous urography; Tumor staging.

Resources

PERIODICALS

Good, Brian. "Battle Against Bladder Cancer." *Men's Health* 18 (December 2003): 32.

Grossman, H. Barton, et al. "Neoadjuvant Chemotherapy Plus Cystectomy Compared With Cystectomy Alone for Locally Advanced Bladder Cancer." *The New England Journal of Medicine* August 28, 2003: 859.

"HRT Increases Risk of Gallbladder, Breast, Endometrial, and Bladder Cancer." *Women's Health Weekly* July 17, 2003: 31.

Lamm, D. L., and M. Allaway. "Current trends in bladder cancer treatment." *Annales Chirurgiae et Gynaecologiae* 89 (2000): 234-241.

Lockyer, C. R., and D. A. Gillatt. "BCG immunotherapy for superficial bladder cancer." *Journal of the Royal Society of Medicine* 94 (March 2001): 119-23.

Oosterlinck, W. "The management of superficial bladder cancer." *BJU International* 87 (January 2001): 135-40.

Petrovich, Z., G. Jozsef, and L. W. Brady. "Radiotherapy for carcinoma of the bladder: a review." *American Journal of Clinical Oncology* 24 (February 2001): 1-9.

Ryan, C. W., and N. J. Vogelzang. "Gemcitabine in the treatment of bladder cancer." *Expert Opinions in Pharmacotherapy* 1 (March 2000): 547-53.

"Tocosol Paclitaxel Receives Expedited Review for Bladder Cancer Indication." *Biotech Week* November 26, 2003: 443.

OTHER

"Bladder Cancer." *American Cancer Society's Urinary Bladder Cancer Resource Center.* 2000. [cited June 26, 2001]. <http://www3.cancer.org/cancerinfo/res_home.asp?ct=44>.

"Bladder Cancer: FAQ." *American Cancer Society*. [cited July 11, 2000 and June 26, 2001]. <http://www3.cancer.org/cancerinfo>.

"Staging: Stages of cancer of the bladder." *University of Pittsburgh Cancer Institute.* June 2001. [cited June 28, 2001]. http://www.upci.upmc.edu/internet/prostate/cancer/bladder/stage.cfm.

"Taking Part in Clinical Trials: What Cancer Patients Need To Know (NIH Publication #97 4250)." *National Institutes of Health & National Cancer Institute*. May 1998. [cited June 26, 2001]. http://www.cancernet.nci.nih.gov/peb/taking_part_treatment/index.html.

Lata Cherath, Ph.D.
Monique Laberge, Ph.D.

Bleomycin

Definition

Bleomycin (Blenoxane) kills **cancer** cells by damaging the genetic material known as DNA, thus preventing cells from repairing themselves.

Purpose

Bleomycin is used in the treatment of a number of different cancers, including cancer of the head and neck, skin, esophagus, lung, testis, penis, vulva, cervix, and genitourinary tract. In addition, it is used in the treatment of **Hodgkin's disease** and non-Hodgkin's lymphomas. It may also be used to treat **Kaposi's sarcoma**.

Because bleomycin is used in the treatment of so many different cancers, only a sampling of its uses can be provided here. In the treatment of Hodgkin's disease, one **chemotherapy** regimen used is the so-called ABVD, which consists of **doxorubicin**, bleomycin, **vinblastine**, and **dacarbazine**. Another regimen is called MOPP/ABV, which consists of **mechlorethamine**, **vincristine**, prednisone, **procarbazine**, doxorubicin, bleomycin, and vinblastine.

A treatment used for stage III and IV **non-Hodgkin's lymphoma** is the CHOP-bleomycin regimen, which consists of **cyclophosphamide**, hydroxydaunomycin, vincristine, prednisone, and bleomycin. Another approach to the same illness involves the m-BACOD chemotherapy regimen, which consists of **methotrexate**, bleomycin, doxorubicin, cyclophosphamide, vincristine, and **dexamethasone**. Yet another approach to treating this disease is called ProMACE-CytaBOM, and consists of cyclophosphamide, doxorubicin, **etoposide**, prednisone, **cytarabine**, bleomycin, vincristine, methotrexate, and **leucovorin**.

KEY TERMS

DNA—DNA is a nucleic acid found inside of cells that carries genetic information.

Raynaud's phenomenon— Raynaud's phenomenon, which affects the fingers and toes, may involve pain, pale color, and abnormal sensation (e.g., burning or prickling).

Description

Bleomycin is an antitumor antibiotic that fights cancer by attacking the DNA in cancerous cells, thus interfering with cell growth.

Recommended dosage

A dose of 0.25–0.50 units/kg (10–20 units per square meter) is given once or twice a week either intravenously, intramuscularly, or subcutaneously. A small test dose should be given first to test for a possible severe allergic reaction.

Precautions

Patients who receive certain forms of oxygen therapy while taking bleomycin or who receive anesthesia while taking bleomycin are at increased risk for developing serious lung problems.

Patients given bleomycin may develop an acute allergic reaction that may be fatal in rare cases. Therefore, a patient should only receive a small test dose of bleomycin the first time the drug is administered. After this initial dose the patient is observed carefully for one hour. Assuming no further problems appear, the patient may then receive a standard dose.

The likelihood that lung damage will occur increases if a patient receives more than 450–500 units of the drug during an entire lifetime. So, it is prudent to limit the amount of this medication given. Furthermore, it may be unwise to give bleomycin in regimens containing cyclophosphamide, as this combination also increases the likelihood that lung damage will occur.

Side effects

Lung problems are a serious side effect affecting some patients who receive bleomycin. While lung problems can appear regardless of how much of the medicine is given, they are more likely to appear if a patient receives more than a certain amount of the

medicine—250 units according to some authorities and 450–500 units according to others. The appearance of a dry cough may indicate the development of lung problems. Lung damage can be assessed by measuring the rate at which the patient is able to transfer gas across the lung membranes (D$_{LCO}$ or diffusion lung capacity).

Other side effects of bleomycin may include skin problems and alteration of skin color, allergic reactions, Raynaud's phenomenon, and hair loss (**alopecia**). In addition, headache, and **nausea and vomiting** may occur. Rheumatoid arthritis may worsen during bleomycin therapy. Patients with testicular tumors who receive multiple chemotherapy agents including bleomycin may develop Raynaud's phenomenon and cardiovascular disease. Raynaud's phenomenon, which affects the fingers and toes, may involve pain, pale color, and abnormal sensation (for instance, burning or prickling).

Approximately one out of every 100 patients who takes bleomycin experiences a reaction that involves chills, **fever**, wheezing, low blood pressure, and mental confusion. Unlike many other cancer drugs, bleomycin is not likely to cause any damage to the bone marrow.

Patients may be given steroids before bleomycin therapy is started in an effort to reduce the side effects of the drug.

Interactions

Bleomycin is often given in combination with with other **anticancer drugs**, for example **cisplatin**, vinblastine, and etoposide. Such combinations have been found to be more effective than single drug therapy.

Bob Kirsch

Blood dyscrasias *see* **Multiple myeloma; Waldenstrom's macroglobulinemia**
Blood transfusion *see* **Transfusion therapy**

Body image/self image
Description

Body image refers to a person's internal picture of his or her external physical appearance. Self image is a broader category that refers to one's inner perception of his or her physical, mental, interpersonal, and spiritual characteristics and abilities. The distinction is important because cultures vary significantly regarding the amount of emphasis given to body image as one aspect of self image. In Japan, for example, body image is a much smaller part of most people's self-image than it is in the United States. Both forms of self-perception, however, may be affected by **cancer** treatment.

Specific body image or self image concerns vary according to age and gender. Children being treated for cancer have different issues from adults because their self and body images are still being formed. Children and adolescents with cancer sometimes internalize a pictureof themselves as disfigured or unattractive, or as physically weak and incompetent. Even when the cancer has been successfully treated, the child's self image may still reflect feelings of being "sick" or "damaged." A distorted self image in turn can cause difficulties in social relationships as the child grows older. The Candlelighters programs offer practical advice and social support for children with cancer and their families.

Self image problems in adults tend to reflect (and reinforce) American society's patterns of gender socialization. Studies indicate that many women tend to be openly concerned about damage to their external appearance caused by cancer treatments. For many women, anxiety about losing their looks is directly related to fear of losing their husband or partner. Men's concern about outward appearance is less obvious but may be expressed as a need to look "healthy" in order to keep their job. Although there are not as many studies of men's reactions to cancer treatment as there are of women's, recent research indicates that men are still more concerned about losing physical strength or specific physical abilities required by their work than about their looks as such.

Causes

Cultural context

It is important to situate body image/self image issues related to cancer treatment within the larger context of contemporary emphasis on physical perfection. Advertising in the mass media encourages people to feel dissatisfied with their bodies. One study of the effects of television advertising on college youth found that as little as half an hour of ideal-body commercials has a negative impact on a person's body image. Another study found that a majority of American adults, men as well as women, believe that people are judged on the basis of appearance first and talent or personality second. In a cultural setting in which healthy people often feel they cannot measure up to media standards of attractiveness, it is not surprising

that cancer patients are concerned about the effects of therapy on their appearance.

In addition to concerns about appearance, some cancer patients experience a loss of adult identity related to the need to relearn bowel and bladder habits. Patients with colorectal cancer and others who have stomas must undergo a second period of toilet training as adults. Many of these patients report that their ability to travel, work, or socialize with others is significantly impaired by their problems with bowel control. According to a Swedish study, these difficulties often affect the patient's spouse as well in terms of limitations on the couple's social life.

Surgery

Surgery on the face or the parts of the body associated with sexual performance or attractiveness has a more severe impact on self image than surgery on the hands, feet, or back. Breast surgery in women and surgical treatment of **prostate cancer** in men are often accompanied by changes in the patient's self image, particularly with respect to sexual relations. Sexual responsiveness can also be affected if the surgeon has had to remove tissue containing nerve endings that are sensitive to touch.

Radiation and chemotherapy

Radiation and **chemotherapy** can affect a cancer patient's body image because they often cause hair loss, radiation burns, and unattractive changes in the patient's complexion. While hair loss caused by chemotherapy is usually a temporary condition, hair loss caused by radiation treatment may be permanent. In addition, both radiation and chemotherapy can cause **nausea**, **vomiting**, **fatigue**, **depression**, and other reactions that affect the patient's sense of competence as well as their relationships with others. Self image often suffers when a person feels that job performance and valued relationships are being strained by these side effects of cancer treatment.

Treatments

Cosmetic

Since 1989, the American Cancer Society, the Cosmetic, Toiletry, and Fragrance Association Foundation, and the National Cosmetology Association have sponsored the "Look Good... Feel Better" (LGFB) program, which offers classes in a number of medical centers. These classes help female cancer patients with self image issues as well as teaching them special grooming techniques to manage the side effects of cancer therapy. LGFB has been available in Canada since 1992.

Hair loss can be covered by a variety of wigs, partial hairpieces, and scarves or turbans. The American Hair Loss Council offers more detailed information about these and other ways to cope with hair loss caused by cancer treatment. Doctors who specialize in plastic surgery can suggest ways to treat facial scars or other types of surgical disfigurement, including the loss of body parts. A prosthesis, which is an artificial replacement for a missing or damaged body part, can be made to order for the patient.

Counseling and support

Cancer patients who are experiencing serious emotional problems related to changes in appearance may benefit from counseling or support groups. Individual psychotherapy guides people to look at the reasons for focusing on their looks as well as ways to cope with the changes. Pastoral or spiritual counseling can help remind patients that they are more than just their bodies. Support groups for cancer patients are good places to share feelings and useful tips about dress and grooming with others who are in the same situation.

Alternative and complementary therapies

Alternative and complementary therapies may help patients to deal with changes in self and body image through developing a fuller self image, finding new interests, or learning new skills. Meditation and prayer can help patients put physical appearance inside a larger framework of values. Some cancer patients find yoga, t'ai chi, and dance or movement therapy are interesting to learn as well as good forms of exercise. In addition, a group of researchers at Brown Medical School reported in early 2004 that cancer survivors who exercise regularly have higher levels of energy and self-esteem, and lower levels of depression and other mood disturbances, than survivors who do not exercise.

Also, massage, calming or uplifting music, and aromatherapy allow patients to balance the side effects of cancer treatment with relaxing and pleasant experiences.

See also Alopecia; Sexuality.

Resources

PERIODICALS

Carter, J., D. S. Chi, N. Abu-Rustum, et al. "Brief Report: Total Pelvic Exenteration—A Retrospective Clinical Needs Assessment." *Psychooncology* 13 (February 2004): 125–131.

Persson, E., E. Severinsson, and A. L. Hellstrom. "Spouses' Perceptions of and Reactions to Living with a Partner Who Has Undergone Surgery for Rectal Cancer Resulting in a Stoma." *Cancer Nursing* 27 (January-February 2004): 85–90.

Pinto, B. M., and J. J. Trunzo. "Body Esteem and Mood among Sedentary and Active Breast Cancer Survivors." *Mayo Clinic Proceedings* 79 (February 2004): 181–186.

Rosman, S. "Cancer and Stigma: Experience of Patients with Chemotherapy-Induced Alopecia." *Patient Education and Counseling* 52 (March 2004): 333–339.

Rosmovits, L., and S. Ziebland. "Expressions of Loss of Adulthood in the Narratives of People with Colorectal Cancer." *Qualitative Health Research* 14 (February 2004): 187–203.

OTHER

"For Women:Body Image Issues." *Gillette Women's Cancer Connection.* 1999. [cited March 16, 2001]. http://www.gillettecancerconnect.org.

Rebecca J. Frey, Ph.D.

Bone marrow aspiration and biopsy

Definition

Bone marrow aspiration, also called bone marrow sampling, is the removal by suction of fluid from the soft, spongy material that lines the inside of most bones. Bone marrow **biopsy**, or needle biopsy, is the removal of a small piece of bone marrow.

Purpose

Bone marrow aspiration is used to:

- pinpoint the cause of abnormal blood test results
- confirm a diagnosis or check the status of severe anemia (abnormally low numbers of red blood cells in the bloodstream) of unknown cause, or other irregularities in the way blood cells are produced or become mature
- evaluate abnormalities in the blood's ability to store iron
- diagnose infection

Bone marrow biopsy is used to:

- obtain intact bone marrow for laboratory analysis
- diagnose and stage some types of cancer or anemia and other blood disorders
- identify the source of an unexplained fever
- diagnose fibrosis of bone marrow or myeloma (a tumor composed of cells normally found in the

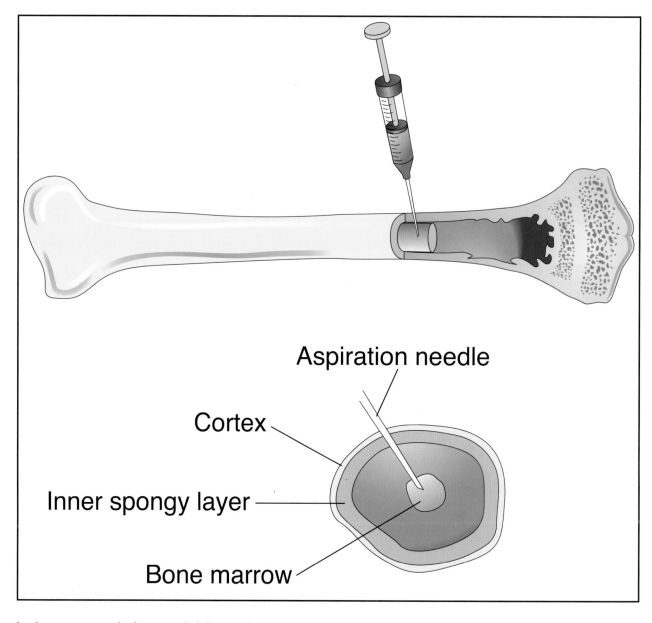

Aspiration needle

Cortex

Inner spongy layer

Bone marrow

In a bone marrow aspiration, a needle is inserted beneath the skin and rotated until it penetrates the cortex, or outer covering, of the bone. A small amount of marrow is suctioned out of the bone by a syringe attached to the needle. *(Illustration by Electronic Illustrators Group. Cengage Learning, Gale.)*

bone marrow) when bone marrow aspiration has failed to provide an appropriate specimen

Bone marrow aspiration and bone marrow biopsy are also used to gauge the effectiveness of **chemotherapy** and other medical treatments. These procedures are often used together to ensure the availability of the best possible bone marrow specimen.

Precautions

Allergies or previous adverse reactions to medications should be discussed with the doctor. Any current medications, including herbal or nutritional supplements, should be evaluated for the potential to interfere with proper coagulation (clot formation). These would include coumadin, aspirin, and other agents used as blood thinners. Caution should be used when the herbs gingko, ginger, garlic, or ginseng have been utilized as supplements, due to a risk of bleeding.

Pregnancy, lactation (production and secretion of milk), and preexisting platelet or bleeding disorders should be evaluated before either procedure is undertaken.

Description

Bone marrow aspiration and biopsy should be performed by a physician or nurse clinician. Each procedure takes about 20 to 30 minutes and is usually performed on an outpatient basis, but can be done in a hospital if necessary.

The skin covering the biopsy site is cleansed with an antiseptic, and the patient may be given a mild sedative. A local anesthetic is administered. The hematologist or nurse clinician performing the procedure will not begin until the anesthetic has numbed the area from which the specimen is to be extracted. In both adults and children, aspiration and biopsy are most commonly performed on the rear bone of the hip (posterior iliac crest). In adults, sampling from the sternum (breastbone) is sometimes done. The latter location is technically easier, but is somewhat more painful for the patient and presents the risk of heart injury. On rare occasions, a long bone of the leg (tibia) may be used as a sample site for an infant.

In a bone marrow aspiration, a special needle is inserted beneath the skin and rotated until it penetrates the cortex, or outer covering of the bone. At least half a teaspoon of marrow is withdrawn from the bone by a syringe attached to the needle. The patient may experience discomfort when the needle is inserted or when the marrow is aspirated. If more marrow is needed, the needle is repositioned slightly, a new syringe is attached, and a second sample is taken. The samples are transferred from the syringes to slides and vials, then sent to a laboratory for analysis.

Bone marrow biopsy may be performed immediately before or after bone marrow aspiration. The procedure utilizes a special large-bore needle that is used to drill out a core of marrow. In bone marrow biopsy, the needle is inserted, rotated from side to side, withdrawn, and reinserted at a different angle. This procedure is repeated if needed until a small core, about 0.4 inches (1 cm) long, is separated from the bone marrow. The needle is again removed, and a piece of fine wire threaded through its tip transfers the specimen onto sterile gauze. The patient may feel discomfort or pressure when the needle is inserted and experience a brief, pulling sensation when the marrow is withdrawn. Unlike aspiration specimens, which are smeared, these samples contain structurally intact bone marrow. Microscopic examination can show what material its cells contain and how they are alike or different from one another. The bone may either be embedded intact in paraffin (a type of wax), or be decalcified (a process which takes place overnight) for a different type of staining and examination. Each type of preparation has certain advantages.

Preparation

A current history and physical are obtained from the patient, along with proper consent. The patient is generally placed in a prone position (lying face down) for preparation, and local anesthetic, with or without sedation, is administered.

Aftercare

After the needle is removed, the biopsy site will be covered with a clean, dry bandage. Pressure is applied to control bleeding. The patient's pulse, breathing, blood pressure, and temperature are monitored until they return to normal, and the patient may be instructed to remain in a supine position (lying face up) for half an hour before getting dressed.

The patient should be able to leave the clinic and resume normal activities immediately. Patients who have received a sedative often feel sleepy for the rest of the day; driving, cooking, and other activities that require clear thinking and quick reactions should therefore be avoided.

The biopsy site should be kept covered and dry for several hours. Walking or taking prescribed pain medications usually ease any discomfort felt at the biopsy site, and ice can be used to reduce swelling.

A doctor should be notified if the patient:

- Feels severe pain more than 24 hours after the procedure.
- Experiences persistent bleeding or notices more than a few drops of blood on the wound dressing.
- Has a temperature above 101°F (38.3°C). Inflammation and pus at the biopsy site and other signs of infection should also be reported to a doctor without delay.

Risks

Bleeding and discomfort often occur at the biopsy site. **Infection** and hematoma may also develop. In rare instances, the heart or a major blood vessel is pierced when marrow is extracted from the sternum during bone marrow biopsy. This can lead to severe hemorrhage.

Normal results

Healthy adult bone marrow contains yellow fat cells, connective tissue, and red marrow that produces blood. The bone marrow of a healthy infant is primarily red due to active production of red cells necessary for growth.

Abnormal results

Culture of bone marrow aspirate may yield information about an infectious agent. Microscopic examination of bone marrow can reveal granulomas, **myelofibrosis**, lymphomas, leukemias, or other cancers. Analyzing specimens can help doctors diagnose iron deficiency, vitamin B_{12} deficiency, and folate deficiency, as well as **anemia**.

Obesity can affect the ease with which a bone marrow biopsy can be done, and the results of either procedure can be affected if the patient has had **radiation therapy** at the biopsy site.

Maureen Haggerty

Bone marrow transplantation

Definition

The bone marrow—the sponge-like tissue found in the center of certain bones—contains stem cells that are the precursors of white blood cells, red blood cells, and platelets. These blood cells are vital for normal body functions, such as oxygen transport, defense against **infection** and disease, and clotting. Blood cells have a limited lifespan and are constantly being replaced; therefore, healthy stem cells are vital.

In association with certain diseases, stem cells may produce too many, too few, or otherwise abnormal blood cells. Also, medical treatments may destroy stem cells or alter blood cell production. The resultant blood cell abnormalities can be life threatening.

Bone marrow transplantation involves extracting bone marrow containing normal stem cells from a healthy donor, and transferring it to a recipient whose body cannot manufacture proper quantities of normal blood cells. The goal of the transplant is to rebuild the recipient's blood cells and immune system and hopefully cure the underlying ailment.

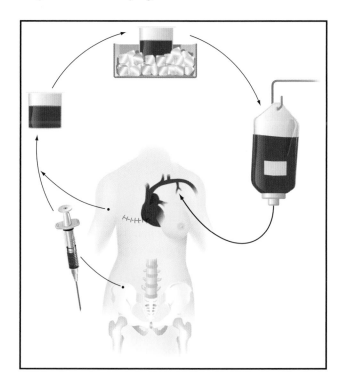

In autologous bone marrow transplantation, stem cells are collected. Once the patient has undergone chemotherapy, the cells are replaced in the blood via an intravenous catheter. The cells return to the bone marrow and begin producing healthy new cells. *(Illustration by Argosy Publishing. Cengage Learning, Gale.)*

Treatment of acute leukemia by bone marrow transplant.
(Photo Researchers, Inc. Reproduced by permission.)

Purpose

A person's red blood cells, white blood cells, and platelets may be destroyed or may be abnormal due to disease. Also, certain medical therapies, particularly **chemotherapy** or **radiation therapy**, may destroy a person's stem cells. The consequence to a person's health is severe. Under normal circumstances, red blood cells carry oxygen throughout the body and remove carbon dioxide from the body's tissues. White blood cells form the cornerstone of the body's immune system and defend it against infection. Platelets limit bleeding by enabling the blood to clot if a blood vessel is damaged.

A bone marrow transplant is used to rebuild the body's capacity to produce these blood cells and bring their numbers to normal levels. Illnesses that may be treated with a bone marrow transplant include both cancerous and noncancerous diseases.

Cancerous diseases may or may not specifically involve blood cells; but, **cancer** treatment can destroy the body's ability to manufacture new blood cells. Bone marrow transplantation may be used in conjunction with additional treatments, such as chemotherapy, for various types of leukemia, **Hodgkin's disease**, **lymphoma**, breast and **ovarian cancer**, and other cancers. Noncancerous diseases for which bone marrow transplantation can be a treatment option include aplastic **anemia**, sickle cell disease, thalassemia, and severe immunodeficiency.

Precautions

Bone marrow transplants are not for everyone. Transplants are accompanied by a risk of infection, transplant rejection by the recipient's immune system, and other complications. The procedure has a lower success rate the greater the recipient's age. Complications are exacerbated for people whose health is already seriously impaired as in late-stage cancers. Therefore, a person's age or state of health may prohibit use of a bone marrow transplant. The typical cut-off age for a transplant ranges from 40 to 55 years; however, a person's general health is usually the more important factor.

Even in the absence of complications, the transplant and associated treatments are hard on the recipient. Bone marrow transplants are debilitating. A person's ability to withstand the rigors of the transplant is a key consideration in deciding to use this treatment.

Description

Autologous and allogeneic transplants

Two important requirements for a bone marrow transplant are the donor and the recipient. Sometimes, the donor and the recipient may be the same person. This type of transplant is called an autologous transplant. It is typically used in cases in which a person's bone marrow is generally healthy but will be destroyed due to medical treatment for diseases such as **breast cancer** and Hodgkin's disease. Most bone marrow transplants are autologous. If a person's bone marrow is unsuitable for an autologous transplant, the bone marrow must be derived from another person in an allogeneic transplant.

Allogeneic transplants are more complicated because of proteins called human lymphocyte antigens (HLA) that are on the surface of bone marrow cells. If the donor and the recipient have very dissimilar antigens, the recipient's immune system regards the donor's bone marrow cells as invaders and launches

KEY TERMS

ABO antigen—Protein molecules located on the surfaces of red blood cells that determine a person's blood type: A, B, or O.

AML—Acute myelogenous leukemia, also called acute myelocytic leukemia. Malignant disorder where myeloid blast cells accumulate in the marrow and bloodstream.

Allogeneic—Referring to bone marrow transplants between two different, genetically dissimilar people.

Anemia—Decreased red cell production which results in deficiency in oxygen-carrying capacity of the blood.

Antigen—A molecule that is capable of provoking an immune response.

Aplastic anemia—A disorder in which the body produces inadequate amounts of red blood cells and hemoglobin due to underdeveloped or missing bone marrow.

Autologous—Referring to bone marrow transplants in which recipients serve as their own donors.

Blank—If an individual has inherited same HLA antigen from both parents, the HLA typing is designated by the shared HLA antigen followed by a "blank"(–)

Blast cells—Blood cells in early stage of cellular development.

Blast crisis—Stage of chronic myelogenous leukemia where large quantities of immature cells are produced by the marrow and is not responsive to treatment.

Bone marrow—A spongy tissue located within flat bones, including the hip and breast bones and the skull. This tissue contains stem cells, the precursors of platelets, red blood cells, and white blood cells.

Bone marrow transplant—Healthy marrow is infused into people who have had high-dose chemotherapy for one of the many forms of leukemias, immunodeficiencies, lymphomas, anemias, metabolic disorders, and sometimes solid tumors.

Chemotherapy—Medical treatment of a disease, particularly cancer, with drugs or other chemicals.

Chronic myelogenous leukemia (CML)—Also called chronic myelocytic leukemia, malignant disorder that involves abnormal accumulation of white cells in the marrow and bloodstream.

Cytomegalovirus (CMV)—Virus that can cause pneumonia in post bone marrow transplant patients

Conditioning—Process of preparing patient to receive marrow donation, often through the use of chemotherapy and radiation therapy

Confirmatory typing—Repeat tissue typing to confirm the compatibility of the donor and patient before transplant

Donor—A healthy person who contributes bone marrow for transplantation.

Graft versus host disease—A life-threatening complication of bone marrow transplants in which the donated marrow causes an immune reaction against the recipient's body.

a destructive attack against them. Such an attack negates any benefits offered by the transplant.

HLA matching

There are only five major HLA classes or types—designated HLA–A,–B,–C,–D, and class III—but much variation within the groupings. For example, HLA–A from one individual may be similar to, but not the same as, HLA–A in another individual; such a situation can render a transplant from one to the other impossible.

HLA matching is more likely if the donor and recipient are related, particularly if they are siblings; however, an unrelated donor may be a potential match. Only in rare cases is matching HLA types between two people not an issue: if the recipient has an identical twin. Identical twins carry the same genes; therefore, the same antigens. A bone marrow transplant between identical twins is called a syngeneic transplant.

Peripheral blood stem cell transplants

A relatively recent development in stem cell transplantation is the use of peripheral blood stem cells instead of cells from the bone marrow. Peripheral blood stem cells (PBSCs) are obtained from circulating blood rather than from bone marrow, but the amount of stem cells found in the peripheral blood is much smaller than the amount of stem cells found in the bone marrow. Peripheral blood stem cells can be

Histocompatibility—The major histocompatibility determinants are the human leukocyte antigens (HLA) and characterize how well the patient and donor are matched.

HLA (human leuckocyte antigen)—A group of protein molecules located on bone marrow cells that can provoke an immune response. A donor's and a recipient's HLA types should match as closely as possible to prevent the recipient's immune system from attacking the donor's marrow as a foreign material that does not belong in the body.

Hodgkin's disease—A type of cancer involving the lymph nodes and potentially affecting nonlymphatic organs in the later stage.

Immunodeficiency—A disorder in which the immune system is ineffective or disabled either due to acquired or inherited disease.

Leukemia—A type of cancer that affects leukocytes, a particular type of white blood cell. A characteristic symptom is excessive production of immature or otherwise abnormal leukocytes.

Lymphoma—A type of cancer that affects lymph cells and tissues, including certain white blood cells (T cells and B cells), lymph nodes, bone marrow, and the spleen. Abnormal cells (lymphocyte/leukocyte) multiply uncontrollably.

Match—How similar the HLA typing, out of a possible six antigens, is between the donor and the recipient.

Mixed lymphocyte culture (MLC)—Test that measures level of reactivity between donor and recipient lymphocytes.

Neuroblastoma—Solid tumor in children, may be treated by BMT.

Platelets—Fragments of a large precursor cell, a megakaryocyte found in the bone marrow. These fragments adhere to areas of blood vessel damage and release chemical signals that direct the formation of a blood clot.

Recipient—The person who receives the donated blood marrow.

Red blood cells—Cells that carry hemoglobin (the molecule that transports oxygen) and help remove wastes from tissues throughout the body.

Sickle cell disease—An inherited disorder characterized by a genetic flaw in hemoglobin production. (Hemoglobin is the substance within red blood cells that enables them to transport oxygen.) The hemoglobin that is produced has a kink in its structure that forces the red blood cells to take on a sickle shape, inhibiting their circulation and causing pain. This disorder primarily affects people of African descent.

Syngeneic—Referring to a bone marrow transplant from one identical twin to the other.

Thalassemia—A group of inherited disorders that affects hemoglobin production. (Hemoglobin is the substance within red blood cells that enables them to transport oxygen.) Because hemoglobin production is impaired, a person with this disorder may suffer mild to severe anemia. Certain types of thalassemia can be fatal.

White blood cells—A group of several cell types that occur in the bloodstream and are essential for a properly functioning immune system.

used in either autologous or allogeneic transplants. The majority of PBSC transplants are autologous. However, recent clinical studies indicate that PBSCs are being used more frequently than bone marrow for allogeneic bone marrow transplantation.

The advantages of PBSC transplants when compared to bone marrow transplants are: in allogeneic transplantation, haematopoietic and immune recovery are faster with PBSCs. In autologous transplantation, the use of PBSCs can result in faster blood count recovery. Also, some medical conditions exist in which the recipient cannot accept bone marrow transplants, but can accept PBSC transplants. Some possible disadvantages to PBSC transplant versus bone marrow transplantation are: so much more fluid volume is necessary to collect enough PBSCs that, at the time that the new stem cells are infused into the recipient, the fluid can collect in the lungs. Also, the time commitment for the donor for a PBSC transplant is considerable. When the PBSCs are being collected, several outpatient sessions are needed and each session lasts approximately two–four hours.

The transplant procedure

BONE MARROW TRANSPLANTATION. The bone marrow extraction, or harvest, is the same whether for an autologous or allogeneic transplant. Harvesting is done under general anesthesia (i.e., the donor sleeps through the procedure), and discomfort is usually minimal afterwards. Bone marrow is drawn from the iliac crest (the part of the hip bone to either side of the lower back) with a special needle and a syringe. Several punctures are usually necessary to collect the needed amount of bone marrow, approximately 1–2 quarts. (This amount is only a small percentage of the total bone marrow and is typically replaced within four weeks.) The donor remains at the hospital for 24–48 hours and can resume normal activities within a few days.

If the bone marrow is meant for an autologous transplant, it is stored at –112 to –320°F (–80 to –196°C) until it is needed. Bone marrow for an allogeneic transplant is sometimes treated to remove the donor's T cells (a type of white blood cell) or to remove ABO (blood type) antigens; otherwise, it is transplanted without modification.

The bone marrow is administered to the recipient via a catheter (a narrow, flexible tube) inserted into a large vein in the chest. From the bloodstream, it migrates to the cavities within the bones where bone marrow is normally stored. If the transplant is successful, the bone marrow begins to produce normal blood cells once it is in place, or engrafted.

PERIPHERAL BLOOD STEM CELL TRANSPLANTATION.
Before collection for a PBSC transplant, donors receive daily four injections of the drug G-CSF, or **filgrastim**. (Patients can give it to themselves at home if need be.) These pretreatments stimulate the body to release stem cells into the blood. After these pretreatments, the donors' experience is similar to that of a whole blood donor's experience—PBSC donors' blood is collected at a clinic or hospital as an outpatient procedure. The differences are that several sessions will be needed over days or weeks and the blood is collected in a process called apheresis. The blood travels from one arm into a blood cell separator that removes only the stem cells, and the rest of the blood is returned back to the donor, in the other arm. The cells are then frozen for later use.

The PBSCs are administered to the recipient using the same methods as those used in bone marrow transplantation. As stated, the amount of fluid with PBSCs infused into the recipient's body can be an issue.

Costs

Bone marrow transplantation is an expensive procedure. (Bone marrow donors are volunteers and do not pay for any part of the procedure.) Insurance companies and health maintenance organizations (HMOs) may not cover the costs.

Preparation

A bone marrow transplant recipient can expect to spend 4–8 weeks in the hospital. In preparation for receiving the transplant, the recipient undergoes "conditioning"—a preparative regimen in which the bone marrow and abnormal cells are destroyed. Conditioning rids the body of diseased cells and makes room for the marrow to be transplanted. It typically involves chemotherapy and/or radiation treatment, depending on the disease being treated. Unfortunately, this treatment also destroys healthy cells and has many side effects such as extreme weakness, **nausea**, **vomiting**, and **diarrhea**. These side effects may continue for several weeks.

Aftercare

A two- to four-week waiting period follows the marrow transplant before its success can begin to be judged. The marrow recipient is kept in isolation during this time to minimize potential infections. The recipient also receives antibiotic medications and blood and platelet transfusions to help fight off infection and prevent excessive bleeding. Further side effects, such as **nausea and vomiting**, can be treated with other medications. Once blood counts are normal and the side effects of the transplant abate, the recipient is taken off **antibiotics** and usually no longer needs blood and platelet transfusions.

Following discharge from the hospital, the recipient is monitored through home visits by nurses or outpatient visits for up to a year. For the first several months out of the hospital, the recipient needs to be careful in avoiding potential infections. For example, contact with other people who may be ill should be avoided or kept to a minimum. Further blood transfusions and medications may be necessary, but barring complications, the recipient can return to normal activities about six to eight months after the transplant.

Risks

Bone marrow transplants are accompanied by serious and life-threatening risks. Furthermore, they are not always an absolute assurance of a cure for the underlying ailment; a disease may recur in the future. Approximately 30% of people receiving allogeneic transplants do not survive. Autologous transplants have a much better survival rate—nearly 90%—but are not appropriate for all types of ailments requiring a bone marrow transplant. Furthermore, they have a higher failure rate with certain diseases, specifically leukemia.

In the short term, there is the danger of **pneumonia** or other infectious disease, excessive bleeding, or liver disorder caused by blocked blood vessels. The transplant may be rejected by the recipient's immune system, or the donor bone marrow may launch an immune-mediated attack against the recipient's tissues. This complication is called acute graft-versus-host disease, and it can be a life-threatening condition. Characteristic signs of the disease include **fever**, rash, diarrhea, liver problems, and a compromised immune system.

Approximately 25–50% of bone marrow transplant recipients develop long-term complications. **Chronic graft-vs-host disease** symptoms include skin changes such as dryness, altered pigmentation, and thickening; abnormal liver function tests; dry mouth and eyes; infections; and **weight loss**. Other long-term complications include cataracts (due to radiation treatment), abnormal lung function, hormonal abnormalities resulting in reduced growth or hypothyroidism, secondary cancers, and infertility.

Normal results

In a successful bone marrow transplant, the donor's marrow migrates to the cavities in the recipient's bones and produces normal numbers of healthy blood cells. Bone marrow transplants can extend a person's life, improve quality of life, and may aid in curing the underlying ailment.

Resources

PERIODICALS

Dreger, P., and N. Schmitz. "Allogeneic transplantation of blood stem cells: coming of age?" *Annals of Hematology* 80, no. 3 (March 2001): 127-36.

Nuzhat, Iqbal, Donna Salzman, Audrey J. Lazenby, et al. "Diagnosis of Gastrointestinal Graft-Versus-Host Disease." *The American Journal of Gastroenterology* 95 (November 2000): 3034- 3038.

ORGANIZATIONS

American Society for Blood and Marrow Transplantation (ASBMT). 85 W. Algonquin Road, Suite 550 Arlington Heights, IL 60005. (847) 427-0224. mail @asbmt.org. Founded in 1990, a national professional association that promotes advancement of the field of blood and bone marrow transplantation in clinical practice and research.

Blood & Marrow Transplant Newsletter (Formerly BMT Newsletter). 2900 Skokie Valley Road, Suite B, Highland Park, IL 60035 (847) 433-3313. 1-888-597-7674. help@bmtinfonet.org. <http://www2.bmtnews.org>. Blood & Marrow Transplant Newsletter is a not-for-profit organization that provides publications and support services to bone marrow, peripheral blood stem cell, and cord blood transplant patients and survivors.

BMT Information. http://www.bmtinfo.org/. Website, sponsored by a variety of other bone marrow transplant organizations, lists basic information and resources about bone marrow transplants.

Health Resources and Services Administration. 5600 Fishers Lane, Rm. 14-45, Rockville, MD 20857, 301-443-3376, comments@hrsa.gov. http://www.hrsa.gov. HRSA manages contracts for the Organ Procurement and Transplantation Network, Scientific Registry of Transplant Recipients and National Marrow Donor Program and provides public education and technical assistance to increase donation. HRSA also monitors the performance of the nation's transplant centers and provides potential transplant recipients with survival rates and other vital information.

International Bone Marrow Transplant Registry/Autologous Blood and Marrow Transplant Registry N. America. Health Policy Institute, Medical College of Wisconsin, 8701 Watertown Plank Road, P.O. Box 26509, Milwaukee, WI 53226 USA, 414-456-8325, ibmtr@mcw. edu. Voluntary organizations of more than 400 institutions in 47 countries that submit data on their allogeneic and autologous blood and marrow transplant recipients to the IBMTR/ABMTR Statistical Center at the Medical College of Wisconsin in Milwaukee.

Leukemia & Lymphoma Society, Inc. 1311 Mamaroneck Avenue White Plains, NY 10605, 914-949-5213 http://www.leukemia-lymphoma.org/. National voluntary health agency dedicated to curing leukemia, lymphoma, Hodgkin's disease and myeloma, and to improving the quality of life of patients and their families.

National Marrow Donor Program. Suite 500, 3001 Broadway Street Northeast, Minneapolis, MN 55413-1753. (800) MARROW-2. http://www.marrow.org. Founded in 1986, The National Marrow Donor Program (NMDP) is a non-profit international leader in the facilitation of unrelated marrow and blood stem cell transplantation.

National Organ and Tissue Donation Initiative. http://www.organdonor.gov/ Created by Health Resources and Services Administration (HRSA) Department of Health and Human Services (DHHS) http://www.os.dhhs.gov/. Provides information and resources on organ donation and transplantation issues.

Julia Barrett
Laura Ruth, Ph.D.

Bone pain

Description

Bone pain represents one of the most debilitating side effects of the metastases (distant spread) of many cancers such as breast, prostate, lung, and **multiple myeloma** (myelomatosis). Severe bone pain is frequent, reported by greater than 65% of patients suffering with bone metastases. The most common sites affected include the pelvis, femur, skull, and vertebra. The patient often describes the pain as dull and aching, localized at the site affected; however, some patients experience short, shooting pain that radiates out from the torso to the extremities. Movement typically aggravates the pain. Bone pain can signal disease progression, a new **infection**, or a complication from treatment. Pain is a reliable early indicator of complications from metastases — osteoporosis, **hypercalcemia**, fractures, and **spinal cord compression**. These conditions not only adversely affect the patient's quality of life, but in some cases may create such a decline that death results not from the **cancer**, but from bone- and skeletal-related complications. When a patient complains of bone pain, it require confirmation, usually by imaging. Plain-film radiography may detect typical lesions, but may not be sensitive enough to detect certain complications. In these cases, radionuclide scintigraphy and **magnetic resonance imaging** (MRI) are the preferred diagnostic tools.

Causes

Bone pain may be the result of direct tumor involvement. Pain is produced when the tumor pushes against or enters the bone. The tumor may compress surrounding blood vessels, nerves, and soft tissue, or may activate nociceptors (pain receptors) located at the site. Pain also may result from tissue compression caused by fibrosis (a condition caused by an increase in tissue) after the patient has undergone **radiation therapy**. A major source of bone pain in the cancer patient is pathologic fracture and osteoclast-induced bone resorption by the tumor. This condition promotes bone loss and, at the same time, provides growth factors for the tumor to increase in size.

Treatments

There are several options for **pain management** for bone metastases. The primary treatment for the majority of patients is external beam radiation therapy. These treatments provide excellent pain relief. Localized radiation treatments target specific sites for pain relief, promote healing, and help prevent fractures. Spinal cord compression from vertebral collapse requires immediate and localized radiation therapy, possibly in conjunction with surgical intervention to prevent paralysis or loss of life. Wide-field radiation therapy treats multiple disease sites and is appropriate for more diffuse bone pain. One half of the body receives radiation in a single treatment. Studies report relief of bone pain in 55%–100% of patients. A 2003 study reported that external beam radiation therapy treatments provided significant pain relief for two-thirds of patients with bone mestastases from breast and **prostate cancer**.

Analgesics (pain relievers) are typically given in conjunction with radiotherapy. Severity of the bone pain and general health of the patient will determine the prescribed medication. The medications prescribed range from over-the-counter pain medicine to **opioids** for extreme bone pain management.

Radiopharmaceuticals may be an effective choice for bone pain management. Iodine-131 is used in the treatment of multiple bone metastases from **thyroid cancer**. Phosphorus-32 orthophosphate has a success rate of about 80% in bone pain management in patients suffering with breast and prostate cancer. Strontium-89 provides partial or complete pain relief in approximately 65% of patients. Other radiopharmaceuticals are being tested internationally but have not yet received FDA approval for use in the United States. In treatments for bone resorption-induced pain, a group of chemical agents, known as **bisphosphonates** and **calcitonin**, acts to strongly block the bone resorption process. These agents are used in the management of hypercalcemia and have the added effect of reducing the prescribed amount of analgesics and shortening the duration of bone pain.

Alternative and complementary therapies

Comprehensive management of bone pain includes non-clinical choices. Patients should be encouraged to participate in complementary therapies, and some patients may choose to investigate more alternative therapies. More conventional complementary therapies may include relaxation and imagery therapy, cognitive distraction and reframing, support group and pastoral counseling, skin stimulation, biofeedback, nerve blocks, immobilization and stabilization techniques, and surgical intervention. Less well-defined alternative therapies may include acupuncture, body massage with pressure and vibration techniques, hypnosis, menthol preparations, and holistic or herbal medical practices. No conclusive data exist on the effectiveness of these therapies used alone; however, in conjunction with conventional methods of bone pain management, they do not appear to hinder therapy and may provide the patient with increased goodwill and a positive outlook.

Resources

PERIODICALS

Coleman, Robert E. "Management of Bone Metastases." *The Oncologist* 5 (September 2000): 463-470.

"External Beam Radiation Effective in Providing Bone Metasteses Pain Relief." *Medical Devices & Surgical Technology Week* November 16, 2003: 137.

Jane Taylor-Jones, M.S.

Bone survey

Definition

A bone survey is an x ray to check the health and status of a person's bones. It is an important tool for diagnosing the presence of **multiple myeloma** lesions in bone.

Purpose

The bone survey is the standard method for determining if there is bone involvement in multiple **myeloma**. Multiple myeloma lesions may not show up in other bone studies. However, if the lesions are present, they are likely to appear on a bone survey, making this an important diagnostic tool.

In patients who have been treated for multiple myeloma, bone surveys should be repeated to see if the disease has responded to treatment, or if it has progressed further. While the repeated bone survey may show that bone healing has occurred, this is not usually the case. Only 30% of patients whose multiple myeloma is responding to treatment show an improvement on their bone surveys. Multiple myeloma patients whose disease is progressing, or who have new areas of **bone pain**, can benefit from repeat bone surveys because this procedure can locate sites of potential fractures that may then be prevented by radiation or surgery.

Precautions

The dose of radiation in diagnostic **x rays** is very small, and this procedure is considered relatively safe. However, x rays are generally not advised for pregnant women. These women should inform their physician or the x-ray technician of their pregnancy (or suspected pregnancy) prior to the procedure.

Description

A bone survey in people with multiple myeloma includes x rays of the skull, spine, pelvis, and long bones of the legs and arms because the disease may spread to these particular areas. The procedure may be done in the radiology department of a hospital (for inpatients or outpatients) or in an imaging facility.

Patients may be given a hospital gown and asked to remove clothing that could interfere with the image, such as buttons or snaps. A lead shield for protection from radiation may be placed over the parts of the body that are not undergoing an x ray.

An x ray creates a two-dimensional (flat) image shown on film. Since the human body is three-dimensional, at least two different angles of the same area will be x-rayed. The radiology technician helps the patient achieve the proper position. Most imaging centers have special tables that help position the patient.

When the patient is properly positioned, the technician will leave the room to activate the x-ray machine. It is important that the patient remain completely still while the x ray is being taken. The x ray does not cause any pain or other sensation, and gives off no smell, sound, or taste, although it is penetrating the body. The patient may hear a sound, but this is the equipment and not the x ray itself.

The x ray creates shadows on film, and the film is viewed by a physician (radiologist) who specializes in **imaging studies**. The film will have contrasts that appear as varying shades of gray.

Preparation

Because the procedure in non-invasive, no specific preparation is necessary.

Aftercare

Bone surveys do not require any aftercare.

Risks

While radiation in high doses may present a **cancer** risk, the dosage for diagnostic purposes is very low. New technology has increased the safety of radiologic procedures. As in any procedure, the risk must be weighed against the benefit. In patients with multiple myeloma, the bone survey is needed to determine bone involvement, which could then dictate treatment. Pregnant women generally do not receive x rays, and should discuss this with their physician.

Normal results

Bone structure that is free of disease, fracture, or other problem areas is a normal result.

Abnormal results

Areas where multiple myeloma is present show up as destructive bone lesions. Parts of the bone may appear moth-eaten, and fractures may be present.

Resources

BOOKS

Helms, Clyde A. "Malignant Bone and Soft-Tissue Tumors" In *Fundamentals of Diagnostic Radiology*, edited by W. Brant and C. Helms, 2nd ed. Philadelphia: Williams & Wilkins, 1999, pp. 991–3.

Kyle, Robert A., and Joan Blade. "Multiple Myeloma and Related Disorders." In *Clinical Oncology*, edited by M. Abeloff, et al. Philadelphia: Churchill Livingstone, 2000, pp. 2601–3.

Vescio, Robert A., and James R. Berenson. "Myeloma, Macroglobulinemia, and Amyloidosis." In *Cancer Treatment*, edited by C. Haskell, 5th ed. Philadelphia: W. B. Saunders, 2001, pp. 1503-4.

Wolbarst, Anthony Brinton. *Looking Within: How X-Ray, CT, MRI, Ultrasound, and Other Medical Images Are Created and How They Help Physicians Save Lives.* Berkeley, CA: University of California Press, 1999.

Rhonda Cloos, R.N.

Bone metastasis *see* **Metastasis**

Bone scan *see* **Nuclear medicine scans**

Bortezomib

Definition

Bortezomib is an anti-cancer drug that is marketed under the name Velcade by Millenium Pharmaceuticals. It is approved for use in two types of blood **cancer**,

mantle cell lymphoma and **multiple myeloma**. Bortezomib belongs to a class of drugs known as proteasome inhibitors.

Purpose

Multiple **myeloma** is a cancer of bone marrow immune system cells called plasma cells. Plasma cells are formed in the bone marrow and travel in the blood and lymphatic system. Plasma cells form antibodies against infectious molecules encountered in the body. In multiple myeloma, a gene mutation causes an abnormal overproduction of plasma cells. The malignant plasma cells cause multiple medical issues, such as bone damage and kidney failure, as well as increased infections due to a dysfunctional immune system. In 2008, bortezomib was approved by the FDA as first-line treatment for multiple myeloma in combination with other drugs. First-line drug therapy is a term used to describe the drug or combination of drugs that have been evaluated as the most effective treatment for a given disease, and therefore the drug of choice in the absence of factors that would prohibit its use.

The FDA has also approved bortezomib for use in mantle cell **lymphoma** patients who have already been treated with at least one other cancer drug regimen. Mantle cell lymphoma is a type of cancer involving white blood cells known as lymphocytes and usually originates in lymph nodes. Relative to some other forms of lymphoma, mantle cell lymphoma is a rare form. While it is thought to be caused by a gene mutation, it is not a genetic disease that is inherited. In Mantle cell lymphoma, lymphocytes develop in an abnormal manner into dysfunctional cells that accumulate and do not support immune function, eventually decreasing the ability of the immune system to function. The disease also frequently impacts the bone marrow and gastrointestinal tract.

Description

Bortezomib is a proteasome inhibitor. Proteasomes are enzymes that are responsible for the degradation of proteins and a part of normal regulatory bodily processes. They are present in normal cells as well as cancer cells. In normal cells proteasomes dispose of damaged or unnecessary proteins, thereby keeping that cell in a healthy enough state that it remains alive. This allows cell division and growth of that group of replicating cells. If damaged proteins are not degraded by proteasomes, the cell does not remain healthy, and the cell will undergo a process of cell death known as apoptosis in which damaged cells are not allowed to replicate. Proteasomes help keep cells healthy, alive, and replicating. In cancer cells proteasomes are working to allow replication of the abnormal cancerous cells and growth of a tumor. Inhibiting proteasomes in cancer cells stops tumors from growing and induces apoptosis. For reasons that are not yet clearly understood, proteasome inhibitor drugs are more selective for the cancerous cells in mantle cell lymphoma and multiple myeloma than for other cancer types or normal cells. This fortunate relative specificity allows bortezomib to be used in clinical treatment.

Bortezomib decreases tumor growth and increases time to tumor progression, median survival time, and overall survival. Median survival time is a term used to describe the time from either diagnosis or treatment at which half of the patients with a given disease are expected to still be alive. In a clinical trial designed to test out a cancer drug in humans, median survival time is one way to measure how effective a treatment is. The term time to tumor progression describes a period of time from when disease is diagnosed (or treated) until the disease starts to get worse.

Recommended dosage

Bortezomib was the first therapeutic proteasome inhibitor used in humans for **chemotherapy**. It is administered as an injection into a vein by a health care professional. The dose that is used varies from patient to patient and is affected by the medical condition and the individual's response to treatment. In general, bortezomib may be given on a rotating schedule that includes 2 weeks during which bortezomib is given twice a week and 10 days without bortezomib. During the weeks that bortezomib is given, doses will always be at least 72 hours apart. The rotating schedule may continue for up to nine cycles. After that, a doctor may decide to continue treatment, but will administer bortezomib less often.

An example of a specific dosage regimen is the clinical scenario of bortezomib used in combination with the drugs **melphalan** and prednisone for the first-line treatment of multiple myeloma. In this case the regimen may administered in nine 6-week cycles. During the first four cycles the recommended adult dosage is 1.3 mg/m2 (a dose that is based on the patient approximate body surface area). This dose is given by IV injection over three to five seconds twice a week during weeks 1, 2, 4, and 5 (days 1, 4, 8, 11, 22, 25, 29, and 32 of the 6-week cycle). After this section of the regimen there is a 10-day rest period (days 33–42). For the remaining cycles (five through nine), the same dose of drug is administered once a week during weeks 1, 2, 4, and 5 (days 1, 8, 22, and 29) followed by a 13-day rest period. In all nine cycles, the other drugs used in the combination treatment are administered in their own regimen.

Precautions

Bortezomib is not recommended for use in pregnant women. Birth control is recommended while on this drug. Bortezomib is a pregnancy Category D drug. Category D describes drugs in which there is evidence of potential human fetal risk based on adverse reaction data from investigational or marketing experience or studies in humans, but potential benefits may warrant use of the drug in pregnant women despite potential risks. For Category D drugs, medical necessity must be great enough to warrant risking harm to the fetus. Bortezomib is not recommended for use in breast feeding women. It is not known whether bortezomib is excreted in breast milk, and there are potential toxic effects for a nursing infant. Bortezomib is only used in adults as the safety for use in patients less than 18 years of age has not been established.

Caution must be used in patients greater than 65 years of age, as bortezomib may cause increased toxic side effects in this age group. All patients taking bortezomib must remain well hydrated. Bortezomib may not be suitable for patients with a history of **neuropathy** (nerve damage), heart disease, low blood pressure, pulmonary hypertension, diabetes, liver disease, severe kidney disease, herpes infections, or shingles. Bortezomib may not be used in patients who are currently in a state of dehydration or **pneumonia**, or with allergies to boron or mannitol.

Because bortezomib causes dizziness, patients should be cautious when rising from lying down. Caution should be used when considering driving a car or operating machinery. Patients should not have any vaccinations while taking bortezomib without the consent of their treating physician. Patients taking bortezomib should avoid being around people who have recently had the oral polio vaccine.

Side effects

Bortezomib is used when the medical benefit is judged to be greater than the risk of side effects. Potential side effects include dizziness, abdominal cramping, **nausea and vomiting**, lightheadedness, headache, loss of appetite, altered taste in the mouth, **diarrhea** and constipation, **fatigue** and weakness, and blurred vision. Back pain, muscle pain, **bone pain**, joint pain, **fever**, and chills may occur. Bortezomib may cause nerve damage in the arms or legs known as peripheral neuropathy, which may be painful. The immune system may be suppressed, resulting in increased susceptibility to **infection** that may limit the dose that can be used in an individual patient. Infections such as pneumonia or general upper respiratory infections may occur. Patients on bortezomib may have a greater risk for developing shingles, which is reactivation of the chicken pox virus that lies dormant in nerves over many years, causing patches of painful blisters. Bortezomib may cause itchy skin and rash, **anemia**, insomnia, anxiety, and psychiatric disturbances. Generally the side effects seen with bortezomib treatment are tolerable enough that it may make a better treatment alternative than other therapeutic options such as bone marrow transplant.

Interactions

Patients should make their doctor aware of any and all medications or supplements they are taking before using bortezomib. Bortezomib interacts with many other drugs. Some drug interactions may make bortezomib unsuitable for use, while others may be monitored and attempted. Medications for diabetes or high blood pressure may not be suitable for use with bortezomib. Drugs that may cause peripheral neuropathy such as amiodarone, isoniazid, nitrofurantoin, and the antiviral acyclovir may have an additive effect with bortezomib for this side effect. Green tea extract reduces the effectiveness of bortezomib as a cancer treatment. Combining bortezomib with some other drugs such as the anti-cancer agent **thalidomide** may increase its potency.

Bortezomib is metabolized by a set of liver enzymes known as CYP450 subtype 3A4. Drugs that induce, or activate these enzymes increase the metabolism of bortezomib. This results in lower levels of therapeutic bortezomib, thereby negatively affecting treatment of cancer. For this reason drugs that induce CYP450 subtype 3A4 may not be used with bortezomib. This includes some anti-epileptic drugs such as **carbamazepine**, some anti-inflammatories such as **dexamethasone**, anti-tuberculosis drugs such as rifampin, and the herb St. John's Wort.

Drugs that act to inhibit the action of CYP450 subtype 3A4 may cause undesired increased levels of bortezomib in the body. This could lead to toxic doses. Some examples are **antibiotics** such as clarithromycin, antifungal drugs such as ketoconazole, antiviral drugs such as indinavir, antidepressants such as fluoxetine, and some cardiac agents such as verapamil. Grapefruit juice may also increase the amount of bortezomib in the body. Eating grapefruit or drinking grapefruit juice is not advised while taking bortezomib.

Resources

BOOKS

Goodman and Gilman's The Pharmacological Basis of Therapeutics, Eleventh Edition McGraw Hill Medical Publishing Division, 2006.

Tarascon Pharmacopoeia Library Edition Jones and Bartlett Publishers, 2009.

OTHER

Medscape *Bortezomib IV.*<http://www.medscape.com.>
RxList *Bortezomib.*<http://www.rxlist.com.>

ORGANIZATIONS

Cancer Support Groups, http://www.cancernews.com/support.html.

FDA U.S. Food and Drug Administration. 10903 New
Hampshire Ave, Silver Spring, MD 20993. (888)INFO-
FDA <http://www.fda.gov.>
National Cancer Institute. 6116 Executive Boulevard, Room
3036A, Bethesda, MD 20892-8322. (800)4-CANCER
<http://www.cancer.gov.>

Maria Basile, Ph.D.

Bowen's disease

Definition

Bowen's disease is a superficial precancerous squamous cell **cancer**, slow-growing (i.e. has not started spreading) skin malignancy. It is named for John Templeton Bowen (1857–1941), an American dermatologist. Bowen's disease is also called precancerous dermatosis.

Description

Red-brown, scaly or crusty patch on the skin that resembles psoriasis, dermatitis or eczema that can occur on any part of the body.

Demographics

Bowen's disease affects both males and females. Women are affected in the genital area three times as often as men. The disease can occur at any age, but is rare in children.

Close-up of a dark, bruise-like lesion on the leg of an elderly woman, caused by Bowen's disease. *(© Dr. P. Marazzi, Science Source/Photo Researchers, Inc. Reproduced by permission.)*

KEY TERMS

Cancer—General term for abnormally growing (malignant) cells.

Dermatitis—Inflammation of the skin that may be due to an allergic reaction.

Melanoma—Abnormal growth in melanin cells which are most commonly found in the skin or in the eye.

Paget's disease of the breast—Cancer of breast nipples that occurs in both men and women. Paget's is characterized by oozy and crusty skin inflammation (dermatitis).

Precancerous dermatosis—Another name for Bowen's disease.

Psoriasis—Common inherited condition that is characterized by reddish, silvery-scaled maculopapules, predominantly on the elbows, knees, scalp, and trunk.

Squamous cell carcinoma—Type of skin cancer

Causes and symptoms

The exact cause of Bowen's disease is unknown. Like many forms of cancer, long-term sun exposure may be a cause. The skin usually indicates sun damage, such as wrinkling, changes in pigmentation, and loss of elasticity. Ingestion of arsenic has been associated with cases of Bowen's disease found in skin areas unexposed to light or mucous membranes. Human papillomavirus 16 DNA is found repeatedly in Bowen's disease lesions, which suggests that this virus might be a cause. The role of heredity is not well understood. There are cases of Bowen's disease for which a cause cannot be determined.

Symptoms

The symptoms of Bowen's disease include:

- plaque located on or within the skin (intraepidermal)
- open sore that bleeds and crusts and persists for weeks
- wart-like growth that crusts and occasionally bleeds
- persistent, scaly red patch with irregular borders that sometimes crusts or bleeds
- pinkish or brownish raised areas of skin

Diagnosis

Bowen's disease can be confused with such other common skin disorders as psoriasis or types of dermatitis.

Paget's disease of the breast and malignant **melanoma** are other types of cancer which may be confused for Bowen's disease. A medical history, physical examination, and **biopsy** establish the diagnosis.

Clinical staging, treatments, and prognosis

Treatment usually involves surgical removal of the lesion. Curettage and cautery methods,which include carbon dioxide lasers, liquid nitrogen, and topical **fluorouracil** (5-fluorouracil, FU) compose the most efficient treatment for management of small solitary lesions.

There can be difficulties with the liquid nitrogen, 5-FU (Efudex, fluoroplex), scraping and burning because Bowen's lesions can hide deep in pores, and cells may extend into the surrounding area where the lesion is visible.

Newer treatments for Bowen's disease include acitretin (Soriatane), an oral medication originally developed to treat psoriasis; and imiquimod (Aldara), an **immune response** modifier available as a 5% topical cream. Imiquimod has been reported to give good results in treating Bowen's disease of the penis as well as large facial lesions.

Clinical trials

Dr. Colin Morton and colleagues at the Western Infirmary in the UK have been developing a **photodynamic therapy** using topical 5-aminolaevulinic acid(5-ALA).

Dr. Lee and colleagues at the University College of Medicine in Korea have been developing a specially designed radioactive skin patch.

Prevention

As with most skin cancers, prolonged exposure to the sun can increase the risk of developing the disease.

Special concerns

All treatment options for Bowen's disease have a recurrence rate of 5–10%, and no treatment modality seems superior for all clinical situations.

Resources

BOOKS

Beers, Mark H., MD, and Robert Berkow, MD, editors. "Bowen's Disease." Section 10, Chapter 126 In *The Merck Manual of Diagnosis and Therapy*. Whitehouse Station, NJ: Merck Research Laboratories, 2002.

Beers, Mark H., MD, and Robert Berkow, MD, editors. "Penile Cancer." Section 17, Chapter 233 In *The Merck Manual of Diagnosis and Therapy*. Whitehouse Station, NJ: Merck Research Laboratories, 2002.

PERIODICALS

Ahmed, I., J., S. Berth-Jones, Charles Holmes, C. J. O. Callaghan, and A. Ilcyhyshyn. "Comparison of Cryotherapy with Curettage in the Treatment of Bowen's Disease: A Prospective Study." *British Journal of Dermatology* 143 (2000): 759–766.

Chung, Y. L., J. D. Lee, D. Bang, J. B. Lee, K. B. Park, and M. G. Lee. "Treatment of Bowen's disease with a specially designed radioactive skin patch." *European Journal Nuclear Medicine* 27, no. 7 (July 2000): 842–6.

Cox, N. H. "Bowen's Disease: Where Now with Therapeutic Trials?" *British Journal of Dermatology* 143 (2000):699–700.

Danielsen, A. G., C. Sand, and K. Weismann. "Treatment of Bowen's Disease of the Penis with Imiquimod 5% Cream." *Clinical and Experimental Dermatology* 28 (November 2003) (Supplement 1): 7–9.

Khandpur, S., and V. K. Sharma. "Successful Treatment of Multiple Premalignant and Malignant Lesions in Arsenical Keratosis with a Combination of Acitretin and Intralesional 5-Fluorouracil." *Journal of Dermatology* 30 (October 2003): 730–734.

Kossard, S. "Treatment of Large Facial Bowen's Disease: Case Report." *Clinical and Experimental Dermatology* 28, Supplement 1 (November 2003): 13–15.

Morse, L. G., C. Kendrick, D. Cooper, et al. "Treatment of Squamous Cell Carcinoma with Intralesional 5-Fluorouracil." *Dermatologic Surgery* 29 (November 2003): 1150–1153.

Morton, Colin, A., Colin Whitehurst, John H. McColl, James V. Moore, and Rona M. MacKie."Photodynamic Therapy for Large or Multiple Patches of Bowen Disease and Basal Cell Carcinoma." *Archives Dermatology* 137 (March 2001): 319–324.

Nouri, K., C. O'Connell, and M. P. Rivas. "Imiquimod for the Treatment of Bowen's Disease and Invasive Squamous Cell Carcinoma." *Journal of Drugs in Dermatology* 2 (December 2003): 669–673.

OTHER

Skincancerinfo.com Detailed summary of information about Bowen's disease. [cited 2 July 2001]. http://www.skincancerinfo.com/sectionc/bowen.html.

ORGANIZATIONS

American Cancer Society, Inc. 1599 Clifton Road NE, Atlanta, GA 30329, (404)320-3333, http://www.cancer.org. The American Cancer Society (ACS) is a nationwide community-based voluntary health organization dedicated to eliminating cancer as a major health problem and the largest source of private, nonprofit cancer funds. The ACS hopes to prevent cancer, save lives, and diminish suffering from cancer, through research, education, advocacy, and service. 2 July 2001.

National Organizations of Rare Disorders (NORD). PO Box 8923, Fairfield, CT, 06812-8923, (800)999-6673; [cited July 2, 2001]. http://www.rarediseases.org. NORD is a voluntary health organization dedicated to helping people with rare diseases and assisting the organizations that serve them.

NIH/National Arthritis and Musculoskeletal and Skin Diseases Information Clearinghouse. One AMS Circle, Bethesda, MD, 20892-3675.(301)495-4484. http://www.nih.gov/niams. The NIAMS conducts and supports basic, clinical, and epidemiologic research and research training and disseminates information on diseases that include many forms of arthritis and diseases of the musculoskeletal system and the skin. [cited July 2, 2001].

NIH/National Cancer Institute (NCI) Office of Communications-Public Inquiries Office, Building 31, Rm 10A03, 9000 Rockville Pike, Bethesda, MD 20892.(800)422-6237. [cited July 2, 2001]. http://www.cancer.gov. Specializes in different aspects of cancer which includes cancer biology, cancer control and population sciences, cancer epidemiology and genetics, cancer prevention, and cancer treatment and diagnosis.

Skin Cancer Foundation. 245 Fifth Avenue, Suite 1403, New York, NY 10016.(212)725-5176. [cited July 2, 2001]. http://www.skincancer.org. National and international organization that is concerned exclusively with skin cancer.

Laura Ruth, Ph.D.
Rebecca J. Frey, PhD

Brain and central nervous system tumors

Definition

Like all other parts of the body, the brain and central nervous system are made up of cells that ordinarily grow and divide to create new cells as needed. This is usually an orderly process; but when cells lose their ability to grow normally or to die off naturally, they divide too often and produce tumors that are made up of these extra cells.

Brain and Central nervous system tumors	
Gliomas	**Non-glial tumors**
Astrocytomas	Medulloblastomas
Brain stem gliomas	Meningiomas
Ependymomas	Schwannomas
Oligodendrogliomas	Craniopharyngiomas
	Germinomas
	Pineal region tumors

(Table by GGS Creative Resources. Reproduced by permission of Cengage Learning, Gale.)

A diagram of a brain scan revealing a tumor (shown in red) in the right hemisphere. *(Illustration by Argosy, Inc. Cengage Learning, Gale.)*

Description

The brain and spinal cord together comprise what is known as the central nervous system (CNS). Like all tumors in the body, CNS tumors are either benign or malignant. Benign tumors are called non-cancerous because they have precise borders, are not invasive, and the cells that make up the growth are similar to other normal cells and grow relatively slowly. However, benign CNS tumors can press on a specific region

KEY TERMS

Angiogram—A diagnostic test that makes it possible for blood vessels to be seen on film by filling them with a contrast substance or dye that appears on x rays.

Anti-convulsant drugs—A group of medications used in the treatment of seizures.

Brain scan—A general term that can include CT scans, MRIs, seldom-used radionuclide scanning (use of radioactive isotopes), or ultrasounds.

Computerized tomography (CT) scan—The combined use of a computer and x rays that are passed through the body to produce clear, cross-sectional images.

Magnetic resonance imaging (MRI)—An imaging technique that produces good cross-sectional images without x rays or other radiation sources.

Myelogram—X-ray examination of the spinal cord after injection of a contrast substance or dye that shows up on x rays.

Neurological exam—A physical examination that focuses on the patient's nerves, reflexes, motor and sensory functions, and muscle strength and tone.

Seizures—Sudden, uncontrolled electrical activity in the brain resulting in characteristic twitching, or spastic, movements that may be accompanied by loss of consciousness.

Steroids—A group of drugs that are similar to the hormones produced by the cortex of the adrenal gland.

Ventricles of the brain—The four fluid-filled chambers, or cavities, found in the two cerebral hemispheres of the brain, at the center of the brain, and between the brain stem and cerebellum, and linked by channels, or ducts, allowing cerebral fluid to circulate through them.

of the spinal cord or brain and, thereby, cause symptoms. However, when such a benign tumor develops in an area that interferes with essential nervous system functioning, it is treated as malignant.

Malignant, or cancerous, tumors of the central nervous system are likely to be fast-growing, are invasive into surrounding healthy tissue, and the cells are very different from normal cells. These tumors can create a life-threatening situation by stopping vital functions of the brain. Some cancerous CNS tumors do not put out roots nor do they grow rapidly. These tumors are described as being encapsulated.

Another way that brain and central nervous system tumors are classified is by site of origin. Those that actually develop in the brain or spinal cord are called primary CNS tumors. **Metastasis** to the brain or spinal cord is, for the most part, a one-way street, meaning these tumors almost never metastasize to other areas in the body. The tumors that develop elsewhere in the body and metastasize, or spread, to the central nervous system are considered to be secondary CNS tumors. Such metastatic cells do not resemble other CNS cells. Instead, they have the same appearance as the **cancer** cells at the original cancer site elsewhere in the body.

Frequently observed signs of a brain tumor are the following:

- severe headaches
- an ataxic, or stumbling, gait
- nausea and vomiting
- lack of coordination
- unusual drowsiness
- weakness or loss of feelings in the arms and legs
- changes in personality or memory
- changes in speech
- changes in vision or abnormal eye movements
- seizures

Approximately 1 1/2% of all diagnosed cancers are CNS cancers, and they account for about 2 1/2% of all cancer deaths. The American Cancer Society (ACS) estimates that in 2009 22,070 malignant tumors of the brain or spinal cord will be diagnosed in adults and children in the United States. Of those people diagnosed, ACS projects that 12,920 will die from malignant CNS tumors.

Typically, diagnosis of CNS tumor is made by a physician who does a complete physical examination, including a family history and neurological examination. Computerized tomography (CT) scans, **magnetic resonance imaging** (MRI) scans, skull **x rays**, brain scans, angiograms, or myelograms are among the means of visualizing the brain or spinal cord to search for tumors.

General categories of treatment methods for CNS tumors include surgery, **radiation therapy**, and **chemotherapy**, with surgery being the single most commonly used therapy. Steroids are usually given prior to treatment to decrease swelling, and anti-convulsant drugs may be given to prevent seizures.

Types of cancers

Primary brain tumors are also classified by their site of origin. Gliomas, occurring in the glial, or supportive tissues around the brain, are the most common. Gliomas are further broken down into the following variations:

- Astrocytomas are named for the star-shaped, small cells that they are comprised of. Children may develop these in their brain stem, cerebrum, or cerebellum, while adults commonly develop them in the cerebrum.
- Brain-stem gliomas are usually astrocytomas that originate in the bottom, stem-like portion of the brain. Because this area controls many essential bodily functions, such tumors often cannot be removed.
- Ependymomas occur in the linings of the four brain ventricles, or chambers, or along the spinal cord. These are more common in children.
- Oligodendrogliomas are very rare and, when seen, are usually found in middle-aged adults. They grow slowly and ordinarily do not invade surrounding brain or spinal cord tissue. They originate in the cells responsible for the manufacture of myelin, a fatty covering for nerve tissue.

Other CNS tumors do not originate in glial tissue. Among these are:

- Medulloblastomas, tumors of the cerebellum, are most common in male children. Studies have shown these to originate in primitive nerve cells that normally would have disappeared soon after birth.
- Meningiomas are usually benign. They develop in the meninges, or brain linings, and grow very slowly. Because of this slow growth, they may go undetected for years. Meningiomas are more common in women between the ages of 30 and 50.
- Schwannomas are also benign tumors, specific to the myelin-producing cells (Schwann cells) for the acoustic, or hearing, nerve. These, too, are more common in women than men.
- Craniopharyngiomas are usually benign, but because of their location near the pituitary gland and hypothalmus, they can easily affect vital functions and are therefore treated as if malignant. They occur more frequently in children and teenagers.
- Germinomas, or germ cell tumors, develop from primitive sex cells called germ cells.
- Pineal-region tumors originate in the area near the pineal gland, a small central brain gland that secretes melatonin, a brain chemical. These can be either fast-growing pineoblastoma, or slow-growing pineocytoma.

Resources

ORGANIZATIONS

The American Cancer Society's Resource Center for Brain/Central Nervous System Tumors in Children. (800) ACS-2345.

Cancer Care, Inc. (800) 813-4673. http://www.cancercare.org.

National Cancer Institute. http://cancernet.nci.nih.gov.

Joan Schonbeck, R.N.

Brain metastasis *see* **Metastasis**

BRCA 1 & 2

Definition

BRCA 1 and BRCA 2 are genes that encode for proteins that help prevent breast and ovarian cancers.

Description

Family histories of breast/ovarian cancers

Breast cancer is the second most commonly diagnosed **cancer** among women and the second leading cause of cancer death in women. An estimated 192,370 new breast cancer cases were diagnosed in the United States in 2009 and about 40,170 women died of breast cancer. About 5–10% of women with breast cancer have an inherited susceptibility. After gender and age, a family history of breast or **ovarian cancer** is the single best predictor of the likelihood that a woman will develop these cancers.

Family histories that suggest a hereditary predisposition for breast and ovarian cancer include:

- multiple affected family members, particularly a mother, sister, or daughter
- cancers occurring 5–15 years earlier than sporadic cancers (those not associated with a genetic risk)
- two or more primary cancers in a single individual, such as breast and ovarian cancers or bilateral breast cancer (separate cancers in each breast)
- male breast cancer
- other multiple cancers in the family, especially prostate cancer
- an Ashkenazi (eastern and central European) Jewish background.

BRCA gene alterations

BRCA stands for BReast CAncer or breast cancer susceptibility. After a long search for changes in DNA sequences that were common in breast-cancer-prone families, particularly Ashkenazi Jews, BRCA 1 was discovered in 1994 and BRCA 2 in 1995. Inherited alterations (mutations) in the DNA sequences of these genes account for 5–10% of all breast cancers.

BRCAs are inherited as autosomal dominant genes. This means that an altered BRCA gene can be passed from either a mother or a father to a son or a daughter. Humans have 23 pairs of chromosomes that carry genes. One member of each chromosome pair is inherited from the father and the other member of the pair is inherited from the mother, so that a person has two copies of each gene. If either parent has an altered BRCA, their children each have a 50% chance of inheriting the altered BRCA. Because the altered BRCA is dominant over the normal gene inherited from the other parent, a child who inherits one altered BRCA is at an increased risk for breast and/or ovarian cancer. Males with an altered BRCA gene, especially BRCA 2, are at increased risk for breast and prostate cancers.

With the exception Ashkenazi Jews, the likelihood of a BRCA mutation is:

- 0.5% in the general population
- 2% in women with breast cancer
- 9% in women under 40 with breast cancer
- 5% in men with breast cancer
- 10% in women with ovarian cancer.

The likelihood of a BRCA mutation in Ashkenazi Jews is:

- 2.5% in the general population
- 10% in women with breast cancer
- 30–35% in women under 40 with breast cancer
- 19% in men with breast cancer
- 36–41% in women with ovarian or primary peritoneal or pelvic cancers.

Among Ashkenazi Jews, 1% have an alteration called 185delAG in BRCA 1; 0.1% have a mutation called 5382insC in BRCA 1; and 1.4% have a mutation called 6174delT in BRCA 2. Each of these three mutations carries a similar breast cancer risk. Various other ethnic groups, including Norwegians, Dutch, and Icelanders, have different specific BRCA mutations.

Although more than 2,000 mutations and DNA sequence variations have been found in BRCAs, most of them do not increase an individual's risk of developing cancer. However 0.1%–0.6% of the general population may carry a potentially damaging BRCA 1 mutation.

Not everyone with an altered BRCA gene will develop cancer. An altered BRCA increases a woman's risk of developing breast cancer during her lifetime from 13.2% to 36–85%. In the general population most breast cancers occur in post-menopausal women over age 50. Women with BRCA mutations most often are diagnosed with breast cancer in their 40s. An altered BRCA increases a woman's lifetime risk of developing ovarian cancer from 1.7% to 16–60%. Women with a BRCA 1 mutation have about a 40% chance of developing ovarian cancer by age 70. Women with a BRCA 2 mutation have about a 20% risk of developing ovarian cancer by age 70. BRCA 2 mutations also double a man's risk for **prostate cancer**.

Not all breast or ovarian cancers in cancer-prone family are due to BRCA mutations. Mutations in BRCA 1 account for breast or ovarian cancers in 45% of families with a history of breast cancer and up to 90% in families with a history of both breast and ovarian cancers. BRCA 2 mutations account for breast cancer in about 35% of families with a history of breast cancer.

BRCA mutations also appear to be involved in fallopian tube cancers and in peritoneal cancers. Cancer of the peritoneum that surrounds the organs of the pelvis is similar to ovarian cancer.

BRCA 1-related breast cancer appears to be more aggressive than other types of breast cancer and has a poorer prognosis. Most BRCA 1-related ovarian cancers also are of a particular invasive type.

BRCAs are believed to code for tumor suppressor proteins that interact with one another. They are thought to be involved in repairing DNA following damage caused by radiation or other factors that might otherwise lead to cancer. BRCA proteins are very large and deleterious mutations in their genes usually result in a shortened, nonfunctional, or missing protein.

Genetic testing

Genetic testing for BRCA mutations that increase the risk of breast and ovarian cancers have been available since 1996; as of 2004 between 26% and 78% of at-risk women had chosen to be tested. Genetic counseling by a trained professional is a very important part of making the decision to be tested.

Results

For BRCA testing blood is drawn at a laboratory, doctor's office, clinic, or hospital and sent to a laboratory. The results may not be available for several weeks or months. Many laboratories offer screening for specific BRCA mutations that occur in certain families or ethnic groups. Although technically much simpler to perform, these tests may not detect other potentially significant BRCA mutations.

It often is best to first test for a BRCA mutation in a family member who has breast or ovarian cancer. If that person has an altered BRCA gene, it becomes a known mutation and other family members can be tested for that specific mutation. A positive test for that mutation indicates that the person is at an increased risk for cancer. A negative test for that mutation—called a true negative—indicates that the person is unlikely to have an increased risk for cancer.

If there is no known BRCA mutation to screen for, a negative test can be a false negative because the test may have missed the mutation. An ambiguous or uncertain test result means that a BRCA alteration was found but has not been associated with cancer in other people. One study found that about 10% of women undergoing BRCA testing had this type of ambiguous result. Altered genes other than BRCAs, as well as various inherited conditions, also are associated with an increased risk for breast and other cancers. These will not be detected with genetic screening for BRCA.

Deciding to be tested

A number of factors may influence the decision to be tested:

- Testing costs several hundred to several thousand dollars. Although some health plans cover genetic testing, many people do not want their insurance companies to know that they are even thinking about being tested for a genetic condition or predisposition.
- Many people want to know about any inherited risks for their children and other family members.
- Tests may give false negative or ambiguous results.
- Test results may influence important clinical decisions.

The results of genetic testing can have an impact on:

- emotions
- social relationships
- finances
- medical choices

- family relationships, since the tests can reveal information about other family members
- personal choices such as marriage and childbearing

A negative test result may:

- provide a sense of relief
- cause guilt over avoiding a disease that affects other family members
- eliminate the need for special preventative exams, tests, and surgeries
- provide a false sense of security, since the person still has the same cancer risk as the general population.

A positive test result may:

- provide relief from uncertainty
- cause anxiety, anger, or depression
- provide the opportunity to make informed decisions about the future
- force a choice concerning preventative measures that may have serious long-term implications with no guarantee of protection

Genetic discrimination

A positive test result for a BRCA mutation may put a person at risk for discrimination. Clinical test results usually are included in an individual's medical file, although some physicians choose not to include the results of genetic testing. However information about a person's genetic profile sometimes can be obtained from a family medical history. Medical records may be available to medical, life, and disability insurance companies, as well as employers.

A positive genetic test result may cause a person to be:

- denied medical coverage for expenses relating to their genetic condition
- dropped by their health plan
- unable to qualify for insurance

The Health Insurance Portability and Accountability Act (HIPPA) of 1996 prohibits employer-based group health plans from denying coverage on a genetic basis if the person does not have the disease. However employers can refuse to offer health coverage to that individual. Although several states prohibit genetic discrimination by employers and **health insurance** companies, decisions made in one state may have repercussions if the person moves to a different state.

Preventive measures

There are numerous risk factors for the development of breast and ovarian cancers. Most of these risk factors have not been evaluated in people carrying BRCA mutations.

Even thought mammograms do not detect some breast cancers, particularly in younger women such as those at-risk due to BRCA mutations, early diagnosis is very important for the prognosis of breast cancer. Women with a BRCA mutation should use augmented breast cancer surveillance techniques:

- monthly breast self-examinations beginning at age 18
- clinical breast examinations performed by a physician or nurse breast specialist every 6–12 months beginning at age 18
- mammograms every 6–12 months, beginning at age 25–35, or at least five years before the youngest age that breast cancer was diagnosed in a family member

Although it is unclear whether early detection of ovarian cancer increases survival rates, increased surveillance for ovarian cancer should begin at age 25–35, or 5–10 years before the youngest age that ovarian cancer was diagnosed in a family member. Surveillance includes:

- a pelvic examination every 6–12 months
- testing for CA-125—a blood protein marker for ovarian cancer— once or twice per year
- transvaginal or pelvic ultrasound once or twice per year

Chemoprevention includes treatment of a healthy at-risk woman with **tamoxifen** or other selective estrogen receptor modulators (SERMs). One study found that tamoxifen treatment reduced the incidence of breast cancer by 62% in women with an altered BRCA 2 gene but had no effect on women with an altered BRCA 1.

Risk-reducing, prophylactic, or preventive masectomy—the removal of the breasts and as much at-risk tissue as possible—in healthy women with a BRCA mutation reduces the risk of breast cancer by 90%. However it is not clear whether women undergoing this procedure are at any less risk of dying from breast cancer as compared with women who use careful surveillance methods.

Prophylactic or risk-reducing salpingo-**oophorectomy** (RRSO)—the removal of the fallopian tubes and ovaries—is estimated to reduce the risk of ovarian cancer by 95% in women with BRCA mutations. Surgical removal of the ovaries in pre-menopausal, high-risk women reduces their chance of developing breast cancer by about 50%. RRSO is recommended for high-risk women who have completed childbearing. Tubal ligation—the tying-off of the fallopian tubes—also may reduce the risk of developing ovarian cancer to a lesser extent. Unlike RRSO, tubal ligation does not result in the onset of menopause.

However not all at-risk tissue can be removed by these procedures. Some women still develop breast, ovarian, or peritoneal cancers despite prophylactic surgery.

Resources

BOOKS

Ross, Jeffrey S., and Gabriel N. Hortobagyi, editors. *Molecular Oncology of Breast Cancer*. Sudbury, MA: Jones and Bartlett, 2005.

PERIODICALS

Kauff, N. D., et al. 'Risk-Reducing Salpingo-Oophorectomy in Women with a BRCA1 or BRCA2 Mutation.' *New England Journal of Medicine* 346, no. 21 (2002): 1609–15.

King, M., et al. 'Tamoxifen and Breast Cancer Incidence Among Women with Inherited Mutations in BRCA1 and BRCA2.' *Journal of the American Medical Association* 286, no. 18 (2001): 2251–6.

King M. C., et al. 'Breast and Ovarian Cancer Risks Due to Inherited Mutations in BRCA1 and BRCA2.' *Science* 302, no. 5645 (2003): 643–6.

Rebbeck, T. R., et al. 'Prophylactic Oophorectomy in Carriers of BRCA1 or BRCA2 Mutations.' *New England Journal of Medicine* 346, no. 21 (2002): 1616–22.

OTHER

"Background." *Breast Imaging Study*. National Cancer Institute. March 30, 2005. http://breastimaging.cancer.gov/background.html.

"Genetic Testing for BRCA1 and BRCA2: It's Your Choice." *Cancer Facts*. February 6, 2002. National Cancer Institute. March 30, 2005. http://cis.nci.nih.gov/fact/3_62.htm.

"Genetics of Breast and Ovarian Cancer (PDQ)". December 21, 2004. National Cancer Institute. March 30, 2005. http://cancernet.nci.nih.gov/cancertopics/pdq/genetics/breast-and-ovarian.

"Questions and Answers About Estimating Cancer Risk in Ashkenazi Jews." *Cancer Facts*. August 10, 2000. National Cancer Institute. March 30, 2005. http://cis.nci.nih.gov/fact/3_60.htm.

ORGANIZATIONS

American Cancer Society. PO Box 102454, Atlanta, GA 30368-2454. 800-ACS-2345. http://www.cancer.org. Information, research, and patient support.

Cancer Genetics Network. Division of Cancer Control and Population Sciences, National Cancer Institute. 6130 Executive Boulevard, Executive Plaza North, Rockville, Maryland 20852. 301-594-6776. <http://epi.grants.cancer.gov/CGN>. A database and national network of centers for individuals and families and for research on genetic predispositions to cancer.

Margaret Alic, Ph.D.

Breast cancer

Definition

Breast **cancer** is caused by the development of abnormal cells in the breast. The abnormal cells originate in the lining of the either the milk glands or the ducts of the breast (ductal epithelium), defining this malignancy as a cancer. Cancer cells are characterized by uncontrolled division leading to abnormal growth and the ability of these cells to invade normal tissue locally or to spread throughout the body, a process called **metastasis**.

Demographics

The American Cancer Society estimated that about 192,370 new cases of breast cancer and 62,280 cases of cancer in situ would be diagnosed in the United States in 2009. About 40,000 American women die of breast cancer each year; breast cancer is the second leading cause of cancer death in women. However, in the United States, there 2.5 million breast cancer survivors. Both deaths from breast cancer and the number of newly diagnosed cases have declined in recent years in the United States. This is thought to be the result of earlier diagnosis from screening mammograms, improving therapies, and a dramatic decrease in the use of hormone replacement therapy (HRT) in post-menopausal women.

Male breast cancer is rare and accounts for less than 1% of all breast cancers. The American Cancer Society estimated that in 2009 1,910 new cases of

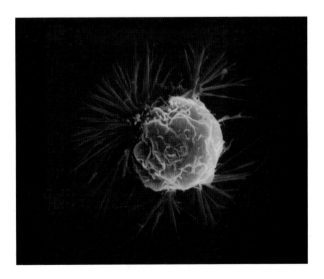

A picture of a breast cancer cell. *(Phototake Kunkel/Phototake NYC. Reproduced by permission.)*

The woman in this illustration has breast cancer. The tumor is visible in the breast, and the axillary lymph nodes reveal cancer as well. *(Custom Medical Stock Photo. Reproduced by permission.)*

invasive breast cancer would be diagnosed in men and about 400 men would die from the disease.

Description

Breast cancer often arises in the milk-producing glands of the breast tissue. Groups of glands in normal breast tissue are called lobules. The products of these glands are secreted into a ductal system that leads to the nipple. Depending on where in the glandular or ductal unit of the breast the cancer arises, it will develop certain characteristics that are used to sub-classify breast cancer into types. Ductal **carcinoma** begins in the ducts, and lobular carcinoma has a pattern involving the lobules or glands. The pathologist will note the subtype at the time of evaluation with the microscope. The more important classification is related to the evaluated tumor's capability to invade, as this characteristic defines the disease as a true cancer. The stage before invasive cancer is called "in situ," meaning that the early malignancy has not yet become

capable of invasion. Thus, ductal carcinoma in situ is considered a minimal breast cancer.

How breast cancer spreads

The primary tumor begins in the breast itself, but once it becomes invasive, it may progress beyond the breast to the regional lymph nodes or travel (metastasize) to other organ systems in the body and become systemic in nature. Lymph is the clear, protein-rich fluid that bathes the cells throughout the body. Lymph works its way back to the bloodstream via small channels known as lymphatics. Along the way, the lymph is filtered through cellular stations known as lymph nodes. Nearly all organs in the body have a primary lymph node group filtering fluid that comes from that organ. In the breast, the primary lymph nodes are under the armpit, or axilla. Classically, the primary tumor begins in the breast and the first place to which it is likely to spread is the regional lymph nodes. Cancer, as it invades in its place of origin, may also work its way into blood vessels. If cancer gets into the blood vessels, the blood vessels provide yet another route for the cancer cells to spread to other organs of the body.

Breast cancer follows this classic progression, although it often becomes systemic or widespread early in the course of the disease. By the time one can feel a lump in the breast it is often 0.4 inches (1 cm) in size and contains roughly one million cells. Research suggests that a tumor of this size may take one to five years to develop. During that time, the cancer may metastasize, or spread by lymphatics or blood to areas elsewhere in the body.

When primary breast cancer spreads, it may first go to the axillary nodes. If this occurs, regional metastasis exists. If it proceeds elsewhere either by lymphatic or blood-borne spread, the patient develops systemic metastasis that may involve a number of other organs in the body. Favorite sites of systemic involvement for breast cancer are the lung, bones, liver, skin, and soft tissue. As it turns out, the presence of, and the actual number of, regional lymph nodes containing cancer remains the single best indicator of whether or not the cancer has become widely metastatic. Because tests to discover metastasis in other organs may not be sensitive enough to reveal minute deposits of cancer cells, the evaluation of the lymph nodes under the armpit for regional metastasis becomes very important in making treatment decisions for this disease.

If breast cancer spreads to other major organs of the body, its presence will compromise the function of those organs. Death is the result of extreme compromise of vital organ function.

Risk factors

Every woman is at risk for breast cancer. If she lives to be 85, there is a one in eight chance (12%) that she will develop breast cancer sometime during her life. The rate is slightly higher for white women and slightly lower for black women. As a woman ages, her risk of developing breast cancer rises dramatically regardless of her ethnicity or family history. The breast cancer risk of a 25-year-old woman is only one out of 19,608; by age 45, it is one in 93. In fact, fewer than 5% of cases are discovered before age 35 and the majority of all breast cancers are found in women over age 50.

There are a number of other risk factors for the development of breast cancer; however, among experts there is some disagreement about how important each of these factors is. Risk factors include:

- a family history of breast cancer in mother or sister.
- carrying the BRCA1 and BRCA2 genes. Women with these genes account for 5–10% of breast cancer cases and have an 80% chance of developing breast cancer at some time during their life.
- history of abnormal breast biopsies or previous history of breast cancer.
- having first menstruation before age 12 or entering menopause after age 55.
- having no children or having a first child after age 30.
- daily alcohol consumption of two drinks or more.
- obesity and a high fat diet.
- breast exposure to radiation (e.g., in treatment of other cancers).
- postmenopausal hormone replacement therapy (HRT) with a combination estrogen/progesterone drug. Estrogen alone does not appear to increase risk. The longer a woman used HRT, the more her risk increases.

HRT provides significant relief of menopausal symptoms, prevention of osteoporosis, and possibly protection from cardiovascular disease and stroke. While physicians have long known a small increased risk for breast cancer was linked to use of HRT, a landmark study released in 2003 proved the risk was greater than thought. The Women's Health Initiative found that even relatively short-term use of estrogen plus progestin is associated with increased risk of breast cancer, diagnosis at a more advanced stage of the disease, and a higher number of abnormal mammograms.

Causes and symptoms

All cancer is thought to occur because of small changes (mutations) in genes. A gene is a small packet of deoxyribonucleic acid (DNA), the genetic master molecule of all cells that is inherited from each parent. Genes control all aspects of development and metabolism. Small changes in the structure of genes can cause changes in proteins that regulate metabolic functions. In healthy cells, cell division is controlled by proteins regulated by genes. Specific genes make proteins that signal healthy cells when to stop dividing. In cancer, the controlling gene(s) is damaged or mutated and does not produce the proteins necessary to signal cells to stop dividing. The mutations that cause breast cancer do not have a single cause. Genetic, environmental, and lifestyle factors all play a role in determining who gets breast cancer.

Of all the risk factors listed above, family history appears to be the most important. Some studies have found that about half of all familial breast cancer cases (families in which there is a high breast cancer frequency) have mutations affecting the genes BRCA1 or BRCA2. Other genes (e.g., ATM, CHEK2, p53, PTEN) have been identified that may influence the development of breast cancer, but their impact is much less than the BRCA genes. Nevertheless, breast cancer due to heredity accounts for only a small proportion of breast cancer cases; only 5%–10% of all breast cancer cases will be women who inherited a high susceptibility through their genes.

Although there are many recognized risk factors, it is important to note that more than 70% of women who get breast cancer have no known risk factors. Having several risk factors may increase a woman's chance of developing breast cancer, but the interplay of predisposing factors is complex. In addition to those accepted factors listed above, some studies suggest that high-fat diets, obesity, or the use of alcohol can contribute to the risk profile.

Not all lumps detected in the breast are cancerous. Fibrocystic changes in the breast are extremely common. Also known as **fibrocystic condition of the breast**, fibrocystic changes are a leading cause of noncancerous lumps in the breast. Fibrocystic changes also cause symptoms of pain, swelling, or discharge and may become evident to the patient or physician as a lump that is either solid or filled with fluid. Complete diagnostic evaluation of any significant breast abnormality is mandatory because, although women commonly develop fibrocystic changes, breast cancer also is common, and the signs and symptoms of fibrocystic changes overlap with those of breast cancer. Certain benign changes in the breast also may be linked to increased risk for breast cancer.

Diagnosis

The diagnosis of breast cancer is accomplished by the **biopsy** of any suspicious lump or mammographic abnormality that has been identified. (A biopsy is the removal of tissue for examination by a pathologist. A mammogram is a low-dose, 2-view, x-ray examination of the breast.) The patient may be prompted to visit her doctor upon finding a lump in a breast, or she may have noticed skin dimpling, nipple retraction, or discharge from the nipple. A patient may not have noticed a symptom or abnormality, before a lump was detected by a screening mammogram.

When a patient has no signs or symptoms

Screening involves the evaluation of women who have no symptoms or signs of a breast problem. **Mammography** has been helpful in detecting breast cancer that cannot be identified on physical examination. More than 90% of all breast cancers are detected by mammogram screening. However, about 10% of breast cancer does not show up on mammography, and a similar number of patients with breast cancer have an abnormal mammogram and a normal physical examination. These figures emphasize the need for regular examination as part of the screening process.

Screening

All women are encouraged to do regular, monthly breast self-examinations. This involves feeling the breasts for any abnormal lumps or pain. If an uncertainty or a lump is found, evaluation by an experienced physician and a mammogram is recommended. The American Cancer Society (ACS) has made recommendations for the use of mammography on a screening basis. In 2009, the ACS guidelines recommended that women should begin annual screening at age 40 For women at high risk for breast cancer, the ACS recommends beginning screenings at an earlier age, having screening at more frequent intervals, and having **magnetic resonance imaging** (MRI) screening in addition to a standard mammogram. A list of conditions considered to put women at high risk for breast cancer can be found on the ACS Web site.

Because of the greater awareness of breast cancer in recent years, screening evaluations by examinations and mammography are performed much more frequently than in the past and is likely to be paid for by **health insurance**. As a result, the number of breast cancers diagnosed has increased, but the disease is being diagnosed at an earlier stage than previously. The earlier the stage of disease at the time it is discovered, the better the long-term outcome (prognosis) becomes.

When a patient has physical signs or symptoms

A common finding that leads to diagnosis is the presence of a lump within the breast. Skin dimpling, nipple retraction, or discharge from the nipple is less frequent initial findings prompting biopsy. Though bloody nipple discharge is distressing, it is most often caused by benign disease. Skin dimpling or nipple retraction in the presence of an underlying breast mass on examination is a more advanced finding. Actual skin involvement, with swelling (edema) or ulceration of the skin, are late findings.

The presence of a breast lump is a common sign of breast cancer. If the lump is suspicious and the patient has not had a mammogram by this point, a study should be done on both breasts before anything else so that the original characteristics of the lesion can be studied. The opposite breast should also be evaluated mammographically to determine if other problems exist that were undetected by physical examination.

Whether an abnormal screening mammogram or one of the signs mentioned above followed by a mammogram prompted suspicion, the definitive diagnosis is established by obtaining tissue by biopsy of the area. There are different types of biopsies, each used with its own indication. If signs of widespread metastasis are already present, biopsy of the metastasis itself may establish diagnosis.

Biopsy

Depending on the situation, different types of biopsy may be performed. The types include incisional and excisional biopsies. In an incisional biopsy, the physician takes a sample of tissue, and in excisional biopsy, the mass is removed. Fine needle aspiration biopsy and core needle biopsy are kinds of incisional biopsies.

FINE NEEDLE ASPIRATION BIOPSY. In a fine needle aspiration biopsy, a fine-gauge needle may be passed into the lesion and cells from the area suctioned into the needle can be quickly prepared for microscopic evaluation (**cytology**). (The patient experiencing nipple discharge also can have a sample taken of the discharge for cytological evaluation.) Fine needle aspiration is a simple procedure that can be done under local anesthesia, and will tell if the lesion is a fluid-filled cyst or whether it is solid. The sample obtained will yield much diagnostic information. Fine needle aspiration biopsy is an excellent technique when the lump is palpable and the physician can easily hit the target with the needle. If the lesion is a simple cyst, the fluid will be evacuated and the mass will disappear. If it is solid, the diagnosis may be obtained. Care must be taken, however, because if the mass is solid and the specimen is non-malignant, a complete removal of the lesion may be appropriate to be sure.

CORE NEEDLE BIOPSY. Core needle biopsies also are obtained simply under local anesthesia. The larger piece of tissue obtained with its preserved architecture may be helpful in confirming the diagnosis short of open surgical removal. An open surgical incisional biopsy is rarely needed for diagnosis because of the needle techniques. If there remains question as to diagnosis, a complete open surgical biopsy may be required.

EXCISIONAL BIOPSY. When performed, the excisional (complete removal) biopsy is a minimal outpatient procedure often done under local anesthesia.

NON-PALPABLE LESIONS. As screening increases, non-palpable lesions (abnormalities that can not be felt by hand examination) demonstrated only by mammography are becoming more common. The use of **x rays** and computers to guide the needle for biopsy or to place markers for the surgeon performing the excisional biopsy are commonly employed. Some benign lesions can be fully removed by multiple directed core biopsies. These techniques are very appealing because they are minimally invasive; however, the physician needs to be careful to obtain a good sample.

Other tests

If a lesion is not palpable and has simple cystic characteristics on mammography, ultrasound may be used both to determine that it is a cyst and to guide its evacuation. Ultrasound may also be used in some cases to guide fine needle or core biopsies of the breast.

Computed tomography (CT) scans are used only rarely in the evaluation of breast lesions. MRI is recommended for high-risk women and to follow up on suspicious findings from mammograms or for certain patients.

Staging

Once diagnosis is established and before treatment is begun, more tests are done to determine if the cancer has spread beyond the breast. These tests include a chest x ray and blood count with liver function tests. Along with the liver function measured by the blood sample, the level of alkaline phosphatase, an enzyme from bone, is also determined. A radionuclear bone scan may be ordered. This test looks at the places in the body to which breast cancer usually metastasizes. A CT scan also may be ordered. The physician will do a careful examination of the axillae to assess likelihood of regional metastasis. Sometimes, the physician will remove all of the axillary lymph nodes to assess breast cancer stage. However, recent studies

show great success with **sentinel lymph node biopsy**. This technique removes the sentinel lymph node, or that lymph node that receives fluid drainage first from the area where the cancer is located. If this node is free of cancer, staging can be assigned accordingly. This method saves women the discomfort and side effects associated with removing additional lymph nodes in her armpit.

Using the results of these studies, the stage of cancer is defined for the patient. This helps establish a treatment protocol and prognosis. In the United States, formal staging is done using the TNM system. This system considers the tumor size and how much it has grown (T), whether the cancer has spread to the lymph nodes (N), and whether it has metastasized (M) to distant sites in the body. Stages are summarized below.

- Stage I. The cancer is no larger than 2 cm and no cancer cells are found in the lymph nodes.
- Stage II. The cancer is no larger than 2 cm but has spread to the lymph nodes or is larger than 2 cm but has not spread to the lymph nodes.
- Stage IIIA. Tumor is larger than 5 cm and has spread to the lymph nodes or is smaller than 5 cm, but has spread to the lymph nodes, which have grown into each other.
- Stage IIIB. Cancer has spread to tissues near the breast or to lymph nodes inside the chest wall, along the breastbone.
- Stage IV. Cancer has spread to skin and lymph nodes near the collarbone or to other organs of the body.

Treatment

Surgery, radiation, and **chemotherapy** all may be used in the treatment of breast cancer. Depending on the stage, they will be used in different combinations or sequences to effect an appropriate strategy for the type and stage of the disease being treated.

Surgery

Historically, surgical removal of the entire breast and axillary lymph nodes, along with the muscles down to the chest wall (radical **mastectomy**), was performed as the preferred therapy for breast cancer. In the past 30 years, surgery remains a primary option, but other therapies have risen in importance. Recent studies have suggested that breast conserving treatment (as opposed to radical mastectomy) improves the quality of life for women without compromising survival. Ultimately, the extent of surgery depends on the type of breast cancer, whether the disease has spread, and the patient's age and health.

If the tumor is less than 1.5 (4 cm) in size and located so that it can be removed without destroying the reasonable cosmetic appearance of the residual breast, just the primary tumor and a rim of normal tissue will be removed. The axillary nodes will still be removed for staging purposes, usually through a separate incision. Because of the risk of recurrence in the remaining breast tissue, **radiation therapy** is used to lessen the chance of local recurrence. This type of primary therapy is known as **lumpectomy**, (or segmental mastectomy), and **axillary dissection**.

Sentinel **lymph node biopsy**, a technique for identifying which nodes in the axilla drain the tumor, has been developed to provide selective sampling and further lessen the degree of surgical trauma the patient experiences.

When patients are selected appropriately based on the preoperative clinical stage, all of these surgical approaches have been shown to produce similar results. In planning primary surgical therapy, it is imperative that the operation is tailored to fit the clinical circumstance of the patient.

The pathologic stage of the cancer is evaluated after surgical treatment and defines additional treatment. In addition to stage, other tests may be necessary to aid in decisions regarding additional adjuvant therapies. Adjuvant therapies are treatments used after the primary treatment to help ensure that no microscopic disease exists and to help prolong patients' survival time or reduce pain.

Radiation therapy

Like surgical therapy, radiation therapy is a local modality—it treats only the specific tissue exposed to radiation and not the rest of the body. Radiation is usually given post-operatively after surgical wounds have healed. The pathologic stage of the primary tumor is now known and this aids in treatment planning. The extent of the local surgery also influences the planning. Radiation may not be needed at all after **modified radical mastectomy** for stage I disease but is usually used when breast-preserving surgery is performed. If the tumor was extensive or if multiple nodes were involved, the field of tissue exposed will vary accordingly. Radiation is used as an adjunct to surgical therapy and is considered important to gaining local control of the tumor. In the past, radiation was used as an alternative to surgery on occasion. However, now that breast-preserving surgical protocols have been developed, primary radiation treatment of the tumor is no longer performed. Radiation also has an important role in the treatment of the patient with widespread (disseminated) disease, particularly if it involves the skeleton. Radiation therapy can affect pain control and prevention of fracture in this circumstance.

Chemotherapy

Survival after breast cancer surgery is improved by the addition of postoperative chemotherapy. Postsurgical chemotherapy therapy in patients who have no evidence of residual disease is now performed on the basis that some patients have metastases that are too small to be detectable. This occurs because it is unlikely that the surgeon has removed every single cancerous cell. Loose cancer cells, if not killed by chemotherapy, may travel through the circulatory system and form new tumors elsewhere. Chemotherapy may also be given in some circumstances before surgery. Chemotherapy is administered either orally or by injection into a blood vessel and usually involves multiple drugs. It is given in cycles, followed by a period of time for recovery, followed by another course of drugs.

Chemotherapy can produce significant side effects, including **nausea and vomiting**, temporary hair loss, mouth or vaginal sores, **fatigue**, weakened immune system, and infertility. Complementary therapies are often helpful in reducing some of these side effects.

Hormone therapy

Many breast cancers, particularly those originating in post-menopausal women, are responsive to hormones. These cancers have receptors on their cells for the hormone estrogen. Part of the post-surgery primary tumor assessment is evaluation for the presence of estrogen and progesterone receptors. If they are present on the cancer cells, altering the hormone status of the patient will slow tumor growth and have a positive impact on survival. Hormonal status may be changed with drug therapy. The drug **tamoxifen** binds to estrogen receptors on the cancer cells, so that hormones cannot interact with the cells and stimulate their growth. If the patient has these receptors present, tamoxifen is commonly prescribed for five years as an adjunct to primary treatment. In women whose cancer cells have estrogen receptors, tamoxifen reduces the chance of breast cancer reoccurring by about 50%.

Toremifene (Fareston) and fulvestrant (Faslodex) are drugs similar to tamoxifen in that they target hormone receptors on cancer cells. They are often used when cancer cells are unresponsive to tamoxifen. In addition, a new group of drugs called **aromatase**

inhibitors that block the enzymes that produce estrogen in postmenopausal (but not premenopausal) women have been used to treat both early and late advanced breast cancer. These drugs include drugs are letrozole (Femara), anastrozole (Arimidex), and exemestane (Aromasin). Because of these agents, there is rarely any need for surgical removal of hormone-producing glands, such as the ovary or adrenal, that was sometimes necessary in the past.

Biotherapeutics

Biotherapeutics are a type of targeted therapy. Large amounts of antibodies of a single type (called **monoclonal antibodies**) that react with specific receptors on cancer cells are made in the laboratory. When given to the patient, they inactivate or destroy those cells containing that specific receptor, but do not react with other cells. **Trastuzumab (Herceptin)** and **Lapatinib** (Tykerb) target cells that contain a growth protein known as HER/2. Between 15% and 25% of women have breast cancer that responds to these drugs. **Bevacizumab** (Avastin) is a biotherapeutic used to treat breast cancer that has metastasized. It helps prevent tumors from becoming established by interfering with the growth of blood vessels into the tumor. Without access to nutrients in the blood, the tumors cannot increase in size. Biotherapeutics are normally used in addition to chemotherapy drugs.

Complementary treatments

Complementary treatments are alternative therapies used along with conventional medicine. They often are successful in moderating side effects of conventional treatment and improving the patient's quality of life. For example, acupuncture and guided imagery may be useful tools in treating pain symptoms and side effects of chemotherapy associated with breast cancer. Acupuncture involves the placement of a series of thin needles into the skin at targeted locations on the body, known as acupoints, in order to harmonize the energy flow within the human body. Guided imagery involves creating a visual mental image of pain. Once the pain can be visualized, the patient can adjust the image to make it more pleasing, and thus more manageable.

Many herbal remedies are available to lessen pain symptoms and chemotherapy side effects such as **nausea**, and to promote relaxation and healing. However, breast cancer patients should consult with their healthcare professional before taking any herbal treatments. Depending on the preparation and the type of herb, these remedies may interact with and enhance or diminish the effects of other prescribed medications. One herb that is generally regarded as helpful in

relieving the nausea that accompanies chemotherapy, is ginger (*Zingiber officinale*).

Prognosis

The prognosis for breast cancer depends on the type and stage of cancer. Lymph node involvement is one of the best indicators of breast cancer survival rates. According to the American Cancer Society, As of 2009, the five-year survival rate for American women with carcinoma in situ and stage I breast cancer was 100%. The five-year survival rate for women with stage II breast cancer 86% About 53% of stage III patients survive five years, and about 20% of stage IV patients do so.

Prevention

Breast cancer cannot be prevented, but making lifestyle choices that eliminate the risk factors listed above is both prudent and promotes general health and well being. While regular breast exams and screening mammograms will not prevent breast cancer, they significantly aid in its early detection and treatment, thus increasing the chances of survival.

Resources

BOOKS

Hirshaut, Yashar and Peter Pressman. *Breast Cancer: The Complete Guide*, 5th ed. New York: Bantam Books, 2008.
Lewis, Shelley. *Five Lessons I Didn't Learn From Breast Cancer (And One Big One I Did)*. New York: Penguin Books, 2008.

QUESTIONS TO ASK YOUR DOCTOR

- Has my cancer spread?
- What is the stage of my cancer? What does that mean?
- What treatment choices do I have?
- What treatment do you recommend? Why?
- What are the advantages and disadvantages of this treatment?
- Will I lose my hair? If so, what can be done about it?
- What are the chances my cancer will come back after this treatment?
- What should I do to be ready for treatment?
- What should I tell my family about my cancer?
- Can you refer me to a support group for women with breast cancer?

Link, John S. *Breast Cancer Survival Manual: A Step-by-Step Guide for the Woman With Newly Diagnosed Breast Cancer*, 4th ed. New York: H. Holt, 2007.

Miller, Kenneth D. *Choices in Breast Cancer Treatment: Medical Specialists and Cancer Survivors Tell You What You Need to Know*. Baltimore: Johns Hopkins University Press, 2008.

OTHER

"Breast Cancer." MedlinePlus. September 22, 2009 [September 23, 2009]. http://www.nlm.nih.gov/medlineplus/breastcancer.html.

"Breast Cancer." Centers for Disease Control and Prevention. July 6, 2009 [September 22, 2009]. http://www.cdc.gov/cancer/breast.

"What You Need to Know About Breast Cancer." National Cancer Institute. November 1, 2007 [September 22, 2009]. http://www.cancer.gov/cancertopics/wyntk/breast.

ORGANIZATIONS

American Cancer Society, 1599 Clifton Rd., NE, Atlanta, GA, 30329, (404) 320-3333, (800) ACS-2345, http://www.cancer.org.

Breast Cancer Network of Strength Headquarters, 135 S. LaSalle Street, Ste 2000, Chicago, IL, 60603, (312) 986-8338, (800) 221-2141 (English); (800) 986-9505 (Español), (312) 294-8597, http://www.networkofstrength.org.

Cancer Research and Prevention Foundation, 1600 Duke Street, Suite 500, Alexandria, VA, 22314, (703) 836-4412, (800) 227-2732, info@preventcancer.org, http://www.preventcancer.org.

National Cancer Institute Public Inquires Office., 6116 Executive Boulevard, Room 3036A, Bethesda, MD, 20892-8322, (800) 4-CANCER. TTY (800) 332-8615, http://www.cancer.gov.

Richard A. McCartney, MD
Tish Davidson, A.M.

Breast reconstruction

Definition

Breast reconstruction consists of a series of surgical procedures performed to recreate a breast. Reconstructions are commonly begun after portions of one or both breasts are removed as a treatment for **breast cancer**. A breast may have to be refashioned for other reasons such as trauma or to correct abnormalities that occur during breast development.

Purpose

Many experts consider reconstruction to be an integral component of the therapy for breast **cancer**.

A naturally appearing breast offers a sense of wholeness and normalcy, which can aid in the psychological recovery from breast cancer. It eliminates the need for an external prosthesis (false breast), which many women find to be physically uncomfortable as well as inconvenient.

Demographics

Breast surgery, including reconstruction, is the second most commonly performed cosmetic surgical procedure practiced on women in the United States. According to the American Society of Plastic and Reconstructive Surgeons, more than 200,000 breast augmentation or reconstruction procedures are performed each year.

Presently, more than 2.1 million, or approximately 8%, of women in the United States have breast implants. The majority of breast implant recipients are Caucasian women (95%), followed by African-American women (4%). The remaining women that have breast implants are Asian (0.5%) and other non-specified races (0.5%).

Description

Breast reconstruction is performed in two stages, with the ultimate goal of creating a breast that looks and feels as natural as possible. It is important to remember that while a good result may closely mimic a normal breast, there will inevitably be scars and some loss of sensation. The reconstructed breast cannot exactly match the original.

The first step is to create a structure called a breast mound. This can be accomplished using artificial materials called breast implants, or by using tissues from other parts of the woman's body. The second step involves creating a balance between the newly constructed breast and the breast on the opposite side. The nipple and areolar complex (darker area around the nipple) are recreated. This is usually done several months after the mound is created, to allow swelling to subside. Other procedures may be necessary, such as lifting the opposite breast (mastopexy) or making it larger or smaller to match the reconstructed breast.

Immediate or delayed reconstruction

While immediate reconstruction (IR) is not recommended for women with breast cancer who need to undergo other, more important treatments, breast reconstruction can be done almost anytime. It can be delayed, or it can be completed during the same procedure as the **mastectomy**. There are psychological benefits to IR. The ability to return to normal

Breast reconstruction

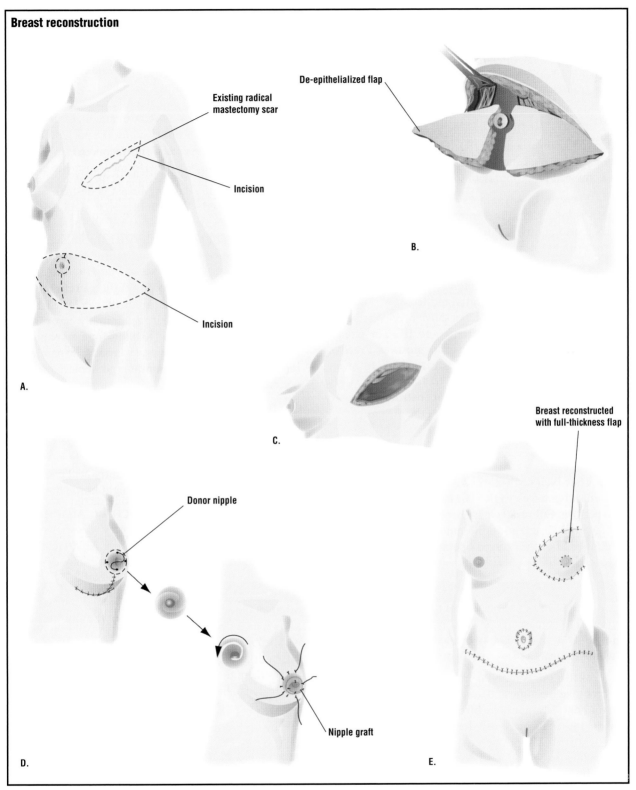

Existing radical
mastectomy scar

Incision

Incision

A.

De-epithelialized flap

B.

C.

Donor nipple

Nipple graft

D.

Breast reconstructed
with full-thickness flap

E.

Breast reconstruction is often performed after a mastectomy. In an autologous procedure, a section of tissue from the patient's abdomen (B) is used to create a natural-looking new breast. In a separate procedure, a layer of the patient's existing nipple can be grafted onto the new breast (D). *(Illustration by GGS Information Services. Cengage Learning, Gale.)*

activities and routines is often enhanced when reconstruction follows immediately after mastectomy. A better final appearance may result from IR. There is less skin removal, often resulting in a shorter scar. The surgeon is better able to preserve the normal boundaries of the breast, so it is easier to more closely match the opposite breast.

The cost of IR is generally lower than the cost of delayed reconstruction (DR). There is one less operation and hospital stay. Surgeon's fees may be lower for a combined procedure than for two separate surgeries.

There are disadvantages of IR as well. The surgery itself is longer, resulting in more time under anesthesia. Postoperative pain and recovery time will be greater than for mastectomy alone.

Other authorities contend that delayed reconstruction (DR) offers different physical and psychological advantages. The initial mastectomy procedure alone takes less time, and has a shorter recovery period and less pain than mastectomy and IR. The woman has more time to adjust to her diagnosis and recover from additional therapy. She is better able to review and evaluate her options and to formulate realistic goals for reconstruction. Some **reconstructive surgery** requires blood transfusions. With DR, the patient can donate her own blood ahead of time (autologous blood donation), and/or arrange to have family and friends donate blood for her use (directed donation).

The psychological stress of living without a breast is a disadvantage of DR. The extra procedure needed to perform DR results in higher costs. Although initial recovery is faster, an additional recuperation period is required after the delayed operation.

Type of reconstruction

There are two basic choices for breast reconstruction. The breast tissue can be replaced with an implant, or the breast is created using some of the woman's own tissues (autologous reconstruction).

ARTIFICIAL IMPLANTS. In general, implant procedures take less time and are less expensive than autologous ones. Implants are breast-shaped pouches. They are made of silicone outer shells, which may be smooth or textured. The inside contains saline (salt water). Implants made prior to 1992 were filled with silicone gel. In 1992, the U.S. Food and Drug Association (FDA) discontinued the use of silicone as a filling material. In 2006, the FDA again allowed silicone gel for use in implants.

An implant may be a fixed-volume type, which cannot change its size. Implants that have the capacity

to be filled after insertion are called tissue expanders. These may be temporary or permanent.

The initial procedure for any implant insertion uses the mastectomy incision to make a pocket of tissue, usually underneath the chest wall muscle. In DR, the mastectomy scar may be reopened and used for this purpose, or a more cosmetic incision may be made. The implant is inserted into the pocket, the skin is stretched as needed, and sutured closed.

If there is inadequate tissue to achieve the desired size, or a naturally sagging breast is desired, a tissue expander is used. It resembles a partially deflated balloon, with an attached valve or port through which saline can be injected. After the initial surgical incision is healed, the woman returns to the doctor's office on a weekly or bi-weekly basis to have small amounts of saline injected. Injections can continue for about six to eight weeks, until the preferred size is obtained. In some cases, it may initially be overfilled and later partially deflated to allow for a more pliable, natural result. A temporary tissue expander is removed after several months and replaced with a permanent implant.

IR surgery using an implant takes approximately two to three hours, and usually requires up to a three-day hospital stay. Implant insertion surgery that is accomplished as part of DR takes one to two hours and can sometimes be done as an outpatient procedure. Alternatively, it may entail overnight hospitalization.

AUTOLOGOUS RECONSTRUCTION. Attached flap and free flap are two types of surgery where a woman's own tissue is used in reconstruction. An attached flap uses skin, muscle, and fat, leaving blood vessels attached to their original source of blood. The flap is maneuvered to the reconstruction site, keeping its original blood supply for nourishment; this is also known as a pedicle flap. The second kind of surgery is called a free flap, which also uses skin, muscle, and fat, but the surgeon severs the blood vessels and reattaches them to other vessels where the new breast is to be created. The surgeon uses a microscope to accomplish the delicate task of sewing blood vessels together (anastomosis). Sometimes, the term microsurgery is used to refer to free flap procedures. Either type of surgery may also be called a myocutaneous flap. This refers to the skin and muscle used.

The skin and muscle used in autologous reconstruction can come from one of several possible places on the body, including the abdomen (tummy tuck flap), the back (latissimus dorsi flap), or the buttocks (gluteus maximus free flap).

Finishing the reconstruction

Other procedures may be necessary to achieve the goal of symmetrical breasts. It may be necessary to make the opposite breast larger (augmentation), smaller (reduction), or higher (mastopexy). These, or any other refinements, should be completed before the creation of a nipple and areola. Tissue to form the new nipple may come from the reconstructed breast itself, the opposite breast, or a more distant donor site such as the inner thigh or behind the ear. The nipple and areolar construction is usually accomplished as an outpatient procedure. A final step, often done in the doctor's office, is tattooing the new nipple and areola to match the color of the opposite nipple and areola as closely as possible.

Insurance

Insurance coverage varies widely for breast reconstruction. Some policies will allow procedures on the affected breast, but refuse to pay for alterations to the opposite breast. Other plans may cover the cost of an external prosthesis or reconstructive surgery, but not both. The Women's Health and Cancer Rights Act of 1998 requires group health plans and health issuers to provide medical and surgical benefits with respect to mastectomy and to cover the cost of reconstructive breast surgery for women who have undergone a mastectomy.

Implants may pose additional insurance concerns. Some companies will withdraw coverage for women with implants, or add a disclaimer for future implant-related problems. Careful reading of insurance policies, including checking on the need for pre-approval and a second opinion, is strongly recommended.

Diagnosis and preparation

The diagnosis for breast reconstruction is almost always made on a visual basis. The underlying medical reasons include replacing all or part of breast tissue that has been removed during the course of cancer treatment, replacing breast mass that has been lost due to injury, or equalizing otherwise normal breasts that are markedly different in size. Underlying cosmetic reasons include personal preference for larger breasts among genetic females or the creation of breasts in male-to-female transsexuals.

Routine preoperative preparations, such as having nothing to eat or drink the night before surgery, are needed for reconstructive procedures. Blood transfusions are often necessary for autologous reconstructive surgeries. The patient may donate her own blood and/or have family and friends donate blood for her use several weeks prior to the surgery.

Emotional preparation is also important. Breast reconstruction will not resolve a psychological problem the woman had before mastectomy, nor make an unstable relationship strong. An expectation of physical perfection is also unrealistic. A woman who cites any of these reasons for reconstruction shows that she has not been adequately informed or prepared. Complete understanding of the benefits and limitations of this surgery are necessary for a satisfactory result.

Not all women are good candidates for breast reconstruction. Overall poor physical health, or specific problems such as cigarette smoking, obesity, high blood pressure, or diabetes will increase the chance of complications. Also, a difficult or prolonged recovery period or failure of the reconstruction may be a result. A woman's physical ability to cope with major surgery and recuperation should also be considered.

Aftercare

The length of the hospital stay, recovery period, and frequency of visits to the doctor after surgery vary considerably with the different types of reconstruction. In general, autologous procedures require longer hospitalization and recovery times than implant procedures. For all surgical procedures, bandages and drainage tubes remain in place for at least a day. Microsurgical or free flap procedures are most closely monitored in the first day or two after surgery. The circulation to the breast may be checked as often as every hour. Complete breast reconstruction requires at least one additional surgery to create a nipple and areola. Scars may remain red and raised for a month or longer. They will fade to their final appearance within one to two years. The true, final appearance of the breasts usually will not be visible for at least one year.

Risks

Some women have reported various types of auto-immune-related connective tissue disorders, which they attribute to their implants—usually involving silicone gel implants. Lawsuits have been filed against the manufacturers of these implants. In 1992, FDA issued guidelines to greatly curtail the use of silicone implants, restricting their use to women who had to replace an existing silicone gel-filled implant. The order required recipients to sign a consent form that details the potential risks of silicone gel-filled implants and become enrolled in a long-range study. Saline became the filling of choice for breast implants.

Saline-filled implants were permitted for all uses, although manufacturers were ordered to continue to collect data on possible risks.

The FDA issued "A Status Report on Breast Implant Safety" in 1995, and revised it in March 1997. It noted that studies have not shown a serious increase in the risk of recognized autoimmune diseases in women with silicone gel-filled breast implants. It also addressed concerns about other complications and emphasized the need for further study of this issue.

In 2006, the FDA once again approved silicone gel-filled implants for breast reconstruction in women of all ages and breast augmentation in women aged 22 and older. The FDA required both approved manufacturers to study 40,000 women each for 10 years to assess potential health problems.

There are a number of risks common to any surgical procedure, such as bleeding, **infection**, anesthesia reaction, or unexpected scarring. Hematoma (accumulation of blood at the surgical site), or seroma (collection of fluid at the surgical site) can delay healing if they are not drained. Any breast reconstruction also poses a risk of asymmetry and the possible need for an unplanned surgical revision. Persistent pain is another potential complication of all types of breast reconstruction.

Implants have some unique problems that may develop. A thick scar, called a capsule, forms around the implant as part of the body's normal reaction to a foreign substance. Capsular contracture occurs when the scar becomes firm or hardened. This may cause pain accompanied by changes in the texture or appearance of the breast. Implants can rupture and leak, deflate, or become displaced. The chances of capsular contracture or rupture increase with the age of the implant. These complications can usually be remedied with outpatient surgery to loosen the capsule and remove or replace the implant as needed. There is some evidence that using implants with textured surfaces may decrease the incidence of these problems. An implant tends to remain firm indefinitely. It will not grow larger or smaller as a woman's weight changes. Asymmetry can develop if a woman gains or loses a large amount of weight.

The autologous procedures all carry a risk of flap failure, which is a loss of blood supply to the tissue forming the new breast. If a large portion of the flap develops inadequate blood supply, another reconstructive technique may be necessary. Tummy tuck flap procedures can result in decreased muscle tone and weakness in the abdomen, or lead to an abdominal hernia. Arm weakness may occur after latissimus dorsi flap surgery.

WHO PERFORMS THE PROCEDURE AND WHERE IS IT PERFORMED?

Breast reconstruction is normally performed by a surgeon with advanced training in plastic and reconstructive procedures. It is commonly, but not exclusively, performed as an outpatient procedure.

Normal results

A normal result of breast reconstruction depends on the woman's goals and expectations. It will not be the same as the breast it replaces. In general, the reconstructed breast should be similar in size and shape to the opposite breast, but will have less sensation and be less mobile than a natural breast. A reconstruction using an implant will usually be firmer and rounder than the other breast. It may feel cooler to the touch, depending on the amount of tissue over it. Scars are unavoidable, but should be as inconspicuous as possible.

Morbidity and mortality rates

Normal scar formation should be expected. With any silicone prosthesis, a capsule usually forms around it; however, in some instances, a mild form of capsular contraction may develop. Mild ridges that can be felt under the skin categorize this condition. If the capsule contracts, as occasionally occurs, it results in a hardening of the breast. There is no way to predict who will excessively scar. Other risks include infection, excessive bleeding, problems associated with anesthesia, rupturing of the implant, and leakage. There have been a total of 120,000 reports of ruptured silicone implants. Approximately 50,000 reports of breakage have been received for saline implants. Most studies have failed to link implants to serious or chronic diseases such as cancer and lupus, but questions remain over how often the implants rupture and what happens if the silicone enters the body. One of the approved manufacturers reported that its implants have a 14 percent likelihood of rupturing over a 10-year period. The other conducted a three-year study and reported that the rupture rate after three years was negligible.

Deaths associated with breast reconstruction are extremely rare. Most post-surgical mortality has been attributed to anesthesia errors or overdoses of pain medications.

QUESTIONS TO ASK THE DOCTOR

- What will be the resulting appearance?
- Is the surgeon board certified in plastic and reconstructive surgery?
- How many procedures has the surgeon performed?
- What is the surgeon's complication rate?

Alternatives

Alternatives to breast reconstruction surgery include using external breast forms that fit into brassiere cups or are attached to the skin of the chest. Creams that allege to increase breast size usually produce no noticeable results. The use of creams containing hormones can lead to long-term hormonal imbalances. Reputable experts do not generally recommend these preparations for breast enlargement.

Resources

BOOKS

Disa, J. J., and M. C. Kuechel. *100 Questions and Answers About Breast Surgery*. Sudbury, MA: Jones and Bartlett, 2005.

Dixon, J. M. *Breast Surgery: A Companion to Specialist Surgical Practice*, 3rd ed. Philadelphia: Saunders, 2006.

Freund, R. M., and A. VanDyne. *Cosmetic Breast Surgery: A Complete Guide to Making the Right Decision—From A to Double D*. New York: Marlowe & Company, 2004.

Mang, W., K. Lang, F. Niedel, N. S. Mackowski, N. Rossman, and M. Stock. *Manual of Aesthetic Surgery 2*. New York: Springer, 2005.

Spear, S. L., S. C. Willey, G. L. Robb, D. C. Hammond, and N. Y. Nahabedian. *Surgery of the Breast: Principles And Art*, 2nd ed. Philadelphia: Lippincott Williams & Wilkins, 2005.

Steligo, K. *The Breast Reconstruction Guidebook*, 2nd ed. San Carlos, CA: Carlo Press, 2005.

PERIODICALS

Dehn, T. "The timing of breast reconstruction." *Annals of the Royal College of Surgeons of England* 89, no. 8 (November 2007): 754–759.

Guyomard, V., S. Leinster, and M. Wilkinson. "Systematic review of studies of patients' satisfaction with breast reconstruction after mastectomy." *Breast* 16, no. 6 (December 2007): 547–567.

Yano, K., K. Hosokawa, T. Masuoka, K. Matsuda, A. Takada, T. Taguchi, Y. Tamaki, and S. Noguchi. "Options for immediate breast reconstruction following skin-sparing mastectomy." *Breast Cancer* 14, no. 4 (2007): 406–413.

OTHER

"Breast Implants." U.S. Food and Drug Administration, Centers for Devices and Radiological Health. November 17, 2006. http://www.fda.gov/cdrh/breastimplants/ (December 23, 2007).

"Breast Implants on Trial." *Frontline*. Public Broadcasting System. http://www.pbs.org/wgbh/pages/frontline/implants/ (December 23, 2007).

"Breast Reconstruction." American Society of Plastic Surgeons. 2008. http://www.plasticsurgery.org/patients _consumers/procedures/BreastReconstruction.cfm? CFID = 92081034 &CFTOKEN = 88819197 (December 23, 2007).

"Breast Reconstruction." Medline Plus. March 21, 2008. http://www.nlm.nih.gov/medlineplus/breastreconstruction.html (December 23, 2007).

"Breast Reconstruction After Mastectomy." American Cancer Society. September 6, 2007. http://www.cancer. org/docroot/CRI/content/CRI_2_6X_Breast_ Reconstruction_After_Mastectomy_5.asp (December 23, 2007).

"Breast Reconstruction After Mastectomy." Mayo Clinic. August 18, 2006. http://www.mayoclinic.com/health/breast-reconstruction/WO00083 (December 23, 2007).

"Breast Reconstruction Guide for Patients." M. D. Anderson Cancer Center, University of Texas. 2008. http://www.mdanderson.org/Diseases/BreastCancer/reconstruction/ (December 23, 2007).

ORGANIZATIONS

American Board of Plastic Surgery, Seven Penn Center, Suite 4001635 Market Street, Philadelphia, PA, 19103-2204, (215) 587-9322, http://www.abplsurg.org.

American College of Surgeons, 633 North Saint Claire Street, Chicago, IL, 60611, (312) 202-5000, http://www.facs.org.

American Society for Aesthetic Plastic Surgery, 11081 Winners Circle, Los Alamitos, CA, 90720, (888) 272-7711, http://www.surgery.org/.

American Society of Plastic Surgeons, 444 E. Algonquin Rd., Arlington Heights, IL, 60005, (847) 228-9900, http://www.plasticsurgery.org.

L. Fleming Fallon, Jr., M.D., Dr.P.H.

Breast self-exam

Definition

Breast self-examination (BSE) is a diagnostic technique regularly performed by a woman, independent from a physician, both by feeling for anything suspicious in her breasts and by observing any changes through the use of a mirror.

Woman examining her breast for abnormalities. *(© Francoise Sauze, Science Source/Photo Researchers, Inc. Reproduced by permission.)*

Purpose

BSE should be performed monthly in order to discover changes in breast tissue, discharge from the nipple, or the onset of pain in the breast area. While 80% of lumps are not cancerous, such discoveries can ultimately lead to the detection of **breast cancer**.

Precautions

BSE is an effective self-diagnostic procedure, but it must not take the place of having a mammogram and having a health care provider check the breasts for abnormal changes. Make sure to schedule an annual clinical breast examination with a licensed medical care provider to supplement the BSE.

Description

It is important that BSEs are performed routinely so that a woman knows what her breasts normally feel and look like, resulting in quicker identification of anything abnormal. Self-exams take less than five minutes to perform and should be done a few days after the end of menstruation. Women that menstruate irregularly should choose a day of the month that is easy to remember, such as the date of their birth, and perform the exams on the same day each month.

The first phase of the BSE is to disrobe and stand in front of a mirror, observing the breast area in four different positions. First, with the arms down to the sides, look at the color, shape, outline, and direction of the breasts and nipples, taking note of anything atypical. Then, press the hands on the hips in order to flex the chest muscles, making the same observations. Next, observe the breasts while leaning forward. Finally, raise the arms overhead and notice anything abnormal such as color changes, dimpling of the skin, or nipple discharge.

The second phase of the BSE is performed lying down. First, put a pillow under the right shoulder and place the right hand under the head so that the elbow is positioned at a 90-degree angle. This is done in order to flatten the breast as much as possible, making the examination easier and more effective.

Then, using the pads of the fingers of the left hand, press firmly around the breast using a small circular motion about the size of a penny. A small amount of lotion or petroleum jelly can make it easier to feel for lumps. Three types of pressure should be used. The first pressure should be enough to examine the surface, typically just to move the skin and feel for changes in the top layer of tissue. The second level of pressure is a deeper pressure, probing into the tissue. The final pressure level is applied deep into the breast tissue so that the rib cage can be felt and a minor amount of discomfort is experienced. Choose a comfortable pattern such as circles, lines, or wedges to make sure that the entire breast and armpit area are thoroughly examined with each level of pressure.

Finally, tenderly squeeze the area around the nipple and check for fluid discharge. After the right breast has been thoroughly examined, repeat the above steps on the left breast.

Although it is uncommon, forms of breast **cancer** can also occur in men. The breast self-exam can be modified to be effective for men. Men can utilize the visual exam and can also feel for any changes in the tissue.

Preparation

Since the patient performs BSE in the comfort of her own home, there are not many preparations that need to be made. The patient should remove any distractions that could interfere with the performance of a thorough exam. It is also advisable to disrobe and to use lotion or lubricant when palpating the breast area.

Aftercare

BSE is not an invasive procedure. Therefore there is not any significant aftercare that needs to take place. Individuals should simply remember to perform the exam monthly and inform their doctor of any changes.

Risks

There are no known risks associated with the breast self-exam as long as the individual schedules regular exams with a physician and immediately reports anything unusual.

Normal results

Patients who perform BSE regularly know what their breast tissue normally feels like. Typically, there will not be any detectable anomalies in their breast tissue, unless they carry out the exam just prior to menstruation or during pregnancy when breasts may seem more lumpy and tender. In these cases, it is likely that abnormal lumps and tenderness are not associated with cancerous tumors. However, if a woman finds anything that makes her uneasy, she should consult with her physician.

Abnormal results

Women should consult with their physician if they notice dimpling of the skin, any change in outline or shape of their breasts, unusual lumps, areas of thickening, or pain during the palpation of the breasts. If milky white or bloody discharge from the nipple is observed, then the patient should call the doctor. Generally, if there are any observations that make a person uneasy, it is advisable to contact a doctor.

Resources

OTHER

"Breast Self-Exam (BSE) Why, When and How." *Breast Cancer Information Service*. April 2001. [cited June 29, 2001]. <http://trfn.clpgh.org/bcis/GeneralInfo/bse.html>.

"Breast Self Examination: Your Key to Better Breast Health." *Y-ME National Breast Cancer Organization* April 2001. [cited June 27, 2001]. http://www.y-me.org/images/breast_self_exam.pdf.

"BSE Breast Self Examination." *Info Breast Cancer* April 2001. [cited June 28, 2001]. http://www.infobreastcancer.cyberus.ca/bse2.htm.

"An Ounce of Prevention...How to Do Self-Exams." *Sister: Columbia University's Feminist Magazine* April 2001. [cited June 27, 2001]. http://www.columbia.edu/cu/sister/SelfExams.html.

Sally C. McFarlane-Parrott

Breast ultrasound

Definition

Breast ultrasound (or sonography) is an imaging technique for diagnosing breast disease, such as **cancer**. It uses harmless, high-frequency sound waves to

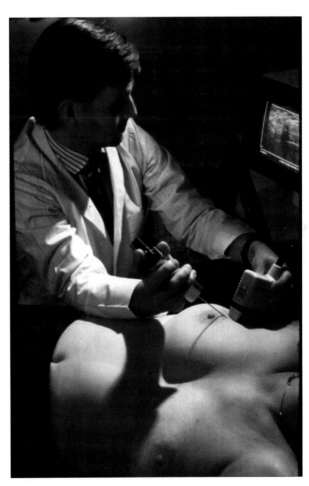

This woman is having her breast scanned by ultrasound while a tissue biopsy is being taken. In breast scanning, ultrasound is used to distinguish between solid lumps and fluid-filled cysts. *(Photo by Geoff Tompkinson. Photo Researchers, Inc. Reproduced by permission.)*

form an image (sonogram). The sound waves pass through the breast and bounce back or echo from various tissues to form a picture of the internal structures. It is not invasive and involves no radiation.

Purpose

Breast ultrasound may be used in several ways. The most common application is to investigate a specific area of the breast where a problem is suspected. A palpable lump and/or a lump or density discovered by x ray (mammogram) can be further evaluated by ultrasound. It is especially helpful in distinguishing between a fluid-filled cyst and a solid mass. It can also identify small lesions that are too tiny to be felt.

Breast ultrasound is often the first study performed to evaluate masses in women under 35 whose mammograms can be difficult to interpret due to the density of their breast tissue. In 2003, a new study found that ultrasound was more accurate than **mammography** at diagnosing **breast cancer** in women under age 45. However, mammography still works as a screening tool, with breast ultrasound as the follow-up examination. Another study in that year found that combining ultrasound with **magnetic resonance imaging** (MRI) direction greatly improved diagnostic decisions about breast cancer lesions. The lesions detected by MRI could also be localized using ultrasound needle guidance for follow-up **biopsy**.

The lack of radiation used with ultrasound makes it ideal for studying breast abnormalities in women who are pregnant. Assessing breast implants for leakage or rupture is another way ultrasound is used. Breast inflammation, where pockets of **infection** or abscesses may form, can be diagnosed and monitored by ultrasound.

Thickened and swollen breast skin may be a sign of inflammatory breast cancer. Ultrasound can sometimes identify a cancerous growth within the breast causing

the thickened skin. These cases are usually followed by a core biopsy guided by ultrasound (described below).

Breast ultrasound is employed to observe and guide a needle for several interventional procedures. These include cyst aspiration, fine needle aspiration, large core needle biopsy (as a first step in determining treatment for a lesion that is likely to be cancerous), and needle localization in surgical breast biopsy. Biopsies guided by ultrasound have distinct advantages. Patients usually find that the procedure is less traumatic and more comfortable than surgical biopsies. Ultrasound is known for its accuracy in determining how far a cancerous growth extends into the surrounding tissue in lesions that cannot be felt. Biopsies guided by ultrasound are generally less costly than surgical biopsies. Additionally, if the abnormality that requires biopsy can be seen on both a mammogram and ultrasound, an ultrasound-guided biopsy is often more comfortable for the patient as no compression is necessary.

Description

Ultrasound can be done in a doctor's office or another outpatient setting, such as a hospital or imaging center.

The patient removes her clothing from the waist up and puts on a hospital gown, open in the front. She lies on her back or side on an examining table. A gel that enhances sound transmission is spread over the area to be examined. The technologist then places a transducer, an instrument about the size of an electric shaver, against the skin. The images from reflected sound waves appear on a monitor screen.

A physician called a radiologist interprets the images obtained from ultrasound imaging. In 2003, it was reported that new computer-aided diagnosis (CAD) technology that had recently been widely added to mammography may help improve ultrasound as well. The CAD system uses computer algorithms applied to a three-dimensional ultrasound image to assign scores to mass characteristics. Though the technology will not replace human observation and judgment, it may soon be added to support the radiologist's interpretation.

A good ultrasound study is difficult to obtain if the patient is unable to remain quietly in one position. Obesity may hinder clear viewing of internal structures, and the accuracy of an ultrasound study is highly dependent on the skill of the person performing the examination. The images recorded vary with the angle and pressure of the transducer and the equipment settings. The examination may take from 30 to 45 minutes. Most insurance plans cover the cost of an ultrasound examination.

Normal results

An ultrasound examination may reveal either normal tissue or a benign condition such as a cyst. Ultrasound can confidently diagnose a benign structure that has certain characteristics of a simple cyst. In the case of a simple cyst with no symptoms, additional treatment beyond continued observation is usually not needed.

Abnormal results

A potentially malignant mass can be identified by breast ultrasound. Abnormal results fall into the following categories: benign fibrous nodule, complex cyst, suspicious lesion, and lesion highly suggestive of cancer. In cases where ultrasound shows the presence of a complex cyst or fibrous nodule, a biopsy is justified because 10% to 15% of these growths are malignant. Lesions falling into the last two categories (suspicious or highly suggestive of cancer) have a higher chance of being cancerous, and should be investigated further, either by biopsy or surgery.

Breast cancers such as the following may be identified on ultrasound: ductal **carcinoma**, infiltrating lobular carcinoma, medullary carcinoma, mucinous (colloid) carcinoma, tubular carcinoma, and papillary carcinoma. On ultrasound, the shape of a lesion and the type of edges it has can sometimes indicate if it is benign or cancerous, but there are exceptions. For example, benign fibroadenomas are usually oval, and some cancers can be similarly shaped. Cancerous tumors usually have jagged edges, but some benign growths can have these edges as well. Ultrasound is not a definitive test. Tissue diagnosis is often required.

See also Biopsy; Breast cancer; Breast self–exam.

Resources

PERIODICALS

"Breast Ultrasound Wins in Younger Women." *Diagnostic Imaging* 33 (July 1, 2003): 22.

"CAD Software Improves Breast Ultrasound, Digital Mammograms." *Cancer Weekly* December 23, 2003: 13.

Rubin, Eva, et al. "Reducing the Cost of Diagnosis of Breast Carcinoma: Impact of Ultrasound and Imaging–Guided Biopsies on a Clinical Breast Practice." *Cancer* 91 (January 2001) 324-31.

Smith, LaNette F., et al. "Intraoperative Ultrasound–guided Breast Biopsy." *The American Journal of Surgery* 180 (December 2000): 419-23.

Trevino, Merlino. "MR-directed US Provides Economical Breast Diagnosis — Ultrasound Characterizes Indeterminate Lesions Already Found by MRI." *Diagnostic Imaging* April 1, 2003: 59.

Velez, Nitzet, et al. "Diagnostic and Interventional Ultrasound for Breast Disease." *The American Journal of Surgery* 180 (October 2000): 284-7.

Ellen S. Weber, M.S.N.

Bronchoalveolar lung cancer

Definition

Bronchoalveolar lung **cancer**, also known as bronchioloalveolar lung cancer or BAC, is a type of **non-small cell lung cancer**. The World Health Organization (WHO) classifies BAC as a subtype of **adenocarcinoma**.

Demographics

Lung cancer is leading cause of cancer deaths in the United States. The American Cancer Society predicted about 219,440 new cases of lung cancer (all types) would develop in 2009. Lung cancer occurs primarily in people over age 45, and is slightly more likely to occur in men than in women. The average age at diagnosis for lung cancer is 71 years. More than 400,000 people alive today in the U.S. have been diagnosed with lung cancer at some point in their lives.

Lung cancer remains a highly lethal cancer. The highest survival from lung cancer occurs in the United States. However, the 5-year survival rate for lung cancer in the U.S. is only 14%. In comparison, the overall 5-year survival rate for lung cancer in Europe is a dismal 8%.

Adenocarcinoma accounts for about 40% of all lung cancers, up from about 13% in 1965. The number of lung cancer cases attributed to adenocarcinoma is increasing rapidly in the United States and Europe, especially in women, although cases are also increasing among men. Bronchoalveolar cancer is thought to account for between 2% and 14% of all cases of lung cancer. About 85% of lung cancers can be attributed to smoking tobacco. However, although smoking **cigarettes** increases the risk of developing bronchoalveolar cancer, it is the most common type of lung cancer found among individuals who have never smoked cigarettes.

Description

When a person breathes, air enters the trachea (windpipe). In the chest, the trachea splits into two passageways called bronchi. One goes to the right lung and the other to the left lung. The bronchi then subdivide into smaller tubes called bronchioles. These bronchioles end in tiny air sacs called alveoli. A diagram of the respiratory system resembles an upside down tree with the trachea as the tree trunk and the alveoli as the leaves. Exchange of gasses between the lungs and the blood occurs in the alveoli.

Lung cancer, like all cancers, is the result of uncontrolled cell growth. The specific characteristics of each cancer depend on which cells are growing out of control and where they are located. There are two distinct types of lung cancer each with its own characteristics and treatment strategies—small cell lung cancer (SCLC) and non-small cell lung cancer (NSCLC).

NSCLC can develop from several different types of lung cells, so it is further categorized as either squamous cell **carcinoma**, adenocarcinoma, or large-cell lung cancer. Bronchoalveolar lung cancer is a subtype of adenocarcinoma.

Bronchoaveolar lung cancer is a primary malignant cancer of the lungs, meaning that the lungs are the first place this cancer develops; it does not migrate to the lungs from elsewhere in the body. Bronchoalveolar cancer usually develops in the outer (peripheral) regions of the lungs in gland-like cells that secrete mucus. It spreads along the membranes that separates the alveoli from each other. This subtype may occur as a solitary nodule, as multiple nodules in the lungs or as a rapidly progressing pneumonic form of the cancer which can spread rapidly from one lobe of the lung to other lobes.

Bronchoalveolar lung cancer is comprised of three subtypes: mucinous, nonmucinous, and a mixed mucinous/nonmucinous or indeterminate subtype.

Typically, BAC does not metastasize to other parts of the body outside of the lung. However, BAC does have the propensity to spread within the lungs.

Risk factors

Major risk factors associated with the development of lung cancers in general include:

- history of smoking
- exposure to tobacco smoke
- exposure to asbestos fibers and other workplace chemicals
- exposure to radon gas
- a personal or family history of lung cancer

A specific risk factor linked to the development of BAC is the use of low-tar, unfiltered cigarettes.

Causes and symptoms

In general, lung cancers develop because of acquired changes that occur in the genes of lung cells when they are exposed to carcinogens such as tobacco smoke. These changes either turn on genes that cause cells to grow uncontrollably (oncogenes) or turn off genes that cause cells to die at the appropriate time (tumor suppressor genes) or both.

Because bronchoalveolar cancer is the most likely lung cancer to develop among people who have never smoked, its exact cause is somewhat unclear. Like all lung cancers, smoking tobacco or marijuana, exposure to asbestos, and inhalation certain workplace chemicals (e.g. radon gas, arsenic, beryllium, vinyl chloride, coal products, gasoline exhaust) increases the risk of developing bronchoalveolar cancer. However, since this type of cancer is increasing and is common among non-smokers, some other yet to be determined factors seem to play a role in its development.

More recent research findings indicate that the dramatic increase in BAC in recent decades may be due to the introduction of low-tar, filtered cigarettes. People who smoke this type of cigarette, draw tiny particles deep into the lungs which may precipitate cancerous changes in the lungs over time.

Lung cancer symptoms tend to develop only after the cancer is far advanced and possibly has even spread (metastasized) to other placed in the body such as the liver, adrenal glands, bones, or brain. Bronchoalveolar cancer is no exception. When symptoms do occur, they include:

- coughing
- difficulty breathing
- chest pain
- weight loss

Bronchoalveolar lung cancer causes the cells lining the lungs to produce large amounts of watery mucus. When examined by a doctor, the lungs may have an abnormal dead or dull sound because of the amount of mucus they contain. Severity of symptoms, however, is not well correlated to the severity or stage of this cancer.

Diagnosis

Examination

Initially, a history and physical will be conducted by the health care practitioner. The practitioner will determine the performance status of the patient and whether the patient has experienced a **weight loss** of greater than 5%. The physician will also determine the presence of symptoms such as voluminous, watery mucus which is a sign indicative of BAC.

Tests and procedures

Diagnostic tests are the same as for any suspected lung cancer, beginning with a chest x ray and moving on to other **imaging studies** such as **computed tomography** (CT) scan, **magnetic resonance imaging** (MRI), ultrasound, and **positron emission tomography** (PET) scans. Initial tests determine the presence and extent of suspected cancer in the lungs, while later tests such as bone scans are done to determine if the cancer has metastasized to other sites. A sample of sputum (coughed up mucus) may be examined for cancer cells, but the definitive diagnosis is made by taking a **biopsy** of lung tissue.

Other tests which may be conducted include a complete blood count (CBC)as well as tests of electrolyte, liver and renal function.

Treatment

The staging, treatment, and prognosis for bronchoalveolar lung cancer is the same as for other NSCLS. The stage of the cancer is based on the TNM system. This considers the tumor size and how much it has grown (T), whether the cancer has spread to the lymph nodes (N) and whether it has metastasized (M) to distant sites in the body.

Stage IA

T1 N0 M0. The tumor is no larger than 3 cm (about 1.2 in) with no sign of lymph node involvement or **metastasis**. Treatment at this stage is likely to involve only surgery to remove the tumor. Surgery can remove one lobe of the lung (**lobectomy**) or a part of a lobe (wedge resection or **segmentectomy**). The estimated five-year survival rate when NSCLC is treated at this stage is 75%, however lung cancer is rarely diagnosed this early.

Stage IB

T2 NO MO. The tumor is larger than 3 cm, but cancer has not spread beyond the lung. Treatment is usually surgery. Sometimes **radiation therapy** is recommended following surgery. The estimated five-year survival rate when NSCLC is treated at this stage is 55%.

Stage II A

T1 N1 MO. The tumor is smaller than 3 cm, but cancer has spread locally to the lymph nodes, although it has not metastasized to distant sites. Treatment at this stage is usually surgery to remove a lobe of the lung or sometimes the entire lung. (Individuals can survive well with a single lung.) Radiation therapy may follow surgery. Supplemental **chemotherapy** at this stage is being studied in **clinical trials**. The estimated five-year survival rate when NSCLC is treated at this stage is 50%.

Stage II B

T2 N1 MO or T3 N0 M0. Either the individual's condition is the same as in stage IIA except that the tumor is larger than 3 cm, or the tumor has grown into the membrane surrounding the lungs, the chest cavity, diaphragm, or membrane surrounding the heart. Treatment is similar to stage IIA. The estimated five-year survival rate when NSCLC is treated at this stage is 40%.

Stage III A

T1-3 N2 M0 or T3 N1 M0. The tumor can be any size, but cancer has spread to additional, more distant lymph nodes, but has not metastasized to distant sites. Alternately, the tumor is growing into the surrounding membranes or muscles, but only local lymph nodes are involved. Treatment at this stage depends on where in the lung the cancer is located. Most bronchoalveolar cancers are located on the edges of the lung. Surgery of the lung and lymph nodes may be performed depending on where the tumor is located, but chemotherapy and radiation therapy are also required. The estimated five-year survival rate when NSCLC is treated at this stage is 10–35% depending in part on whether the tumor is operable.

Stage III B

Any T4 or N3 and M0. The tumor has invaded nearby organs such as the esophagus, trachea, large blood vessels or heart or the cancer has spread to large and diverse lymph nodes, although it has not metastasized to distant organs. Surgery at this stage will not remove the cancer. Individuals in good health undergo chemotherapy and radiation therapy. The estimated five-year survival rate when NSCLC is treated at this stage is less than 5%.

Stage IV

Any M1. Cancer has metastasized to distant organs. Stage IV cancer is almost incurable. The goal of treatment is to improve the quality of life or extend life. Aggressive chemotherapy with cisplatin-based therapy may be used for individuals in otherwise good health. Alternately, care may be given to make the individual as comfortable as possible. The estimated five-year survival rate when NSCLC is treated at this stage is about 2%.

Recent data suggest that the drugs **gefitinib** (Iressa) and **erlotinib** (Tarceva) may be effective in treating BAC because of a mutation in the epidermal growth factor receptor (EGFR) in some types of lung cancer.

Prognosis

People diagnosed with BAC tend to have a more favorable prognosis than individuals diagnosed with other subtypes of adenocarcinoma, however, prognosis is dependent upon stage at diagnosis.

Estimated overall lung cancer 5-year survival rates by stage are:

- Stage 1A – 75%
- Stage IB – 55%

QUESTIONS TO ASK YOUR DOCTOR

- What type of lung cancer do I have?
- What stage is my cancer?
- Why do you recommend this particular treatment and what are the alternatives?
- What kind of side effects can I expect from treatment?
- Are there any clinical trials that might be appropriate for me?

- Stage IIA – 50%
- Stage IIB – 40%
- Stage IIIA – 10 to 35%
- Stage IIIB – less than 5%
- Stage IV – less than 5%

The overall 5-year survival rate for all stages and types of lung cancer remains a dismal 14% in the United States.

Prevention

Avoiding smoking is the best way to prevent all lung cancers. Between 85% and 90% of people who develop lung cancer are smokers. No matter how long or how much an individual has smoked, the chance of getting lung cancer decreases and general health improves by quitting smoking.

Other ways to prevent all lung cancers include avoiding breathing gasoline and diesel fuel fumes and exposure to asbestos and other airborne chemicals known to be carcinogens. Maintaining a healthy weight, exercising regularly, and eating a diet high in vegetables and fruits are other positive steps individuals can take. However, all these diet and exercise precautions are of minor importance when compared to the preventative effects of not smoking.

Resources

PERIODICALS

Jackman, D.M., Chirieac, L.R., & Janne, P.A. "Bronchioloalveolar Carcinoma: A Review of the Epidemiology, Pathology and Treatment." *Semin Respir Crit Care Med*, 26, no. 3 (2005):342–353.

Miller, V.A., Riely, G.J., Zakowski, M.F., et al. "Molecular Characteristics of Bronchioloalveolar Carcinoma and Adenocarcinoma, Bronchioloalveolar Carcinoma Subtype, Predict Response to Erlotinib." *J Clin Oncol* 26(2008):1472–8.

ORGANIZATIONS

American Cancer Society. 1599 Clifton Road NE, Atlanta
GA 30329-4251. 1-800-ACS-2345. http://
www.cancer.org.
National Cancer Institute Information Line 1-800-4-
CANCER (1-800-422-6237) http://www.cancer.gov.
cancergovstaff@mail.nih.gov.

OTHER

American Cancer Society. *Non Small Cell Lung Cancer*, 10/
24/08 [September 20, 2009]. http://www.cancer.org/
docroot/CRI/content/CRI_2_4_1X_What_Is_Small_
Cell_Lung_Cancer.asp?sitearea = .
Huq,S., Maghfoor, I., & Perry, M. *Lung Cancer, Non-Small
Cell* July 30,2009 [cited September 20, 2009]. http://
www.emedicine.medscape.com/article/279960.

Tish Davidson, A.M.
Melinda Granger Oberleitner, R.N., D.N.S.,
A.P.R.N., D.N.S.

Bronchoscope

Bronchoscopy is a procedure in which a hollow, flexible tube is inserted into the airways, allowing the physician to visually examine the lower airways, including the larynx, trachea, bronchi, and bronchioles. It can also be used to collect specimens for bacteriological culture to diagnose infectious diseases such as tuberculosis. *(Illustration by Electronic Illustrators Group. Cengage Learning, Gale.)*

Bronchoscopy

Definition

Bronchoscopy is a procedure in which a cylindrical fiberoptic scope is inserted into the airways. This scope contains a viewing device that allows the visual examination of the lower airways.

Purpose

During a bronchoscopy, a physician can visually examine the lower airways, including the larynx, trachea, bronchi, and bronchioles. The procedure is used to examine the mucosal surface of the airways for abnormalities that might be associated with a variety of lung diseases. Its use includes the visualization of airway obstructions such as a tumor, or the collection of specimens for the diagnosis of **cancer** originating in the bronchi of the lungs (bronchogenic cancer). It can also be used to collect specimens for culture to diagnose infectious diseases such as tuberculosis. The type of specimens collected can include sputum (composed of saliva and discharges from the respiratory passages), tissue samples from the bronchi or bronchioles, or cells collected from washing the lining of the bronchi or bronchioles. The instrument used in bronchoscopy, a bronchoscope, is a slender cylindrical instrument containing a light and an eyepiece. There are two types of bronchoscopes, a rigid tube that is sometimes referred to as an open-tube or ventilating bronchoscope, and a more flexible fiberoptic tube. This tube contains four smaller passages—two for light to pass through, one for

seeing through and one that can accommodate medical instruments that may be used for **biopsy** or suctioning, or that medication can be passed through.

Bronchoscopy may be used for the following purposes:

- to diagnose cancer, tuberculosis, lung infection, or other lung disease
- to examine an inherited deformity of the lungs
- to remove a foreign body in the lungs, such as a mucus plug, tumor, or excessive secretions
- to remove tissue samples, also known as biopsy, to test for cancer cells, help with staging the advancement of the lung cancer, or to treat a tumor with laser therapy
- to allow examination of a suspected tumor, obstruction, secretion, bleeding, or foreign body in the airways
- to determine the cause of a persistent cough, wheezing, or a cough that includes blood in the sputum
- to evaluate the effectiveness of lung cancer treatments

Precautions

Patients not breathing adequately on their own due to severe respiratory failure may require mechanical ventilation prior to bronchoscopy. It may not be appropriate to perform bronchoscopy on patients with an unstable heart condition. All patients must be constantly monitored while undergoing a bronchoscopy so that any abnormal reactions can be dealt with immediately.

Description

There are two types of bronchoscopes, a rigid tube and a fiberoptic tube. Because of its flexibility, the fiberoptic tube is usually preferred. However, if the purpose of the procedure is to remove a foreign body caught in the windpipe or lungs of a child, the more rigid tube must be used because of its larger size. The patient will either lie face-up on his/her back or sit upright in a chair. Medication to decrease secretions, lessen anxiety, and relax the patient are often given prior to the procedure. While breathing through the nose, anesthesia is sprayed into the mouth or nose to numb it. It will take 1-2 minutes for the anesthesia to take effect. Once this happens, the bronchoscope will be put into the patient's mouth or nose and moved down into the throat. While the bronchoscope is moving down the throat, additional anesthesia is put into the bronchoscope to numb the lower parts of the airways. Using the eyepiece, the physician then observes the trachea and bronchi, and the mucosal lining of these passageways, looking for any abnormalities that may be present.

If the purpose of the bronchoscopy is to take tissue samples or biopsy, forceps or a bronchial brush are used to obtain cells. If the purpose is to identify an infectious agent, a bronchoalveolar lavage (BAL) can be used to gather fluid for culture purposes. Also, if any foreign matter is found in the airways, it can be removed.

Another procedure using bronchoscopy is called fluorescence bronchoscopy. This can be used to detect precancerous cells present in the airways. By using a fluorescent light in the bronchoscope, precancerous tissue will appear dark red, while healthy tissue will appear green. This technique can help detect lung cancer at an early stage, so that treatment can be started early.

Alternative procedures

Depending upon the purpose of the bronchoscopy, alternatives might include a **computed tomography** scan (CT) or no procedure at all. Bronchoscopy is often performed to investigate an abnormality that shows up on a chest x ray or CT scan. If the purpose is to obtain biopsy specimens, one option is to perform surgery, which carries greater risks. Another option is percutaneous (through the skin) biopsy guided by computed tomography.

Preparation

The doctor should be informed of any allergies and all the medications that the patient is currently taking. The doctor may instruct the patient not to take medications like aspirin or anti-inflammatory drugs, which interfere with clotting, for a period of time prior to the procedure. The patient needs to fast for 6 to 12 hours prior to the procedure and refrain from drinking any liquids the day of the procedure. The bronchoscopy takes about 45 to 60 minutes, with results usually available in one day. Prior to the bronchoscopy, several tests may be done, including a chest x ray and blood work. Sometimes a bronchoscopy is done under general anesthesia. Patients usually have an intravenous (IV) line in the arm. Most likely, the procedure will be done under local anesthesia, which is sprayed into the nose or mouth. This is necessary to decrease the gag reflex. A sedative may also be used to help the patient relax. It is important that the patient understands that at no time will the airway be blocked and that oxygen can be supplied through the bronchoscope. A signed consent form is necessary for this procedure.

Aftercare

After the bronchoscopy, the patient will be monitored for vital signs such as heart rate, blood pressure, and breathing, while resting in bed. Sometimes patients have an abnormal reaction to anesthesia. All saliva should be spit into a basin so that it can be examined for the presence of blood. If a biopsy was taken, the patient should not cough or clear the throat as this might dislodge any blood clot that has formed and cause bleeding. No food or drink should be consumed for about two hours after the procedure or until the anesthesia wears off. Diet is gradually progressed from ice chips and clear liquids to the patient's regular diet. There will also be a temporary sore throat and hoarseness that may last for a few days.

Risks

Minor side effects arise from the bronchoscope causing abrasion of the lining of the airways. This results in some swelling and inflammation, as well as hoarseness caused from abrading the vocal cords. If this abrasion is more serious, it can lead to respiratory difficulty or bleeding of the airway lining. A more serious risk involved in having a bronchoscopy performed is the occurrence of a pneumothorax, due to puncturing of the lungs, which allows air to escape into the space between the lung and the chest wall. These risks are greater with the use of a rigid bronchoscope than with a fiberoptic bronchoscope. If a rigid tube is used, there is also a risk of chipped teeth.

Normal results

Normal tracheal appearance consists of smooth muscle with C-shaped rings of cartilage at regular intervals. The trachea and the bronchi are lined with a mucous membrane.

Abnormal results

Abnormal bronchoscopy findings may involve abnormalities of the bronchial wall such as inflammation, swelling, ulceration, or anatomical abnormalities. The bronchoscopy may also reveal the presence of abnormal substances in the trachea and bronchi. If samples are taken, the results could indicate cancer, disease-causing agents or other lung disease. Other abnormalities include constriction or narrowing (stenosis), compression, dilation of vessels, or abnormal branching of the bronchi. Abnormal substances that might be found in the airways include blood, secretions, or mucous plugs. Any abnormalities are discussed with the patient.

Resources

BOOKS

Fauci, Anthony S. *Harrison's Principles of Internal Medicine.* 14th ed. New York: McGraw-Hill, 2000.

Cindy L. Jones, Ph.D.

Burkitt's lymphoma

Definition

Burkitt's **lymphoma** (BL) is a type of **non-Hodgkin's lymphoma** (NHL) that is sometimes called a B-cell lymphoma or small noncleaved cell lymphoma. It is an endemic (characteristic of a specific place) disease in central Africa but sporadic (occurring in scattered instances) in other countries. Burkitt's lymphoma

African child with facial disfigurement caused by Burkitt's lymphoma. *(Custom Medical Stock Photo. Reproduced by permission.)*

KEY TERMS

Ann Arbor system—A system of tumor staging used to classify non-Hodgkin's lymphomas in adults. It specifies four stages, which can be further defined by the use of letters to identify general physical symptoms and the parts of the body affected by the lymphoma. The corresponding staging system in children is the St. Jude Children's Research Hospital system.

B cell—A type of lymphocyte that produces antibodies. Burkitt's lymphoma is a cancer of the immune system in which the B cells multiply at an extremely fast rate.

Endemic—Natural to or characteristic of a specific place. In central Africa, Burkitt's lymphoma is an endemic disease.

Epstein-Barr virus (EBV)—A type of herpesvirus (human herpesvirus 4), first identified in 1964, that causes infectious mononucleosis. It is found in most patients with the endemic form of Burkitt's lymphoma, though its role in the disease is still unclear.

International Prognostic Index (IPI)—A system for predicting the prognosis of lymphoma patients on the basis of five factors.

Intrathecal chemotherapy—A form of treatment in which the drug is injected directly into the patient's spinal fluid. It is given to prevent a lymphoma from spreading to the brain and spinal cord, or to treat one that has already spread.

Lymphatic system—The system of glands, tissues, and vessels in the body that produces lymphocytes and circulates them through the body in a clear, yellowish fluid called lymph.

Lymphocyte—A type of white blood cell involved in the production of antibodies.

Monoclonal antibody—An antibody produced in the laboratory from a cloned cell rather than in the body.

Non-Hodgkin's lymphoma (NHL)—One of two major subdivisions of lymphomas. Burkitt's lymphoma is a subcategory of NHL.

Oncogene—A gene that causes the uncontrolled cell growth characteristic of cancer.

Sporadic—Occurring in isolated or scattered instances. Burkitt's lymphoma is a sporadic disease in most countries.

Translocation—The movement of a gene or group of genes from one chromosome to another. Burkitt's lymphoma is associated with a genetic translocation.

is one of the most rapidly growing forms of human **cancer**. In addition, the number of new cases of this tumor is rising in most countries.

Description

Burkitt's lymphoma was first described in 1957 by Denis Parsons Burkitt, an Irish surgeon. While this type of lymphoma is still relatively rare in the United States, it is responsible for 50% of cancer deaths in children in Uganda and central Africa. The endemic form of Burkitt's lymphoma is characterized by rapid enlargement of the patient's jaw, loosening of the teeth, protruding eyeballs, or an abdominal tumor in the region of the kidneys or ovaries.

In the sporadic form of Burkitt's, the patient may have a facial tumor but is much more likely to have an abdominal swelling, often in the area of the ileocecal valve (the valve between the lower portion of the small intestine and the beginning of the large intestine). About 90% of American children with Burkitt's have abdominal tumors. Others may develop tumors in the testes, ovaries, skin, nasal sinuses, or lymph nodes. In adults, Burkitt's lymphoma frequently produces a bulky abdomen and may involve the liver, spleen, and bone marrow.

Demographics

In Western countries, Burkitt's lymphoma is more common in male than in female children. While the average age of patients with endemic Burkitt's is seven years, outside Africa the average age is closer to 11 years. In the United States, the non-Hodgkin's lymphomas as a group account for about 7% of cancers in persons under 20 years of age. Between 40% and 50% of these cases are Burkitt's lymphoma.

In adults, Burkitt's lymphoma is again more common in males than in females. It is 1,000 times more common in persons with AIDS than in the general population. Currently, about 2% of AIDS patients develop Burkitt's lymphoma. The majority of these patients have stage IV disease by the time the tumor is diagnosed.

Causes and symptoms

Causes

ONCOGENES. Burkitt's lymphoma affects a part of the immune system known as the lymphatic or lymphoid system. The lymphatic system is a network of tissues, glands, and channels that produces lymphocytes, a type of white blood cell. Some lymphocytes remain in clusters within the lymph nodes, while others circulate throughout the body in the bloodstream or in the lymph, which is a clear yellowish fluid carried by the lymphatic channels. Lymphocytes fall into two groups: T cells, which regulate the immune system; and B cells, which produce antibodies. Burkitt's lymphoma involves the B-cell lymphocytes. In 1982, researchers discovered an oncogene (a gene that can release cells from growth constraints, possibly converting them into tumors) in 90% of patients with Burkitt's lymphoma. Called the C-*myc* oncogene, it is responsible for the uncontrolled production of B-lymphocytes. It results from a translocation, or exchange, of genetic material between the long arm of human chromosome 8 and the long arm of human chromosome 14. In a smaller number of patients with Burkitt's, the translocation involves chromosomes 2 and 22 or chromosomes 2 and 8.

In the summer of 2000, researchers reported that a gene called the HMG-I/Y gene is also involved in the development of Burkitt's lymphoma. The C-*myc* oncogene appears to stimulate the HMG-I/Y gene, which then triggers the changes in normal B cells that cause them to multiply rapidly and form tumors.

VIRUSES. In addition to translocations of genetic material, Burkitt's lymphoma is also associated with oncogenic viruses—the **Epstein-Barr virus** (EBV) in endemic Burkitt's and human immunodeficiency virus (HIV) in the sporadic form. EBV, or human herpesvirus 4, is the virus that causes infectious mononucleosis. The presence of EBV in patients with endemic Burkitt's has been interpreted as a side effect of the high rates of malaria in central Africa. African children may have immune systems that cannot fight off **infection** with EBV because they have been weakened by malaria. The children's B-lymphocytes then reproduce at an unusually high rate. Currently, however, the precise role of EBV in Burkitt's lymphoma is still being investigated, because the virus is less common in patients

outside Africa. In the United States, about 25% of children and 40% of adult AIDS patients with Burkitt's have the Epstein-Barr virus.

Symptoms

In children, symptoms may appear as soon as four to six weeks after the lymphoma begins to grow. The more common symptom pattern is a large tumor in the child's abdomen accompanied by fluid buildup, pain, and **vomiting**. If the lymphoma begins in the blood marrow, the child may bleed easily and become anemic.

In adults, the first symptoms of Burkitt's lymphoma may include swelling in a lymph node in the upper body or a swollen and painful abdomen. If the tumor is located in the chest, it may put pressure on the airway and cause difficulty in breathing. There may be unexplained **itching** or **weight loss**. Other patients may have more general symptoms, such as **fever** or a loss of energy. Adults with AIDS often have tumors developing in several different locations in the body by the time they are diagnosed.

Diagnosis

Burkitt's lymphoma is usually diagnosed by examining a piece of tissue from a surgical **biopsy** of a swollen area in the patient's body—often the jaw area in endemic Burkitt's or the abdomen in the sporadic form. The tissue is examined under a microscope by a pathologist, who is a physician with special training in the study of tissue or body fluid samples. In Burkitt's lymphoma, the tumor cells will show a very high rate of cell division and a characteristic "starry sky" pattern. The pathologist may also test the tissue sample for the presence of EBV, which is found in about 30% of patients diagnosed with Burkitt's lymphoma in the United States.

In addition to a tissue biopsy, the patient is also given a complete blood count (CBC) test, a platelet count, and a **lumbar puncture** (spinal tap). A small sample of bone marrow is usually taken as well. Most cases of Burkitt's lymphoma do not require extensive **x rays**, although CT (**computed tomography**) scans of the chest and abdomen are usually taken, as well as a **gallium scan**. This scan involves being injected with the radioactive isotope gallium, which is attracted to cancerous cells. Thus, when technicians scan images the body, they are able to pinpoint those cells.

Treatment team

Because cancer in children and adolescents is rare, young people with cancer should be referred to pediatric cancer centers with multidisciplinary teams that specialize in treating cancers in this age group. The specialty teams usually include primary care doctors, pediatric oncologists (pediatricians who specialize in the treatment of **childhood cancers**), radiation oncologists, social workers, pediatric nurses, and rehabilitation specialists.

Adult AIDS patients who develop Burkitt's lymphoma require specialists in treating HIV infection on their treatment team as well as oncologists, radiologists, and nursing specialists.

Clinical staging, treatments, and prognosis

Staging

The most common system of staging for non-Hodgkin's lymphomas in adults, including Burkitt's lymphoma, is the Ann Arbor system. It specifies four stages as follows:

- Stage I: The lymphoma is either limited to one group of lymph nodes either above or below the diaphragm, or is in an organ or part of the body other than the lymph nodes, but has not spread to other organs or lymph nodes.
- Stage II: The lymphoma is either in two or more lymph node groups on the same side of the diaphragm, or is in only one organ or site other than the lymph nodes but has spread to the lymph nodes near that organ or site.
- Stage III: The lymphoma is present in groups of lymph nodes on both sides of the diaphragm. It may involve an organ or site outside the lymph nodes, the spleen, or both.
- Stage IV: The lymphoma is disseminated (spread) throughout one or more organs outside the lymph nodes. There may or may not be involvement of lymph nodes that are remote from the affected organs.

At each stage, the patient's condition may be described in more detail by using letters to denote the presence of specific general symptoms and/or the body organs that have been affected by the disease. A is used to designate patients who do not have general symptoms; B is used for patients with any of the following:

- unexplained loss of more than 10% of body weight in the last six months
- unexplained fever higher than 38 degrees C (101 degrees F)
- drenching night sweats

The letter E is added if the patient has developed malignancies outside the lymph nodes in areas of the body other than the lymphatic system. Other sites in the body are identified with additional letters, such as D for the skin or H for the liver.

The most commonly used staging system for NHL in children is that of the St. Jude's Children's Research Hospital. It separates patients with a single tumor or diseased lymph node (Stage I) or two or more tumors or diseased lymph nodes on the same side of the diaphragm (Stage II) from those with a large chest or abdominal tumor (Stage III) or involvement of the bone marrow and central nervous system (Stage IV).

Treatment

Because of the rapid rate of tumor growth in this lymphoma, it is important to begin treatment as soon as possible after diagnosis. Bulky abdominal tumors or chest tumors are sometimes removed surgically before the patient begins **chemotherapy**.

Children with Burkitt's lymphoma are treated with chemotherapy and **radiation therapy**. The drug used most often to treat endemic Burkitt's is **cyclophosphamide** (Cytoxan), a drug that suppresses the immune system but has severe side effects. It may be given orally or intravenously. Radiation therapy is used to treat lymphomas that affect the jaw and the area around the eyes. Children with sporadic Burkitt's are treated with a short course of high-dose chemotherapy, usually cyclophosphamide in combination with **methotrexate** (MTX), **vincristine** (Oncovin), prednisone (Meticorten), and **doxorubicin** (Adriamycin). To prevent the spread of the lymphoma to the central nervous system, the patient's head and spine may be treated with radiation therapy and intrathecal methotrexate. In **intrathecal chemotherapy**, the drug is injected directly into the patient's spinal fluid.

Adults with sporadic Burkitt's lymphoma are treated with a combination of radiation therapy and chemotherapy. A newer high-dose chemotherapy regimen called CODOX-M/IVAC, which is a combination of cyclophosphamide, vincristine, doxorubicin, methotrexate, **ifosfamide** (Ifex), **etoposide** (VePesid), and **cytarabine** (ARA-C), appears to produce good results. Adults with AIDS are usually given low-dose chemotherapy because their immune systems are already damaged. They do not respond as well to treatment as patients without HIV infection.

Newer methods of treatment include bone marrow or stem cell transplantation and **monoclonal antibodies** (antibodies produced by cloned mouse cells grown in a laboratory). One monoclonal antibody, **rituximab** (Rituxan), has been approved by the FDA for treatment of non-Hodgkin's lymphomas, including Burkitt's lymphoma. **Clinical trials** in France indicate that rituximab combined with standard chemotherapy improves the rates of remission and survival in high-risk patients.

Prognosis

The prognosis for children with Burkitt's lymphoma is generally good, as this type of lymphoma responds well to chemotherapy. Children with African Burkitt's often show a significant improvement after only one dose of cyclophosphamide. In the United States, 80% of children treated for early-stage Burkitt's lymphoma remain free from relapse three years after treatment. The newer CODOX-M/IVAC combination chemotherapy has been credited with a cure rate above 90% in both children and adults.

The prognosis for adults depends on a number of factors. In recent years, the International Prognostic Index, or IPI, has been used to predict a specific patient's chance of recurrence and length of survival on the basis of five factors. Each of the following factors is given one point:

- age over 60 years
- the lymphoma is classified as Stage III or Stage IV
- the lymphoma has spread to more than one site outside the lymph nodes
- high levels of lactate dehydrogenase (an enzyme used to measure tumor burden)
- poor general health

An IPI score of 0 or 1 is associated with a 70% rate of disease-free survival at the end of five years and an overall survival rate of 73% at the end of five years. An IPI score of 5, on the other hand, is associated with five-year rates of 40% disease-free survival and 26% overall survival respectively.

In patients with AIDS, the factors that affect the prognosis include: the CD4 lymphocyte count; the presence of opportunistic infections (AIDS-defining illnesses); involvement of the bone marrow; spread of the lymphoma beyond the lymph nodes; age; and the patient's overall strength. A history of opportunistic infections, a CD4 count below 200, age above 35, and being too weak to walk indicate a poor prognosis. The average length of survival of HIV-positive patients with Burkitt's lymphoma is six months.

Alternative and complementary therapies

Alternative and complementary treatments that have been reported as helpful to lymphoma patients include yoga, therapeutic massage, meditation, creative visualization, acupuncture, Reiki, journaling, and art therapy.

Coping with cancer treatment

Adults being treated for Burkitt's lymphoma are most likely to be affected by the side effects of chemotherapy (**nausea**, hair loss, etc.). Patients with AIDS have the additional concern of increased vulnerability to other AIDS-related infections (**thrush**, **pneumonia**, etc.).

Children

Children being treated for Burkitt's lymphoma share many of the concerns of children with other types of cancer, such as changes in appearance (hair loss caused by chemotherapy), continuing a normal schedule (school, sports participation), and coping with such other side effects of treatment as nausea or **fatigue**. One useful resource is the Candlelighters programs, which offer support and practical information to the parents of children with cancer.

Clinical trials

As of 2001, 39 clinical trials of treatments for AIDS-related lymphomas in adults were being conducted at research centers in the United States. Because Burkitt's lymphoma is relatively rare in children, the National Cancer Institute (NCI) requests that all children with Burkitt's (or other non-Hodgkin's lymphomas) be considered as possible subjects for clinical trials. Information about current clinical trials is available at (800) 4-CANCER or http://www.cancernet.nci.nih.gov/trialsrch.

Prevention

Prevention of the endemic form of Burkitt's lymphoma is complicated by the high incidence of malaria in central Africa combined with inadequate medical care. In other countries, some risk factors associated with the sporadic form can be lowered, most particularly lifestyle behaviors that increase the risk of HIV infection. In addition, patients with Burkitt's lymphoma may want to consider genetic counseling because of the role of the C-*myc* oncogene in their disorder.

Special concerns

Patients diagnosed with Burkitt's lymphoma should be followed up at regular intervals after chemotherapy because of the possibility of long-term relapse. Follow-up examinations should include a general physical examination, a complete blood count, and radiologic examinations.

See also AIDS-related cancers; Alopecia; Chromosome rearrangements; Nausea and vomiting.

Resources

BOOKS

Beers, Mark H., MD, and Robert Berkow, MD, editors. "Hematology and Oncology." In *The Merck Manual of Diagnosis and Therapy*. Whitehouse Station, NJ: Merck Research Laboratories, 2007.

OTHER

Lymphoma Information Network. [cited June 27, 2001]. http://www.lymphomainfo.net.

Oncology Channel. [cited June 21, 2001]. http://www.oncologychannel.com.

ORGANIZATIONS

American Cancer Society (ACS). 1599 Clifton Road, NE, Atlanta, GA 30329. (404) 320-3333 or (800) ACS-2345. Fax: (404) 329-7530. http://www.cancer.org.

Candlelighters Childhood Cancer Foundation. 7910 Woodmont Avenue, Suite 460, Bethesda, MD 20814. (301) 657-8401 or (800) 366-CCCF.

National Cancer Institute, Office of Cancer Communications. 31 Center Drive, MSC 2580, Bethesda, MD 20892-2580. (800) 4-CANCER. TTY: (800) 332-8615. http://www.nci.nih.gov.

NIH National Center for Complementary and Alternative Medicine (NCCAM) Clearinghouse. P.O. Box 8218, Silver Spring, MD 20907-8218. TTY/TDY: (888) 644-6226. Fax: (301) 495-4957.

Rebecca J. Frey, Ph.D.

Buserelin

Definition

Buserelin is a synthetic analog of natural gonadotropin-releasing hormone and is used to treat **prostate cancer**. Buserelin, also called buserelin acetate, is sold under the brand name Suprefact in Canada. It is not commercially available in the U.S. for human use.

Purpose

Androgens, particularly **testosterone**, appear to play a major role in prostate **cancer**. Buserelin inhibits production of luteinizing hormone from the pituitary gland which decreases the levels of testosterone. Prostate cancer is often sensitive to testosterone levels, thus, a reduction in testosterone may influence the rate of cancer growth progression and affect the size of the tumor. Hormone therapy with buserelin cannot cure prostate cancer but may decrease symptoms and improve the quality of life for most patients.

Breast cancer may also treated with buserelin. A research study examined combined treatment with buserelin and **tamoxifen** in women with premenopausal metastatic breast cancer. Together, these drugs were more effective and resulted in longer overall survival than treatment with either drug alone.

Description

Buserelin indirectly decreases the testosterone levels in the body. Testosterone is produced in the testes and the adrenal glands, but the testes will only produce testosterone if adequate levels of luteinizing hormone are present. Buserelin reduces the production of luteinizing hormone, thus causing a drop in testosterone levels. When buserelin administration is started, a brief increase in the hormone levels in the first few days or weeks may occur.

Recommended dosage

Two dosage forms of buserelin are available. Either as an injection (1 mg/mL multidose vial) or as an intranasal spray (100 mcg/spray).

A dose of 500 mcg (0.5 milligrams [mg]) is injected under the skin three times per day for seven days every eight hours. The doctor may lower the dose to 200 micrograms (mcg) or 0.2 mg once a day with time if required. Treatment with the nasal spray form of the drug is administered at 200 mcg, (2 sprays) into each nostril every eight hours. The doctor determines the duration of treatment.

Precautions

Buserelin induces a temporary rise in sex hormones at the start of treatment, but they usually remain within the normal range. This rise may be associated with an increase in disease symptoms in some patients. Symptoms such as **bone pain**, impaired urination, and muscular weakness in the legs may occur with the temporary increase in tumor activity. These symptoms usually ease gradually, although they can be avoided altogether by prescribing an antiandrogen such as cyproterone acetate or flutamide at the same time.

Due to these effects, it is advisable for patients to also take an antiandrogen with buserelin if a temporary increase in the size of the tumor may lead to: urinal tract obstruction, increased intracranial pressure (in rare cases with brain metastases), or paresis (slight or incomplete paralysis) due to increased pressure on the spinal cord. Antiandrogen treatment should be started about five days before buserelin and for three to four weeks along with buserelin therapy until the sex hormones have returned to an acceptable level.

Buserelin causes sterility in men and menopause in women which may be permanent. It is not known if buserelin is safe to use during pregnancy. Due to the secretion into breast milk, breast-feeding is not recommended. In addition, it is not known if buserelin is mutagenic or carcinogenic.

Alert doctors or dentists about buserelin therapy before receiving any treatment.

Side effects

Many people have very few side effects with buserelin, while others may experience more.

The most common side effects are:

- Nasal irritation.
- Skin reaction at the injection site. The injection may be slightly uncomfortable, and redness might occur at the injection site following administration.
- Hot flushes.
- Headache (when administered through the nasal passage).
- Burning, swelling, and/or itching at place of injection.
- Loss of libido and impotence during treatment.

- Breast tenderness or fullness. Slight breast swelling and tenderness may occur. This side effect can be reduced with medication.
- Weight gain.
- Fatigue.
- Depressive moods.
- Feelings of sickness and diarrhea. They are usually mild and controlled easily.
- Dry nose (when administered through the nasal passage).
- Tumor flare. Because buserelin may temporarily increase testosterone levels for the first few days or weeks of treatment, an increase in symptoms may be experienced. Serious disease flare reactions may occur such as an increase in bone pain, spinal cord compression, or urinary tract obstruction.
- Thrombosis with pulmonary embolism.
- Calcium loss in the skeleton (women).

Interactions

There are no known interactions between buserelin and any other medication reported to date.

Crystal Heather Kaczkowski, M.S.

Busulfan

Definition

Busulfan (also known by the brand name Myleran) is a **chemotherapy** medicine used to treat **cancer** by destroying cancerous cells.

Purpose

Busulfan is approved by the Food and Drug Administration (FDA) to treat chronic myelogenous leukemia (also called **chronic myelocytic leukemia**). It has also been less commonly used for other **acute leukemias** and a blood disease known as polycythemia vera, in which there are too many red blood cells. Busulfan is also used in combination with other chemotherapy drugs for a procedure known as **bone marrow transplantation**.

Description

Busulfan a member of the group of chemotherapy drugs known as alkylating agents. Alkylating agents interfere with the genetic material (DNA) inside the cancer cells and prevent them from further dividing and producing more cancer cells. Busulfan is taken orally and comes in tablet form.

Recommended dosage

Busulfan can be taken following several different dosing schedules, depending on the disease. Busulfan is a 2 mg oral tablet, and patients may need to take more than one tablet at a time depending on the dose. The induction or starting dose is 4 mg up to 12 mg per day. This may then be decreased to 1–3 mg per day as a maintenance dose. The dose of busulfan for use in combination with other chemotherapy drugs before a bone marrow transplant is much larger than leukemia dosing. Busulfan, when used for bone marrow transplants, is dosed by patient body weight. Busulfan is usually given at a dose of 4 mg per kilogram of body weight each day for 4 days before a bone marrow transplant.

Precautions

Blood counts are monitored regularly while on busulfan therapy. During a certain period of time after receiving busulfan, there is an increased risk of contracting infections. Caution should be taken to avoid unnecessary exposure to bacteria and viruses. All patients should increase their daily fluid intake while receiving this drug.

Patients who are pregnant or are trying to become pregnant should notify their physician before taking busulfan (or any chemotherapy medication). Busulfan causes a high incidence of sterility in males, and has been known to cause sterility in females as well.

Patients with a known previous allergic reaction to chemotherapy drugs, or who suffer from gout, thalassemia, or seizure problems, should notify their physician before beginning treatment. The physician should also be consulted before receiving live virus **vaccines** while on chemotherapy.

Side effects

The most common side effect expected from taking busulfan is low blood counts, referred to as **myelosuppression**. Lowering of the white count, or **neutropenia**, is common and lasts for some time before the white count returns to normal levels. When the white blood cell count is low, patients are at an increased risk of developing a **fever** and infections. The platelet blood count can also be decreased due to busulfan administration. Platelets are blood cells in the body that cause clots to form; the purpose of these clots is to control bleeding. When the platelet count is low, patients are at an increased risk for both bruising and bleeding. If the platelet count remains too low, a platelet blood transfusion may be an option for treatment. Busulfan also causes low red blood cell counts, or **anemia**. Low red counts make patients feel tired, dizzy, and fatigued. **Erythropoietin** is a drug that can be used to increase red blood cell count.

In bone marrow transplant patients, the dose of busulfan that is given in combination with other chemotherapy drugs is intended to cause complete bone marrow destruction prior to bone marrow transplant.

Nausea, **vomiting**, loss of appetite, mouth sores, and **diarrhea** are rare side effects from busulfan at normal doses, but are common at the higher doses used for bone marrow transplant. If **nausea and vomiting** are a problem, patients can be given medications known as **antiemetics** before receiving busulfan to help prevent or decrease these side effects. Taking busulfan on an empty stomach may also decrease nausea and vomiting.

Damage to nerves and nervous system tissues is uncommon with standard busulfan therapy. However, at high doses, some reports do exist of seizures, dizziness, confusion, and visual disturbances.

Busulfan can also cause severe lung problems known as "busulfan lung". Symptoms include a non-stop cough, shortness of breath, fever, and difficulty breathing.

Less common side effects caused by busulfan include skin rashes or reactions (including darkening of the skin), dryness of the skin, **itching**, and hair loss (**alopecia**).

Although it is uncommon, severe liver problems may occur due to busulfan administration at higher doses. Rare reactions to busulfan include: lung problems, cataracts, **fatigue**, heart problems, low blood pressure, development of another type of cancer or leukemia, enlarged breast tissue (referred to as gynecomastia), and increased uric acid levels (which can lead to kidney problems and gout).

Any side effects experienced by a patient should be reported to his or her physician.

Interactions

Busulfan used for transplant purposes, when given in high doses with the chemotherapy drug **cyclophosphamide**, caused an increase in serious heart problems.

Patients who have taken busulfan with the drug **thioguanine** over long periods of time have shown an increase in enlarged veins in the esophagus and liver problems.

Nancy J. Beaulieu, RPh.,BCOP

C

Calcitonin

Definition

Calcitonin is a hormone involved in regulating calcium metabolism. The hormone calcitonin is produced by the thyroid gland. A synthetic human product, sold as Calcimar or Miacalcin, is available in the United States. A third brand called Fortical applied for U.S. Food and Drug Administration (FDA) approval in 2003 for marketing in the United States.

Purpose

Calcitonin is often ordered for **cancer** patients experiencing **bone pain** due to **metastasis**. Calcitonin is also used to treat Paget's disease, post-menopausal osteoporosis, and increased levels of calcium in the blood.

Description

Calcitonin reduces breakdown of bone. It causes less bone tissue to be reabsorbed. It slows the rate of bone destruction and decreases the amount of calcium released into the blood. Most calcitonin ordered for patients is derived from salmon. Calcitonin is not effective when given orally, and is available for injection or in a nasal spray.

Recommended dosage

The usual dose for patients receiving calcitonin-salmon for bone metastases is 200 IU given through the vein twice daily. It is important to take this drug exactly as ordered. If a dose is missed and is noticed within two hours, the drug should be taken. If it is not noted until later, the patient should skip the dose and return to the regular schedule. Patients should not take additional or double doses. When using calcitonin to lower calcium levels, therapy is limited to approximately five days. Extended use of calcitonin results in a loss of calcium-lowering effect.

Precautions

Calcitonin-salmon solution should be stored in the refrigerator, not frozen. Patients should allow a new bottle of nasal spray to warm to room temperature. It may be kept at room temperature for two to four weeks. The nasal spray pump should be primed before using. Patients should push the plunger until a mist is observed, usually within several pushes. Before using, the patient should blow his or her nose. The patient should alternate nostrils with each dose. The head should be kept upright. The pump should be pressed toward the bottle one time. The patient should not inhale when spraying. The patient should then inhale through the nose and exhale through the mouth. The nosepiece should be wiped clean after each use. Patients giving themselves an injection should check that the contents are clear. Patients should not inject medication that is colored or grainy.

Calcitonin should be used cautiously when breast feeding, as it may decrease the amount of available milk. Its use during pregnancy has not been adequately studied. However, animal studies indicated a risk for low birth weight offspring.

Side effects

Calcitonin is a protein. It may cause a severe allergic reaction. The doctor should be notified if a rash or hives develop. Patients should have supplies on hand to manage an allergic reaction. Skin testing may be done prior to treatment. Allergic reactions are rarer in the human product than in the salmon product.

Diarrhea, red skin, poor appetite, **nausea, vomiting**, stomach pain, and back and joint pain are common side effects. Other side effects include increased or decreased appetite, gas, constipation, or an unusual taste in the mouth. Nausea is usually mild and

Cancer

temporary. Giving calcitonin at bedtime may decrease **nausea and vomiting**. Patients may experience dizziness, difficulty sleeping, anxiety, headache, agitation, palpitations, or other heart problems. Redness, swelling, and soreness may occur at the injection site. Patients using the nasal spray may develop crusting or patches in the nose, as well as nasal dryness, redness, swelling, or irritation. Less often, those using the nasal spray may experience difficulty with urination, breathing problems, loss of smell, or cold symptoms. Some patients injecting the drug may develop frequent urination, chills, dizziness, headache, chest pressure, a congested nose, tingling or discomfort in the hands and feet, difficulty breathing, or weakness. Patients should notify the doctor if side effects occur. Side effects may subside as the patient's body becomes accustomed to the drug. Patients should receive regular medical checks and lab work to assess for adverse reactions and changes in urine content.

Interactions

At present, there are no known interactions with other drugs.

Resources

PERIODICALS

Boersig, Charles. "Nasal Calcitonin in Greece." *Med Ad News* November 2003: 14.

Debra Wood, R.N.
Teresa G. Odle

Cancer

Definition

Cancer is not just one disease, but a large group of over 100 diseases. Its two main characteristics are uncontrolled growth of the cells in the human body and the ability of these cells to migrate from the original site and spread to distant sites. If the spread is not controlled, cancer can result in death.

Demographics

About 1.5 million Americans are diagnosed with cancer annually. One out of every four deaths in the United States is from cancer. More than 562,000 people in the United States are anticipated to die of cancer in 2009. This equates to more than 1,500 deaths from cancer per day. Overall, cancer death rates for both men and women have decreased since 2004. However, cancer ranks as the number one cause of death in persons under the age of 85 and ranks second only to heart disease as a cause of death overall in the United States.

Since the occurrence of cancer increases as individuals age, most of the cases are seen in adults, middle-aged or older. Seventy-seven percent of all cancers are diagnosed in people who are older than 55 years of age. The probability of an American male developing an invasive cancer or dying from cancer in his lifetime is one in two; for American females the probability is one in three. The most common cancers are **skin cancer**, lung cancer, **colon cancer**, **breast cancer** (in women), and **prostate cancer** (in men). In addition, cancer of the kidneys, ovaries, uterus, pancreas, bladder, rectum, and blood and lymph node cancer (leukemias and lymphomas) are also included among the 12 major cancers that affect most Americans.

Although most cancer occurs in adults, in the United States cancer is still responsible for more deaths in children under age 20 than any other disease. Each year, about 12,500 new cases of cancer are diagnosed in children compared to 1.5 million new cases annually in adults. About 2,300 children die of cancer in the U.S. each year. In general, children respond better to cancer treatment than adults do. Advances in treatment have resulted in better outcomes and increased long-term survival rates for children. Eighty percent of children newly diagnosed with cancer now live at least five years, compared to about 60% in the mid-1970s. However, the incidence of cancer in children, especially **acute lymphocytic leukemia** and brain cancer, has increased steadily for the past 30 years.

Description

Cancer, by definition, is a disease of the genes. A gene is a small part of DNA, which is the master molecule of the cell. Genes make proteins, which are the ultimate workhorses of the cells. These protein allow the body to carry out the many processes that permits an individual to function, breathe, think, and move.

Throughout people's lives, the cells in their bodies are growing, dividing, and replacing themselves. Many genes produce proteins that are involved in controlling the processes of cell growth and division. An alteration (mutation) to the DNA molecule can disrupt the genes and produce faulty proteins. This causes the cell to become abnormal and lose its restraints on growth. The abnormal cell begins to divide uncontrollably and eventually forms a new growth known as a tumor or neoplasm (medical term for cancer meaning "new growth").

In a healthy individual, the immune system can recognize the neoplastic cells and destroy them before they get a chance to divide. However, some mutant cells may escape immune detection and survive to become tumors or cancers.

Tumors are of two types, benign or malignant. A benign tumor is not considered cancer. It is typically slow-growing, does not spread or invade surrounding tissue, and once it is removed, does not usually recur. A malignant tumor, by contrast, is cancer. It invades surrounding tissue and spreads to other parts of the body. If the cancer cells have spread to the surrounding tissues, even after the malignant tumor is removed, it generally recurs.

A majority of cancers are caused by changes in the cell's DNA because of damage to the environment. Environmental factors that are responsible for causing the initial mutation in the DNA are called carcinogens, of which there are many types.

Some cancers have a genetic or inherited basis. In other words, individuals can inherit faulty DNA from a parent, which could predispose the person to getting cancer. While there is scientific evidence that both factors (environmental and genetic) play a role, less than 10% of all cancers are strictly linked to hereditary factors. Cancers that are known to have a hereditary link are breast cancer, colon cancer, **ovarian cancer**, and uterine cancer. Besides genes, certain physiological traits could also be inherited and contribute to cancers. For example, inheriting fair skin makes a person more likely to develop skin cancer, but only if that person has prolonged exposure to intensive sunlight.

There are several different types of cancers:

- Carcinomas are cancers that arise in the epithelium (the layer of cells covering the body's surface and lining the internal organs and various glands). Ninety percent of human cancers fall into this category. Carcinomas can be subdivided into two types: adenocarcinomas (those that develop in an organ or a gland) and squamous cell carcinomas (those that originate in the skin).

- Melanomas also originate in the skin, usually in the pigment cells (melanocytes).
- Sarcomas are cancers of the supporting tissues of the body, such as bone, muscle, and blood vessels.
- Cancers of the blood and lymph glands are called leukemias and lymphomas, respectively.
- Gliomas are cancers of the nerve tissue.

Risk factors

The major risk factors for cancer are related to: tobacco and alcohol use, dietary factors, sexual and reproductive behavior, exposure to infectious agents, family history, occupation, and environmental factors including pollution.

Causes and symptoms

According to estimates of the American Cancer Society (ACS), approximately 40% of cancer deaths in 2009 were anticipated to be due to tobacco and excessive alcohol use. An additional one-third of the deaths were expected to be related to being overweight, being obese, lacking physical activity, and having poor nutrition. Many of the one million skin cancers diagnosed in 2009 were believed to be a direct result of over-exposure to ultraviolet light from the sun's rays.

Tobacco

Eighty to ninety percent of lung cancer cases occur in smokers. Smoking has also been shown to be a contributory factor in cancers of the upper respiratory tract, esophagus, larynx, bladder, pancreas, and probably liver, stomach, breast, and kidney as well. In the 2000s, scientists also confirmed that secondhand smoke (or passive smoking) can increase one's risk of developing cancer.

Alcohol

Excessive consumption of alcohol is a risk factor in certain cancers, such as **liver cancer**. Alcohol, in combination with tobacco, significantly increases the chances that an individual will develop mouth, pharynx, larynx, and esophageal cancers.

Diet

Thirty-five percent of all cancers are due to dietary causes. Excessive intake of fat leading to obesity has been associated with cancers of the breast, colon, rectum, pancreas, prostate, gall bladder, ovaries, and uterus.

Sexual and reproductive behavior

The human papillomavirus (HPV), which is sexually transmitted, has been shown to cause cancer of the cervix. Having multiple sexual partners and becoming sexually active at an early age have been shown to increase one's chances of contracting HPV. In addition, it has also been shown that women who do not have children or have children later in life have an increased risk for both ovarian and breast cancer.

Infectious agents

Between 1985 and 2005, scientists obtained evidence to show that approximately 15% of the world's cancer deaths can be traced to viruses, bacteria, or parasites.

Family history

Certain cancers such as breast, colon, ovarian, and uterine cancer recur generation after generation in some families. A few cancers, such as the eye cancer **retinoblastoma**, a type of colon cancer, and a type of breast cancer known as early-onset breast cancer, have been shown to be linked to certain genes that can be tracked within a family. It is, therefore, possible that inheriting particular genes makes a person susceptible to certain cancers.

Occupational hazards

There is evidence to show that certain occupational hazards account for 4% of all cancer deaths. For example, asbestos workers have an increased incidence of lung cancer. Similarly, a higher likelihood of getting **bladder cancer** is associated with dye, rubber, and gas workers; skin and lung cancer with smelters, gold miners, and arsenic workers; leukemia with glue and varnish workers; liver cancer with PVC manufacturers; and lung, bone, and bone marrow cancer with radiologists and uranium miners.

Environment

Radiation is believed to cause 1 to 2% of all cancer deaths. Ultraviolet radiation from the sun accounts for a majority of **melanoma** deaths. Other sources of radiation are **x rays**, radon gas, and ionizing radiation from nuclear material.

Pollution

Several studies have shown a link between asbestos and cancer. Chlorination of water may account for a small rise in cancer risk. However, the main danger from pollution occurs when dangerous chemicals from industries escape into the surrounding environment. It has been estimated that 1% of cancer deaths are due to air, land, and water pollution.

Symptoms

Cancer is a progressive disease and goes through several stages. Each stage may produce a number of symptoms. Some symptoms are produced early and may occur due to a tumor that is growing within an organ or a gland. As the tumor grows, it may press on the nearby nerves, organs, and blood vessels. This causes pain and some pressure, which may be the earliest warning signs of cancer.

Despite the fact that there are over 100 different types of cancers, producing very different symptoms, the American Cancer Society (ACS) has established the following seven symptoms as possible warning signals of cancer:

- changes in the size, color, or shape of a wart or a mole
- a sore that does not heal
- persistent cough, hoarseness, or sore throat
- a lump or thickening in the breast or elsewhere
- unusual bleeding or discharge
- chronic indigestion or difficulty in swallowing
- any change in bowel or bladder habits

Many other diseases besides cancer can produce the same symptoms. However, it is important to have these symptoms checked, as soon as possible, especially if they linger. The earlier a cancer is diagnosed and treated, the better the chance of a cure. Many cancers such as breast cancer may not have any early symptoms. Therefore, it is important to undergo routine screening tests such as breast self-exams and mammograms.

Diagnosis

Examination

Diagnosis of many cancers begins with a thorough physical examination and a complete medical history. The doctor will observe, feel, and palpate (apply pressure by touch) different parts of the body in order to identify any variations from the normal size, feel, and texture of the organ or tissue.

As part of the physical exam, the doctor will inspect the patient's mouth. By focusing a light into the mouth, the physician will look for abnormalities in color, moisture, surface texture, or presence of any thickening or sore in the lips, tongue, gums, the hard palate on the roof of the mouth, and the throat. To detect **thyroid cancer**, the doctor will observe the front of the neck for swelling. He may gently manipulate the neck and palpate the front and side surfaces of the thyroid gland (located at the base of the neck) to detect any nodules or tenderness. As part of the physical examination, the doctor will also palpate the lymph nodes in the neck, under the arms, and in the groin. Many illnesses and cancers cause a swelling of the lymph nodes.

The doctor may conduct a thorough examination of the skin to look for sores that have been present for more than three weeks and that bleed, ooze, or crust; irritated patches that may itch or hurt; and any change in the size of a wart or a mole.

Examination of the female pelvis is used to detect cancers of the ovaries, uterus, cervix, and vagina. In the visual examination, the doctor looks for abnormal discharges or the presence of sores. Then, using gloved hands the physician palpates the internal pelvic organs such as the uterus and ovaries to detect any abnormal mass. Breast examination includes visual observation where the doctor looks for any discharge, unevenness, discoloration, or scaling. The doctor palpates both breasts to feel for masses or lumps.

For males, inspection of the testicles, rectum and the prostate is also included in the physical examination. The doctor inserts a gloved finger into the rectum and rotates it slowly to feel for any growths, tumors, or other abnormalities. The doctor also conducts an examination of the testes, in which the doctor observes the genital area and looks for swelling or other abnormalities. The testicles are palpated to identify any lumps, thickening, or differences in the size, weight, and firmness.

Tests

The doctor may order diagnostic tests if an abnormality has been detected on physical examination, or if the patient has some symptom that could be indicative of cancer.

Laboratory studies of sputum (sputum **cytology**), blood, urine, and stool can detect abnormalities that may indicate cancer. Sputum cytology is a test in which the phlegm that is coughed up from the lungs is microscopically examined. It is often used to detect lung cancer. Many blood tests used for cancer detection are typically easy to perform. The blood sample is obtained by a lab technician or a doctor by inserting a needle into a vein and is relatively painless. Blood tests can be either specific or non-specific. Often, in certain cancers, the cancer cells release particular proteins (called **tumor markers**), and blood tests can be used to detect the presence of these tumor markers. However, with a few exceptions, tumor markers are not used for routine screening of cancers, because several non-cancerous conditions also produce positive results. Blood tests are generally more useful in monitoring the effectiveness of the treatment, or in following the course of the disease and detecting recurrent disease.

Imaging tests such as **computed tomography** scans (CT scans), **magnetic resonance imaging** (MRI), ultrasound, and fiberoptic scope examinations help the doctors determine the location of the tumor even if it is deep within the body. Conventional x rays are often used for initial evaluation because they are relatively cheap, painless, and easily accessible. In order to increase the information obtained from a conventional x ray, air or a dye (such as barium or iodine) may be used as a contrast medium to outline or highlight parts of the body.

The most definitive diagnostic test is the **biopsy**, wherein a piece of tissue is surgically removed for microscope examination. Besides confirming a cancer, the biopsy also provides information about the type of cancer, the stage it has reached, the aggressiveness of the cancer, and the extent of its spread. Since a biopsy provides the most accurate analysis, it is considered the gold standard of diagnostic tests.

Screening examinations conducted regularly by healthcare professionals can result in the detection of cancers of the breast, colon, rectum, cervix, prostate, testes, tongue, mouth, and skin at early stages, when treatment is more likely to be successful. Some of the routine screening tests recommended by the ACS are **sigmoidoscopy** (for colorectal cancer), **mammography** (for breast cancer), pap smear (for **cervical cancer**), and the PSA test (for prostate cancer). Self-examinations for cancers of the breast, testes, mouth, and skin can also help in detecting the tumors before the symptoms become serious.

A revolution in molecular biology and **cancer genetics** has contributed a great deal to the development of several tests designed to assess the risk of getting cancers. These new techniques include **genetic testing**, in which molecular probes are used to identify mutations in certain genes that have been linked to particular cancers. As of 2009, however, there remain some limitations to genetic testing and its utility appeared ambiguous, emphasizing the need to develop better strategies for early detection.

Treatment

Treatment and prevention of cancers continued to be the focus of a great deal of research as of 2009. Research into new cancer therapies included cancer-targeting gene therapy, cancer **vaccines**, and other targeted therapies such as **monoclonal antibodies**. Most new therapies take years of clinical testing and research.

The aim of cancer treatment is to remove all or as much of the tumor as possible and to prevent the recurrence or spread of the primary tumor. While devising a treatment plan for cancer, the likelihood of curing the cancer has to be weighed against the side effects of the treatment. If the cancer is very aggressive and a cure is not possible, then the treatment should be aimed at relieving the symptoms and controlling the cancer for as long as possible.

Cancer treatment can take many different forms, and is typically tailored to the individual patient. The decision as to which type of treatment is the most appropriate depends on the type and location of cancer; the extent to which it has already spread; and the patient's age, sex, general health status, and personal treatment preferences. The major types of treatment are: surgery, radiation, **chemotherapy**, biological therapy, targeted therapy, hormone therapy, and bone marrow and stem cell transplantation.

Surgery

Surgery is the removal of a visible tumor and is the most frequently used cancer treatment. It is most effective when a cancer is small and/or confined to one area of the body.

Surgery can be used for many purposes:

- Treatment. Treatment of cancer by surgery involves removal of the tumor to cure the disease. This is typically done when the cancer is localized to a discrete area. Along with the cancer, some part of the normal surrounding tissue is also removed to ensure that no cancer cells remain in the area. Since cancer usually spreads via the lymphatic system, adjoining lymph nodes may be examined and sometimes are removed as well.
- Prevention. Preventive or prophylactic surgery involves removal of an abnormal looking area that is likely to become malignant over time. For example, 40% of people with a colon disease known as ulcerative colitis ultimately die of colon cancer. Rather than live with the fear of developing colon cancer, these people may choose to have the colon removed, which reduces the risk of developing colon cancer significantly.
- Diagnostic purposes. The most definitive tool for diagnosing cancer is a biopsy. Sometimes, a biopsy can be performed by inserting a needle through the skin. However, at other times, the only way to obtain a tissue sample for biopsy is by performing a surgical operation.

Specific types of surgery include:

- Cytoreductive surgery, a procedure in which the doctor removes as much of the cancer as possible and then treats the remaining area with radiation therapy or chemotherapy or both.
- Palliative surgery, which is aimed at minimizing symptoms associated with cancer. Usually, in such cases, the tumor is so large or has spread so much that removing the entire tumor is not an option. For example, a tumor in the abdomen may be so large that it may press on and block a portion of the intestine, interfering with digestion and causing pain and vomiting.
- Debulking surgery, which can be used to remove a part of the blockage and to relieve associated symptoms. In tumors that are dependent on hormones, removal of the organs that secrete the hormones is an option. For example, in prostate cancer, the release of testosterone by the testicles stimulates the growth of cancerous cells. Hence, a man may undergo an orchiectomy (removal of testicles) to slow the progress of the disease. Similarly, in a type of aggressive breast cancer, removal of the ovaries (oophorectomy) stops the synthesis of hormones from the ovaries and may slow the progression of the cancer.

Radiation therapy

Radiation kills tumor cells. Radiation is used alone in cases in which a tumor is unsuitable for surgery. More often, it is used in conjunction with surgery and chemotherapy. Radiation can be either external or internal. In the external form, the radiation is aimed at the tumor from outside the body. In internal radiation (also known as brachytherapy), a radioactive substance in the form of pellets or liquid is placed at the cancerous site by means of a pill, injection, or insertion in a sealed container.

Chemotherapy

Chemotherapy is the use of drugs to kill cancer cells. It destroys the hard-to-detect cancer cells that have spread and are circulating in the body. Chemotherapeutic drugs can be given in many forms. The most common administration methods include oral (by mouth) or intravenous administration. Chemotherapy may be given alone or in conjunction with surgery, radiation, or both.

When chemotherapy is used before surgery or radiation, it is known as primary chemotherapy or neoadjuvant chemotherapy. An advantage of neoadjuvant chemotherapy is that since the cancer cells have not been exposed to anti-cancer drugs, they are especially vulnerable. It can, therefore, be used effectively to reduce the size of the tumor for surgery or target it for radiation. The more common use of chemotherapy is adjuvant therapy, which is given to enhance the effectiveness of other treatments. For example, after surgery, **adjuvant chemotherapy** is given to destroy any cancerous cells that still remain in the body.

Biological and targeted therapies

Biological and targeted therapies use the body's own immune system to destroy cancer cells. As of 2009, this form of treatment was being intensively studied in **clinical trials**. Many newer agents are used to treat a variety of cancers. The various agents being tested in clinical trials and used as treatment modalities included substances produced by the body (such as the **interferons**, interleukins, and growth factors), monoclonal antibodies, and vaccines. Unlike traditional vaccines, cancer vaccines do not prevent cancer. Instead, they are designed to treat people who already have the disease. Cancer vaccines work by boosting the body's immune system and training the immune cells to specifically destroy cancer cells.

Hormone therapy

Hormone therapy is standard treatment for some types of cancers that are hormone-dependent and grow faster in the presence of particular hormones. These include cancer of the prostate, breast, and uterus. Hormone therapy involves blocking the production or action of these hormones. As a result, the growth of the tumor slows, and survival may be extended.

Bone marrow, stem cell, and cord blood transplantation

The bone marrow is the tissue within the bone cavities that contains blood-forming cells. Healthy bone marrow tissue constantly replenishes the blood supply and is essential to life.

A bone marrow transplant is the removal of marrow from one person and the transplant of the blood-forming cells either to the same person or to someone else. Bone marrow transplantation, while not a therapy in itself, is often used to "rescue" patients, by allowing those with cancer to undergo aggressive therapy. Stem cell transplants have been performed to replace bone marrow that has been destroyed by cancer, chemotherapy, or **radiation therapy**. Stem cells are specialized cells in the bone marrow from which the body receives a constant source of blood cells. Stem cells may also be harvested from umbilical

cords, a process which is referred to as cord blood transplant. Some cancers in which stem cell transplants may be used include leukemia, **lymphoma**, and **multiple myeloma**.

Alternative treatment

There are a multitude of alternative treatments available to help the person with cancer. They can be used in conjunction with, or separate from, surgery, chemotherapy, and radiation therapy. Alternative treatment of cancer is a complicated arena and a trained health practitioner should be consulted.

Although the effectiveness of complementary therapies such as acupuncture in alleviating cancer pain has not been clinically proven, many cancer patients find it safe and beneficial. Bodywork therapies such as massage and reflexology ease muscle tension and may alleviate side effects such as **nausea and vomiting**. Homeopathy and herbal remedies used in Chinese traditional herbal medicine also have been shown to alleviate some of the side effects of radiation and chemotherapy and are recommended by many doctors.

Certain foods, including many vegetables, fruits, and grains, are believed to offer protection against various cancers. However, isolation of the individual constituent of vegetables and fruits that are anticancer agents has proven difficult. In laboratory studies, **vitamins** such as A, C, and E, as well as compounds such as isothiocyanates and dithiolthiones found in broccoli, cauliflower, and cabbage, and beta-carotene found in carrots, have been shown to protect against cancer. Studies have shown that eating a diet rich in fiber as found in fruits and vegetables reduces the risk of colon cancer. Exercise and a low-fat diet help control weight and reduce the risk of endometrial, breast, and colon cancer.

Cancer treatment team

Many different specialists generally work together as a team to treat cancer patients. An oncologist is a physician who specializes in cancer care. The oncologist provides chemotherapy, hormone therapy, and any other non-surgical treatment that does not involve radiation. The oncologist often serves as the primary physician and coordinates the patient's treatment plan.

The radiation oncologist specializes in using radiation to treat cancer, whereas the surgical oncologist performs the operations needed to diagnose or treat cancer. Gynecologist-oncologists and pediatric-oncologists, as their titles suggest, are physicians involved with treating women's and children's cancers, respectively. Many other specialists also may be involved in the care of a cancer patient. For example, radiologists specialize in the use of x rays, ultrasounds, CT scans, MRI imaging and other techniques that are used to diagnose cancer. Hematologists specialize in disorders of the blood and are consulted in case of blood cancers and bone marrow cancers. The samples that are removed for biopsy are sent to a laboratory, where a pathologist examines them to determine the type of cancer and extent of the disease. There are many other specialties, and virtually any type of medical or surgical specialist may become involved with care of the cancer patient should it become necessary.

Prognosis

Lifetime risk is the phrase that cancer researchers use to refer to the probability that an individual over the course of a lifetime will develop cancer or die from it. In the United States, men have a one in two lifetime risk of developing cancer, and for women the risk is one in three. Overall, African Americans are more likely to develop cancer than whites. African Americans are also 30% more likely to die of cancer than whites.

Many cancers are curable if detected and treated in their early stages. A cancer patient's prognosis is affected by many factors, particularly the type of cancer the patient has, the stage of the cancer, the extent to which it has metastasized, and the aggressiveness of the cancer. In addition, the patient's age, general health status, and the effectiveness of the treatment being pursued are important factors.

To help predict the future course and outcome of the disease and the likelihood of recovery from the disease, doctors often use statistics. The five-year survival rates are the most common measures used. The number refers to the proportion of people with cancer who are expected to be alive five years after initial diagnosis compared with a similar population that is free of cancer. It is important to note that while statistics can give some information about the average survival experience of cancer patients in a given population, they cannot be used to indicate individual prognosis because no two patients are exactly alike.

Prevention

According to nutritionists and epidemiologists from leading universities in the United States, a person can reduce the chances of getting cancer by following some simple guidelines:

- eating plenty of vegetables and fruits
- exercising vigorously for at least 30 minutes on five or more days every week; 45–60 minutes of moderate to vigorous physical activity is preferable
- avoiding excessive weight gain
- avoiding tobacco (even secondhand smoke)
- decreasing or avoiding consumption of animal fats and red meats
- avoiding excessive amounts of alcohol
- avoiding the midday sun (between 11 a.m. and 3 p.m.) when the sun's rays are the strongest
- avoiding risky sexual practices
- avoiding known carcinogens in the environment or work place

Resources

BOOKS
Bradbury, Robert H., ed. *Cancer.* New York: Springer, 2007.
Geffen, Jeremy R. *The Journey Through Cancer: Healing and Transforming the Whole Person.* New York: Three Rivers Press, 2006.
Visel, Dave. *Living With Cancer: A Practical Guide.* New Brunswick, NJ: Rutgers University Press, 2006.
Weinberg, Robert A. *The Biology of Cancer.* New York: Garland Science, 2007.

PERIODICALS
Jemal, A., Siegel, R., Ward, E., et al. "Cancer Statistics 2009." *CA: A Cancer Journal for Clinicians* 59(2009): 225–249.

OTHER
"Cancer Facts and Figures 2009." http://www.cancer.org/downloads/STT/500809web.pdf. [cited September 20, 2009].

ORGANIZATIONS
American Cancer Society, 250 Williams Street, Atlanta, GA, 30303-1002, (800) ACS-2345, http://www.cancer.org/.
National Cancer Institute, 6116 Executive Blvd., Room 3036A, Bethesda, MD, 20892-8322, (800) 422-6237, http://www.cancer.gov.

National Coalition for Cancer Survivorship, 1010 Wayne Avenue, 5th Floor, Suite 300, Silver Spring, MD, 20910, (888) 650-9127, http://www.canceradvocacy.org/.

Rosalyn Carson-DeWitt, MD
Teresa G. Odle
Melinda Oberleitner, R.N., D.N.S.

Cancer biology

Definition

Cancer is the second leading cause of death in the United States, with one out of every three Americans falling victim to it at some point in their lives. It is a disease of unregulated cell growth. The knowledge gained in cancer biology over the past 20 years has allowed for the discovery of new, highly targeted drugs to treat cancer.

Causes of cancer

The molecular cause of cancer involves mutations in the nuclear DNA (the genetic material in cells) that can be caused by chemicals, viruses, radiation, or spontaneous mutations. Although much importance has been put on chemicals and environmental pollutants as carcinogens (agents that cause cancer), it actually turns out that the predominant factors in determining cancer are associated with lifestyle. For instance, cigarette smoking accounts for 30% of cancers in males. Dietary factors are associated with another 35% of all human cancers. It is estimated that with dietary improvements there could be a 50% reduction in colon and rectal cancers, a 25% reduction in **breast cancer**, and 15% reductions each in prostate, endometrial and gallbladder cancers. Other cancers that might

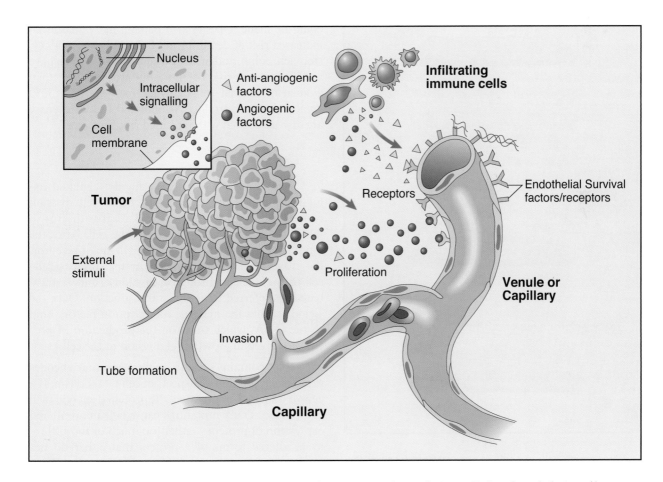

Angiogenesis. To keep up with the demand for blood vessels, the tumor releases factors called angiogenic factors. (An individual tumor cell is shown in the inset.) These factors initiate the growth of more blood vessels into the tumor. The rich supply of blood vessels also gives the tumor more opportunity to metastasize (spread) to distant sites by traveling through the blood. *(Illustration by Argosy Publishing. Cengage Learning, Gale.)*

Factors that help to protect the body from cancer
Genetic resistance
Nutrition
Metabolism
DNA repair
Tumor suppressor genes
Cell differentiation
Death of damaged tissue
Programmed cell death
Immune system

(Table by GGS Creative Resources. Cengage Learning, Gale.)

Factors that favor the progression of cancer
Genetic susceptibility
Age
Mutations
Abnormal cell growth
Aneuploidy (abnormal numbers of chromosomes)
Growth and survival factors
Angiogenesis
Loss of heterozygosity (Having only one version of a gene instead of the usual two different versions)
Gene amplification

(Table by GGS Creative Resources. Cengage Learning, Gale.)

be decreased by dietary improvements include cancer of the stomach, esophagus, pancreas, ovaries, liver, lung, and urinary bladder. This adds up to a 9% reduction in overall deaths. It is estimated that if Americans doubled their intake of fruits and vegetables and fiber and decreased their fat intake by 25%, significant advances could be made. Obesity also puts an individual at an increased risk of death for uterus, gallbladder, kidney, stomach, colon, and breast cancers. Obese women have a 55% greater risk of mortality from cancer than women of normal weight, while men are at a 33% greater risk of mortality. Alcohol and lack of exercise are also associated with increased risk for cancer.

Cell growth

Normal growth of cells is a highly regulated cellular function. The stimulus to begin cell division comes from a growth factors that react with growth factor receptors on the surface of the cell. After the binding of a growth factor to a growth factor receptor, the growth message is carried from the surface of the cell to the nucleus through a cascade of biochemical reactions referred to as signal transduction. Once the signal reaches the nucleus, transcription factors bind to the DNA, which turns on the production of proteins involved in growth and division of the cells.

DNA contains genetic information that encodes proteins involved in all aspects of cell metabolism. If a gene is damaged or mutated, the protein it encodes will be affected. DNA mutations can result in an altered expression of protein—either too much or too little—or in altered forms of a protein that either do not perform their function or perform it differently. Damage to genes that encode for proteins regulating cell growth such as oncogenes, tumor suppressor genes, and DNA repair genes can result in alterations in cell growth and thus cancer.

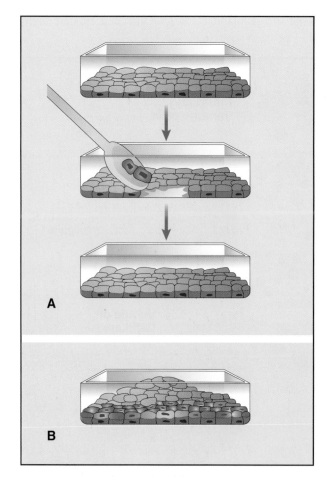

A. When normal cells in a culture plate are scraped away, the cells on the plate divide to replace them. The cells on the plate grow until they touch a neighboring cell and receive a signal to stop growing. B. Cancer cells do not receive this signal and grow on top of each other, forming piles of cells, or tumors.
(Illustration by Argosy Publishing. Cengage Learning, Gale.)

Oncogenes

Oncogenes are altered forms of normal genes called proto-oncogenes. There have been over 100 oncogenes identified so far. Their primary role in the cell is in regulation of growth. They encode growth factors, growth factor receptors, transcription factors that regulate the manufacturing of new proteins, and signal transduction proteins. Signal transduction refers to the process of transmitting a signal from the outside layer of the cell through the cytoplasm into the nucleus of the cell, and it begins with growth factor and receptor interaction. Cancer cells sometimes have altered levels of growth factors or their receptors, or factors involved in signal transduction. For example, the K-*ras* oncogene is an example of a mutated signal transduction protein involved in cancers such as colon and lung cancer, and the HER2/neu oncogene is a mutated receptor associated with breast cancer. Finally, this series of biochemical reactions reaches the nucleus to affect gene transcription, or the reading of genes into RNA and protein. This occurs via transcription factors. Mutations in transcription factors result in abnormal levels of certain proteins that can result in cancer. *Myc* is an example of a transcription factor mutated in lung cancer.

Tumor suppressor genes

Also called anti-oncogenes, tumor suppressor genes code for proteins that halt cell growth. In the normal cell, when DNA has become damaged, the cell stops growing to devote time to repairing DNA. Factors responsible for allowing this repair to take place are tumor suppressor genes. If tumor suppressor genes malfunction, the cells do not stop dividing when DNA is damaged and the mutation is then carried over to the daughter cells after cell division. This increases the risk of developing cancer. In hereditary cancers it is often a malfunctioning tumor suppressor gene that is inherited. Although there are two copies of each tumor suppressor gene, the second gene can take over the role if it is not mutated. A mutation in the second copy of the gene is required for total loss of tumor suppressor function. There are dozens of tumor suppressor genes identified that are involved in cancer including p53 (identified with many cancers) and APC in **colon cancer**, and BRCA1 in breast cancer.

Characteristics of cancer cells

Cancer cells appear differently than normal cells do under the microscope. Their nucleus is much larger than in normal cells, their chromosomes are irregular in distribution, and the nucleoli in the nucleus are very prominent. When cancer cells are grown in culture in the lab they also appear different than normal cells. Rather than growing in neat single-layer sheets with one next to the other they grow more haphazardly. They have long processes that extend from the cells, they overlap one another, and their shape is more rounded. Normal cells will continue to divide and grow in a culture plate until they touch a neighboring cell where they receive a signal to stop growing. Cancer cells, on the other hand, do not receive this signal and grow on top of each other forming piles of growing cells that resemble a tumor.

Normal cells require growth factors added to their growth medium to enable them to grow in culture. Cancer cells do not require the same amount of growth factors, possibly because they are able make their own growth factors. Normal human cells will grow for a short amount of time in culture and then die, while cancer cells tend to keep on growing. The term given for this ability is immortalization. Cancer cells in culture are immortalized or have unlimited growth potential.

Cancer cells also have a more immature appearance compared to normal cells. This is referred to as dedifferentiation, or the lack of differentiation. As an embryo matures and develops, its cells differentiate. This means they take on more specific roles that are reflected in their appearance—kidney cells begin to look different than skin cells or breast cells. Cancer cells look less and less like the tissue they are part of and more like embryonic cells. They also produce embryonic proteins that are used as **tumor markers** such as carcinoembryonic antigen (CEA) and alpha fetoprotein (AFP).

Pathology

Tumors are either malignant or benign depending upon their invasiveness. Benign tumors are less aggressive, less likely to invade the surrounding tissue, less likely to metastasize (spread), and are slower growing. Although it sounds as if they pose no threat to the individual, this is not always the case. A tumor in the brain especially can be life threatening and put pressure on the brain as it grows. A benign tumor may also secrete hormones that in high levels can be toxic to the individual.

A malignant tumor is more aggressive, more invasive into the surrounding tissue, faster growing, and more likely to metastasize. Malignant tumors usually kill the individual if they are not removed. The diagnosis as to whether a tumor is benign or malignant is done on a small sample of the tumor, called a **biopsy**. A pathologist will microscopically examine a thin, stained slice of the tissue. The tumor is graded, or given a number from 1–4 that corresponds to its degree of malignancy, with 4 being the most malignant and 1 being benign. The more malignant the tumor, the less organized the cells of the tissue are and the more anaplastic or dedifferentiated they appear.

The tumor is also staged, which refers to the amount it has spread. This is done both by gross examination of the patient and by microscopic examination of the tissue. The staging relates to the patient's prognosis. The best prognosis is if the tumor is confined to the epithelial layer of an organ and not spread into the basement membrane. The prognosis is worse if the tumor cells have spread to adjacent lymph nodes. As a tumor grows, it becomes capable of both invasion and **metastasis**.

An organ of the body consists of epithelial cells that are supported by a basement membrane. (Epithelial cells are cells that form the tissue that covers internal and external surfaces of the body and is found on skin and mucosal surfaces.) The basement membranes separate the epithelial cells from connective tissues that are rich in blood vessels. As the tumor enlarges, it can grow into the surrounding tissue, through the basement membrane, and into blood or lymph vessels. This is a critical point in the growth of a tumor. Now, a small piece of tumor can break off and travel through the circulation until it receives a signal to attach to the vessel wall. It can then move through the vessel, into the tissue bed, where it grows to become a secondary tumor. This is termed metastasis. Two common locations for metastasizing tumors are the lungs and the liver.

Cancer can also involve the immune system and individuals with weakened immune systems are often at increased risk for developing cancer. AIDS patients, for example, are at increased risk for developing some cancers, such as **Kaposi's sarcoma**. As a cell becomes cancerous, it develops different antigens on its cell surface that may be recognized by the immune system and removed. However, the disposal of cancerous cells by the immune system does not occur consistently. Presently, scientists do not understand why this happens occasionally but not consistently. There have been documented cases of spontaneous tumor regression that may be due to activation of the immune system.

These unique antigens expressed on the surface of cancer cells can be used to the patient's advantage in treating cancer. **Monoclonal antibodies** are proteins produced in the laboratory from a single clone of a B cell, the type of cells of the immune system that make antibodies. Antibodies, also known as immunoglobulins, are proteins that help identify foreign substances to the immune system, such as bacteria or a virus. Antibodies work by binding to the foreign substance to mark it as foreign. The substance that the antibody binds to is called an antigen. Monoclonal antibodies that can recognize and attach to the specific antigens found on cancer cells are now being used to target cancer cells directly.

Unfortunately, cancer may go undiagnosed until it is quite advanced. This is because the body has many ways to adapt itself to damage and so symptoms are reduced for some time. Metastasis may be present by the time cancer is diagnosed. Symptoms of cancer include pain emanating from the organ being stretched, as well as **fever** and weakness. As the disease progresses, cachexia (the wasting that occurs due to starvation and debilitation caused by the cancer) may occur. The patient becomes unable to mount an anti-inflammatory response and infections occur. These infections become the cause of death in most cancer patients.

Carcinogenesis

How does a cancer cell become a cancer cell? Most scientists agree that cancer is a "multi-hit" process—a process that requires a series of genetic mutations that occur either spontaneously, are inherited, or are caused by specific carcinogens. There are several stages in the development of cancer: initiation, promotion, and progression.

- Initiation. During initiation, a carcinogen interacts with and damages the DNA. Repair can occur after this point and the process can be reversed.
- Promotion. Promotion causes reproduction or proliferation of these damaged cells, forming a mass of cells or a benign adenoma. This stage is still reversible and removal of the promoting agent can stop the expansion of the tumor mass.
- Progression. Progression is irreversible and involves a number of sequential mutations in genes including oncogenes and tumor suppressor genes. The end result of progression is a late adenoma that eventually converts to a malignant carcinoma.

This entire process can take 20 years or more.

A specific multistep **carcinogenesis** scheme has been outlined for colon cancer that involves the following sequence of events:

- mutation of the APC tumor suppressor gene causing loss of its function
- activation of the K-*ras* oncogene

- loss of function of the DCC ("Deleted for Colon Cancer") tumor suppressor gene followed by loss of function of the p53 tumor suppressor gene

Such defining of the process of carcinogenesis can identify tumor markers used for diagnosis and monitoring of cancers. Also, an understanding of pathways involved in carcinogenesis can provide information to better design and target drugs, making them more specific to decrease their effects on normal cells. Information gained on carcinogenesis pathways can also be used to research targets for gene replacement therapy.

Angiogenesis

As the tumor grows, its need for a blood supply increases. A tumor larger than 1 mm diameter (0.03 in) cannot continue to grow without access to circulation. Blood supplies the nutrients the tumor requires and can remove the toxic metabolites that are built up in the tumor tissue. To keep up with the demand for blood vessels, the tumor releases factors called angiogenic factors. One such factor is termed vascular endothelial growth factor (VEGF). These factors initiate the growth of more blood vessels into the tumor. This process of increased blood vessel growth is termed angiogenesis. The rich supply of blood vessels also gives the tumor more opportunity to metastasize to distant sites by traveling through the blood. Using drugs that can block angiogenesis is a newly developing field of cancer treatment.

Apoptosis

Apoptosis is a way the organism has of removing genetically damaged cells from itself to prevent cancer. It is different from another process of death called necrosis where damaged tissue dies for various reasons. When DNA damage occurs to the cell, the body has many opportunities to repair this damage and thus to prevent cancer. If the DNA repair does not occur, however, the last chance the organism has to protect itself from cancer is to eradicate the entire cell. This programmed cell death, or selective destruction of a cell, is called apoptosis. Precancerous cells receive signals that activate this self-destruct program. Genes that are involved in apoptosis include bcl-2 (breast cancer tumor suppressor genes 1 and 2) and p53. When these genes are mutated, apoptosis is limited and the risk of a cell becoming cancerous is increased. Some anti-cancer drugs act by stimulating the apoptotic pathway.

Tumor markers

Tumor markers may be soluble factors secreted by cancer cells, altered proteins retained by cancer cells, or mutated genes in the cancer cells. They are typically identified in the blood of patients but sometimes tissue from a biopsy is necessary. Tumor markers can be used as an aid in diagnosing cancer but, more importantly, they can give information on the prognosis of the cancer and aid the clinician in determining appropriate treatment. For instance, if the tumor marker HER-2/neu associated with breast cancer is identified in a patient, specific **chemotherapy** that is directly targeted to the HER-2/neu protein can be used, giving the patient a better prognosis. Some tumors secrete high levels of hormones that are used as tumor markers to help identify the cancer. For instance, choriocarcinoma (a malignancy that originates inside the uterus) produces large amounts of human chorionic gonadotropin (hCG). The presence of hCG in the blood helps identify the tumor. Other common tumor markers include prostate-specific antigen (PSA) associated with **prostate cancer** and CA 125 associated with **ovarian cancer**.

Genetics

Cancer is basically thought of as a genetic disease. (That is not to say, however, that all cancers are inherited.) Genes are sequences of DNA located on chromosomes within the nucleus. The genes contain information that encodes proteins involved in all aspects of cell metabolism. Genes involved in cell growth and division are the most important in regards to cancer. These genes are oncogenes, tumor suppressor genes, and DNA repair genes. Before science had the ability to identify specific genes it was noted that some cancers were associated with chromosomal abnormalities. For instance, chronic myeloid leukemia (CML) is associated with a fragmented chromosome termed the Philadelphia chromosome. The Philadelphia chromosome results from a translocation of part of chromosome 22 to chromosome 9. Using newer molecular techniques, we now know that this translocation results in a fusion between two oncogenes: *bcr* and *abl*.

We now know of many hereditary conditions that result in an increased risk of cancer. Although hereditary cancers are actually quite rare, they are notable because individuals who inherit a predisposition for cancer become afflicted with cancer at a much earlier age than those without an inherited susceptibility. Cancer results from a series of genetic mutations that may take 20 years or more to accumulate. If one of these mutations is inherited, it shortens the time for cancer to develop. Individuals with hereditary predispositions tend to get cancer at a much earlier age than those who get non-hereditary cancer.

Familial colon cancer and breast cancer are two widely known examples of inherited cancers. One percent of individuals with colon cancer has an inherited condition called familial adenomatous polyposis (FAP). Individuals with FAP inherit a mutation of the adenomatous polyposis coli (APC) gene, a tumor suppressor gene that is involved in apoptosis. Patients with FAP tend to have many benign polyps of the colon and are likely to develop colon cancer by the age of 40. Mutation of the APC gene is an early event in non-hereditary colon cancer as well. The difference is that in non-hereditary colon cancer, this mutation is a spontaneous event, and the accumulation of mutations that result in cancer occur later in life than with hereditary colon cancer.

There are two genes associated with hereditary breast cancer, the **BRCA1** gene and the **BRCA2** gene. About 80% of families with cases of early onset breast cancer have mutations in the BRCA1 gene. This gene is also associated with increased risk of ovarian cancer. The BRCA2 gene, associated with hereditary breast cancer, is related to ovarian cancer to a lesser extent than BRCA1. Both genes act as tumor suppressor genes.

The **Li-Fraumeni syndrome** is a hereditary syndrome that puts individuals at an increased risk for a number of cancers including breast cancer, soft tissue sarcomas, osteosarcomas, **brain tumors**, leukemias, and adrenocortical carcinomas. Individuals with this syndrome have mutations in the tumor suppressor gene p53. Mutations in this gene are associated with 50% of all cancers. The protein associated with p53 is found in the nucleus of the cell and regulates cell functions such as cell cycle, DNA repair, and apoptosis. Mutations in p53 are also noted in colon cancer.

Other hereditary cancer syndromes include **retinoblastoma**, in which a mutated Rb gene is inherited, and neurofibromatosis, in which a mutated NF1 gene is inherited. The K-*ras* gene is an oncogene that is commonly mutated in many types of cancer including colon and lung cancer. Individuals who are part of families with high rates of these types of cancers can choose to be genetically tested to determine if they are at an elevated risk for developing cancer.

Treatment

Most cancer treatments center around three modalities: surgical removal of the tumor, radiotherapy, and chemotherapy to kill the cancer cells. If the cancer has not spread and is isolated, surgery is the best option as it can physically remove the entire tumor. The location of all tumor tissue must be able to be identified for this procedure, however. There are

risks of surgery that include those associated with anesthesia and **infection**.

Radiation therapy uses **x rays** directed at the tumor to cause damage that kills the cells. Radiation therapy will also affect normal tissue that lies in the radiation field. These side effects will vary depending upon the part of the body undergoing treatment.

Chemotherapy involves using drugs that circulate through the body to affect the tumor. The first drugs that were used to treat cancer are the antimetabolite drugs such as **methotrexate** and **mercaptopurine**. These drugs were designed to interfere in cell division and kill rapidly dividing cells. Unfortunately, they cannot differentiate between rapidly dividing tumor cells and rapidly dividing normal cells. The toxic effects on non-tumor cells account for many of the side effects of chemotherapy, including loss of hair and gastrointestinal problems. Calculating the correct dosage of these drugs is very important to minimize side effects. Although these drugs cause more side effects because they are delivered to the entire body, this is the only way to treat tumors that have metastasized from the main tumor.

Knowledge gained about cancer over the past 20 years or so has brought about cancer therapies more directly targeted at proteins known to be involved in carcinogenesis. For instance, small molecules that can specifically inhibit signal transduction proteins can slow cancer growth. A new drug known as **imatinib mesylate** (formerly known as STI-571) deactivates the enzyme called tyrosine kinase, which allows the growth of **chronic myelocytic leukemia** cells.

Monoclonal antibodies can be made in the lab that are able to recognize specific antigens on cancer cells. These antibodies can in turn be joined to cancer drugs and be used to deliver the drug directly to the cancer cell. Being able to deliver the cytotoxic drug to the cancer cell decreases the side effects on normal tissue.

New categories of cancer treatment have also evolved including hormone therapy and immunotherapy, also called biological therapy or **biological response modifiers**. Biological therapy takes advantage of the body's own immune system to recognize the cancer and remove it. Cytokines are immunoregulatory substances secreted by the cells of the immune system. Immunotherapy can use cytokines that are naturally produced by the body and affect immune cells and blood cells. These cytokines include **interferons**, interleukins, and colony stimulating factors such as **filgrastim** and **sargramostim**. For instance, interferon-alpha and interleukin-2 are now used to treat metastatic **melanoma**.

Hormonal treatment of cancer aims to interfere with some hormonal action on cancer cells. This therapy is mostly used on breast cancer and prostate cancer. Some breast cancers grow in response to estrogen. The anti-estrogen **tamoxifen** can reduce the amount of growth in breast cancer. Prostate cancer grows in response to **testosterone**. Drugs can be used to decrease the amount of testosterone produced by the testes.

Finally, gene therapy has potential to directly target genetic abnormalities found in cancer cells. The tumor suppressor protein p53 is found mutated in a large number of cancers. By introducing the appropriate DNA sequence into a cell, this protein can be replaced bringing back the ability of the cancer cell to undergo apoptosis.

Tumor growth

A tumor that can be clinically identified is typically at least one gram in size and has undergone 30 population doublings. It is before this point that tumor growth has been its fastest and now growth has slowed down significantly. This growth curve of cancer is expressed mathematically by the Gompertzian equation. According to this growth curve, most tumors originate two years before detection. Why does tumor cell growth slow down after it reaches the one-gram size? Factors that contribute to this decline in growth include lack of oxygen, decreased availability of nutrients, accumulation of toxic metabolites, and lack of communication between cells.

Understanding the Gompertzian growth curve mathematics can help with decisions about cancer treatment. Most chemotherapy drugs target fast-growing cells and so they work best when a tumor is growing quickly. If at the time a tumor is detected, its cells are growing slower, then chemotherapy is less effective. If initial treatment involves surgery or radiation therapy, then the number of tumor cells will be decreased enough that cells will begin to reproduce again at a faster rate of growth. This makes chemotherapy more effective following surgery or radiation therapy to reduce the tumor load. This might also explain why some patients seem to go into remission only to have their cancer recur later. During remission, the cell number was too low to be detected, but cell growth was rapid during that period.

Many times a patient's response to chemotherapy is very good only to be followed by a relapse with a drug-resistant tumor. Combination chemotherapy, or the use of more than one drug at a time, is often more effective that single drug therapy. This is because cancer cells can spontaneously mutate and become resistant to drugs. This ability to mutate was mathematically explained by Goldie and Coldman and named the Goldie-Coldman model. The model predicts that spontaneous mutations in cancer cells that are capable of leading to **drug resistance** occur every 10,000 to 1,000,000 cell divisions. This implies that smaller tumors are less likely to be drug-resistant and are easier to cure. By treating tumors early and aggressively, the chance of recurrence with a drug-resistant cancer decreases. The combination of active drugs is also more effective in reducing the initial cancer.

This model of combination chemotherapy has proven useful in treating childhood **acute lymphocytic leukemia**, **Hodgkin's disease**, and **testicular cancer**. However, it has not proven useful in treating some solid tumors. These tumors seem to have a much higher capacity to develop drug resistance. The drugs used to treat these cancers are actually capable themselves of promoting resistance in the tumors. Resistance to one of these drugs often results in resistance to another drug and is referred to as multi-drug resistance. Multi-drug resistance is due to a decreased uptake and increased elimination of the drugs from the tumor cells. A specific pump has been identified in cancer cells that is responsible for multi-drug resistance.

Resources

PERIODICALS

Gibbs, Jackson B. "Mechanism-Based Target Identification and Drug Discovery in Cancer Research." *Science* 2000; 287:1969-1973.

Lowe Scott W., and Athena W. Lin. "Apoptosis in Cancer." *Carcinogenesis* 21 (2000): 485-495.

OTHER

DeNittis, Albert, Thomas J. Dilling, Joel W. Goldwein. "The Biology of Cancer." *OncoLink, University of Pennsylvania.* [cited December 21, 2000]. http://www.oncolink.upenn.edu/specialty/med_onc/nature_cancer1.htm.

Mellors, Robert C. "Etiology of Cancer: Carcinogenesis." *Neoplasia.* Weill Medical College of Cornell University, July 1999. http://edcenter.med.cornell.edu/CUMC_PathNotes/Neoplasia/Neoplasia_04.html.

"Oncogenes and Tumor Suppressor Genes." *Cancer Resource Center, American Cancer Society.* [cited January 19, 2001]. http://www3.cancer.org.

ORGANIZATIONS

American Cancer Society. 1599 Clifton Road NE, Atlanta, GA, 30329. (800) 227-2345. http://www.cancer.org.

American Society of Clinical Oncology. 225 Reinekers Lane, Suite 650, Alexandria, VA 22314. (703) 299-0150. http://www.asco.org.

National Cancer Institute. 9000 Rockville Pike, Building 31, Bethesda, MD 20892. (800) 4-CANCER. http://www.nci.nih.gov.

Cindy L. A. Jones, Ph.D.

Cancer cluster

Definition

The National Cancer Institute (NCI) defines a cancer cluster as "the occurrence of a greater than expected number of cases of [cancer] within a group of people, a geographical area, or a period of time." Cancer is not the only disease that sometimes occurs in clusters: AIDS, SARS, and certain types of food poisoning are other examples.

Cancer clusters are also defined by a primary cancer of a specific tissue or organ; cases involving metastases to that part of the body are not included in evaluations of suspected clusters.

Description

Although some cancer clusters have received considerable publicity through books and films about their investigation, they are much less common than many people think. Epidemiologists and toxicologists in the United States receive about 1,500 requests every year to investigate suspected clusters; however, very few of these turn out to be genuine clusters. A suspected cluster has a greater chance of being a true cluster when all of the following factors are present:

- All the reported cases of cancer belong to one type or closely related types.
- The cancer is an uncommon type.
- The type of cancer affects members of a group that does not usually develop this form of cancer, as when young people develop a type of cancer usually seen in the elderly.

There are several reasons why it is hard to prove that a group of cancer cases is a true cluster:

- Cancer is not a single disease but a term that covers over 100 different diseases, each with its own set of causes, risk factors, demographic patterns, and characteristic symptoms.
- The causes of cancer include a variety of external and internal factors ranging from chemicals or radiation in

KEY TERMS

Carcinogen—Any substance that causes cancer.

Epidemiology—The branch of medicine concerned with studying outbreaks of disease in large groups of people, the factors that affect the frequency or spread of disease, and detection of the sources or causes of epidemics.

Toxicology—The branch of medicine concerned with the effects of poisonous substances and treatment of these effects. Toxicologists are often involved in investigations of cancer clusters.

the environment to inherited genetic mutations and hormone levels in the body. Lifestyle differences (occupation, nutritional status, use of tobacco and alcohol, etc.) and racial and ethnic differences also affect an individual's risk of developing cancer. All these risk factors and environmental exposures interact in complex ways that are not fully understood as of the early 2000s.

- Cancer takes a relatively long time to develop, often 10 years or even longer following exposure to an environmental trigger.
- Many reported clusters involve only a small number of cases, which complicates statistical analysis. Another way of putting the problem is that having a relatively small number of cases makes it harder to exclude the possibility of simple chance or coincidence.
- It is not always easy for doctors to determine the primary site of a patient's cancer, which in turn makes it hard to decide whether the patient should be counted as part of a cancer cluster.
- The so-called "sharpshooter's fallacy." Sharpshooter's fallacy refers to a story about a man who fires a gun at random into a target and then draws a circle around the bullet holes, thus creating the appearance of a bull's-eye that does not really exist. In investigating a suspected cancer cluster, some observers tend to expand the geographical boundaries of the cluster to include new cases as they appear, thus creating the illusion of a cancer cluster. This particular fallacy was involved in the theory—which was publicized in the mid-1990s by articles in the *New Yorker* and other popular magazines—that exposure to the electromagnetic fields surrounding high-voltage power lines causes cancer clusters in neighborhoods around the transmission towers.

Causes

As cancer is not a contagious disease, true cancer clusters result from a combination of genetic factors that increase some individuals' susceptibility to specific types of cancer, combined with exposure to environmental carcinogens. Environmental factors known to be related to cancer include sunlight and other forms of radiation as well as toxic chemicals and atmospheric pollutants.

Special concerns

Possible clusters of cancers that primarily affect children are given priority by public health investigators. It is noteworthy that two well-known cases concerned childhood leukemia—the cluster of cases in Woburn, Massachusetts, in the 1970s, and a newer cluster first reported in 1999 in Churchill County, Nevada. The Bureau of Environmental Health Assessment (BEHA) of the Commonwealth of Massachusetts maintains a frequently updated website about the Woburn cluster. The Nevada cluster is still under investigation as of early 2005.

Reporting a cancer cluster

Prior to 1990, the Centers for Disease Control and Prevention (CDC) had primary responsibility for investigating suspected cancer clusters. Since that date, departments of public health at the state or local level have conducted initial evaluations of cancer clusters. Persons who think there may be a cancer cluster in their neighborhood or workplace should first contact their local health department or their state's cancer registry. Contact information for state health departments and cancer registries is available through the CDC website. The CDC and such other national agencies as the National Center for Environmental Health (NCEH) and the National Institute of Environmental Health Sciences (NIEHS) will join the investigation if the state health department requests their help.

Investigating a cancer cluster

When a possible cancer cluster is reported, the state health department will take the following steps:

- Ask the person reporting the cluster for information about the type of cancer involved, number of cases, suspected time period or geographic area, etc. Information will also be requested about each case in the cluster (patient's contact information, the length of time they have lived in the area, etc.) and diagnostic information about the cancer (patient's age at diagnosis, whether the cancer is primary or metastatic, etc.) Between 75 and 80% of reports are closed at this point because the basic information indicates that the group of cases is not a true cluster.

- If the cluster seems to require a closer look, the investigators will contact the patients to verify diagnoses and obtain medical records; compare the number of cases with information from cancer registries and data banks to determine whether the cluster represents an unusually high rate of occurrence; and consult the relevant medical literature for reports of possible occupational or environmental factors linked to the type of cancer.

- If necessary, the state health department will contact the CDC and other federal agencies to help conduct a comprehensive study. Fewer than 4% of reported clusters are investigated at this level.

Interested readers may wish to test their own skills in medical investigation by playing a game called "Cluster Busters," listed under Resources below. The game, which can be downloaded from the NIEHS website, was originally developed to teach health sciences students at the University of Arizona.

Interpreting the findings

If a comprehensive investigation does indicate that a reported cancer cluster is a true cluster, this finding does not necessarily mean that the cases resulted from one single risk factor or environmental cause. The investigators may arrive at any of the following conclusions:

- The cluster resulted from chance.
- The expected number of cancer cases in the group of people defined as being at risk was calculated incorrectly.
- The cancers have a known cause (such as smoking).
- The cancers have a cause that is still unknown.

See also Leukemia.

Resources

BOOKS

Harr, Jonathan. *A Civil Action.* New York: Vintage Books, 1996. The classic book-length account of the cluster of childhood leukemia cases in Woburn, Massachusetts, and the court case that grew out of the medical investigation.

PERIODICALS

Costas, K., R. S. Knorr, and S. K. Condon. "A Case-Control Study of Childhood Leukemia in Woburn, Massachusetts: The Relationship between Leukemia Incidence and Exposure to Public Drinking Water." *Science of the Total Environment* 300 (December 2, 2002): 23–35.

Steinmaus, C., M. Lu, R. Todd, and A. H. Smith. "Probability Estimates for the Unique Childhood Leukemia Cluster in Fallon, Nevada, and Risks Near Other U. S.

Military Aviation Facilities." *Environmental Health Perspectives* 112 (May 2004): 766–771.

Waller, L. A. " *A Civil Action* and Statistical Assessments of the Spatial Pattern of Disease: Do We Have a Cluster?" *Regulatory Toxicology and Pharmacology* 32 (October 2000): 174–183.

OTHER

Centers for Disease Control and Prevention, National Center for Environmental Health (NCEH). *Cancer Clusters.* http://www.cdc.gov/nceh/clusters/about_clusters.htm.

Hines, Stefani, MS, John King, MS, and Joanna K. Norman, PhD. *Cluster Busters: A Game of Disease Mystery Solving.* Tucson, AZ: University of Arizona Center for Toxicology, 1999. http://www.niehs.nih.gov/health/docs/disease-solve.pdf.

National Cancer Institute (NCI). *Cancer Facts: Cancer Clusters.* Bethesda, MD: NCI, 2004. http://cis.nci.nih/gov/fact/3_58.htm.

United States Environmental Protection Agency (EPA), Region 2. *Cancer Clusters.* http://www.epa.gov/Region2/health/cancer_clusters.htm.

ORGANIZATIONS

Centers for Disease Control and Prevention, National Center for Environmental Health (NCEH). Hotline: (888) 232-6789. http://www.cdc.gov/nceh/Information/contact.htm.

Commonwealth of Massachusetts Department of Public Health, Bureau of Environmental Health Assessment (BEHA). 250 Washington Street, 7th Floor, Boston, MA 02108. (617) 624-5757. Woburn cancer cluster website: http://www.mass.gov/dph/beha/cau/reports/woburn/woburn.htm.

National Institute of Environmental Health Sciences (NIEHS). P. O. Box 12233, Research Triangle Park, NC 27709. (919) 541-3345. http://www.niehs.nih.gov.

United States Environmental Protection Agency (EPA). Ariel Rios Building, 1200 Pennsylvania Avenue NW, Washington, DC 20460. (202) 272-0167. http://www.epa.gov. Contact information for the EPA's 10 regional offices is available on the main EPA website.

Rebecca Frey, PhD

Cancer genetics

Definition

Cancer genetics is the study of the process in which multiple alterations occur in genes, changing cell structure and leading to cancer. Cancerous cells continuously divide and change, leading to uncontrolled division and proliferation (duplication) of cells. These genetic alterations are referred to as mutations, which are changes in the normal DNA sequence of a particular gene. Mutations may include deletions, chromosomal translocations, inversions, amplifications, or point mutations.

Cancer genetics is the understanding of the genetic processes underlying the actual disease. This understanding plays a significant role in early detection, therapy, prevention, and prognosis.

Description

Nearly all cancers originate from a single cell and are the result of genetic alterations, although most of them are not inherited. Individuals who are genetically predisposed to a particular cancer will not necessarily develop the disease in the absence of somatic mutations. Somatic mutations occur in non–sex determining cells, meaning they will not be passed on to offspring. These mutations can be influenced by environment and other causes, such as an individual's habits (e.g., smoking). A single genetic error or mutation in a cell does not typically cause malignancy; instead it develops after a series of mutations over a period of time.

Regulation of cell death and survival

A balance between cell division and death of the old, degenerated cells is essential for proper cellular functioning of any organism. Cells that can no longer duplicate or that have sustained injuries (like hypoxia, heat, extreme cold, or ultraviolet radiation) are candidates for cell death. Alternatively, cells can be killed if infected by intracellular organisms (pathogens), or damaged cells may be engulfed by a host's lymphocytes (white blood cells involved in cellular defense mechanisms). Another form of cell death in the disease process is a suicide mechanism initiated by cells known as apoptosis. In this process, extracellular or intracellular signals may trigger the degradation of nuclear material resulting in cell death. Some of the apoptotic genes like bcl2 family members (bcl-X, A1, bax, bad) are likely involved in various cancers. Studies to alter the activity of bcl2 family members and related genes will be of potential use in designing cancer therapies.

Oncogenes and tumor suppressor genes

The constant cell proliferation in cancer may either be due to over-activation of a specific gene that promotes cell division or the improper functioning of a gene that will otherwise restrain growth. Genes that promote cell division are proto-oncogenes—positive regulators of cell division. Overexpression of proto-oncogenes results in uncontrolled cell growth. Genes that suppress or restrain growth are tumor suppressor genes. Loss of their function results in unregulated cell division. An alteration in

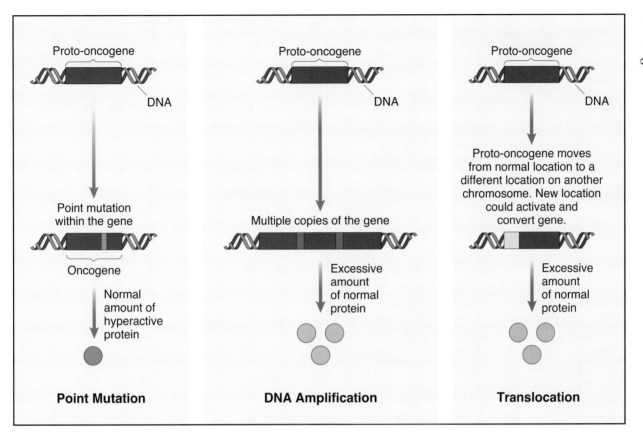

Point mutation, DNA amplification, and chromosomal alterations (like translocations) are three examples of mutations that can turn proto-oncogenes into oncogenes. *(Illustration by Argosy Publishing. Cengage Learning, Gale.)*

Chromosomes and cancer

Cancer type	Associated gene mutation
Chronic myelocytic leukemia	translocation resulting in the Philadelphia chromosome (Ph[1])
Burkitt's lymphoma	translocation involving the c-*myc* proto-oncogene
Retinoblastoma	mutation in chromosome 13; mutation can be inherited
Wilms' tumor	mutation in chromosome 11; mutation can be inherited
Colon cancer (occurs sporadically, but also occurs as a familial cancer syndrome)	mutation in adenomatous polyposis coli (APC) gene followed by further mutations
Breast cancer (occurs sporadically and also as a familial cancer syndrome)	mutation affecting the gene *BRCA1*, or mutation in *BRCA2*

(Table by GGS Creative Resources. Cengage Learning, Gale.)

the function of genes in each of these classes is due to a change, or mutation, in the DNA within the cell. The different types of mutations include point mutations, amplifications, and chromosomal alterations.

Point mutations

DNA is composed of a string of nucleotides, each containing a phosphate group, deoxyribose, and one of four bases: adenine (A), guanine (G), cytosine (C), and thymine (T). These bases are paired as either A-T or C-G and the pairs compose the "rungs" in the double helix structure of DNA. The order of the bases creates the genetic code for development. A sample genetic code is CAG-TAA-CCA-GCG, etc. These triplets code for synthesis of specific proteins.

A point mutation is a single nucleotide change in a DNA strand. This may alter the genetic code, thus altering the function of the protein. In the above example, a point mutation in the thymine base of the second triplet would look like: CAG-AAA-CCA-GCG. Changing the code from TAA to AAA could alter the function of a protein and thus could cause a predisposition to disease such as cancer. One example of a point mutation that has been identified is the *ras* family of oncogenes (such as H*ras*, K-*ras*, N-*ras*), present in 15% of all human cancers.

Childhood cancers associated with congenital syndromes or malformations

Syndrome or Anomaly	Tumor
Aniridia	Wilms' tumor
Hemihypertrophy	Wilms' tumor
	Hepatoblastoma
	Adrenocortical carcinoma
Genito-urinary abnormalities (including undescended testicles)	Wilms' tumor
	Ewing's sarcoma
	Nephroblastoma
	Testicular cancer
Beckwith-Wiedmann syndrome	Wilms' tumor
	Neuroblastoma
	Adrenocortical carcinoma
Dysplastic nevus syndrome	Melanoma
Nevoid basal cell carcinoma syndrome	Basal cell carcinoma
	Medulloblastoma
	Rhabdomyosarcoma
Poland syndrome	Leukemia
Trisomy-21 (Down syndrome)	Leukemia
	Retinoblastoma
Bloom syndrome	Leukemia, gastrointestinal carcinoma
Severe combined immune deficiency disease	EBV-associated B-lymphocyte lymphoma/leukemia
Wiscott-Aldridge syndrome	EBV-associated B-lymphocyte lymphoma
Ataxia telangiectasia	EBV-associated B-lymphocyte lymphoma
	Gastric carcinoma (stomach cancer)
Retinoblastoma	Wilms' tumor
	Osteosarcoma
	Ewing's sarcoma
Fanconi anemia	Leukemia
	Squamous cell carcinoma
Multiple endocrine neoplasia syndromes (MEN I, II, III)	Adenomas of islet cells, pituitary, parathyroids, and adrenal glands
	Submucosal neuromas of the tongue, lips, eyelids
	Pheochromocytomas
	Medullary carcinoma of the thyroid (thyroid cancer, a specific type)
	Malignant schwannoma
	Non-appendiceal carcinoid
Neurofibromatosis (von Recklinghausen syndrome)	Rhabdomyosarcoma
	Fibrosarcoma
	Pheochromocytomas
	Optic glioma
	Meningioma

(Table by GGS Creative Resources. Reproduced by permission of Gale, a part of Cengage Learning.)

DNA amplification

Another mechanism of oncogene activation—DNA amplification—results in an increase in the amount of DNA in the cell. A large number of genes are amplified in human cancers.

DNA amplification can be detected by cytological staining (a method in which the amplified DNA is stained), or by another fluorescent technique called comparative genomic hybridization (CGH). CGH allows the specific recognition of regions of gene amplifications in tumor DNA and is a more sensitive diagnostic tool.

Chromosomal alteration

Chromosomal alteration may involve translocations and is often seen in lymphoid tumors. Translocation is the transfer of one part of a chromosome to another chromosome during cell division and may involve transcription factors (i.e., nuclear factors), signal transduction proteins, and cellular regulatory molecules.

DNA repair genes

In addition to oncogenes and tumor suppressor genes, DNA repair genes may lead to cancer. DNA repair genes are capable of correcting the errors that occur during cell division. Malfunction of these repair genes, either through inherited mutation or acquired mutation, may affect cell division resulting in malignancies.

RNA and DNA viruses

Malignancies are known to be associated with RNA or DNA viruses. A retrovirus is an RNA virus that possesses a single-stranded RNA as its genetic material, in contrast to the double-stranded DNA. Retroviruses are known to induce malignancies in animals, and one known human malignancy is T-cell **lymphoma** or leukemia caused by human T-cell lymphotropic virus (HTLV) type I.

DNA viruses are implicated in human malignancies more often than RNA viruses. **Human papilloma virus** is related to human **cervical cancer**, and hepatitis B and C are related to hepatocellular **carcinoma** (**liver cancer**). In addition, the **Epstein-Barr virus** that causes the commonly known infectious mononucleosis also causes **Burkitt's lymphoma** in Africa and nasopharyngeal carcinoma in parts of Asia.

Mendelian cancer syndromes

Some forms of cancer are classified as hereditary cancers, or familial cancers, because they follow the Mendelian pattern of inheritance, the more familiar form of inheritance in which genetic material is passed from the mother or father to the offspring during reproduction. Cancer-related genes may be inherited as autosomal dominant, autosomal recessive, or x-linked traits.

About 100 syndromes have been identified as hereditary cancers although not all of them are common. Some of the known tumor suppressor genes responsible for **familial cancer syndromes** are **BRCA1**, which is associated with breast, ovarian, colon, or prostate cancers; **BRCA2** involved in **breast**

KEY TERMS

Autosomal dominant—A pattern of genetic inheritance where only one abnormal gene is needed to display the trait or disease.

Autosomal recessive—A pattern of genetic inheritance where two copies of an abnormal gene must be present to display the trait or disease.

Gene—A building block of inheritance that contains the instructions for the production of a particular protein and is made up of a molecular sequence found on a section of DNA. Each gene is found on a precise location on a chromosome.

Hypoxia—Lack of oxygen to the cells that may lead to cell injury and ultimately cell death.

Infectious mononucleosis—A common viral infection caused by Epstein-Barr virus with symptoms of sore throat, fever, and fatigue. This infection is not in any way related to cancer.

Malignant—A tumor that tends to spread to local or distant tissues, usually cancerous.

Nucleotides—Building blocks of genes, which are arranged in specific order and quantity.

Oncogene—Genes that allow the uncontrolled division and proliferation of cells that lead to tumor formation and usually to cancer.

Translocation—The transfer of one part of a chromosome to another chromosome during cell division. A balanced translocation occurs when pieces from two different chromosomes exchange places without loss or gain of any chromosome material. An unbalanced translocation involves the unequal loss or gain of genetic information between two chromosomes.

X-linked traits—Genetic conditions associated with mutations in genes on the X chromosome. A male carrying such a mutation will contract the disorder associated with it because he carries only one X chromosome. A female carrying a mutation on just one X chromosome, with a normal gene on the other chromosome, will not be affected by the disease.

---

cancer, **male breast cancer**, and **ovarian cancer**; *TSC2* associated with angiofibroma; and *RB* associated with **retinoblastoma** and **osteosarcoma**. The discovery of these genes that are associated with hereditary cancer syndromes is also beneficial in understanding the normal control of cell growth.

Complex inherited cancer syndromes

Several types of cancer do not follow a simple Mendelian pattern of inheritance. In many instances, environmental factors can affect the outcome of disease expression in conjunction with genetic alterations. One such example is lung cancer. Cigarette smoke is an environmental factor that may result in lung cancer for individuals frequently exposed to the toxins in the smoke. However, individuals who possess a gene that predisposes them to lung cancer are genetically more susceptible than the rest of the population to these toxins, and may develop cancer with less exposure or none at all. Individuals without a predisposing gene may not develop the cancer as readily.

It is estimated that less than 10% of breast and ovarian cancers are the result of mutations in the BRCA1 or BRCA2 genes. The remaining 90% of breast cancer incidences are not usually dependent on inherited factors, although family history should be investigated.

Genetic mapping and research

In 2002, researchers completed the first draft of the Human Genome Project. The project undertook identifying all of the genes in the human body. By identifying and scientifically mapping our genetic code, scientists can better explore causes, treatments, and possible **vaccines** for diseases such as cancer. Since the project was completed, rapid developments have occurred in identifying chromosomes on genes responsible for various diseases. For example, in 2003, scientists discovered a third breast cancer gene called EMSY. Late in 2003, scientists announced that measurement of new genes at diagnosis of acute lymphoblastic leukemia in children, made possible by the Human Genome Project, may help predict their outcome. Researchers have introduced a urine-based genetic test for **prostate cancer**. Scientists have been pushing for a tumor classification system to be added to the current cancer staging system that would be based on genetics.

Genetic counseling

Genetic counselors comprehend the medical aspects of hereditary cancer syndromes and can educate the affected family regarding available management options. Counselors communicate the risk for disease development to individuals and their families and actively participate in guiding the course of action from an unbiased perspective. Genetic counselors also aid in providing updated information regarding **genetic testing** for cancer risk, especially with the discovery of hereditary cancer–associated genes. Genetic counseling efforts may involve a team of health professionals anchored by the genetic counselor, which includes a medical geneticist with appropriate background, a mental health professional, a physician specializing in cancer (oncologist), and a surgeon (if the type of cancer requires surgery).

Genetic testing

Genetic testing examines the genetic information contained inside an individual's DNA to determine if that person has a certain disease, is at risk to develop a certain disease, or could pass a genetic alteration to his or her offspring. Individuals who seek genetic testing are usually family members believed to have a predisposition or susceptibility to cancer as known from the personal family medical history. The identification of genes associated with certain types of cancers, such as BRCA1, BRCA2, HNPCC (**colon cancer**), and RB, improves the accuracy of DNA testing to predict cancer risk.

Often a positive test result indicates that the individual carries the abnormal gene and is more likely to get the disease for which the test was performed than the rest of the population. A negative test result can signify the absence of the abnormal gene and a lesser chance of developing the disease. However, a negative test result cannot guarantee that the person will never develop cancer at any point in his or her lifetime. This is because many mutations are induced by environmental factors and accumulate over a period of time.

It is necessary for the individual undergoing genetic testing to know that assessing the mutations is challenging and false-positive results are possible. False-positive results are those that indicate the presence of an abnormal gene that may not really exist, or the abnormal gene may result in a disorder other than the one for which the testing was performed. If the tests administered are not sensitive and specific, they may detect sequence variations that could be benign variants rather than the disease-causing mutations.

Genetic testing is recommended for individuals at higher risk of cancer based on the family medical history.

Genetic testing also is performed for individuals who have survived cancer at an earlier time in their lives. It may be performed to determine one or more of the following:

- risk to offspring

- necessity of prophylactic surgery in appropriate cases
- surveillance purposes
- personal cancer etiology (cause of disease)

Genetic counseling professionals can assist in the decision to perform genetic testing and in understanding the associated risks. Some individuals find it difficult to cope with the knowledge of their own genetic predisposition. These patients should consider addressing these issues with appropriate health care professionals.

See also Cancer biology; Carcinogenesis; Chromosome rearrangements.

Resources

PERIODICALS

"A Genetically Based Tumor Classification System Will Soon be Possible." *Cancer Weekly* October 28, 2003: 163.

"Genetic Test for Prostate Cancer Introduced." *Health & Medicine Week* October 2003: 616.

"Hereditary Common Cancers: Molecular and Clinical Genetics." *Anticancer Research* 20 (November-December 2000): 4841-4851.

"New Human Breast and Ovarian Cancer Gene Described." *Biotech Week* December 31, 2003: 89.

"Newly Identified Genes May Help Predict Outcome in Childhood Leukemia." *Cancer Weekly* December 30, 2003: 5.

Venter, J. Craig, et al. "The Sequence of the Human Genome." *Science* 291 (February 16, 2001): 1304-1351.

OTHER

American Academy of Family Physicians. *Genetic Testing: What you should know.* http://family doctor.org/handouts/462.htm. (Rev. June 2001).

National Cancer Institute. "Cancer genetics." *CancerNet.* http://cancernet.nci.nih.gov/prevention/genetics. shtml. (December 1999).

Kausalya Santhanam, PhD

Cancer prevention

Definition

Preventing the incidence of **cancer** is complex and involves many factors that ultimately work by avoiding or limiting exposure to carcinogens. Known carcinogens in humans include physical, chemical, viral, and bacterial carcinogens. Physical carcinogens include the hydrocarbon byproducts of cigarette smoke, radiation, and asbestos. Benzene and vinyl chloride are examples of chemical carcinogens. The human papillomaviruses, which play a role in the development of **cervical cancer**, are viral carcinogens. A bacterial carcinogen is the bacteria *Helicobacter pylori*, which has been linked to the cancer B-cell **lymphoma**, unique to the gastric mucosa. Familial (hereditary) **carcinogenesis** plays a role in as many as 15% of all human cancers and has been implicated as the cause of some cases of **melanoma**, breast, colon, and other cancers.

Some factors that place individuals at high risk for the development of cancer can be modified to decrease risk for development. For example, people can make lifestyle and environmental changes to decrease risk. Behavior modification such as dietary changes, exercise, and avoiding exposure to known carcinogens are primary prevention measures that everyone should adopt.

An evolving field, **chemoprevention**, is the use of **vitamins** or medicines to prevent cancer development. In 2003, the U.S. Preventive Services Task Force released a report stating that evidence was insufficient to recommend for or against use of vitamin supplements to help prevent cancer. The task force recommended against supplementation with beta-carotene because of higher incidence of lung cancer among those who used certain levels of beta-carotene supplements.

Chemopreventive agents have the ability to potentially delay and even reverse the sequence of events at the cellular level that change a normal cell to a cancer cell. An example of a chemopreventive agent is **tamoxifen**, a drug that is effective in preventing **breast cancer** in women who are at high risk for developing breast cancer. **Vaccines** for Hepatitis B virus will not only prevent primary Hepatitis B and liver failure, but also **liver cancer**.

Preventive surgery may be an option for those individuals who are considered to be at high risk of developing cancer because of a genetic or inherited predisposition. Examples of preventive surgery are prophylactic (preventive) **mastectomy** to reduce risk for breast cancer, and colon polyp removal in individuals at high risk for the development of **colon cancer**.

In 2009 the American Cancer Society (ACS) estimated that 30% of cancer deaths were caused by cigarette smoking alone and some 169,000 deaths could be attributed to tobacco use. All cancers caused by smoking **cigarettes** and by excessive use of alcohol can be completely prevented. **Alcohol consumption** is another risk factor for cancer. According to the ACS, up to one-third of the more than 562,340 cancer deaths in the United States in 2009 were related to poor nutrition or insufficient physical exercise. A recent study reported that women of average weight who walked briskly at least one and one-fourth hours per week

had a 30% lower risk of breast cancer than women who did not exercise. Many of the more than one million skin cancers that develop annually could be prevented by adopting protective measures from ultraviolet radiation caused by the sun.

Different cancers are associated with different risk factors. While modification of risk factors plays an important role in the prevention of cancer, it is known that some individuals who have one or more risk factors never develop cancer. Others, however, who have no known risk factors are eventually diagnosed with cancer. Research aimed at identifying additional risk factors for specific cancers continues.

Lifestyle and cancer

Nutrition

The relationship between food intake and cancer is complex and not well understood. Research seems to indicate that certain foods may have either protective or promoting effects on the development of cancer. Foods that have a protective effect seem to play a role in the prevention of certain types of cancers. Foods that have promoting effects are associated with an increased risk of developing certain types of cancers. According to the American Cancer Society, the single most important dietary intervention to lower risk for cancer is eating five or more servings of fruits and vegetables daily. Adopting a diet rich in plant sources provides phytochemicals that possess health protective benefits. Dietary recommendations related to reducing risk of cancer include the recommendation to choose most foods from plant sources such as fruits and vegetables. Five or more servings of fruits and vegetables should be consumed every day. Fruits and vegetables should be eaten at every meal and as snacks. Other foods from plant sources that should be included in the diet several times a day include breads, cereals, grain products (preferably whole grain), rice, and pasta. Beans should be eaten as an alternative to meat. The foods and herbs with the highest anticancer activity include garlic, soybeans, cabbage, ginger, licorice root, and the umbelliferous vegetables such as carrots. Citrus foods also contain a host of active phytochemicals.

A diet rich in foods from plant sources may reduce the risk for development of cancers of the gastrointestinal tract, respiratory tract, and colon. Vegetables that seem to play a strong role in protecting against colon cancer include green and dark yellow vegetables, vegetables in the cabbage family, soy products, and legumes. Increased consumption of fruits and vegetables reduce risk for lung cancer, even for those individuals who smoke. Forms of fruits and vegetables that appear to provide the greatest protection include foods in fresh, frozen, canned, dried, or juice forms. Extractions from fruits and vegetable do not provide protective effects.

Diets high in fat have been associated with some increased risk for colon, rectal, prostate, and endometrial (uterine) cancers. The association between high-fat diets and the development of breast cancer is much weaker. Specific dietary recommendations are to replace high-fat foods with fruits and vegetables, eat smaller portions of high-fat foods, and limit consumption of meats, especially those that are considered high in fat.

Foods from animal sources remain a staple in American diets. Consumption of meat, especially red meats such as beef, pork, and lamb, have been associated with increased risk of colon and **prostate cancer**. Cooking methods also have been linked to the development of cancer. Mutagenic compounds are produced when proteins such as meat protein are cooked at high temperatures. These compounds may be responsible for the association between meat consumption and increased risk for colon cancer.

Obesity has been linked to cancers at several sites including colon and rectum, prostate, and kidney, as well as endometrial and breast cancer in postmenopausal women.

Physical activity

Recommendations related to physical exercise include engaging in moderate levels of activity for at least 30 minutes most days of the week. Studies have revealed an association between physical activity and a reduced risk of the development of certain types of cancers, including colon, breast, and prostate cancer. For example, physical activity is thought to stimulate the movement of stool through the bowel, resulting in less exposure of the bowel lining to mutagens in the stool.

Consumption of alcohol

Drinking alcohol has been linked to increased risk of developing cancers of the mouth, esophagus, pharynx, larynx, and liver in both men and women, and increases the risk of breast cancer in women. Cancer risk increases as the amount of alcohol consumed increases. An individual who both smokes and drinks alcohol greatly increases the risk of developing cancer when compared to either smoking or drinking alone. Risk increases significantly for cancers of the mouth, esophagus, and larynx when more than two drinks per day are consumed. A drink is defined as 5 ounces

(141.75 grams) of wine, 12 ounces (340.20 grams) of regular beer, or 1.5 ounces (42.52 grams) of 80-proof distilled spirits. Women who drink are at increased risk for the development of breast cancer. Studies have shown that the risk of breast cancer increases with just a few drinks per week.

Consumption of tobacco

Smoking-related illnesses account for more than 400,000 deaths each year in the United States. These deaths occur 12 years earlier than would be expected on average. Tobacco is known as one of the most potent human carcinogens. Tobacco causes more than 148,000 deaths each year in the form of various cancers. Most of the cancers of the lung, trachea, bronchus, larynx, pharynx, oral cavity, and esophagus diagnosed each year are caused by tobacco. Smoking is also associated with cancers of the pancreas, kidney, bladder, and cervix. Smoking is known to affect the health of nonsmokers through environmental or secondhand smoke, which is implicated in causing lung cancer. Cigarette smoking is more common among men; however, because of the increase in the number of women who smoke, more women die from lung cancer each year than from breast cancer. Mortality from lung cancer for men appears to have peaked and has been declining since the 1980s. This decline in mortality is attributed to a decrease in tobacco product use among men.

Substantial health benefits occur once an individual stops smoking. If a smoker stops smoking before the age of 50 years, his or her risk of dying in the next 15 years is half of that for a continuing smoker. Even if the smoker stops smoking after the age of 70 years, the risk of dying is still reduced substantially. After 10 years of not smoking, an ex-smoker's risk of lung cancer is reduced by 30–50%. After five years of not smoking, an ex-smoker's risk of oral and **esophageal cancer** is reduced by 50%. Risk for cervical and **bladder cancer** is also reduced once smoking is stopped.

The three treatment elements identified as particularly effective in **smoking cessation** treatment include pharmacotherapy, such as nicotine replacement patches and gums; social support from physicians and other clinicians; and skills training and problem solving, particularly in the areas of smoking cessation and abstinence techniques.

Radiation exposure

Only high-frequency radiation such as ionizing radiation (IR) and ultraviolet (UV) radiation has been proven to cause cancer in humans. A source of ultraviolet radiation is sunlight. Prolonged, unprotected exposure to UV radiation is the major cause of basal and squamous cell skin cancers. UV radiation is also a major cause of melanoma. Disruption of the earth's ozone layer by pollution is thought to result in increasing levels of UV radiation reaching the earth's surface, which has been linked to the rise in the incidence of skin cancers and melanomas.

IR has cancer-causing capability as proven by studies on atomic bomb survivors and other groups. Virtually any part of the body can be affected by IR, but the areas most affected are the bone marrow and the thyroid gland. IR is released in very low levels from diagnostic equipment such as medical and dental x-ray equipment. Much higher levels of IR are released from machines delivering **radiation therapy**. Great precautions are taken during treatment not to expose patients or staff unnecessarily to the effects of IR. Another occupational group affected by IR includes uranium miners. Exposure to radon, a naturally occurring gas which is a form of IR, can increase risk for lung cancer, especially among smokers.

See also Antioxidants; Familial cancer syndromes; Occupational exposures and cancer.

Resources

BOOKS

Yarbro, J.W. "Carcinogenesis." *Cancer Nursing Principles and Practice*, edited by C.H. Yarbro, M.H. Frogge, M. Goodman, and S.L. Groenwald. Boston: Jones and Bartlett, 2000, pp.48-59.

PERIODICALS

"A Brisk Walk for Breasts." *Nutrition Action Newsletter* December 2003: 10.
Craig, W., and L. Beck. "Phytochemicals: Health Protective Effects." *Canadian Journal of Dietetic Practice and Research* 60 (1999): 78-84.
"Routine Vitamin Supplementation to Prevent Cancer and Cardiovascular Disease: Receommendations and Rationale." *American Family Physician* 68 (December 15, 2003): 2422.

OTHER

"Cancer Prevention and Early Detection." *American Cancer Society, Inc.* 2009 [cited December 10, 2009]. http://www.cancer.org/downloads/STT/860009.web-6-4-09.pdf.
"Prevention of Cancer PDQ." *CancerNet*. 2000. National Cancer Institute. [cited June 29, 2001]. http://cancernet.nci.nih.gov.

Melinda Granger Oberleitner, RN, DNS

Cancer screening guidelines for men

Definition

Cancer screening guidelines delineate the examinations, laboratory tests, and/or procedures that some or all men should have for detecting common and potentially deadly cancers at early stages when there are no symptoms and the cancers are most treatable. These include screening guidelines for colorectal cancer and possibly prostate and skin cancers. Government agencies, professional organizations, and cancer centers differ somewhat in their screening guidelines.

Purpose

Colorectal cancer (CRC) is a cancer of the colon or rectum. It is the fourth most common cancer diagnosed in the United States and the third-leading cause of cancer-related deaths. It is estimated that 52,010 men will be diagnosed with **colon cancer** in 2009 in the United States and 23,580 men will be diagnosed with **rectal cancer**. It is expected that 25,240 men will die of CRC in 2009. Although colorectal cancer may have no early-warning signs or symptoms, it is often curable if detected early. Studies have indicated that one-third of colorectal cancer deaths could be prevented with early screening. More than 90% of people diagnosed with colorectal cancer are over the age of 50 and the risk increases with age.

Screening also may prevent colorectal cancer. The majority of colorectal cancers begin as the growth of abnormal tissue, called a polyp, on the wall of the colon. It usually takes about 10–15 years for colorectal cancer to develop from the first abnormal cells. Polyps and lesions can be removed before they become malignant, thereby preventing colorectal cancer.

Prostate cancer is the second most common cause of cancer deaths in American men. About one man in six will be diagnosed with prostate cancer during his lifetime. It is estimated that in the United States in 2009 about 192,280 men will be diagnosed with prostate cancer and 27,360 will die of the disease. Most cases of prostate cancer are diagnosed in men aged 65 and older and it is rarely diagnosed in men under 40. It is more common in African-American men and in those with a family history of prostate cancer.

Since the introduction of blood tests for prostate-specific antigen (PSA) in the 1990s, more prostate cancers are being detected before they spread to other organs and become difficult to treat. However

Colorectal cancer screening guidelines for men over 50

Type of exam	Occurrence
Fecal immunochemical test	Annually
Fecal occult blood test	Annually
Flexible sigmoidoscopy	Every 5 years
Virtual colonoscopy	Every 5 years
Colonoscopy	Every 10 years
Double-contrast barium enema	Every 10 years
Stool DNA test	Unknown

(Table by GGS Creative Resources. Reproduced by permission of Gale, a part of Cengage Learning.)

screening for prostate cancer is controversial for several reasons:

- The available tests do not detect all prostate cancers.

- About one-third of positive test results are not cancer.

- The majority of prostate cancers are slow-growing and may never affect a man's health or life expectancy.

- Side effects of prostate cancer treatment, including impotence and incontinence, can be more harmful than the cancer.

Description

Colorectal cancer

There are a variety of screening tests and procedures for CRC and/or polyps and lesions that may develop into CRC. These screens vary greatly in sensitivity and convenience:

- Fecal occult blood testing (FOBT)—also called stool occult blood, hemoccult, or guaiac smear test (gFOBT)—detects occult (hidden) blood in the stool from damaged blood vessels on the surfaces of larger polyps or cancers. The test cannot distinguish between blood from the colon and elsewhere in the gastrointestinal tract, such as the stomach.

- Fecal immunochemical testing (FIT)—sometimes called immunochemical FOBT or immunoassay FOBT (iFOBT)—also detects blood in the stool. Unlike FOBT, food and drugs do not interfere with FIT, sample collection is easier, and FIT is less likely than FOBT to detect bleeding from the upper digestive tract. Like FOBT, FIT may not detect a cancerous tumor that is not bleeding.

- The stool DNA test (sDNA) detects abnormal DNA in the stool from cancer or polyp cells. It is more expensive than FOBT or FIT.

- Flexible sigmoidoscopy uses a flexible lighted tube with a small video camera at the end to examine the inside of the rectum and the lower third of the colon to visualize polyps and lesions and possibly remove them.

- Double-contrast barium enemas are x rays of the rectum and colon.

- Colonoscopy is similar to sigmoidoscopy but examines the entire length of the colon.

- Computed tomographic colonography (CTC) or virtual colonoscopy visualizes the rectum and colon by combining multiple x-ray pictures.

FOBT, FIT, and sDNA primarily detect cancer. Simoidoscopy and **colonoscopy** can detect cancer and can also detect and remove lesions and polyps that may develop into cancer. Colonoscopy is the most sensitive method for detecting and removing lesions, polyps, and cancerous tumors. It is also the most invasive and the most expensive and requires sedation. **Sigmoidoscopy**, barium enemas, colonoscopy, and CTC all require bowel preparation, which many people find both inconvenient and unpleasant; in contrast, stool tests are usually performed at home using a simple kit that is sent to a laboratory for developing. An FOBT performed by a physician during a digital rectal exam (DRE) is not an adequate screen for CRC. Polyps or cancers that are detected by any method other than colonoscopy will require a follow-up colonoscopy.

The U.S. Preventive Services Task Force CRC screening guidelines are as follows:

- People of average risk aged 50–75 should be screened by FOBT or FIT annually and by sigmoidoscopy every five years or colonoscopy every ten years.

- People at higher risk for CRC require more frequent screening.

- Continued screening for those aged 76–85 depends on the patient's health, previous screening results, and life expectancy.

- People over the age of 85 should not be screened.

The American Cancer Society (ACS) guidelines stress the importance of tests that are most likely to find and remove polyps for preventing colorectal cancer. The ACS guidelines for those at average risk for CRC call for one of the following tests beginning at age 50:

- flexible sigmoidoscopy every five years
- colonoscopy every ten years
- double-contrast barium enema every five years
- CTC every five years
- a take-home multiple-sample FOBT every year
- a take-home multiple-sample FIT every year

- an sDNA test, although the appropriate interval is not known

The American College of Gastroenterology guidelines call for a screening colonoscopy every 10 years beginning at age 50 for those at normal risk for CRC or, alternatively, an annual stool blood test and a flexible sigmoidoscopy every three to five years. Those at high risk for CRC should have colonoscopic surveillance, also called screening colonoscopy, at more frequent intervals. Medicare provides for surveillance colonoscopy every two years for those at high risk.

The American College of Gastroenterology calls for African Americans to be screened by colonoscopy every 10 years beginning at age 45. Those with additional risk factors, such as a family history, should be screened more frequently. This is because African Americans tend to be diagnosed with CRC at a younger age and survive for a shorter period of time. There also is some evidence indicating that African Americans have more right-sided polyps and cancers, making colonoscopy of greater benefit.

The University of Texas M. D. Anderson Medical Center guidelines call for one of the following beginning at age 50, in order of preference:

- colonoscopy every ten years
- an annual take-home multiple-sample FOBT or FIT and a flexible sigmoidoscopy every five years
- an annual FOBT or FIT
- flexible sigmoidoscopy every five years
- double-contrast barium enema every five years

People at higher risk for CRC require more frequent and/or more sensitive screening, beginning as early as age 40. Risk factors for CRC include:

- a history of polyps in the colon and/or rectum
- a history of CRC
- a history of inflammatory bowel disease, Crohn's disease, or ulcerative colitis
- a family history (parent, sibling, or child) of CRC, polyposis coli syndrome (numerous colonic polyps), or hereditary CRC syndromes such as familial adenomatous polyposis (FAP) or hereditary non-polyposis colorectal cancer (HNPCC)

Individuals with a significant family history of colorectal polyps or cancer, especially FAP or HNPCC, may have **genetic testing** for known gene mutations that can cause CRC. People with FAP have a lifetime risk of developing CRC of almost 100%, usually before the age of 40. People who test positive for a FAP gene mutation should begin colonoscopy screening as teenagers. People with HNPCC have a

---

QUESTIONS TO ASK YOUR DOCTOR

- Should I be screened for colorectal cancer?
- Is a stool test an adequate screening for me?
- How do I prepare for a colonoscopy?
- Do you recommend that I be screened for prostate cancer?

---

lifetime risk of developing CRC that may be as high as 80%. Members of families known to carry an HNPCC gene mutation who have not been tested or who test positive for the mutation should begin colonoscopy screening during their early 20s.

Prostate cancer

The American Urological Association, the National Comprehensive Cancer Network, and the American Cancer Society advise screening for prostate cancer with both a PSA test and a digital rectal exam (DRE). Blood levels of PSA are often high in men with prostate cancer; however, other prostate conditions can also cause high PSA. A DRE is a physical examination of the lower rectum by a physician, to feel for lumps or other abnormalities in the prostate.

Guidelines for prostate cancer screening vary:

- The National Cancer Institute, the U.S. Preventive Services Task Force, the American College of Preventive Medicine, and the American Academy of Family Physicians have not made recommendations for or against routine prostate cancer screening for low-risk men.
- The American Cancer Society recommends that men 50 years of age and older who have a life expectancy of at least 10 years be offered both a PSA test and a DRE every year.
- The U.S. Preventive Services Task Force has suggested that testing every other year is probably sufficient. They further recommend that both PSA and DRE screening be discontinued at age 75 or in men with a chronic medical condition or a life expectancy of less than 10 years, since the potential harm associated with screening outweighs the benefits for such men.
- For men who decide to be screened, the American Cancer Society and the American Urological Association guidelines call for testing beginning at age 50 for men with average risk and beginning in one's 40s for men with risk factors.

- The National Comprehensive Cancer Network suggests that men who want screening, especially those at increased risk, have a baseline PSA test at age 40.

Men of African descent and those with a father or brother diagnosed with prostate cancer at an early age are considered to be at increased risk. Men with more than one relative affected at an early age are considered to be at high risk.

Skin cancer

Guidelines for **skin cancer** screening involve consulting a physician with regard to any:

- suspicious skin areas
- non-healing sores
- changes in a freckle or mole

Risks

Most cancer screenings carry some risks:

- Stool tests for CRC and the PSA test can yield false positive or false negative results.
- Because sigmoidoscopy and colonoscopy are invasive procedures, there is a small risk of tearing tissue or causing infection. There is also a very small risk of significant bleeding or puncture of the colon or rectum. Rarely, puncture may require surgical repair. Colonoscopy carries more risk of complications than sigmoidoscopy.
- Detection of prostate cancer may not improve health or life expectancy if the cancer has spread to other parts of the body.
- Some prostate cancers may never cause symptoms or become life-threatening, yet treatment for them can result in serious side effects.

See also Testicular self-exam.

Resources

BOOKS

Bellenir, Karen. *Cancer Sourcebook*, 5th ed. Detroit: Omnigraphics, 2007.

Cramer, Scott D. *Prostate Cancer*. New York: Chelsea House, 2007.

Liu, Davis. *Stay Healthy, Live Longer, Spend Wisely: Making Intelligent Choices in America's Health Care System*. Sacramento, CA: Stetho, 2008.

Stokes, Mark. *Colon Cancer: Current and Emerging Trends in Detection and Treatment*. New York: Rosen, 2006.

Walsh, Patrick C., and Janet Farrar Worthington.
Dr. Patrick Walsh's Guide to Surviving Prostate Cancer, 2nd ed. New York: Warner Wellness, 2007.

PERIODICALS

Smith, Robert A., Vilma Cokkinides, and Otis Webb Brawley. "Cancer Screening in the United States, 2008: A Review of Current American Cancer Society Guidelines and Cancer Screening Issues." *Ca: A Cancer Journal for Clinicians* 58, no. 3: 161.

Song, Kyung M. "New Colon-Cancer-Screening Guidelines; Colonoscopies or Similar Exams Recommended/Grant Covers Cost for Some Uninsured." *Seattle Times* (March 31, 2008): B2.

U.S. Preventative Services Task Force. "Screening for Colorectal Cancer: U.S. Preventive Services Task Force Recommendation Statement." *Annals of Internal Medicine* 149, no. 9 (November 4, 2008): 627-637.

OTHER

"Can Colorectal Cancer Be Prevented?" *Cancer Reference Information*. http://www.cancer.org/docroot/CRI/content/CRI_2_4_2X_Can_colon_and_rectum_cancer_be_prevented.asp

"Can Colorectal Cancer and Polyps Be Found Early?" *Cancer Reference Information*. http://www.cancer.org/docroot/CRI/content/CRI_2_4_3X_Can_colon_and_rectum_cancer_be_found_early.asp?rnav=cri

"Cancer Screening Guidelines." *The University of Texas M. D. Anderson Cancer Center*. http://www.mdanderson.org/patient-and-cancer-information/cancer-information/cancer-topics/prevention-and-screening/cancer-screening-guidelines/index.html_early.asp?rnav=cri

"Colon Cancer Prevention & Screening." *American College of Gastroenterology*. http://www.gi.org/patients/women /colon.asp

"Colorectal Cancer Screening." *National Cancer Institute*. http://www.cancer.gov/cancertopics/pdq/screening/colorectal/Patient/page3

"Government Colorectal Cancer Screening Guidelines Updated." *Lab Tests Online*. http://labtestsonline.org/news/colon_screen081117.html

"Prostate Cancer Screening." *National Cancer Institute*. http://www.cancer.gov/cancertopics/pdq/screening/prostate/Patient/page3

"Prostate Cancer Screening: A Decision Guide." *U.S. Centers for Disease Control and Prevention*. http://www.cdc.gov/cancer/prostate/pdf/prosguide.pdf

"Prostate Cancer Screening: A Decision Guide for African Americans." *U.S. Centers for Disease Control and Prevention*. http://www.cdc.gov/cancer/prostate/pdf/aaprosguide.pdf

"Screening Tests for Adults (50 and Up)." *Lab Tests Online*. http://labtestsonline.org/understanding/wellness/e_over50_1.html

ORGANIZATIONS

American Cancer Society, 1599 Clifton Road NE, Atlanta, GA, 30329-4251, (800) ACS-2345, http://www.cancer.org.

American College of Gastroenterology, PO Box 342260, Bethesda, MD, 20827-2260, (301) 263-9000, http://www.acg.gi.org.

American Urological Association, 1000 Corporate Boulevard, Linthicum, MD, 21090, (410) 689-3700, (866) RING AUA (746-4282), (410) 689-3800, aua@AUAnet.org, http://www.auanet.org.

National Cancer Institute, NCI Public Inquiries Office, 6116 Executive Boulevard, Room 3036A, Bethesda, MD, 20006, (800) 4-CANCER, http://www.cancer.gov.

National Comprehensive Cancer Network, 275 Commerce Dr, Suite 300, Fort Washington, PA, 19034, (215) 690-0300, (215) 690-0280, http://www.nccn.org.

U.S. Centers for Disease Control and Prevention, 1600 Clifton Road, Atlanta, GA, 30333, (888) 232-6348, (301) 563-6595, cdcinfo@cdc.gov, http://www.cdc.gov.

Margaret Alic, PhD

Cancer screening guidelines for women

Definition

Cancer screening guidelines outline the examinations, laboratory tests, and/or procedures that some or all women should have for detecting common and potentially deadly cancers at early stages when there may be no symptoms and the cancers are most treatable. The screening guidelines are for breast, cervical, ovarian, colorectal, endometrial, and skin cancers. Government agencies, professional organizations, and cancer centers differ somewhat in their screening guidelines.

Purpose

Almost one in eight women, or 12% of all women, will develop invasive **breast cancer** at some point in their lives. It is estimated that 192,370 cases of invasive breast cancer will be diagnosed in American women in 2009, as well as 62,280 new cases of early-stage non-invasive breast cancer. Breast cancer is the second leading cause of cancer deaths in American women. About 40,170 women will die of the disease in 2009. It is estimated that 16% of breast cancer deaths could be prevented by regular mammogram screenings of women aged 40 and older. Mammograms can detect breast lumps from one to three years before they can be felt.

Before the advent of the Pap test **cervical cancer** was one of the most common causes of cancer deaths among American women; however, most cervical cancer deaths can now be prevented by regular screenings. Cervical cancer is most often diagnosed in women over age 40 and can take several years to develop. Routine screening can identify the cancer at early stages when it is highly curable. Screening also can detect **human papilloma virus** (HPV) **infection**, which is a major risk factor for cervical cancer. HPV types 16 and 18 cause about 70% of all cervical cancers in the United States. Screening also detects precancerous lesions that can be removed, thereby preventing cervical cancer.

Breast and cervical cancer screening guidelines

Type of exam	Recommended age	Occurrence
Breast cancer		
Breast self-exam	20 and older	Regularly
Clinical breast exam	20–39	Every 1–3 years
Mammogram and clinical exam	40 and older	Annually
Cervical cancer		
Liquid-based Pap test	21, or 3 years after first intercourse	Every 2 years
Older-style Pap test	21, or 3 years after first intercourse	Annually
Pap test with HPV DNA test	30 and older	Every 3 years

(Table by GGS Creative Resources. Reproduced by permission of Gale, a part of Cengage Learning.)

Colorectal cancer (CRC) is cancer of the colon or rectum. It is the fourth most common cancer diagnosed in the United States and the third leading cause of cancer-related deaths. It is estimated that 54,090 American women will be diagnosed with **colon cancer** in 2009 and 17,290 women will be diagnosed with **rectal cancer**. It is expected that 24,680 American women will die of CRC in 2009. Colorectal cancer may have no early warning signs or symptoms, but it is often curable if detected early. Studies have indicated that one-third of colorectal cancer deaths could be prevented with early screening. More than 90% of people diagnosed with colorectal cancer are over the age of 50 and the risk increases with age.

Screening can also prevent CRC. The majority of colorectal cancers begin as the growth of abnormal tissue, called a polyp, on the wall of the colon. It usually takes about 10–15 years for CRC to develop from the first abnormal polyp cells. Polyps and lesions can be removed before they become malignant, thereby preventing colorectal cancer.

Description

Breast cancer

General breast cancer screening guidelines are as follows:

- All women should be familiar with the appearance and feel of their breasts and should consult their physicians immediately upon noticing any changes.

- The American Cancer Society (ACS) guidelines include breast self-examinations as an option for women beginning in their twenties.

- All women between the ages of 20 and 39 should have a clinical breast exam performed by a healthcare provider every one to three years.
- Women aged 40 and older should have an annual mammogram and clinical breast exam, preferably at the same time, continuing for as long as they remain in good health. The U.S. Preventive Services Task Force guidelines call for women aged 40 and older to have a screening mammogram, with or without a clinical breast exam, every one to two years.
- Women at increased risk for breast cancer may need to begin mammogram screening at an earlier age, have more frequent exams, or have additional screenings such as ultrasound or magnetic resonance imaging (MRI) of the breasts. Women with a 20% or greater lifetime risk should have alternating mammograms and MRIs every six months. The ACS suggests that women at moderately increased lifetime risk (15–29%) should discuss with their physicians adding an MRI to their yearly mammogram.
- The ACS guidelines call for older women to continue with regular mammograms for as long as they are healthy enough to be candidates for breast cancer treatment.

Women are at increased risk for breast cancer if they:

- have had previous breast cancer
- have a family history of breast cancer
- have a known genetic predisposition for breast cancer

Women with a family history of breast cancer may choose to have genetic screening to determine whether they carry mutations in genes that increase their risk for the disease. The most common genetic causes of breast cancer are mutations in the BRCA1 and BRCA2 genes. Some mutations in these genes can increase a woman's risk of breast cancer to 80%. Breast cancers caused by these mutations tend to occur at an earlier age and in both breasts. Women with these mutations are at higher risk for **ovarian cancer** as well. Genetic screening also can be performed for mutations in certain other genes that increase a woman's risk for breast cancer.

Cervical cancer

General cervical cancer screening guidelines are as follows:

- Women at average risk for cervical cancer should have a liquid-based Pap test every two years, beginning three years after their first vaginal intercourse or at age 21, whichever comes first. If the older-type Pap test is used, screening should be on an annual basis.
- Beginning at age 30, women should have a Pap test and an HPV DNA test every three years.
- Women at higher risk for cervical cancer should be screened annually for as long as they remain in good health.
- Women at lower-than-average risk may be screened less frequently.
- Many older women can stop having Pap and HPV tests altogether. However, most women should continue to have annual pelvic examinations.

Women at higher risk for cervical cancer should be screened more frequently. The ACS guidelines call for annual screenings to continue as long as the woman remains in good health. Women at higher risk include those who:

- have developed new risk factors
- have had abnormal Pap test or HPV test results within the past three years
- were exposed to diethylstilbestrol (DES) before birth
- have had previous cervical cancer
- are infected with HIV or have an otherwise compromised immune system due to an organ transplant, chemotherapy, or chronic steroid use

Women at lower-than-average risk for cervical cancer include those aged 70 or older who have had three consecutive normal Pap tests and no abnormal Pap test results in the past 10 years. Women who have had a total hysterectomy (removal of the cervix and uterus) that was not performed for cancer or precancer of the cervix usually can forego Pap tests as well.

Ovarian cancer

Women with a hereditary ovarian cancer syndrome should have annual or semi-annual pelvic exams, CA-125 blood tests, and possibly **transvaginal ultrasound**, which can detect a mass in the ovaries.

Colorectal cancer

There are a variety of screening tests and procedures for CRC and/or polyps and lesions that may develop into CRC. These screens vary greatly in sensitivity and convenience:

- Fecal occult blood testing (FOBT)—also called stool occult blood, hemoccult, or guaiac smear test (gFOBT)—detects occult (hidden) blood in the stool from damaged blood vessels on the surfaces of larger polyps or cancers. The test cannot distinguish between blood from the colon and elsewhere in the gastrointestinal tract, such as the stomach.

- Fecal immunochemical testing (FIT)—sometimes called immunochemical FOBT or immunoassay FOBT (iFOBT)—also detects blood in the stool. Unlike FOBT, food and drugs do not interfere with FIT, sample collection is easier, and FIT is less likely than FOBT to detect bleeding from the upper digestive tract. Like FOBT, FIT may not detect a cancerous tumor that is not bleeding.
- The stool DNA test (sDNA) detects abnormal DNA in the stool from cancer or polyp cells. It is more expensive than FOBT or FIT.
- Flexible sigmoidoscopy uses a flexible lighted tube with a small video camera at the end to examine the inside of the rectum and the lower third of the colon to visualize polyps and lesions and possibly remove them.
- Double-contrast barium enemas are x rays of the rectum and colon.
- Colonoscopy is similar to sigmoidoscopy but examines the entire length of the colon.
- Computed tomographic colonography (CTC), or virtual colonoscopy, visualizes the rectum and colon by combining multiple x-ray pictures.

FOBT, FIT, and sDNA primarily detect cancer. Simoidoscopy and **colonoscopy** can detect cancer and also can detect and remove lesions and polyps that may develop into cancer. Colonoscopy is the most sensitive method for detecting and removing lesions, polyps, and cancerous tumors. It also is the most invasive and the most expensive and it requires sedation. **Sigmoidoscopy**, barium enemas, colonoscopy, and CTC all require bowel preparation, which many people find both inconvenient and unpleasant; in contrast, stool tests are usually performed at home using a simple kit that is sent to a laboratory for developing. An FOBT performed by a physician during a digital rectal exam (DRE) is not an adequate screen for CRC. Polyps or cancers that are detected by any method other than colonoscopy will require a follow-up colonoscopy.

The U.S. Preventive Services Task Force CRC screening guidelines are as follows:

- People of average risk aged 50–75 should be screened by FOBT or FIT annually and by sigmoidoscopy every five years or colonoscopy every ten years.
- People at higher risk for CRC require more frequent screening.
- Continued screening for those aged 76–85 depends on the patient's health, previous screening results, and life expectancy.
- People over the age of 85 should not be screened.

The ACS guidelines stress the importance of tests that are most likely to find and remove polyps for preventing CRC. The ACS guidelines for those at average risk for CRC call for one of the following tests beginning at age 50:

- flexible sigmoidoscopy every five years
- colonoscopy every ten years
- double-contrast barium enema every five years
- CTC every five years
- a take-home multiple-sample FOBT every year
- a take-home multiple-sample FIT every year
- an sDNA test, although the appropriate interval is not known

The American College of Gastroenterology guidelines call for a screening colonoscopy every 10 years beginning at age 50 for those at normal risk for CRC or, alternatively, an annual stool blood test and a flexible sigmoidoscopy every three to five years. Those at high risk for CRC should have colonoscopic surveillance, also called screening colonoscopy, at more frequent intervals. Medicare provides for surveillance colonoscopy every two years for those at high risk.

The American College of Gastroenterology calls for African Americans to be screened by colonoscopy every 10 years beginning at age 45. Those with additional risk factors, such as a family history, should be screened more frequently. African Americans tend to be diagnosed with CRC at a younger age and survive for a shorter period of time. There also is some evidence indicating that African Americans have more right-sided polyps and cancers, making colonoscopy of greater benefit.

The University of Texas M. D. Anderson Medical Center guidelines call for one of the following beginning at age 50, in order of preference:

- colonoscopy every ten years
- an annual take-home multiple-sample FOBT or FIT and a flexible sigmoidoscopy every five years
- an annual FOBT or FIT
- flexible sigmoidoscopy every five years
- double-contrast barium enema every five years

People at higher risk for CRC require more frequent and/or more sensitive screening, beginning as early as age 40. Risk factors for CRC include:

- a history of polyps in the colon and/or rectum
- a history of CRC
- a history of inflammatory bowel disease, Crohn's disease, or ulcerative colitis

• a family history (parent, sibling, or child) of CRC, polyposis coli syndrome (numerous colonic polyps), hereditary CRC syndromes such as familial adenomatous polyposis (FAP) or hereditary non-polyposis colorectal cancer (HNPCC)

Individuals with a significant family history of colorectal polyps or cancer, especially FAP or HNPCC, may have **genetic testing** for known gene mutations that can cause CRC. People with FAP have a lifetime risk of developing CRC of almost 100%, usually before the age of 40. People who test positive for a FAP gene mutation should begin colonoscopy screening as teenagers. People with HNPCC have a lifetime risk of developing CRC that may be as high as 80%. Members of families known to carry a HNPCC gene mutation who have not been tested or who test positive for a mutation should begin colonoscopy screening during their early 20s.

Endometrial (uterine) cancer

Women with HNPCC or at high risk for HNPCC should have an annual endometrial **biopsy** beginning at age 35 to screen for uterine (endometrial) cancer. The ACS further urges that all women at the time of menopause be informed about the risks for and symptoms of **endometrial cancer** and told to immediately report any unexpected bleeding or spotting.

Skin cancer

Guidelines for **skin cancer** screening include consulting a physician about any:

• suspicious skin areas

• non-healing sores

• changes in a freckle or mole

Risks

Most cancer screening tests carry some risks:

• Mammograms sometimes fail to detect cancerous tissue or detect lumps that are normal breast tissue.

• Pap tests, HIV DNA tests, and stool tests for CRC can yield false positive or false negative results.

• Because sigmoidoscopy and colonoscopy are invasive procedures, there is a small risk of tearing tissue or causing infection. There also is a very small risk of significant bleeding or puncture of the colon or rectum. Rarely, puncture may require surgical repair. Colonoscopy carries more risk of complications than sigmoidoscopy.

QUESTIONS TO ASK YOUR DOCTOR

• How often should I have a mammogram?

• What is my risk of developing breast cancer?

• Should I have additional screenings for breast cancer?

• How often should I have a Pap test?

• What type of Pap test do you perform?

• Should I have an HPV DNA test?

• Should I be screened for ovarian cancer?

• Should I be screened for colorectal cancer?

• Is a stool test an adequate screening for me?

• How do I prepare for a colonoscopy?

Resources

BOOKS

Bellenir, Karen. *Cancer Sourcebook,* 5th ed. Detroit: Omnigraphics, 2007.

Liu, Davis. *Stay Healthy, Live Longer, Spend Wisely: Making Intelligent Choices in America's Health Care System.* Sacramento, CA: Stetho, 2008.

Sutton, Amy L. *Cancer Sourcebook for Women,* 3rd ed. Detroit: Omnigraphics, 2006.

PERIODICALS

Saslow, D., et al., for the American Cancer Society Breast Cancer Advisory Group. "American Cancer Society Guidelines for Breast Screening with MRI as an Adjunct to Mammography." *Ca: A Cancer Journal for Clinicians* 57 (2007): 75-89.

Smith, Robert A., Vilma Cokkinides, and Otis Webb Brawley. "Cancer Screening in the United States, 2008: A Review of Current American Cancer Society Guidelines and Cancer Screening Issues." *Ca: A Cancer Journal for Clinicians* 58, no. 3 (2008): 161.

Song, Kyung M. "New Colon-Cancer-Screening Guidelines; Colonoscopies or Similar Exams Recommended/Grant Covers Cost for Some Uninsured." *Seattle Times* (March 31, 2008): B2.

U.S. Preventative Services Task Force. "Screening for Colorectal Cancer: U.S. Preventive Services Task Force Recommendation Statement." *Annals of Internal Medicine* 149, no. 9 (November 4, 2008): 627-637.

OTHER

"American Cancer Society Guidelines for the Early Detection of Cancer." *American Cancer Society.* http://www.cancer.org/docroot/PED/content/PED_2_3X_ACS_Cancer_ Detection_Guidelines_36.asp?sitearea = PED

"Can Colorectal Cancer Be Prevented?" *Cancer Reference Information.* http://www.cancer.org/docroot/CRI/

content/CRI_2_4_2X_Can_colon_and_rectum_
cancer_be_prevented.asp

"Can Colorectal Cancer and Polyps Be Found Early?"
Cancer Reference Information. http://www.cancer.org/
docroot/CRI/content/CRI_2_4_3X_Can_colon_and
rectum cancer_be_found_early.asp?rnav = cri

"Cancer Screening Guidelines." *The University of Texas M. D.
Anderson Cancer Center.* http://www.mdanderson.org/
patient-and-cancer-information/cancer-information/
cancer-topics/prevention-and-screening/cancer-
screening-guidelines/index.html_early. asp?rnav = cri

"Colon Cancer Prevention & Screening." *American College
of Gastroenterology.* http://www.gi.org/patients/
women/colon.asp

"Colorectal Cancer Screening." *National Cancer Institute.*
http://www.cancer.gov/cancertopics/pdq/screening/
colorectal/Patient/page3

"Government Colorectal Cancer Screening Guidelines
Updated." *Lab Tests Online.* http://labtestsonline.org/
news/colon_screen081117.html

"High-Risk Women Should Stagger Breast Tests."
University of Texas M. D. Anderson Cancer Center.
http://www.mdanderson.org/publications/cancerwise/
archives/2009-march/cancerwise-high-risk-women-
should-stagger-breast-tests.html

"Screening Tests for Adults (50 and Up)." *Lab Tests Online.*
http://labtestsonline.org/understanding/wellness/
e_over50_1.html

ORGANIZATIONS

American Cancer Society, 1599 Clifton Road NE, Atlanta,
GA, 30329-4251, (800) ACS-2345, http://www.cancer.org.

American College of Gastroenterology, PO Box 342260,
Bethesda, MD, 20827-2260, (301) 263-9000, http://
www.acg.gi.org.

National Cancer Institute, NCI Public Inquiries Office, 6116
Executive Boulevard, Room 3036A, Bethesda, MD,
20006, (800) 4-CANCER, http://www.cancer.gov.

Margaret Alic, PhD

Cancer of unknown primary

Definition

Cancer of unknown primary (CUP), also called
carcinoma of unknown primary origin or occult (hidden) primary cancer, is a cancer that has spread or
metastasized to one or more sites in the body, but its
site of origin or **primary site** is unknown.

Demographics

Only about 2–5% of all cancers are of unknown
primary. In the United States every year several thousand people are diagnosed with metastatic CUP. The
exact number is unknown because CUP often is not
reported as a separate category. Furthermore, as diagnostic techniques improve, the incidence of CUP continues to fall.

Description

Cancers are identified by their primary site—the
part of the body where they originated—regardless of
where in the body they have metastasized. Treatment
and prognosis depend, at least in part, on the primary
site. However, in the case of a CUP, the site of origin is
unknown. Often further examinations and tests reveal
the origin of the cancer and it is then renamed and
treated as a cancer of that type. Diagnostic techniques,
especially microscopic techniques, have improved so
dramatically in recent years that the primary cancer
site can now be determined in about 80% of cancers
that are first diagnosed as a CUP. In these cases the
primary cancer site is most often the lung or pancreas,
but it sometimes is the breast, prostate, colon, or
rectum. However, in some cases of CUP, the primary
site is never determined, even by autopsy after death.

Cancers can be classified according to their cell
type as well as their site of origin, and the cell type
may suggest the site of origin. Adenocarcinomas and
squamous cell cancers are the most common types.
Adenocarcinomas develop from gland cells. These are
cells that secrete substances and are found in many
organs of the body. Most cancers of the stomach and
intestines and about 40% of lung cancers are adenocarcinomas. Squamous cell carcinomas are formed by flat
cells resembling cells on the surface of the skin or linings
of some organs. These cancers can start in the mouth,
throat, esophagus, lungs, anus, vagina, and some other
organs. Other types of cancer cells include:

- lymphomas from immune system cells in the lymph
nodes and other organs
- melanomas from the cells that produce skin color
- sarcomas from connective tissue cells such as those in
the tendons, ligaments, muscles, and fat
- germ cell tumors from the testes, ovaries, and parts
of the body where these organs developed in the fetus

Cancer cells also are classified as poorly or well
differentiated. Cancer cells that are very similar to
normal cells of the originating organ are well differentiated. CUPs are often poorly differentiated, meaning that the cancer cells are quite different from
normal cells. Poorly differentiated cancers may be
either lymphomas or **germ cell tumors**. Lymphomas
originate in the lymphatic system (lymph glands and
lymph vessels). Germ cell tumors usually originate in
the ovaries or testes.

CUPs initially are identified as being in one of five broad categories:

- Adenocarcinomas from gland cells account for 60% of CUPs. Common primary sites for adenocarcinomas are the lung, pancreas, breast, prostate, stomach, liver, and colon.
- Poorly differentiated carcinomas, in which the cells are too irregular to identify, account for 30% of CUPs.
- Squamous cell cancers resemble cells on the surface of the skin or lining certain organs. These cancers can start in the mouth, throat, esophagus, lungs, anus, vagina, and some other organs.
- Poorly differentiated malignant neoplasms are cancer cells that are too irregular to identify, but which usually turn out to be lymphomas or carcinomas.
- Neuroendocrine carcinomas are rare cancers that are somewhat similar to nerve and/or endocrine cells that secrete hormones. These account for a small number of CUPs, including some poorly differentiated cancers.

Risk factors

Since CUP encompasses a very diverse group of cancers and the exact cell type is unknown, specific risk factors for CUP have not been identified. However, smoking appears to be an important risk factor, since more than 50% of CUP patients have a history of smoking. Furthermore, autopsies have revealed that many CUPs originate in the lungs, kidneys, pancreas, throat, larynx, or esophagus. Smoking is a risk factor for all such cancers. Some other CUPs have been found to originate in the stomach, colon, rectum, or ovaries. These types of cancers have all been linked to diet, nutrition, and weight. Some cases of CUP are melanomas, an aggressive **skin cancer** for which ultraviolet radiation from sunlight is a major risk factor.

Causes and symptoms

Because CUP includes so many different cancers, it is difficult to define the cause. Cancers often are caused by acquired mutations or changes in DNA—the genetic material of the cell—that occur during a person's lifetime. Acquired mutations that may cause CUP can occur through exposure to tobacco smoke, ultraviolet light, cancer-causing chemicals, radiation, or for no known reason.

Symptoms of CUP depend on the organs to which the cancer has spread. Most often the cancer is first discovered in the lymph nodes, liver, lung, or bone. Possible symptoms of CUP include:

- swollen, firm lymph nodes
- a mass in the abdomen that can be felt or a feeling of "fullness" in the abdomen
- shortness of breath
- chest or abdominal pain
- bone pain
- skin tumors or bumps on the skin, which are often the first sign of metastasized CUP to be noticed
- weakness, fatigue, poor appetite, or weight loss

Diagnosis

Examination

The physician will take a complete medical history including family history, symptoms, and risk factors, followed by a complete physical examination, focusing on parts of the body with symptoms. The pattern of cancer spread often suggests the location of the primary site. If the metastatic cancer is in the upper part of the body, the primary site is likely to be above the diaphragm, such as in the breast or lung. If the metastatic cancer first appears in the lower part of the body, the primary site is likely to be below the diaphragm, such as the liver or pancreas.

Tests

Urine, stool, and blood tests are usually performed. Blood tests may be used to:

- count the different types of blood cells
- measure the levels of various chemicals in the blood to determine the functioning of different organs
- measure the levels of specific serum tumor markers: prostate-specific antigen (PSA) for prostate cancer; CA-125 for ovarian cancer; human chorionic gonadotropin (HCG) for a germ cell tumor; alpha-fetoprotein (AFP) for a germ cell tumor or liver cancer

Tests performed on tumor tissue obtained from a **biopsy** may reveal the primary cancer site:

- Immunohistochemistry can be used to identify certain types of cancer cells. Antibodies that bind to specific proteins on the surfaces of some types of cancer cells are applied to a very thin slice of tissue on a microscope slide. If the protein is present on the cells, the bound antibody changes color.
- Flow cytometry is often used to determine whether cancer in a lymph node is lymphoma and, if so, which type of lymphoma. The cancer cells are treated with specific antibodies and passed by a laser beam. Antibodies that have bound to cancer cells give off a colored light that can be measured.

- Cytogenetic testing examines the cells for chromosomal changes that can cause cancer. The cells must first be grown in the laboratory for about two weeks. Fluorescence in situ hybridization (FISH) uses special fluorescent dyes that recognize specific chromosomal abnormalities and can be performed much faster than standard cytogenetic testing.
- Molecular genetic testing of the DNA in chromosomes uses the polymerase chain reaction (PCR) to find specific chromosomal changes that are too small to be detected by cytogenetic testing.
- Gene expression profiling compares the gene activity in the CUP sample to the gene activities of known cancer cell types to try to identify the type of cancer.
- Electron microscopy, which is hundreds of times more powerful than conventional microscopy, is sometimes used to see miniscule details that may identify the type of cancer cell.

Procedures

Biopsies are usually performed to remove a bit of the tumor for examination under a microscope. The type of biopsy depends on where the tumor is located and other factors:

- fine needle aspiration (FNA) biopsy
- core needle biopsy
- a CT-guided needle biopsy
- excisional biopsy
- incisional biopsy
- thoracentesis for fluid in the chest
- paracentesis for fluid in the abdomen
- bone marrow aspiration and biopsy

After the pathologist has classified the CUP into one of the five broad categories on the basis of test results, a variety of further tests and procedures may be performed to try to classify the cancer more precisely and determine its origin. Diagnostic procedures also are used to stage the cancer or determine how far it has spread and to determine the effectiveness of treatments. These further diagnostic procedures may include:

- x rays
- computed tomography (CT) scans
- magnetic resonance imaging (MRI)
- ultrasound
- positron emission tomography (PET) scans
- endoscopy, in which a tube-like instrument is used to examine the inside of the body

Staging

Since the staging system depends on the type of cancer, it is not possible to stage a cancer of unknown primary. However, since all CUPs have spread beyond their primary site, they are at least stage II and most are stage III or IV.

Based on where in the body the cancer is found, where it is believed to have originated, histology of the cancer cells, and other factors, CUP is sometimes classified into one of the following groups:

- cancer in the cervical lymph nodes of the neck area
- poorly differentiated carcinomas
- metastatic melanoma spread to lymph nodes in only one part of the body, called a single nodal site
- cancer spread only to the lymph nodes in the area of the armpits, called isolated axillary metastasis
- cancer spread to the lymph nodes in the groin area, called inguinal node metastasis
- cancer spread to several different parts of the body, called multiple involvement

Treatment

Traditional

Treatment of a CUP is based on the appearance of the cancer under a microscope (the histology), the results of lab tests, and the organs to which the cancer has spread. If the cancer is confined to the lymph nodes or a single organ, a CUP may be treated with surgery. Surgery may be followed by **radiation therapy** and possibly **chemotherapy**. For cancer that has spread extensively, radiation therapy may be used to relieve symptoms.

Drugs

Chemotherapy is often used to treat CUP. For advanced CUP, chemotherapy may be the primary treatment. If the CUP is likely to be a germ cell tumor or certain types of **lymphoma**, chemotherapy may successfully shrink or destroy the tumors. In other cases chemotherapy is used to relieve symptoms. Combination chemotherapy is usually used to treat CUP:

- Adenocarcinomas and poorly differentiated cancers are usually treated with a platinum drug (cisplatin or carboplatin) and a taxane drug (paclitaxel or docetaxel). Gemcitabine, etoposide, and irinotecan also may be used.
- Squamous cell cancer is usually treated with cisplatin, 5-fluorouracil (5-FU), and a taxane (paclitaxel or docetaxel).
- Neuroendocrine carcinomas are usually treated with a platinum drug (cisplatin or carboplatin) and etoposide.

QUESTIONS TO ASK YOUR DOCTOR

- Should I have extensive testing to categorize or identify my CUP?
- What type of CUP do you believe I have?
- How extensive is my cancer?
- What are my treatment options?
- What treatment do you recommend and why?
- Are there clinical trials that may be appropriate for me?
- What will my treatment involve?
- What are the likely side effects of my treatment?
- What is my prognosis?

If the CUP is likely to be a breast or **prostate cancer** it may be treated with hormone therapy. **Breast cancer** hormone therapy utilizes drugs such as **tamoxifen** and **aromatase inhibitors** (anastrozole, letrozole, and exemestane), which either lower estrogen levels or prevent the cancer cells from utilizing estrogen. Luteinizing hormone-releasing hormone (LHRH) agonists, such as leuprolide and goserelin, and anti-androgens, such as flutamide and bicalutamide, are used to treat prostate cancer. These drugs either lower **testosterone** levels or prevent the cancer cells from utilizing testosterone.

Pain is an important concern with CUP. For most patients morphine or other opioid drugs can relieve pain without interfering significantly with normal daily functioning.

Prognosis

Because CUP includes so many different types of cancer, it is difficult to make a prognosis. Some CUPs can be treated effectively and even cured; however, most CUPs are so advanced that treatment is unlikely to be effective in the long term. Including all types of CUP, the average survival time is 9–12 months from diagnosis. Individual survival time varies greatly depending on the cancer cell type, the degree of **metastasis**, the patient's general health, and response to treatment.

CUPs tend to be particularly dangerous cancers because:

- They have already metastasized at diagnosis, so curative treatments are often not available.
- Since the exact type of cancer is unknown, it can be difficult to choose the best treatment.
- They are often fast-growing and/or fast-spreading cancers.

Prevention

By definition CUP is never diagnosed at an early stage. Although screening tests are available for a few of the cancers that can lead to CUP, there are no early screening tests for lung, pancreatic, stomach, or kidney cancers—the most common causes of cancer of unknown primary.

Since CUP includes so many different types of cancer, there are no specific preventions. However, lifestyle changes can reduce one's risk for many types of cancer, including CUP. One out of three cancer deaths are believed to be the direct result of smoking, and not smoking reduces the risk for many cancers, including CUP. Approximately one out of three cancer deaths also are caused by factors linked to body weight, nutrition, and physical activity. Maintaining a healthy weight, a healthy diet emphasizing plant-based foods, physical activity, and limited consumption of alcohol reduces the risk of CUP, as well as other cancers.

Resources

BOOKS

Bellenir, Karen. *Cancer Sourcebook*, 5th ed. Detroit: Omnigraphics, 2007.

Fizazi, Karim. *Carcinoma of an Unknown Primary Site*. New York: Taylor & Francis, 2006.

Greco, F. A., and J. D. Hainsworth. "Cancer of Unknown Primary Site." In: Devita, V. T., T. S. Lawrence, and S. A. Rosenberg, eds. *DeVita, Hellman, and Rosenberg's Cancer: Principles and Practice of Oncology*, 8th ed. Philadelphia: Lippincott Williams & Wilkins, 2008.

Wick, Mark R., ed. *Metastatic Carcinomas of Unknown Origin*. New York: Demos, 2008.

PERIODICALS

Hainsworth, J. D., et al. "Phase II Trial of Bevacizumab and Erlotinib in Carcinomas of Unknown Primary Site: The Minnie Pearl Cancer Research Network." *Journal of Clinical Oncology* 25 (2007): 1747-1752.

Pollack, Andrew. "Genetic Tests May Pinpoint Cancers' Sources." *International Herald Tribune* (March 12, 2009): 8.

Seve, P., et al. "The Influence of Comorbidities, Age, and Performance Status on the Prognosis and Treatment of Patients with Metastatic Carcinomas of Unknown Primary Site." *Cancer* 106 (2006): 2058-2066.

OTHER

"Cancer of Unknown Primary Origin." *National Cancer Institute*. http://www.cancer.gov/cancertopics/factsheet/Sites-Types/unknownprimary (accessed November 3, 2009).

"Carcinoma of Unknown Primary Treatment (PDQ)." *National Cancer Institute*. http://www.cancer.gov/cancertopics/pdq/treatment/unknownprimary/patient/#Section_2 (accessed November 3, 2009).

"Detailed Guide: Cancer of Unknown Primary." *American Cancer Society* (October 15, 2009) http://www.cancer.org/docroot/cri/content/cri_2_4_1x_what_is_cancer_of_unknown_primary_58.asp?sitearea = cri (accessed November 3, 2009).

ORGANIZATIONS

American Cancer Society, 1599 Clifton Road NE, Atlanta, GA, 30329-4251, (800) ACS-2345, http://www.cancer.org.

National Cancer Institute, NCI Public Inquiries Office, 6116 Executive Boulevard, Room 3036A, Bethesda, MD, 20006, (800) 4-CANCER, http://www.cancer.gov.

Margaret Alic, PhD

Cancer therapy, palliative

Definition

Palliative **cancer** therapy is treatment specifically designed to help improve symptoms at the end of life associated with advanced and/or terminal cancer. Palliative care has evolved to become an integral component of cancer care and is typically provided by a team of multidisciplinary health care professionals.

Demographics

Currently, it is estimated that approximately 40% of patients diagnosed with cancer—about 550,000 people per year in the United States—will die from their cancer. The end-of-life care of many of these patients will be delivered by professionals skilled in hospice or palliative cancer care.

Description

Palliative care is directed at improving symptoms associated with advanced and incurable cancer. The five major precepts of palliative care, which were delineated as part of the Robert Wood Johnson Foundation-funded Last Acts campaign to improve quality of care at the end of life, include:

- respect for patient wishes and goals related to end-of-life decisions
- provision of comprehensive end-of-life care
- integration of care delivery from a multidisciplinary perspective
- incorporating the caregiver in to the plan of care at the end of life
- developing adequate support systems for the patient, caregiver, and family

Palliative care can include surgery, **radiation therapy**, **chemotherapy**, hormone therapy, and other specialized therapies, as well as treatment of symptoms resulting from cancer, and providing relief from side effects of treatment. The primary objective of palliative care is to improve the quality of the remainder of a patient's life. Treatment usually involves a combination of modalities (multimodality approach) and numerous specialists typically are involved in the treatment planning process. Therapeutic planning usually involves careful coordination with the treatment team. The approach to palliative care also involves easing psychosocial problems and typically incorporates an emphasis on the patient's family.

Causes and symptoms

Some signs of advanced cancer include extreme **fatigue** and weakness that is progressive, unexplained **weight loss**, pain, and shortness of breath, especially if the cancer has spread to the lungs.

There is the potential for a wide range of symptoms as the cancer progresses to the advanced or terminal phase. These symptoms include pain, myoclonus, dyspnea, anxiety, delirium, and noisy breathing or "rattle" among a variety of other symptoms.

Pain is one of the common symptoms associated with cancer. Approximately 75% of terminal cancer patients have pain. Pain is a subjective symptom and thus it cannot be measured using technological approaches. Pain can be assessed using numeric scales (from 1 to 10, 1 is rated as no pain while 10 is severe) or by rating specific facial expressions associated with various levels of pain. The majority of cancer patients experience pain as a result of tumor mass that compresses neighboring nerves, bone, or soft tissues, or from direct nerve injury (neuropathic pain). Pain can occur from affected nerves in the ribs, muscles, and internal structures such as the abdomen (cramping type pain associated with obstruction). Many patients also experience various types of pain as a direct result of follow-up tests, treatments (surgery, radiation, and chemotherapy) and diagnostic procedures (i.e., **biopsy**).

Diagnosis

Patients typically are informed that their diagnosis is terminal and treatments are directed to improve quality of life and ease suffering at the end of life.

Examination

The physician may perform a physical examination to help confirm advanced cancer based on the signs and symptoms the patient is experiencing.

Results of this physical exam may include evidence of fluid in the lungs or abdominal area. An enlarged liver may be palpated by the physician, or external lumps that are comprised of tumor may be able to be seen and palpated on various areas of the body.

Tests

Blood test results that may confirm advanced cancer include elevated levels of **tumor markers** in the blood, elevated liver function tests and liver enzymes, and elevated or decreased white blood cells, red blood cells, and/or platelets, among other findings.

Imaging tests such as x rays and CT, MRI, PET, bone, and ultrasound scans may be conducted to determine the location and spread of the cancer.

A comprehensive palliative care assessment should be conducted to evaluate the following:

- benefits and risks associated with continuing treatments and therapies directed at controlling the cancer
- physical symptoms and problems such as pain, anorexia, dyspnea, nausea/vomiting, constipation, fatigue, weakness, alterations with sleep, and delirium, as well as other problems
- psychosocial symptoms and problems including spiritual needs
- the patient's and family's goals and wishes related to end-of-life care
- educational level to determine information needs and requirements
- the impact of cultural beliefs on preferences related to end-of-life care

Treatment

Surgery can be utilized for palliation after careful evaluation and planning. The use of surgery in these cases may reduce the tumor bulk and help improve the quality of life by relieving pain, alleviating obstruction, or controlling bleeding. Radiation therapy for terminal cancer patients can also alleviate pain, bleeding, and obstruction of neighboring areas. A combination of radiation therapy and bisphosphanates offers palliative relief to patients with metastatic bone disease (metastatic disease is cancer that has spread beyond the original site or organ to other areas of the body). Chemotherapy may be helpful to reduce tumor size and provide some reduction to metastatic disease. Long-term chemotherapy patients develop **drug resistance**, a situation that renders chemotherapeutic treatments ineffective. If this occurs, patients usually are given a second-line medication or, if admission criteria are met, they may participate in an experimental research protocol. Palliative

treatments and terminal cancer in combination can cause many symptoms that can become problematic. These symptoms commonly include pain, **nausea**, **vomiting**, difficulty breathing, constipation, dehydration, agitation, and delirium. The palliative treatment-planning goal focuses on reducing these symptoms.

Surgery for tumor removal, biopsy, or size reduction is associated with postoperative pain and local nerve damage, which may be both severe and difficult to alleviate. Chemotherapy and radiation therapy also can produce nerve damage and severe pain. Additionally, patients with malignant cancer are susceptible to infections such as herpes, **pneumonia**, urinary tract infections, and wound abscess, all of which can cause severe pain. Pain associated with cancer and/or treatments can significantly impair the patient's abilities to perform daily tasks and hence impair quality of life. These complications may negatively impact the patient's psychological well-being.

Drugs

Drugs that may be used in palliative care include:

- opioids, benzodiazepines, glycopyrrolate, and scopolamine—used to treat dyspnea in advanced cancer
- appetite stimulants such as megestrol acetate, medroprogesterone acetate, and steroids—used to ameliorate the effects of anorexia/cachexia
- antiemetics such as prochlorperazine, haloperidol, metoclorpramide, 5-HT3 receptor antagonists, and others—used to treat nausea and vomiting

- biscodyl, glycerine suppositories, polyethylene glycol, lactulose, magnesium hydroxide, magnesium cirate, and/or methylnaltrexone—used to treat constipation in advanced cancer
- haloperidol, risperidone, olanzapine, or quetiapine fumarate—used in the treatment of delirium at the end of life

Prognosis

Palliative cancer care is typically offered to patients with six months to one year of life expectancy.

Prevention

Currently, the only way to prevent a cancer from spreading and developing into an advanced or incurable cancer is to detect the cancer prior to metastatic spread and to initiate treatment for the cancer as soon as possible after diagnosis.

Resources

BOOKS

Esper, P. "Principles and Issues in Palliative Care." In *Cancer Nursing Principles and Practice,* Yarbro, C.H., Frogge, M.H., & Goodman, M. 6th Ed. Boston, MA: Jones and Bartlett Publishers, 2005.

Paice, J. "Delivery of Comfort Care." In *Cancer Nursing Principles and Practice, Yarbro, C.H.,* Frogge, M.H., & Goodman, M. 6th Ed. Boston, MA: Jones and Bartlett Publishers, 2005.

PERIODICALS

"Bisphosphanates, Radiation Therapy Can be Used for Metastatic Bone Disease." *Cancer Weekly* October 28, 2003: 112.

Cimino, James E. "The Role of Nutrition in Hospice and Palliative Care of the Cancer Patient." *Topics in Clinical Nutrition* July-September 2003: 154–158.

Chochinov, H.M. "Dying, Dignity, and New Horizons in Palliative End-of-Life Care." *CA: A Cancer Journal for Clinicians* 56(2006):84–103.

Holland, J.C., Andersen, B., & Breitbark, W.S., et al. "Distress Management." *Journal of the National Comprehensive Cancer Network* 5(2007): 66–98.

OTHER

"Overview: Advanced Cancer." *American Cancer Society Cancer Reference Information.* February 26, 2009. http://www.cancer.org/docroot/CRI/content/CRI_2_2_3X_Advanced_Cancer_Overview [cited September 7, 2009].

"Palliative Care." *National Comprehensive Cancer Network Practice Guidelines in Oncology – v.1.2009.* http://www.nccn.org./professionals/physician_gls/PDF/palliative.pdf [cited September 7, 2009].

ORGANIZATIONS

American Cancer Society. http://www.cancer.org.

American Pain Society. http://www.ampainsoc.org.

National Cancer Institute. http://www.cancer.gov.

Laith Farid Gulli, M.D.
Nicole Mallory, M.S.
Melinda Granger Oberleitner, R.N., D.N.S., A.P.R.N., C.N.S.

▌Capecitabine

Definition

Capecitabine (brand name Xeloda) is a drug that interferes with the growth of **cancer** cells.

Purpose

Capecitabine is used to treat **breast cancer** and cancer of the colon and rectum (colorectal cancer) that has spread to other parts of the body (metastasized).

Description

Capecitabine is a type of medicine known as an antimetabolite because it interferes with the metabolism and growth of cells. Capecitabine is an unusual anti-cancer drug in that it is most active in cancer cells; normal cells are exposed to far lower concentrations of the drug. Cancer cells convert capecitabine into another anti-cancer drug called 5-fluorouracil (**fluorouracil**). This substance prevents cells from growing and reproducing by interfering with the production of DNA and RNA. Eventually the cells die.

Capecitabine has been approved by the U.S. Food and Drug Administration for the treatment of metastasized breast cancer that is resistant to standard **chemotherapy**. Capecitabine may be used in combination with the drug **docetaxel** (Taxotere). A recent study found that the combination of docetaxel and capecitabine improves survival in women with metastatic breast cancer without a significant increase in treatment-related side effects.

An earlier study found that capecitabine is as effective as 5-fluorouracil for treating metastasized colorectal cancer, and has fewer and less severe side effects. However, it does not increase the average survival time of approximately 13 months.

Recommended dosage

The dosage of capecitabine depends on a number of factors including body size. The average dosage is

2,500 mg per square meter of body surface area per day. Capecitabine is a pill that is taken with water within 30 minutes after a meal. It may be taken every 12 or 24 hours. For colorectal cancer, capecitabine may be administered for two weeks, followed by one week off, for a total of 30 weeks.

Precautions

Capecitabine can temporarily reduce the number of white blood cells, thus reducing the body's ability to fight **infection**. It is very important to avoid exposure to infections and to receive prompt medical treatment if exposed. Immunizations (vaccinations) should be avoided during or after treatment with capecitabine. It also is important to avoid contact with individuals who have recently taken an oral polio vaccine.

Capecitabine may temporarily reduce the number of blood platelets that are necessary for blood clotting. The risk of bleeding may be reduced by:

- using caution when cleaning teeth
- avoiding dental work
- avoiding cuts, bruises, or other injuries

Capecitabine can cause birth defects and fetal death in animals. Therefore, this drug should not be taken by pregnant women or by either a man or woman at the time of conception. Because capecitabine may cause serious side effects, women usually are advised against breast-feeding while taking this drug.

Some individuals may have an allergic reaction to capecitabine. Allergies to foods, preservatives, or dyes, or to the drug 5-fluorouracil, must be considered before this drug is prescribed.

Side effects

Common side effects of capecitabine may include:

- loss of appetite (**anorexia**)
- **diarrhea**
- **nausea and vomiting**
- stomach or abdominal pain
- swelling, peeling, redness, or blistering of hands and feet
- numbness, pain, itching, or tingling in hands and feet

- pain, swelling, or sores in the mouth or on the lips
- rashes or dry skin
- fatigue or weakness due to reduced red blood cell count

The treatment is stopped if side effects are severe enough to interfere with eating or other normal activities.

Less common or rare side effects of capecitabine may include:

- constipation
- cough or hoarseness
- difficulty swallowing
- shortness of breath
- chest pain
- blood pressure changes
- fast or irregular heartbeat
- pain or swelling of the ankles, legs, or stomach
- poor coordination, dizziness
- changes in fingernails or toenails
- headache
- heartburn
- sensitivity to sunlight
- muscle pain
- eye irritation
- insomnia
- lower back or side pain
- painful or difficult urination
- loss of fingerprints

Side effects of capecitabine may include symptoms of infection, such as **fever**, chills, sore throat, or swollen glands, or symptoms of liver malfunction. Side effects also may include unusual bleeding or bruising due to the reduction in blood platelets.

Other diseases or medical conditions may increase the side effects associated with capecitabine. Chicken pox or shingles (**Herpes zoster**) may become severe and spread to other parts of the body. If heart, kidney, or liver disease is present, the side effects related to these organs may be more severe. In addition, in the presence of liver disease, the amount of capecitabine in the body may be higher. Individuals over the age of 80 often experience more severe side effects with capecitabine.

Interactions

Other drugs that may interact with capecitabine include:

- Amphotericin B (Fungizone)
- Antithyroid drugs that are used to treat an overactive thyroid

- Azathioprine (Imuran)
- Chloramphenicol (Chloromycetin)
- Colchicine
- Flucytosine (Ancobon)
- Ganciclovir (Cytovene)
- Interferon (Intron A, Roferon-A)
- Plicamycin (Mithracin)
- Zidovudine (AZT, Retrovir)

Coumadin-type anticoagulants that are used to thin the blood and medicines containing aspirin can increase the chances of bleeding. **Folic acid**, alone or in a multivitamin, may increase the side effects of capecitabine. Finally, capecitabine can increase the effects on the blood of other cancer medicines or **radiation therapy**.

Resources

PERIODICALS

"Docetaxel and Capecitabine Improve Survival in Metastatic Breast Cancer." *Drug Week* October 10, 2003: 57.

"Fingerprints May Vanish with Cancer Drug." *U.S. News & World Report*, May 27, 2009. http://health.usnews.com/articles/health/healthday/2009/05/27/Fingerprints-may-vanish-with-cancer-drug.html.

Margaret Alic, Ph.D.

Capsaicin

Definition

Capsaicin is the active ingredient in chili peppers, the substance that gives chili and cayenne its heat. In its purified form it is a crystalline alkaloid.

Purpose

Research on the use of capsaicin for **cancer** patients has focused on several areas:

- its ability to decrease pain
- its potential to be carcinogenic
- any chemoprotective capacity
- any antimicrobial and detoxification properties

Description

Folk accounts of capsaicin's medicinal properties in the form of cayenne have included aiding digestion, promoting the sweating process to create cooling (for reducing a **fever**), fighting infections, and stimulating the

KEY TERMS

Alkaloid—Any of a large group of bitter-tasting alkaline substances containing nitrogen that are found in plants. Capsaicin is an example of an alkaloid.

Bioavailability—A term used in describing the amount of a medication taken that is actively available to the targeted body area. Bioavailability can be affected by factors such as the rate at which a tablet or capsule dissolves, binding products used in formulating the medication, and the person's ability to break down and use the medication.

Carcinogenic—A substance that can cause cancer to develop.

Mucositis—An inflammation of the lining of the digestive tract, often accompanied by mouth and throat lesions.

Neuropathic pain—Pain that is felt near the surface of the skin, along nerve pathways.

Neurotoxic—A substance that is harmful to the nervous system.

function of the kidneys, lungs, stomach, and heart. Research on capsaicin's ability to decrease pain has been in the areas of chronic pain, arthritic pain, migraine pain, sports injuries, and neuropathic cancer pain. It appears to interfere with chemicals that facilitate pain messages to the brain. Capsaicin has a hyperemic effect, which means that it increases blood flow similar to when an area is inflamed. When applied to the skin in cream form, the area becomes red, warm, and may become slightly swollen. Many individuals experience a localized burning sensation when a cream containing capsaicin is applied to the skin. However, with repeated use, the burning sensation usually disappears, and pain relief is noted. The burning or stinging sensation may last a few weeks for some. Capsaicin appears to work through a mechanism that initially causes a hypersensitivity to pain, and then ends in pain relief.

Several clinical studies performed on the effectiveness of various formulations of capsaicin have demonstrated that a majority of patients experience a reduction in pain and few or minor side effects. Capsaicin has been reported to have an effect against *H. pylori*, and also some antimicrobial properties. It appears to protect the lining of the digestive tract from harm due to aspirin use. Capsaicin has also showed an inhibitory effect on skin **carcinogenesis** in mice and a suppression of proliferation of human cancer cells.

Early studies on capsaicin raised the concern that capsaicin could be carcinogenic. However, further studies reported that capsaicin was not carcinogenic, and in fact might have chemoprotective properties. Studies investigating its potential to promote tumor development indicate it does not have this ability.

Recommended dosage

The Physician's Desk Reference (PDR) for Herbal Medicines indicates the availability of the following dosages of cayenne:

- Capsules: 400, 445, 450, 455, and 500 mg strengths
- Cream containing 0.25% and 0.75% capsaicin
- Liquid alcohol-based extract

The average daily dose in capsule form for cayenne (capsicum annum) is 30 to 120 mg. Individuals wishing to use capsaicin should do so under the guidance of a practitioner knowledgeable about its properties, to ensure proper monitoring for any adverse reactions.

Precautions

Capsaicin's fiery nature requires some precautions to be used when handling it in its natural form or when applying it topically as a cream. Thorough hand washing after contact with it is necessary, as it can cause an intense burning or stinging sensations. Avoid any contact with mucous membranes, such as eyes or mouth, or any open wounds, until hands have been washed. Bottles storing capsaicin or cayenne should be well sealed and kept out of the light. It should not be refrigerated.

The National Cancer Institute (NCI) cautions that it is not known whether capsaicin used by a breast-feeding mother will pass into the breast milk. Individuals who have had an allergic reaction to hot peppers should speak to their health care provider before using capsaicin. Some individuals may experience a prolonged burning sensation with topical capsaicin. However, the NCI states that reducing the number of doses per day will not result in decreasing the sensation and may prolong the time period over which the sensation is experienced. In addition, a reduction in the number of doses may also reduce the degree of pain relief. Patients taking capsaicin should not double-up on a dose if a dose is missed.

Side effects

Research on capsaicin is still in the early stages, but the following side effects have been reported:

- hypersensitivity reaction such as anaphylaxis and rhinoconjunctivitis
- abnormal blood clotting ability

- an increase in bowel function, leading to diarrhea
- blister formation on the skin
- contact dermatitis
- increase in cough with extended exposure to chili peppers
- long-term use of high dosages can lead to kidney and liver damage, chronic gastritis, and neurotoxic effects

Interactions

If aspirin and capsicum annum extract (in the form of 100 mg of capsaicin) are taken at the same time, decreased bioavailability of aspirin may occur. This treatment may interfere with MAO inhibitors and antihypertensive therapy. As with any medication, patients should notify their physician of any prescription, over-the-counter, or herbal remedies they are taking prior to receiving treatment.

Resources

BOOKS

Beers, Mark H., MD, and Robert Berkow, MD, editors. "Neuropathic Pain." Section 14, Chapter 167 In *The Merck Manual of Diagnosis and Therapy*. Whitehouse Station, NJ: Merck Research Laboratories, 2002.

PERIODICALS

Annals of the New York Academy of Sciences 889 (1999): 157–92.
Bolin, D. J. "Transdermal Approaches to Pain in Sports Injury Management." *Current Sports Medicine Reports* 2 (December 2003): 303–309.
Cancer Letters 164, no. 2 (March 26, 2001): 119–26.
Mutation Research 428, no. 1–2 (July 16, 1999): 305–27.
Rock, E., and A. DiMichele. "Nutritional Approaches to Late Toxicities of Adjuvant Chemotherapy in Breast Cancer Survivors." *Journal of Nutrition* 133, no. 11, Supplement 1 (November 2003): 3785S–3793S.

Esther Csapo Rastegari, R.N., B.S.N., Ed.M.
Rebecca J. Frey, PhD

Carbamazepine

Definition

Carbamazepine (Tegretol, Carbatrol) may be administered to **cancer** patients as a pain medicine.

Purpose

Carbamazepine is given to cancer patients primarily as a pain medication. The drug may, for example, be

KEY TERMS

Anticonvulsant—A type of medication given to prevent seizures. Carbamazepine is an anticonvulsant.

Bipolar disorder—A mood disorder in which the patient experiences both periods of mania and periods of depression.

Bone marrow— The spongy tissue found in the large bones of the body.

Trigeminal neuralgia—A nerve problem associated with pain.

prescribed for stabbing pain that moves along a nerve. For noncancer patients, it is often used to treat epilepsy or bipolar disorder (manic-depressive illness). Carbamazepine is classified as an anticonvulsant because it is often given to control seizures.

Description

Carbamazepine suppresses some of the activities of the nerves. It does this by delaying the amount of time it takes for certain passageways in the nerves to recover after they have sent out a message.

Recommended dosage

Carbamazepine comes in several forms. There are 200 mg tablets, 100 mg chewable tablets, and a liquid containing 20 mg per milliliter that may be swallowed. There are extended-release tablets of carbamazepine containing 100, 200, or 400 mg and extended release capsules of the medication containing 200 and 300 mg.

Some authorities recommend starting with 100 to 200 mg twice a day. This strategy helps to minimize side effects. Then, the dose may be gradually increased every week. Adults may eventually receive 600 to 1,200 mg a day, while 20 to 30 mg per kg of body weight per day is appropriate for children.

Side effects

Carbamazepine may exhibit side effects to the nervous system, such as, drowsiness, dizziness, blurred vision, unsteadiness, **depression**, impaired concentration, and headache. Patients should be cautious about operating machinery or performing tasks requiring alertness until tolerant of the side effects. After several weeks of treatment, these side effects may disappear. To minimize these side effects, doctors may start carbamazepine at a low dose and may recommend that it be taken before bedtime. As carbamazepine may cause

stomach upset and **nausea**, the medicine should be taken with meals.

Effects of carbamazepine may include bone marrow suppression, which involves a low white blood cell and platelet count, but this is usually not severe. Very rarely, a dangerous **anemia** may occur during carbamazepine therapy. Blood counts should be monitored for patients using this drug. Some patients with previously diagnosed depression of the bone marrow should not be given carbamazepine.

Carbamazepine may cause birth defects and should be avoided in women who are pregnant. In addition, women sometimes develop hypersensitivity reactions to carbamazepine during pregnancy. An appropriate contraceptive method should be used while on carbamazepine. Carbamazepine can cross into breast milk and should be avoided in women who are breast-feeding. Carbamazepine may also cause rash or sensitivity to the sun.

Interactions

Carbamazepine may affect the activity of other medicines, including oral contraceptives, **warfarin**, theophylline, doxycycline, haloperidol, **corticosteroids**, valproate, clonazepam, ethosuximide, lamotrigine, felbamate, and thyroid hormones. Oral contraceptives may become less effective if a patient is taking carbamazepine. Some doctors recommend that the form of birth control pill be altered or that a different method of contraception be used. If **phenytoin** and phenobarbital are taken at the same time as carbamazepine, the capacity of carbamazepine to interact with additional medications may increase. Side effects may occur if a patient is taking carbamazepine and one of the following medications simultaneously: **danazol**, dextropropoxyphene, erythromycin, clarithromycin, isoniazid, verapamil, or diltiazem. Due to the numerous potential of interactions with other drugs, patients should consult with their physician or pharmacist prior to starting any new medications either bought over the counter or initiated by another physician. Patients taking carbamazepine should not drink grapefruit juice.

Carbamazepine sometimes complicates the treatment of **brain tumors** because it can lower the blood level of other drugs given to stop the growth of the tumor. Researchers are currently exploring the use of newer anticonvulsant drugs in treating patients with brain tumors.

Carbamazepine has also been reported to interact with certain herbs, including evening primrose (*Oenothera biennis*), gingko (*Gingko biloba*), and wormwood (*Artemisia pontica*). Patients should always tell their doctor about any herbal preparations they may be taking as well as other prescription medications.

Resources

PERIODICALS

Deering, S. H., K. Thompson, J. Taylor, and N. Hueppchen. "Anticonvulsant Hypersensitivity Reaction in Pregnancy." *Obstetrics and Gynecology* 102 (November 2003): 1215–1217.

Misra, U. K., J. Kalita, and C. Rathore. "Phenytoin and Carbamazepine Cross-Reactivity: Report of a Case and Review of Literature." *Postgraduate Medical Journal* 79 (December 2003): 703–704.

Vecht, C. J., G. L. Wagner, and E. B. Wilms. "Treating Seizures in Patients with Brain Tumors: Drug Interactions Between Antiepileptic and Chemotherapeutic Agents." *Seminars in Oncology* 30 (December 2003): 49–52.

Wang, P. W., T. A. Ketter, O. V. Becker, and C. Nowakowska. "New Anticonvulsant Medication Uses in Bipolar Disorder." *CNS Spectrums* 8 (December 2003): 930–2, 941–7.

ORGANIZATIONS

United States Food and Drug Administration (FDA). 5600 Fishers Lane, Rockville, MD 20857-0001. (888) INFO-FDA (463-6332). http://www.fda.gov.

Bob Kirsch
Rebecca J. Frey, PhD

Carboplatin

Definition

Carboplatin is a chemotherapeutic agent used to treat **cancer** by interfering with the growth of cancer cells. At the molecular level, carboplatin causes cancer cells to destroy themselves through the mechanism of apoptosis. Carboplatin is marketed under the brand name Paraplatin; it may also be referred to as CBDCA, JM-8, or carboplatinum.

Purpose

Carboplatin was approved in 1989 by the Food and Drug Administration (FDA) for the palliative treatment of **ovarian cancer**. The term palliative means that the treatment is not intended to cure but only to relieve symptoms. Carboplatin has also been used to treat other types of cancer, including head and neck cancer, **cervical cancer**, lung cancer, **endometrial cancer**, **testicular cancer**, hormone-refractory **prostate cancer**, and **brain tumors**.

More recently, carboplatin has been investigated in **clinical trials** as a possible treatment for squamous cell skin cancers and malignant **melanoma**.

Description

Carboplatin is a member of the group of **chemotherapy** drugs known as heavy metal-like alkylating agents. Alkylating agents interfere with the genetic material (deoxyribonucleic acid, or DNA) inside the cancer cells and prevent them from further dividing and growing more cancer cells.

Recommended dosage

The dose of carboplatin can be calculated using several methods. A carboplatin dose can be determined using a mathematical calculation that measures a person's body surface area (BSA). This number is dependent upon a patient's height and weight: the larger the person, the greater the body surface area. BSA is measured by the square meter (m^2). The body surface area is calculated and then multiplied by the drug dosage in milligrams per square meter (mg/m^2). This calculates the actual dose a patient is to receive.

A common dosage of carboplatin alone for the treatment of patients with recurrent ovarian cancer is 360 mg/m^2 given on day one into a vein every four weeks. When given in combination with the chemotherapeutic agent **cyclophosphamide** for the treatment of recurrent ovarian cancer, a dose of 300 mg/m^2 administered intravenously is typical. This combination is repeated every four weeks for six cycles.

The second way to determine the dose of carboplatin is for the physician to measure or estimate how well the patient's kidneys work. The patient may be asked to collect all of their urine in a bottle for a 24-hour period. The sample will then be sent to a laboratory and analyzed. A mathematical calculation is performed to determine how well the patient's kidneys are working and subsequently to determine the carboplatin dose.

Precautions

Blood counts will be monitored regularly while on carboplatin therapy. During a certain time period after receiving carboplatin there is an increased risk of getting infections. Caution should be taken to avoid unnecessary exposure to infectious agents. Patients should also check with their doctors before receiving live virus **vaccines** while on chemotherapy.

Patients who may be pregnant or trying to become pregnant should talk to their doctor before receiving carboplatin. Men and women undergoing chemotherapy are at risk of becoming sterile.

Patients with known previous allergic reactions to chemotherapy drugs should notify their doctors.

Side effects

Most of the side effects of carboplatin are due to its induction of apoptosis in tumor cells. **Nausea and vomiting** are among the most common side effects from receiving carboplatin. **Nausea** and **vomiting** can begin up to six hours after treatment and can last as long as 24 hours. Patients are given medicines known as **antiemetics** before receiving carboplatin to help prevent or decrease this side effect. **Diarrhea**, loss of appetite, constipation, pain, and weakness have also been reported to occur.

Myelosuppression, or a suppression of bone marrow activity resulting in a low blood cell count, is expected to occur following carboplatin administration. When a patient's white blood cell count drops below normal (leukopenia), there is an increased risk of developing a **fever** and infections. Neupogen, a drug used to increase the white blood cell count, may be administered.

A decrease in platelet count is most notable following carboplatin administration. Platelets are blood cells that aid for the formation of clots. When the platelet count becomes abnormally low, patients are at an increased risk for bruising and bleeding. If the platelet count remains too low a platelet blood transfusion is an option. Low red blood cell counts (**anemia**) may also occur following many cycles of carboplatin administration; during the first cycles this is usually not a common problem. Low red blood cell counts may result in dizziness and **fatigue** and can be treated with the drug **erythropoietin**.

A less common side effect of carboplatin is damage to nerves and nervous system tissues. Patients may feel tingling and numbness of the fingers and toes. This side effect is more common in patients over 65 years of age or those who have previously received the chemotherapy drug **cisplatin**. Other less common side effects include rash, **itching**, hair loss (**alopecia**), mouth sores, hearing problems, kidney problems, liver problems, vision problems, swelling, redness and pain at the site of injection, allergic reactions, heart problems, and breathing problems.

Carboplatin may cause the body to waste certain normal electrolytes that circulate in the body. Low levels of magnesium, calcium, phosphate, or sodium can be found in patients who have received carboplatin. These rarely cause difficulties and are monitored by the doctor.

Some patients develop hypersensitivity or allergic reactions to carboplatin that may include difficulty breathing, rash, itching, redness in the face, dizziness, an increased heart rate, and a drop in blood pressure. The risk of such reactions is increased in patients who have had more than six cycles of treatment with the drug. A group of researchers in Ohio has developed a skin test to evaluate patients for possible hypersensitivity reactions to carboplatin, and a second team is working on a desensitization regimen that will allow patients who have become hypersensitive to the drug to continue to benefit from treatment with it.

Interactions

Patients being treated with carboplatin should avoid other drugs that may cause damage to the kidneys or hearing.

Resources

PERIODICALS

Boulikas, T., and M. Vougiouka. "Cisplatin and Platinum Drugs at the Molecular Level." *Oncology Reports* 10 (November-December 2003): 1663–1682.

Markman, M., K. Zanotti, G. Peterson, et al. "Expanded Experience with an Intradermal Skin Test to Predict for the Presence or Absence of Carboplatin

Hypersensitivity." *Journal of Clinical Oncology* 21 (December 15, 2003): 4611–4614.

Markman, M. "Toxicities of the Platinum Antineoplastic Agents." *Expert Opinion on Drug Safety* 2 (November 2003): 597–607.

McElroy, T. M., V. E. Gruenigen, and S. E. Waggoner. "A Case of Prolonged Carboplatin Therapy in a Patient with Carboplatin Hypersensitivity." *Gynecologic Oncology* 91 (November 2003): 435–437.

Moosman, P., F. Egli, R. A. Stahel, and L. Jost. "Weekly Paclitaxel and Carboplatin Combination Chemotherapy in Patients with Advanced Squamous Cell Carcinoma of the Head and Neck." *Onkologie* 26 (December 2003): 568–572.

Oh, W. K., S. Halabi, W. K. Kelly, et al. "A Phase II study of Estramustine, Docetaxel, and Carboplatin with Granulocyte-Colony-Stimulating Factor Support in Patients with Hormone-Refractory Prostate Carcinoma: Cancer and Leukemia Group B 99813." *Cancer* 98 (December 15, 2003): 2592–2598.

Strauss, S. J., M. Marples, M. P. Napier, et al. "A Phase I (Tumour Site-Specific) Study of Carboplatin and Temozolomide in Patients with Advanced Melanoma." *British Journal of Cancer* 89 (November 17, 2003): 1901–1905.

ORGANIZATIONS

United States Food and Drug Administration (FDA). 5600 Fishers Lane, Rockville, MD 20857-0001. (888) INFO-FDA (463-6332). http://www.fda.gov.

Nancy J. Beaulieu, RPh.,BCOP
Rebecca J. Frey, PhD

Carcinogenesis

Definition

Also called tumorigenesis, carcinogenesis is the molecular process by which **cancer** develops.

Description

The development of cancer is a complicated process in which a large number of factors interact to disrupt normal cell growth and division. Cancer can be caused by a number of internal factors such as heredity, immunology, and hormones as well as external factors such as chemicals, viruses, diet, and radiation. Although attention is often focused on environmental chemicals (such as asbestos and coal tar) as a cause of cancer, only 5% of cancers can be linked to chemical exposure. We now know that the chief causes of cancer are lifestyle factors such as diet, cigarette smoke, alcohol, and sun exposure. In fact, dietary factors are associated with 35% of all human cancers and cigarette smoke for another 30%.

Whatever the cause of cancer, its development is a multi-stage process involving damage to the genetic material of cells (deoxyribonucleic acid, or DNA). This damage occurs in genes regulating normal cell growth and division. Because several stages or several mutations are required for cancer to develop, there is usually a long latent period before cancer appears.

Carcinogens

Agents that cause cancer (carcinogens) can be classified as genotoxic or nongenotoxic (also referred to as epigenetic). Genotoxins cause irreversible genetic damage or mutations by binding to DNA. Genotoxins include chemical agents like N-methyl-N-nitrosourea (MNU) or non-chemical agents such as ultraviolet light and ionizing radiation. After the carcinogen enters the body, the body makes an attempt to eliminate it through a process called biotransformation (a series of reactions in which the chemical structure of a compound is altered). The purpose of these reactions is to make the carcinogen more water soluble so that it can be removed from the body, but these reactions can also convert a less toxic carcinogen into a more toxic one. Certain viruses can also act as carcinogens by interacting with DNA.

Nongenotoxins do not directly affect DNA but act in other ways to promote growth. These include hormones and some organic (carbon-based) compounds.

Stages of carcinogenesis

Cancer develops through four definable stages: initiation, promotion, progression, and malignant conversion. These stages may progress over many years. The first stage, initiation, involves a change in the genetic makeup of a cell. This may occur randomly or when a carcinogen interacts with DNA causing damage. This initial damage rarely results in cancer because the cell has in place many mechanisms to repair damaged DNA. However, if repair does not occur and the damage to DNA is in the location of a gene that regulates cell growth and proliferation, DNA repair, or a function of the immune system, then the cell is more prone to becoming cancerous.

During promotion, the mutated cell is stimulated to grow and divide faster and becomes a population of cells. Eventually a benign tumor becomes evident. In human cancers, hormones, cigarette smoke, or bile acids are substances that are involved in promotion. This stage is usually reversible as evidenced by the fact that lung damage can often be reversed after smoking stops.

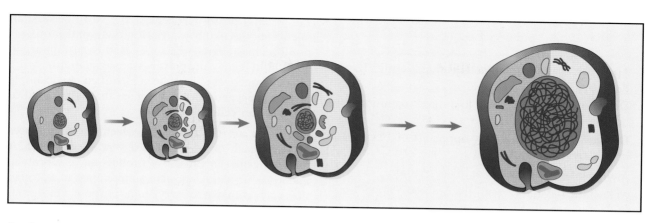

Carcinogenesis. After several mutations, a normal cell becomes cancerous. The first stage of carcinogenesis, called initiation, involves a change in the genetic makeup of a cell. This may occur randomly or when a carcinogen interacts with DNA causing damage. This initial damage rarely results in cancer because the cell has in place many mechanisms to repair damaged DNA. However, if repair does not occur and the damage to DNA is in the location of a gene that regulates cell growth and proliferation, DNA repair, or a function of the immune system, then the cell is more prone to becoming cancerous. *(Illustration by Argosy Publishing. Cengage Learning, Gale.)*

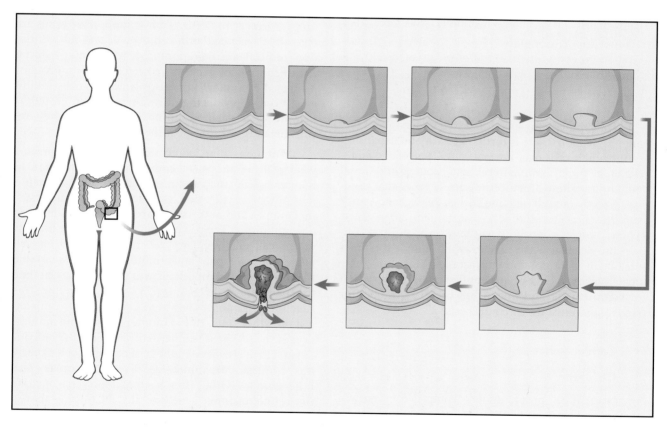

Colon cancer has become a model for studying multi-stage carcinogenesis. Four distinct sequential mutations have been described in the development of colon cancer: mutations of the APC (adenomatous polyposis coli), K-ras, DCC (deleted in colon cancer), and p53 genes. With each mutation, progressive changes are seen in the colonic epithelium (the cells on the internal surface of the colon). Normal epithelium is shown in first panel. Mutation of APC typically occurs early and is sometimes inherited. Mutations in APC lead to dysplasia or formation of a polyp (panel 2). When one cell in this polyp develops a second mutation, in the K-ras gene, it grows at a faster rate resulting in a benign Class I adenoma (panel 3). Subsequent mutations in DCC and p53 genes lead to late adenoma (panels 4 and 5) and finally carcinoma (panel 6). Once cancer forms, it can eventually break through the colon's cellular surface (panel 7) and spread through blood to other sites in the body. *(Illustration by Argosy Publishing. Cengage Learning, Gale)*

The progression phase is less well understood. During progression, there is further growth and expansion of the tumor cells over normal cells. The genetic material of the tumor is more fragile and prone to additional mutations. These mutations occur in genes that regulate growth and cell function such as oncogenes, tumor suppressor genes, and DNA mismatch-repair genes. These changes contribute to tumor growth until conversion occurs, when the growing tumor becomes malignant and possibly metastatic. Many of these genetic changes have been identified in the development of **colon cancer** and thus it has become a model for studying multi-stage carcinogenesis.

Cancer genes

Oncogenes

Normal cell proliferation is controlled by growth factors and cytokines (mediating proteins) that act on the cell membrane, triggering a cascade of biochemical signals (a process called signal transduction). These signals control, among others, the genes that regulate cell growth and division. Oncogenes are altered forms of normal cellular genes called proto-oncogenes that are involved in this cascade of events. They may mutate spontaneously, through interaction with viruses, or by chemical or physical means.

When a proto-oncogene is altered to become an oncogene, the pathway of cell growth and proliferation becomes altered. This may lead to the abnormal growth of cells (neoplastic transformation). More than 100 oncogenes have been identified. An example of an oncogene is the K-ras gene that is mutated in colon cancer cells.

Genes are the means by which a cell produces proteins, each of which have a very specific role. A mutated gene can cause overproduction of a protein, underproduction of a protein, or alteration of a protein that may be unable to carry out its purpose. Oncogenes typically produce more of their protein product when mutated, while tumor suppressor genes typically produce less of their protein product when mutated.

Tumor suppressor genes

Both the activation of oncogenes and the inactivation of tumor suppressor genes appear to be necessary for cancer to occur. Tumor suppressor genes are typically associated with cell growth and differentiation and cell suicide (apoptosis). More than a dozen tumor suppressor genes have been identified. Proteins produced by tumor suppressor genes typically inhibit a cell from reproducing during times when growth is inappropriate such as during DNA repair; they are considered the "brakes" of the cell.

Mutations that inactivate the tumor suppressor gene p53 are the most common mutations seen in human cancers, accounting for about 50%. Carcinomas of the breast, colon, stomach, bladder and testis; **melanoma**; and **soft tissue sarcoma** all are linked to p53 mutations. The p53 protein is found in the nucleus of the cell and regulates cell functions such as cell growth, DNA repair, and apoptosis. The most notable role for p53 is to halt cell growth to allow the cell time to repair damaged DNA. If p53 is mutated, it loses this function, apoptosis does not occur, and unregulated cell growth results. In **Li-Fraumeni syndrome** a mutation of the p53 gene is inherited. This puts the individual at a high risk for a number of cancers such as early onset breast **carcinoma**, childhood sarcomas, and other tumors. Other tumor suppressor genes include the **retinoblastoma** gene and the DCC gene that is mutated in colon cancer.

DNA mismatch-repair genes

This more recently discovered class of cancer susceptibility genes is associated with the genetic instability of cancer cells that allows for multiple mutations to occur. This instability hastens the course of cancer. The normal function of these genes is to repair damage to the DNA. Mutations in DNA mismatch-repair genes are most notable in hereditary non-polyposis colorectal cancer (HNPCC).

Apoptosis

Apoptosis, also called cell suicide, refers to the death of a damaged cell. It is not random but occurs in cells with damaged DNA. When a cell becomes mutated and does not repair itself, it can be sacrificed to prevent that mutation from being passed on to the next generation of cells. Inhibition of apoptosis can be an essential step in carcinogenesis. Two genes involved in apoptosis are the tumor suppressor gene p53 and the bcl-2 proto-oncogene.

Colon carcinogenesis

Colon cancer has become a model for studying multi-stage carcinogenesis. Four distinct sequential mutations have been described in the development of colon cancer. These are mutations of the APC (adenomatous polyposis coli), K-ras, DCC (deleted in colon cancer), and p53 genes. With each mutation, progressive changes are seen in the colonic epithelium (the cells on the internal surface of the colon).

Mutation of APC typically occurs early and is sometimes inherited. Mutations in APC lead to dysplasia (abnormalities in adult cells) or polyp formation (usually benign growths on the surface of mucous membranes). These polyps can remain dormant for many decades. When one cell in this polyp develops a second mutation, in the K-ras gene, it grows at a faster rate resulting in a larger tumor or intermediate **adenoma**. Subsequent mutations in DCC and p53 lead to late adenoma and finally carcinoma.

These mutations result in both the overexpression of oncogenes and the deletion of anti-oncogenes, the combination of which results in cancer. This is, however, just a model and not all genes are altered in all cases of colon cancer; additional mutations are likely. Individuals with the hereditary predisposition to colon cancer known as familial adenomatous polyposis (FAP) typically have inherited mutations of the APC gene, the first step of colon cancer. Only 15% of colon cancer cases are due to hereditary factors, however, with 85% due to sporadic mutations.

Resources

PERIODICALS

Weinstein, I. Bernard. "Disorders in Cell Circuitry During Multistage Carcinogenesis: The Role of Homeostasis." *Carcinogenesis* 21 (2000): 857-64.

OTHER

Mellors, Robert C. "Etiology of Cancer: Carcinogenesis." *Neoplasia*. Weill Medical College of Cornell University. July 1999. [cited June 27, 2001]. http://edcenter.med.cornell.edu/CUMC_PathNotes/Neoplasia/Neoplasia_04.html.

Cindy L. A. Jones, Ph.D.

Carcinoid tumors, gastrointestinal

Definition

Gastrointestinal carcinoid tumors are rare malignancies in which **cancer** develops in hormone-producing cells that line the appendix, bronchus, esophagus, intestines, liver, ovary, pancreas, rectum, stomach, testes, and thymus.

Description

Gastrointestinal carcinoid tumors are also called:

- carcinoids
- endocrine tumors, carcinoid type
- metastatic carcinoid tumors
- neuroendocrine tumors
- neuroendocrine cancers

Colored transmission electron micrograph of a cancer cell from a carcinoid tumor of the human gut. The large oval is the cell nucleus. The red patch inside it is the nucleolus, often prominent in cancer cells. The small red granules in the cytoplasm are packed with the hormone serotonin. High levels of this hormone can cause symptoms like wheezing and diarrhea. *(Copyright Science Photo Library/Photo Researchers, Inc. Photo reproduced by permission.)*

Types of gastrointestinal carcinoids

Doctors describe gastrointestinal carcinoids according to the part of the gastrointestinal tract in which they originate. Foregut tumors start in the cells of the esophagus, bronchus, thymus, and stomach.

Midgut tumors originate in the: appendix, liver, ovary, small intestine, and parts of the large intestine.

Hindgut tumors originate in the rest of the colon or in the rectum.

About 75% of all carcinoid tumors originate in the digestive system. Most of them develop in the:

- small intestine (ileum)
- appendix
- rectum

Atypical tumor behavior

Most cancers cause symptoms in the organs in which they start or to which they spread (metastasize), but carcinoids can release chemicals (hormones) that travel through the bloodstream and cause symptoms in many parts of the body. These substances can damage heart valves, causing weakness, heart murmur, and shortness of breath.

Some gastrointestinal carcinoids stimulate the adrenal glands to produce abnormally high levels of the hormones that regulate the balance of water and salt in the body. Overproduction of these hormones causes weakness, weight gain, secondary diabetes, and excessive facial and body hair.

Carcinoid syndrome

Although gastrointestinal carcinoids behave differently in different people, tumors that originate in the

appendix don't usually spread to other organs. Tumors that develop in the colon or rectum hardly ever produce hormones. Tumors that originate in the small intestine or other parts of the gastrointestinal tract and spread to the liver generally cause carcinoid syndrome. Flushing of the face and neck is the most common symptom of this rare malignant disease that affects the small intestine, stomach, and pancreas, and fewer than 10% of patients with gastrointestinal carcinoids.

Carcinoid syndrome is also characterized by:

- abdominal cramps
- breathlessness
- cyanosis
- diarrhea
- rapid heart beat (tachycardia)
- swelling around the eyes
- tearing
- wheezing

Stress, strenuous exercise, eating spicy foods, or drinking alcohol can intensify these symptoms.

Disease progression

Gastrointestinal carcinoids originate as small growths called tumorlets. These miniature tumors grow very slowly and few of them develop into carcinoid tumors.

The hormones that gastrointestinal carcinoids release generally cause more problems than the tumors themselves. Death usually results from heart or liver failure or from complications associated with tumor growth.

Demographics

About 2,500 carcinoids are diagnosed in the United States every year. African Americans develop carcinoids more often than Caucasians, and African-American women develop them more often than African-American men. Caucasian men and women are equally likely to develop these tumors.

The average age of patients diagnosed with carcinoid tumor of the appendix is 40. The average age of patients diagosed with carcinoid tumor of the stomach, small intestine, colon, and rectum is 55–65.

Causes and symptoms

The cause of gastrointestinal carcinoids is unknown, but some risk factors have been identified. The risk factors that increase a person's risk of developing gastrointestinal carcinoids include:

- Having certain diseases that damage the stomach and decrease production of stomach acid. Some of these diseases include chronic atrophic gastritis associated with pernicious anemia, chronic gastric infection with the *H. pylori* bacteria, auto-immune gastritis, or AIDS.

- Having a family history of multiple endocrine neoplasia, type 1. The multiple endocrine neoplasia (MEN) syndromes are three related disorders in which two or more of the hormone-secreting (endocrine) glands of the body develop tumors. Commonly affected glands are the thyroid, parathyroids, pituitary, adrenals, and pancreas. Patients diagnosed with this syndrome are at a higher risk for developing a variety of cancers, and require more frequent monitoring than the average patient might.

Symptoms

Early-stage gastrointestinal carcinoids rarely cause symptoms. About half of these tumors are discovered during tests or surgical procedures performed to diagnose or treat other diseases of the digestive system.

The most common early symptom of gastrointestinal carcinoids is uncomfortable flushing of the face and neck. Most people who have gastrointestinal carcinoids eventually experience:

- abdominal cramps
- changes in bowel habits
- other symptoms similar to those of other intestinal cancers

Some gastrointestinal carcinoids cause:

- intestinal bleeding
- asthmatic wheezing
- impotence
- loss of interest in sex (libido)

Most patients develop abnormal connective tissue on the right side of the heart (endocardial fibrosis).

Diagnosis

If a patient has any abnormality that could be a symptom of a gastrointestinal carcinoid, the doctor asks about other symptoms that could be associated with carcinoid syndrome or caused by a tumor in the stomach, intestines, or rectum.

Diagnostic techniques

Doctors use a variety of diagnostic techniques to locate gastrointestinal carcinoids and determine how far the disease has spread:

- barium enemas and x rays highlight abnormalities in the lining of the esophagus, stomach, and intestines
- blood and urine tests measure amounts of substances that carcinoids secrete
- colonoscopy provides a view of the entire length of the colon
- endoscopic ultrasound shows how deeply tumors have penetrated the wall of the esophagus, stomach, intestines, or rectum and whether they have spread to nearby tissues
- octreoscan detects the spread of gastrointestinal carcinoids by using a special camera to track the path of injected radioactive hormone-like substances that are attracted to these tumors

Provocative testing designed to cause the patient to flush can help doctors diagnose some gastrointestinal carcinoids, but it can also provoke potentially serious reactions and must be performed in a hospital, under close medical supervision.

Biopsy

Diagnostic tests can indicate that a patient has a gastrointestinal carcinoid, but only **biopsy** can confirm the diagnosis. Endoscopic biopsy is the most common way to remove a sample of a suspected gastrointestinal carcinoid.

A doctor performs this procedure by passing a flexible lighted tube topped with a tiny video camera (endoscope) down the patient's throat or up through the anus to examine the lining of the organs of the digestive tract. After locating a tumor, the doctor manipulates pincers or tongs (biopsy forceps) through the endoscope to remove a tissue sample.

Clinical staging, treatments, and prognosis

Staging

Doctors divide gastrointestinal carcinoids into three categories.

- Localized cancer is found in the appendix, colon, rectum, small intestine, and stomach, but has not spread beyond the wall of the organ in which it originated.
- Regional spread describes tumors that have penetrated the wall of the organ in which they originated and have involved nearby fat cells, ligaments, muscles, and lymph nodes.
- Distant spread, or metastatic disease, refers to gastrointestinal carcinoids that have spread to the liver, bones, lungs, or other tissues or organs far from the original tumor.

Recurrent gastrointestinal carcinoid is disease that has returned after having been treated. Recurrent disease can develop at the site of the original tumor or in another part of the body.

Treatment

Treatment of gastrointestinal carcinoids is based on:
- where the tumor originated
- whether the cancer has spread beyond the gastrointestinal system
- the patient's general health

Surgery

Surgery cures most gastrointestinal carcinoids. What type of operation a patient undergoes depends on the size and location of the tumor, whether the patient has serious disease of any other organ, and whether the tumor is causing carcinoid syndrome.

TREATING LOCALIZED GASTROINTESTINAL CARCINOIDS. A surgeon can usually remove all of a tumor that has not spread (is localized). This procedure, called local excision, consists of removing the tumor and nearby normal tissue, and sewing together the affected ends of the remaining tissue.

If a carcinoid originates in the appendix, doctors usually remove the appendix (appendectomy). If the tumor is larger than 3/4" (cm) and the patient is under the age of 60 and otherwise in good health, the doctor may also remove the third of the colon closest to the appendix, and nearby blood vessels and lymph nodes.

When a carcinoid tumor originates in the small intestine, doctors usually remove part of the bowel, and may remove nearby lymph nodes to see if they contain cancer cells. Local excision is used to remove carcinoids that are not much larger than 3/8" (cm). Surgery for larger tumors removes a greater amount of normal surrounding tissue and some nearby blood vessels and lymph nodes.

Doctors usually treat localized carcinoids that originate in the stomach, pancreas, and colon by removing the affected organ.

Local excision is used to treat carcinoids that are limited to areas of the large intestine other than the appendix or to the rectum. Doctors use a flexible lighted instrument (colonoscope) to remove small tumors from these sites and remove larger tumors through an incision in the patient's abdomen.

Electrofulguration, a surgical procedure sometimes used to cure rectal carcinoids, destroys the tumor by heating it with electrical current. Doctors use electrofulguration to burn away rectal carcinoids no larger than 3/8". Tumors measuring 3/4" or more are apt to grow and metastasize and must be surgically removed.

Segmental colon resection (also called hemicolectomy) removes between one-third and one-half of the large intestine, and blood vessels and lymph nodes near the affected tissue.

Abdominoperineal resection is used for very large or very invasive carcinoids of the lower rectum. A patient who has this operation also has a **colostomy**. Deeply invasive rectal carcinoids that measure less than 3/4" are treated like larger tumors. Mildly invasive tumors of comparable size are treated with local excision and careful monitoring to check for recurrence.

Lower anterior resection is used for some carcinoids in the upper part of the rectum. This procedure removes some of the rectum before the remaining ends are sewn together, and has little lasting effect on the digestive system.

TREATING REGIONAL SPREAD. When a gastrointestinal carcinoid has spread to organs or tissues close to the original tumor (regional spread), doctors usually remove the affected organ. Some nearby organs and tissues may also be removed.

If it is not possible to completely remove a gastrointestinal carcinoid that has spread to another part of the body, surgeons remove as much of the cancer as they can without damaging vital organs or causing severe side effects. Surgery cannot cure gastrointestinal carcinoids that have spread to parts of the body far from the original tumor, but it can relieve symptoms and slow the progression of the disease.

Liver resection removes one or more metastases (secondary tumors) from the liver. This procedure does not cure cancer but can relieve symptoms of carcinoid syndrome. Doctors destroy gastrointestinal carcinoids that have spread to the liver by:

- using images generated by a CT scan (computed tomography scan) to guide a long thin needle into tumors and injecting them with concentrated alcohol
- cooling the needle with liquid nitrogen to freeze carcinoid tumor cells (cryosurgery)

TREATING METASTATIC DISEASE. Doctors treat gastrointestinal carcinoids that have spread to distant parts of the body by:

- freezing and killing cancer cells
- performing surgery or administering radiation or chemotherapy to relieve symptoms
- using biological therapy to stimulate the patient's immune system to attack tumor cells

Neither radiation nor **chemotherapy** can cure gastrointestinal carcinoids. Doctors sometimes use external beam radiation to treat patients who are too ill or frail to withstand surgery, and to relieve pain caused by tumors that have spread to the bones.

Doctors may use several different chemotherapy drugs or combine a chemotherapy drug with other medication to slow tumor growth and relieve symptoms. Chemotherapy is generally used only for gastrointestinal carcinoids that have spread to other organs, cause severe symptoms, and have not responded to other treatments.

Doctors sometimes treat gastrointestinal carcinoids that have spread to the liver by injecting chemotherapy drugs directly into the artery that supplies blood to the liver (hepatic artery). This technique (intra-arterial chemotherapy):

- exposes liver tumors to high doses of cancer-killing drugs
- prevents side effects by shielding healthy tissues from these powerful medications

When doctors also inject material that blocks the hepatic artery, this treatment is called **chemoembolization**.

Octreotide is a hormone-like drug that can prevent or relieve flushing, wheezing, **diarrhea**, and other symptoms that sometimes occur during surgery or when gastrointestinal carcinoids release high levels of hormones. Octreotide can temporarily shrink these tumors but does not cure the cancer. Some patients experience pain at the site where the medication is injected, cramps, **nausea and vomiting**, dizziness, and **fatigue**.

Doctors also prescribe other medications to relieve specific symptoms.

Biological therapy or interferon-alpha therapy may stimulate the patient's immune system to attack the tumor, shrink metastatic gastrointestinal carcinoids, and may relieve symptoms of carcinoid syndrome.

This technique, which is also called immunotherapy, is sometimes used to treat tumors that have not responded to chemotherapy or octreotide, but can cause severe flu-like side effects.

TREATING RECURRENT DISEASE. Treatment of recurrent disease depends on where the new tumor is located and what treatment the patient has already received.

TREATING CARCINOID SYNDROME. Treatments for carcinoid syndrome include surgically removing the cancer, blocking the hepatic artery or injecting chemotherapy drugs into it, medication to relieve symptoms, and stimulating the patient's immune system to attack the tumor.

LONG-TERM SURVEILLANCE. After completing treatment, patients with certain types of gastrointestinal carcinoids must continue to have regular physical examinations, **x rays**, and blood and urine tests to help doctors detect recurrence during the earliest stages of disease.

Because some gastrointestinal carcinoids recur many years after initial treatment, high-risk patients should continue to see their doctor regularly. Any patient who has had a gastrointestinal carcinoid should immediately notify the doctor of any new symptoms. These symptoms could be side effects of treatment or a sign that the cancer has returned.

Prognosis

The only way to cure gastrointestinal carcinoids is to remove the tumors surgically. But because these cancers grow so slowly, it is not unusual for a patient to survive 10–15 years after being diagnosed with metastatic disease.

5-YEAR SURVIVAL RATES. For patients whose carcinoid tumor originates in the stomach, the 5-year survival rate is:

- 64% for localized disease
- 40% for regional spread
- 10% for mestatatic disease

When tumors originate in the small intestine, the 5-year survival rate is:

- 65% for localized disease
- 66% for regional spread
- 36% for metastatic disease

For carcinoids that originate in parts of the colon other than the appendix, the 5-year survival rate is:

- 71% for localized disease
- 44% for regional spread
- 21% for metastatic disease

For carcinoids that originate in the appendix, the 5-year survival rate is:

- 94% for localized disease
- 85% for regional spread
- 34% for metastatic disease

For carcinoids that originate in the rectum, the 5-year survival rate is:

- 81% for localized disease
- 47% for regional spread
- 18% for metastatic disease

Having a gastrointestinal carcinoid increases a patient's risk of developing other cancers in the digestive system.

Clinical trials

Researchers are investigating:

- how changes in cells transform normal tissues into gastrointestinal carcinoid tumors
- how effectively specific chemotherapy drugs and surgical procedures treat gastrointestinal carcinoids
- new ways of slowing or preventing growth of gastrointestinal carcinoids by blocking or shrinking the blood vessels that nourish them
- how nuclear medicine can contribute to early detection of gastrointestinal carcinoids

Prevention

There is no known way to prevent gastrointestinal carcinoids or to reduce the risk of developing them, but avoiding the following can prevent symptoms of carcinoid syndrome from becoming more intense:

- alcoholic drinks
- hot, spicy foods
- strenuous exercise
- stress

See also Cryotherapy; Gastrointestinal cancers; Hepatic arterial infusion; Neuroendocrine tumors.

Resources

BOOKS

Goldman, Lee, and J. Claude Bennett. *Cecil Textbook of Medicine.* Vol. 2. 21st ed. Philadelphia: W.B.Saunders Company, 2000.

OTHER

"Carcinoid May Be Rare—But If You have It, You Are Not Alone." *National Carcinoid Suport Group.* 15 May 1999. [cited March 31, 2001]. http://members.aol.com/thencsg.

"Carcinoid Research: There Is Hope." *National Carcinoid Support Group.* [cited March 31, 2001]. http://members.aol.com/thencsg.

"Carcinoid Treatment: More Than One Option to Consider." *National Carcinoid Support Group.* [cited March 31, 2001]. http://members.aol.com/thencsg/treatment.html.

"Gastrointestinal Carcinoid Tumor." *CancerNet.* November 2000. [cited March 31, 2001]. http://cancernet.nci.nih.gov.

"Gastrointestinal Carcinoid Tumors." *Gastrointestinal Carcinoid Tumors Resource Center.* 12 February 1999. [cited April 2001]. http://www3.cancer.org.

National Carcinoid Support Group. *Questions & Answers About Carcinoid.* [cited March 31, 2001]. http://members.aol.com/thencsg/info.html.

ORGANIZATIONS

Carcinoid Cancer Foundation, 333 Mamaroneck Ave., # 492, White Plains, NY 10605. (888)-722-3132. http://www.carcinoid.org.

Maureen Haggerty

Carcinoid tumors, lung

Definition

Lung carcinoid tumors are rare malignant growths that develop from cells that help regulate the flow of air and blood through the lungs. These growths are also known as neuroendocrine lung tumors, pulmonary carcinoids, and lung carcinoids.

Lung carcinoid, spindle cell form. *(Copyright Parviz M. Pour, Science Source/Photo Researchers, Inc. Photo reproduced by permission.)*

KEY TERMS

Acromegaly—Hormonal disorder causing progressive enlargement of hands and feet and elongation of the face, headache, muscle pain, and visual and emotional distrbances in middle-aged men and women.

Carcinoid syndrome—Rare malignant disease characterized by facial flushing, abdominal cramps, diarrhea, breathlessness, and other symptoms. Affects fewer than 10% of patients with carcinoid tumor.

Cushing's syndrome—Hormonal disorder characterized by a round face, mental or emotional instability, high blood pressure, weight gain, or abnormal growth of facial and body hair in women.

Emphysema—Abnormal lung condition characterized by breathing problems, cough, and rapid heartbeat. Later stages are characterized by restlessness, weakness, confusion, and increased breathlessness, and the condition may cause fluid to collect around the lungs (pulmonary edema) and congestive heart failure.

Hypercalcemia—Abnormally high levels of calcium in the blood, causing muscle pain and weakness and loss of appetite. Severe cases can result in kidney failure.

Description

These cancers account for 1% to 3% of all lung tumors. Most lung carcinoids measure between slightly less than 1/4" (0.63 cm) and slightly more than 3/4" (1.9 cm). These tumors usually develop in the right lung.

Doctors classify lung carcinoids according to what tumor cells look like under a microscope, and where in the lung the tumor is located. Typical lung carcinoids occur about nine times as often as atypical tumors. They grow slowly and rarely spread beyond the lungs. Atypical lung carcinoids grow somewhat faster than typical tumors and are more likely to spread to other organs. In their most invasive form, atypical lung carcinoids look and behave like small-cell lung cancers.

About 80% of lung carcinoids are central carcinoids. Located in the walls of the large airways in the center of the lungs, where the neuroendocrine cells that form them are most concentrated, these tumors are almost always typical tumors. Carcinoids that develop in the narrower airways, close to the edges of the lungs, are called peripheral carcinoids. Most are typical tumors.

Demographics

Lung carcinoids usually develop between the ages of 45 and 55. These tumors are equally common in men and women and rarely affect children.

Causes and symptoms

Lung carcinoids are not caused by smoking or by exposure to chemicals at work or in the environment. Doctors believe that central carcinoids develop from glands beneath the surface of the large air passages. Lung biopsies performed to diagnose or treat other conditions sometimes reveal microscopic clusters of neuroendocrine cells. These carcinoid tumorlets look like tiny peripheral carcinoids. They are most common when disease has caused scar tissue to form in the lungs, and may grow to be carcinoid tumors.

Patients who have peripheral or small central carcinoids don't usually show symptoms, but some patients who have central carcinoids cough, wheeze, or cough up blood (**hemoptysis**).

A large carcinoid that blocks part or all of an airway can cause post-obstructive **pneumonia**. Doctors may not consider the possibility of a carcinoid until **antibiotics** fail to cure this lung **infection**.

About 10% to 20% of lung carcinoids produce hormone-like substances that release into the bloodstream. These substances can cause symptoms such as **Cushing's syndrome**, acromegaly, or **hypercalcemia**. They may also cause carcinoid syndrome, which is a constellation of symptoms including facial flushing, abdominal cramps, **diarrhea**, and breathlessness, among others.

Diagnosis

A thorough physical examination will detect symptoms of syndrome health problems associated with these tumors. If a patient has one or more symptoms that suggest the presence of a lung carcinoid, the doctor will inquire about:

- chest pain
- cough
- blood-tinged sputum
- asthma
- wheezing
- pneumonia not cured by antibiotics
- recent weight gain
- facial flushing
- diarrhea

The doctor will use one or more methods to determine whether the patient has a lung tumor. Lung carcinoids that do not cause symptoms usually show up on chest **x rays** taken during a routine physical or as a result of other health problems.

Chest x rays cannot detect tumors that are very small or hidden by other organs in the chest. A doctor who suspects a lung carcinoid may order additional **imaging studies** in order to make a more detailed search.

About 75% of lung carcinoids can be seen through a long, lighted tube called a bronchoscope. Doctors also use CT scans, octreoscans, or MIBG (metaiodobenzyl-guanidine) scans to locate lung carcinoids and determine how far they have spread. CT scans provide a detailed view of the lungs. Octreoscans and MIBG scans trace the path of radioactive substances that are attracted to lung carcinoids.

Also called indium-111-labeled DTPA-octreotide scintigraphy, octreoscan involves injecting a small amount of a radioactive hormone-like substance into the patient's vein. Carcinoid tumors attract this substance, and a special camera locates tumors by pinpointing the area where the radioactive material accumulates.

Doctors perform MIBG scans by attaching radioactive iodine to a chemical absorbed by carcinoid tumors. This compound is injected into the patient's bloodstream, drawn to carcinoid tumor cells, and tracked by a special scanner.

Although diagnostic procedures can indicate that a patient might have a lung carcinoid, **biopsy** is the only way to confirm the diagnosis. Doctors use several different techniques to remove samples of these tumors.

BRONCHOSCOPIC BIOPSY. To obtain a sample of a tumor in one of the large airways, the doctor uses a bronchoscope to examine the lining of these organs. When a tumor is located, the doctor manipulates pincers or tongs (biopsy forceps) through the bronchoscope to remove a small sample of tissue. The patient leaves the hospital a few hours after undergoing this outpatient procedure. If serious bleeding occurs, the doctor narrows or seals the blood vessels by injecting drugs or aiming a laser beam.

BRUSHING SAMPLE. A doctor who performs a bronchoscopic biopsy may also wipe a tiny brush over the surface of the tumor. Tumor cells extracted in this way (brushing sample) are examined under a microscope. A brushing sample can add useful information to the results of bronchoscopic biopsy.

NEEDLE BIOPSY. Doctors often use needle biopsy to obtain samples of tumors that are not close to the large airways. Guided by a **computed tomography** scan (CT scan) image, a long needle is passed between the ribs and into the lung to remove a small piece of the tumor. Because carcinoid tumors are usually small, localization using a needle biopsy may be difficult or impossible.

THORACOTOMY. If neither bronchoscopic biopsy nor needle biopsy yields enough tissue to identify the tumor type, the doctor may open the patient's chest (**thoracotomy**) to remove a tissue sample. A doctor who feels certain that a tumor is a carcinoid may perform a thoracotomy and remove the entire tumor without having taken a biopsy sample.

Treatment team

Lung carcinoids are treated by thoracic and cardiothoracic surgeons.

Clinical staging, treatments, and prognosis

Staging

Once lung carcinoids have been diagnosed, more tests are done to find out if the **cancer** has spread from the lung to other parts of the body (staging). A doctor needs to know the stage to plan treatment. Doctors stage lung carcinoids the same way they stage non-small cell lung cancers:

- Stage 0: Cancer is only found in a local area and only in a few layers of cells. It has not grown through the top lining of the lung.
- Stage I: The cancer is only in the lung, and normal tissue is around it.
- Stage II: Cancer has spread to nearby lymph nodes.
- Stage III: Cancer has spread to the chest wall or diaphragm near the lung, or the cancer has spread to the lymph nodes in the area that separates the two lungs (mediastinum), or to the lymph nodes on the other side of the chest or in the neck. Stage III is further divided into stage IIIA (usually can be operated on) and stage IIIB (usually cannot be operated on).
- Stage IV: Cancer has spread to other parts of the body.

Treatment of lung carcinoids

Doctors consider tumor size and location, and whether the patient has additional lung problems or serious disease affecting any other organ, in order to determine the most appropriate treatment for lung carcinoids.

SURGERY. Removing the tumor (surgical resection) is the treatment of choice for these cancers because most lung carcinoids:

- can be cured by surgery alone
- do not respond to chemotherapy or radiation
- must be removed in order to prevent airway obstruction and other complications of tumor growth

If the tumor is located in a large airway, the surgeon may remove the tumor and normal tissue above and below it, then sew together the remaining lung tissue. This procedure is a sleeve resection.

If tumor size or location makes sleeve resection impossible, the surgeon removes the affected lobe of the lung (**lobectomy**). In rare cases, the surgeon removes the entire right or left lung (**pneumonectomy**).

Surgeons use lobectomy to remove peripheral carcinoids located at the edges of the lungs farthest from the large airways. If the tumor is very small, the surgeon may remove it and a wedge-shaped piece of lung tissue surrounding it (wedge resection).

Surgeons who remove lung carcinoids usually remove some of the lymph nodes near the lungs because:

- About 10% of typical carcinoids and 30% to 50% of atypical carcinoids have spread to lymph nodes by the time the disease is diagnosed.
- Not removing lymph nodes might increase the risk of cancer spreading to other organs.
- Surgery alone cannot cure lung carcinoids that have spread to other organs.
- Examining lymph nodes can indicate the likelihood that cancer will recur.

Surgeons who remove lung carcinoids try to preserve the patient's lung function by removing the smallest possible amount of normal lung tissue.

PALLIATIVE TREATMENT. A patient who has severe emphysema, chronic bronchitis, heart disease, or other medical problems may not be able to withstand the stress of surgery to cure lung carcinoids or to cope with breathing difficulties resulting from removal of normal lung tissue.

Doctors use a bronchoscope and a laser to burn away (vaporize) most of the tumor in a patient who is too ill to withstand surgery. These palliative treatments can relieve most symptoms associated with lung carcinoids, but cannot cure the disease. They are often supplemented by radiation administered externally or directly into the air passages (intrabronchial radiation).

MEDICAL TREATMENTS. Guidelines issued in 2001 by the National Comprehensive Cancer Network recommend the use of radiation following surgery to remove carcinoid lung tumors, and **chemotherapy** and radiation following surgery to remove atypical lung carcinoids.

Injected into a vein or taken by mouth, chemotherapy drugs are also used to treat lung carcinoids that have spread to other organs, are causing severe symptoms, or have not responded to other medications. Doctors may combine two or more chemotherapy drugs or add them to other medications to relieve symptoms of lung carcinoids that have spread to other organs.

Octreotide controls wheezing, flushing, and other symptoms of carcinoid syndrome. This medication may temporarily shrink lung carcinoids but does not cure them.

Alpha-interferon can shrink some lung carcinoids that have spread to other parts of the body and relieve symptoms of carcinoid syndrome. Doctors can prescribe other medications to relieve specific symptoms.

Radiation may be an option for patients who are too frail or ill to undergo surgery but is not a very effective treatment for lung carcinoids. High doses of radiation can damage lung tissue, create scar tissue, cause breathing problems, and make the patient more susceptible to infection.

PROGNOSIS. Five-year survival rates for patients with lung carcinoids are 90% to 100% for typical tumors, and 40% to 76% for atypical tumors. Ten-year survival rates are about 10% lower than five-year rates for both types of tumors. The prognosis is worse for lung carcinoids that measure 1 1/4" (3.2 cm) or larger or have spread to lymph nodes.

Some patients who have had lung carcinoids must continue to have regular x rays and blood tests to help doctors detect recurrent disease in its earliest stages. Any patient who has had a lung carcinoid should notify the doctor whenever new symptoms develop. These symptoms could be side effects of treatment or signs that the disease has recurred. A patient who has recovered from surgery should ask the doctor about an exercise routine to restore energy and reduce shortness of breath.

Clinical trials

Researchers are currently investigating whether:

- new methods of delivering radiation can shrink lung carcinoids that have not responded to treatment

- inhaling chemotherapy drugs can shrink advanced lung carcinoids
- biological therapy can starve lung carcinoids by cutting off the flow of blood that nourishes them and stimulate patients' white blood cells to kill cancer cells
- new methods of delivering chemotherapy can kill cancer cells without harming normal cells
- new combinations of chemotherapy drugs can prevent cancer cells from multiplying
- chemotherapy drugs combined with radioactive substances can locate and kill cancer cells without harming normal cells

Information about **clinical trials** is available from the National Institute of Health's National Cancer Institute.

Prevention

There are no known risk factors for lung carcinoids, and no methods of prevention are known.

See also Bronchoscopy; Neuroendocrine carcinomas.

Resources

PERIODICALS

"New NCCN Recommendations for Small-Cell Lung Cancer." *Oncology News International* 10, no. 4 (April 2001).

OTHER

"Lung Carcinoid Tumor." *Lung Carcinoid Tumor Research Center*. [cited May 23, 2000, April 2, 2001, and July 2, 2001]. <http://www3.cancer.org>.

"Lung Tumors: A Multidisciplinary Database." *Virtual Hospital*. August 1999. [cited May 27, 2001 and July 2, 2001]. http://www.vh.org/Providers/Textbooks/Lung Tumors/TitlePage.html.

National Cancer Institute. *CancerNet*. [cited May 28, 2001]. http://cancernet.nci.nih.gov.

ORGANIZATIONS

Carcinoid Cancer Foundation, 333 Manaroneck Ave., # 492, White Plains, NY 10605. (888)-722-3132. http://www.carcinoid.org.

Maureen Haggerty

Carcinoma

Definition

A malignant tumor that arises from epithelial cells, which line the internal and external surfaces of the body.

X ray showing presence of carcinoma. *(Photo Researchers, Inc. Reproduced by permission.)*

Carcinomas are most commonly found in the lining of body organs, such as the breast, prostate, lung, stomach, or bowel. Most human cancers are carcinomas.

See also Cancer of Unknown Primary.

Kate Kretschmann

Carcinomatous meningitis

Definition

Carcinomatous meningitis, also called meningeal carcinomatosis, neoplastic meningitis, or leptomeningeal carcinomatosis (LC), is a complication of a metastatic **cancer** that has spread to the lining of the brain and spinal cord—the parts of the body that make up the central nervous system.

Demographics

Once thought to be a rare complication of cancer, carcinomatous meningitis is increasing in frequency. This increase may be because people with cancer are living longer, giving the cancer a chance to spread to the central nervous system. Another possibility is that the disorder is being diagnosed more often; first identified in 1870, leptomeningeal carcinomatosis (LC) was underdiagnosed for many years. The number of people who develop carcinomatous meningitis is difficult to determine because the condition is often overlooked at autopsy. As of 2009, it is thought that between 1% and 8% of patients diagnosed with cancer develop LC. Frequently, people who develop tumors in the leptomeninges also develop them in other parts of the brain.

The lungs are the most common origin of LC (30–70% of cases), followed by the breasts (10–30%), the digestive tract (2–20%), and malignant melanomas (2–15%). Because of the different frequencies of these cancers, however, most patients diagnosed with LC are **breast cancer** patients.

Leptomeningeal carcinomatosis is equally common in both sexes and in all racial and ethnic groups. Older adults are somewhat more likely to develop LC with metastatic cancer than younger adults.

LC is more common in adults than in children. When it does occur in children, it is most likely to be found in those with **acute lymphocytic leukemia** (ALL) and primary **brain tumors**, particularly ependymomas, medulloblastomas, and germ-cell tumors.

Description

The meninges are membranes that cover the brain and spinal cord. There are two types of meninges, thin membranes called the pia-arachnoid or leptomeninges, and firmer, tougher membranes called the dura or pachymeninges. Carcinomatous meningitis is a cancer-related disorder of the leptomeninges. These membranes are bathed in and help contain cerebrospinal fluid (CSF).

Carcinomatous meningitis is a complication of metastatic cancer. The cancer cells that form tumors on the leptomeninges have come from other places in the body. Cancer cells break off from the primary tumor and circulate through the blood stream. When they enter the CSF, they act like seeds, attaching to many sites on the leptomeninges and developing into many tumors. The most common cancers that metastasize to carcinomatous meningitis are leukemia, **lymphoma**, **melanoma**, breast, lung, and **gastrointestinal cancers**.

Causes and symptoms

Carcinomatous meningitis is caused by the spread of other types of cancer to the central nervous system. There are many symptoms, including:

- headache
- decrease in mental abilities
- memory loss
- confusion
- disturbances in the ability use the legs and arms
- back pain
- weakness
- burning or prickling sensations
- loss of feeling in the face
- problems with vision (seeing double), hearing, or swallowing
- increased pressure in the brain due to the accumulation of fluid
- fecal or urinary incontinence

Pain and seizures, however, are the most common initial symptoms of LC. It is rare for these symptoms, however, to be the first signs of cancer in a patient. Most patients who develop leptomeningeal carcinomatosis have already been diagnosed with widespread cancer.

Diagnosis

Magnetic resonance imaging (MRI) scans of the brain and spinal cord may be done as part of the diagnosis for carcinomatous meningitis. However, the definitive diagnosis comes from removing a sample of cerebrospinal fluid, looking at it under the microscope, and finding cancer cells. This procedure is called a **lumbar puncture**. A lumbar puncture may also be performed to rule out meningitis caused by fungi or other disease organisms. It is common for doctors to have to do several lumbar punctures before a firm diagnosis of LC can be made.

Tests

The doctor will usually order one or more imaging tests of the patient's head or neck, most commonly a contrast-enhanced CT scan or a gadolinium-enhanced MRI. These tests do not usually confirm a diagnosis of LC but are useful in ruling out other causes of the patient's symptoms and in detecting additional metastases.

Procedures

In a few cases the doctor may order a **biopsy** of the leptomeninges if no evidence can be found of a primary tumor elsewhere in the body.

Treatment

The treatment team for a patient with carcinomatous meningitis usually involves an oncologist (cancer specialist), a radiation oncologist (specialist in **radiation therapy**), radiation technicians, nurses with special training in cancer care, a social worker, and possibly a surgeon.

Traditional

Carcinomatous meningitis is treated with either radiation or **intrathecal chemotherapy**. In radiation therapy, high-energy, penetrating waves or particles such as **x rays**, gamma rays, or proton rays are aimed at the spot where the tumor is located. The goal is to destroy the cancer cells or keep them from reproducing. There is no wide agreement on the best treatment for LC as of 2009 because of the lack of large controlled **clinical trials** for the condition.

Drugs

Drug treatment for carcinomatous meningitis takes the form of intrathecal **chemotherapy**, which involves injecting chemotherapy drugs directly into the CSF. Drugs are injected either through a lumbar puncture or through an **Ommaya reservoir** located on the skull below the scalp. The goal is for the drugs to kill the cancer cells, although some normal cells are also killed. The drugs most often used are **methotrexate** (Folex PFS), **cytarabine** (Cytosar-U), and **thiotepa**.

Alternative

Alternative and complementary therapies range from herbal remedies, vitamin supplements, and special diets to spiritual practices, acupuncture, massage, and similar treatments. When these therapies are used in addition to conventional medicine, they are called complementary therapies. When they are used instead of conventional medicine, they are called alternative therapies.

No specific alternative therapies have been directed toward carcinomatous meningitis. However, good nutrition and activities such as yoga, meditation, and massage, which reduce stress and promote a positive view of life, have no unwanted side effects and may help improve the quality of life. Alternative and experimental treatments are usually not covered by insurance.

QUESTIONS TO ASK YOUR DOCTOR

- What kind of changes in my body can I expect to see from this cancer?
- What is the treatment plan?
- What are the likely side effects of the treatment plan?
- How long am I likely to survive?
- How many patients have you treated for this complication of metastatic cancer?

Prognosis

Carcinomatous meningitis has a grim prognosis. It is a complication of cancer that usually leads to degeneration of the nervous system and then to death. A person who has developed carcinomatous meningitis is likely to have tumors in other places in the body as well. The chance of recovery is very slight; the median survival time is 7 months for patients with LC from breast cancers, 4 months for patients with LC from small cell lung cancers, and 3.6 months for patients with LC from melanomas.

Coping with cancer treatment

Carcinomatous meningitis is almost always fatal. In addition, radiation and chemotherapy cause **fatigue**, **nausea and vomiting**, and other uncomfortable side effects. Emotions are intense and often conflicting. In this extremely stressful time, it is often helpful for both the patient and loved ones to have the support of a therapist, religious leader, or other counselor. Hospice staff members or hospital social workers or chaplains can direct patients and family members to resources that address their individual needs.

Clinical trials

In 2009, there were five clinical trials related to new chemotherapy drugs for carcinomatous meningitis. Current information on what clinical trials are available and where they are being held can be found by entering the search term "carcinomatous meningitis" at the following websites:

- National Cancer Institute: http://www.cancer.gov/clinicaltrials or (800) 4-CANCER
- National Institutes of Health Clinical Trials: http://clinicaltrials.gov
- Center Watch: A Clinical Trials Listing: http://www.centerwatch.com

Prevention

Carcinomatous meningitis arises from the spread of other cancers. The best form of prevention is immediate and thorough treatment of the primary cancer.

Resources

BOOKS

Booth, Sara, ed. *Palliative Care Consultations in Advanced Breast Cancer*. New York: Oxford University Press, 2006.

Yang, Andrew V., ed. *Brain Cancer Therapy and Surgical Interventions*. New York: Nova Biomedical Books, 2006.

PERIODICALS

Bidard, F.C., et al. "Meningeal Carcinomatosis in HER2-overexpressing Breast Cancers." *Journal of Neuro-oncology* 93 (June 2009): 287–88.

Bruna, J., et al. "Leptomeningeal Carcinomatosis: Prognostic Implications of Clinical and Cerebrospinal Fluid Features." *Cancer* 115 (January 15, 2009): 381–389.

Gaviani, P., et al. "Neoplastic Meningitis from Breast Carcinoma with Complete Response to Liposomal Cytarabine: Case Report." *Neurological Sciences* 30 (June 2009): 251–54.

Raj, K. P., et al. "Need for a New Treatment Strategy: Leptomeningeal Carcinomatosis from Gastric Cancer." *Anticancer Drugs* 20 (April 2009): 301–04.

Silvestris, N., et al. "Rapidly Progressive Coma in Leptomeningeal Carcinomatosis from Undiagnosed Bronchioloalveolar Carcinoma." *Journal of Clinical Oncology* 27 (August 20, 2009): 65–66.

So, T., et al. "Gefitinib and a Ventriculo-peritoneal Shunt to Manage Carcinomatous Meningitis from Non-small-cell Lung Cancer: Report of Two Cases." *Surgery Today* 39 (July 2009): 598–602.

OTHER

American Brain Tumor Association (ABTA). *Metastatic Brain Tumors*. http://www.abta.org/siteFiles/sitePages/7F67D9EF28C67A64B50A7D42670EC586.pdf.

Sewell, R. Andrew, and Lawrence D. Recht. "Leptomeningeal Carcinomatosis." *eMedicine*, August 30, 2007. http://emedicine.medscape.com/article/1156338-overview.

ORGANIZATIONS

American Brain Tumor Association (ABTA), 2720 River Road, Des Plaines, IL, 60018, 847-827-9910, 800-886-2282, 847-827-9918, info@abta.org, http://www.abta.org/.

American Cancer Society, 250 Williams Street NW, Atlanta, GA, 30303, 800-ACS-2345 (227-2345), www.cancer.org.

American Society of Clinical Oncology (ASCO), 2318 Mill Road, Suite 800, Alexandria, VA, 22314, 571-483-1300, 888-282-2552, membermail@asco.org, http://www.asco.org/ASCOv2?edition=default.

The Childhood Brain Tumor Foundation (CBTF), 20312 Watkins Meadow Drive, Germantown, MD, 20876, 301-515-2900, 877-217-4166, cbtf@childhoodbraintumor.org, http://www.childhoodbraintumor.org/.

National Cancer Institute, 6116 Executive Blvd., Room 3036A, Bethesda, MD, 20892-8322, 800-422-6237, cancergovstaff@mail.nih.gov, www.cancer.gov.

National Institute of Neurological Disorders and Stroke (NINDS), P.O. Box 5801, Bethesda, MD, 20824, 800-352-9424, 301-496-5751, http://www.ninds.nih.gov/index.htm.

Tish Davidson, A.M.
Rebecca J. Frey, PhD

Cardiomyopathy

Definition

Cardiomyopathy is a type of heart disease in which the heart muscle is abnormally enlarged, thickened and/or stiffened. As a result, the heart muscle's ability to pump blood is usually impaired.

Description

When the heart muscle enlarges and is unable to pump effectively, its function declines. This is called congestive heart failure. Congestive heart failure results in a reduction in oxygen delivery to the tissues and a backup of fluid into those tissues. Fluid in the lungs can cause shortness of breath with exertion and a

Colored chest x ray of a patient suffering from cardiomyopathy (heart failure), showing enlargement of the left ventricle of the heart. *(Photo Researchers, Inc. Reproduced by permission.)*

need to sleep with the head elevated. Fluid buildup in other areas can manifest itself as swelling of the feet and ankles or swelling and pain in the liver. Congestive heart failure once carried a grim prognosis, but new advances in medical treatment have improved that prognosis significantly.

People with cardiomyopathy can develop an abrupt buildup of fluid in the lungs, called acute pulmonary edema. This is a medical emergency. In addition to intravenous medications that remove fluid, support blood pressure, and strengthen the heart's pumping function, acute pulmonary edema is also treated with oxygen and sometimes the temporary use of a respirator.

Almost anything that can damage the heart muscle fibers can produce cardiomyopathy and congestive heart failure. Long-standing high blood pressure, diabetes, heart attacks, alcohol, drugs, and certain viruses are all causes of cardiomyopathy.

In a person with **cancer**, cardiomyopathy and its symptoms are generally due to the adverse effects of treatment.

Causes

Among the causes of cardiomyopathy in cancer patients is **radiation therapy** to the chest, which is often employed for **breast cancer**, cancer of the esophagus, or **lymphoma**. Children who receive radiation therapy to the spinal column can suffer late effects to their hearts. The radiation can damage the heart muscle, leading to cardiomyopathy and heart failure.

It can also damage the coronary arteries, leading to angina or a heart attack.

More commonly, cardiomyopathy in a cancer patient is an adverse effect of **chemotherapy**. Among the chemotherapeutic drugs known to be toxic to the heart are:

- Doxorubicin
- Daunorubicin
- Mitoxantrone
- Cyclophosphamide
- 5-Fluorouracil (fluorouracil)
- Vincristine
- Vinblastine
- Busulfan
- Mitomycin C
- Cisplatin
- Amsacrine
- Paclitaxel
- Docetaxel
- Interferons
- Aldesleukin
- Trastuzumab

The drugs most frequently associated with cardiotoxicity are **doxorubicin** and **daunorubicin**, which are anthracyclines. The total cumulative dose of anthracyclines a person receives determines the likelihood of developing chronic cardiomyopathy. In a few cases, these agents will cause an acute cardiotoxic effect, with symptoms such as abnormal heart rhythms and electrocardiogram changes.

Patients receiving anthracyclines have nuclear imaging scans of their hearts before starting treatment, during treatment, and after treatment, since the adverse effects can be delayed. These studies measure the heart's ejection fraction, which is the percentage of blood volume pumped with each heartbeat. A normal ejection fraction is around 60%. In other words, 60% of the blood that collects in the heart between heartbeats is pumped out with each beat. Anthracyclines can cause a significant reduction in ejection fraction and therefore in heart function.

Often used for colon, breast, and **head and neck cancers**, 5-fluorouracil can cause cardiotoxicity, mostly in those patients with existing coronary artery disease or those who are also receiving radiation therapy to the chest. **Cyclophosphamide**, often used in those who have had bone marrow transplants, is another cause of cardiomyopathy. The taxanes, paclitaxel and **docetaxel**, are newer agents often used for breast and ovarian cancers. Taxanes can cause slowing of the heart rate, but this is not usually serious or prolonged.

Trastuzumab is a monoclonal antibody used in some patients with breast cancer. About 30% of women have overexpression of human epidermal growth factor receptors, called HER-2, on the surface of their cancer cells. Trastuzumab selectively attacks those receptors. Heart muscle also has some HER-2 receptors, which is believed to be the reason that trastuzumab can cause cardiomyopathy. Trastuzumab is often used in conjunction with anthracyclines or taxanes, both of which have effects on the heart, and patients on these drugs must be carefully monitored for signs of heart disease.

The diagnosis of cardiomyopathy is made on the basis of the patient's history and physical examination, along with tests of heart function. Occasionally, biopsies of the heart muscle are performed to confirm the diagnosis.

Other forms of damage to the heart can occur with cancer and its treatments. Some cancers can metastasize to the heart muscle or the valves within the heart. Cancers that spread to the pericardium, the outer lining of the heart, can induce fluid collections called pericardial effusions.

High-output cardiac failure is an unusual form of heart failure that results when the body senses a lowered total blood volume. This can occur with **anemia**, a side effect of many treatments, or with large tumors that have large numbers of blood vessels, drawing blood away from the general circulation.

Amyloidosis is a condition in which abnormal proteins are deposited in tissues throughout the body, including the heart. Amyloidosis is seen with **multiple myeloma**.

Abnormal heart rhythms can occur due to toxic effects of chemotherapeutic drugs and perhaps radiation treatments on the electrical conducting system of the heart.

Treatments

The treatment of cardiomyopathy in cancer patients consists of removing the cause when possible and using cardiac medications to reduce symptoms.

Since the most common cause of cardiomyopathy in cancer patients is due to the use of anthracyclines, oncologists keep a careful record of the total dose administered to patients over the course of their treatment, and stop the drug before the known toxic dose has been reached.

Newer forms of anthracyclines have been formulated which are called liposome encapsulates. These have been shown to be less toxic to the heart and still effective against cancer. Administering anthracyclines weekly, rather than every three to four weeks, and giving the dose more slowly both seem to reduce the cardiac toxicity. The simultaneous administration of drugs that might protect the heart is under study, but their use is not yet recommended routinely.

The treatment of established cardiomyopathy and heart failure due to cancer treatment is a combination of medications that are used for heart failure of any origin. One of these is digoxin, which improves the heart's pumping function in addition to other beneficial effects. Diuretics, often called water pills, flush water and salt from the body and are used to reduce swelling. Angiotensin-converting enzymes or ACE inhibitors comprise the third group of drugs useful for heart failure. These relax the arteries, which reduces the work that the heart must do to effectively pump blood. The fourth group of medications includes beta-blockers, which slow the heart rate and reduce its workload. This combination of medications has significantly improved the prognosis for people with heart failure.

Lifestyle changes can reduce symptoms of heart failure. Reducing salt and fluid intake and avoiding alcohol are beneficial. A judicious exercise plan can increase stamina without overtaxing a failing heart. Many people who have undergone cancer treatment also have coronary artery disease, which can aggravate the symptoms of heart failure caused by chemotherapy toxicity. Patients whose cancer prognosis is good can sometimes benefit from treatment of their coronary artery disease.

Some patients whose cancer is cured but whose cardiomyopathy progresses despite medication are candidates for heart transplant.

Alternative and complementary therapies

Naturopaths might prescribe hawthorn for symptoms of congestive heart failure. No studies have demonstrated either benefit or harm from this preparation.

Acupuncture and acupressure are sometimes beneficial in reducing symptoms of shortness of breath and may offer some relief to those with heart failure due to cardiomyopathy. The pressure point for the heart is said to be on the palm of the hand, over the bones between the fourth and fifth fingers.

Resources

BOOKS

Moore, Katen, and Libby Schmais. *Living Well with Cancer: A Nurse Tells You Everything You Need to Know About Managing the Side Effects of Your Treatment.* New York: Putnam Publishing Group, 2001.

PERIODICALS

Ginsburg, A.D. "Doxorubicin-induced Cardiomyopathy." *New England Journal of Medicine* 340, no. 8 (February, 1999): 654.

OTHER

Heart Center Online Home Page. [cited June 6, 2001]. http://www.heartcenteronline.com/. This website serves cardiologists and their patients and has sections on pericardiocentesis, pericarditis, and tamponade.

Marianne Vahey, M.D.

Carmustine

Definition

Carmustine is an antineoplastic drug, meaning that it inhibits the growth of **cancer**. It does this by disrupting DNA and synthesis, which leads to cell death. Carmustine is often referred to as BCNU, and along with other chemically similar drugs (**lomustine, semustine**, and **streptozocin**) is classified as a nitrosourea. Brand names for carmustine in the United States include BiCNU and Gliadel Wafers.

Purpose

Because it readily crosses the blood-brain barrier, carmustine is used to treat several types of **brain tumors**, including **astrocytoma, ependymoma**, glioblastoma, brainstem glioma, **medulloblastoma**. It is usually given intravenously, but it is also available as a wafer that is implanted in the brain during surgery. Carmustine is also used in the treatment of **multiple myeloma** and **melanoma**, usually in combination with other agents. It is also used in high does for patients undergoing bone marrow or stem cell transplants. Patients with non-Hodgkin's or Hodgkin's **lymphoma** whose disease has either relapsed or not responded to initial therapy may be treated with carmustine used in combination with other drugs.

Description

Carmustine was approved for use by the U.S. Food and Drug Administration (FDA) in 1977. Carmustine comes in vial, in a powder form, and is reconstituted with sterile water according to the manufacturer's instructions. It may be used as a single agent, meaning it is administered alone, or it may be used with other drugs. It is further diluted in a larger volume of fluid and given slowly into a vein over a one- to two-hour period. Faster administration may

KEY TERMS

Antiemetic—A drug that prevents or alleviates nausea and vomiting.

Body surface area—A measurement based on height and weight that is expressed in square meters. It is used to determine chemotherapy dosages.

Myelosuppression—Suppression of bone marrow function that results in decreased platelets, red blood cells, and white blood cells.

cause a burning sensation in the vein, as well as facial flushing. The wafer is implanted surgically.

Carmustine is excreted by the kidneys during urination, and the lungs during expiration. Studies have shown that within four days, up to 70% of the drug is excreted in the urine, while an additional 10% is excreted in exhaled carbon dioxide. No one is certain what happens to the remaining 20% of the drug.

Recommended dosage

Because carmustine can have delayed toxic effects on the bone marrow, doses should be given at least four to six weeks apart. If carmustine is given in conjunction with other drugs that also suppress the bone marrow, dosages may be reduced. Blood tests are performed frequently during and after treatment, and their results may require dosage adjustments. Currently, there is no known remedy for a carmustine overdose.

Chemotherapy dosages are based on a person's body surface area (BSA), which is calculated in square meters using height and weight measurements. Drug dosages are ordered in milligrams per square meter (mg/m^2). Carmustine doses vary, but common doses include 75–250 mg/m^2 every four to six weeks, and 80 mg/m^2 daily for three days every six weeks. Higher doses are used for patients undergoing bone marrow or stem cell transplants. The specific dose should be verified for each patient. Continued doses after the first course of carmustine depend on the patient's response and on toxicity. Sometimes doses are adjusted because of toxicity or low blood counts.

Precautions

Carmustine may be damaging to an unborn fetus. Women of child-bearing potential should take measures to prevent pregnancy and women receiving carmustine should not breast-feed.

Side effects

Carmustine should be used after careful consideration of the risks and benefits involved, as there can be serious adverse side effects.

Myelosuppression

Effects on the bone marrow can lead to reduced numbers of platelets and white blood cells, which can have potentially life-threatening results, including bleeding and **infection**. These effects are first seen from four to six weeks after treatment is started, are cumulative, and are related to the amount of the drug given. A patient taking carmustine who develops a **fever** or notices an increased tendency to bleed or bruise may have dangerously low blood counts, and should be evaluated by a physician.

Pulmonary damage

Patients taking carmustine are at risk for damage to the lungs marked by pulmonary fibrosis. The main symptom of pulmonary fibrosis is shortness of breath. Pulmonary fibrosis can lead to heart failure. It is most likely to develop in patients with total cumulative doses greater than 1,400 mg/m^2, although lower doses may also cause damage.

Individuals with underlying lung disease, such as chronic obstructive pulmonary disease, may be more likely to develop carmustine-associated pulmonary injury. Prior to initiating treatment with carmustine, a doctor will usually evaluate how well the lungs function by performing pulmonary function tests (PFTs). Patients are more likely to develop lung damage if portions of these tests are abnormal. PFTs may be repeated during treatment to monitor for adverse effects of carmustine. If carmustine is used in conjunction with other drugs that have toxic effects on pulmonary function, there may be a greater risk of lung damage.

Nausea and vomiting

Like many antineoplastic drugs, carmustine can cause **nausea and vomiting**. Before carmustine is administered, medications called **antiemetics** should be given to prevent or minimize **nausea**. Patients who experience severe nausea, or nausea that is uncontrolled with antiemetics, should notify their doctor.

Organ damage

Carmustine may cause damage to the kidneys. With careful monitoring and frequent blood tests, this damage can be prevented or reversed. Kidney damage is more likely to occur in individuals who have received prolonged therapy with large cumulative doses. Blood tests to evaluate renal function should be performed routinely. Carmustine may be discontinued or reduced depending on these results.

Secondary malignancies

Although carmustine is used to treat cancer, it may also cause secondary malignancies when used long term.

Carmustine wafers

Intracranial implantation of carmustine wafers has been associated with abnormal wound healing after surgery, brain edema or accumulation of fluid, infection, and the formation of cysts near the site of implantation.

Interactions

Patients should tell their doctor about medications they are taking in addition to their cancer treatment, as these medications may interact with carmustine. For example, cimetidine, a drug used to treat heartburn and ulcers, may increase the toxic effects of carmustine on the bone marrow. Carmustine, on the other hand, may decrease blood levels of **phenytoin**, a drug used in the treatment of patients with seizures. If blood levels are too low, seizures may not be prevented.

Patients undergoing treatment for cancer with carmustine should talk to their doctor prior to taking any **vaccines**. Live vaccines, in particular, can increase the likelihood of complications.

Aspirin and ibuprofen, which are found in many over-the-counter products, should be avoided. These drugs can increase the potential for bleeding in people who may already have decreased platelet counts due to carmustine therapy.

Tamara Brown, R.N.

Cartilage supplements

Description

Cartilage is a type of dense connective tissue found in humans and other animals. Bluish-white or gray in color, the semi-opaque tissue has no nerve or blood supply of its own. Cartilage supplements come from such animal sources as cattle, sharks, sheep, and chickens, with cattle and sharks being the predominant sources. Bovine cartilage supplements are derived from the windpipes of cows, while the cartilage from the heads and fins of sharks is used for shark supplements.

General use

Both bovine and shark cartilage supplements have been proposed as treatments for **cancer**. In addition, a compound derived from cartilage called chondroitin has been publicized as a useful treatment for osteoarthritis. Cartilage preparations are available as pills, powders, or liquids for oral dosage. They can also be given as enemas, topical applications, or intravenous or intramuscular injections.

Bovine cartilage supplements

Beginning in the 1950s, the physician John F. Prudden noticed that bovine cartilage could enhance wound healing in animals. Prudden then injected an extract of bovine cartilage into a **breast cancer** patient whose tumor had ulcerated her skin. The patient's tumor ultimately disappeared, and she lived for 12 years before dying of other causes. In 1985, Prudden published the first of several scientific papers on the subject.

Prudden believed that the anticancer ingredients in bovine cartilage are mucopolysaccharides, which are complex sugar molecules that help fight cancer by stimulating the patient's immune system. Prudden also states that these large sugar molecules act on tumor cell membranes by blocking mitosis (cell division). Other proposed explanations of the effectiveness of bovine cartilage include the inhibition of protease, which is an enzyme that helps to break down proteins, and inhibited formation of enzymes that break down collagen proteins. Numerous bovine cartilage supplements have been made available for immunostimulation or to fight off cancer cells. Most reports on tumor response and the survival of cancer patients after cartilage treatment, however, are anecdotal.

In 2001, researchers at Georgetown University in Washington D.C. reported on the isolation of a compound, which they named *metastatin*, from bovine cartilage. Metastatin was able to block the formation of tumor nodules in the lungs of mice inoculated with b16bl6 **melanoma** or Lewis lung **carcinoma** cells. They concluded that metastatin is a potentially useful anti-tumor agent. Variations in study results may, in part, be due to variations in concentration and availability of metastatin.

Shark cartilage supplements

The use of shark cartilage to treat cancer is based on the claim that it blocks angiogenesis, or the development of new blood vessels that tumors need to survive. A researcher at Harvard Medical School in the 1970s, Judah Folkman, developed the theory of angiogenesis. Folkman's proposal that tumors, much like a normal organ or mass of cells, require a supply of blood to deliver nutrients for growth, has since become closely linked to the treatment of cancer with shark cartilage.

In 1983, William Lang, motivated by Folkman's research, began investigating the possible link between shark cartilage and its ability to starve tumors with an antiangiogenetic mechanism. In 1993, Lane published his book *Sharks Don't Get Cancer*, making shark cartilage one of the leading alternative cancer therapies, with 99% of the cartilage market in 1997 comprised of shark cartilage.

The use of shark cartilage as an alternative treatment has been opposed by wildlife experts who say that use of the substance threatens the shark population. A study discussed at a cancer research meeting in 2000 documented about a dozen cases of apparent cancer in sharks, including cancer of the cartilage.

Both shark and bovine cartilage have been used to treat a wide variety of cancers, including tumors of the breast, ovary, cervix, prostate, rectum, colon, stomach, kidney, and brain. The U.S. Food and Drug Administration (FDA) maintains that both types of cartilage can be tested as potential cancer therapies in **clinical trials** but must be sold strictly as dietary supplements. Dietary supplement manufacturers as of 2005 are also prohibited from making specific claims that the supplements can cure disease.

Chondroitin sulfate

Chondroitin is best known to the general public as a remedy for osteoarthritis, which is a form of arthritis caused by wearing away or degeneration of the cartilage that cushions the ends of bones. It is thought that the drying out of cartilage tissue in osteoarthritis is a major cause of tissue destruction. Chondroitin sulfate is given together with glucosamine, a compound that is a building block of cartilage. The chondroitin helps to attract and hold fluid within cartilage tissue. Tissue fluid keeps cartilage healthy in two ways: it acts as a shock absorber within the joints of the body, thus protecting cartilage from being worn away by the bones, and it carries nutrients to the cartilage. Studies have shown that combining glucosamine and chondroitin works better than either alone in preventing cartilage damage, but results are varied.

Preparations

Shark and bovine cartilage supplements are available in capsule form, while shark is also sold as a powder and liquid. Shark supplements are made from ground-up shark skeletons (mainly the fins and head), while bovine supplements are prepared from the cartilage taken from cow bones. Chondroitin sulfate can be taken orally as a pill, powder, or liquid. It can also be administered by injection. Oral preparations of chondroitin, by itself or in combination with glucosamine, are available in the United States as over-the-counter (OTC) dietary supplements. They can be purchased over the Internet and at pharmacies, health food stores, or even some grocery stores.

Precautions

While cartilage supplements do not appear to be harmful, persons who are considering them as a cancer treatment should not use them as their sole form of therapy and should consult their doctor before taking them. Persons who are considering chondroitin as a treatment for joint pain should be careful not to diagnose themselves. They should check with their physician to be sure that the pain is caused by osteoarthritis. Some conditions, including Lyme disease, gout, bursitis, and rheumatoid arthritis, can also cause pain in the joints. Although chondroitin appears to be helpful in treating osteoarthritis, it is not useful for these other conditions. Chondroitin has not been studied in children or in pregnant or nursing women.

Side effects

Both shark and bovine cartilage supplements show little or no side effects when taken at the appropriate dosage levels. Some patients have reported an allergic reaction to traces of bovine protein or other side effects that include a bad taste in the mouth, **fatigue**, and **nausea**. Shark cartilage can cause **hypercalcemia** (excessive amounts of calcium in the body) when taken at the recommended daily dose of 70 g per day, 14 times the amount of calcium recommended by the United States Recommended Daily Allowance (USRDA). Some patients taking chondroitin have been known to experience nausea and gas or bloating.

Interactions

Chondroitin sulfate is not known to cause any significant interactions with other medications.

Resources

PERIODICALS

Theodosakis, Jason. "Relief for your Painful Joints (Wellness)." *Better Nutrition* (May 2002): 32.

OTHER

Center for Alternative Medicine Research in Cancer Home Page [cited January 17, 2001]. http://www.sph.uth.tmc.edu/utcam/therapies/crtlg.htm.

ORGANIZATIONS

National Cancer Institute. (800)332-8615. http://www.cancernet.nci.nih.gov.

NIH National Center for Complementary and Alternative Medicine (NCCAM). NCCAM Clearinghouse. PO Box 8218, Silver Spring, MD 20907-8218. (888)644-6226. www.nccam.nih.gov.

Beth Kapes

CAT scan, CT scan, Computerized axial tomography *see* **Computed tomography**

Cefepime *see* **Antibiotics**

Ceftazidime *see* **Antibiotics**

Ceftriaxone *see* **Antibiotics**

Celecoxib *see* **Cyclooxygenase 2 inhibitors**

Cellcept *see* **Mycophenolate mofetil**

Central nervous system carcinoma

Definition

A central nervous system **carcinoma** is a malignant tumor arising in the cells of the brain or spinal cord.

Description

The central nervous system (CNS) is comprised of the brain and spinal cord. The CNS takes its name from the crucial role it plays in maintaining physical and mental well-being (homeostasis). The brain controls and monitors the body's activity, while the spinal cord conveys information to the body from the brain, and vice versa. Consequently, a tumor in the CNS disrupts motor (e.g., standing, walking, writing) and sensory (e.g., seeing, tasting, hearing) activities.

KEY TERMS

Biopsy—Tissue sample taken from body for microscopic examination.

Carcinoma—A cancer that originates in cells that developed from epithelial tissue, a tissue that forms layers and often specializes to cover and protect organs.

Computed tomography (CT)—X rays aimed at sections of the body (by rotating equipment). The images appear as slices. Results are assembled with a computer to give a three-dimensional image.

Homeostasis—Self-regulating mechanisms are working, body is in equilibrium, no uncontrolled cell growth.

Magnetic resonance imaging (MRI)—Magnetic fields and radio frequency waves are used to make images of the inside of the body.

Meninges—The three layers of tissue that cover the brain and spinal cord.

Pineal—A very small gland in the center of the brain that is sensitive to light.

Pituitary—A gland at the base of the brain that produces hormones.

Positron emission tomography (PET)—A nuclear medicine procedure in which small amounts of radioactive materials are placed in the patient's body, usually by injection. Then a special camera and computer reconstruct a three-dimensional image.

QUESTIONS TO ASK THE DOCTOR

- Which type of CNS carcinoma do I have?
- With this type of carcinoma, what is the five-year survival rate for a person of my age and gender? What is the one-year survival rate?
- Is there a center that specializes in treating this type of cancer?
- Are there any clinical trials in which I might be eligible to participate?
- Does this health care institution have a support group for individuals with my type of carcinoma?
- What is your approach to relieving pain?

The two major components of brain tissue are neurons (nerve cells) and glial cells. About half of all malignant CNS tumor growth starts in glial cells. Long thought to be mere space-holders, glial cells have been found to be extremely important. These cells actually protect and nourish the neurons, and may also help them transmit information. There are many different types of glial carcinomas, or gliomas.

The three layers of membrane (meninges) that cover the brain and spinal cord and the pituitary and pineal parts of the brain are common sites for tumor growth. About 40% of benign (noncancerous) CNS tumors occur in the meninges and the pituitary and pineal glands.

Some cancers that originate in organs, such as the kidneys, spread (metastasize) to the brain and spinal cord. These metastases differ from CNS carcinomas, however.

Demographics

About 35,000 cases of CNS carcinoma are diagnosed each year. The Central Brain Tumor Registry of the United States (CBTRUS) puts the incidence of CNS tumors at 12.8 per 100,000 person-years. The rate is slightly higher in males and slightly lower in females. Over a lifetime the chance a man will be diagnosed with and die from a CNS tumor is 1 in 200 and for a woman the rate is 1 in 263.

The older a person is the more likely he or she is to be diagnosed with CNS carcinoma. According to CBTRUS, the pediatric (individuals ages 0-19 years) incidence of CNS tumors is significantly lower, or about 3.8 per 100,000 person-years. People under the age of 20 years also have a higher survival rate. They are five times more likely to live at least five years with a CNS tumor than are people between the ages of 45 and 64 years.

In addition to the diagnosis of primary CNS tumors (those that originate in the brain and spinal cord) is the diagnosis of metastatic **cancer**. Metastatic cancers are those that have spread from other primary sites, such as the breast, prostate, lungs, and colon. For every person diagnosed with a primary CNS tumor, at least four other individuals will be diagnosed with cancer that has metastasized to the brain and spinal cord. Occasionally, the identification of a metastatic brain cancer leads a physician to discover a cancer in another organ, or the **primary site**.

Causes and symptoms

The cause of CNS carcinoma is unknown. Important factors might include heredity, genetic make-up, and exposure to radiation and chemicals. Head injury might lead to meningiomas (carcinoma of the meninges). Extra or missing chromosomes or other genetic abnormalities are linked to the development of some CNS tumors. In 2004, researchers identified a gene that may be linked to development of gliomas, the most common type of brain tumor. In one study a group of researchers led by T. Ballard showed that pilots and flight attendants are at greater risk for CNS carcinoma, perhaps because of their frequent exposure to high levels of cosmic radiation.

Many individuals display no symptoms of CNS carcinoma until the tumor has grown large enough to exert pressure on part of the CNS. Because the skull covers the brain and the vertebral column protects the spinal cord, a growing tumor soon pushes up against a barrier of bone. The bone limits the expansion of the tumor and the cancerous and adjacent parts of the CNS become distorted. The meninges then swell in response to the distortion, producing symptoms.

Symptoms include:

- headache
- muscle weakness
- exhaustion
- nausea and vomiting
- changes in vision
- seizures

When a tumor is in the spinal cord, symptoms include back pain and **incontinence** (inability to control defecation and urination). Paralysis on one side of the body (hemiparesis), which often indicates a stroke in an elderly person, sometimes occurs because of a brain tumor.

Diagnosis

Seizures and difficulties with walking, speech, sight, or other day-to-day activities usually cause patients with CNS carcinoma to consult a physician. The techniques a physician uses to diagnose CNS carcinoma begin with an examination and medical history. Some combination of blood tests, x ray, **computed tomography** (CT), and **magnetic resonance imaging** (MRI) is used. In recent years, another form of imaging called **positron emission tomography**, (PET) has been used increasingly to diagnose and monitor treatment of CNS carcinoma and other cancers. If a tumor is detected with a CT or MRI scan a **biopsy** is usually done to determine the type of tumor.

Treatment team

A CNS carcinoma requires attention from several different types of physician specialists. A neurologist, a physician specializing in the nervous system, does the initial assessment. A radiologist interprets **x rays** and CT and MRI images. A hematologist or oncologist evaluates the results of blood tests. A pathologist studies the tissue from a biopsy. The surgery team typically is led by a neurosurgeon. At premier cancer centers teams of physicians work collaboratively with one person, usually an oncologist, taking the lead. Physical and occupational therapists help with rehabilitation following treatment and surgery, and registered nurses who administer **chemotherapy** are also part of the team.

Clinical staging, treatments, and prognosis

By studying tissue from the tumor and surrounding cells the oncologist determines whether the tumor is growing and, if so, how fast. A precise system assigns stages and grades to the tumors. Staging and grading helps physicians compare cases, monitor treatment, and determine prognosis. Staging depends on things such as which part of the brain was served by the glial cell(s) in which the tumor began.

A plan for treatment is based on the location, size, and rate of growth of the tumor. Surgical removal of the tumor, radiation, and chemotherapy are all used. Method of treatment depends on the type of CNS carcinoma. In some cases the treatment is strictly palliative (provides comfort) and is not expected to halt the course of the cancer. Drugs, such as steroids, are often given to reduce swelling and, correspondingly, reduce pain and other symptoms.

About three-fourths of all individuals diagnosed with CNS carcinoma die before attaining a five-year survival rate.

Alternative and complementary therapies

Relaxation techniques may help to relieve pain from swelling.

Coping with cancer treatment

Being an active participant in the treatment team, something that specialized cancer centers encourage, is one way to cope. Joining a support group also may help.

Clinical trials

The National Cancer Institute at the National Institutes of Health operates an information service that provides the most up-to-date information about **clinical trials**. The number is (800) 4-CANCER ([800] 422-6237).

Prevention

Limiting exposure to cosmic radiation and chemicals might lower the risk. However, experts have no specific recommendations for prevention.

Special concerns

Psychological changes as simple as mood swings and as severe as major changes in personality are possible. Sensory impairment is also possible. **Advance directives**, or written instructions for the care a person wants at each juncture of treatment, should be prepared and legalized as early in the therapeutic process as possible. Such directives make the patient's choices clear should he or she become unable to express them as the cancer progresses. Doing so relieves loved ones of the responsibility for making those decisions, which can become extremely difficult.

See also Brain and central nervous system tumors.

Resources

PERIODICALS

Ballard, T., et al. "Cancer Incidence and Mortality Among Flight Personnel: A Meta-Analysis." *Aviation, Space, and Environmental Medicine* 71 (March 2000): 216-24.

"Brain Cancer Gene Identified." *Drug Week* April 9, 2004: 211.

Brice, James. "PET Agents Offer New Ways to Monitor Brain Cancer—F-18 FLT and F-18 FDOPA Eliminate Uncertainties Associated With Popular Diagnostic Techniques." *Diagnostic Imaging* June 1, 2004: 11.

Huncharek, M., et al. "Chemotherapy Response Rates in Recurrent/Progressive Pediatric Glioma; Results of a Systematic Review." *Anticancer Research* 19 (July-August 1999): 3569-74.

OTHER

"Facts and Statistics from the American Brain Tumor Association" *CancerWise.org* [cited March 28, 2001 and July 6, 2001]. http://www.cancerwise.org/archive/august/facts_figures/ff_brain.html.

"Year 2000 Standard Report" *Central Brain Tumor Registry of the United States* [cited March 28, 2001 and July 6, 2001]. http://www.cbtrus.org/2000/y2kstats_report.htm.

ORGANIZATIONS

American Brain Tumor Association. 2720 River Road, Des Plaines, IL 60018 (800) 886-2282 http://www.abta.org.

The Brain Tumor Society. 124 Watertown Street, Suite 3-H, Watertown, MA 02472. (617) 924-9997 http://www.tbts.org.

Diane M. Calabrese
Teresa G. Odle

Central nervous system lymphoma

Definition

Central nervous system **lymphoma**, now often called primary central nervous system lymphoma (PCNSL), is a fatal **cancer** that originates in the brain, spinal cord, or meninges. This cancer arises from the abnormal growth and development of lymphocytes, a type of white blood cell that normally functions as part of the immune system. Occasionally PCNSL begins in the eye (ocular lymphoma)

Demographics

PCNSL is rare in people with healthy immune systems, making up only about 2% of central nervous system (CNS) tumors in those people. PCNSL is more common in people with compromised immune systems, most especially those with HIV/AIDS. Some estimates put the incidence of PCNSL at 51 per 10,000,000 per year in people with HIV **infection**, while other estimates suggest that between 6% and 20% of people with HIV infection will eventually develop PCNSL.

The median age of diagnosis in non-immunocompromised individuals is 55 years. However, in HIV-infected individuals the median age at diagnosis is much younger, at about 35 years. In the non-immunocompromised population, men develop PCNSL twice as often as women. In the HIV-positive population, 95% of people with this cancer are male.

Description

PCNSL affects the brain and the spinal cord, the two components of the central nervous system. The brain and spinal cord work together to control, monitor, and interpret all the physical and mental processes of the body. They make possible the activities a person takes for granted, such as walking, talking, thinking, and remembering. A malignancy (neoplasm) in the brain or spinal cord interferes with vital functions of the nervous system.

Lymphoma is the uncontrolled growth of immune system cells called lymphocytes. About 90% of cases of PCNSL are caused by abnormal B lymphocytes (B cells); the remaining 10% of cases are caused by abnormal T lymphocytes (T cells). Under normal conditions these cells would help the body resist invasion by foreign substances and organisms by assisting in immune system response. In PCNSL, these cells form lesions that destroy nerve tissue.

PCNSL is an aggressive cancer that is always fatal. It tends to form a primary tumor and then spread rapidly throughout the brain and spinal cord, although it rarely spreads beyond the central nervous system. In most cases, it does not produce multiple defined tumors. Instead, as the cancer spreads, lesions, which are places where tissue breaks down, develop.

Risk factors

Infection with the HIV virus is by far the greatest risk factor for developing PCNSL. People who have received organ transplants and are taking immuno-suppressive drugs are also at higher risk.

Causes and symptoms

The specific cause of PCNSL is not known.

Symptoms of PCNSL include:

- change in personality
- headache
- nausea and vomiting
- seizures
- weakness
- numbness, particularly in the face
- sensory problems (cannot hear, see)
- difficulty swallowing

Diagnosis

Symptoms such as those listed above cause a person to consult a physician. The initial assessment often is made using **computed tomography** (CT) or **magnetic resonance imaging** (MRI). To confirm a diagnosis and rule out other possible diseases, the physician does a variety of tests. These may include a physical examination of lymph nodes, chest x ray, blood and urine tests, HIV testing, eye exam, and **bone marrow biopsy**. Some of the tests are done to rule out other kinds of lymphoma. Definitive diagnosis may require a **lumbar puncture**, which is a procedure in which a small amount of cerebrospinal fluid is removed from the lower spine so that it can be examined under the microscope for cancer cells.

Treatment

PCNSL requires care from a team of physician specialists. A neurologist—a physician specializing in the nervous system—does the initial assessment. A radiologist interprets **x rays**, CT scans, and MRI images. A hematologist or oncologist evaluates the results of blood tests. A pathologist studies the tissue from a **biopsy**. If there is surgery, and in many cases there is not, a surgery team removes the tumor. At premier cancer centers, teams of physicians work collaboratively, with one person (usually an oncologist) taking the lead. Physical and occupational therapists help with rehabilitation following treatment and surgery, and registered nurses who administer **chemotherapy**, if needed, are also part of the team.

Traditional

PCNSL is a fatal cancer that is very difficult to treat, in part because the blood-brain barrier makes it difficult to get therapeutic medication into the brain. Treatment often is palliative (designed to provide relief from symptoms and make a patient comfortable) rather than curative, although successful treatment can, in some cases, prolong life for about three years. Surgery is sometimes used to eliminate a well-defined mass that is causing pressure in the brain and spinal cord. This pressure causes the symptoms, such as headache and numbness, because it contributes to swelling and dislocation. However, because PCNSL generally spreads diffusely throughout the brain and spinal cord, surgery is usually not a treatment choice.

Radiation alone can keep patients alive an average of 18 months. Radiation with chemotherapy can increase this to three years; however, about half the patients receiving chemotherapy with radiation develop severe dementia. As of late 2009, there was no standard protocol for treating PCNSL. **Clinical trials** are ongoing. The National Cancer Institute at the National Institutes of Health, Bethesda, MD, offers a Cancer Information Service that can connect people with clinical trials. The toll free number for the service is 1-800-4-CANCER (1-800-422-6237).

Alternative

Relaxation programs, such as biofeedback or yoga, often help a patient deal with the poor prognosis, pain, and symptoms of PCNSL.

Prognosis

The prognosis (outlook for recovery) for a patient with PCNSL is very poor. Untreated, the disease usually results in death within a few weeks. If treated aggressively, life can be extended by perhaps 18 months and occasionally longer. Those who live longer often develop problems with memory and cognitive function related to treatment, thus their quality of live can be severely compromised. In addition, most people who develop PCNSL are HIV positive, which presents an additional set of health problems and treatment challenges.

Because PCNSL is invariably fatal, and usually within a short time, patients must make decisions about end-of-life care including whether to end their life at home, in a hospice, or in a hospital. They must decide who will make decisions when they are no longer able to state their preferences. An advance medical directive stating how a person wishes the medical team to respond at each juncture of the illness, should be completed and witnessed as soon as possible after a diagnosis is made.

Prevention

There is no definitive method of prevention; however, taking steps to remain HIV-free greatly reduces the likelihood of PCNSL developing.

Resources

OTHER

"Primary Central Nervous System CNS Lymphoma." LymphomaNet [September 14, 2009]. http://www.lymphomainfo.net/nhl/types/cns.html.

"Primary Central Nervous System Lymphoma (PDQ)." National Cancer Institute. June 18, 2008 [September 14, 2009]. http://www.cancer.gov/cancertopics/pdq/treatment/primary-cns-lymphoma/patient.

Ramachandran, Tarakad S. "Primary CNS Lymphoma." June 22, 2009 [September 14, 2009]. http://emedicine.medscape.com/article/1157638-overview.

ORGANIZATIONS

American Cancer Society, 1599 Clifton Rd., NE, Atlanta, GA, 30329, (404) 320-3333, (800) ACS-2345, http://www.cancer.org.

Cancer Research and Prevention Foundation, 1600 Duke Street, Suite 500, Alexandria, VA, 22314, (703) 836-4412, (800) 227-2732, info@preventcancer.org, http://www.preventcancer.org.

National Cancer Institute Public Inquires Office., 6116 Executive Boulevard, Room 3036A, Bethesda, MD, 20892-8322, (800) 4-CANCER. TTY (800) 332-8615, http://www.cancer.gov.

Diane M. Calabrese
Tish Davidson, A.M.

Central nervous system tumors *see* **Brain/Central nervous system tumors**
Cerebrospinal fluid analysis, spinal tap *see* **Lumbar puncture**

Cervical cancer

Definition

Cervical **cancer** is a disease in which the cells of the cervix become abnormal and start to grow uncontrollably, forming tumors.

Description

In the United States, cervical cancer is the fifth most common cancer among women aged 35-54, and the third most common cancer of the female reproductive tract. In some developing countries, it is the most common type of cancer. It generally begins as an abnormality in the cells on the outside of the cervix. The cervix is the lower part or neck of the uterus (womb). It connects the body of the uterus to the vagina (birth canal).

Approximately 90% of cervical cancers are squamous cell carcinomas. This type of cancer originates in the thin, flat, squamous cells on the surface of the ectocervix, the part of the cervix that is next to the

A biopsied section of the cervix indicating a carcinoma in situ. (*Custom Medical Stock Photo, Inc. Reproduced with permission.*)

KEY TERMS

Adenocarcinoma—Cervical cancer that originates in the mucus-producing cells of the inner or endocervix.

Biopsy—Removal of a small sample of tissue for examination under a microscope; used for the diagnosis and treatment of cervical cancer and precancerous conditions.

Carcinoma in situ—Cancer that is confined to the cells in which it originated and has not spread to other tissues.

Cervical intraepithelial neoplasia (CIN)—Abnormal cell growth on the surface of the cervix.

Cervix—Narrow, lower end of the uterus forming the opening to the vagina.

Colposcopy—Diagnostic procedure using a hollow, lighted tube (colposcope) to look inside the cervix and uterus.

Conization—Cone biopsy; removal of a cone-shaped section of tissue from the cervix for diagnosis or treatment.

Dysplasia—Abnormal cellular changes that may become cancerous.

Endocervical curettage—Biopsy performed with a curette to scrape the mucous membrane of the cervical canal.

Human papilloma virus (HPV)—Virus that causes abnormal cell growth (warts or papillomas); some types can cause cervical cancer.

Hysterectomy—Removal of the uterus.

Interferon—Potent immune-defense protein produced by viral-infected cells; used as an anti-cancer and anti-viral drug.

Laparoscopy—Laparoscopic pelvic lymph node dissection; insertion of a tube through a very small surgical incision to remove lymph nodes.

Loop electrosurgical excision procedure (LEEP)—Cone biopsy performed with a wire that is heated by electrical current.

Lymph nodes—Small round glands, located throughout the body, that filter the lymphatic fluid; part of the body's immune defense.

Pap test—Pap smear; removal of cervical cells to screen for cancer.

Pelvic exenteration—Extensive surgery to remove the uterus, ovaries, pelvic lymph nodes, part or all of the vagina, and the bladder, rectum, and/or part of the colon.

Squamous cells—Thin, flat cells of the surfaces of the skin and cervix and linings of various organs.

Squamous intraepithelial lesion (SIL)—Abnormal growth of squamous cells on the surface of the cervix.

Vaginal stenosis—Narrowing of the vagina due to a build-up of scar tissue.

---

vagina. (Squamous cells are the thin, flat cells of the surfaces of the skin and cervix and linings of various organs.) Another 10% of cervical cancers are of the **adenocarcinoma** type. This cancer originates in the mucus-producing cells of the inner or endocervix, near the body of the uterus. Occasionally, the cancer may have characteristics of both types and is called adenosquamous **carcinoma** or mixed carcinoma.

The initial changes that may occur in some cervical cells are not cancerous. However, these precancerous cells form a lesion called dysplasia or a squamous intraepithelial lesion (SIL), since it occurs within the epithelial or outer layer of cells. These abnormal cells can also be described as cervical intraepithelial neoplasia (CIN). Moderate to severe dysplasia may be called carcinoma in situ or non-invasive cervical cancer.

Dysplasia is a common condition and the abnormal cells often disappear without treatment. However, these precancerous cells can become cancerous. This may take years, although it can happen in less than a year. Eventually, the abnormal cells start to grow uncontrollably into the deeper layers of the cervix, becoming an invasive cervical cancer.

Although cervical cancer used to be one of the most common causes of cancer death among American women, in the past 40 years there has been a 75% decrease in mortality. This is primarily due to routine screening with Pap tests (Pap smear) to identify precancerous and early-invasive stages of cervical cancer. With treatment, these conditions have a cure rate of nearly 100%.

Demographics

Worldwide, there are more than 400,000 new cases of cervical cancer diagnosed each year. The American Cancer Society (ACS) estimated 11,270 new cases of invasive cervical cancer in the United States in 2009.

Older women are at the highest risk for cervical cancer. Although girls under the age of 15 rarely develop this cancer, the risk factor begins to increase in the late teens. Rates for carcinoma in situ peak between the ages of 20 and 30. In the United States, the incidence of invasive cervical cancer increases rapidly with age for African American women over the age of 25. The incidence rises more slowly for Caucasian women. However, women over age 65 account for more than 25% of all cases of invasive cervical cancer.

The incidence of cervical cancer is highest among poor women and among women in developing countries. In the United States, the death rates from cervical cancer are higher among Hispanic, Native American, and African American women than among Caucasian women. These groups of women are much less likely to receive regular Pap tests. Therefore, their cervical cancers usually are diagnosed at a much later stage, after the cancer has spread to other parts of the body.

Causes and symptoms

Human papillomavirus

Infection with the common human papillomavirus (HPV) is a cause of approximately 90% of all cervical cancers. There are more than 80 types of HPV. About 30 of these types can be transmitted sexually, including those that cause genital warts (papillomas). About half of the sexually transmitted HPVs are associated with cervical cancer. These "high-risk" HPVs produce a protein that can cause cervical epithelial cells to grow uncontrollably. The virus makes a second protein that interferes with tumor suppressors that are produced by the human immune system. The HPV-16 strain is thought to be a cause of about 50% of cervical cancers.

More than six million women in the United States have persistent HPV infections, for which there are no cure. Nevertheless, most women with HPV do not develop cervical cancer.

Symptoms of invasive cervical cancer

Most women do not have symptoms of cervical cancer until it has become invasive. At that point, the symptoms may include:

- unusual vaginal discharge
- light vaginal bleeding or spots of blood outside of normal menstruation
- pain or vaginal bleeding with sexual intercourse
- post-menopausal vaginal bleeding

Once the cancer has invaded the tissue surrounding the cervix, a woman may experience pain in the pelvic region and heavy bleeding from the vagina.

Diagnosis

The Pap test

Most often, cervical cancer is first detected with a Pap test that is performed as part of a regular pelvic examination. The vagina is spread with a metal or plastic instrument called a speculum. A swab is used to remove mucus and cells from the cervix. This sample is sent to a laboratory for microscopic examination.

The Pap test is a screening tool rather than a diagnostic tool. It is very efficient at detecting cervical abnormalities. The Bethesda System commonly is used to report Pap test results. A negative test means that no abnormalities are present in the cervical tissue. A positive Pap test describes abnormal cervical cells as low-grade or high-grade SIL, depending on the extent of dysplasia. About 5-10% of Pap tests show at least mild abnormalities. However, a number of factors other than cervical cancer can cause abnormalities, including inflammation from bacteria or yeast infections. A few months after the infection is treated, the Pap test is repeated.

Biopsy

Following an abnormal Pap test, a colposcopy is usually performed. The physician uses a magnifying scope to view the surface of the cervix. The cervix may be coated with an iodine solution that causes normal cells to turn brown and abnormal cells to turn white or yellow. This is called a Schiller test. If any abnormal areas are observed, a colposcopic **biopsy** may be performed. A biopsy is the removal of a small piece of tissue for microscopic examination by a pathologist.

Other types of cervical biopsies may be performed. An endocervical curettage is a biopsy in which a narrow instrument called a curette is used to scrape tissue from inside the opening of the cervix. A **cone biopsy**, or conization, is used to remove a cone-shaped piece of tissue from the cervix. In a cold knife cone biopsy, a surgical scalpel or laser is used to remove the tissue. A loop electrosurgical excision procedure (LEEP) is a cone biopsy using a wire that is heated by an electrical current. Cone biopsies can be used to determine whether abnormal cells have invaded below the surface of the cervix. They also can be used to treat many precancers and very early cancers. Biopsies may be performed with a local or general anesthetic. They may cause cramping and bleeding.

Diagnosing the stage

Following a diagnosis of cervical cancer, various procedures may be used to stage the disease (determine how far the cancer has spread). For example, additional pelvic exams may be performed under anesthesia.

There are several procedures for determining if cervical cancer has invaded the urinary tract. With **cystoscopy**, a lighted tube with a lens is inserted through the urethra (the urine tube from the bladder to the exterior) and into the bladder to examine these organs for cancerous cells. Tissue samples may be removed for microscopic examination by a pathologist. **Intravenous urography** (intravenous pyelogram or IVP) is an x ray of the urinary system, following the injection of special dye. The kidneys remove the dye from the bloodstream and the dye passes into the ureters (the tubes from the kidneys to the bladder) and bladder. IVP can detect a blocked ureter, caused by the spread of cancer to the pelvic lymph nodes (small glands that are part of the immune system).

A procedure called proctoscopy or **sigmoidoscopy** is similar to cystoscopy. It is used to determine whether the cancer has spread to the rectum or lower large intestine.

Computed tomography (CT or CAT) scans, ultrasound, or other imaging techniques may be used to determine the spread of cancer to various parts of the body. With a CT scan, an x-ray beam rotates around the body, taking images from various angles. It is used to determine if the cancer has spread to the lymph nodes. **Magnetic resonance imaging** (MRI), which uses a magnetic field to image the body, sometimes is used for evaluating the spread of cervical cancer. Chest **x rays** may be used to detect cervical cancer that has spread to the lungs.

Treatment team

Pap smears usually are performed by a women's health specialist, a nurse practitioner, a family practice physician, or a gynecologist. These practitioners may treat precancerous conditions. Procedures for diagnosing cervical cancer are performed by a gynecologist. A pathologist examines the biopsied tissue for cancer cells. Following diagnosis, a specialist in cancers of the female reproductive system, known as a gynecological oncologist, as well as a radiation oncologist and a surgeon may join the team.

Clinical staging, treatments, and prognosis

Following a diagnosis of cervical cancer, the physician takes a medical history and performs a complete physical examination. This includes an evaluation of symptoms and risk factors for cervical cancer. The lymph nodes are examined for evidence that the cancer has spread from the cervix. The choice of treatment depends on the clinical stage of the disease.

The FIGO system of staging

The International Federation of Gynecologists and Obstetricians (FIGO) system usually is used to stage cervical cancer:

- Stage 0: Carcinoma in situ; non-invasive cancer that is confined to the layer of cells lining the cervix.
- Stage I: Cancer that has spread into the connective tissue of the cervix but is confined to the uterus.
- Stage IA: Very small cancerous area that is visible only with a microscope.
- Stage IA1: Invasion area is less than 3 mm (0.13 in) deep and 7 mm (0.33 in) wide.
- Stage IA2: Invasion area is 3–5 mm (0.13-0.2 in) deep and less than 7 mm (0.33 in) wide.
- Stage IB: Cancer can be seen without a microscope or is deeper than 5 mm (0.2 in) or wider than 7 mm (0.33 in).
- Stage IB1: Cancer is no larger than 4 cm (1.6 in).
- Stage IB2: Stage IB cancer is larger than 4 cm (1.6 in).

- Stage II: Cancer has spread from the cervix but is confined to the pelvic region.
- Stage IIA: Cancer has spread to the upper region of the vagina, but not to the lower one-third of the vagina.
- Stage IIB: Cancer has spread to the parametrial tissue adjacent to the cervix.
- Stage III: Cancer has spread to the lower one-third of the vagina or to the wall of the pelvis and may be blocking the ureters.
- Stage IIIA: Cancer has spread to the lower vagina but not to the pelvic wall.
- Stage IIIB: Cancer has spread to the pelvic wall and/or is blocking the flow of urine through the ureters to the bladder.
- Stage IV: Cancer has spread to other parts of the body.
- Stage IVA: Cancer has spread to the bladder or rectum.
- Stage IVB: Cancer has spread to distant organs such as the lungs.
- Recurrent: Following treatment, cancer has returned to the cervix or some other part of the body.

In addition to the stage of the cancer, factors such as a woman's age, general health, and preferences may influence the choice of treatment. The exact location of the cancer within the cervix and the type of cervical cancer also are important considerations.

Treatment of precancer and carcinoma in situ

Most low-grade SILs that are detected with Pap tests revert to normal without treatment. Most high-grade SILs require treatment. Treatments to remove precancerous cells include:

- cold knife cone biopsy
- LEEP
- cryosurgery (freezing the cells with a metal probe)
- cauterization or diathermy (burning off the cells)
- laser surgery (burning off the cells with a laser beam)

These methods also may be used to treat cancer that is confined to the surface of the cervix (stage 0) and other early-stage cervical cancers in women who may want to become pregnant. They may be used in conjunction with other treatments. These procedures may cause bleeding or cramping. All of these treatments require close follow-up to detect any recurrence of the cancer.

Surgery

A simple hysterectomy is used to treat some stages of 0 and IA cervical cancers. Usually only the uterus is removed, although occasionally the fallopian tubes and ovaries are removed as well. The tissues adjoining the uterus, including the vagina, remain intact. The uterus may be removed either through the abdomen or the vagina.

In a radical hysterectomy, the uterus and adjoining tissues, including the ovaries, the upper region (1 in) of the vagina near the cervix, and the pelvic lymph nodes, are all removed. A radical hysterectomy usually involves abdominal surgery. However it can be performed vaginally, in combination with a laparoscopic pelvic **lymph node dissection**. With **laparoscopy**, a tube is inserted through a very small surgical incision for the removal of the lymph nodes. These operations are used to treat stages IA2, IB, and IIA cervical cancers, particularly in young women. Following a hysterectomy, the tissue is examined to see if the cancer has spread and requires additional radiation treatment. Women who have had hysterectomies cannot become pregnant, but complications from a hysterectomy are rare.

If cervical cancer recurs following treatment, a pelvic **exenteration** (extensive surgery) may be performed. This includes a radical hysterectomy, with the additional removal of the bladder, rectum, part of the colon, and/or all of the vagina. Such operations require the creation of new openings for the urine and feces. A new vagina may be created surgically. Often the clitoris and other outer genitals are left intact.

Recovery from a pelvic exenteration may take six months to two years. This treatment is successful with 40-50% of recurrent cervical cancers that are confined to the pelvis. If the recurrent cancer has spread to other organs, radiation or **chemotherapy** may be used to alleviate some of the symptoms.

Radiation

Radiation therapy, which involves the use of high-dosage x rays or other high-energy waves to kill cancer cells, often is used for treating stages IB, IIA, and IIB cervical cancers, or in combination with surgery. With external-beam radiation therapy, the rays are focused on the pelvic area from a source outside the body. With implant or internal radiation therapy, a pellet of radioactive material is placed internally, near the tumor. Alternatively, thin needles may be used to insert the radioactive material directly into the tumor.

Radiation therapy to the pelvic region can have many side effects:

- skin reaction in the area of treatment
- fatigue
- upset stomach and loose bowels

- vaginal stenosis (narrowing of the vagina due to build-up of scar tissue) leading to painful sexual intercourse
- premature menopause in young women
- problems with urination

Chemotherapy

Chemotherapy, the use of one or more drugs to kill cancer cells, is used to treat disease that has spread beyond the cervix. Most often it is used following surgery or radiation treatment. Stages IIB, III, IV, and recurrent cervical cancers usually are treated with a combination of external and internal radiation and chemotherapy. The common drugs used for cervical cancer are **cisplatin**, **ifosfamide**, and **fluorouracil**. These may be injected or taken by mouth. The National Cancer Institute recommends that chemotherapy with cisplatin be considered for all women receiving radiation therapy for cervical cancer.

The side effects of chemotherapy depend on a number of factors, including the type of drug, the dosage, and the length of the treatment. Side effects may include:

- nausea and vomiting
- fatigue
- changes in appetite
- hair loss (alopecia)
- mouth or vaginal sores
- infections
- menstrual cycle changes
- premature menopause
- infertility
- bleeding or anemia (low red blood cell count)

With the exception of menopause and infertility, most of the side effects are temporary.

Alternative and complementary therapies

Biological therapy sometimes is used to treat cervical cancer, either alone or in combination with chemotherapy. Treatment with the immune-system protein interferon is used to boost the **immune response**. Biological therapy can cause temporary flu-like symptoms and other side effects.

Some research suggests that vitamin A (carotene) may help to prevent or stop cancerous changes in cells such as those on the surface of the cervix. Other studies suggest that **vitamins** C and E may reduce the risk of cervical cancer.

Prognosis

For cervical cancers that are diagnosed in the pre-invasive stage, the five-year-survival rate is almost 100%. When cervical cancer is detected in the early invasive stages, approximately 91% of women survive five years or more. Stage IVB cervical cancer is not considered to be curable. The five-year-survival rate for all cervical cancers combined is about 70%. The death rate from cervical cancer continues to decline by about 2% each year. Women over age 65 account for 40-50% of all deaths from cervical cancer.

Coping with cancer treatment

Medications can ease some of the side effects of radiation and chemotherapy, such as **nausea** and menopausal symptoms. Premature menopause may require estrogen-replacement therapy; however, in 2003, a large study called the Women's Health Initiative documented several health problems with hormone replacement therapy, so women should check with their physicians. Vaginal dilators and lubricants can relieve the effects of vaginal stenosis. A nutritious diet, rest, and a strong emotional support system help with recovery from treatment.

Following treatment for cervical cancer, additional tests are conducted to check for recurrence. These tests include frequent Pap smears, biopsies, and blood tests. X rays, CT or MRI scans, or other **imaging studies** such as ultrasound also may be used.

Clinical trials

There are many **clinical trials**, ongoing throughout the United States, for the treatment of most stages of cervical cancer. These include the testing of new chemotherapy drugs, new methods of radiation therapy, and new combinations of surgery and radiation or chemotherapy. New methods for performing Pap tests also are being studied.

A new test for HPV, called the Hybrid Capture HPV test, is being studied. Results suggest that this test may be useful for determining which women with abnormal Pap test results should have colposcopy. Various types of HPV **vaccines** are also being tested. These include vaccines that prevent HPV infection, vaccines for women infected with HPV, and vaccines for women with advanced cervical cancer. In 2006, Gardasil became the first FDA-approved HPV vaccine. A second vaccine, cervarix, was approved in 2009.

Prevention

Viral infections

Most cervical cancers are preventable. More than 90% of women with cervical cancer are infected with HPV. HPV infection is the single most important risk factor. This is particularly true for young women because the cells lining the cervix do not fully mature until age 18. These immature cells are more susceptible to cancer-causing agents and viruses.

Since HPV is a sexually transmitted infection, sexual behaviors can put women at risk for HPV infection and cervical cancer. These behaviors include:

- sexual intercourse at age 16 or younger
- partners who began having intercourse at a young age
- multiple sexual partners
- sexual partners who have had multiple partners ("high-risk males")
- A partner who has had a previous sexual partner with cervical cancer

HPV infection may not produce any symptoms, so sexual partners may not know that they are infected. Condoms do not necessarily prevent HPV infection. In 2003, a new DNA **screening test** was approved by the FDA to test for HPV at the same time as the Pap test.

Infection with the human immunodeficiency virus (HIV) that causes acquired immunodeficiency syndrome (AIDS) is a risk factor for cervical cancer. Women who test positive for HIV may have impaired immune systems that cannot correct precancerous conditions. Furthermore, sexual behavior that puts women at risk for HIV infection, also puts them at risk for HPV infection. There is some evidence suggesting that another sexually transmitted virus, the genital herpes virus, also may be involved in cervical cancer.

Smoking

Smoking may double the risk of cervical cancer. Chemicals produced by tobacco smoke can damage the DNA of cervical cells. The risk increases with the number of years a woman smokes and the amount she smokes. A 2003 study also linked smoking to poorer outcomes and survivals in cervical cancer patients.

Diet and drugs

Diets that are low in fruits and vegetables increase the risk of cervical cancer. A 2003 study also linked obesity to increased risk for cervical adenocarcinoma. Even women who were overweight had a higher incidence of the disease. The link appears to be increased levels of estrogen. Excessive fat tissue influences levels of estrogen and other sex hormones. Women also have an increased risk of cervical cancer if their mothers took the drug diethylstilbestrol (DES) while they were pregnant. This drug was given to women between 1940 and 1971 to prevent miscarriages. Some statistical studies have suggested that the long-term use of oral contraceptives may slightly increase the risk of cervical cancer.

Pap tests

Most cases of cervical cancers are preventable, since they start with easily detectable precancerous changes. Therefore, the best prevention for cervical cancer is a regular Pap test. The ACS revised its guidelines for regular screening in late 2002. In brief, women should begin having Pap tests about three years after having sexual intercourse, but no later than 21 years of age. Women should continue screening every year with regular Pap tests until age 30. Once a woman has had three normal results in a row, she may get screened every two to three years. A doctor may suggest more frequent screening if a woman has certain risk factors for cervical cancer. Women who have had total hysterectomies including the removal of the cervix and those over age 70 who have had three normal results generally do not need to continue having Pap tests under the new guidelines.

The National Breast and Cervical Cancer Early Detection Program provides free or low-cost Pap tests and treatment for women without **health insurance**, for older women, and for members of racial and ethnic minorities. The program is administered through individual states, under the direction of the Centers for Disease Control and Prevention.

Special concerns

If a woman is diagnosed with very early-stage (IA) cervical cancer while pregnant, the physician usually will recommend a hysterectomy after the baby is born. For later-stage cancers, the pregnancy is terminated or the baby is removed by cesarean section as soon as it can survive outside the womb. This is followed by a hysterectomy and/or radiation treatment. For the most advanced stages of cervical cancer, treatment is initiated despite the pregnancy.

Many women with cervical cancer have hysterectomies, which are major surgeries. Although normal activities, including sexual intercourse, can be resumed in four to eight weeks, a woman may have emotional problems following a hysterectomy. A strong support system can help with these difficulties.

See also Gynecologic cancers.

Resources

BOOKS

Holland, Jimmie C., and Sheldon Lewis. *The Human Side of Cancer: Living with Hope, Coping with Uncertainty.* New York: HarperCollins, 2000.

Runowicz, Carolyn D., Jeanne A. Petrek, and Ted S. Gansler. *Women and Cancer: A Thorough and Compassionate Resource for Patients and their Families.* New York: Villard Books, 1999.

PERIODICALS

"American Cancer Society Issues New Early Detection Guidelines." *Women's Health Weekly* December 19, 2002: 12.

"Get Ready to Take Cervical Cancer Screening to the Next Level: Newly Approved Human Papillomavirus Test Offers 2-in-1 Package." *Contraceptive Technology Update* June 2003: 61–64.

"Obesity Linked to Cervical Adenocarcinoma, a Hormone-Dependent Cancer." *Cancer Weekly* July 29, 2003: 59.

"Study: HPV Test Is more Effective than Pap Smear for Cervical Cancer Screening." *Biotech Week* December 31, 2003: 143.

Van Kessel, Katherine, and Koutsky, Laura. "The HPV Vaccine: Will it One Day Wipe Out Cervical Cancer?" *Contemporary OB/GYN* November 2003: 71–75.

Walgate, Robert. "Vaccine Against Cervical Cancer Passes Proof of Principle." *Bulletin of the World Health Organization* January–February 2003: 73–81.

Worcester, Sharon. "Smoking Tied to Poorer Outcomes in Cervical Ca: Locally Advanced Disease." *Family Practice News* May 15, 2003: 29–31.

OTHER

"Cancer of the Cervix." *CancerNet.* Dec. 12, 2000. National Cancer Institute. NIH Publication No. 95-2047. [cited Apr. 3, 2001.] http://cancernet.nci.nih.gov/wyntk_pubs/cervix.htm#2.

"Cervical Cancer." *Cancer Resource Center.* American Cancer Society. Mar. 16, 2000. [cited Apr. 3, 2001.] http://www3.cancer.org/cancerinfo/load_cont.asp?ct=8&doc=25&Language=English.

"Cervical Cancer." *National Institutes of Health Consensus Development Conference Statement.* 1-3 Apr. 1996. [cited Apr. 3, 2001.] http://text.nlm.nih.gov/nih/cdc/www/102txt.html.

"Cervical Cytology: Evaluation and Management of Abnormalities." *American College of Obstetricians and Gynecologists (ACOG) Techincal Bulletin.* Number 183. August 1993.

ORGANIZATIONS

American Cancer Society. 1599 Clifton Road, N.E., Atlanta, GA 30329. (800) ACS-2345. http://www.cancer.org. Information, funds for cancer research, prevention programs, and patient services, including educational and support programs for patients and families and temporary accommodations for patients.

Centers for Disease Control and Prevention. National Center for Chronic Disease Prevention and Health Promotion. Mail Stop K-64. 4770 Buford Highway NE, Atlanta, GA 30341-3717. (770) 488-4751. (888) 842-6355. http://www.cdc.gov/cancer. Research and public education and outreach for disease prevention under the U.S. Department of Health and Human Services.

EyesOnThePrize.Org. 446 S. Anaheim Hills Road, #108, Anaheim Hills, CA 92807. http://www.eyesontheprize.org. On-line information and emotional support for women with gynecologic cancer.

Gynecologic Cancer Foundation. 401 North Michigan Avenue, Chicago, IL 60611. (800) 444-4441. (312) 644-6610. http://www.wcn.org/gcf/. Research, education, and philanthropy for women with gynecologic cancer.

National Cancer Institute. Public Inquiries Office, Building 31, Room 10A31, 31 Center Drive, MSC 2580, Bethesda, MD 20892-2580. (800)-4-CANCER. http://www.nci.nih.gov/. Research, information, and clinical trials.

National Cervical Cancer Coalition. 16501 Sherman Way, Suite #110, Van Nuys, CA 91406. (800) 685-5531. (818) 909-3849. http://www.nccc-online.org/. Information, education, access to screening and treatment, and support services; sponsors the Cervical Cancer Quilt Project.

Lata Cherath, Ph.D.
Margaret Alic, Ph.D.
Teresa G. Odle

▌Cetuximab

Definition

Cetuximab is an anti-cancer chemotherapeutic used to treat colorectal **cancer** and malignant tumors of the head and neck.

Purpose

Cetuximab is used to treat a type of colorectal cancer called colorectal **carcinoma** with epidermal growth factor receptor (EGFR) expression. This type of colorectal cancer has a receptor on the cell surface for a type of growth factor involved in tumor cell development and replication. Cetuximab is used only for this type of colorectal cancer cell. Patients enrolled in clinical studies examining cetuximab treatment were required to have immunohistochemical evidence (process of labeling proteins with antibodies to identify them) of EGFR expression on their tumor cells. Cetuximab is used for treatment of EGFR expressing colorectal cancer that has failed treatment with other chemotherapeutic agents. Cetuximab may be used in combination with other chemotherapeutic agents such as the drug **irinotecan** to treat metastatic colorectal cancer that does not respond to other agents or to irinotecan alone.

Cetuximab is used to treat malignant tumors of the head and neck. The EGFR has been detected in nearly all **head and neck cancers**, therefore patients enrolled in clinical studies done for cetuximab use in head and neck cancer did not need immunohistochemical evidence of EGFR expression. Cetuximab is used in combination with **radiation therapy** for the initial treatment of locally or regionally advanced squamous cell carcinoma of the head and neck, especially in patients who cannot tolerate platinum-based chemotherapies with radiation therapy.

Description

Cetuximab is marketed by Bristol-Myers Squibb under the trade name Erbitux. In **clinical trials** cetuximab treatment was shown to increase median survival time compared to placebo. Median survival time is a term used to describe the time from either diagnosis or treatment at which half of the patients with a given disease are expected to still be alive. In a clinical trial designed to test out a cancer drug in humans, median survival time is a way to measure how effective a treatment is.

Cetuximab specifically targets the EGFR expressed by cancer cells to prevent cancer cell growth and replication. The EGFR is a type of chemical receptor that sits on the outer membrane of both normal cells and cancer cells. Chemical receptors in the body activate a sequence of cellular events known as a chemical cascade or signaling pathway. It is these signaling pathways that are responsible for many normal body functions. Drugs or natural chemicals that bind to and activate the receptor signaling pathway are known as receptor agonists. Drugs or natural chemicals that bind to the receptor and block them from creating a signaling pathway are known as receptor antagonists, because they antagonize the effects of that receptor. EGFR are receptors that bind growth factors to create signaling cascades that are a natural part of cell development and necessary for normal cell growth. The agonist that normally binds to the EGFR is epidermal growth factor (EGF). When EGF binds to the EGFR, it initiates chemical

---

KEY TERMS

Angiogenesis—Physiological process involving the growth of new blood vessels from pre-existing blood vessels, process used by some cancers to create their own blood supply.

Colorectal cancer—Cancer involving both the colon and the rectum of the gastrointestinal tract.

Cytochrome P450— Enzymes present in the liver that metabolize drugs.

Epilepsy—Neurological disorder characterized by recurrent seizures.

Immunohistochemical technique—Scientific laboratory technique in which proteins present in or on a cell are identified using antibodies to identify them.

Interstitial pneumonitis—Type of lung disease caused by inflammation of the tissue and space around the air sacs of the lungs.

Metastasize—The process by which cancer spreads from its original site to other parts of the body.

Pulmonary fibrosis—Disease in which there are deposits of fibrous tissue in the tissue and space around the air sacs of the lungs.

QT prolongation—Potentially dangerous heart condition that affects the rhythm of the heart beat and alters the ECG reading of the heart.

Tuberculosis—Potentially fatal infectious disease that commonly affects the lungs, is highly contagious, and is caused by an organism known as mycobacterium.

---

signals that tell the cell how to grow and replicate. Some cancer cells have a mutated form of the EGFR that can be targeted by drugs that differentiate between the normal and mutated EGFR. Cetuximab antagonizes the mutant EGFR by binding and prevent the signaling pathway for growth from happening. Cetuximab mainly acts on cancer cells instead of normal cells because it targets the mutated form of the EGFR.

Cetuximab is a chimeric (fusion) mouse and human monoclonal antibody used to treat metastatic colorectal cancer and malignant head and neck cancer. Drugs like cetuximab are made in mice for experimental purposes but need to be humanized to eliminate or reduce the chance that patients will mount an immune reaction to the antibody when administered in therapy. Cetuximab binds to and blocks the EGFR to fight tumor cells, and in some cases has also been shown to be directly toxic to tumor cells. By blocking EGFR, cetuximab blocks the biological signal that promotes tumor growth and **metastasis**. The biological signal also promotes new blood vessel formation in the process of angiogenesis. Once a solid tumor reaches a certain size, it needs blood vessels in order for its cells to remain alive, and to continue to grow. Blood vessels that grow in tumors in the process called angiogenesis also contribute to its metastasis to other parts of the body. All of these components are critical to the ongoing survival of the tumor and are blocked by cetuximab.

Recommended dosage

Cetuximab is administered intravenously. It is not given as a rapid infusion or as a bolus (one larger dose at one time). The maximum infusion rate should not exceed 10 mg/min. The initial dose is given over two hours, with the remainder of doses given once weekly over one hour each.

For previously treated EGFR-expressing metastatic colorectal cancer, cetuximab may either be used as a single agent or in combination with the chemotherapeutic drug irinotecan. The initial dose of cetuximab is 400 mg/m², given as an infusion over two hours. The remainder treatments are a dose of 250 mg/m² given as an infusion over one hour once a week. Treatment is continued until disease progression occurs or until unacceptable toxicity from side effects occurs, whichever comes first.

For the treatment of locally or regionally advanced squamous cell cancer of the head and neck, cetuximab may be used in combination with radiation therapy. The initial dose of cetuximab is 400 mg/m², given as an infusion over two hours. The initial dose is given one week prior to the initiation of radiation therapy. Radiation therapy is given over six to seven weeks. During that time cetuximab is given at a dose of 250 mg/m² as an infusion over one hour once a week. Administration of cetuximab must be completed one hour prior to radiation therapy during this time.

Cetuximab intravenous therapy is associated with severe infusion reactions, ranging from skin inflammation and **itching**, to life-threatening drop in blood pressure, difficulty breathing, heart attack, collapse of the blood vessels, and shock. To help prevent infusion reactions 50 mg intravenous diphenhydramine (Benadryl) is given 30 to 60 minutes prior to the cetuximab infusion for the initial dose. Further doses of diphenhydramine may be given in later doses if clinically indicated.

Precautions

Cetuximab is a pregnancy category C drug. Pregnancy category C drugs are drugs in which animal studies show adverse effects on the fetus but there is not sufficient data in humans. However, if the potential benefits to the patient are determined to outweigh the potential risks to the fetus the drug may be used during pregnancy. Cetuximab is contraindicated with breastfeeding both during treatment and within 60 days of the last dose. Cetuximab has not been approved for use in patients less than 18 years of age. Cetuximab may not be appropriate for use in patients who have a form of respiratory inflammation known as interstitial pneumonitis, or patients with a respiratory disorder known as pulmonary fibrosis.

Cetuximab intravenous therapy is associated with severe infusion reactions, including life-threatening conditions such as severe drop in blood pressure, respiratory arrest, heart attack, collapse of the blood vessels, and shock. Cetuximab treatment has caused fatal respiratory disease, cardiac arrest, and sudden death. Fatal toxic skin infections and kidney failure have also been reported.

Side effects

Cetuximab is used when the potential benefits to the patient are considered greater than the potential risks of side effects. Some potential side effects seen with cetuximab treatment are abdominal pain and cramping, abnormal liver function tests, acne, hair loss, **anemia**, loss of appetite, back pain, conjunctivitis, **diarrhea**, constipation, cough, difficulty breathing, dizziness, **depression**, **fever**, **nausea**, **vomiting**, **weight** loss, headache, insomnia, weakness, increased infections, itchiness, rash, dry mouth, dry skin, difficulty swallowing, sore throat, and kidney failure.

Interactions

Patients should make their doctor aware of any and all medications or supplements they are taking before using cetuximab. Cetuximab interacts with many other drugs. Some drug interactions may make cetuximab unsuitable for use, while others may be monitored and attempted. Certain combinations of cancer treatments including cetuximab have been associated with heart toxicity and death. The combination of cetuximab, the drug **cisplatin**, and radiation therapy have caused both these sequelae. Cetuximab treatment used at the same time as radiation therapy as opposed to in staggered doses is associated with formation of a moderate to severe rash. The incidence of late radiation toxicity is higher in patients receiving both cetuximab and radiation therapy than in those receiving radiation therapy alone.

Resources

BOOKS

Brunton, Laurence L., et al. *Goodman and Gilman's The Pharmacological Basis of Therapeutics, Eleventh Edition.* McGraw Hill Medical Publishing Division, 2006.

Hamilton, Richard J., editor. *Tarascon Pharmacopoeia Library Edition.* MA: *Jones and Bartlett Publishers, 2009.*

OTHER

Epocrates, *Cetuximab.* http://www.epocrates.com.

Medscape, *Cetuximab.* http://www.medscape.com.

RxList, *Cetuximab.* http://www.rxlist.com.

ORGANIZATIONS

National Cancer Institute. 6116 Executive Boulevard, Room 3036A, Bethesda, MD 20892-8322. (800)4-CANCER http://www.cancer.gov.

FDA U.S. Food and Drug Administration. 10903 New Hampshire Ave, Silver Spring, MD 20993. (888)INFO-FDA http://www.fda.gov.

Maria Basile, Ph.D.

Chemoembolization

Definition

Utilized to treat tumors in the liver, chemoembolization is the process of injecting **chemotherapy** directly into the blood vessels that feed the tumor.

Purpose

Chemoembolization is a treatment that can be focused on cancerous cells that have spread to the liver but does not expose the rest of the body to the effects of chemotherapy. It is not a cure but does offer relief (palliative) and preserves the quality of life. The technique is minimally invasive and approximately 70% of patients will experience improvement in liver function and survival time.

Precautions

The referring physician will probably recommend several tests prior to the procedure, such as, liver function blood tests and a CAT scan or an MRI of the liver. These tests insure there is no blockage of the portal vein in the liver; there is no cirrhosis of the liver; and there is no blockage of the bile ducts. Any of these complications may prevent the procedure from being performed.

Description

A radiologist performs this procedure in a hospital under x-ray guidance by inserting a small catheter (tiny tube) through a hollow needle into the femoral artery, located in the groin. It is then threaded up through the aorta and into the artery in the liver that feeds the tumor. During chemoemolization, three chemotherapy drugs are injected directly into this artery and it is then "embolized" or blocked off with a mixture of oil and tiny particles. Since the drugs are injected directly into the tumor, the dosage is 20-200 times greater than that received with standard treatment via

QUESTIONS TO ASK THE DOCTOR

- Am I a good candidate for this procedure?
- Do I have any contraindications that should be considered before having the procedure?
- Will I experience any improvement in my quality of life?
- What are the advantages and disadvantages of the procedure?
- Does the physician performing the procedure do this often or just once in awhile?

a vein in the arm. Since the tumor is blocked off, the drugs stay in it for a much longer time. Also, with the blood supply blocked, the tumor is deprived of oxygen and nutrients, which serves to hasten its destruction. The liver has two blood supplies, a hepatic artery and a large portal vein so it can still function with one blocked off.

The procedure takes approximately three hours to perform, occurs while the patient is under conscious sedation, and usually involves an overnight stay in the hospital. It is usually performed on a monthly basis with three sessions being the average treatment regimen.

Preparation

The evening before the procedure nothing may be taken by mouth after dinner. Generally, a patient must arrive at the hospital early in the morning to permit the infusion of large amounts of fluids by an intravenous (IV) line placed in the arm. These fluids contain **antibiotics** and other medications needed prior to the procedure. The patient is then taken to the Department of Radiology for the treatment.

Aftercare

Immediately following the injection of the chemotherapy mixture, the patient is returned to a hospital room and must lie flat in bed for at least six hours. More IV fluids are provided during this time as well as overnight. Most patients are discharged the next day. It is important to spend as much time as possible in bed one to two days following the procedure in order to improve blood flow to the liver.

Risks

Serious complications are extremely rare from this procedure. Some statistics have quoted that in less than 3% of the procedures, the liver tumor that was destroyed became infected and abscessed. Others have noted approximately one fatality per 100 procedures due to liver failure.

Normal results

The patient may experience varying degrees of pain, **fever**, and **nausea**, following the treatment, which may last anywhere from a few hours to a few days. Pain or high fevers the first few days following the treatment are a result of the tumor breaking down and is normal. Frequently, a medication (a laxative) called Lactulose is given to help the body rid itself of metabolic waste usually eliminated by the liver. This may cause loose stools for several days. Extreme **fatigue** is a common problem for three to four weeks after the procedure. With the tumor now blocked, liver function should improve and thus, the quality of life.

Follow-up scans may be performed in order to determine any changes in the tumor and to look for the appearance of any new tumors. Chemoembolization can be repeated many times over a period of many years depending on the status of the patient.

Abnormal results

A sudden change in the degree of pain and/or fever that persists after the first week should be reported to a physician. Any unusual changes should be communicated immediately.

Resources

BOOKS

Wilkes, Gail M., and Terri B. Ades. *American Cancer Society's Consumers Guide to Cancer Drug,* 2nd ed. Jones and Bartlett, 2004.

OTHER

Montgomery, Sue. *Chemotherapy Delivered Directly to Liver Tumors Doubles Life Expectancy.* University of Pennsylvania Cancer Center. [cited April 13, 2001].

ORGANIZATIONS

American Cancer Society. P.O. Box 102454, Atlanta, GA 30368-2454. http://www.cancer.org.

American Society of Clinical Oncology,1900 Duke Street, Suite 200, Alexandria, VA 22314. Phone: 703-299-0150. http://www.asco.org.

Linda K. Bennington, C.N.S., M.S.N.

Chemoprevention

Definition

Chemoprevention is the attempt to prevent **cancer** from developing by using substances that interfere in the process of **carcinogenesis**.

Purpose

Clinical trials are currently investigating chemoprevention for people at high risk of certain cancers. For instance, to prevent **breast cancer** in the second breast of women who have already been treated for breast cancer, or women who have never had breast cancer but are determined to be at high risk; or to prevent **colon cancer** in people with a genetic predisposition for the cancer. Individuals not at a particularly high risk can use behavioral and dietary modifications for chemoprevention. Since the 1980s, the National Cancer Institute has identified more than 1,000 natural and synthetic chemicals with some degree of cancer preventive activity. Currently, more than 400 potential agents are under investigation for their ability to prevent cancer and at least 40 compounds or combinations are undergoing human clinical trials.

Chemopreventive agents have been identified that interact with all stages of carcinogenesis: initiation, promotion and progression. They work by inactivating carcinogens (cancer-causing agents), inducing enzymes, or as **antioxidants**. Later in the process they may inhibit tumor growth by acting as suppressors or stimulating apoptosis.

Description

Chemoprevention differs from **chemotherapy** in that it is used long before cancer develops to prevent cancer or to inhibit pre-cancer, possibly in at-risk individuals. Chemotherapy, on the other hand, seeks to kill cells that already have become cancerous. Chemoprevention uses natural products from foods or synthetic preparations. Because chemoprevention is used long term, it must be non-toxic, effective, easy to administer, and inexpensive. Few specific agents are currently advised for widespread clinical use since clinical trials that last up to 15 years are still ongoing.

Strategies for chemoprevention change often based on clinical trial results and scientific discoveries. For example, scientists completed the first map of the human genome (genetic makeup) in mid-2002. Since that time, cancer research has evolved rapidly. Epigenetic events, or the alterations in gene expressions

without certain DNA involvement, may lead to cancer chemopreventive drug development aimed at tumor suppressor genes.

Dietary factors and lifestyle changes are important areas in chemoprevention. It is estimated that through dietary improvements there could be a 50% reduction in colon and rectal cancers, a 25% reduction in breast cancer and a 15% reductions each in prostate, endometrial, and gallbladder cancers. Cancers of the stomach, esophagus, pancreas, ovaries, liver, lung, and bladder also may be affected by dietary factors. However, these improvements probably should come from the diet rather than from dietary supplements. In 2003, the U.S. Preventive Services Task Force released a report stating that evidence was insufficient to recommend for or against use of vitamin supplements to help prevent cancer. The task force recommended against supplementation with beta carotene because of higher incidence of lung cancer among those who used certain levels of beta carotene supplements.

Phytochemicals from food are a source of many chemopreventive agents. Garlic alone contains 30 cancer-preventing compounds including selenium. Broccoli contains indole-3-carbinol as well as phenethylisothiocyanate, a sulfur-containing compound. Soy products contain phytoestrogens such as genistein. Tea, both black and green, contains an abundance of polyphenols such as the catechins that have antioxidant and anti-cancer activity. Compounds in tea also have antiestrogen activity and can modulate detoxification enzymes. Curcumin from the spice turmeric is gaining attention as a chemopreventive agent. It is both an anti-inflammatory agent and an antioxidant. In laboratory animals curcumin has shown inhibition toward colon, breast, and **stomach cancer**.

Chemoprevention of breast cancer

Antiestrogens can counteract the growth effect estrogen has on some breast cancers. Two antiestrogens, **tamoxifen** and **raloxifene**, have been shown in clinical trials to prevent breast cancer in women at high risk for the disease. As a result of these trials, tamoxifen has been approved by the FDA as a preventive therapy as well as a treatment. Other antiestrogens, including soy isoflavones, are still under investigation. The synthetic retinoid, fenretinide, also shows promise in preventing breast cancer. Also under investigation are indole-3-carbinol from broccoli.

Chemoprevention of colon cancer

Because there are more identifiable **tumor markers** known for colon cancer, the evaluation of chemopreventive agents can be a shorter process. The recurrence of polyps rather than the development of malignant cancer can be used as an endpoint. Inflammation has been linked to cancer for some time and the anti-inflammatory agents sulindac and sulindac sulfone as well as specific cyclooxygenase-2 inhibitors are proving useful in preventing colon cancer. Adding fruits and vegetables to the diet also appears from epidemiological studies to have a protective effect on colon cancer.

Chemoprevention of prostate cancer

Antiandrogens and antiestrogens are both important in preventing **prostate cancer**. Finasteride is under investigation as an anti-estrogen to prevent prostate cancer in at-risk men. Finasteride is a drug that can reduce the levels of dihydrotestosterone, which is associated with prostate enlargement and possibly cancer. It has been used to treat enlarged prostate and is currently being investigated to prevent prostate cancer in men over the age of 55 years. Men at an increased risk for prostate cancer include those with a history of prostate cancer, those with a high-fat diet, increasing age, and those of African American descent. Soy products and indole-3-carbinol may also be effective for this reason. Lycopene, a vitamin A-like compound found in tomatoes and other red fruits and vegetables is associated with a decreased risk of prostate cancer. Both selenium and tea may also have chemopreventive effects on prostate cancer.

Chemoprevention of skin cancer

The incidence of **skin cancer** has dramatically increased in recent years, probably due to the popularity of sun tanning. Compounds under investigation for the prevention of skin cancer include compounds from tea, silymarin from milk thistle, vitamin A, and coumarins found in a number of plants.

Recommendations

Changes in lifestyle can significantly affect an individual's risk for cancer. It is estimated that 32%

of colon cancers are related to physical inactivity, which may also play a part in other cancers. Tobacco accounts for 30% of all cancers, not just lung cancer. **Alcohol consumption** is related to cancers of the oral cavity, pharynx, larynx, esophagus, and liver, and possibly colorectal and breast cancers. The combination of alcohol and tobacco is especially dangerous. The main cause of skin cancers is exposure to UV radiation. Fair skinned individuals are at an increased risk. Obesity puts an individual at an increased risk of death from uterus, gallbladder, kidney, stomach, colon, breast, and prostate cancers.

The lifestyle recommendations from the American Cancer Society for preventing cancer include:

- Maintain a desirable body weight
- Eat a variety of foods
- Include both fruits and vegetables in the daily diet
- Eat more high-fiber foods
- Cut down on total fat intake
- Limit consumption of alcoholic beverages
- Limit consumption of salt-cured, smoked and nitrite preserved foods

Risks

Because chemopreventive agents can be administered in high doses and for long periods of time, the risk of side effects is increased. During the 1980s, the CARET study found that beta-carotene actually increased the risk of lung cancer in male smokers. Studies of tamoxifen to prevent breast cancer show the drug can increase the risks of uterine cancer, and cause other serious side effects. Long-term use of nonsteroidal anti-inflammatory drugs to prevent colon cancer can result in gastrointestinal problems and liver toxicity. Current recommendations are to increase consumption of fruits, vegetables, and fiber in the diet rather than taking supplements.

Resources

BOOKS

American Institute for Cancer Research. *Stopping Cancer Before it Starts.* New York: Golden Books, 1999.
Kelloff, Gary J, James A. Crowell, Vernon E. Steele, Ronald A. Lubet, et. al. "Progress in Cancer Chemoprevention." In *Cancer Prevention: Novel Nutrient and Pharmaceutical Developments.* Annals of The New York Academy of Sciences, vol. 889, edited by H. Leon Bradlow, Jack Fishman, and Michael P. Osborne. New York: The New York Academy of Sciences, 1999.

PERIODICALS

Koplevich, Levy, James A. Crowell, and Judith R. Fay. "The Epigenome as a Target for Cancer

Chemoprevention." *Journal of the National Cancer Institute* December 3, 2003.

Rao, Chinthalapally V., Abraham Rivenson, Barbara Simi, and Bandaru S. Reddy. "Chemoprevention of Colon Cancer by Dietary Curcumin." 768 *Annals New York Academy of Sciences* 1995: 201–204.

"Routine Vitamin Supplementation to Prevent Cancer and Cardiovascular Disease: Receommendations and Rationale." *American Family Physician* 68 (December 15, 2003): 2422.

OTHER

Dresbach, Sereana Howard and Amy Rossi. "Chemoprevention—The Answer to Cancer?" *Ohio State University Extension Fact Sheet, Family and Consumer Science* [cited 4 July 2001]. http://www.ag.ohio-state.edu/~ohioline/hyg-fact/5000/5051.html.

Greenwald, Peter and Sharon S. McDonald. "Cancer Prevention: The Roles of Diet and Chemoprevention." *Cancer Control Journal.* [cited 4 July 2001]. http://www.moffitt.usf.edu/providers/ccj/v4n2/article2.html.

Cindy L. A. Jones, Ph.D.

Chemotherapy

Routes of delivering chemotherapy

Routes of delivering chemotherapy	Some common drugs used
Oral	Capecitabine
Intravenous	Fluorouracil (5–FU)
	Doxorubicin
Intra-arterial (into the arteries)	Floxuridine
	Fluorouracil
	BUDR
	FCNU
	Doxorubicin
	Mitomycin-C
	Cisplatin
	Streptomycin
Intralesional (directly into the tumor)	Vinblastine
	Vincristine
Intraperitoneal (into the cavity surrounding the abdominal organs)	Cisplatin
	Paclitaxel
	Floxuridine
	Fluorouracil
	Mitoxantrone
	Carboplatin
	Alpha interferon
Intrathecal (into the spinal fluid)	Methotrexate
	Cytarabine
Topical (applied to skin)	Fluorouracil

(Table by GGS Creative Resources. Cengage Learning, Gale.)

Chemotherapy

Definition

Chemotherapy is the systemic (whole body) treatment of **cancer** with **anticancer drugs**.

Purpose

The main purpose of chemotherapy is to kill cancer cells. It can be used as the primary form of treatment or as a supplement to other treatments. Chemotherapy is often used to treat patients with cancer that has spread from the place in the body where it started (metastasized), but it may also be used to keep cancer from coming back (adjuvant

therapy). Chemotherapy destroys cancer cells anywhere in the body. It even kills cells that have broken off from the main tumor and traveled through the blood or lymph systems to other parts of the body.

Chemotherapy can cure some types of cancer. In some cases, it is used to slow the growth of cancer cells or to keep the cancer from spreading to other parts of the body. When a cancer has been removed by surgery, chemotherapy may be used to keep the cancer from coming back (adjuvant therapy). It is also helpful in reducing the tumor size prior to surgery (primary [neo-adjuvant] chemotherapy). Chemotherapy can ease the symptoms of cancer (palliate), helping some patients have a better quality of life.

Types of chemotherapy

Chemotherapy may be used as the first line of treatment or it may be started after a tumor is removed. A variety of factors, including the type and stage of cancer, will determine the type of chemotherapy used.

Adjuvant chemotherapy

Adjuvant chemotherapy refers to giving patients anticancer drugs after the primary tumor has been removed and there is no evidence that cancer remains in the body. It was first studied in the 1950s. This form

Types of chemotherapy

Type	Definition
Adjuvant	Given to improve survival when cancer is no longer evident
Primary (formerly called neo-adjuvant)	Use of chemotherapy drugs as main treatment, or as a treatment prior to surgery or radiation
Induction	Initiation of chemotherapy with plans for further treatments
Combination	Use of two or more chemotherapy drugs together

(Table by GGS Creative Resources. Cengage Learning, Gale.)

A woman receiving Adriamycin (doxorubicin) chemotherapy. *(Custom Medical Stock Photo. Reproduced by permission.)*

of treatment initially gained popularity because it showed promise in improving the survival for patients with certain cancers. The theory was that adjuvant chemotherapy would attack microscopic cancer cells that remained after tumor removal. Adjuvant chemotherapy may be effective in some types of cancers, including **breast cancer**, colorectal cancer, osteogenic **sarcoma**, and **Wilms' tumor**.

A patient's response to adjuvant therapy is determined by a variety of factors, including drug dosage, schedule of drug therapy, and **drug resistance**. Toxic side effects and cost-effectiveness are other important issues. This area is undergoing further investigation.

Primary (neoadjuvant) chemotherapy

Primary chemotherapy, also sometimes called neoadjuvant chemotherapy or induction chemotherapy, is the use of anticancer drugs as the main form of treatment. Chemotherapy can be the primary treatment with cancers such as these: certain lymphomas, childhood and some adult forms of **Hodgkin's disease**, Wilms' tumor, embryonal **rhabdomyosarcoma**, and **small cell lung cancer**.

Primary chemotherapy can also be used to treat tumors prior to surgery or radiation. In some cases, the tumor may be so large that surgery to remove it would destroy major organs or would be quite disfiguring. Primary neoadjuvant chemotherapy may reduce the tumor size, making it possible for a surgeon to perform a less traumatic operation. Examples of cancers in which primary chemotherapy may be followed-up with less extensive surgeries include: **anal cancer**, **bladder cancer**, breast cancer, **esophageal cancer**, **laryngeal cancer**, osteogenic sarcoma, and **soft tissue sarcoma**.

An advantage of primary chemotherapy is that the blood vessels are intact since they have not been exposed to surgery or radiation. Therefore, drugs can easily travel through the bloodstream toward the tumor. In fact, the therapy can improve the tumor's blood flow, making it more receptive to the impact of radiation. In addition, the use of chemotherapy before surgical removal of cancer allows the physician to assess the responsiveness of the tumor to the drug(s) used. Since not all chemotherapy regimens are equally effective, knowing how a particular tumor responds to the chemotherapy regimen prescribed can be an advantage in treating the disease.

Primary chemotherapy does have drawbacks. Some cancer cells may be drug-resistant, making the therapy ineffective. (Although discovering that the drug is ineffective minimizes the number of cycles of the drug that the patient must undergo.) The drug may not significantly reduce tumor size, or the tumor may continue to grow despite treatment. Furthermore, the initial use of a drug may lead to higher toxicity when chemotherapy is given later in the course of treatment.

Primary chemotherapy is becoming the norm in treating some patients with certain cancers, such as specific types of lymphomas, some small cell lung cancers, **childhood cancers**, **head and neck cancers**, and locally advanced breast cancer. Additional research using this type of chemotherapy is underway.

Combination chemotherapy

In most cases, single anticancer drugs cannot cure cancer alone. The use of two or more drugs together is often a more effective alternative. This approach is called combination chemotherapy. Scientific studies of different drug combinations help doctors learn which combinations work best for various types of cancers.

Combination chemotherapy provides a higher chance of destroying cancerous cells. An oncologist decides which chemotherapy drug or combination of drugs will work best for each patient. Different drugs attack cancer cells at varying stages of their growth cycles, making the combination a stronger weapon against cancerous cells. Furthermore, using a combination of drugs may reduce the chance of drug resistance.

When selecting the combination of drugs, a variety of factors are examined. It is important for each drug to be effective against the particular tumor being targeted. Toxicity must also be studied to be sure that each different drug used in a combination is not toxic for the same organ. For example, if two drugs are each toxic to the liver, the combination could be more damaging to that organ.

How chemotherapy is given

Chemotherapy medications enter a person's body in different ways, depending on the drugs to be given and the type of cancer.

The goal is for the chemotherapy drug to reach the tumor. Some areas of the body are less accessible for anticancer drugs, and this is considered when the doctor determines the route of administration. For example, the blood-brain barrier refers to the inability of some anticancer drugs to travel through the bloodstream and enter the brain or the fluid surrounding the brain. Areas of the body that are inaccessible to a particular drug create a phenomenon called the sanctuary effect. In other words, the tumor is safe because the chemotherapy cannot reach it. To overcome a problem such as this one, the doctor must consider the route that will most effectively deliver the drug to the cancerous cells. Chemotherapy may be given by one or more of the following methods:

- oral (by mouth)
- injection (intramuscular or subcutaneous)
- intravenous (IV)
- intra-arterial (into the arteries)
- intralesional (directly into the tumor)
- intraperitoneal (into the peritoneal cavity)
- intrathecal (into the spinal fluid)
- topically (applied to the skin)

Orally

Oral chemotherapy is given by mouth in the form a pill, capsule, or liquid. This is the easiest method and can usually be done at home.

Injection

Intramuscular (IM) chemotherapy is injected into a muscle. Chemotherapy given by intramuscular injection is absorbed into the blood more slowly than IV chemotherapy. Because of this, the effects of IM chemotherapy may last longer than chemotherapy given intravenously. Chemotherapy may also be injected subcutaneously (SQ or SC), which means under the skin.

Intravenous

Intravenous (IV) chemotherapy is the most common way to deliver anticancer drugs into a person's body. The drug is injected directly into a vein. A small needle is inserted into a vein on the hand or lower arm.

Chemotherapy may also be given by a catheter or port inserted into a central vein or body cavity, where it can remain for an extended period of time. A port is a small reservoir or container that is placed in a vein or under the skin in the area where the drug will be given. These methods eliminate the need for repeated injections and may allow patients to spend less time in the hospital while receiving chemotherapy. A common location for a permanent catheter is the external jugular vein in the neck. Catheters and ports require meticulous care and cleaning to avoid complications, such as blood clots or **infection**. They may be inserted using a surgical procedure.

Chemotherapy given by the IV method may be administered intermittently or continuously. The main reasons for a continuous flow are to increase effectiveness against the tumor or to lower toxicity. Some drugs perform more effectively when exposed to the cancer over a period of time, making a continuous flow more desirable. A drug that is commonly used to treat colorectal cancer in continuous infusions is 5-fluorouracil, also known as 5-FU or **fluorouracil**. A drug that has less toxicity to the heart with continued infusion is **doxorubicin**, also known as Adriamycin. In some cases, toxicity occurs when the drug reaches a peak level. Offering a continuous infusion prevents the drug from reaching this level, thus lowering the chance of toxic side effects.

Intra-arterial

Cancerous tumors require a supply of blood and oxygen so that they can grow. They get these essentials from the arteries that supply organs with their blood and oxygen. Putting chemotherapy drugs into the arteries provides good access to the cancerous tumor. Intra-arterial chemotherapy is not designed for all patients. The tumor must be confined to one specific organ and the blood supply to the tumor must be accessible. The liver is the most common organ targeted in this type of chemotherapy, although it is also effective in certain brain cancers. Its use in head and **neck cancers** remains controversial. Further use of this type of chemotherapy is being investigated.

A catheter is inserted using radiologic techniques or surgery. Surgical insertion is the most common. Although it is less costly and less stressful, radiologic insertion results in a catheter that cannot stay in place as long as one inserted surgically. A radiologically inserted catheter stays in place for weeks compared to surgically inserted catheters designed to stay in place from weeks to years. In the long run, the surgically implanted arterial catheter has fewer complications, such as thrombosis or infection, and is more highly acceptable to the patient.

The radiologically placed catheter is initially inserted into an artery in the person's arm or leg, and then it is guided to its final destination near the tumor, where it can remain for an extended period.

The catheters require meticulous care to keep them clean and securely in place, which lessen the chance of complications. Problems associated with catheters include movement of the tip, blood clots, and infection.

Pumps may be used to move the drug through the artery and into the tumor. A pump may be external or internally planted. External pumps range from large machines found in hospitals to portable wallet-sized devices. Implanted pumps give patients greater freedom, and are safe and effective. Some internal pumps deliver a constant flow of drugs, while others are programmed to deliver intermittent doses.

Drugs used for intra-arterial chemotherapy include FUDR (**floxuridine**), fluorouracil, mitomycin, **cisplatin**, and streptomycin. Less frequently, doxorubicin has been used intra-arterially for treating certain cancers of the breast, bladder, stomach, and other areas.

Intralesional

Intralesional chemotherapy is the injection of anticancer drugs directly into a tumor that is in the skin, under the skin, or in an organ inside the body. Some examples involving the use of intralesional chemotherapy include **melanoma** and **Kaposi's sarcoma**. This type of chemotherapy shows promise for other malignancies such as laryngeal cancers, and further uses are under investigation.

Intraperitoneal

Intraperitoneal (IP) chemotherapy is administered into the abdominal cavity through a catheter or port that is put into place by surgery.

Ovarian cancer is sometimes treated with IP chemotherapy because this type of cancer usually stays within a confined area. This type of therapy is only suitable for some patients. Ovarian cancer patients whose tumors have a diameter greater than two centimeters may not receive this therapy because the anticancer drug does not reach very far into the tumor. Also, patients whose cancers are resistant to certain drugs may not undergo IP therapy. Patients with smaller tumors, or those who show response to chemotherapy are better candidates.

Drugs used in IP chemotherapy include cisplatin, paclitaxel, floxuridine, 5-FU, **mitoxantrone**, **carboplatin**, and alfa-interferon.

Intrathecal

Intrathecal chemotherapy is the injection of anticancer drugs into the spinal fluid. This method is used primarily in treating **acute lymphocytic leukemia**. It is effective in placing the anticancer drug directly into the cerebrospinal fluid that surrounds the spinal cord and the brain. A spinal tap, also called **lumbar puncture**, is the procedure usually used to gain access to the spinal fluid. If many treatments are needed, a device called an **Ommaya reservoir** may be used. This device is inserted under the scalp and allows injection of anticancer drugs throughout the spinal fluid via the reservoir. Patients can go home with the Ommaya reservoir in place. Common drugs used intrathecally include **methotrexate** and **cytarabine**, which are usually given by a doctor with a nurse's assistance. Some leukemia patients receive IV treatments at the same time they are having intrathecal treatments.

Topical chemotherapy

Topical chemotherapy is given as a cream or ointment applied directly to the cancer. This method is more common in the treatment of certain types of **skin cancer**. An example is fluorouracil, also known as 5-FU, which is a topical anticancer cream.

Chemotherapy drugs

More than 50 chemotherapy drugs are currently available to treat cancer and many more are being tested for their ability to destroy cancer cells. About 30% of anticancer drugs come from or are derived from natural sources. Most chemotherapy drugs interfere with the cell's ability to grow or multiply. Although these drugs affect all cells in the body, many useful treatments are most effective against rapidly growing cells. Cancer cells grow more quickly than most other body cells. Other cells that grow fast are cells of the bone marrow that produce blood cells, cells in the stomach and intestines, and cells of the hair follicles. Therefore, the most common side effects of chemotherapy are linked to their effects on other fast growing cells. Some tumor cells are resistant to drugs, making them more difficult to target.

Alkylating agents

Alkylating drugs kill cancer cells by directly attacking DNA, the genetic material of the genes. By attacking the DNA, the drug prevents the cell from forming new cells. Nitrogen mustards, which were the first nonhormonal chemicals with anticancer abilities, are alkylating drugs. **Cyclophosphamide** and Mustargen are two alkylating agents. Cyclophosphamide, the most common alkylating agent, is often used in combination with other drugs to treat breast cancer, lymphomas, and other tumors in both children and adults. Mustargen is part of the treatment for Hodgkin's disease.

Platinum drugs

Drugs containing platinum are useful in treating a number of malignant tumors. Examples of these drugs include cisplatin, carboplatin, and oxaliplatin. Cisplatin is more toxic than the other two, and it is subject to resistance by the cancerous tumors. In fact, it was cisplatin's high toxicity that prompted the discovery of the other two platinum drugs, which are less toxic and more effective. Carboplatin has been shown to cause less **nausea and vomiting** than cisplatin, and it has replaced cisplatin in many treatment regimes. New platinum drugs are being investigated.

Antimetabolites

Antimetabolites interfere with the production of DNA and keep cells from growing and multiplying. They are used to treat a variety of cancers including breast cancer, leukemia, **lymphoma**, colorectal cancer, head and neck cancer, osteogenic sarcoma, choriocarcinoma (a rare uterine cancer), and urothelial cancer. Some drug resistance has occurred with these types of drugs. Examples of antimetabolites are 5-fluorouracil (5-FU), Tegafur, and Uracil.

Antitumor antibiotics

Antitumor **antibiotics** are made from natural substances such as fungi in the soil. They interfere with important cell functions, including production of DNA and cell proteins. Doxorubicin, **daunorubicin**, **idarubicin**, **epirubicin**, **dactinomycin**, and **bleomycin** belong to this group of chemotherapy drugs.

Topoisomerase inhibitors

Topoisomerase inhibitors are effective in treating a number of cancers. Topoisomerase is an enzyme necessary for the replication of DNA within the cell. The topoisomerase inhibitors act on this enzyme, and the cell eventually dies. Drugs in this class include **etoposide** and **teniposide**.

Camptothecin analogues are also classed as topoisomerase inhibitors. Specific drugs are **topotecan** and **irinotecan**.

Anthracyclines are topoisomerase inhibitors such as daunorubicin, doxorubicin, epirubicin, and idarubicin. A drawback of the anthracyclines is their toxicity to the heart. Because of this, there have been efforts to develop synthetic drugs similar to the anthracyclines. Mitoxantrone and losoxantrone are two examples of synthetics.

Dactinomycin is another drug acting on the DNA of the cell. It is an effective drug for treating a variety of cancers including **Ewing's sarcoma**, Wilms' tumor, embryonal rhabdomyosarcoma, and gestational choriocarcinoma (rare uterine cancer). It has also been used to treat cancer of the testicles, lymphoma, and Kaposi's sarcoma.

Antimicrotubule Agents

A microtubule is an important part of a cell, and is the target of a class of anticancer drugs.

Vinca alkaloids, which attack the cell's microtubules, are found in very small amounts in the periwinkle plant. Three types of vinca alkaloids are **vincristine**, **vinblastine,** and **vinorelbine**. Vincristine is used more frequently in treating childhood, rather than adult, cancers. It is used in combination chemotherapy for the treatment of acute lymphocytic leukemia and Hodgkin's and **non-Hodgkin's lymphoma**, as well as other cancers. Vinblastine is used in combination chemotherapy for Kaposi's sarcoma, as well as cancers of the bladder, brain, and breast. It is also used in the treatment of advanced cases of lymphoma and germ cell cancers.

The taxanes are another group of antimicrotubule agents. They are from the Pacific yew tree, and were first isolated in 1963. In 1971, paclitaxel was found to be an active ingredient in the bark of this tree. Paclitaxel has shown promising results in people with cancers of the ovaries or breasts. It is also used for AIDS patients who have Kaposi's sarcoma, and in combination with cisplatin in the treatment of **non-small cell lung cancer**. Paclitaxel is also part of the chemotherapy treatment in breast cancer patients whose cancer has spread to the lymph nodes. A related drug, **docetaxel** is used for treating advanced cases of breast cancer as well as certain non-small cell lung cancers.

Estramustine phosphate is related to nitrogen mustard. This drug acts on the microtubule of the cell, and has been effective in treating certain prostate cancers.

Hormones

Steroid hormones slow the growth of some cancers that depend on hormones. For example, **tamoxifen** is used to treat breast cancers that depend on the hormone estrogen for growth. Additionally, androgen suppression therapy is used in the treatment of **prostate cancer**. The goal of this therapy is to lower the levels of male hormones (androgens), especially **testosterone**, that can cause prostate cancer cells to grow. Lutenizing hormone-releasing hormone (LHRH) analogs lower testosterone levels by decreasing the androgens produced by the testicles. Two LHRH analogs available in the United States are **leuprolide acetate** and goserelin.

Treatment location and schedule

Patients may take chemotherapy at home, in the doctor's office, or as an inpatient or outpatient at the hospital. Most patients stay in the hospital when first beginning chemotherapy, so their doctor can check for any side effects and change the dose if needed. A very important part of chemotherapy is determining the appropriate dose. To do this, the doctor must consider the person's size as well as any toxic side effects the drug may have.

How often and how long chemotherapy is given depends on the type of cancer, how patients respond to the drugs, the patients' health and ability to tolerate the drugs, and the types of drugs given. Chemotherapy administration may take only a few minutes or may last as long as several hours. Chemotherapy may be given daily, weekly, or monthly. A rest period may follow a course of treatment before the next course begins. In combination chemotherapy, more than one drug may be given at a time, or they may be given alternately, one following the other.

Precautions

There are many different types of chemotherapy drugs. Oncologists, doctors who specialize in treating cancer, determine which drugs are best suited for each patient. This decision is based on the type of cancer, the patient's age and health, and other drugs the patient is taking. Some patients should not be treated with certain chemotherapy drugs. Age and other conditions may affect the drugs with which a person may be treated. Heart disease, kidney disease, and diabetes are conditions that may limit the choice of treatment drugs. Pregnancy is another precaution because of the anticancer drug's impact on fetal development.

Preparation

A number of medical tests are done before chemotherapy is started. The oncologist will determine how much the cancer has spread from the results of **x rays** and other imaging tests and from samples of the tumor taken during surgery.

A patient's complete medical history will be taken, including any past chemotherapy. The patient will be asked to sign a consent form, and will be told about the drugs and procedures involved with chemotherapy. It is essential that the patient understand both the risks and benefits of treatment.

The nurse explains what will take place during the treatment, and what side effects to expect. In addition to the physical side effects, the stress of chemotherapy will be discussed. Patients who are better prepared tend to have fewer side effects and a higher emotional ability to handle the chemotherapy treatments.

Blood tests give the doctor important information about the function of the blood cells and levels of chemicals in the blood. A complete blood count (CBC) is commonly done before and regularly during treatment. The CBC shows the numbers of white blood cells, red blood cells, and platelets in the blood. Because chemotherapy affects the bone marrow, where blood cells are made, levels of these cells often drop during chemotherapy. The white blood cells and platelets are most likely to be affected by chemotherapy. A drop in the white blood cell count means that the immune system cannot function properly. Low levels of platelets can cause a patient to bleed easily from a cut or other wound. A low red blood cell count can lead to **anemia** (deficiency of red blood cells) and **fatigue**.

When a chemotherapy treatment takes a long time, the patient may prepare for it by wearing comfortable clothes. Bringing a book to read or a tape to listen to may help pass the time and ease the stress of receiving chemotherapy. Some patients bring a friend or family member to provide company and support during treatment.

Sometimes, patients taking chemotherapy drugs known to cause **nausea** are given medications called **antiemetics** before chemotherapy is administered. Antiemetic drugs help to lessen feelings of nausea. Two anti-nausea medications that may be used are Kytril and Zofran.

Other ways to prepare for chemotherapy and help lessen nausea are:

- Regularly eat nutritious foods and drink lots of fluids
- Eat and drink normally until about two hours before chemotherapy
- Eat high-carbohydrate, low-fat foods and avoid spicy foods

Aftercare

To control side effects after chemotherapy, patients should:

- Follow any instructions given by the doctor or nurse
- Take all prescribed medications
- Eat small amounts of bland foods
- Drink lots of fluids
- Get plenty of rest

Some patients find it helps to breathe fresh air or get mild exercise, such as taking a walk.

Risks

Chemotherapy drugs are toxic to normal cells as well as cancer cells. A dose that will destroy cancer cells will probably cause damage to some normal cells. Doctors adjust doses to do the least amount of harm possible to normal cells. Some patients feel few or no side effects, and others may have more serious side effects. In some cases, a dose adjustment is all that is needed to reduce or stop a side effect.

A person may experience a side effect right away or the reaction may be delayed. Side effects are classified as follows:

- acute, develops within 24 hours of treatment
- delayed, develops after 24 hours but within six to eight weeks of treatment
- short-term, combination of acute and delayed
- late/long-term, develops months or years after treatment, or lasts for an extended period of time
- expected, a side effect that develops in three-quarters of patients
- common, occurs in 25–75% of patients
- uncommon/occasional, occurs in less than a quarter of patients

- rare, occurs in 5% of patients
- very rare, occurs in less than 1% of patients

Certain chemotherapy drugs have more side effects than others. While some drugs have immediate effects, other effects are delayed. Patients are encouraged to discuss the potential for side effects with their doctor. They must seek immediate medical attention if they are experiencing any unusual symptoms. Some of the most common side effects are discussed in this section.

Nausea and vomiting/loss of appetite

Nausea and **vomiting** are common, but can usually be controlled by taking antinausea drugs, drinking enough fluids, and avoiding spicy foods. Loss of appetite (**anorexia**) may be due to nausea or the stress of undergoing cancer treatment. Drugs that have a high likelihood of causing nausea or vomiting include cisplatin, **mechlorethamine**, **streptozocin**, **dacarbazine**, **carmustine**, and dactinomycin. Those with moderate nausea-inducing potential include cyclophosphamide, doxorubicin, carboplatin, mitomycin, and L-asparaginase. Anticancer drugs with a low chance of causing nausea or vomiting include fluorouracil, methotrexate, etoposide, vincristine, and bleomycin.

Hair loss

Some chemotherapy drugs cause hair loss, but it is almost always temporary. Hair regrowth may not begin until several weeks have passed since the final treatment. This is the most common impact that chemotherapy has on the outer surfaces of the body. In some patients, an ice wrap, called an ice turban, can reduce hair loss. The effectiveness will depend on factors such as the type of drug, dose, and treatment schedule. This preventive treatment must be avoided by patients with leukemia, lymphoma, **mycosis fungoides,** or by those with scalp tumors. People should use with caution if they have conditions such as vasculitis, cryoglobulinemia, or a history of radiation to the head. Patients should discuss the ice turban treatment with their doctor before trying it.

Anemia and fatigue

Low blood cell counts caused by the effect of chemotherapy on the bone marrow can lead to anemia, infections, and easy bleeding and bruising. Patients with anemia have too few red blood cells to deliver oxygen and nutrients to the body's tissues. Anemic patients feel tired and weak. If red blood cell levels fall too low, a blood transfusion may be given.

Infections

Patients receiving chemotherapy are more likely to get infections. This happens because their infection-fighting white blood cells are reduced. The level of reduction can vary depending on the dose and schedule of treatments, and whether the drug is used alone or in combination with other anticancer agents.

It is important for chemotherapy patients to avoid infection. When the white blood cell count drops too low, the doctor may prescribe medications called colony stimulating factors that help white blood cells grow. Neupogen and Leukine are two colony stimulants used as treatments to help fight infection.

Easy bleeding and bruising

Platelets are blood cells that make the blood clot. When patients do not have enough platelets, they may bleed or bruise easily, even from small injuries. Patients with low blood platelets should take precautions to avoid injuries. Medicines such as aspirin and other pain relievers can affect platelets and slow down the clotting process.

Sores in the mouth

Chemotherapy can cause irritation and dryness in the mouth and throat. An inflammation in the mouth is called **stomatitis**. Painful sores may form that can bleed and become infected. Precautions to avoid this side effect include getting dental care before chemotherapy begins, brushing the teeth and gums regularly with a soft brush, and avoiding mouth washes that contain salt or alcohol. Good oral hygiene is important. It is helpful for some patients to chew on ice chips for half an hour during chemotherapy treatments, but this should be discussed with the doctor before it is done.

Neuropathy and other damage to the nervous system

Cancer patients may develop neurological problems due to the cancer or the anticancer drugs. A variety of problems can develop, including altered mental alertness, changes in taste and smell, seizures, and peripheral **neuropathy** (tingling and burning sensations and/or weakness or numbness in the hands and/or feet). Different drugs can lead to different types of neurological disorders. Patients should discuss neurological symptoms with the doctor.

Heart damage

Some anticancer drugs are damaging to the heart. In these cases, the dosage is closely monitored in an attempt to avoid heart damage. Specific drugs that may be toxic to the heart include doxorubicin, daunorubicin, high doses of cyclophosphamide, and, in some cases, 5-FU. Patients experiencing chest pain or any cardiac symptoms should seek immediate medical help.

Kidney damage

A number of anticancer drugs can damage the kidney. Examples include high doses of methotrexate or 6-MP, as well as regular doses of L-asparaginase, cisplatin, mithramycin, streptozocin, and mitomycin C. Some kidney problems can be lessened by taking in adequate amounts of fluids. A secondary danger of kidney damage is that a less functional kidney can be more susceptible to further toxicity caused by other anticancer drugs that the patient is taking.

Respiratory problems

Cancer patients who have had radiation in the chest area are more susceptible to respiratory complications. Nitrosourea or bleomycin cause the most common type of respiratory toxicity, called pulmonary fibrosis. Patients should get immediate medical assistance if they have difficulty breathing.

Sexual function

Some drugs can lead to impaired sexual function. Alkylating agents and **procarbazine** may result in the absence of sperm in a man and the lack of menstruation in a woman. Patients of child-bearing age are usually told to refrain from conceiving while undergoing chemotherapy because of the defects it can cause in the fetus.

Vision problems

Some anticancer drugs can impact a person's vision. High doses of cyclophosphamide can cause blurred vision in children, while some alkylating agents can cause cataracts. Tamoxifen may be damaging to the retina, and cisplatin can damage the optic nerve. Conjunctivitis, commonly called pinkeye, is a treatable problem that occurs with many anticancer drugs.

Results

The main goal of chemotherapy is to cure cancer. Many cancers are cured by chemotherapy. The chemotherapy treatment may be used in combination with surgery to keep a cancer from spreading to other parts of the body. Some widespread, fast-growing cancers are more difficult to treat. In these cases, chemotherapy may slow the growth of the cancer cells.

Doctors can tell if the chemotherapy is working by the results of medical tests. Physical examination, blood tests, and x rays are all used to check the effects of treatment on the cancer.

The possible outcomes of chemotherapy are:

- Complete remission or response. The cancer completely disappears for at least one month. The course of chemotherapy is completed and the patient is tested regularly for a recurrence.
- Partial response. The cancer shrinks in size by at least 30–50%, the reduction in size is maintained for at least one month, and no new lesions are found during treatment. The same chemotherapy may be continued or a different combination of drugs may be used.
- Minor response. The cancer shrinks 1–29%.
- Stabilization. The cancer does not grow or shrink. Other therapy options may be explored. A tumor may stay stabilized for many years.
- Progressive disease. The cancer continues to increase in size by at least 25%, or new lesions are noted. Other therapy options may be explored.
- A secondary malignancy may develop from the one being treated, and that second cancer may need additional chemotherapy or other treatment.

See also Cancer biology; Clinical trials; Complementary cancer therapies; Fatigue; Fertility issues; Infection and sepsis; Memory change; Metastasis; Nutritional support; Pregnancy and cancer; Radiation therapy; Second cancers; Sexuality; Taste alteration; Vascular access.

Resources

BOOKS

DeVita, Vincent T., et al, editors. *Cancer: Principles and Practice of Oncology.* 6th ed. Philadelphia, PA: Lippincott, Williams & Wilkins, 2001.

Haskell, Charles M. *Cancer Treatment.* 5th ed. Philadelphia, PA: W.B. Saunders Company, 2001.

OTHER

American Cancer Society. "How Will the Chemotherapy Be Administered?" [cited May 28, 2001]. http://www3. cancer.org.

American Cancer Society. Laryngeal and Hypopharyngeal Cancer Resource Center. "How Are Laryngeal and Hypopharyngeal Cancers Treated?" [cited May 28, 2001]. http://www3.cancer.org.

Cuesta-Romero, Carlos, and Grado-Pena, Jesus de. "Intralesional Methotrexate in Solitary Keratoacanthoma." *Archives of Dermatology,* April 1998 [cited May 28,

2001]. http://archderm.ama-assn.org/issues/v134n4/ffull/dIt0498-6.html.

National Cancer Institute. National Institutes of Health. "Chemotherapy and You: A Guide to Self-Help During Treatment." http://www.cancernet.nci.nih.gov/chemotherapy/chemoint.html.

OncoLink. "Introduction to Chemotherapy." University of Pennsylvania Cancer Center, 1998. http://www.oncolink.upenn.edu/specialty/chemo/general/chemo_intro.html.

OncoLink. "What is Chemotherapy?" University of Pennsylvania Cancer Center, September 1997. http://www.oncolink.upenn.edu/specialty/chemo/general/whatis_chemo.html.

Toni Rizzo
Rhonda Cloos, R.N.

Chest x ray *see* **X ray**

Childhood cancers

Definition

Childhood cancers are malignant diseases that affect children under the age of 18 years. The types of cancers diagnosed in children are different from the most common cancers that affect adults. The most common cancers diagnosed in children include leukemias, brain and central nervous system cancers, lymphomas, bone cancers, sarcomas, kidney cancers, and cancers of the eye.

Demographics

According to the American Cancer Society, approximately 11,000 new cases of **cancer** will be diagnosed in children under the age of 15 years in the United States in 2009. Another 2,000-3,000 cases are diagnosed in teenagers over 15 years of age, but these are often recorded with adult diagnoses. The number of cases of childhood cancer has remained steady for a number of years. Researchers estimate that 1 of every 333 children will be diagnosed with cancer before the age of 20 years.

Cancer remains the leading cause of death from disease among children under the age of 15 years. Almost 1,400 American children will die from cancer in 2009. One-third of the deaths from childhood cancers is from leukemia.

Survival rates for all types of childhood cancers combined have increased dramatically in the last four decades with the five-year overall survival rate increasing from less than 50% to over 80% during that time period. The overall 10-year childhood cancer survival rate approaches 75%.

Leukemia accounts for 33% of the cancers in children, with about three-quarters of those being **acute lymphocytic leukemia** and the other one-fourth mostly acute myelogenous leukemia. Central nervous system (CNS) cancers, commonly lumped together as **brain tumors**, are the next largest group, constituting another 21% of childhood cancers. **Lymphoma**, both Hodgkin's and non-Hodgkin's, accounts for 8% of childhood cancers. The rest of the diagnoses are divided among what are referred to as solid tumors, such as **neuroblastoma**, **retinoblastoma**, **Wilms' tumor**, **rhabdomyosarcoma**, and bone cancers.

These statistics are similar in other parts of the developed world. In Africa, the most common form of childhood cancer is **Burkitt's lymphoma**, which is associated with the Epstein-Barr viral **infection**.

Description

Cancer in children (pediatric cancers) differs from cancer in adults in several important ways. The most important difference is that children have generally better prognoses than do adults. Two-thirds of children with cancer are cured of the disease. Still, despite enormous progress in the treatment of childhood cancer since the 1960s, it is the second-most common cause of death in children older than one year, with accidents being the first.

One difference between pediatric and adult cancer is found in the cells in which the cancers originate. Many adult cancers begin in specific organs, such as a lung, the breast, or the colon. Childhood cancer, except for leukemias and brain tumors, often arise in connective tissues such as bone and muscle.

Childhood cancer is often more aggressive than adult cancers. It grows faster and is frequently metastatic (has moved to other parts of the body or to the major organs) by the time of diagnosis. Thus, surgery alone is less likely to cure a child. Nevertheless, the cancers children develop tend to be more responsive to **chemotherapy** and radiation than those of adults.

The median age for children at the time of a cancer diagnosis is six years; for adults it is 67 years. Most children with cancer are otherwise healthy; many adults have conditions, such as heart disease, that make their treatment and recovery more difficult. Another important difference is that screening tests are available for some adult cancers, such as mammograms for **breast cancer** and Pap smears for **cervical cancer**. There are no useful screening tests for childhood cancers. Not infrequently, the diagnosis is made at a routine pediatric visit.

An extremely important factor in the improved prognosis of children with cancer has been the enrollment of the majority of children with cancer in research trials. Although only 2% of all cancers diagnosed in the United States occur in children, more than 70% of those children are enrolled in formal research protocols. By contrast, although adults have 98% of all cancers diagnosed in the United States, only 3% enroll in trials. Research protocols permit rapid collection of data on the effectiveness of treatment; they recognize adverse effects quickly, and foster valuable communication and collaboration among pediatric oncologists throughout the country and the world.

In 1998, the four major pediatric research consortia in the United States joined forces. The Pediatric Oncology Group, the Children's Cancer Group, the Intergroup Rhabdomyosarcoma Study Group, and the National Wilms' Tumor Study Group combined to form the Children's Oncology Group—to the great benefit of children with cancer. Most American children who are diagnosed with cancer are treated in a treatment center that is a member of the Children's Oncology Group (COG). All members of COG are affiliated with a university or with a hospital which specializes in treating children.

Risk factors

Risk factors related to cancers that are commonly diagnosed in adults are often lifestyle related. For example, common risk factors for adult cancers include smoking, drinking alcohol, obesity, and lack of exercise. Lifestyle factors play little to no role in the development of childhood cancers.

Causes and symptoms

The causes of most childhood cancers are unknown, but some associations are recognized. The risk of childhood leukemia is increased in children with Down syndrome, in boys, in whites, and in those of higher socioeconomic status. Exposure to radiation *in utero* increases the risk as well. Central nervous system cancers are also more common in boys, in whites, and in those who have received radiation treatments for other cancers.

A number of inherited and developmental conditions are associated with an increased risk of childhood cancer. These include neurofibromatosis, Bloom's syndrome, ataxia-telangiectasia, and tuberous sclerosis. A family history of **Hodgkin's disease** increases its

likelihood, and a family history of retinoblastoma in both eyes confers a 50% chance of an offspring carrying the gene. Ninety percent of children carrying the gene will develop the disease.

Symptoms of cancer in children vary by cancer type and are often vague and non-specific in the early stages. Parents are encouraged to bring their children to regularly scheduled medical appointments.

Some signs and symptoms in children which indicate the need for further evaluation by a medical professional include:

- unusual or easy bruising
- paleness and complaints of fatigue or tiredness
- any unusual lumps or swelling of a body part
- frequent headaches especially if associated with vomiting
- sustained complaints of pain
- limping or complaints of pain in the legs while running or walking
- complaints of changes in vision
- unexplained loss of weight
- persistent fever
- illnesses that recur or do not resolve as expected

Special concerns

Family

Few situations test a family or a marriage like a diagnosis of cancer in a child. One day, parents have a healthy child with unlimited potential and a bright future; the next day, they have a child with a possibly fatal disease.

With a diagnosis of cancer in a child, parents must begin to negotiate complicated medical, social, family, and financial issues. Because children are generally best treated in centers that have pediatric oncologists, and because such centers can be far from a family's home, whole families can be uprooted, parents forced to spend weeks apart, and siblings left home with other relatives for long stretches of time.

Guilt can consume parents. They often assume they are responsible for their child's illness, they feel guilty if finances or insurance coverage issues force both to remain employed during their child's illness, and they worry that they are neglecting their other children.

One of the most difficult aspects of dealing with a diagnosis of cancer in a child is deciding what to tell that child and when. For infants and toddlers, this is not a concern, but older children need to know that they are ill, that they need these painful and unpleasant treatments, and—importantly—that they are not being punished for some misdeed, which is a common fear.

School

More than 80% of children with cancer miss at least some school during their treatments. Some children must miss school for prolonged periods. Federal law requires all states to provide education to handicapped children, and children with cancer are considered handicapped under the law. An individual education plan must be developed and an education provided, even for those who are homebound due to illness. Hospital social workers can be good resources for parents to explore their children's rights under their state's laws.

Completion of treatment

One of the surprisingly difficult aspects of cancer treatment comes when the treatment itself is completed. Parents, and certainly older children, can find the loss of the routine of regular treatment and the comfort of knowing that something active is being done to keep the cancer at bay quite frightening. Some parents and children become excessively focused on minor symptoms, fearful of recurrence. Occasionally, children who survive cancer become risk-takers as they grow, engaging in dangerous sports or hobbies.

Death

Though the survival rates for children with cancer continue to improve, the tragic truth is that some children will die of their disease. For parents, the day they learn that no further treatment is available is even harder than the day they learned their child's diagnosis. No decision is more difficult than stopping futile treatment and turning to care that is palliative (aimed solely at making the child comfortable).

Hospice care can be a valuable part of the end-of-life treatment for a child with cancer. Though not all inpatient hospice facilities accept children, they do provide home hospice care. Most families find that bringing their terminally ill child home, letting the child die in familiar surroundings with their loved ones at their side, offers them the only comfort to be had in a time of great sadness.

Grief for the death of a parent or spouse can last for months or even years, but most adults eventually come to accept those losses. Grief for the death of a child is lifelong. One of the hardest tasks for a parent

in mourning can be offering the necessary support and love to their other surviving children. Some parents who lose a child to cancer can find some solace from support groups. Such groups are available through hospitals, hospices, churches, counseling, and cancer organizations. Other parents prefer solitude and time to face their loss.

Diagnosis

The diagnosis of childhood cancer varies by type of cancer but will typically involve a history and physical examination by a medical professional. A variety of blood and imaging tests will be ordered to rule out or confirm a diagnosis of cancer. Procedures such as biopsies may also be used to confirm the diagnosis.

Treatments

The treatment of childhood cancer depends on the specific disease, what tissues are affected, and how extensively it has spread at the time of diagnosis.

Acute lymphoblastic leukemia and acute myelocytic leukemia

Leukemia accounts for about one-third of all childhood cancer cases. Acute lymphoblastic, or lymphocytic, leukemia (ALL) is the most common form of cancer in children, occurring about three times as often as acute myelocytic leukemia (AML). AML is diagnosed in about 20% of children with leukemia. Peak incidence of ALL is from three to five years. Leukemia of either type causes symptoms such as fevers, pallor, **fatigue**, bleeding or bruising, swollen glands, and bone pain— which can manifest itself as a limp or refusal to walk.

The diagnosis is made based on blood tests and bone marrow studies. The treatment is similar for both types. ALL has a very good prognosis, with a cure rate of about 80%; AML has a poorer prognosis, with about 60% of children with AML achieving long-term remission with chemotherapy or hematopoietic stem cell transplants.

Treatment for ALL requires prolonged chemotherapy, consisting of remission induction, consolidation or intensification therapy, and maintenance. An essential component of the successful treatment of ALL is prophylactic (preventative) treatment to the CNS, a common site of relapse. In the past, children received radiation to the CNS, but this carried a risk of later brain tumors and significant neurologic and psychiatric deficits. Only the highest risk children now receive CNS radiation; the rest receive **intrathecal chemotherapy**, which means that the medications are introduced directly into the spinal fluid during spinal taps.

Chemotherapy is typically stopped after two to three years of treatment for ALL. Hematopoietic stem cell transplantation is an option for very high-risk cases and for those whose disease relapses early after treatment.

Similar treatment strategies are used in children diagnosed with AML. Chemotherapy is the most common form of therapy for children with AML. Allogeneic stem cell transplants (using stem cells from a donor) with cells harvested from bone marrow, cord blood, or peripheral blood are used in children who are at high risk for relapse or who have disease that is resistant to other treatment.

Non-Hodgkin's lymphoma

Non-Hodgkin's lymphoma constitutes about 55% of the lymphomas in children, and 4% of all childhood cancers. A rare childhood cancer, approximately nine in one million children under age 15 will develop non-Hodgkin's lymphoma each year. It is a cancer of the lymphatic system, which includes the spleen and lymph nodes. It is more common in boys than in girls, and other risks for the development of non-Hodgkin's lymphoma include conditions that depress the immune system, such as AIDS or immune suppressive treatment after organ or bone marrow transplant. Many such cases are Burkitt's lymphomas, and are associated with the presence of the **Epstein-Barr virus**. These often manifest as masses in the jaw.

Non-Hodgkin's lymphoma has survival rates of 80–90%, depending upon the stage at which it is diagnosed. Lymphoma might be found at a routine examination, with nothing but swollen lymph nodes or an enlarged spleen as early signs. Some children do experience fevers or drenching **night sweats**, while others complain of persistent **itching**. Like adults, some teenagers will experience unexplained abdominal pain with alcohol ingestion, but might never report this symptom to parents for fear of consequences for underage drinking.

Non-Hodgkin's lymphoma is treated with chemotherapy using a combination of drugs. Because of the effectiveness of treatment with chemotherapy, **radiation therapy** is used infrequently to treat non-Hodgkin lymphoma in children.

Hodgkin's disease

Hodgkin's disease is rare in young children but becomes more common in the teen years. Peak incidence in the United States and Europe is in the 20s with another peak later in adulthood. The virus that causes mononucleosis, the Epstein-Barr virus, is implicated in the development of some cases of Hodgkin disease. Early Hodgkin's disease is one of the most curable of all cancers, with a cure rate as high as 95%. Even in advanced disease, the survival rate is as high as 70 to 90%. Early disease is often treated with chemotherapy alone, while more advanced disease is often treated with both chemotherapy and low-dose radiation.

Central nervous system cancers

CNS tumors account for about 21% of all childhood cancers. Several major categories of brain cancers are found in children.

MEDULLOBLASTOMA. This is the most common brain tumor found in children. Its symptoms can appear as headaches, **nausea and vomiting**, and it can also cause gait disturbances and damage to the cranial nerves (those nerves that control such functions as eye movement and facial muscle control).

Medulloblastoma, also known as primitive neuroectodermal tumor, is treated by surgical removal of the tumor and postoperative chemotherapy and radiation therapy. The goal of surgery is to remove as much tumor as possible. With today's precise surgical and radiologic techniques, most tumors can be completely removed. Patients whose tumors are able to be totally removed and which have not spread are treated with reduced-dose radiation therapy to the brain and spinal cord. The radiation is then followed by chemotherapy. Results of a recent national study indicated that 80% of children treated this way survived. Patients whose tumors have spread to other areas of the brain, spinal cord, and/or bone marrow are treated with higher doses of radiation which is then followed by treatment with chemotherapy.

GLIOMA. These arise most often in the brainstem, at the base of the brain. Those that arise in the segment of the brain known as the pons have the poorest prognosis. Many gliomas produce gait abnormalities and cranial nerve problems such as double vision, and swallowing and speech disorders. Their location makes them difficult to reach surgically, so the primary treatment is radiation therapy. Most trials of chemotherapy have not shown benefit, but newer agents are being explored.

High-grade malignant gliomas include astrocytomas and glioblastomas. Treatment is determined by the grade of the tumor. Low-grade astrocytomas may be able to be surgically removed and no further treatment may be needed. If the tumor cannot be completely removed and the child has not finished growing, chemotherapy may be administered and radiation therapy delayed until is the child is older because of the long-term side effects of radiation therapy on younger children.

High-grade astrocytomas can rarely be totally removed surgically. All patients with high-grade astrocytomas receive radiation and chemotherapy regardless of age.

EPENDYMOMA. These cancers arise in the cells that line spaces within the brain—known as the ventricles—or the spinal column. In addition to **nausea**, **vomiting**, and headache, an **ependymoma** can cause head tilting and hearing loss. Treatment consists of surgery to remove the tumor followed by radiation.

Neuroblastoma

Neuroblastoma, which accounts for about 7-10% of all childhood cancers, is far more common in infants than in older children. Most cases of neuroblastoma are diagnosed by age two. It originates in the sympathetic nervous system, a complicated system involving nerves and the adrenal glands, which produce hormones such as epinephrine and norepinephrine (also called adrenaline and noradrenaline). Most neuroblastomas arise in the adrenal glands, and are noticed as a mass in the abdomen. However, they can arise anywhere in the sympathetic nervous system, appearing as masses in the neck, the chest, or the pelvis.

Symptoms are usually related to whatever organs are compressed by the growing tumors. Thus, abdominal masses produce discomfort, vomiting or loss of appetite. Neck masses can press on certain nerves and cause an eyelid to droop, the pupil to constrict, and the eye to stop producing tears. Masses in the pelvis can cause constipation or urinary retention. Because these cancers arise in tissues that produce epinephrine and similar substances, symptoms may be related to high levels of those substances. Children might be noted to sweat, flush, become pale, complain of palpitations or a rapid heartbeat, or develop high blood pressure.

Neuroblastomas are staged based on the age at diagnosis, location of the tumor, and degree of spread. Children considered at low or intermediate risk have the best prognoses, with up to 90% achieving long-term survival. Treatment consists of surgery to remove as much tumor as possible, chemotherapy, and often radiation therapy.

Wilms' tumor

Wilms' tumor, or nephroblastoma, is a cancer that arises in the kidney. It accounts for 5% of all cancers in children. Signs and symptoms of Wilms'

tumors include abdominal masses, abdominal pain or swelling, high blood pressure, and blood in the urine—either visible or in microscopic examination. Treatment consists of removal of the tumor followed by chemotherapy. If the tumor is difficult to remove or if there is tumor in both kidneys, chemotherapy will be administered prior to surgery. Radiation therapy is reserved for patients with advanced disease. Wilms' tumors diagnosed at the very earliest stages have extremely favorable prognoses, with as high as a 98% cure rate.

Sarcomas

Soft tissue sarcomas are broadly divided into rhabdomyosarcoma and nonrhabdomyosarcoma soft tissue sarcomas. These are cancers of connective tissue. Rhabdomyosarcomas constitute about half of these types of cases. It is the fourth-most common solid tumor in children, after brain tumors, neuroblastoma, and Wilms' tumor. It begins most commonly in sites in the head and neck, but can also arise in the urinary tract and the extremities. Symptoms can vary depending on the site of origin but, most often, rhabdomyosarcoma develops as a painless mass.

The nonrhabdomyosarcomas arise in a variety of different cell types. Among those cell types are the cells of the linings of peripheral nerves, the linings of joints, and other fibrous tissue. The most common sites of origin are the arms and the legs.

The prognosis of both types of sarcomas varies with the extent of spread at the time of diagnosis and the type of cell from which the cancer arose. About 90% of children with early stage sarcomas can be cured, while only 20% of those with the most advanced disease at the time of diagnosis can be cured. Treatment for rhabdomyosarcoma consists of surgery followed by chemotherapy. Some cases may require radiation therapy. Treatment for nonrhabdomyosarcoma includes surgical removal of the tumor. Patients whose tumors cannot be completely excised may be given radiation therapy. Patients with high-risk disease may be administered chemotherapy.

Osteosarcoma

This is the most common form of bone cancer in children and adolescents. In the past, all such cancers were treated with **amputation**. Now, **limb salvage** surgery can be performed in 95% of cases of localized **osteosarcoma** limited to the extremity. Chemotherapy and surgery combined have improved the prognosis for this disease to a 65% five-year survival rate.

Ewing's sarcoma

Ewing's sarcoma is a rare bone cancer that usually occurs in teenagers. It is more common in girls than in boys, and often starts in the femur (thighbone). About two-thirds of children diagnosed with localized Ewing's **sarcoma** will survive long-term; if the disease has spread to other parts of the body, survival rates are less than 30%.

Retinoblastoma

Retinoblastoma is a cancer that arises in the cells of the retinas of the eyes. It is a disease of young children and has been diagnosed at birth. It can occur in both eyes in an inherited syndrome, and siblings of children with retinoblastoma in both eyes need to be screened. First symptoms include a sudden onset of squinting or crossed eyes.

Treatment depends on whether the tumor affects one eye, both eyes, or if the disease has spread outside of the eye to other parts of the body. Patients with tumor in one eye are usually treated with removal of the eye (enucleation). Following this treatment, most patients do not require further treatment. If the tumor has spread, the child may be treated with chemotherapy after surgery. Children with more extensive spread will require more intensive chemotherapy which usually includes a bone marrow transplant. The eye is seldom removed in children with multiple disease sites or disease that involves both eyes. These children typically receive chemotherapy in an attempt to shrink the size of the tumors. The tumors are then treated with laser therapy, freezing treatments, or the use of radioactive discs while the child is under anesthesia. If the tumors are advanced or unresponsive to these treatments, radiation therapy or removal of the eye may be necessary.

Germ cell cancers

These include teratomas, choriocarcinomas, embryonal carcinomas, and germinomas. These are all cancers of stem cells—cells that represent the earliest, or embryonal, stages of cell development and that have the potential to develop into mature cells. Some **germ cell tumors** are benign; others are malignant. They arise in the ovaries, testes, or sites along the midline of the interior of the body. Symptoms vary with the site of origin. Testicular masses are usually painless; ovarian masses can be accompanied by abdominal pain and swelling. Midline germ cell cancers can cause constipation or urinary retention as they grow and block internal organs. They are treated with surgery and chemotherapy,

and long-term survival rates are as high as 80% percent for patients diagnosed with localized tumors.

Hepatic cancers

Hepatic (liver) cancers are rare but not unheard of in children. There are two types of **liver cancer** in children. Hepatoblastoma, which accounts for about two-thirds of these, is associated with familial polyposis, an inherited disease of multiple polyps in the colon. It has also been associated with fetal alcohol syndrome. Its incidence has risen since the 1970s.

The second type is hepatocellular **carcinoma**, which accounts for about one-third of the cases of liver cancer in children, and its incidence has been falling. Hepatocellular carcinoma has been associated with hepatitis B and C, exposure to anabolic steroids, aflatoxins (food contaminants), pesticides, and vinyl chloride.

Treatment of both of these cancers includes surgical removal of the cancer. Hepatoblastoma is more responsive to chemotherapy than is hepatocellular carcinoma. Hepatocellular carcinoma is not very responsive to currently utilized chemotherapeutic agents.

Alternative and complementary therapies

Alternative and complementary treatments have not been studied extensively in children, and some have been proven harmful. Herbal remedies can be particularly dangerous, in that children have very different metabolisms from adults and relatively benign treatments for adults can be fatal in children. For example, *jin bu hua*, a traditional Chinese medicine, can produce heart problems or difficulty breathing. Life root or comfrey might cause fatal liver damage in children.

Techniques such as guided imagery can be adapted for children. Providing favorite toys or videotapes can serve as focal points for children to distract them from painful or frightening procedures.

Late effects of treatment

Currently, there are more than 10 million cancer survivors alive in the United States. Of these, at least 270,000 individuals were originally diagnosed and treated when they were under age 21. In addition, advances in the care and treatment of children diagnosed with cancer mean that almost 80% of those children will be alive at least five years after diagnosis.

The high cure rates for children with cancer have not come without a price. While chemotherapeutic drugs and radiation are highly toxic to cancer cells, they are highly toxic to healthy cells and organs, as well. Most organ systems can be affected by cancer treatment, and children who have been cured of cancer frequently face lifelong consequences of those treatments.

Organ systems

CENTRAL NERVOUS SYSTEM. Children who receive radiation therapy to their brains often experience a decline in scores on cognitive tests. More than one-half of the children who receive high-dose brain radiation have IQ scores below 90. Children with acute leukemia who are given chemotherapeutic agents directly into their spinal fluid are also at risk for developing learning disabilities and other neurologic effects.

EYES AND VISION. Both radiation to the brain and chemotherapy can cause damage to vision. If the eyes are included in a radiation field, the child can develop radiation cataracts. The long-term use of steroids, which are part of most chemotherapeutic regimens and used after bone marrow transplant, can also cause cataracts.

HEARING. Both radiation and the drug, **cisplatin**, can cause hearing loss.

TEETH AND SALIVARY GLANDS. Radiation therapy to the head and neck can damage permanent teeth and salivary glands. The chemotherapy administered to very young children with acute lymphoblastic leukemia can also cause damage to the teeth.

HEART. Heart damage can occur from the toxic effects of radiation therapy and from certain chemotherapeutic drugs. That damage can be centered in the heart muscle, the pericardium (lining) of the heart, or the coronary arteries. The drugs most noted for causing heart damage are **daunorubicin** and **doxorubicin**. They do particular damage to the left ventricle, the main pumping chamber of the heart. This can lead to congestive heart failure, in which the heart fails to pump blood effectively throughout the body. This might not appear until later in life, precipitated by such stressors as vigorous exercise or pregnancy. Some survivors of childhood (and adult) cancers eventually come to require heart transplant.

LUNGS. Bleomycin and **carmustine**, two chemotherapeutic drugs, can cause inflammation of the lungs with later scarring and decrease in lung function. Radiation treatment of the chest can also impair lung function.

KIDNEYS. The kidneys can be damaged by radiation therapy to the abdomen or by a number of chemotherapeutic drugs. Some of those drugs are cisplatin, BCNU, **ifosfamide**, **methotrexate**, **vinblastine**, and bleomycin. Children treated for Wilms' tumors can develop kidney disease in the unaffected kidney years after treatment.

BLADDER. Radiation to the pelvis combined with the drug **cyclophosphamide** can produce a cystitis or bladder inflammation.

LIVER. Liver damage can occur with radiation or with chemotherapy. The agents used to treat leukemias are particularly known for their liver toxicity. BCNU is another agent with known liver toxicity.

Because so many children receive transfusions of blood products, they are at risk for developing transfusion-related hepatitis, which can progress to cirrhosis in a few cases. Blood products are now screened for the presence of hepatitis B and C viruses, but many older surviving children received transfusions before the screening tests were available.

SMALL INTESTINE. Radiation can cause an acute inflammation of the intestines with vomiting and **diarrhea**. Some children go on to develop scarring of the intestines that can lead to blockages requiting surgical repair.

MUSCULOSKELETAL SYSTEM. Radiation to the spine, sometimes used for children with Hodgkin's disease or medulloblastoma, can produce curvature of the spine, in the form of kyphosis, or hunchback, or scoliosis, an S-shaped curve of the spine. Radiation to the hips can cause damage to the hipbones. The two most common forms of that damage are slipped capital femoral epiphysis and avascular necrosis, both of which involve damage to the end of the thighbone where it meets the pelvic bones.

Loss of the necessary minerals within the bones can be seen in children who have been treated for brain cancers, acute lymphoblastic leukemia, lymphoma, and some solid tumors. Long term use of steroids or methotrexate is a common cause of this. These children are at risk of fractures.

ENDOCRINE SYSTEM. The endocrine system is the group of glands responsible for the production of hormones. Almost any gland can be affected.

Pituitary gland: Brain radiation can cause growth hormone deficiency. Even when normal levels of growth hormone are found, children who have undergone brain radiation are often obese and fail to achieve their expected height. Those whose levels are low will grow when growth hormone injections are administered.

Thyroid gland: The thyroid gland can be damaged by radiation treatment that involves the neck, typically becoming underactive. This might not occur until several years after treatment, and is treated with oral thyroid hormone.

Reproductive function: Radiation therapy and chemotherapy can both damage the ovaries, causing loss of hormones, lack of periods, and infertility. The testes are less easily damaged and adult male survivors often have normal hormonal levels and sexual function, but might be sterile. Adolescents might be offered the opportunity to bank sperm before treatment to ensure that they might have future children through artificial insemination. Those who have had surgery to remove internal nodes involved in **testicular cancer** might be impotent as adults due to damage to the nerves that control sexual function.

Concerns have been raised that since chemotherapeutic agents can cause genetic mutations, those survivors whose fertility has been preserved might be at risk of giving birth to children with birth defects. This has not been observed yet, but children of women treated for Wilms' tumors often have low birth weights.

Second cancers

The most serious late effect of successful treatment for childhood cancer is a second cancer. **Second cancers** are a different type and are related to either inherited factors or, far more often, to late effects of treatments.

GENETIC CAUSES. About 50% of those who have been treated for the hereditary form of retinoblastoma develop a second cancer at some point in their lives.

SURGICAL TREATMENT. Children with cancers that obstruct the flow of urine sometimes require a procedure called ureterosigmoidostomy. In this, the ureter, which carries urine from the kidney to the bladder, is attached instead to the sigmoid colon. Such children have a significant risk of developing **adenocarcinoma** of the colon at the site of the connection in adulthood.

RADIATION THERAPY. Radiation to the neck can cause later **thyroid cancer**. Radiation to the brain can cause later brain tumors, such as meningiomas or gliomas. This was once fairly common in children treated for leukemia and given prophylactic radiation therapy to prevent central nervous system relapse. Bone sarcomas are possible after radiation treatment of retinoblastomas or Ewing's sarcoma. The risk of later breast cancer is increased in those who were treated with radiation for Hodgkin's disease in childhood.

CHEMOTHERAPY. Etoposide and **teniposide**, chemotherapeutic drugs known as epipodophyllins, are associated with a risk of developing acute myelogenous leukemia in the years after initial treatment for cancer. These are used in treatment of some germ cell tumors, ALL, and non-Hodgkin's lymphoma.

IMMUNE SUPPRESSION. To prevent rejection, children who undergo bone marrow transplant receive drugs to suppress their immune systems. Long-term use of these medications is associated with a risk of developing cancer that originates in the white blood cells known as B cells.

Prognosis

The overall five-year survival rate for childhood cancers has climbed significantly to over 80% in the last forty years due to major advances in treatment modalities. As of January 1, 2005, there were an estimated 328,652 childhood cancer survivors in the United States. Of those, 24% had survived thirty or more years since diagnosis.

Projected 10-year survival rates for children diagnosed with some of the more commonly diagnosed childhood cancers between 2005-2009 are:

- acute lymphoblastic leukemia (ALL) – 88%
- acute non-lymphoblastic leukemia – 64%
- non-Hodgkin's lymphoma – 91%
- Hodgkin's lymphoma – 94%

However, results of the National Cancer Institute's Childhood Cancer Survivor Study, which was started in 1993 and which Followed more than 14,000 childhood cancer survivors who were originally diagnosed between 1970 and 1986 in the United States and Canada, indicates that at least 60% of childhood cancer survivors have substantial morbidities resulting from the treatment of their cancers.

A number of potential late effects have been identified as a result of studying the first cohort of 14,000 childhood cancer survivors including incidence of premature menopause, stroke, and second cancers. These survivors received close, long-term follow-up from physicians experienced in dealing with the late effects of cancer treatment. Another group of 14,000 childhood cancer survivors who were diagnosed between 1987 and 1999 were recruited beginning in 2007. The second group will also be followed for at least five years. Incidence of late effects of treatment for childhood cancer from both groups will be compared.

Prevention

Currently, there are no known avoidable risk factors associated with the development of childhood cancers.

QUESTIONS TO ASK YOUR DOCTOR

- What type of cancer does my child have?
- What course of therapy do you recommend?
- What medications will you use and what side effects should we anticipate?
- Will my child require surgery?
- Will my child need radiation therapy?
- Will my child need to be hospitalized for treatments?
- Should my child be enrolled in a clinical trial?
- Should my child be treated at a pediatric oncology center?
- Can my child continue to go to school?

See also Cancer genetics; Extragonadal germ cell tumor; Osteosarcoma.

Resources

BOOKS

Chester, M. & Eldridge, S. *You Are Not Alone.* Candlelighters Childhood Cancer Foundation.

Janes-Hodder, Honna, and Nancy Keene. *Childhood Cancer: A Parent's Guide to Solid Tumor Cancers.* Candlelighters Childhood Cancer Foundation.

Keene, Nancy. *Childhood Leukemia: A Guide for Families, Friends & Caregivers, 3rd Ed.* Candlelighters Childhood Cancer Foundation.

Keene, Nancy, Kathy Ruccione, and Wendy L. Hobbie. *Childhood Cancer Survivors: A Practical Guide to Your Future.* Candlelighters Childhood Cancer Foundation.

PERIODICALS

Mariotto, A.B., Rowland, J.H., Yabroff, K.R., Scoppa, S., Hachey, M., Ries, L., & Feuer, E.J. "Long-term Survivors of Childhood Cancers in the United States." *Cancer Epidemiol Biomarkers* 18(2009):1033–40.

Patel, S.K., Katz, E.R., Richardson, R., Rimmer, M., & Killan, S. "Cognitive and Problem-Solving Training in Children with Cancer." *Journal of Pediatric Hematology/Oncology* 31(2009):670–7.

Pulte, D., Gondos, A., Brenner, H. "Trends in 5- and 10-Year Survival After Diagnosis With Childhood Hematologic Malignancies in the United States, 1990-2004." *Journal of the National Cancer Institute* 100(2008):1301–9.

Wayne, A.S., Reaman, G.H., & Helman, L.J. "Progress in the Curative Treatment of Childhood Hematologic Malignancies." *Journal of the National Cancer Institute* 100(2008):1271–3.

OTHER

National Cancer Institute. Clinical Trials [cited December 11, 2009]. http://www.cancer.gov/clinicaltrials.

National Children's Cancer Society [cited July 1, 2001]. http://www.children-cancer.com.

Patient-centered Guides. [cited July 1, 2001]. http://www.patientcenters.com/leukemia/.

PDQ (Physician Data Query). (800)4-CANCER [cited July 1, 2001]. <http://cancernet.nci.nih.gov>.

Why, Charlie Brown, Why? Videotape. Topper Books, 1990.

ORGANIZATIONS

American Cancer Society. 1599 Clifton Road, Atlanta, GA, 30329. (800)ACS-2345. http://www.cancer.org.

Cancer Care, Inc. 275 Seventh Ave., New York, NY 10001. (212)712-8400 or (800)813-4673. http://www.cancercare.org.

Candlelighters Childhood Cancer Foundation. 10400 Connecticut Ave., Suite 205 Bethesda, MD 20895. (800)366-CCCF. http://www.candlelighters.org.

Childhood Cancer Ombudsman Program. P.O. Box 595, Burgess, VA 22432. Fax: (804)580-2502.

The Leukemia and Lymphoma Society of America (formerly The Leukemia Society of America). 1311 Mamaroneck Avenue, Suite 310, White Plains, NY 10605. (800) 955-4572. http://www.leukemia-lymphoma.org/.

The National Cancer Institute. Cancer Information Service. 6116 Executive Blvd., Room 3036A, Bethesda, MD 20892-8322. (800)422-6237. http://www.cancer.gov/help.

National Childhood Cancer Foundation. 440 E. Huntington Drive, Suite 400, Arcadia, CA 91066-3776. (800)458-6223. http://www.curesearch.org.

National Marrow Donor Program. Suite 100, 3001 Broadway Street NE, Minneapolis, MN 55413-1753. (800)MARROW2 (800-627-7692). http://www.marrow.org/.

Marianne Vahey, M.D.
Melinda Granger Oberleitner, R.N., D.N.S., A.P.R.N., C.N.S.

Chlorambucil

Definition

Chlorambucil (marketed under the brand name Leukeran) is a **chemotherapy** medicine used to treat **cancer** by interfering with the growth of cancer cells.

Purpose

Chlorambucil is approved by the Food and Drug Administration (FDA) to treat **chronic lymphocytic leukemia** and malignant lymphomas. It has also been less commonly used for other types of cancer including **breast cancer**, **ovarian cancer**, and choriocarcinoma. Chlorambucil is not used with the intent to cure the cancer but to improve symptoms of the disease.

Chlorambucil

KEY TERMS

Anemia—A reduction in the normal number of red blood cells in the blood.

Chemotherapy—Specific drugs that are used to treat cancer.

Cystitis—An irritation of the bladder lining.

DNA—Deoxyribonucleic acid; genetic material inside of cells.

Food and Drug Administration—A government agency that oversees public safety in relation to drugs and medical devices. The FDA gives the approval to pharmaceutical companies for commercial marketing of their products.

Intravenous—Entering the body through a vein.

Leukopenia—A reduction in the normal number of white blood cells in the blood.

Metastatic—Cancer that has spread to one or more parts of the body.

Description

Chlorambucil is a member of the group of chemotherapy drugs known as alkylating agents. Alkylating agents interfere with the genetic material (deoxyribonucleic acid, or DNA) inside the cancer cells and prevent them from further dividing and growing more cancer cells. Chlorambucil is a tablet that is taken orally.

Recommended dosage

Chlorambucil can be taken according to several different dosing schedules, depending on the disease to be treated. Chlorambucil is a 2mg oral tablet, and patients may need to take more than one tablet at a time depending on the dose. The dose is based on a patient's weight in kilograms. Patients with leukemia take chlorambucil daily for three to six weeks at a dose of 0.1 to 0.2 mg/kg/day (milligram per kilogram of body weight per day).

Precautions

Patients who have received a full course of **radiation therapy** or chemotherapy generally should not receive chlorambucil until four weeks after the radiation or chemotherapy has been completed. Heath care providers should be notified if patients have had any previous allergic reactions to chemotherapy treatment. Patients should also increase the amount of fluids that they drink while on this medicine.

Blood counts will be monitored regularly while on chlorambucil therapy. During a certain time period after receiving chlorambucil there may be an increased risk of getting infections. Caution should be taken to avoid unnecessary exposure to infectious agents. Patients should check with their doctors before receiving live virus **vaccines** while on chemotherapy.

Patients who may be pregnant or trying to become pregnant should tell their doctor before receiving chlorambucil. Men and women undergoing chemotherapy are at risk of becoming sterile.

Side effects

The most common side effect from taking chlorambucil is **myelosuppression**, a suppression of bone marrow activity resulting in a low blood cell count. Myelosuppression is usually the goal when treating leukemia with chlorambucil. When the white blood cell count is lower than normal (leukopenia), patients are at an increased risk of developing a **fever** and infections.

The platelet count can also be decreased due to chlorambucil administration. Platelets are blood cells normally found in large numbers that aid in clot formation. When the platelet count is low, patients are at an increased risk for bruising and bleeding. If the platelet count remains too low, a platelet blood transfusion is an option for treatment. More rarely, chlorambucil causes a condition called **anemia** in which the number of circulating red blood cells drops, resulting in dizziness and/or **fatigue**. **Erythropoietin** is a drug that can be used to increase the red blood cell count.

Less common side effects from chlorambucil include **nausea**, **vomiting**, loss of appetite, mouth sores, skin rashes, and **diarrhea**. **Antiemetics** may be given to patients before taking chlorambucil to help prevent or reduce **nausea and vomiting**. Liver problems may occur due to chlorambucil administration, but they are typically mild and resolve when the drug is stopped.

Damage to nerves and nervous system tissues is uncommon with chlorambucil therapy. Some reports do exist of nerve damage that has resulted in seizures, muscle twitching, muscle shaking, confusion, visual hallucinations, irritability, and loss of muscle control. Other rare reactions to chlorambucil include hair loss (**alopecia**), **itching**, fever, lung problems, eye problems, tingling of the hands and feet, cystitis (bladder **infection**), and the development of another type of cancer or leukemia.

Interactions

There are no significant drug interactions associated with taking chlorambucil.

Nancy J. Beaulieu, RPh.,BCOP

Cholangiocarcinoma *see* **Bile duct cancer**

Chondrosarcoma

Definition

Chondrosarcoma is a malignant tumor that arises from cells that produce cartilage, the rubbery tissue around joints. Therefore, it is a type of **sarcoma** that is predominantly found in the area around bones.

Description

Sarcomas of the bone are rare and represent about 0.2% of all new **cancer** cases each year. The two most common forms of bone cancer are **osteosarcoma** and **Ewing's sarcoma**. Among the less common are chondrosarcoma, **fibrosarcoma**, and **malignant fibrous histiocytoma**, all of which arise from spindle cell neoplasms.

An x ray revealing a chondrosarcoma. *(Custom Medical Stock Photo, Inc. Reproduced by permission.)*

KEY TERMS

Carcinogen—An agent that is capable of causing cancer.

Epiphysis—The end of long tubular bones such as femur in the leg and the humerus in the arm. Initially separated from the main bone by a layer of cartilage that eventually allows the parts to fuse.

Spindle cells—Spindle-shaped cells typically found in connective tissue.

Chondrosarcomas arise from chondroblasts, cells that form cartilage. Cartilage is the matrix found at the tip of the nose and ears. However, cancer that develops from chondroblasts is usually observed on the surface of the pelvis, in the femur of the upper leg, around the shoulder, in the humerus of the upper arm, and in the ribs.

Depending on the type and location of the chondrosarcoma, the tumor can either be high grade and aggressive or low grade and not as invasive. There are two different categories of chondrosarcomas—classic chondrosarcomas and variant chondrosarcomas. Together they have five main types.

Central chondrosarcoma and peripheral chondrosarcoma are both classic chondrosarcomas. Central chondrosarcoma occurs within a bone, and peripheral chondrosarcoma develops on the surface of a bone. Both can develop as a primary tumor or as a secondary tumor to an existing tumor elsewhere in the body. Most, however, are primary tumors. Seventy-six percent of primary chondrosarcomas occur centrally within a bone.

There are three variant chondrosarcomas: clear cell chondrosarcoma, mesenchymal chondrosarcoma, and dedifferentiated chondrosarcoma. Clear cell chondrosarcoma is the most rare form of chondrosarcoma. It is a low grade, slow growing tumor that typically occurs locally in the epiphysis, or end part, of long tubular bones such as the femur and humerus, meaning that it does not normally invade into surrounding soft tissue. As the name implies, cells biopsied from this type of chondrosarcoma appear clear with many large vacuoles.

Mesenchymal chondrosarcoma is another rare variant. However, as opposed to clear cell chondrosarcoma, it is highly malignant and frequently metastasizes, commonly to the lungs, lymph nodes, and other bones. This variant has a tendency to develop in flat bones such as vertebra, the pelvis, or the skull, as opposed to long tubular bones. Under a microscope, the cells appear round and contain spindle cell elements and neoplastic cartilage formation.

Dedifferentiated chondrosarcoma is also rare and is the most malignant form of chondrosarcoma. It is characterized by the presence of a mix of low-grade chondrosarcoma and has undergone malignant degeneration, producing a fully malignant soft tissue mass that is no longer identifiable as cartilage. These cancers occur most commonly in the flat bones of individuals over the age of 60. Despite varied treatments, they are almost always fatal.

Due to the location of chondrosarcoma tumors, the result is often a decrease in the range of motion of limbs, especially tumors occurring on the epiphysis of bones such as those seen in clear cell chondrosarcoma.

Demographics

Although there are exceptions, chondrosarcomas occur mainly in older adults 40 to 60 years old and typically occur more in men than in women. Chondrosarcomas are rarely seen in infants and children. Dedifferentiated chondrosarcomas predominantly arise in the elderly over the age of 60, equally between males and females. Mesenchymal chondrosarcoma develops in the young adult population between the ages of 20 and 40 years old, and it is slightly more common in females. Classic chondrosarcomas usually develop in people over the age of 40. However, when they occur in younger age groups, they have a propensity to be highly malignant, capable of **metastasis**.

Causes and symptoms

As of 2005, there is little known about what causes chondrosarcomas. However, researchers have discovered that chondrosarcomas are sometimes associated with underlying benign bone tumors. They can also result as a side effect from previous **radiation therapy** for unrelated primary cancer treatment. Individuals with other bone diseases such as Maffucci's syndrome and Ollier's disease are at a higher risk for developing chondrosarcomas.

There are many symptoms associated with the onset of chondrosarcomas. They tend to develop slowly in most cases, except when the cancer is aggressive. The following is a list of the main symptoms that may present:

- pain
- swelling
- firm lump
- broken bone
- impeded normal range of motion
- urinary frequency (seen in pelvic chondrosarcomas)
- urinary obstruction (seen in pelvic chondrosarcomas)

The above symptoms are not always indicators of the presence of chondrosarcoma. Any one of these symptoms could be related to another, less serious condition. A doctor should be seen to diagnose the problem properly.

Diagnosis

In order to diagnose bone cancer, a doctor will take the patient's history and conduct a thorough physical exam. Blood tests will be performed to rule out other conditions and identify cancer markers.

The most revealing initial exam is an x ray. It can show the location, size, and shape of the tumor. If a malignant tumor is present, the x ray will expose a soft tissue mass with ill-defined edges. This procedure takes less than an hour and can be performed in the doctor's office. Depending on the medical facilities, the results can be returned the same day after being interpreted by a physician, and perhaps a consulting oncologist and radiologist.

Once there is evidence of a tumor, one or more of several other procedures may be performed, including CT scans, MRI (**magnetic resonance imaging**), angiograms, and **biopsy**.

Treatment team

If the patient is seeing a primary care provider, the provider may perform the initial diagnostic tests. However, in order to comprehensively diagnose and treat chondrosarcomas, the primary care provider will refer the patient to an orthopaedic oncologist (bone cancer specialist). Radiologists, pathologists, and orthopaedic surgeons will also be involved to read **x rays**, examine tissue samples, and remove the tumor if necessary.

Many other individuals will be involved with the treatment of chondrosarcoma. For example, nurses and dieticians are available to explain side effects of treatment and offer suggestions on eating healthy meals to help fight the side effects. If a limb is totally or partially removed, a physical therapist or vocational therapist will assist the patient in learning how to use a prosthetic limb.

Clinical staging, treatments, and prognosis

After the physician makes the diagnosis, it is important to determine the stage of the cancer. This will help reveal how far the cancer has progressed and how much tissue has been affected.

A new system of staging was adopted in 1980 by the Musculoskeletal Tumor Society. It is based on the fact that differing tissue types associated with the bone behave similarly when cancerous. This classification system uses grade (G), location (T), and lymph node involvement and metastasis (M).

Surgical grade (G) refers to how aggressive the cancer is. For example, G0 represents a benign tumor and G2 represents a highly aggressive tumor. The anatomical location (T) establishes whether or not the tumor is inside the bone (T1) or outside the bone (T2). If metastases are present, then the tumor is classified as M0; and if metastases are not present, the tumor is classified as M1. The following is a list of stages and their indications:

- Stage IA (G1, T1, M0): low grade within the bone, without metastasis
- Stage IB (G1, T2, M0): low grade outside the bone, without metastasis
- Stage IIA (G2, T1, M0): high grade within the bone, without metastasis
- Stage IIB (G2, T2, M0): high grade outside the bone, without metastasis
- Stage IIIA (G1 or G2, T1, M1): inside the bone, with metastasis
- Stage IIIB (G1 or G2, T2, M1): outside the bone, with metastasis

Physicians can employ several courses of treatment to remove chondrosarcomas. The most effective treatment is surgical removal. When performing the surgery, the doctor will remove the tumor and some healthy tissue or bone around it to ensure that the tumor does not recur near the original site. The physician may replace the removed bone with a metal device. In children, the metal device can be lengthened as the child grows, but this will require further surgeries. The fact that most chondrosarcomas tend to be low grade and slow-progressing makes this procedure one that does not necessitate entire limb removal except in extreme cases when the tumor is large.

Even individuals with low-grade chondrosarcoma that have undergone surgery experience a moderate risk of local recurrence. To combat recurrence, **chemotherapy** (the use of one or more cancer killing drugs) and radiation therapy (the use of high energy rays) have also been used to complement surgery. Employing chemotherapy or radiation therapy individually (without surgery) is much less effective. In fact, chondrosarcomas are generally resistant to chemotherapy alone.

Low stage chondrosarcomas (Stages IA and IB) have greater one and five-year survival rates than the high stages (Stages IIIA and IIIB). High-grade tumors are more aggressive and highly metastatic than lower grade tumors, and therefore they have a lower survival rate. Not only is the grade of the tumor (the estimate of its aggressiveness) important in determining prognosis, but the age of the patient is also crucial. Generally, chondrosarcomas that occur in childhood and infancy have a higher mortality rate than those that occur in adults.

Metastases appear later in the development of chondrosarcomas. The lungs are the sites of primary metastasis. Once metastasis to the lungs has occurred, survival rate decreases.

Coping with cancer treatment

Chemotherapy often results in several side effects, depending on the drug used and the patient's individual tolerance. Patients may have to deal with **nausea**, **vomiting**, loss of appetite, and hair loss. Often, chemotherapy and radiation therapy are better handled if the patient is eating well. Nurses and dieticians can aid in choosing healthful foods to incorporate into the patient's diet.

If the chondrosarcoma necessitates limb **amputation**, the patient will need to learn how to cope with a prosthetic device. Both physical and vocational therapists can help the patient adjust and learn to use prosthetic devices to perform daily activities in new ways.

Clinical trials

Since chondrosarcomas are rare forms of cancer, there is still much to be learned. Clearly, surgery is the most effective treatment. New techniques in cryosurgery are being developed in various institutions across the country.

Chemotherapy trials have shown improved results with more intense regimens. Such drugs that are under study include **methotrexate**, **leucovorin**, **vincristine**, **bacillus Calmette Guérin**, **doxorubicin**, or a combination of two or three of these.

Patients should consult with their physicians or contact the American Cancer Society to learn what procedures are currently in **clinical trials**. In some cases, insurance companies will not cover clinical trial procedures. Patients should talk with their doctor and insurance company to determine which procedures are covered.

Prevention

Since little is known about what causes chondrosarcomas, there is also little known about how to prevent them. In general, the prevention of cancer can be assisted by avoiding known chemical carcinogens such as alpha-naphthylamine, carbon tetrachloride, and benzene. Another way to avoid developing cancer— especially bone cancer—is to minimize exposure to penetrating radiation such as x rays and radioactive elements. Medical x rays revolutionized the field of medicine and are used to detect and treat many diseases. In most cases, the benefits of medical x rays outweigh the risks.

Special concerns

Cancer treatments, especially surgical amputation, can take a physical and psychological toll on cancer patients and their families. To deal with the psychological impact, many different support groups and psychotherapists are available to help. Some therapists will consider amputation a post-traumatic stress disorder and treat it accordingly. Faith practices are also beneficial for cancer patients in dealing with their condition. Patients should discuss all options with their physician to determine what is available to them.

Once the cancer has been treated, patients should make sure to schedule follow-up appointments with their physicians. Physicians will want to monitor the patient for side effects or possible recurrence that may develop years after treatment.

See also Limb salvage; Tumor grading; Tumor staging.

Resources

BOOKS

Rosen, Gerald, M.D. "Neoplasms of the Bone and Soft Tissue." In *Cancer Medicine*, edited by Robert C. Bast, Jr., M.D., et al. London: BC Decker, Inc., 2000, pp.1870-95.

PERIODICALS

Lee, Francis, M.D., et al. "Chondrosarcoma of Bone: An Assessment of Outcome." *The Journal of Bone and Joint Surgery* March 1999: 326-38.

Mitchell, A.D., et al. "Experience in the Treatment of Dedifferentiated Chondrosarcoma." *The Journal of Bone and Joint Surgery* January 2000: 55-61.

ORGANIZATIONS

American Cancer Society. http://www.cancer.org.
National Cancer Institute. http://cancer.gov.

Sally C. McFarlane-Parrott

Chordoma

Definition

Chordomas are rare tumors of the central nervous system (brain and spinal cord).

Description

Chordomas are slow-growing tumors that invade bone and tissue surrounding the spinal column. They

Colored 3-D computed tomography (CT) scan of the spine and ribcage of a male patient, showing cancer of the spine. The front of the body is at top, and at bottom left and right are the shoulder blades. The vertebral bone of the spine appears yellow and to the left of the vertebra is the cancerous tumor. *(Copyright Simon Fraser, Science Source/Photo Researchers, Inc. Reproduced by permission.)*

rarely spread to other parts of the body, but they can cause considerable damage or death because they destroy bone and soft tissue and often grow along the roots of nerves, putting pressure on the nerves and disrupting their function.

Chordomas appear at the base of the skull about 60% of the time and in the sacrum, located at the base of the spine, about 30% of the time. The other 10% of chordomas can occur anywhere else along the spinal column.

Demographics

Chordomas are very rare, accounting for between 1–4% of tumors of the brain and spinal column. Chordomas that occur at the base of the skull are most common in adults between 30 and 40 years of age. Those tumors that arise at the sacrum, located at the base of the spine, most commonly appear in older adults between the ages of 50 and 70. Chordomas are about twice as common in men as they are in women.

Causes and symptoms

During the fourth through sixth week of fetal development, a group of cells come together to form a structure called the notochord. The notochord defines the vertical mid-line of the body, and the spinal column develops around it. Normally, as development progresses, the notochord degenerates and disappears, except for small bits that become part of the disks between the spinal vertebrae. Chordomas are believed to develop from pieces of notochord that, for some reason, do not break down as they should. Over many years, these harmless bits of notochord transform and become malignant, forming chordomas.

Symptoms of chordoma depend on where the tumor is located. They are often vague and similar to symptoms of other tumors or even other conditions. Tumors located at the base of the skull may cause headaches, difficulty swallowing, or seizures depending on how much they have invaded the bones of the skull. Tumors located on the sacrum can cause general low back pain or difficulty with bowel and bladder control.

Diagnosis

Diagnosis has two parts: first, determining that the patient has a central nervous system tumor and where it is located, and second, determining what type of tumor it is. It is not easy to diagnose either of these.

A battery of tests is used to diagnose chordomas. A basic neurological examination tests the patient's reflexes, vision, hearing, senses of touch and smell, mental acuity, orientation, memory, and head and neck movements. If the results of the test indicate central nervous system dysfunction, the patient is usually referred to a neurologist (specialist in the central nervous system).

Several different scans are done to locate the tumor. Two of the most common are the **computed tomography** (CT or CAT) scan and **magnetic resonance imaging** (MRI). A CT scan uses x-ray images taken from many angles and computer reconstruction to show parts of the body in cross section. This helps to locate and estimate the size the tumor, and provides information on whether it can be surgically removed. MRI uses magnets and radio waves to create more detailed cross-sectional scans than computed tomography. There are many variations on these two scans that use dyes or radioactive materials to provide information about blood flow around the tumor and help determine whether the tumor can be surgically removed.

Treatment team

A neurosurgeon (a surgeon that specializes in the nervous system) will most likely lead the treatment team. A radiologist that specializes in nervous system radiology will interpret CT and MRI scans. Depending on the treatment plan, other members of the team may include a radiation oncologist (a specialist in **radiation therapy**), radiation technicians, and nurses with special training in assisting **cancer** patients.

Clinical staging, treatments, and prognosis

Staging of chordomas is less important in developing a treatment plan than it is for some other cancers, since chordomas rarely spread from their original location. If the tumor is in a location where it can safely be removed without damaging other nerves or structures, surgery is the preferred treatment.

But chordomas can be difficult to treat because the location of the tumor often makes it inoperable or impossible to remove completely. This is especially true of chordomas located at the base of the skull. When the tumor is inoperable, radiation therapy is the preferred treatment. Proton therapy, also called charged particle therapy, is a type of radiation treatment that spares the tissues around the tumor. For this reason, it is sometimes recommended for chordoma around the skull. One drawback of proton therapy is that the procedure is only offered at a few sites around in the United States. It is always appropriate to get a second opinion before agreeing to any treatment plan. Some insurers require second opinions before surgery.

The success of the treatment plan depends almost entirely on the location of the tumor. Chordomas can recur after either surgery or radiation therapy. They rarely spread (metastasize) to other parts of the body.

Alternative and complementary therapies

Alternative and complementary therapies range from herbal remedies, vitamin supplements, and special diets to spiritual practices, acupuncture, massage, and similar treatments. When these therapies are used in addition to conventional medicine, they are called complementary therapies. When they are used instead of conventional medicine, they are called alternative therapies.

No specific alternative therapies have been directed toward chordoma. However, good nutrition and activities such as yoga, meditation, and massage, which reduce stress and promote a positive view of life, have no unwanted side effects and appear to be beneficial. Alternative and experimental treatments are normally not covered by insurance.

Coping with cancer treatment

Cancer treatment, even when successful, has many unwanted side effects. Radiation therapy may cause **fatigue**, and **nausea and vomiting**. Bladder control and sexual function may be impaired after surgery on sacral chordomas. Mental functions may be impaired because of inoperable chordomas near the brain.

Discovering one has cancer is a traumatic event. Not only is one's health affected, one's whole life suddenly revolves around trips to the doctor for cancer treatment and adjusting to the side effects of these treatments. As this is a stressful time for both the cancer patient and family members, support groups and psychological counseling may be helpful. Many national organizations that support cancer education can provide information either in person or through online support and education groups.

Clinical trials

Chordoma is a rare tumor. Current information on what **clinical trials** are available and where they are being held can be found by entering the search term "chordoma" at the following websites:

- National Cancer Institute: http://cancer.gov/clinical trials or (800) 4-CANCER
- National Institutes of Health Clinical Trials: http:// clinicaltrials.gov
- Center Watch: A Clinical Trials Listing: http:// www.centerwatch.com

Prevention

There is no way to prevent chordoma. There appear to be no environmental factors that affect the development of this tumor.

Resources

ORGANIZATIONS

American Brain Tumor Association. 2720 River Road, Des Plaines, IL 60018. (847) 827-9910. Patient line (800) 886-2282. http://www.abta.org.

Tish Davidson, A.M.

Choriocarcinoma *see* **Gestational trophoblastic tumors**

▌ Choroid plexus tumors

Definition

Choroid plexus tumors (CPTs) are rare abnormal growths on a part of the brain called the choroid plexus. The choroid plexus is the structure in the brain that produces the cerebrospinal fluid that coats the brain and spinal cord.

KEY TERMS

Choroid plexus—Tissues of the brain that produce the fluid that coats the brain and spinal cord.

Choroid plexus carcinoma (CPC)—A malignant tumor of the choroid plexus that often invades the underlying brain tissues and can spread to other parts of the body.

Choroid plexus papilloma (CPP)—A benign tumor of the choroid plexus that does not invade the underlying brain tissues and does not spread to other parts of the body.

Intracranial hypertension—A higher than normal pressure of the fluid in the skull.

Spinal fluid shunt—A small tube that is surgically implanted to allow excess spinal fluid to drain directly into the abdominal cavity.

QUESTIONS TO ASK THE DOCTOR

- Which type of CPT do I have?
- Is my tumor operable?
- What is the likelihood of my type of CPT coming back?
- How often should I seek follow-up examinations?

Description

There are two types of CPT: choroid plexus papilloma (CPP) and choroid plexus **carcinoma** (CPC). CPPs account for the majority of all CPTs.

A CPP is a benign, slow-growing, wart-like tumor that tends to grow on the surface of the choroid plexus. CPPs can spread by growing and by multiplying, just like warts, but they do not spread (metastasize) to organs that are not directly attached to the brain. A CPC is a malignant slow-growing tumor that tends to invade healthy brain tissue. CPCs can metastasize to distant parts of the body.

A primary brain tumor is a tumor that begins in the brain, as opposed to a secondary (or metastatic) brain tumor, which begins in another organ and metastasizes to the brain. CPPs make up approximately 1% of primary **brain tumors** in adults and 3% of primary brain tumors in children.

Demographics

CPTs occur in approximately two of every one million people. CPTs can occur in people of any age, but greater than 70% of all CPTs occur in children younger than two years of age. When CPPs occur in children, they tend to be located in the uppermost portion of the spinal fluid pathway (the lateral ventricles). When they occur in adults, they tend to be located in the lower portion of the spinal fluid pathway in the brain (the fourth ventricle). CPCs occur almost exclusively in children, most under the age of

two years, and are almost always located in the lateral ventricles.

CPTs occur with equal frequency in members of all races and ethnic groups. There does not appear to be any relationship of CPTs to any geographic region. Males and females are affected in equal numbers by CPTs.

Causes and symptoms

The cause, or causes, of CPTs are not known. In the early 2000s, ongoing investigations attempted to determine if environmental factors, genetic factors, viruses, or other factors caused primary brain tumors. Primary brain tumors are not contagious.

The symptoms of CPTs are the result of increased pressure in the fluid within the skull (intracranial hypertension). These symptoms include:

- nausea
- vomiting
- irritability
- headache
- vision disturbances
- enlargement of the head
- seizures

CPCs may also be accompanied by:

- bleeding (hemorrhage) at the site of the tumor
- weakness or paralysis on the side of the body opposite to the side of the brain where the tumor is located.

Diagnosis

The diagnosis of CPTs begins in the doctor's office. After taking a complete medical history, the doctor will perform a basic neurological examination. This examination involves:

- testing eye reflexes, eye movement, and pupil reactions
- testing hearing with a tuning fork or ticking watch

- reflex tests with a rubber hammer
- balance and coordination tests
- pin-prick and cotton ball tests for sense of touch
- sense of smell tests with various odors
- facial muscle tests: smiling, frowning, etc.
- tongue movement and gag reflex tests
- head movement tests
- mental status tests: asking what year it is, who the president is, etc.
- abstract thinking tests: asking for the meaning of a common saying, such as "every cloud has a silver lining."
- memory tests: asking to have a list of objects repeated, asking for details of what a patient ate for dinner last night, etc.

If the doctor suspects a brain tumor may be present, further diagnostic tests will be ordered. These tests are performed by a neurological specialist. Imaging tests that may be ordered include:

- computed tomography (CT scan)
- magnetic resonance imaging (MRI)

Other tests may include:

- a lumbar puncture, or spinal tap, to examine the cerebrospinal fluid
- an electroencephalogram (EEG), which measures the electrical activity of the brain

Treatment team

Treatment of any primary brain tumor, including the CPTs, is different from treating tumors in other parts of the body. Brain surgery requires much more precision than most other surgeries. Also, many medicinal drugs cannot cross the blood-brain barrier. Therefore, the therapies that are used to treat CPTs, and the side effects of these therapies, are quite complex.

The most up-to-date treatment opportunities are available from experienced, multidisciplinary medical professional teams made up of doctors, nurses, and technologists who specialize in **cancer** (oncology), neurology, medical imaging, drug or **radiation therapy**, and anesthesiology.

Clinical staging, treatments, and prognosis

CPTs and other primary brain tumors are diagnosed, or staged, in grades of severity from I to IV. Grade I tumors have cells that are not malignant and are nearly normal in appearance. Grade II tumors have cells that appear to be slightly abnormal. Grade III tumors have cells that are malignant and clearly abnormal. Grade IV, the most severe type of brain tumor, contains fast-spreading and abnormal cells. The standard treatment for all grades of CPTs is surgery to completely remove the tumor or tumors. This surgery is generally aided by an image guidance system that allows the surgeon to determine the most efficient route to take to the location of the tumor.

Approximately one-half of CPT patients gain relief of the increased intracranial pressure after complete removal of their tumors. The other half require a spinal fluid shunt to allow drainage of the excess fluid.

In some instances of CPC, the tumor is inoperable. Patients with inoperable CPCs are generally treated with radiation therapies. CPPs are highly resistant to radiation treatment, so these therapies are not used for CPPs.

As of 1999, 8.6% of patients who had surgery to remove CPTs died within five years of the surgery. One-half of these patients (4.3%) died during the surgery itself.

Alternative and complementary therapies

There are no effective alternative treatments for CPTs other than surgery and radiation therapies in the case of inoperable CPCs.

Coping with cancer treatment

Most patients who undergo brain surgery to remove their tumors can resume their normal activities within a few days of the operation.

Clinical trials

There were 35 **clinical trials** underway in 2009 aimed at the treatment of CPTs. More information on these trials, including contact information, may be found by conducting a clinical trial search at the website of the National Cancer Institute: http:// www. cancer.gov.

Prevention

Because the causes of CPTs are not known, there are no known preventions.

Special concerns

Repeat surgery may be necessary for CPTs because these tumors sometimes redevelop. Careful monitoring by the medical team will be required.

Resources

OTHER

Tavares, Marcio P. *Choroid Plexus Tumors—MEDSTU-DENTS—Neurosurgery.* (25 March 2001) [cited July 1, 2001]. http://www.medstudents.com.br/neuroc/neuroc5.htm.

ORGANIZATIONS

The Brain Tumor Society. 124 Watertown Street, Suite 3-H. Watertown, MA 02472. Telephone (617)924-9997. Fax (617)924-9998. http://www.tbts.org.

National Brain Tumor Foundation. 785 Market Street, Suite 1600, San Francisco, CA 94103. Telephone (415)284-0208. http://www.braintumor.org.

Paul A. Johnson, Ed.M.

Chromic phosphate P32 *see*
Radiopharmaceuticals

Chromosome rearrangements

Definition

A chromosome rearrangement is a structural change in a chromosome such as a deletion, translocation, inversion, or gene amplification. Chromosome rearrangements can contribute to the transformation of a normal cell into a cancerous cell and are therefore found in many **cancer** cells.

Description

Chromosomes and genes

A chromosome is a microscopic structure that is composed of proteins and DNA and is found in every cell of the body. Each cell of the body, except for the egg and the sperm cells, contains 23 pairs of chromosomes and 46 chromosomes in total. All cells of the body except for the egg and sperm cells are called the somatic cells. The egg and sperm cells each contain 23 chromosomes. Both males and females have 22 pairs of chromosomes, called the autosomes, that are numbered 1 to 22 in order of decreasing size. The final pair of chromosomes, called the sex chromosomes, determine the sex of the individual. Women possess two identical chromosomes called the X chromosomes while men possess one X chromosome and one Y chromosome.

Each type of chromosome contains different genes that are found at specific locations along the chromosome. Men and women possess two of each type of autosomal gene since they inherit one of each type from each parent. Each gene contains the instructions for the production of a particular protein. The proteins produced by genes have many functions and work together to create the traits of the human body, such as hair and eye color, and are involved in controlling the body's basic functions. Some genes produce proteins that are involved in controlling the growth cycle of the cell and are therefore involved in preventing the development of cancer.

Types of chromosome rearrangements

Sometimes a spontaneous break or breaks occur in a chromosome or chromosomes in a particular cell and can result in a deletion, inversion, or translocation. If the break or breaks result in the loss of a piece of chromosome, it is called a deletion. An inversion results when a segment of chromosome breaks off, is reversed (inverted), and is reinserted into its original location. When a piece of one chromosome is exchanged with a piece from another chromosome it is called a translocation.

Sometimes a small segment of chromosome is amplified, which results in the presence of multiple copies of that section of the chromosome. In most cases the segment of the chromosome that is duplicated contains only one gene, although it is possible for more than one gene to be amplified. Sometimes

A. Normal chromosomes. B. Breakage occurs near a proto-oncogene on chromosome 9. C. Translocation chromosomes. This translocation, called the Philadelphia chromosome, can result in chronic myelocytic leukemia.
(Illustration by Argosy Publishing. Cengage Learning, Gale.)

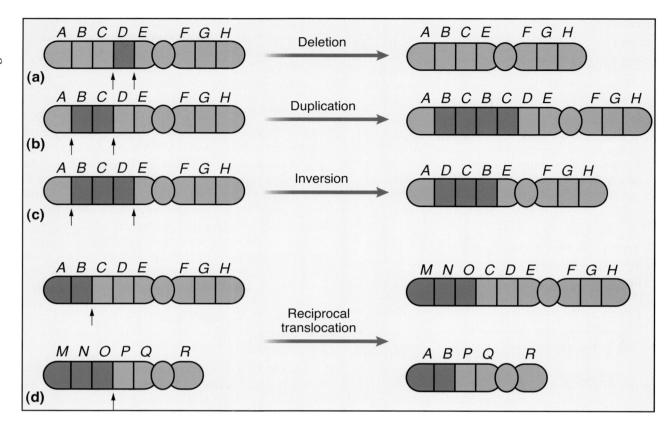

Four kinds of chromosome rearrangements. Arrows indicate where chromosomes break, and dark green indicates the genes affected. (a) A deletion removes a chromosome segment. (b) Duplication repeats a segment. (c) Inversion reverses the order of a segment. (d) A translocation moves a segment from one chromosome to another. Each chromosome contains genes found at specific locations along the chromosome, and each gene contains the instructions for the production of a protein. If a gene produces proteins involved in controlling the cell's growth cycle, and this gene is affected by a chromosome rearrangement, uncontrolled cell growth (cancer) could result. *(Illustration by Argosy Publishing. Cengage Learning, Gale.)*

amplified genes form a separate and unique chromosome and sometimes they are located within an otherwise normal chromosome.

Chromosome rearrangements and cancer

A chromosome rearrangement can delete or disrupt the functioning of genes that are located on the chromosomal pieces involved. Chromosome rearrangements that delete or disrupt genes that regulate the cell cycle can contribute to the transformation of a normal cell into a cancerous cell. That is why chromosomal rearrangements are found in many cancers.

THE TRANSFORMATION OF A NORMAL CELL INTO A CANCEROUS CELL. The process by which a normal cell is transformed into a cancerous cell is a complex, multi-step process involving a breakdown in the normal cell cycle. Normally a somatic cell goes through a growth cycle during which it produces new cells. The process of cell division is necessary for the growth of

tissues and organs of the body and for the replacement of damaged cells.

Cell division is tightly regulated by genes. Normal cells have a limited lifespan and only go through the cell cycle a certain number of times. Genes regulate the cell cycle by producing regulatory proteins. Different types of regulatory proteins regulate cell growth and division in different types of cells. For example, a skin cell may be regulated by a different combination of proteins than a breast cell or a liver cell.

A cell that loses control of its cell cycle and replicates out of control is called a cancer cell. Cancer cells undergo many cell divisions, often at a quicker rate than normal cells, and do not have a limited lifespan. They also have loss of apoptosis, or cell death, which is characteristic of a normal cell. This allows them to eventually overwhelm the body with a large number of abnormal cells and hurt the functioning of the normal cells.

KEY TERMS

Chromosome—A microscopic structure, made of a complex of proteins and DNA, that is found within each cell of the body.

Deletion—A piece missing from a chromosome.

Gene—A building block of inheritance, made up of a compound called DNA (deoxyribonucleic acid) and containing the instructions for the production of a particular protein. Each gene is found on a specific location on a chromosome.

Gene amplification—When multiple copies of a small segment of chromosome containing one or more genes are present as a separate chromosome or as part of an otherwise normal chromosome.

Inversion—A piece of a chromosome that was removed from the chromosome, inverted, and reinserted into the same location on the chromosome.

Leukemia—Cancer of the blood-forming organs which results in an overproduction of white blood cells.

Lymphoma—Cancer involving cells of the immune system.

Oncogene—A changed proto-oncogene that promotes uncontrolled cell division and growth.

Protein—A substance produced by a gene that is involved in creating the traits of the human body such as hair and eye color or is involved in controlling the basic functions of the human body.

Proto-oncogene—A gene involved in stimulating the normal growth and division of cells in a controlled manner.

Somatic cells—All the cells of the body except for the egg and sperm cells.

Translocation—An exchange of a piece of one chromosome with a piece from another chromosome.

Tumor-suppressor gene—Gene involved in controlling normal cell growth and preventing cancer.

A cell becomes cancerous only after changes or deletions occur in a number of genes that are involved in the regulation of its cell cycle. However, a change or deletion of one regulatory gene can result in the change or deletion of other regulatory genes.

Proto-oncogenes and tumor-suppressor genes are the two most common types of genes involved in regulating the cell cycle. We inherit two of each type of proto-oncogene and two of each type of tumor-suppressor gene. Tumor-suppressor genes produce proteins that are involved in helping to prevent uncontrolled cell growth and division. Only one normal copy of a tumor-suppressor gene needs to be present to maintain its normal role in the regulation of the cell cycle. If both copies of a tumor-suppressor gene are changed, however, then not enough normal tumor-suppressor protein will be produced and the cell is more likely to become cancerous.

Proto-oncogenes produce proteins that are largely involved in stimulating the growth and division of cells in a controlled manner. A change in a proto-oncogene can convert it into an oncogene. An oncogene produces an abnormal protein, which is involved in stimulating uncontrolled cell growth. Only one proto-oncogene of a pair needs to be changed into an oncogene for it to promote the transformation of a normal cell into a cancerous cell.

A chromosome rearrangement involving a tumor-suppressor gene or proto-oncogene can contribute to the transformation of a normal cell into a cancerous cell. Certain types of chromosome rearrangements are found more commonly in cancers of certain types of cells. This is because these chromosome rearrangements involve genes that regulate the cell cycle in those specific cells. More than one chromosome rearrangement is usually present in a particular cancer cell since it is necessary for more than one regulatory gene to be altered during the transformation of a normal cell into a cancerous cell. Different types of chromosome rearrangements contribute to the formation of cancer cells in different ways. Researchers don't always know how a chromosome rearrangement contributes to the development of cancer.

How specific types of rearrangements contribute to the development of cancer

Deletions

A deletion of a piece of chromosome that contains a tumor suppressor gene can contribute to the transformation of a normal cell into a cancerous cell. If both copies of a tumor suppressor gene are deleted or changed then little or no tumor suppressor protein is produced. This in turn can impact the regulation of the cell cycle and contribute to the transformation of the normal cell.

A deletion of a segment of chromosome 13, for example, can result in the loss of a tumor-suppressor gene that helps to prevent an eye cancer called **retinoblastoma**. If both retinoblastoma tumor-suppressor genes are deleted or changed in one of the cells of the eye then that cell can become cancerous.

Translocations

A translocation involving a proto-oncogene can result in its conversion into an oncogene, which can contribute to the development of cancer. A translocation involving a proto-oncogene results in the transfer of the proto-oncogene from its normal location on a chromosome to a different location on another chromosome. Sometimes this results in the transfer of a proto-oncogene next to an activating gene. This activating gene abnormally activates the proto-oncogene and converts it into an oncogene. When this oncogene is present in a cell, it contributes to uncontrolled cell growth and the development of cancer.

For example, the translocation of the c-myc proto-oncogene from its normal location on chromosome 8 to a location on chromosome 14 results in the abnormal activation of c-myc. This type of translocation is involved in the development of a type of cancer called **Burkitt's lymphoma**. The translocated c-myc proto-oncogene is found in the cancer cells of approximately 85% of people with Burkitt's **lymphoma**.

A translocation involving a proto-oncogene can also result in the fusion of the proto-oncogene with another gene. The resulting fused gene is an oncogene that produces an unregulated protein which stimulates uncontrolled cell growth. One example is the Philadelphia chromosome translocation, found in the leukemia cells of greater than 95% of patients with a chronic form of leukemia. The Philadelphia chromosome translocation results in the fusion of the c-abl proto-oncogene, normally found on chromosome 9, to the bcr gene that is found on chromosome 22. The fused gene produces an abnormal protein that is involved in the formation of cancer cells.

Inversions

An inversion, like a translocation, can result in the creation of an oncogene through either the activation of a proto-oncogene or the creation of a fusion gene. An inversion involving a proto-oncogene results in the movement of the gene to another location on the same chromosome. For example, an inversion of chromosome 10 can move a proto-oncogene called RET and cause it to fuse with a gene called ELEI or a gene called H4. The fusion of RET with either of these genes creates an oncogene. When the RET oncogene is present in a thyroid cell it promotes the transformation of that cell into a cancerous cell.

Gene amplification

Gene amplification can also contribute to the development of cancer. Amplification of a segment of chromosome that contains a proto-oncogene can result in the formation of many copies of a proto-oncogene. Each copy of the proto-oncogene produces protein that is involved in stimulating cell growth. This can result in a significant increase in the amount of protein produced, which can promote uncontrolled cell growth. Multiple copies of proto-oncogenes are found in many tumors.

See also Cancer genetics.

Resources

OTHER

"Chromosome Rearrangements" *University of Wisconsin–Madison Department of Genetics*. [cited July 3, 2001]. <http://www1.genetics.wisc.edu/466/Fall98/lect08/index.html>.

"The Genetics of Cancer—an Overview" *Robert H. Lurie Comprehensive Cancer Center of Northwestern University*. 17 Feb. 1999. [cited June 29, 2001]. http://www.cancergenetics.org/gncavrvu.htm.

Lisa Andres, M.S., CGC

Chronic lymphocytic leukemia

Definition

Chronic lymphocytic leukemia (CLL) is a **cancer** of white blood cells. In CLL, mature white blood cells of certain types, called lymphocytes, function abnormally and cause disease.

Bone marrow in chronic lymphocytic leukemia. In this disease, bone marrow is replaced by small, mature lymphoid cells. *(Photo Researchers, Inc. Reproduced by permission.)*

KEY TERMS

Antibodies—Proteins made by the B lymphocytes in response to the presence of infectious agents, such as bacteria or viruses, in the body.

Biopsy—The surgical removal and microscopic examination of living tissue for diagnostic purposes.

Chemotherapy—Treatment with drugs that act against cancer.

Chromosome — Part of the cell that carries genetic material.

Cytokines—Chemicals made by the cells that act on other cells to stimulate or inhibit their function. Cytokines that stimulate growth are called "growth factors."

Immunotherapy—Treatment of cancer by stimulating the body's immune defense system.

Maturation—The process by which stem cells transform from immature cells without a specific function into a particular type of blood cell with defined functions.

Radiation therapy—Treatment using high-energy radiation from x-ray machines, cobalt, radium, or other sources.

Remission—A disappearance of a disease as a result of treatment. Complete remission means that all disease is gone. Partial remission means that the disease is significantly improved by treatment, but residual traces of the disease are still present.

Description

Chronic leukemia is a cancer that starts in the blood cells made in the bone marrow. The bone marrow is the spongy tissue found in the large bones of the body. The bone marrow makes precursor cells called "blasts" or "stem cells" that mature into different types of blood cells. Unlike **acute leukemias**, in which the process of maturation of the blast cells is interrupted, in **chronic leukemias**, most of the cells do mature and only a few remain as immature cells. However, even though the cells appear normal, they do not function as normal cells.

The different types of cells produced in the bone marrow are red blood cells (RBCs), which carry oxygen and other materials to all tissues of the body, and white blood cells (WBCs), which fight **infection**. Platelets play a part in the clotting of the blood. The white blood cells can be further subdivided into three main types: the granulocytes, monocytes, and the lymphocytes.

The granulocytes, as their name suggests, contain granules (particles). These granules contain special proteins (enzymes) and several other substances that can break down chemicals and destroy microorganisms such as bacteria. Monocytes are the second type of white blood cell. They also are important in defending the body against pathogens.

The lymphocytes form the third type of white blood cell. There are two main types of lymphocytes: T lymphocytes and B lymphocytes. They have different functions within the immune system. The B cells protect the body by making "antibodies." Antibodies are proteins that can attach to the surfaces of bacteria and viruses. The occurrence of this attachment sends signals to many other cell types to travel through the blood and destroy the antibody-coated organism. The T cell protects the body against viruses. When a virus enters a cell, it produces certain proteins that are projected onto the surface of the infected cell. T cells recognize these proteins and produce certain chemicals (cytokines) capable of destroying the virus-infected cells. In addition, T cells destroy some types of cancer cells.

Chronic leukemias develop very gradually. The abnormal lymphocytes multiply slowly, and in a poorly regulated manner. These lymphocytes live much longer than normal lymphocytes and, thus, their numbers build up in the body. In CLL, lymphocytes accumulate. The enlarged lymphocyte population congregates in the blood, bone marrow, lymph nodes, spleen, and liver. The two types of chronic leukemias can be easily distinguished under the microscope. Chronic lymphocytic leukemia (CLL) involves the T or B lymphocytes. B-cell abnormalities are more common than T-cell abnormalities. T cells are affected in only 5% of the patients.

Demographics

Ninety percent of CLL cases are seen in people who are 50 years or older, with the average age at diagnosis being 72. Rarely is CLL diagnosed in a patient who is less than 35 years of age. The incidence of the disease increases with age. It is almost never seen in children. According to the estimates of the National Cancer Institute (NCI), approximately 15,490 new cases of CLL were diagnosed in 2009, 9,200 in men and 6,290 in women.

CLL affects both sexes. Among patients younger than 50, the disease is slightly more common in men. However, among patients older than 50 years of age,

CLL appears almost twice as often in men than in women. Within the United States, CLL affects African Americans as frequently as it does Caucasians. However, CLL appears more frequently among Americans than among people living in Asia, Latin America, and Africa.

In the United States and Europe, CLL accounts for more than one-quarter of all diagnosed leukemias. Over the past 50 years, the rate at which CLL has been appearing has increased significantly. However, many doctors think that this increase is not necessarily due to the disease actually being more common than in the past, but instead due to the fact that the disease is now more likely to be diagnosed when it does appear. Fifty years ago, only one out of ten CLL patients was diagnosed during the early stages of the disease. Now, half of all CLL patients are diagnosed during this early stage.

Causes and symptoms

The cause of CLL is unknown. It is certain, however, that CLL is linked to genetic abnormalities and environmental factors. For example, close family members of patients with CLL are twice to seven times as likely to be diagnosed with CLL as people in the general population. For another example, exposure to certain chemicals used in farming and other agricultural occupations may increase the risk that a person will develop CLL. In contrast, CLL is not associated with exposure to radiation known to cause other cancers. As of the early 2000s, doctors were unsure whether people who have had certain virus infections are more likely to develop CLL than are people in the general population. If there does turn out to be such an association, it would not be with all viruses but with two human retroviruses (HTLV-I and HTLV-II) or with **Epstein-Barr virus** (EBV).

The symptoms of CLL are generally vague and non-specific. One out of five patients with CLL has no symptoms at all, and the disease is discovered only through a routine blood test. A patient may experience all or some of the following symptoms:

- chronic fatigue
- weakness
- a general feeling of malaise or of things being not quite right
- swollen lymph nodes
- an enlarged spleen, which could make the patient complain of abdominal fullness
- a general feeling of ill health
- fever
- frequent bacterial or viral infections
- unusually severe response to insect bites
- night sweats
- weight loss not due to dieting or exercise

Diagnosis

There is no **screening test** for CLL. If the doctor has reason to suspect leukemia, he or she will conduct a very thorough physical examination to look for enlarged lymph nodes in the neck, underarm, and pelvic region. In addition, the doctor will look to see whether the liver and spleen are enlarged. Urine and blood tests may be ordered to check for microscopic amounts of blood in the urine and to obtain a complete differential blood count. This count will give the numbers and percentages of the different cells found in the blood. An abnormal blood test might suggest leukemia. Some authorities state that CLL may be diagnosed if the number of lymphocytes in the blood exceeds a certain level.

The doctor may perform a **bone marrow aspiration and biopsy** to confirm the diagnosis of leukemia. During the **bone marrow biopsy**, a cylindrical piece of bone and marrow is removed. The tissue is generally taken out of the hipbone. These samples are sent to the laboratory for examination. In many CLL patients, more than one-fourth of the bone marrow is made up of mature lymphocytes. In addition to diagnosis, bone marrow **biopsy** is also conducted during the treatment phase of the disease to see if the leukemia is responding to therapy.

Some CLL patients have a condition called hypogammaglobulinemia. Immunoglobulins are normal parts of the body's immune system, the system used to fight off infection. Patients with hypogammaglobulinemia have very low levels of all of the various types of immunoglobulins.

The doctor may also conduct immunophenotyping. This involves taking a sample of the blood and looking at what types of cells of the immune system are being affected by the CLL. Approximately 19 out of 20 CLL patients have the B-cell type of CLL. Far more rare is the T-cell type of CLL. In addition, the doctor may look for abnormalities in the chromosomes of the affected cells. Chromosomes are a unit of genetic material within cells. Patients exhibiting no chromosomal abnormalities have a better prognosis than those who do have such abnormalities. If the abnormalities become more complex over time, the patient's prognosis may worsen.

Standard imaging tests such as **x rays**, **computed tomography** scans (CT scans), and **magnetic resonance imaging** (MRI) may be used to check whether the leukemic cells have invaded other organs of the body, such as the bones, chest, kidneys, abdomen, or brain.

Clinical staging, treatments, and prognosis

Staging

Usually one of two systems are used to stage CLL. One of these is the Binet system and the other the Rai system. According to the Rai system, patients at low risk have no enlargement of lymph nodes, spleen, or liver. The occurrence of these marks entry into the intermediate stage, according to Rai. High-risk patients have, in addition, **anemia** and a significant decrease in the number of blood platelets in their blood. Blood platelets help blood to clot. According to the Binet system, a patient's stage depends upon how much hemoglobin (part of red blood cells that carry oxygen) and how many platelets are in the blood, as well as how many other areas the disease has affected. According to both systems, patients at low risk usually survive more than 10 years. Patients at intermediate risk usually survive about six years. Patients at high risk usually survive about two years. Other factors with important implications for prognosis include the pattern at which bone marrow is being affected by the CLL and the amount of time it takes for the number of lymphocytes to double.

Treatment

Because the long-term prognosis for many patients with CLL is excellent, many patients receive no treatment at all at first. Many patients go for years before developing aggressive disease that requires treatment. Treatment for early stage CLL should be started only when one of the following conditions appears:

- Symptoms of the disease are growing worse; for example, there is a greater degree of fever, weight loss, night sweats, and so forth.
- The spleen is enlarging or enlargement of the spleen has become painful.
- Disease of the lymph nodes has become more severe.
- The condition of the bone marrow has deteriorated and there is anemia and a marked reduction in the number of blood platelets.
- There is anemia or reduction in the number of blood platelets for reasons not specifically related to the condition of the bone marrow.
- The population of lymphocytes is rapidly growing.
- The patient is experiencing numerous infections caused by bacteria.

Therapy for CLL usually starts with **chemotherapy**. Depending on the stage of the disease, single or multiple drugs may be given. Drugs commonly prescribed include **fludarabine**, **cladribine**, **chlorambucil** and **cyclophosphamide**. Studies have also provided evidence that a combination of fludarabine and cyclophosphamide is effective. However, this combination has not yet been evaluated over periods of 10 years or more. Another combination now being studied involves fludarabine and **mitoxantrone** (Novantrone). Yet another involves fludarabine and anthracyclines. Low-dose **radiation therapy** may be given to the whole body, or it may be used to alleviate the symptoms and discomfort due to an enlarged spleen and lymph nodes. The spleen may be removed in a procedure called a **splenectomy**.

Bone marrow transplantation (BMT) has produced some positive outcomes in patients with CLL, although it has not been the subject of sufficient systematic study to permit doctors to know how effective it is. In BMT, the patient's diseased bone marrow is replaced with healthy marrow. There are two ways of performing a bone marrow transplant. In an allogeneic bone marrow transplant, healthy marrow is taken from another person (donor) whose tissue is either the same or very closely resembles the patient's tissues. The donor may be a twin, a sibling, or a person who is not related at all. First, the patient's bone marrow is destroyed with very high doses of chemotherapy and radiation therapy. To replace the destroyed marrow, healthy marrow from the donor is given to the patient through a needle in the vein.

In the second type of bone marrow transplant, called an autologous bone marrow transplant, some of the patient's own marrow is taken out and treated with a combination of **anticancer drugs** to kill all the abnormal cells. This marrow is then frozen to save it. The marrow remaining in the patient's body is then destroyed with high-dose chemotherapy and radiation therapy. Following that, the patient's own frozen marrow is thawed and given back to the patient through a needle in the vein. The use of this mode of bone marrow transplant for the treatment of CLL is currently being investigated in **clinical trials**.

Allogeneic BMT has been successfully used with younger patients with CLL who have not responded positively to chemotherapy. Autologous BMT has produced some positive results in older CLL patients. However, BMT is generally not considered an option in treating most patients with CLL because they are too old to be considered good candidates for the procedure.

Other CLL therapies that are being investigated include monoclonal antibody-targeted therapy and **interferons**. **Monoclonal antibodies** (MoAbs) are laboratory-manufactured chemicals that closely resemble parts of the body's natural immune system. Studies of MoAbs-targeted therapies have shown some positive results in CLL, although definitive studies have not been performed at the time of this writing. Interferon is a chemical normally made in the cells of the body. It helps protect the body against viruses and also seems to have some effect against certain cancers. The interferon used as medicine is a laboratory-manufactured copy of the interferon produced by the body. As of this writing, interferon therapy has produced some response in CLL patients. However, interferon therapy has not as yet been shown to be associated with prolongation of remission.

Radiation therapy is very effective for approximately one in three of those CLL patients for whom it is considered appropriate.

Because leukemia cells can spread to all the organs via the blood stream and the lymph vessels, surgery is not considered an option for treating leukemias.

Treatment of CLL and its complications

During therapy for CLL, complications frequently appear. Many patients develop infectious illnesses. Sometimes, two or more infectious diseases attack a patient at the same time. These infections should be treated with great care. Most people whose death has been directly attributed to CLL have actually died from bacterial infections. The patient should be involved in identifying symptoms of infection and reporting these to the doctor without delay. Doing so may save the patient's life.

Many patients develop anemia, which is treated with the drug prednisone. Patients who do not respond to prednisone therapy may have their spleen removed and may receive therapy with immunoglobulin, a component of the blood.

Treatment after transformation of CLL

Between three and ten out of every hundred patients with CLL experiences transformation of the disease into large-cell **lymphoma** (LCL). When this happens it is called Richter's transformation. Its occurrence is often marked by **fever**, **weight loss**, and **night sweats**. Treatments for LCL are being studied, although outcomes have not been very good. Very infrequently, CLL may transform into another disease, called prolymphocytic leukemia. Attempts to develop adequate therapies for this disease are ongoing.

Prognosis

For many CLL patients, the prognosis is excellent. Using the Binet and Rai staging systems, patients at low risk usually survive more than 10 years. Patients at intermediate risk usually survive about six years. Patients at high risk usually survive about two years. The average patient survives approximately nine years following diagnosis. Factors with important implications for prognosis that are not included in the Binet or Rai systems are the pattern at which bone marrow is being affected by the CLL and the amount of time it takes for the number of lymphocytes in the blood to double. It is uncertain whether BMT may prolong the lifespan of CLL patients. Many of the chemotherapy agents used to treat disease do effectively control the leukemia and its effects but, as yet, the more established chemotherapy agents have not been shown to increase the life span of patients.

Coping with cancer treatment

Since many CLL patients die from infection, it is essential that patient be very alert to the signs of infection. If patients perform this role and seek medical attention as soon as symptoms of infection appear, then treatment can be started early. This may save a life.

It is very difficult for some patients to be not only informed that they have leukemia but then to also be told that they do not need treatment. This may be very confusing, unless the patient realizes that treatment may be necessary at some future time and that starting therapies too soon may be counterproductive.

Because nutritional alteration, weight loss, and psychosocial problems may accompany CLL, it may be prudent for patients to consult with a registered dietitian.

Cancer patients need supportive care to help them come through the treatment period with physical and emotional strength in tact. Many patients experience feelings of **depression**, anxiety, and **fatigue**, and many experience **nausea and vomiting** during treatment. Studies have shown that these can be managed effectively if discussed with the attending physician.

Prevention

Although some cancers are related to known risk factors, such as smoking, in leukemias, there are no known risk factors. Therefore, at the present time, there is no way known to prevent the leukemias from developing. Everyone should undergo periodic medical checkups.

Resources

BOOKS

Braunwald, Eugene, et al. *Harrison's Principles of Internal Medicine.* 15th ed. New York: McGraw-Hill, 2001.

Herfindal, Eric T., Dick R. Gourley. *Textbook of Therapeutics: Drug and Disease Management.* 7th ed. Philadelphia: Lippincott Williams & Wilkins, 2000.

Humes, H. David, et al. *Kelley's Textbook of Internal Medicine.* 4th ed. Philadelphia: Lippincott Williams & Wilkins, 2000.

Pazdur, Richard, et al. *Cancer Management: A Multidisciplinary Approach: Medical, Surgical, & Radiation Oncology.* 4th ed. Melville, NY: PRR, 2000.

PERIODICALS

Mauro, F. R., et al. "Clinical characteristics and outcome of young chronic lymphocytic leukemia patients: A single institution study of 204 cases." *Blood* 1999; 94: 448-454.

ORGANIZATIONS

The American Cancer Society publishes useful texts, such as *Adult Chronic Leukemia - Overview, Leukemia - Adult Chronic: Treatment, Leukemia - Adult Chronic: Detection and Symptoms, Leukemia: Adult Chronic FAQ [Frequently Asked Questions],* and *Leukemia - Adult Chronic: Prevention & Risk.* Call 1-800-ACS-2345 or on the Internet at www.cancer.org/

The Leukemia & Lymphoma Society (Formerly Leukemia Society of America) publishes useful texts available through the Internet or by mail, including *Chronic Lymphocytic Leukemia (CLL), Making Intelligent Choices About Therapy, Understanding Blood Counts, Patient Aid Program, Family Support Group,* and *Information Resource Center.* Call 1-800-955-4572 or visit on the Internet at www.leukemia-lymphoma.org/.

The National Cancer Institute publishes useful texts available through the internet or by mail, and answers questions by telephone. Some titles include: *What You Need to Know about Leukemia* and *PDQ - Treatment - Patients: Chronic Lymphocytic Leukemia.* Call 1-800-4 CANCER or visit on the Internet at www.nci.nih.gov/.

National Coalition for Cancer Survivorship. 1010 Wayne Avenue, 7th Floor, Silver Spring, MD 20910-5600. Telephone: (301) 650-9127 and (877) NCCS-YES [877-622-7937]. Website: www.canceradvocacy.org.

Lata Cherath, Ph.D.
Bob Kirsch

Chronic myelocytic leukemia

Definition

Chronic myelocytic leukemia (CML) is a **cancer** of white blood cells in which too many white blood

This spleen was removed from a patient with chronic myelocytic leukemia. The spleen has many functions—it removes old red blood cells, stores blood, and produces lymphocytes and plasma cells. Many blood disorders and cancers (including leukemias and lymphomas) can cause the spleen to enlarge. *(Custom Medical Stock Photo. Reproduced by permission.)*

cells are made in the bone marrow. Chronic myelogenous leukemia and chronic myeloid leukemia are other names for CML and refer to the identical disease. Depending on the type of white blood cell that is involved, chronic leukemia can be classified as **chronic lymphocytic leukemia** or chronic myelocytic leukemia. In chronic myelocytic leukemia, there is an increased proliferation of white blood cells called granulocytes.

Description

Chronic leukemia is a cancer that starts in the blood cells made in the bone marrow. The bone marrow is the spongy tissue found in the large bones of the body. The bone marrow makes precursor cells called "blasts" or "stem cells" that mature into different types of blood cells. Unlike **acute leukemias**, in which the process of maturation of the blast cells is interrupted, in **chronic leukemias**, the cells do mature and only a few remain as immature cells. However, even though the cells appear normal, they do not function as normal cells.

Color-enhanced scanning electron microscope image of leukemia cells. Leukemia cells (left) are compared to healthy bone marrow cells. The leukemia cells are larger and have a higher metabolism than the normal cells.

The different types of cells produced in the bone marrow are red blood cells (RBCs), which carry oxygen and other materials to all tissues of the body; white blood cells (WBCs), which fight **infection**; and

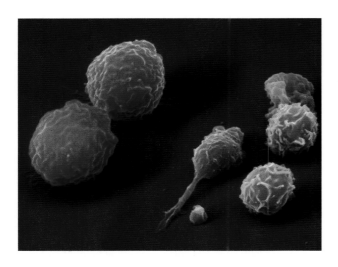

Color-enhanced scanning electron microscope image of leukemia cells. Leukemia cells (left) are compared to healthy bone marrow cells. The leukemia cells are larger and have a higher metabolism than the normal cells. *(Copyright Meckes/ Ottawa, Science Source/Photo Researchers, Inc. Reproduced by permission.)*

platelets, which play a part in the clotting of the blood. The white blood cells can be further subdivided into three main types: the granulocytes, monocytes, and the lymphocytes.

The granulocytes, as their name suggests, have granules (particles) inside them. These granules contain special proteins (enzymes) and several other substances that can break down chemicals and destroy microorganisms such as bacteria. Monocytes are also important in defending the body against pathogens.

The lymphocytes form the third type of white blood cell. There are two main types of lymphocytes: T lymphocytes and B lymphocytes. They have different functions within the immune system. The B cells protect the body by making antibodies. Antibodies are proteins that can attach to the surfaces of bacteria and viruses. This attachment sends signals to many other cell types to come and destroy the antibody-coated organism. The T cell protects the body against viruses. When a virus enters a cell, it produces certain proteins that are projected onto the surface of the infected cell. The T cells can recognize these proteins and produce certain chemicals (cytokines) that are capable of destroying the virus-infected cells. In addition, the T cells can destroy some types of cancer cells.

Chronic leukemias develop very gradually. The abnormal lymphocytes multiply slowly, but in a poorly regulated manner. They live much longer than normal cells and thus their numbers build up in the body. The two types of chronic leukemias can be easily

KEY TERMS

Accelerated phase—The middle one of the three-phase course of CML. However, between 20% and 40% of patients never enter the accelerated phase but, rather, go directly from the chronic to the terminal blastic phase.

Basophil—A type of white blood cell.

Blast—An immature cell.

Bone marrow—Spongy tissue found in the large bones of the body.

Chemotherapy—Treatment with drugs that act against cancer.

Chronic phase—The initial phase of CML.

Hypercellular—Bone marrow is described as being hypercellular if the number of cells present in the bone marrow is unusually great.

Leukapheresis — A procedure to remove or extract excessive white blood cells from the blood.

Philadelphia (Ph) chromosome — The Philadelphia (Ph) chromosome is present if some of the genetic material in two specific parts of two specific genetic units, called chromosomes, have exchanged some content in a particular way.

Remission—Remission of a disease is achieved if the disease becomes diminished for a period.

Terminal blastic phase—The final stage of CML.

distinguished under the microscope. Chronic lymphocytic leukemia (CLL) involves the T or B lymphocytes. In chronic myelocytic leukemia (CML), the cells affected are the granulocytes. In addition, CML involves abnormalities of both the blood platelets, structures that help blood to clot, and the red blood cells, the blood cells that carry oxygen.

Very rarely will CML appear in children. Juvenile CML is a distinct disease of children younger than 14 years of age. There is a decrease in the number of blood platelets, substances that help the blood to clot. And there is an increase in certain white blood cells.

Demographics

Slightly more men than women are affected by CML. The average patient is 66 years of age. However, CML can affect people of any age. Chronic myelocytic leukemia accounts for 10-15 of all leukemias. Chronic myelocytic leukemia is generally seen in people over the age of 65. According to the estimates of the

QUESTIONS TO ASK THE DOCTOR

- How can I obtain supportive care to help my family and I deal with my diseases?
- What sort of benefit and what sort of side effects might each of the available treatment options bring?
- How can I begin forming a treatment plan?
- What is my prognosis?
- Are blasts present?
- Has complete remission or partial remission been achieved?
- What can I do to lower my risk of infection during chemotherapy?

American Cancer Society (ACS), approximately 5,050 new cases of leukemia were diagnosed in the year 2009, 2,930 in men and 2,120 in women. Between 1973 and 1991, the rate at which CML appeared in the United States decreased slightly.

Causes and symptoms

People exposed to nuclear and other radiation are at increased risk for CML. Thus, people who have had higher exposure to radiation for medical reasons are at increased risk of developing this cancer. Parents with CML do not have children who are more than normally likely to develop CML. However, it is possible that people whose immune system exhibits certain characteristics are at increased risk for the disease.

CML develops in a two- or three-stage progression. First, the chronic phase appears. Between 60% and 80% of patients next exhibit the symptoms of what is called the accelerated phase. The final stage of CML is the terminal blastic phase.

Symptoms of chronic phase CML appear in 60–85% of patients. This means 15% to 40% of all the people diagnosed with CML have no symptoms at all and are diagnosed with the disease only because of the results of a routine blood test. Patients who do have symptoms most frequently find themselves to have **fatigue**, **weight loss**, or pain. Some patients have a mass of tissue or an enlarged liver that the doctor is able to feel. Some patients experience strokes, visual problems, a lowering of alertness or responsiveness,

priapism, and ringing in the ear. Many patients in accelerated phase CML have no specific symptoms. However, **fever**, weight loss, and **night sweats** may appear.

Patients with terminal, blastic phase CML often experience symptoms. There may be fever, weight loss, night sweats, and **bone pain**. Many patients develop infections. Many have **anemia** (low counts of red blood cells) and many bleed easily.

Diagnosis

There are no screening tests available for chronic leukemias. The detection of these diseases may occur by chance during a routine physical examination.

People who have CML have an unusually high number of white blood cells. Somewhat less than half of these people also have high numbers of blood platelets. Most patients have mild anemia. The composition of the bone marrow in CML patients also differs from that of a healthy person. The marrow is described as being hypercellular. This means that the number of cells present in the bone marrow is unusually great.

If the doctor has reason to suspect leukemia, he or she will conduct a very thorough physical examination to look for enlarged lymph nodes in the neck, underarm, and pelvic region. Swollen gums, an enlarged liver or spleen, bruises, or pinpoint red rashes all over the body are among the signs of leukemia. Urine and blood tests may be ordered to check for microscopic amounts of blood in the urine and to obtain a complete differential blood count. This count will give the numbers and percentages of the different cells found in the blood.

Standard imaging tests such as **x rays**, **computed tomography** scans (CT scans), and **magnetic resonance imaging** (MRI) may be used to check whether the leukemic cells have invaded other organs of the body, such as the bones, chest, kidneys, abdomen, or brain.

Many doctors consider the presence of the Philadelphia (Ph) chromosome to be a crucial factor in the diagnosis of CML. The Ph chromosome is formed if some of the genetic material in two specific parts of two specific genetic units, called chromosomes, have exchanged some content in a particular way and created an arrangement of genetic material characteristic of CML patients.

Laboratory findings indicate when a patient enters the accelerated phase of CML. There may be more than 15% blasts (immature cells) in the blood.

Alternately, the accelerated phase has started when more than 30% of the blood may be composed of a combination of blasts and promyelocytes. Promyelocytes are immature granulocytes. Another marker for the start of the accelerated phase is when the blood contains more than 20% of another white blood cell, called a basophil. Finally, the accelerated phase may be heralded by there being more than 100,000,000,000 platelets per liter of blood. The terminal, blastic phase of CML is heralded by measurements of 30% or more of blasts in either the bone marrow or the blood.

Clinical staging, treatments, and prognosis

Staging

Several different staging systems are in use. Most of these make use of the fact that a number of factors relevant to patients with CML say something about the patient's prognosis. Among these factors are the patient's age, the white blood cell count, the platelet count, the percentage of blast cells and basophil cells in either the blood or the bone marrow, the size of the liver, the size of the spleen, population of red blood cells that have a central portion called a nucleus, and the evolution of certain cell clones.

Treatment

It is very fortunate that several years ago the American Society of Hematology convened an Expert Panel on Chronic Myeloid Leukemia. This panel reviewed available therapies and published its findings in 1999. The findings were rigorously based upon evidence provided by the best research. The panel, comprised of top doctors from around the world, carefully sifted through all of the studies on treatment for CML and put aside all those studies performed with questionable methodology. This is a most important document relevant to CML therapy.

In 2001, the FDA approved a medicine known as STI571, **Imatinib mesylate**, or Gleevec. A second drug, dasatinib, was approved in 2006 for use in patients with a resistance to Gleevec.

In terms of CML therapy, physicians have the reliable report of the Expert Panel and information about these medications. How the Expert Panel's findings and this information should be integrated with the results of recent studies of imatinib mesylate is an issue that cancer doctors are currently resolving.

The Expert Panel looked at treatment of the chronic phase of CML. One therapy examined by the panel is **busulfan** (BUS). Another is **hydroxyurea** (HU). Both BUS and HU are **chemotherapy** medications. Studies have demonstrated that CML patients in chronic phase given HU live longer than patients given BUS.

Another therapy examined by the expert panel is interferon-alpha. Interferon is a chemical normally made in the cells of the body. It helps protect the body against viruses and also seems to have some effect against certain cancers. The interferon used as medicine is a laboratory-manufactured copy of the interferon produced by the body. The Expert Panel concluded that patients in chronic phase CML who have received interferon live longer than those given HU or BUS. This conclusion applies, in particular, to patients who have had little prior treatment for CML, who start interferon treatment soon after diagnosis, and who have certain other characteristics. However, side effects of interferon therapy are greater than those of therapy with HU or BUS. Patients who develop the side effects of interferon may feel like they have the flu. Patients receiving interferon seem to do better if they also receive chemotherapy with either HU or a medicine called Ara-C, or **cytarabine**.

Bone marrow transplantation (BMT) is an effective treatment for CML. In BMT, the patient's diseased bone marrow is replaced with healthy marrow. There are two ways of doing a bone marrow transplant. In an allogeneic bone marrow transplant, healthy marrow is taken from another person (donor) whose tissue is either the same or very closely resembles the patient's tissues. The donor may be a twin, a sibling, or a person who is not related at all. First, the patient's bone marrow is destroyed with very high doses of chemotherapy and **radiation therapy**. To replace the destroyed marrow, healthy marrow from the donor is given to the patient.

In the second type of bone marrow transplant, called an autologous bone marrow transplant, some of the patient's own marrow is taken out and treated with a combination of **anticancer drugs** to kill all the abnormal cells. This marrow is then frozen to save it. The marrow remaining in the patient's body is then destroyed with high dose chemotherapy and radiation therapy. Following that, the patient's own marrow that was frozen is thawed and given back to the patient.

Allogeneic BMT may be used soon after diagnosis or after a patient has been treated with interferon or chemotherapy. The Expert Panel found that carefully designed, well-controlled, randomized studies have not been conducted on BMT therapy for CML. In the studies that do exist, scientists performed BMT on a group of patients and then observed the results. These studies show that BMT may lead to long-term remission. Remission is achieved if the disease becomes diminished for a period. Patients appear to live longer if they received chemotherapy followed by BMT. But the Expert Panel cautions that the results of these observational studies cannot be relied upon. One problem with them might be, for example, that the patients chosen to receive BMT might have started out being healthier than patients who did not receive BMT. The side effects of BMT may be severe, and a large number of CML patients receiving BMT die as a direct result of the BMT.

Therefore, one important consideration when BMT is being considered is whether the conditions under which the individual patient might receive BMT are favorable. In other words, is a very suitable marrow donor available? Is the patient within two years of CML diagnosis? It is important that patients understand clearly the ptential benefits and risks of BMT. One comment made by the Expert Panel is that younger patients who hope to live a very long time after CML diagnosis are more likely to benefit from allogeneic BMT. Autologous BMT has not achieved superior long-term results.

The recent studies of imatinib mesylate found it very effective in two groups of CML patients. One group was made up of patients who had unsuccessful results with interferon alfa therapy. The other group of CML patients studied were in the blast phase of the disease. Both studies found the medication to be effective and well tolerated. However, studies reporting on the long-term effectiveness of imatinib mesylate were not yet available.

Because leukemia cells can spread to all the organs via the blood stream and the lymph vessels, surgery is not considered an option for treating the leukemias.

The Expert Panel was careful to state that patient preferences should be taken into account as a treatment plan is developed. No approach to CML therapy is perfect. Each provides some benefit and is accompanied by certain side effects and risks. Which therapy or therapies is best for each individual patient depends upon on certain facts, such as the age of the patient and whether the patient is suffering from illnesses other than CML. In addition, the Expert Panel explains that the personal preferences of each patient are an important consideration. For example, some

patients would rather avoid potential severe side effects and would be willing to give up the potential of living another few months or years. Other patients would be entirely unwilling to accept this way of looking at risks and benefits. It is important that health care professionals educate patients as to what treatment options are available and the perfections and imperfections associated with each. The opinions of each patient should be an important factor in deciding which treatment is best for that patient.

In the accelerated and blastic phase of CML, aggressive chemotherapy may be given. Combination chemotherapy, in which multiple drugs are used, is more effective than using a single drug for the treatment. Interferon and BMT may be used, although results are not as good as for patients in the chronic phase of CML.

It should be mentioned that during treatment the doctor may order a procedure called leukapheresis. This lowers the numbers of white blood cells circulating in the patient's body. Also, either before or after therapy, it may be necessary to provide the patient with a transfusion of blood platelets. In addition, **antibiotics** are often used to help prevent infection in leukemia patients.

Prognosis

The most important factor in determining the likelihood that a patient receiving interferon therapy will achieve long-term survival is whether there is a positive response to interferon-alfa. Although experience with imatinib mesylate is being gathered in studies, this drug remains so new that doctors do not know what effect it will have on the prognosis of CML patients. Once the threat of transplantation-related complications has passed, patients receiving BMT may achieve longer survival than patients receiving interferon therapy.

Before the discovery of modern therapies, patients often spent between three-and-a-half and five years in the chronic phase. Then some patients entered an accelerated phase, from which most died within 18 months. Once patients were in the terminal, blastic phase most died within six months. However, all of this has changed with the arrival of newer therapeutic techniques. Just as many patients used to die from heart attack while similar patients may now live for decades, so cancer patients are achieving longer lives.

Coping with cancer treatment

Cancer patients need supportive care to help them come through the treatment period with physical and emotional strength in tact. Many patients experience feelings of **depression**, anxiety, and fatigue, and many experience **nausea and vomiting** during treatment. Studies have shown that these can be managed effectively if discussed with a doctor.

Prevention

Although some cancers are related to known risk factors, such as smoking, in leukemias, there are no definitive risk factors. Therefore, at the present time, there is no way known to prevent the leukemias from developing. People who are at an increased risk for developing leukemia because of proven exposure to ionizing radiation, the organic liquid benzene, or people who have a history of other cancers of the lymphoid system (Hodgkin's **lymphoma**) should undergo periodic medical checkups.

See also Chromosome rearrangements.

Resources

BOOKS

Braunwald, Eugene, et al. *Harrison's Principles of Internal Medicine.* 15th ed. New York: McGraw-Hill, 2001.

Humes, H. David, et al. *Kelley's Textbook of Internal Medicine.* 4th ed. Philadelphia: Lippincott Williams & Wilkins, 2000.

Pazdur, Richard, et al. *Cancer Management: A Multidisciplinary Approach: Medical, Surgical, & Radiation Oncology.* 4th ed. Melville, NY: PRR, 2000.

PERIODICALS

Drucker B. J., et al. "Activity of a specific inhibitor of the BCR-ABL tyrosine kinase in the blast crisis of chronic myeloid leukemia and acute lymphoblastic leukemia with the Philadelphia chromosome." *New England Journal of Medicine* 344 (2001): 1038-1042.

Drucker, B. J., et al. "Efficacy and safety of a specific inhibitor of the BCR-ABL tyrosine kinase in chronic myeloid leukemia." *New England Journal of Medicine* 344 (2001): 1031-1037.

Silver, Richard T., et al. "An evidence-based analysis of the effect of busulfan, hydroxyurea, interferon, and allogeneic bone marrow transplantation in treating the chronic phase of chronic myeloid leukemia: developed for the American Society of Hematology." *Blood,* 94 (1999): 1517-1536.

ORGANIZATIONS

The American Cancer Society publishes useful texts, which include: *Adult Chronic Leukemia - Overview, Leukemia - Adult Chronic: Treatment, Leukemia - Adult Chronic: Detection and Symptoms, Leukemia: Adult Chronic FAQ [Frequently Asked Questions],* and *Leukemia - Adult Chronic: Prevention & Risk.* Telephone:1-800-ACS-2345. Web site: www.cancer.org/.

The Leukemia & Lymphoma Society (Formerly Leukemia Society of America) publishes useful texts available through the Internet or by mail. Some publications include: *Chronic Myelogenous Leukemia (CML), Choosing a Specialist, Choosing a Treatment Facility, Making Intelligent Choices About Therapy, Understanding Blood Counts, Patient Aid Program,* and *Family Support Group.* Telephone:1-800-955-4572. Web site: www.leukemia-lymphoma.org/.

The National Cancer Institute publishes useful texts available through the Internet or by mail, and answers questions by telephone. Some publications include: *Leukemia, What You Need to Know About Leukemia, PDQ - Treatment - Patients: Chronic Myelogenous Leukemia,* and *Complementary & Alternative Therapies for Leukemia, Lymphoma, Hodgkin's Disease, & Myeloma.* Telephone: 1-800-4-CANCER. Web site: www.nci.nih.gov/.

National Coalition for Cancer Survivorship. 1010 Wayne Avenue, 7th Floor, Silver Spring, MD 20910-5600. Telephone: (301) 650-9127 and (877)NCCS-YES [877-622-7937]. Web site: www.canceradvocacy.org.

Lata Cherath, Ph.D.
Bob Kirsch

Chronic myelogenous leukemia *see* **Chronic myelocytic leukemia**

Cigarettes

Description

Farmers were harvesting tobacco crops eight thousand years ago. Its uses since then have ranged from weather forecasting, appetite suppression, and pain relief to the ceremonial smoking of the peace pipe and recreational use. Although tobacco was smoked and chewed in the United States back in the days of Columbus, it was not until the 1880s that smoking cigarettes became a widespread custom. At its peak in 1965, 52% of adult men and 32% of adult women in the United States routinely smoked. By the year 2008, smoking rates in the United States had decreased to 23% in men, and 19% in women; they averaged 21% for all U.S. adults. Unfortunately, rates among young people may be rising again. A survey in Oregon in 2004 showed that by self-report, nearly 21% of girls and 18% of boys had tried smoking by seventh grade.

The potential adverse health effects of smoking were suspected as far back as 1859. It was then that an evaluation of 68 patients with oral cavity **cancer** linked 66 of them with the practice of smoking tobacco through short-stemmed clay pipes. Epidemiological evidence of the potentially harmful effects of cigarette smoking continued to mount over the following years. Finally, in 1962, the Royal College of Physicians of

London officially deemed smoking a serious threat to health; in 1964 the U.S. Surgeon General followed suit.

Health risks of cigarette smoking

An estimated 443,600 Americans die annually from diseases related to cigarette smoking. According to the American Cancer Society, 3,400 nonsmoking adults die each year of lung cancer from the effects of secondhand smoke. Pregnant women who smoke are more likely to give birth to low-weight babies, and smokers have increased rates of heart disease and respiratory problems.

In addition to those health risks, smokers are at a higher risk for the development of many types of cancer. In fact, 38% of all cancer deaths in men and 23% of all cancer deaths in women are believed to be attributed to cigarette smoking. As cigarette smoking becomes more prevalent in developing countries, the incidence of particular diseases, such as lung cancer, has also increased.

Cancers associated specifically with tobacco use include:

- Lung cancer. Smoking is now the primary modifiable risk factor for lung cancer. Tobacco was first linked to lung cancer in 1898, when it was thought to be the cause for several cases of lung cancers in tobacco workers. Since then, studies have continued to document the relationship between smoking and lung cancer. Lung cancer incidence—the number of new cases diagnosed per year—closely follows smoking trends. As more and more women began to smoke, for example, the incidence of lung cancer in women also increased. By the late 1900s, 90% of lung cancer cases in men and 79% in women were believed to be related to smoking. A 2004 study showed that smoking reduced-tar cigarettes did not lower lung cancer risk.
- Head and neck cancer. Smoking increases the risk of head and neck cancers. When tobacco is used in conjunction with alcohol, there is believed to be an even higher risk of these diagnoses. The precise mechanism of this relationship, known as a "synergistic effect," is not yet well understood.
- Esophageal cancer. Smokers, particularly women smokers, are at an increased risk for developing esophageal cancer—a risk that increases with the quantity of cigarettes smoked per day.
- Pancreatic cancer. An estimated 22,000 people die from pancreatic cancer each year, and an alarming 30% of these deaths are related to cigarette smoking.
- Colorectal cancer. Individuals who smoke cigarettes are more likely to develop polyps in the colon, which in turn increases the risk of colon cancer. There is also evidence that the risk of colon and/or rectal cancer increases with pack years for smokers. (Pack years are calculated by multiplying the number of packs of cigarettes smoked a day by the number of years smoked.)
- Stomach cancer. Although some studies have found no existing relationship between smoking and stomach cancer, others have shown an increased risk for smokers over the age of 50 years and a relationship between the disease and pack-years of smoking. More conclusive research is necessary to better understand the role that smoking plays in the development of stomach, or gastric, cancer.
- Bladder cancer. Smoking is believed to be related to 30-40% of all bladder cancers, most of which are of the transitional cell type. The risk of developing bladder cancer is believed to be related to the duration of smoking and inversely related to the age at which smoking began (that is, the younger a person is when he or she starts smoking, the higher the chances of developing bladder cancer).
- Cervical cancer. There appears to be a relationship between smoking and cervical cancer—the higher the "dose," or amount smoked, the higher the likelihood of developing cervical cancer. Estimates show that smoking causes 1,200 cases of cervical cancer annually in Great Britain. Smoking is also associated with human papilloma virus infection, or HPV. Certain types of HPV can cause warts to develop in the genital area and cervix. These types of infections are a major cause of cervical cancer. Because of these overlapping relationships, the exact effect of smoking in cervical cancer needs further study.
- Breast cancer. Smoking was established as a risk factor for breast cancer by a large study of women in California that was published in 2004. Women who were current smokers had a 30% higher risk of breast cancer than women who had never smoked.

Although cancer is not always preventable, avoiding known risk factors, such as smoking, is an important part of prevention. The best approach to prevent disease is not to start smoking at all. However, even individuals who have smoked for years can decrease their risk of cancer and improve their health and well being by breaking the habit. Shortly after quitting smoking, a person will notice an improvement in their sense of taste and smell. Reducing the number of cigarettes smoked can help smokers successfully quit, says a new study from Yale University. However, just cutting back on the number of cigarettes, but continuing to smoke does little to reduce smoking's cancer risks.

After a smoke-free 10 years, lung cancer risk declines by up to 50%. After 15 smoke-free years, an ex-smoker has the same risk of early death than a person who never smoked at all. Although quitting smoking reduces the likelihood of cancer development, the risk depends upon the amount smoked, the number of years smoked, and whether or not a person is ill at the time of **smoking cessation**.

Resources

PERIODICALS

"Breast Cancer Risk in Smokers." *Pulse* January 12, 2004: 7.

Christiani, D. "Smoking and Pulmonary and Cardiovascular Diseases." *Clinics in Chest Medicine* 21 (March 2000): 87-93.

"Cigarette Use in the U.S., 1985–2002." *World Almanac and Book of Facts* Annual 2004: 1417.

"Cutting Down on Cigarettes Promotes Quitting, Yale Study Said." *Health & Medicine Week* February 9, 2004: 6.

"Cutting Down Doesn't Cut Carcinogens." *Pulse* February 2, 2004: 11.

"Girls Before Boys in Cigarette and Alcohol Use: Longitudinal Study." *Pediatric News* March 2004: 29–31.

Leistikow, B. "Smoking and Pulmonary and Cardiovascular Diseases." *Clinics in Chest Medicine* 21 (March 2000): 189-97.

Mitchell, B., et al., "Tobacco Use and Cessation: The Adverse Health Effects of Tobacco and Tobacco-Related Products." *Clinics in Office Practice* 26 (September 1999): 463-98.

"MIT Study: Low-tar Cigarettes Do Not Cut Lung Cancer Risk." *Cancer Weekly* January 27, 2004: 114.

Smith, R. "Epidemiology of Lung Cancer." *Radiologic Clinics of North America* 38 (May 2000): 453-460.

"Smoking's 'Shocking' Effect on Reproductive Health." *Pulse* February 16, 2004: 14.

Tanoue, L. "Cigarette Smoking and Women's Respiratory Health." *Clinics in Chest Medicine* 21 (March 2000): 47-65.

Tamara L. Brown, R.N.
Teresa G. Odle

Cimetidine *see* **Histamine 2 antagonists**
Ciprofloxacin *see* **Antibiotics**

Cisplatin

Definition

Cisplatin, also known by the brand name Platinol-AQ, Cis-platinum, CDDP, or DDP, is a **chemotherapy** medicine used to treat certain types of **cancer** by destroying cancerous cells.

Purpose

Cisplatin is approved by the Food and Drug Administration (FDA) to treat metastatic **testicular cancer** and metastatic **ovarian cancer**. It is also approved for late-stage **bladder cancer** and has been used to treat other types of cancer including head and neck cancer, **esophageal cancer**, **stomach cancer**, lung cancer, **skin cancer**, **prostate cancer**, **lymphoma** and others (breast, **neuroblastoma**, **sarcoma**, bladder, cervical, **myeloma**, **mesothelioma**, **osteosarcoma**).

Description

Cisplatin is a member of the group of chemotherapy drugs known as heavy metal alkylating-like agents. These drugs interfere with the genetic material (DNA) inside the cancer cells and prevent them from further dividing and growing more cancer cells.

Cisplatin has been used to treat cancer for more than 30 years. It can be used alone or in combination with other chemotherapies, including bleomycin-etoposide, **ifosfamide**, **gemcitabine**, paclitaxel, fluorouracil-leucovorin, **vinorelbine**, methotrexate-vinblastine-doxorubicin. Cisplatin may also be given with **radiation therapy**.

Recommended dosage

A cisplatin dose can be determined using a mathematical calculation that measures body surface area (BSA), which depends on a person's overall size. Body surface area is measured in the units known as square meter (m^2). The body surface area is calculated and then multiplied by the drug dosage in milligrams per m^2 (mg/m^2), which gives the proper dosage.

Cisplatin is a clear, colorless solution administered by an infusion into a vein. Infusions can be given once every three to four weeks over a 30 minutes up to two hours. It can also be given continuously over 24 hours a day for several days in a row. One cycle of cisplatin should not be given more frequently than once every three to four weeks. Dosages depend on the cancer being treated.

To treat metastatic testicular cancer

Dosages are 20 mg/m^2 per day administered into a vein every day for five days in a row. This regimen is used in combination with other chemotherapy drugs, mainly **bleomycin** and **etoposide** or **vinblastine**.

To treat metastatic ovarian cancer

Dosages are 50 mg/m^2 to 100 mg/m^2 administered into a vein once every four weeks. This regimen can be combined with the chemotherapy drug **cyclophosphamide** or **doxorubicin**.

To treat advanced bladder cancer

Cisplatin doses range from 50 mg/m^2 to 70 mg/m^2 administered into a vein once every three to four weeks. Cisplatin is usually given alone for bladder cancer.

Before receiving cisplatin large volumes of intravenous fluids are given to keep the kidneys flushed with water. If patients have severe kidney problems the physician will either not use cisplatin or decrease the dose being used.

Normal metal ions found in the body, called electrolytes, can be lost due to administration of cisplatin. These may be added to these intravenous fluids for replacement.

Precautions

When receiving cisplatin, it is important to drink a lot of fluids to help flush the kidneys and prevent kidney damage. Patients also receive additional fluids through their veins before, during, and after receiving cisplatin.

Blood counts will be monitored regularly while on cisplatin therapy. During a certain time period after receiving cisplatin, there is an increased risk of getting infections. Caution should be taken to avoid unnecessary exposure to crowds and people with infections.

Patients with a known previous allergic reaction to chemotherapy drugs or any other medications should tell their doctor.

Patients who may be pregnant or trying to become pregnant should also tell their doctor before receiving cisplatin.

Chemotherapy can cause men and women to be sterile (not able to have children).

Patients should check with their doctors before receiving live virus **vaccines** while on chemotherapy.

An additional difficulty that can arise with cisplatin and other platinum-based **anticancer drugs** is that some tumor cells develop resistance to the drug. These resistant cells can then regrow and multiply. One strategy against **drug resistance** is to develop new drugs that can be used together with cisplatin to target resistant cells. In February 2004 the FDA approved **pemetrexed** (Alimta) for use together with cisplatin in the treatment of certain types of lung cancer. Another strategy for defeating tumor resistance to cisplatin is genetic modification of the resistant tumor cells. This approach in still in the early stages of experimentation as of 2004.

Side effects

Common side effects include **nausea and vomiting**, which can begin from one hour after receiving the drug and last as long as a week. Patients are given medicines known as **antiemetics**, before and after receiving cisplatin to help prevent or decrease this side effect. **Diarrhea** has also been known to occur.

A serious common side effect related to the total dose of cisplatin received is kidney damage, which can occur in up to one-third of patients. Taking fluids before, during, and after receiving cisplatin help prevent this from occurring. In addition, some researchers in Brazil have reported that quercetin, a yellowish plant pigment found in apples and onions, shows promise as a protective treatment against kidney damage related to cisplatin.

Hearing damage can also occur in up to one-third of patients. Patients may experience ringing in the ears and hearing loss of high-pitched frequency. Hearing tests may be requested before and/or after cisplatin therapy. One promising treatment for cisplatin-related hearing damage is vitamin E, which is being studied by a group of researchers in Illinois.

Low blood counts, referred to as **myelosuppression**, are expected due to cisplatin administration. When the white blood cell count is low this is called **neutropenia** and patients are at an increased risk of developing a **fever** and infections. Platelets are blood cells in the body that allow for the formation of clots. When the platelet count is low, patients are at an increased risk for bruising and bleeding. Low red blood cell counts, referred to as **anemia**, may also occur due to cisplatin administration. Low red counts make people feel tired.

Cisplatin can also cause damage to nerves and nervous system tissues. Patients may feel tingling, numbness and sometimes burning of the fingers and toes. This side effect is common and can be severe.

Less common side effects include change of taste sensation, loss of appetite, dizziness, seizures, confusion, muscle cramps, and uncontrolled muscle contractions. Men treated with cisplatin for testicular cancer sometimes develop so-called dry ejaculations. Other side effects include, hair loss (**alopecia**), hiccups, rash, allergic reactions with difficulty breathing, swelling, and a fast heart rate.

Cisplatin may cause the body to waste normal electrolytes that circulate in the body (potassium, magnesium, phosphate, sodium, calcium) resulting in low levels of these electrolytes. These will be monitored by the doctor and replacement drugs will be given if necessary.

All side effects should be reported to the doctor or nurse.

Interactions

Patients should avoid other drugs that may cause damage to the kidneys.

Certain water pills and cisplatin given together may increase the risk of hearing damage. Before starting any medications, patients should notify their doctors.

Cisplatin may make medications that control seizures less effective.

Resources

BOOKS

Karch, A. M. *Lippincott's Nursing Drug Guide*. Springhouse, PA: Lippincott Williams & Wilkins, 2003.

PERIODICALS

Fossa, S. D. "Long-Term Sequelae after Cancer Therapy—Survivorship After Treatment for Testicular Cancer." *Acta Oncologica* 43 (February 2004): 134–141.

Francescato, H. D., T. M. Coimbra, R. S. Costa, and L. Bianchi Mde. "Protective Effect of Quercetin on the Evolution of Cisplatin-Induced Acute Tubular Necrosis." *Kidney and Blood Pressure Research* 27 (March 2004): 148–158.

Funato, T. "Utility of Antioncogene Ribozymes and Antisense Oligonucleotides in Reversing Drug Resistance." *Methods in Molecular Medicine* 106 (2004): 215–234.

Hazarika, M., R. M. White, J. R. Johnson, and R. Pazdur. "FDA Drug Approval Summaries: Pemetrexed (Alimta)." *Oncologist* 9 (March 2004): 482–488.

Kalkanis, J. G., C. Whitworth, and L. P. Rybak. "Vitamin E Reduces Cisplatin Ototoxicity." *Laryngoscope* 114 (March 2004): 538–542.

ORGANIZATIONS

American Society of Health-System Pharmacists (ASHP). 7272 Wisconsin Avenue, Bethesda, MD 20814. (301) 657-3000. www.ashp.org.

United States Food and Drug Administration (FDA). 5600 Fishers Lane, Rockville, MD 20857-0001. (888) INFO-FDA. www.fda.gov.

Nancy J. Beaulieu, RPh., BCOP
Rebecca J. Frey, PhD

Cladribine

Definition

Cladribine, also known by the brand name Leustatin, is a **chemotherapy** medicine used to treat certain types of **cancer** by destroying cancerous cells.

Purpose

Cladribine is approved by the Food and Drug Administration (FDA) to treat active **hairy cell leukemia**. It has also been used to treat other types of leukemias and lymphomas.

Description

A member of the group of chemotherapy drugs known as a purine nucleoside analog, cladribine may also be referred to as 2-CdA, chlorodeoxyadenosine, and 2-chlorodeoxyadenosine. The purine nucleosides interfere with the genetic material (DNA) inside the cancer cells, cause DNA strand breaks, and block RNA synthesis. These traits help prevent cancer cells

KEY TERMS

Anemia—A red blood cell count that is lower than normal.

Chemotherapy—Specific drugs used to treat cancer.

Complete response—No sign of leukemia in the blood or bone marrow.

DNA— Genetic material inside of cells that that carry information to make proteins that are necessary for proper cell functioning.

Food and Drug Administration—A government agency that oversees public safety in relation to drugs and medical devices. The FDA gives approval to pharmaceutical companies for commercial marketing of their products

Intravenous—To enter the body through a vein.

Neutropenia—White blood cell count that is lower than normal.

from further dividing and growing and also may cause the cancer cells to die.

Recommended dosage

Cladribine is a clear solution that is administered through a vein. The dose of cladribine is based on a patient's weight in kilograms. The approved dose for hairy cell leukemia is 0.09 mg per kilogram of body weight administered each day as a continuous intravenous infusion administered over 24 hours each day for seven continuous days. Some patients may receive this treatment in more than one cycle.

Other doses include 0.1 to 0.3 mg per kilogram of body weight per day for seven days administered as a continuous infusion. Patients may also receive cladribine as a two-hour infusion daily for five days in a row.

Precautions

Blood counts will be monitored regularly while on cladribine therapy. During a certain time period after receiving cladribine, there is an increased risk of getting infections. Caution should be taken to avoid unnecessary exposure to crowds and people with **infection**.

Patients with a known previous allergic reaction to chemotherapy drugs should tell their doctor.

Patients who may be pregnant or are trying to become pregnant should tell their doctors before receiving cladribine.

Although chemotherapy can cause men and women to be sterile (not able to have children), it is unknown if cladribine has this effect on humans.

Patients should check with their doctors before receiving live virus **vaccines** while on chemotherapy.

Side effects

The most common side effect from taking cladribine is low blood counts, referred to as **myelosuppression**. When the white blood cell count is lower than normal, referred to as **neutropenia**, patients are at an increased risk of developing a **fever** and infections. The platelet blood count can also be decreased due to cladribine administration, but generally returns back to normal within two weeks after the end of the infusion. Platelets are blood cells in the body that cause clots to form these clots stop bleeding. When the platelet count is low, patients are at an increased risk for bruising and bleeding. Cladribine causes low red blood cell counts, which is referred to as **anemia**. Low red counts make people feel tired and dizzy.

Other common side effects of cladribine include skin rashes or reactions, pain, redness, or swelling at the injection site. Half of patients with hairy cell leukemia experience a rash.

Patients may experience infections, chills, and fever when being treated with cladribine. This may result in treatment with **antibiotics**.

Nausea, vomiting, loss of appetite, abdominal pain, constipation, and **diarrhea** are mild side effects from cladribine. If **nausea and vomiting** are a problem, patients can be given medicines known as **antiemetics** before receiving cladribine to help prevent or decrease these side effects.

Damage to the kidneys and nervous system tissues is uncommon with cladribine, unless given in high doses for bone marrow transplant patients. At high doses, kidney problems and nerve damage have resulted in weakness of the arms and legs.

Less common side effects of cladribine are hair loss, **itching**, a fever from taking the drug, lung problems, cough, inability to sleep, headache, dizziness, fast heart rate, muscle and joint aches, and **fatigue**.

Interactions

Patients should notify their doctors of any medications they are taking. In the case of cladribine, medications to make special note of include antithyroid agents, **azathioprine**, chloramphenicol, flucytosine, ganciclovir, interferon, **plicamycin**, zidovudine, probenecid, sulfinpyrazone.

Patients should tell their doctors if they have a known allergic reaction to **amifostine** or any other medications or substances, such as foods and preservatives. Before taking any new medications, including nonprescription medications, **vitamins**, and herbal medications, the patients should notify their doctors.

Nancy J. Beaulieu, RPh.,BCOP

Clinical trials

Definition

A clinical trial is a research study designed to answer specific medical questions regarding **cancer** care.

Description

The clinical trial is a scientific study that follows a written guideline (protocol) or recipe for treatment. It is the only scientific mechanism designed to test the effectiveness of new and promising therapies. The clinical trial provides intensive testing of new or updated treatment regimens. Almost all standard treatments in the field of oncology (cancer) originated from clinical trials. These trials are conducted by medical, surgical and radiation oncologists (cancer specialists).

Cancer clinical trials are the key to preventing, diagnosing and treating all types of cancer. It is estimated that 60% of all cancer patients in the United States are being cured. Yet, fewer than 3% of adult cancer patients participate in clinical trials. In contrast, about 71% of children enter clinical trials. This has led to major advancements in treatment and high cure rates for many **childhood cancers** such as **Wilms' tumor** (malignant neoplasm of the kidney), **osteosarcoma** (tumor of the bone), and childhood leukemia (cancer of the blood).

Types of clinical trials

Clinical trials that involve new drugs or devices for humans must first be tested in animals. When a new or investigational drug has been discovered that shows anti-tumor activity in laboratory animals, it is tested on a small number of patients with different types of cancer, usually in a university setting. These are called Phase I trials and are designed to test the maximum tolerated dose (MTD) and side effects or toxicities of a new drug. This phase also helps

determine how a new drug should be given (by mouth or by injection). The patients being tested are those with advanced cancer who have exhausted other treatment options. These patients may not personally benefit from participation in the trial.

If the investigational agent or drug continues to show anti-tumor activity and if the side effects are tolerable and not life-threatening, the drug is moved into a Phase II trial for further testing. In a Phase II trial, the drug is offered to a specific group of patients having the same tumor type. The drug is being tested to determine if it regresses tumor growth. Additional information on side effects of the treatment is also evaluated in this phase.

If the drug continues to show response to the patient's cancer, it is moved into a Phase III trial. At this phase, the investigational treatment is compared to the standard cancer therapy. This is to ensure that no one in a study is left without any treatment when standard treatment is available. If there is no standard therapy, a placebo (a pill that looks like the drug being studied but contains no active medication) may be used for comparison. However, researchers must inform potential patients of this possibility before patients decide whether to participate. Patients are usually assigned their treatment by a process called randomization, which is similar to the toss of a coin. Comparison or randomized trials help researchers find the most effective treatment for a specific type of cancer.

The objectives of Phase III trials include tumor response to treatment, survival, and quality of life during therapy. This phase can involve 400-1000 patients. Anti-tumor response by a significant proportion of the involved patients indicates that the investigational drug or treatment is ready to be submitted to the Food and Drug Administration (FDA) for approval. If approved, the drug is released from investigational status and made available for commercial use in patients with the specifically tested type of cancer.

What to expect as part of a clinical trial

Taking part in a clinical trial does not mean that patients are seen as or treated like "guinea pigs," or that they will receive substandard care. Cancer patients who enroll in clinical trials may be the first to receive a new technique or drug that becomes the standard of care. Clinical trials, however, have risks, as well. The treatment or drug being tested is new, and the side effects may be unknown. The cancer patient, his or her loved ones, and the patient's physician must weigh the risks and benefits when deciding whether or not to enroll in a clinical trial.

When patients participate in a clinical trial, they receive treatment in a cancer center, hospital, clinic, and/or doctor's office. Doctors, nurses, social workers, and other health professionals may be part of the treatment team, and will closely monitor progress. Cancer clinical trial patients:

- are, as stated above, under close scrutiny
- are seen frequently by the members of the treatment team
- are tested often
- follow the treatment plan their doctor prescribes and as according to the study's protocol
- and may also have other responsibilities, such as keeping a log or filling out health forms. Some studies continue to check on patients after their treatment is completed.

Resources

BOOKS

Klimaszewski, Angela D., Jennifer L. Aikin, Monica A. Bacon, Susan A. DiStasio, Heidi E. Ehrenberger, and Bertie A. Ford, editors. *Manual for Clinical Trials Nursing*. Pittsburgh: Oncology Nursing Press, Inc., 2000.

OTHER

National Cancer Institute. *Cancer Trials*. [cited July 8, 2001]. <http://cancertrials.nci.nih.gov/>.
National Cancer Institute. *An Introduction to Clinical Trials*. January 2000 National Cancer Institute. [cited July 8, 2001]. <http://cancertrials.nci.nih.gov>.

Phyllis M. Stein, B.S., CCRP

Codeine *see* **Opioids**

Coenzyme Q10

Definition

Coenzyme Q10 is a fat-soluble nutrient also known as CoQ10, or ubiquinone. It is primarily found in the mitochondria, which are small bodies within cells that produce energy for the body. Apart from the important process that provides energy, CoQ10 also stabilizes cell membranes and acts as an antioxidant (a substance that reduces damage that results from oxygen, such as is caused by free radicals).

Purpose

Some people believe, and anecdotal data suggest, that oxygen-derived radicals are involved in the origins and development of **cancer**. Oxygen-derived radicals may cause damage to membranes, mitochondria, and large molecules, including proteins, lipids, and DNA. Accumulation of DNA damage may contribute to the development of cancer. There may be a relationship between oxidative stress and **breast cancer** development. People who subscribe to the belief that **antioxidants** are health-promoting may consume coenzyme Q10 (CoQ10) as one way of maintaining their health. However, as of 2009, this belief has not been conclusively proven by medical institutions.

Increased antioxidant enzyme activities may affect susceptibility of cells to cancer-causing agents and the response of tumor cells to **chemotherapy**. Administration of coenzyme Q10 by nutrition may induce the protective effect of coenzyme Q10 on breast tissue.

Furthermore, coenzyme Q10 is reputed to reduce the toxicity of some types of chemotherapy. **Doxorubicin**, a chemotherapeutic agent, is known to sometimes damage the heart. But use with coenzyme Q10 may reduce this toxic effect. People who are considering taking coenzyme Q10 should discuss its possible benefits of with a nutritionally oriented healthcare provider.

Description

Coenzyme Q10 appears to help ignite the cellular power stations that are necessary to maintain healthy cells, enhancing energy at the cellular level. The powerful antioxidant is highly concentrated in heart muscle cells. Coenzyme Q10 is believed by some to be an immune system booster and antioxidant that may help people avoid getting cancer, and it may be useful in treating it. Apart from its important function of providing energy, CoQ10 also stabilizes cell membranes, and as an antioxidant, it destroys free radicals in the body. These unstable molecules can cause damage to normal cells.

CoQ10 occurs naturally in many foods, which provide approximately half of the body's requirement. Cold-water fish such as mackerel, salmon, sardines, and tuna are particularly high in CoQ10. Meats and vegetable oils are also good sources. The human liver manufactures adequate amounts to fulfill the need not met in the diet. Some whole food nutritionists may believe that people who are deficient in B **vitamins**, selenium, vitamin C, or vitamin E may not be able to make as much coenzyme Q10 as they need since all these nutrients are required in order to produce it. The belief is that liver production and consumption of foods rich in CoQ10 may not provide the amounts needed to treat certain cancers, and for that reason, some people consume the enzyme in supplement form. It can be found formulated as capsules, gel caps, liquids, and tablets. The latter may be the best choice as it generally includes a source of fat that improves absorption. Vitamin E is a helpful stabilizing additive as well.

Coenzyme Q10 was first identified in 1957. Its chemical structure was determined in 1958. Interest in coenzyme Q10 as a potential treatment for cancer began in 1961, when a deficiency of the enzyme was noted in the blood of cancer patients. Low blood levels of coenzyme Q10 have been found in some patients with **myeloma** (a malignant tumor that develops in the blood-cell-producing cells of the bone marrow), **lymphoma** (cancer of the lymph nodes), and cancers of the breast, lung, prostate, pancreas, colon, kidney, and head and neck, according to the National Cancer Institute (NCI).

Recommended dosage

Coenzyme Q10 is usually taken by mouth as a tablet or capsule. It may also be given by injection into a vein. CoQ10 is available in oil-based capsules, powder-filled capsules, tablets, and liquid soft gels. The soft gels are believed to give higher absorption. Therapeutic dosages of CoQ10 for cancer range from 200 to 600 mg per day. As a general nutritional supplement, daily doses of CoQ10 range from 5 to 300 mg. Those who use CoQ10 for periodontal (the tissue around teeth) health may take 100–150 mg daily. The same dose range applies to those who take statin (cholesterol-lowering) drugs for treatment of high cholesterol. CoQ10 is best taken with food. About three weeks of daily dosing are necessary to reach maximum blood concentrations of CoQ10. It comes in the various dosages.

Precautions

Coenzyme Q10 should not be taken by persons who are allergic to it. Symptoms of an allergic reaction include breathing problems or tightness in the throat or chest, chest pain, and skin hives, rash, or itchy or swollen skin. No other known precautions are indicated for normal dosage.

Side effects

No serious adverse side effects have been reported. Some patients using coenzyme Q10 have experienced mild insomnia, elevated levels of liver enzymes, rashes, **nausea**, and upper abdominal pain. Other reported side effects have include dizziness, visual sensitivity to light, irritability, headache, heartburn, and **fatigue**.

Interactions

Patients should talk with their healthcare provider about possible interactions between CoQ10 and prescription drugs they may be taking. Certain drugs, such as those that are used to lower cholesterol or blood sugar levels, may reduce the effects of CoQ10.

CoQ10 may also alter the body's response to **warfarin**, a drug that prevents the blood from clotting, and insulin, used to treat diabetes. The cholesterol-lowering drugs known as statins, such as lovastatin (Mevacor), simvastatin (Zocor), and pravastatin (Pravacol), may decrease CoQ10 levels in humans. It is likely that all statins have this effect. Also, CoQ10 may improve glycemic control in some type II diabetics. If this were to occur, antidiabetic medications might need appropriate adjusting. Some beta-blockers, in particular propanolol, may inhibit some CoQ10-dependent enzymes. Piperine, found in black pepper, may increase levels of CoQ10 in the blood.

Ken R. Wells

Cold sore *see* **Herpes simplex**

Colectomy

Definition

Colectomy is the surgical removal of all or part of the colon, the first part of the large intestine.

Purpose

Doctors perform colectomy to remove large Stage I **colon cancer** lesions or to cure colon **cancer** that: has spread beyond the mucous membrane, has infiltrated or spread beyond the intestinal wall, or is likely to recur.

Doctors also perform this procedure to improve patients' quality of life by relieving pain and preventing bleeding and other symptoms that occur when colon cancer invades organs near the bowel, and also, when non-surgical methods are unsuccessful, to treat diverticulitis, ulcerative colitis, and benign colon polyps.

Precautions

This surgery can significantly diminish bowel control and sexual function.

Description

Colectomy is the preferred therapy for colon cancers that can be cured. Performed in a hospital, under general anesthesia, this procedure involves removing the cancerous part of the colon, a margin of normal bowel, and any tissue or lymph nodes affected by the

disease, and reconnecting the healthy segments of the colon (anastomosis). If **infection** or obstruction make it impossible to reconnect the colon, the surgeon creates an opening (stoma) in the abdominal wall (**colostomy**) through which feces passes from the body into a disposable collection bag.

Colostomy may be:

- temporary, with the ends of the intestines being reconnected at a later time, or

- permanent in patients whose cancer cannot be completely removed.

Open and laparoscopic procedures

Traditional, or open, colectomy is an invasive procedure requiring a wide surgical incision. This surgery allows the surgeon to view the internal organs very clearly.

Laparoscopic colectomy requires only a few small incisions, enables doctors to view the internal organs, and results in a shorter hospital stay and fewer side effects. Studies suggest that laparoscopic colectomy may be safer than open surgery for elderly patients. A clinical trial funded by the National Institutes of Health (NIH) is comparing survival rates for the two procedures.

Types of colectomy

LEFT RADICAL HEMICOLECTOMY. Doctors perform left radical hemicolectomy to remove cancer and other abnormal tissue in the:

- descending colon, which extends from the pelvis to the spleen
- splenic flexure, the place where the descending colon joins the part of the large intestine that extends across the middle of the abdomen (transverse colon)

When cancer is found in the splenic flexure, the surgeon removes the splenic flexure, the first half of the descending colon, and about one-third of the transverse colon

RIGHT RADICAL HEMICOLECTOMY. Doctors perform this procedure to remove tumors and other abnormalities of the:

- section of large intestine nearest the appendix (cecum)
- portion of the large intestine that extends along the right side of the body from the small intestine to the transverse colon (ascending colon)

This procedure involves removing the cecum, descending colon, the hepatic flexure where the ascending colon joins the transverse colon, and the first one-third of the transverse colon. These procedures are considered radical because they involve removing nerves, blood vessels, and lymph nodes near the tumo

TRANSVERSE COLECTOMY. Performed to remove disease in the transverse colon, this procedure includes removing the:

- transverse colon
- and hepatic and splenic flexures

SIGMOID RESECTION. Used to remove cancer in the part of the colon (sigmoid) between the descending colon and rectum, this procedure involves removing the:

- sigmoid colon
- bottom two-thirds of the descending colon

RECTOSIGMOID RESECTION. Used to remove tumors in the part of the colon (rectosigmoid) just above the rectum (sigmoid flexure), this procedure removes:

- the sigmoid colon
- most of the rectum and surrounding rectal tissue (mesorectum)

Because tumors in this part of the colon usually involve the bladder, uterus, or other organs, the surgeon may insert drainage tubes or a catheter to draw urine from the bladder.

ABDOMINOPERINEAL RESECTION (APR). This extensive procedure, which may be performed in two parts or by two surgical teams operating at the same time, involves removing the:

- lower sigmoid colon
- rectum
- anus
- nearby lymph nodes, blood vessels, and nerves

Sphincter-saving APR is designed to minimize loss of bowel control by:

- removing only the tumor
- preserving nerves and blood vessels near the tumor.

These specialized procedures involve repositioning the tumor while removing it, can cause shedding of tumor cells, and may not be available in all hospitals.

After completing any of these procedures, the surgeon uses:

- sutures
- clips
- heat and electrical current (electrothermal bipolar vessel sealer) to tie off the ends of blood vessels before closing the incision.

Preparation

The day before the operation, the patient may consume only clear liquids, and may take nothing by mouth after midnight.

To reduce the possibility of infection, **antibiotics** are given to the patient the night before the operation.

Aftercare

A patient who has had an open colectomy will spend at least a week in the hospital and experience significant postoperative pain.

A patient who has had a laparoscopic colectomy will spend four to five days in the hospital, experience less pain, and resume normal activities within two weeks.

A patient who has had a colostomy must learn to care for the collection bag and keep the area clean. Patients who have had colostomies often worry about:

- not being able to care for themselves
- odors, gas, and leakage from the collection bag
- health problems
- recurrence of cancer

A patient who is depressed about sexual dysfunction, bowel problems, or other aspects of treatment may benefit from professional counseling or from joining a support group.

Risks

Side effects of colectomy include bladder complications, **diarrhea**, bowel irregularities, urinary urgency, and sexual dysfunction.

Normal results

Most patients experience postoperative pain. Patients who have laparoscopic surgery have less pain than patients who have open colectomy. Some patients require temporary colostomy until normal bowel function returns.

Most of these procedures do not affect sexual function, but rectosigmoid resection can make it difficult for a man to achieve erection during intercourse.

Abnormal results

Extensive surgery can cause:

- infection
- severe pain
- fecal incontinence
- prolonged recovery

Resources

OTHER

Colectomy. [cited May 20, 2001]. http://www.medterms.com/script/main/art.asp?articlekey = 12529.

Colorectal Cancer Treatments. [cited May 20, 2001]. http://www.cancerfacts.com.

Laparoscopic Colorectal Surgery. [cited January 20, 2000 and May 21, 2001]. http://www.lapsurgery.com/colectom.htm.

Surgery & Colon Cancer. [cited May 5, 2001]. http://www.colorectal-cancer.net/surgerycoloncancer [cited May 20, 2001]. http://www.colorectal-cancer.net/surgerycoloncancer.htm.

What Are the Latest Treatments of Colon and Rectal Cancers? June 1999. [cited May 20, 2001]. <http://content.health.msn.com/content/dmk/dmk_article_5462002 7>.

Maureen Haggerty

Scanning electron micrograph (SEM) image of the inner surface of the human colon diseased with cancer. *(Copyright Oliver Meckes, Science Source/Photo Researchers, Inc. Reproduced by permission.)*

Scanning electron micrograph (SEM) image of the inner surface of the human colon diseased with cancer. *(Copyright Oliver Meckes, Science Source/Photo Researchers, Inc. Reproduced by permission.)*

Colon cancer

Definition

Cancer of the colon is the disease characterized by the development of malignant cells in the lining or epithelium of the first and longest portion of the large intestine. Malignant cells have lost normal control mechanisms governing growth. These cells may invade surrounding local tissue or they may spread throughout the body and invade other organ systems.

An endoscopic view of a colorectal tumor. *(Custom Medical Stock Photo. Reproduced by permission.)*

Synonyms for the colon include the large bowel or the large intestine. The rectum is the continuation of the large intestine into the pelvis that terminates in the anus.

Description

The colon is a tubular organ beginning in the right lower abdomen. It ascends on the right side of the abdomen, traverses from right to left in the upper abdomen, descends vertically down the left side, takes an S-shaped curve in the lower left abdomen, and then flows into the rectum as it leaves the abdomen for the pelvis. These portions of the colon are named separately though they are part of the same organ.

- cecum, the beginning of the colon
- ascending colon, the right vertical ascent of the colon
- transverse colon, the portion traversing from right to left
- descending colon, the left vertical descent of the colon
- sigmoid colon, the s-shaped segment of colon above the pelvis

These portions of the colon are recognized anatomically based on the arterial blood supply and venous and lymphatic drainage of these segments of the colon. Lymph, a protein-rich fluid that bathes the cells of the body, is transported in small channels known as lymphatics that run alongside the veins of the colon. Lymph nodes are small filters through which the lymph travels on its way back to the bloodstream. Cancer can spread elsewhere in the body by

invading the lymph and vascular systems. Therefore, these anatomic considerations become very important in the treatment of colon cancer.

The small intestine is the continuation of the upper gastrointestinal tract responsible for carrying ingested nutrients into the body. The waste left after the small intestine has completed absorption of nutrients amounts to a few liters (about the same as quarts) of material per day and is directly delivered to the colon (at the cecum) for processing. The colon is responsible for the preservation of fluid and electrolytes as it propels the increasingly solid waste toward the rectum and anus for excretion.

When cells lining the colon become malignant, they first grow locally and may invade partially or totally through the wall of the bowel and even into adjacent structures and organs. In the process, the tumor can penetrate and invade the lymphatics or the capillaries locally and gain access to the circulation. As the malignant cells work their way to other areas of the body, they again become locally invasive in the new area to which they have spread. These tumor deposits, originating from the colon primary tumor, are then known as metastases. If metastases are found in the regional lymph nodes from the primary, they are known as regional metastases, or regional nodal metastases. If they are distant from the primary tumor, they are known as distant metastases. The patient with distant metastases has systemic disease. Thus the cancer originating in the colon begins locally and, given time, can become systemic.

By the time the primary tumor is originally detected it is usually larger than one cm (about 3/8 in) in size and has over one million cells. This amount of growth itself is estimated to take about three to seven years. Each time the cells double in number, the size of the tumor quadruples. Thus like most cancers, the part that is identified clinically is later in the progression than would be desired and screening becomes a very important endeavor to aid in earlier detection of this disease.

Demographics

There are at least 100,000 cases of colon cancer diagnosed per year in the United States. Together, colon and rectal cancers account for 10% of cancers in men and 11% of cancers in women. It is the second most common site-specific cancer affecting both men and women. A 2003 study reported that for unknown reasons, women are more likely to have advanced colon cancer at diagnosis than men. About 49,920 people died from colon and **rectal cancer** in the United States in 2009. In recent years the incidence of this disease has decreased slightly, as has the mortality rate. It is difficult to tell if the decrease in mortality reflects earlier diagnosis, less death related to the actual treatment of the disease, or a combination of both factors.

Cancer of the colon is thought to arise sporadically in about 80% of those who develop the disease. Twenty percent of people are thought to have genetic predisposition, meaning their genes carry a trigger for the disease. Development of colon cancer at an early age, or at multiple sites, or recurrent colon cancer, suggests a genetically transmitted form of the disease as opposed to the sporadic form.

Causes and symptoms

Causes

Causes of colon cancer often are environmental in sporadic cases (80%) and sometimes genetic (20%). Since malignant cells have a changed genetic makeup, this means that in 80% of cases, the environment spontaneously induces change, whereas those born with a genetic predisposition are either destined to get the cancer or less environmental exposure can induce the cancer. Exposure to agents in the environment that may induce mutation is the process of **carcinogenesis** and is caused by agents known as carcinogens (cancer-causing agents). Specific carcinogens have been difficult to identify; however, dietary factors seem to be involved.

Colon cancer is more common in industrialized nations. Diets high in fat, red meat, total calories, and alcohol seem to predispose people to the disease. Diets high in fiber appear to decrease risk. High-fiber diets may help lessen exposure of the colon lining to carcinogens from the environment, as the transit time through the bowel is faster with a high-fiber diet than it is with a low fiber diet.

Age plays a definite role in the predisposition to colon cancer. Two-thirds of all cases occur after age 50 and the average age for those who develop the disease is 62.

There is also a slight increase risk for colon cancer in the individual who smokes.

Patients who suffer from inflammatory diseases of the colon known as ulcerative colitis and Crohn's colitis are also at increased risk.

Researchers know there is a genetic link to many cases of colon cancer, those called familial cases. This is the type of colon cancer that tends to run in families. In late 2003, a team of researchers identified the specific location on a human chromosome by analyzing blood samples from 53 families in which at least one member had a colon cancer or precancerous colon polyp. At least 200 genes exist on the location of chromosome 9, however, so the research will continue to identify the particular gene responsible for the cancer.

The development of polyps of the colon almost always precedes the development of colon cancer by five or more years. Polyps are benign growths of the colon lining. They can be unrelated to cancer, precancerous, or malignant. Polyps, when identified, are removed for diagnosis. If the polyps are benign, the patient should undergo careful surveillance for the development of more polyps or the development of colon cancer.

Symptoms

Colon cancer causes symptoms related to its local presence in the large bowel or by its effect on other organs if it has spread. These symptoms may occur alone or in combination:

- a change in bowel habit
- blood in the stool
- bloating, persistent abdominal distention
- constipation
- a feeling of fullness even after having a bowel movement
- narrowing of the stool—so-called ribbon stools
- persistent, chronic fatigue
- abdominal discomfort
- unexplained weight loss
- and, very rarely, nausea and vomiting

Most of these symptoms are caused by the physical presence of the tumor mass in the colon. Similar symptoms can be caused by other processes; these are not absolutely specific to colon cancer. The key is recognizing that the persistence of these types of symptoms without ready explanation should prompt the individual to seek medical evaluation.

If a tumor develops in the colon, it will begin to cause symptoms as it reaches a certain size. The symptoms are caused by the tumor blocking the opening in the colon. In addition, the tumor commonly oozes blood that is lost in the stool. (Often, this blood is not visible.) This results in **anemia** and chronic **fatigue**. **Weight loss** is a late symptom, often implying substantial obstruction or the presence of systemic disease.

Diagnosis

Screening

In all other cancers (breast and prostate, for example), screening tests look for small, malignant lesions. Screening for colorectal cancers, however, is the search for pre-malignant, benign polyps. This screening can be close to 100% effective in preventing cancer development, not just in detecting small cancers.

Screening involves physical exam, simple laboratory tests, and the visualization of the lining of the colon. To visualize the colon epithelium, clinicians use with **x rays** (indirect visualization) and endoscopy (direct visualization).

The physical examination involves the performance of a digital rectal exam (DRE). The DRE includes manual examination of the rectum, anus and the prostate. During this examination, the physician examines the anus and the surrounding skin for hemorrhoids, abscesses, and other irregularities. After lubricating the gloved finger and anus, the examiner gently slides the finger into the anus and follows the contours of the rectum. The examiner notes the tone of the anus and feels the walls and the edges for texture, tenderness and masses as far as the examining finger can reach. At the time of this exam, the physician checks the stool on the examining glove with a chemical to see if any occult (invisible), blood is present. At home, after having a bowel movement, the patient is asked to swipe a sample of stool obtained with a small stick on a card. After three such specimens are on the card, the card is then easily chemically tested for occult blood also. (The stool analysis mentioned here is known as a **fecal occult blood test**, or FOBT, and, while it can be helpful, it is not 100% accurate—only about 50% of cancers are FOBT-positive.) These exams are accomplished as an easy part of a routine yearly physical exam.

Proteins are sometimes produced by cancers and these may be elevated in the patient's blood. When this occurs, the protein produced is known as a tumor marker. There is a tumor marker for some cancers of the colon; it is known as carcinoembryonic antigen, or CEA. Unfortunately, this protein may be made by other adenocarcinomas as well, or it may not be produced by a particular colon cancer. Therefore, screening by chemical analysis for CEA has not been helpful. CEA has been helpful when used in a follow-up role for patients treated for colon cancer if their tumor makes the protein.

Indirect visualization of the colon may be accomplished by placing barium through the rectum and filling the colon with this compound. Barium produces a white contrast image of the lining of the colon on x ray and thus the contour of the lining of the colon may be seen. Detail can be increased if the barium utilized is thinned and air also introduced. These studies are known as the **barium enema** (BE), and the double contrast barium enema (DCBE).

Direct visualization of the colon lining is accomplished using a scope or endoscope. The physician introduces the instrument through the rectum. Older, shorter scopes were rigid. Today, utilizing fiberoptic technology, the scopes are flexible and can reach much farther. If the left colon only is visualized, it is called flexible **sigmoidoscopy**. When the entire colon is visualized, the procedure is known as **colonoscopy**.

A procedure called virtual colonoscopy has been developed but debate continues on whether or not it is effective as colonoscopy. Virtual colonoscopy refers to the use of imaging, usually with **computed tomography** (CT) scans or **magnetic resonance imaging** (MRI) to produce images of the colon. Studies in late 2003 showed that virtual colonoscopy was as effective as colonoscopy for screening purposes and it offered the advantage of being less invasive and less risky. However, many physicians were unwilling to accept it as a replacement for colonoscopy, particularly since some patients might still require the regular colonoscopy as a follow-up to the virtual procedure if a polyp or abnormality is found that requires **biopsy**.

Unlike the indirect visualizations of the colon (the BE and the DCBE), the endoscopic screenings allow the physician to remove polyps and biopsy suspicious tissue. (A biopsy is a removal of tissue for examination by a pathologist.) For this reason, many physicians prefer endoscopic screening. All of the visualizations, the BE, DCBE, and each type of endoscopy, require pre-procedure preparation (evacuation) of the colon.

The American Cancer Society has recommended the following screening protocol for those at normal risk over 50 years of age:

• yearly fecal occult blood test

• flexible sigmoidoscopy at age 50

• flexible sigmoidoscopy repeated every 5 years

• double contrast barium enema every 5 years

• colonoscopy every 10 years

The American Gastroenterologial Association revised its screening guidelines in 2003 to recommend that people with two or more first-degree relatives with colorectal cancer or a first-degree relative with colon or rectal cancer before age 60 should have a screening colonoscopy beginning at age 40 or beginning 10 years prior to the age of the earlier colon cancer diagnosis in their family (whichever is earliest). Those with a first-degree relative diagnosed with colon cancer after age 60 or two second-degree relative with colon or rectal cancer should begin screening at age 40 with one of the methods listed above, such as annual sigmoidoscopy.

Evaluation of patients with symptoms

If patients have symptoms that could possibly be related to colon cancer, the entire colon will be examined. The combination of a flexible sigmoidoscopy and DCBE may be performed, but the preferred evaluation of the entire colon and rectum is a complete colonoscopy. Colonoscopy allows direct visualization, photography, and the opportunity to obtain a biopsy of any abnormality visualized. If, for technical reasons, the entire colon is not visualized endoscopically, a DCBE should complement the colonoscopy.

The diagnosis of colon cancer is actually made by the performance of a biopsy of any abnormal lesion in the colon. When a tumor growth is identified, it could be either a benign polyp (or lesion) or a cancer; the biopsy resolves the issue. The endoscopist may take many samples to exclude any sampling errors.

If the patient has advanced disease at the time of diagnosis, areas where the tumor has spread (such as the liver) may be amenable to biopsy. Such biopsies are usually obtained using a special needle under local anesthesia.

Once a diagnosis of colon cancer has been established by biopsy, in addition to the physical exam, studies will be performed to assess the extent of the disease. Blood studies include a complete blood count, liver function tests, and a CEA. **Imaging studies** will include a chest x ray and a CAT scan (computed tomography scan) of the abdomen. The chest x ray will determine if the cancer has spread to the lung, the CAT scan will evaluate potential spread to the liver as well as any local spread of the primary tumor. If the patient has any neurologic symptoms, a CAT scan of the brain will be performed, and if the patient is experiencing **bone pain**, a bone scan also will be performed.

Treatment team

The surgeon and the medical oncologist each have a role in therapy that is dictated by the degree of progression of the disease. A radiation oncologist may also play a role on the team; however, radiation treatment is rare in colon cancer.

Clinical staging, treatments, and prognosis

Clinical staging

Once the diagnosis has been confirmed by biopsy, the clinical stage of the cancer is assigned. Using the characteristics of the primary tumor, its depth of penetration through the bowel, and the presence or absence of regional or distant metastases, the stage is derived. Often, the depth of penetration through the bowel or the presence of regional lymph nodes can't be assigned before surgery.

Colon cancer is assigned stages I through IV, based on the following general criteria:

- Stage I: The tumor is confined to the epithelium or has not penetrated through the first layer of muscle in the bowel wall.
- Stage II: The tumor has penetrated through to the outer wall of the colon or has gone through it, possibly invading other local tissue.
- Stage III: Any depth or size of tumor associated with regional lymph node involvement.
- Stage IV: Any of previous criteria associated with distant metastasis.

With many cancers other than colon cancer, staging plays an important pre-treatment role to best determine treatment options. Almost all colon cancers are treated with surgery first, regardless of stage. Colon cancers through Stage III, and even some Stage IV colon cancers, are treated with surgery first, before any other treatments are considered.

Treatments

SURGERY. Surgical removal of the involved segment of colon (**colectomy**) along with its blood supply and regional lymph nodes is the primary therapy for colon cancer. Usually, the partial colectomies are separated into right, left, transverse, or sigmoid sections based on the blood supply. The removal of the blood supply at its origin along with the regional lymph nodes that accompany it ensures an adequate margin of normal colon on either side of the primary tumor. When the cancer lies in a position such that the blood supply and lymph drainage between two of the major vessels, both vessels are taken to assure complete radical resection or removal (extended radical right or left colectomy). If the primary tumor penetrates through the bowel wall, any tissue adjacent to the tumor extension is also taken if feasible.

Surgery is used as primary therapy for stages I through III colon cancer unless there are signs that local invasion will not permit complete removal of the tumor, as may occur in advanced stage III tumors. However, this circumstance is rare, occurring in less than 2% of all colon cancer cases.

After the resection is completed, the ends of the remaining colon are reconstructed; the hook-up is called an anastomosis. Once healing has occurred, there may be a slight increase in the frequency of bowel movements. This effect usually lasts only for several weeks. Most patients go on to develop completely normal bowel function.

Occasionally, the anastomosis is risky and cannot be performed. When the anastomosis cannot be performed, a **colostomy** is performed instead. A colostomy is performed by bringing the end of the colon through the abdominal wall and sewing it to the skin. The patient will have to wear an appliance (a bag) to manage the stool. The colostomy may be temporary and the patient may undergo a hook-up at a later, safer date, or the colostomy may be permanent. In most cases, emergent colostomies are not reversed and are permanent.

RADIATION. **Radiation therapy** is used as an adjunct to surgery if there is concern about potential for local recurrence post-operatively and the area of concern will tolerate the radiation. For instance, if the tumor invaded muscle of the abdominal wall but was not completely removed, this area would be considered for radiation. Radiation has significant dose limits when residual bowel is exposed to it because the small and large intestine do not tolerate radiation well.

Radiation also is used in the treatment of patients with metastatic disease. It is particularly useful in shrinking metastatic colon cancer to the brain.

CHEMOTHERAPY. **Chemotherapy** is useful for patients who have had all identifiable tumor removed and are at risk for recurrence (**adjuvant chemotherapy**). Chemotherapy may also be used when the cancer is stage IV and is beyond the scope of regional therapy, but this use is rare.

Adjuvant therapy is considered in stage II disease with deep penetration or in stage III patients. Standard therapy is treatment with **fluorouracil**, (5FU) combined with **leucovorin** for a period of 6 to 12 months. 5FU is an antimetabolite and leukovorin improves the response rate. (A response is a temporary regression of the cancer from chemotherapy.) Another agent, **levamisole**, (which seems to stimulate the immune system), may be substituted for leucovorin. These protocols reduce rate of recurrence by about 15% and reduce mortality by about 10%. The regimens do have some toxicity but usually are tolerated fairly well.

Similar chemotherapy may be administered for stage IV disease or if a patient progresses and develops metastases. Results show response rates of about 20%. Unfortunately, these patients eventually succumb to the disease, and this chemotherapy may not prolong survival or improve quality of life in Stage IV patients. **Clinical trials** have now shown that the results can be improved with the addition of another agent to this regimen. **Irinotecan** does not seem to increase toxicity but it improved response rates to 39%, added two to three months to disease-free survival, and prolonged overall survival by a little over two months. If the cancer is detected early, surgical removal of the tumor can lead to complete cure in 75%–90% of patients.

Prognosis

Prognosis is the long-term outlook or survival after therapy. Overall, about 50% of patients treated for colon cancer survive the disease. As expected, the survival rates are dependent upon the stage of the cancer at the time of diagnosis, making early detection crucial.

About 15% of patients present with stage I disease and 85-90% survive. Stage II represents 20-30% of cases and 65-75% survive. 30-40% comprise the stage III presentation of which 55% survive. The remaining 20-25% present with stage IV disease and are rarely cured.

Alternative and complementary therapies

Alternative therapies have not been studied in a large-scale, scientific way. Large doses of **vitamins**, fiber, and green tea are among therapies tried. Avoiding **cigarettes** and alcohol may be helpful. Before initiating any alternative therapies, the patient is wise to consult his or her physician to be sure that these therapies do not complicate or interfere with the established therapy.

Coping with cancer treatment

For those with familial syndromes causing colon cancer, genetic counseling may be appropriate. Psychological counseling may be appropriate for anyone having trouble coping with a potentially fatal disease. Local cancer support groups may be helpful and are often identified by contacting local hospitals or the American Cancer Society.

The Colon Cancer Alliance offers online support at the following Web page: http://www. ccalliance.org.

Clinical trials

Clinical trials are scientific studies in which new therapies are compared to current standards in an effort to identify therapies that give better results.

Agents being tested for efficacy in patients with advanced disease include oxaliplatin and CPT-11. Please see the resources section for current information

available from the National Cancer Institute regarding these clinical trials.

Prevention

There is not an absolute method for preventing colon cancer. Still, there are steps an individual can take to dramatically lessen the risk or to identify the precursors of colon cancer so that it does not manifest itself. The patient with a familial history can enter screening and surveillance programs earlier than the general population. High-fiber diets and vitamins, avoiding obesity, and staying active lessen the risk. Avoiding cigarettes and alcohol may be helpful. By controlling these environmental factors, an individual can lessen risk and to this degree prevent the disease.

People who turn age 50, and all of those with a history of colon cancer in their families, should speak with their physicians about the most recent screening recommendations from physician and cancer organizations. They should watch for symptoms and attend all recommended screenings to increase the likelihood of catching colon cancer early.

Special concerns

Polyps are growths of the epithelium of the colon. They may be completely benign, premalignant, or cancerous. The association of colon cancers in patients with certain types of polyps is such that it is thought that many polyps begin as a benign growth and later acquire malignant characteristics. There are two types of polyps, pedunculated and sessile. This terminology comes from their appearance; those that are pedunculated are on a stalk like a mushroom, and the sessile polyps are broad based and have no stalk. Unless a pedunculated polyp gets large, malignant potential is very small. This type may also be easily removed at colonoscopy, by a snaring technique. (A snare is like a lasso introduced through the endoscope to encircle the polyp at its base and amputate it.) The sessile polyp is also known as a villous **adenoma** and as many as one-third of these harbor a malignancy. Therefore, the villous adenoma is considered premalignant. Sessile polyps may or may not be able to be managed with the colonoscope and may need surgical removal because of their pre-malignant nature.

Polyps commonly present with occult blood in the stool. Since they are associated with the development of cancer, patients who have developed polyps need to enter a program of careful surveillance.

There is an occasional patient who develops a pattern of metastatic disease that is isolated to either the liver or the lung and the deposit appears to be solitary. When patients have this type of pattern of metastatic disease, especially if there has been a long interval between the primary management and the development of **metastasis**, they may be considered for surgical resection of the isolated metastasis to effect a cure. In carefully selected patients, long-term survival approaching 20% has been achieved.

When a patient has developed metastatic cancer in the liver alone, a technique of administering chemotherapy directly to the liver is sometimes considered. This is called **hepatic arterial infusion** and requires the placement of a special device into the artery supplying the liver. This method of utilizing chemotherapy has been helpful in carefully selected patients only, and currently is not used as a cure.

Resources

BOOKS

Abelhoff, Martin, MD, James O. Armitage MD, Allen S. Lichter MD, and John E. Niederhuber MD. *Clinical Oncology Library*. Philadelphia: Churchill Livingstone, 1999.

Jorde, Lynn B., PhD, John C. Carey MD, Michael J. Bamshad MD, and Raymond L. White, PhD. *Medical Genetics*. 2nd ed. St. Louis: Mosby, 1999.

PERIODICALS

"Colon Cancer; Facts to Know." *NWHRC Health Center* December 15, 2003.

Golden, William E., and Robert H. Hopkins. "Colon Cancer Screening 2003." *Internal Medicine News* 36 (December 1, 2003): 46.

Greenlee, Robert T., MPH, Mary Beth Hill-Harmon, Taylor Murray, and Michael Thun. "Cancer Statistics 2001." *CA: A Cancer Journal for Clinicians* 51, no. 1 (January-February 2001).

"Professional Organization Recommends Standard Colonoscopy Over Virtual." *Biotech Week* December 31, 2003: 422.

"Researchers Discover New Genetic Link to Common Colon Cancer." *Genomics & Genetics Weekly* November 7, 2003: 29.

Saltz, Leonard, et al. "Irinotecan plus Fluorouracil and Leucovorin for Metastatic Colorectal Cancer." *The New England Journal of Medicine* 343, no. 13 (September 28, 2000).

"Study Shows Virtual Colonoscopy as Effective as Traditional Colonoscopy." *Biotech Week* December 31, 2003.

Wachter, Kerri. "Reasons Unclear for Later Colon Cancer Diagnosis in Women: Regional or Distant Disease More Likely." *Internal Medicine News* 36 (December 1, 2003).

ORGANIZATIONS

American Cancer Society. (800) ACS-2345. http://www.cancer.org.

Cancer Information Service of the NCI. (1-800-4-CANCER). <http://cis.nci.nih.gov>.

Colon Cancer Alliance. http://www.ccalliance.org.

National Cancer Institute Cancer Trials. http://cancertrials.nci.nih.gov/.

Richard A. McCartney, M.D.

Colonoscopy

Definition

Colonoscopy is a medical procedure during which a long, flexible, tubular instrument called the colonoscope is used to view the entire inner lining of the colon (large intestine) and the rectum.

Purpose

A colonoscopy is generally recommended when the patient complains of rectal bleeding or has a change in bowel habits or other unexplained abdominal symptoms. The test is frequently used to test for colorectal **cancer**, especially when polyps or tumor-like growths have been detected using the **barium enema** and other diagnostic tests. Polyps can be removed through the colonoscope and samples of tissue (biopsies) can be taken to test for the presence of cancerous cells.

The test also enables the physician to check for bowel diseases such as ulcerative colitis and Crohn's disease. It is a necessary tool in monitoring patients who have a past history of polyps or **colon cancer**. It also may be used as a screening tool for people at high risk of developing colon cancer, such as those with a strong family history of the disease.

Precautions

Patients who are pregnant or have a history of heart and lung disease and those with blood-clotting problems should tell the doctor about their health history before the procedure. Special precautions may be needed. For instance, a patient with artificial heart valves or a history of **infection** of the lining of the heart may need to take **antibiotics** to prevent infection. Patients also should tell the doctor about all medications they are taking. The doctor may want the patient to stop taking some drugs, such as aspirin, for a period of time before the procedure. Patients with some intestinal conditions should not have a colonoscopy. Examples of these conditions include acute diverticulitis, acute inflamatory bowel disease, a suspected perforation or break in the intestines, and

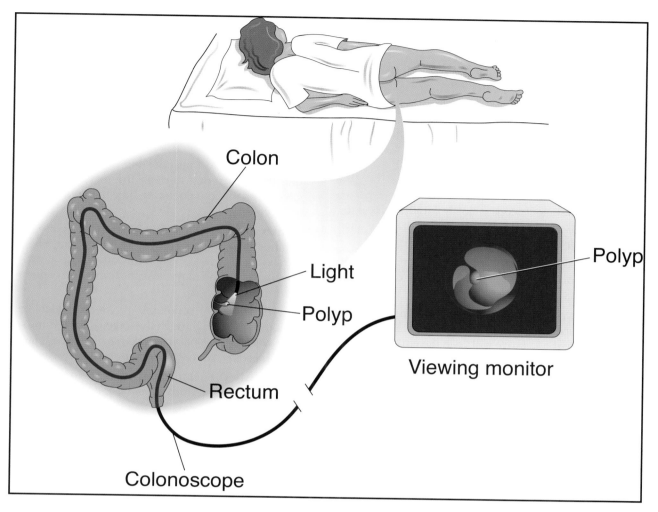

Colonoscopy is a procedure in which a long, flexible, tubular instrument called a colonoscope is inserted into the patient's anus in order to view the lining of the colon and rectum. It is performed to test for colorectal cancer and other bowel diseases and it enables the physician to collect tissue samples for laboratory analysis. *(Illustration by Electronic Illustrators Group. Cengage Learning, Gale.)*

recent abdominal surgery. Patients must be able to cooperate during the procedure.

Description

The procedure can be done either in the doctor's office or in a special procedure room of a local hospital. An intravenous (IV) line will be started in a vein in the arm. Through the IV line, the patient generally receives a sedative and a pain-killer if needed.

During the colonoscopy, the patient will be asked to lie on his/her left side with his/her knees drawn up toward the abdomen. The doctor begins the procedure by inserting a lubricated, gloved finger into the anus to check for any abnormal masses or blockage. A thin, well-lubricated colonoscope then will be inserted into

the anus and it will be gently advanced through the colon. The lining of the intestine will be examined through the scope. Air is pumped through the colonoscope to help clear the path or make it easier to view the lining of the colon. If there are excessive secretions, stool or blood that obstruct the viewing, they will be suctioned out through the scope. The doctor may press on the abdomen or ask the patient to change his/her position in order to advance the scope through the colon.

The entire length of the large intestine can be examined in this manner. If suspicious growths are observed, tiny **biopsy** forceps or brushes can be inserted through the colonoscope and tissue samples can be obtained. Small polyps also can be removed through the colonoscope. Biopsies and the removal of polyps through the colonoscope are both painless procedures. After the procedure, the colonoscope is slowly withdrawn and the instilled air is allowed to escape. The anal area is then cleansed with tissues.

The procedure may take anywhere from 30 minutes to one hour, depending on how easy it is to advance the scope through the colon.

The bowel cleaning preparation may be tiring and often produces **diarrhea** and cramping. During the colonoscopy, the sedative will keep the patient drowsy and relaxed. Most patients complain of minor discomfort, such as cramping or a feeling of fullness. However, the procedure is not painful.

A procedure called virtual colonoscopy has been developed but debate continues on whether or not it is effective as colonoscopy. Virtual colonoscopy refers to the use of imaging, usually with **computed tomography** (CT) scans or **magnetic resonance imaging** (MRI), to produce images of the colon. Studies in late 2003 showed that virtual colonoscopy was as effective as colonoscopy for screening purposes and it offered the advantage of being less invasive and less risky. However, many physicians were unwilling to accept it as a replacement for colonoscopy, particularly since some patients might still require the regular colonoscopy as a follow-up to the virtual procedure if a polyp or abnormality is found that requires biopsy.

Preparation

The doctor should be notified if the patient has allergies to any medications or anesthetics, has any bleeding problems, or if a female patient is pregnant. The doctor should also be informed of all the medications that the patient is currently taking and if he or she has had a barium x-ray examination recently. The doctor may instruct the patient not to take certain medications, like aspirin and anti-inflammatory drugs that interfere with clotting, for a period of time prior to the procedure. If the patient has had heart valves replaced or a history of an inflammation of the inside lining of the heart, the doctor should be

KEY TERMS

Barium enema—An x-ray test of the bowel after giving the patient an enema of a white chalky substance that outlines the colon and the rectum.

Biopsy—Removal of a tissue sample for examination under the microscope to check for cancer cells.

Colonoscope—A thin, flexible, hollow, lighted tube that is inserted through the rectum into the colon to enable the doctor to view the entire lining of the colon.

Crohn's disease—A chronic inflammatory disease resulting from the immune system attacking one's own body. The disease generally affects the gastrointestinal tract and may cause the formation of deep ulcers.

Diverticulosis—A condition in which pouchlike sections that bulge through the large intestine's muscular walls but are not inflamed develop. They may cause bleeding, stomach distress, and excess gas.

Pathologist—A doctor who specializes in the diagnosis of disease by studying cells and tissues under a microscope.

Polyps—Abnormal growths that develop on the inside of a hollow organ such as the colon.

Ulcerative colitis—A chronic condition where recurrent ulcers are found in the colon. It is manifested clinically by abdominal cramping and rectal bleeding.

informed, so that appropriate antibiotics can be administered to prevent any chance of infection. The risks of the procedure will be explained to the patient before performing the procedure and the patient will be asked to sign a consent form.

It is important that the colon be thoroughly cleaned before performing the examination. Before the examination, considerable preparation is necessary to clear the colon of all stool. The patient will be asked to refrain from eating any solid food for 24–48 hours before the test. Only clear liquids such as juices, broth, and gelatin are recommended. The patient is advised to drink plenty of water to avoid dehydration.

The day before the test, the patient will have to drink a special cleansing solution or take a strong laxative that the doctor has prescribed. The patient will also be given specific instructions as to how to use an enema, as a warm water enema may be necessary the next morning.

On the morning of the examination, one or two enemas of warm tap water may have to be taken. Generally, the procedure has to be repeated until the return from the enema is clear of stool particles. The patient is instructed not to eat or drink anything. The preparatory procedures are extremely important because the colon must be thoroughly clean for the exam to be performed.

Aftercare

After the procedure, the patient is kept under observation until the effects of the medications wear off. The patient will not be able to drive immediately after the procedure and can generally resume a normal diet and usual activities unless otherwise instructed. The patient will be advised to drink lots of fluids to replace those lost by **laxatives** and fasting.

For a few hours after the procedure, the patient may feel groggy. There may be some abdominal cramping and a considerable amount of gas may be passed. If a biopsy was performed or a polyp was removed, there may be small amounts of blood in the stool for a few days. If the patient experiences severe abdominal pain or has persistent and heavy bleeding, it should be brought to the doctor's attention immediately.

Risks

The procedure is considered safe. Very rarely (two in 1,000 cases) there may be a perforation (a hole) in the intestinal wall. Heavy bleeding due to the removal of the polyp or from the biopsy site occurs seldom occurs (one in 1,000 cases). Infections due to a colonoscopy are also extremely rare. Patients with artificial or abnormal heart valves are usually given antibiotics before and after the procedure to prevent an infection.

Normal results

The results are said to be normal if the lining of the colon is a pale reddish pink and no abnormal looking masses are found in the lining of the colon.

Abnormal results

Abnormal results would imply that polyps or other suspicious-looking masses were detected in the lining of the intestine. Polyps can be removed during the procedure and tissue samples can be biopsied. If cancerous cells are detected in the tissue samples, then a diagnosis of colon cancer is made. The pathologist analyzes the tumor cells further to estimate the aggressiveness of the tumor and the extent of spread of the disease.

Abnormal findings also could be due to inflammatory bowel diseases such as ulcerative colitis or Crohn's disease. A condition called diverticulosis, in

which many small fingerlike pouches protrude from the colon wall, may also be identified.

Resources

BOOKS

Berkow, Robert, et al., editors. *Merck Manual of Diagnosis and Therapy*. 17th ed. Rahway, NJ: Merck Publishing Group, 1999.

Fauci, Anthony S. "Gastrointestinal Endoscopy." In *Harrison's Principles of Internal Medicine*. 14th ed. New York, NY: The McGraw-Hill Companies, 2000.

Pfenninger, John L. *Procedures for Primary Care Physicians*. 2nd ed. St. Louis: Mosby, Inc. 2000.

PERIODICALS

"Professional Organization Recommends Standard Colonoscopy Over Virtual." *Biotech Week* December 31, 2003: 422.

"Study Shows Virtual Colonoscopy as Effective as Traditional Colonoscopy." *Biotech Week* December 31, 2003.

ORGANIZATIONS

American Cancer Society (National Headquarters). 1599 Clifton Road, N.E. Atlanta, Georgia 30329. (800) 227-2345. http://www.cancer.org.

American Gastroenterological Association. 7910 Woodmont Ave., Seventh Floor, Bethesda, MD 20814. Phone: (301) 654-2055. http://www.gastro.org.

Cancer Research Institute (National Headquarters). 681 Fifth Avenue, New York, N.Y. 10022. (800) 992-2623. http://www.cancerresearch.org.

National Cancer Institute. 9000 Rockville Pike, Building 31, Room 10A31, Bethesda, Maryland, 20892. (800) 422-6237. http://www.nci.nih.gov.

Society of American Gastrointestinal Endoscopic Surgeons (SAGES). 2716 Ocean Park Boulevard, Suite 3000, Santa Monica, CA 90405. (310) 314-2404. http://www.sages.org.

United Ostomy Association, Inc. (UOA). 19772 MacArthur Blvd., Suite 200, Irvine, CA 92612. (800) 826 0826. http://www.uoa.org.

Lata Cherath, Ph.D.

Colorectal cancer *see* **Colon cancer; Rectal cancer**

Colorectal surgery

Definition

Colorectal surgery repairs damage to the colon, rectum, and anus through a variety of procedures that may have little or great long-term consequence to the patient. It may also involve surgery to the pelvic floor to repair hernias.

Colostomy

Omentum

Colon

A.

B.

incision

Fascia

C.

Catheter

Abdominal
wall

Stoma

Colon

D.

To perform a colostomy, a loop of the colon is pulled through the abdominal incision (B); the colon is cut to insert a catheter (C). The skin and tissues are closed around a stoma (D). *(Illustration by GGS Information Services. Cengage Learning, Gale.)*

Purpose

Colorectal surgery is performed to repair damage to the colon, rectum, and anus, caused by diseases of the lower digestive tract, such as **cancer**, diverticulitis, and inflammatory bowel disease (ulcerative colitis and Crohn's disease). Injury, obstruction, and ischemia (compromised blood supply) may require bowel surgery. Masses and scar tissue can grow within the rectum, causing blockages that prevent normal elimination of feces. Other diseases such as diverticulitis and ulcerative colitis can cause perforations in the rectum. Surgical removal of the damaged area or areas can return normal bowel function.

Demographics

Colorectal cancer affects 140,000 people annually, causing 60,000 deaths. Polypectomy (the removal of polyps in the colon), usually performed during a routine diagnostic test (colonscopy or flexible **sigmoidoscopy**), has been a factor in the declining incidence of this cancer. However, incidence of the disease, as reported in the *Journal of the National Cancer Institute* in the early 2000s, differed among ethnic groups, with Hispanics having 10.2 cases per 100,000 people, to African Americans having 22.8 cases per 100,000. Surgery is the optimal treatment for colorectal cancer, resulting in cure in 80% of patients. Recurrence due to surgical failure is low, from 4% to 8%, when surgery is meticulously performed.

Crohn's disease and ulcerative colitis, both chronic inflammatory diseases of the colon, together affect approximately 1,000,000 young adults. Surgery is recommended when medication fails patients with ulcerative colitis. Usually, surgery is drastic, removing the colon and rectum and creating an interior or exterior pouch to collect body wastes. Nearly three-fourths of all Crohn's patients face surgery to removed a diseased section of the intestine or rectum.

Diverticulosis, the growth of pouches in the walls of the intestine, occurs in nearly half of all Americans by the time they reach age 60 and in practically everyone over 80. Sometimes these diverticuli become infected and diverticulitis occurs. Diverticulitis may also require surgery to remove part of the colon if there have been recurrent episodes with complications or perforations.

Description

Colorectal surgery is a necessary treatment option for colorectal cancer, ulcerative colitis, Crohn's disease, and some cases of diverticulitis, often resulting in

---

KEY TERMS

Adjuvant therapy—Treatment that is added to increase the effectiveness of surgery, usually chemotherapy or radiation used to kill any cancer cells that might be remaining.

Anastomosis—The surgical connection of two sections of tubes, ducts, or vessels.

Diverticuli—Pouches in the intestinal wall usually created from a diet low in fiber.

Embolism—Blockage of a blood vessel by any small piece of material traveling in the blood; the emboli may be caused by germs, air, blood clots, or fat.

Enema—Insertion of a tube into the rectum to infuse fluid into the bowel and encourage a bowel movement. Ordinary enemas contain tap water, mixtures of soap and water, glycerine and water, or other materials.

Intestine—Commonly called the bowels, divided into the small and large intestine. They extend from the stomach to the anus.

Ischemia—A compromise in blood supply delivered to body tissues that causes tissue damage or death.

Ostomy—A surgical procedure that creates an opening from the inside of the body to the outside, usually to remove body wastes (feces or urine).

Sigmoid colon—The last third of the intestinal tract that is attached to the rectum.

---

major reconstruction of the intestinal tract. Other bowel conditions that may require surgery to a lesser extent are hemorrhoids, anal fissures (tears in the lining of the anus), rectal prolapse, and bowel **incontinence**. Most of these surgeries repair tears, remove blockages, or tighten sphincter muscles. Patients with anal fissures, for example, experience immediate relief, with more than 90% of them never having the problem recur.

Some colorectal surgeons also treat pelvic floor disorders such as perineal hernia and rectocele (a bulging of the rectum toward the vagina).

Types of surgery

There are a variety of procedures a colorectal surgeon may use to treat intestinal disorders. Until 1990, all colorectal surgery was performed by making large incisions in the abdomen, opening up the intestinal cavity, and making the repair. Most of these repairs involved resection (cutting out the diseased or damaged portion) and anastomosis (attaching the cut ends of the intestine together). Some were tucks to tighten sphincter muscles or repair fissures, and others cut out hemorrhoids. Some colorectal surgeons perform a strictureplasty, a new procedure that widens the intestine instead of making it shorter; this is used with patients with extensive Crohn's disease.

Often colorectal surgery involves creating an ostomy, which is an opening from the inside of the body to the outside, usually to remove body wastes (feces or urine). There are several types of ostomy surgeries that colorectal surgeons do. A **colostomy** is a surgical procedure that brings a portion of the large intestine through the abdominal wall, creating an opening, or stoma, to carry feces out of the body to a pouch. An ileostomy removes the entire colon, the rectum, and the anus. The lower end of the small intestine (the ileum) becomes the stoma.

For all ostomies, a pouch will generally be placed around the stoma on the patient's abdomen during surgery. During the hospital stay, the patient and his or her caregivers will be educated on care of the stoma and the ostomy pouch. Determination of appropriate pouching supplies and a schedule of how often to change the pouch should be established. Regular assessment and meticulous care of the skin surrounding the stoma is important to maintain an adequate surface on which to attach the pouch. Some patients with colostomies are able to routinely irrigate the stoma, resulting in regulation of bowel function; rather than needing to wear a pouch, these patients may need only a dressing or cap over their stoma. Often, an enterostomal therapist will visit the patient in the hospital or at home after discharge to help the patient with stoma care.

Most colostomies and ileostomies are permanent. Temporary colostomies are created to divert stool from injured or diseased portions of the large intestine, allowing rest and healing. Although colorectal cancer is the most common indication for a permanent colostomy, only about 10–15% of patients with this diagnosis require a colostomy.

A new procedure called an ileoanal anastomosis creates an internal reservoir that is sewn to the anus and acts as an artificial rectum. It usually is not used with Crohn's disease patients because their disease often recurs.

Laparoscopic surgery is being used with many diseases of the intestinal tract, including initial cancers. For this surgery, the colon and rectal surgeon inserts a laparoscope (an instrument that has a tiny video camera attached) through a small incision in the abdomen. Other small incisions are made through which the surgeon inserts surgical instruments. This surgery often results in fewer complications, a shorter stay in the hospital, less postoperative pain, a quicker return to normal activities, and less scarring. It is not recommended for patients who have had extensive prior abdominal surgery, large tumors, previous cancer, or serious heart problems.

Diagnosis/Preparation

Some disease or conditions may require a minimally invasive surgery. Other diseases such as inflammatory bowel disease and colorectal cancer may require an ostomy, a more drastic procedure. Determining whether this surgery is necessary is a decision the physician makes based on a number of factors, including patient history, the amount of pain the patient is experiencing, and the results of several diagnostic tests. Due to the lifestyle impact of ostomy surgery, surgeons make that decision with careful input from the patient. Sometimes, though, an immediate decision may be necessary in emergency situations involving injuries or puncture wounds in the abdomen, or intestinal perforations related to diverticulear disease, ulcers, or cancer, which can be life-threatening.

Diagnostic tests

Colonoscopy, flexible sigmoidoscopy, and a lower GI (gastrointestinal) series help determine the condition of the intestinal tract. These tests can identify masses and perforations on bowel walls.

A lower GI series is a series of **x rays** of the colon and rectum, which can identify ulcers, cysts, polyps, diverticuli (pouches in the intestine), and cancer. The patient is given a **barium enema**; the barium coats the intestinal tract, making any signs of disease easier to see on x rays.

Flexible sigmoidoscopy, a flexible tube with a miniature camera, is inserted into the rectum so the physician can examine the lining of the rectum and the sigmoid colon, the last third of the intestinal tract. The sigmoidoscope can also remove polyps or tissue for **biopsy**.

A colonoscopy is a similar procedure to the flexible sigmoidoscopy, except the flexible tube looks at the entire intestinal tract. For the patient's comfort, a sedative is given.

Magnetic resonance imaging (MRI), used both prior to and during surgery, allows physicians to determine the precise margins for resections of the colon, so that they can eliminate all of the diseased tissue. MRI can also identify patients who could most benefit from adjuvant therapy such as **chemotherapy** or radiation.

Preoperative preparation

The doctor will outline the procedure, possible side effects, and what the patient may experience after surgery. As with any surgical procedure, the patient will be required to sign a consent form. Blood and urine studies, along with various x rays and an electrocardiograph (EKG), may be ordered. If necessary, an enterostomal therapist will be contacted to mark an appropriate place on the abdomen for the stoma and offer preoperative education on ostomy management.

In order to empty and cleanse the bowel, the patient may be placed on a restricted diet for several days prior to surgery. A liquid diet may be ordered for at least the day before surgery, with nothing by mouth after midnight. A series of enemas and/or oral preparations (GoLytely, Colyte, or senna) may be ordered to empty the bowel of stool. Oral anti-infectives (neomycin, erythromycin, or kanamycin sulfate) may be ordered to decrease bacteria in the intestine and help prevent postoperative **infection**.

Aftercare

Postoperative care involves monitoring blood pressure, pulse, respiration, and temperature. Breathing tends to be shallow because of the effect of the anesthesia and the patient's reluctance to breathe deeply and experience pain that is caused by the abdominal incision. The patient is instructed how to support the operative site during deep breathing and coughing, and given pain medication as necessary. Fluid intake and output is measured, and the operative site is observed for color and amount of wound drainage.

The patient is usually helped out of bed the evening of the surgery and allowed to sit in a chair. Most patients are discharged in two to four days.

The nasogastric tube will remain in place, attached to low, intermittent suction until bowel activity resumes. For the first 24–48 hours after surgery, the ostomy will drain bloody mucus. Fluids and electrolytes are given intravenously until the patient's diet can gradually be resumed, beginning with liquids only, then adding solids. Usually within 72 hours, passage of gas and stool through the stoma begins. Initially the stool is liquid, gradually thickening as the patient begins to take solid foods. The patient is usually out of bed in eight to 24 hours after surgery and discharged in two to four days.

Risks

Potential risks of colorectal surgery are those of any major surgery and usually occur while the patient is still in the hospital. The patient's general health prior to surgery will also be an indication of the potential for risk. Of special concern are cardiac problems and stressed immune systems.

Psychological complications may result from ostomy surgery because of the fear of the social stigma attached to wearing a colostomy bag. Patients may also be depressed and have feelings of low self-worth because of the change in their lifestyle and their appearance. Some patients may feel ugly and sexually unattractive and may worry that their spouse or significant other will no longer find them appealing. Counseling and education regarding surgery and the inherent lifestyle changes are often necessary.

Normal results

Complete healing is expected without complications. The period of time required for recovery from the surgery may vary, depending on the patient's overall health prior to surgery. Dietary changes may be encouraged to prevent future disorders or to manage a current disease.

Morbidity and mortality rates

Mortality has been decreased from nearly 28% to under 6% through the use of prophylactic **antibiotics** prescribed before and after surgery. Strong indicators of survival outcome or increased complications from surgery for elderly patients are underlying medical conditions. Therefore, the underlying medical conditions of at-risk patients should be controlled prior to a colorectal surgery.

Even among higher risk patients, mortality is about 16%. This rate is greatly reduced (between 0.8% and 3.8%) when the ostomies and resections for cancer are performed by a board-certified colon and rectal surgeon.

The physician and the nursing staff monitor the patient's vital signs and the surgical incision to alert for:

• excessive bleeding
• wound infection
• thrombophlebitis (inflammation and blood clot in the veins in the legs)

- pneumonia
- pulmonary embolism (blood clot or air bubble in the lungs' blood supply)
- cardiac stress due to allergic reaction to the general anesthetic

Symptoms that the patient should report, especially after discharge, include:

- increased pain, swelling, redness, drainage, or bleeding in the surgical area
- flu-like symptoms such as headache, muscle aches, dizziness, or fever
- increased abdominal pain or swelling, constipation, nausea or vomiting, or black, tarry stools

Stomal complications can also occur. They include:

- Death (necrosis) of stomal tissue. Caused by inadequate blood supply, this complication is usually visible 12–24 hours after the operation and may require additional surgery.
- Retraction (stoma is flush with the abdomen surface or has moved below it). Caused by insufficient stomal length, this complication may be managed by use of special pouching supplies; elective revision of the stoma is also an option.
- Prolapse (stoma increases length above the surface of the abdomen). Most often this results from an overly large opening in the abdominal wall or inadequate fixation of the bowel to the abdominal wall; surgical correction is required when blood supply is compromised.
- Stenosis (narrowing at the opening of the stoma). Often this is associated with infection around the stoma or scarring. Mild stenosis can be removed under local anesthesia; severe stenosis may require surgery for reshaping the stoma.
- Parastomal hernia (bulge in the abdominal wall, caused by a section of bowel, next to the stoma). This occurs due to placement of the stoma where the abdominal wall is weak or an overly large opening in the abdominal wall is created. The use of an ostomy support belt and special pouching supplies may be adequate. If severe, the defect in the abdominal wall should be repaired and the stoma moved to another location.

Alternatives

When a colostomy is deemed necessary, there are usually no alternatives to the surgery, though there can be alternatives in the type of surgery involved and adjuvant therapies related to the disease.

WHO PERFORMS THE PROCEDURE AND WHERE IS IT PERFORMED?

Colorectal surgery is performed by general surgeons and board-certified colon and rectal surgeons as in-patient surgeries under general anesthesia.

QUESTIONS TO ASK THE DOCTOR

- Am I a good candidate for laparoscopic surgery?
- What tests will you require?
- What drugs will be given for pain after the surgery?
- What will I need to do to prepare for surgery?
- What will my recovery time be and what restrictions will I have?
- How many of these procedures have you performed?
- What are my risks for this surgery?

Resources

BOOKS

Johnston, Lorraine. *Colon & Rectal Cancer: A Comprehensive Guide for Patients and Families.* Sebastopol, CA: O'Reilly, 2000.

Levin, Bernard. *American Cancer Society Colorectal Cancer.* New York: Villard, 1999.

PERIODICALS

Beets-Tan, R. G. H., et al. "Accuracy of Maganetic Resonance Imaging in Prediction of Tumour-free Resection Margin in Rectal Cancer Surgery." *The Lancet* 357 (February 17, 2001): 497.

"Laparoscopy Could Offer Long-term Survival Benefit over Conventional Surgery." *Cancer Weekly* (July 30, 2002): 14.

Schwenk, Wolfgang. "Pulmonary Function Following Laparoscopic or Conventional Colorectal Resection: A Randomized Controlled Evaluation." *Journal of the American Medical Association* 281 (April 7, 1999): 1154.

Senagore, A. J., and P. Erwin-Toth. "Care of the Laparoscopic Colectomy Patient." *Advances in Skin & Wound Care* 15 (November–December 2002): 277–284.

Walling, Anne D. "Follow-up after Resection for Colorectal Cancer Saves Lives. (Tips from Other Journals)." *American Family Physician* 66 (August 1, 2002): 485.

OTHER

National Digestive Diseases Information Clearinghouse. *Ileostomy, Colostomy, and Ileoanal Reservoir Surgery.* (February 1, 2000): 1.

ORGANIZATIONS

American Board of Colon and Rectal Surgery (ABCRS). 20600 Eureka Road, Suite 713, Taylor, MI 48180. (734) 282-9400. www.fascrs.org.

Mayo Clinic. 200 First St. S.W., Rochester, MN 55905. (507) 284-2511. www.mayoclinic.org.

United Ostomy Association, Inc. (UOA). 19772 MacArthur Blvd., Suite 200, Irvine, CA 92612-2405. (800) 826-0826. http://www.uoa.org.

Wound Ostomy and Continence Nurses Society. 2755 Bristol Street, Suite 110, Costa Mesa, CA 92626. (714) 476-0268. http://www.wocn.org.

Janie F. Franz

Colostomy

Definition

Ostomy is a surgical procedure used to create an opening for urine or feces to be released from the body. Colostomy refers to a surgical procedure in which a portion of the large intestine is brought through the abdominal wall to carry stool out of the body.

Purpose

A colostomy is created as a result of treatment for various disorders of the large intestine, including **cancer**, obstruction, inflammatory bowel disease, ruptured diverticulum, ischemia (compromised blood supply), or traumatic injury. Temporary colostomies are created to divert stool from injured or diseased portions of the large intestine, allowing rest and healing. These temporary colostomies are removed at a later date, with restoration of normal bowel function. Permanent colostomies are performed when the distal bowel (bowel at the farthest distance) must be removed or is blocked and inoperable. Although colorectal cancer is the most common indication for a permanent colostomy, only about 10–15% of patients with this diagnosis require a colostomy.

Description

Surgery will result in one of three types of colostomies:

- End colostomy. The functioning end of the intestine (the section of bowel that remains connected to the upper gastrointestinal tract) is brought out to the surface of the abdomen, forming the stoma by cuffing the intestine back on itself and suturing the end to the skin. A stoma is an artificial opening created to

Colostomy stoma with ring for stoma bag. (Custom Medical Stock Photo. Reproduced by permission.)

the surface of the body. The surface of the stoma is actually the lining of the intestine, usually appearing moist and pink, and it has no pain sensation. The distal portion of bowel (now connected only to the rectum) may be removed, or sutured closed and left in the abdomen. An end colostomy is usually a permanent ostomy, resulting from trauma, cancer or another pathological condition.

- Double–barrel colostomy. This colostomy involves the creation of two separate stomas on the abdominal wall. The proximal (nearest) stoma is the functional end that is connected to the upper gastrointestinal tract and will drain stool. The distal stoma, connected to the rectum and also called a mucous fistula, drains small amounts of mucus material. This is most often a temporary colostomy performed to rest an area of bowel, and to be later closed.

- Loop colostomy. This colostomy is created by bringing a loop of bowel through an incision in the abdominal wall. An incision is made in the bowel to allow the passage of stool through the loop

KEY TERMS

Diverticulum—Pouches that project off the wall of the intestine, visible as opaque on an x ray after the patient has swallowed a contrast (dye) substance.

Embolism—Blockage of a blood vessel by any small piece of material traveling in the blood. The emboli may be caused by germs, air, blood clots, or fat.

Enema—Insertion of a tube into the rectum to infuse fluid into the bowel and encourage a bowel movement. Ordinary enemas contain tap water, mixtures of soap and water, glycerin and water, or other materials.

Intestine—Commonly called the bowels, divided into the small and large intestine. They extend from the stomach to the anus. The small intestine is about 20 ft (6 m) long. The large intestine is about 5 ft (1.5 m) long.

Ischemia—A compromise in blood supply delivered to body tissues that causes tissue damage or death.

Ostomy—A surgically created opening in the abdomen for elimination of waste products (urine or stool).

colostomy. In the past, a plastic rod was used to hold the loop in place, and this supporting rod was removed approximately 7-10 days after surgery, when healing had occurred. The use of the plastic supporting rod is becoming less common. A loop colostomy is most often performed for creation of a temporary stoma to divert stool away from an area of intestine that has been blocked or ruptured.

Preparation

As with any surgical procedure, the patient will be required to sign a consent form after the procedure is explained thoroughly. Blood and urine studies, along with various **x rays** and an electrocardiograph (ECG) may be ordered as the doctor deems necessary. If possible, the patient should visit an enterostomal therapist, who will mark an appropriate place on the abdomen for the stoma, and offer pre-operative education on ostomy management.

In order to empty and cleanse the bowel, the patient may be placed on a low-residue diet for several days prior to surgery. A liquid diet may be ordered for at least the day before surgery, with nothing by mouth after midnight. A series of enemas and/or oral preparations (GoLytely or Colyte) may be ordered to empty the bowel of stool. Oral **antibiotics** (neomycin, erythromycin, or kanamycin sulfate) may be given to decrease bacteria in the intestine and help prevent post-operative **infection**. A nasogastric tube may be inserted from the nose to the stomach on the day of surgery or during surgery to remove gastric secretions and prevent **nausea and vomiting**. A urinary catheter (a thin plastic tube) may also be inserted to keep the bladder empty during surgery, giving more space in the surgical field and decreasing chances of accidental injury.

Aftercare

Post-operative care for the patient with a new colostomy involves monitoring of blood pressure, pulse, respiration, and temperature. Breathing tends to be shallow because of the effect of anesthesia and the patient's reluctance to breathe deeply and experience pain caused by the abdominal incision. The patient is instructed how to support the operative site during deep breathing and coughing, and given pain medication as necessary. Fluid intake and output is measured, and the operative site is observed for color and amount of wound drainage.

Two to three days after the operation, the patient will be able to resume eating. For both open and laparoscopic resections, most patients are discharged from the hospital in five to seven days. Healing may take one to two months.

A colostomy pouch will generally have been placed on the patient's abdomen, around the stoma during surgery. During the hospital stay, the patient and caregivers will be educated about how to care for the colostomy. Determination of appropriate pouching supplies and a schedule of how often to change the pouch should be established. Regular assessment and meticulous care of the skin surrounding the stoma is important to maintain an adequate surface on which to apply the pouch. Some patients with colostomies are able to routinely irrigate the stoma, resulting in regulation of bowel function; rather than needing to wear a pouch, these patients may need only a dressing or cap over their stoma. Often, an enterostomal therapist will visit the patient at home after discharge to help the patient resume normal daily activities.

Risks

Potential complications of colostomy surgery include:

- excessive bleeding
- surgical wound infection

- thrombophlebitis (inflammation and blood clot to veins in the legs)
- pneumonia
- pulmonary embolism (blood clot or air bubble in the lungs' blood supply)

Normal results

Complete healing is expected without complications. The period of time required for recovery from the surgery varies depending on the patient's overall health prior to surgery. The colostomy patient without other medical complications should be able to resume all daily activities once recovered from the surgery.

Abnormal results

The doctor should be made aware of any of the following problems after surgery:

- increased pain, swelling, redness, drainage, or bleeding in the surgical area
- headache, muscle aches, dizziness, or fever
- increased abdominal pain or swelling, constipation, nausea or vomiting, or black, tarry stools

Stomal complications to be monitored include:

- Death (necrosis) of stomal tissue. Caused by inadequate blood supply, this complication is usually visible 12–24 hours after the operation and may require additional surgery.
- Retraction (stoma is flush with the abdomen surface or has moved below it). Caused by insufficient stomal length, this complication may be managed by use of special pouching supplies. Elective revision of the stoma is also an option.
- Prolapse (stoma increases length above the surface of the abdomen). Most often results from an overly large opening in the abdominal wall or inadequate fixation of the bowel to the abdominal wall. Surgical correction is required when blood supply is compromised.
- Stenosis (narrowing at the opening of the stoma). Often associated with infection around the stoma or scarring. Mild stenosis can be removed under local anesthesia. Severe stenosis may require surgery for reshaping the stoma.
- Parastomal hernia (bowel causing bulge in the abdominal wall next to the stoma). Usually due to placement of the stoma where the abdominal wall is weak or creation of an overly large opening in the abdominal wall. The use of an ostomy support belt and special pouching supplies may be adequate. If

severe, the defect in the abdominal wall should be repaired and the stoma moved to another location.

Resources

PERIODICALS

Edwards, D. P., et al. "Stoma -related complications are more frequent after transverse colostomy than loop ileostomy: a prospective randomized clinical trial." *British Journal of Surgery.* 88, no. 3 (March 2001): 360-363.

Whitehead, William E., et al. "Treatment options for Fecal Incontinence." *Diseases of the Colon and Rectum* 44, no. 1 (January 2001): 131-144.

ORGANIZATIONS

The United Ostomy Association, a self-help organization, provides useful information. 36 Executive Park, Suite 120, Irvine, CA 92714. Phone: (800) 826-0826 or (714) 660-8624. uoa@deltanet.com. http://www.uoa.org.

Wound, Ostomy, and Continence Nurses Society. 2755 Bristol Street, Suite 110, Costa Mesa, CA 92626. (714) 476-0268. http://www.wocn.org.

Kathleen Dredge Wright

Complementary cancer therapies

Definition

Alternative and complementary therapies refer to treatments outside the mainstream of Western scientific medicine. They cover a wide variety of approaches, ranging from the medical systems of other cultures to special diets or medications, spiritual practices, herbal remedies, and external energy sources. As a general rule, *complementary* is used to refer to treatments that are offered alongside mainstream methods of **cancer** therapy to relieve the patient's discomfort or contribute to his or her overall sense of well-being. Other terms that are sometimes used for complementary therapies are *adjunctive*, which means helping or assisting, and *supportive*. Complementary or supportive treatments are not considered cures for cancer. When they are given together with mainstream cancer treatments, the combination is called *integrative* therapy.

The word *alternative* refers to treatments used instead of mainstream cancer treatments in an attempt to cure cancer. Some alternative treatments have not yet been tested by scientific researchers while others have been tested and shown not to work. If alternative remedies are used instead of proven cancer treatments, they may harm the patient by allowing the cancer to

KEY TERMS

Adjunctive—Any form of therapy that is considered to help or assist a patient's primary treatment.

Alternative—A form of treatment outside mainstream medicine that is used as a cure instead of standard treatments.

Angiogenesis—The formation of blood vessels. Shark cartilage is undergoing tests on its effects on angiogenesis in tumors.

Anorexia—Loss of appetite. Anorexia is a common side effect of chemotherapy.

Aura—The field of subtle energy that surrounds the human body, according to external energy therapists.

Biologics—Drugs or other medical products made from biological sources.

Cachexia—The wasting away of body tissue.

Complementary—Any form of treatment outside the mainstream that is not considered a cure but is given to ease symptoms or contribute to general well-being.

Detoxification—Ridding the body of digestive wastes considered toxic through fasting, drinking large quantities of juice, or colonic irrigation.

Holistic—Any approach to health care that emphasizes the patient's total well-being, including psychological and spiritual as well as physical aspects.

Integrative—An approach to cancer treatment that combines mainstream therapies with one or more complementary therapies.

Investigational—A drug or therapy that is approved for use in clinical trials but not for regular treatment of patients.

Mantra—A sacred word or phrase, used in some forms of meditation to deepen the meditative state.

Quackery—A fraudulent form of treatment or therapy.

Vegan—A vegetarian who omits all animal products, including eggs and milk, from their diet.

grow and reducing the chances of curing it by standard therapies. Treatments that are still being tested on animals or humans are called research or investigational therapies. In the United States, medications or other methods of treatment must be approved by the Food and Drug Administration (FDA) before they can be considered standard treatments for cancer. In 1991, Congress established the Office of Alternative

Medicine as part of the National Institutes of Health. It includes the National Center for Complementary and Alternative Medicine, or NCCAM. As of October 2009, NCCAM supports 27 specialized research centers that study the safety and effectiveness of various complementary and alternative medicine (CAM) treatments for cancer.

Description

Today there are over two hundred complementary/alternative substances and treatment methods that have been given to cancer patients. They can be grouped for purposes of discussion into ten major categories.

Biologic

Biologic treatments are drugs or other medical products that are derived naturally from plants, animals, or the human body itself. They are thought to help the body fight cancer by restoring its biochemical balance.

Many biologic treatments have already been tested by researchers. They vary widely in their effectiveness:

- Antineoplaston therapy. Antineoplastons, which are extracted from blood serum and urine, are short-chain amino acids that supposedly reprogram the DNA of cancer cells so that the cells reproduce normally instead of uncontrollably. The FDA and National Cancer Institute (NCI) have permitted clinical trials of antineoplastons in cancer patients. However, the clinical trials were closed in 1995 because of small enrollment numbers in the trials and lack of consensus about how to recruit more patients for the trials. Because of the small numbers in the trials, the NCI draws no conclusions about the effectiveness of antineoplastons. Antineoplaston therapy can be used with standard chemotherapy.

- 714X. 714X is a treatment consisting of three 21-day rounds of injections of camphor and organic salts directly into the lymphatic system. It is based on a theory that cancer cells use up large amounts of nitrogen and secrete a poisonous K-cofactor that paralyzes the immune system so that nitrogen can be drawn from healthy cells. Since the camphor in 714X contains nitrogen, the cancer cells do not have to secrete the K-cofactor, which in turn allows the immune system to recover.

- Cancell/Entelev. Cancell/Entelev is a liquid marketed as a treatment for cancer as well as AIDS, epilepsy, lupus, and other diseases. It is also sold as Cantron, Sheridan's Formula, Jim's Juice, and Crocinic Acid. Cancell is a mixture of 12 common chemicals—including nitric acid and sulfuric acid—none of which are known to be effective against cancer. The NCI tested Cancell four times between 1978 and 1991; no benefit to this therapy could be demonstrated, and the NCI decided not to study it further.

- Hydrazine sulfate. Hydrazine sulfate is a chemical that has been used to treat the loss of appetite (anorexia) and wasting away of body tissue (cachexia) that occur in late-stage cancer; it has not been promoted as a cure for cancer. It is available in the United States as a dietary supplement. Hydrazine sulfate has been studied by the Russian government as well as the NCI, but test results are not conclusive. As of 2009, no clinical trials of hydrazine sulfate are being conducted in the United States.

- Laetrile. Laetrile, which is also known as amygdalin or vitamin B_{17}, is a chemical found in fruit pits, lima beans, sorghum, and clover; it contains sugar and produces cyanide. The cyanide is considered to be the primary anti-cancer agent in laetrile. Laetrile has been used by itself to treat cancer and as part of metabolic therapy, but it has not shown any anti-cancer effectiveness in NCI clinical trials. It is not approved for use in the United States but is available in Mexico. When taken by mouth, laetrile can produce side effects resembling the symptoms of cyanide poisoning.

- Hydrogen peroxide therapy. Hydrogen peroxide has been used in the United States and Japan since the 1960s as an adjunctive treatment to radiation therapy. The hydrogen peroxide is diluted in water and injected directly into the patient's arteries. Some researchers think that hydrogen peroxide helps to shrink tumors by making them more sensitive to radiation.

Metabolic therapies

Metabolic therapies combine enzyme treatments, diets, and nutritional supplements with herbal medicines or special formulas. They are based on the belief that cancer results from many factors acting together, and that it should be treated by strengthening the entire body, not just by removing the tumor.

Most of these therapies are considered questionable by mainstream physicians:

- Kelley/Gonzalez therapy. Kelley/Gonzalez therapy focuses on cancer of the pancreas. Its practitioners regard cancer as resulting from inadequate levels of pancreatic enzymes, which help the body to digest protein. Kelley/Gonzalez therapy includes a diet tailored to each individual, nutritional supplements,

digestive aids, enzyme supplements, and colonic irrigation. It is the most promising of the metabolic therapies.

- Gerson therapy. Gerson therapy combines a low-salt vegan diet with large quantities of fruit and vegetable juices, as well as three or four coffee enemas each day to detoxify the body. It is based on the notion that cancer patients have too much sodium in their bodies and not enough potassium. Gerson therapy is not recommended as an alternative to conventional treatment for cancer.

- Issel's whole-body therapy. This form of metabolic therapy originated in Germany. It includes psychotherapy, oxygen therapy, and the removal of amalgam dental fillings (which contain small amounts of mercury) as well as a special diet.

- Revici therapy. Revici therapy is based on the belief that cancer is associated with imbalances in the body's tissue-building and tissue-breakdown processes. These imbalances are treated with intravenous injections of lipids (fatty or waxy organic substances) containing oxygen, copper, calcium, and selenium.

Immune enhancement therapies

Immune enhancement therapies are based on the theory that cancers in humans result from a weakened immune system.

Therapies in this category are not recommended as alternatives to conventional cancer treatment:

- Immuno-augmentative therapy (IAT). IAT is based on the theory that cancer results from an imbalance among four blood protein components, called the tumor antibody, the tumor complement, the blocking protein, and the deblocking protein. Treatment consists of injecting various amounts of these components to restore the proper balance.

- Livingston therapy. Livingston therapy uses a raw-food vegetarian diet combined with nutritional supplements and vaccines to restore the patient's immune system. It is based on a theory that cancer is caused by a bacterium called progenitor cryptocides, found in eggs, milk, poultry, and beef products.

Bodywork/movement therapies

Doctors often recommend bodywork and movement therapies as adjunctive treatments for cancer because they benefit patients emotionally as well as physically. The exercise involved in dance therapy, yoga, and t'ai chi helps to preserve muscle tone and joint flexibility. Therapeutic massage can relieve muscle soreness resulting from emotional stress.

Some common forms of bodywork and movement therapy include:

- Acupuncture and acupressure. Acupuncture is a basic form of treatment in traditional Chinese medicine. It involves the insertion of very thin steel needles into points on the body associated with the flow of vital energy. In acupressure, the energy points are stimulated by finger pressure. These forms of treatment are often combined with massage.
- Chiropractic. A chiropractor treats the patient's nervous system by manipulating or adjusting the segments of the spinal column. Some people find that chiropractic relieves back pain. As of 2009, one of the NCCAM's 27 research centers is specializing in studies of chiropractic.
- Yoga. Yoga is a good form of low-impact exercise for releasing stress and tension. Its stretches and poses can be modified to fit the needs or limitations of individual patients. Cancer patients who have had surgery should consult their doctor before starting a yoga program.
- T'ai chi. T'ai chi is a Chinese system of meditative exercise that involves a series of slow circular or stretching movements. Many patients find it relaxing and calming. In clinical settings, control groups practicing tai chi showed improvements in symptoms and signs such as strength, appetite, weight gain, stamina, and bowel function, hence increasing the ability for self-cure. In addition, t'ai chi and related practices are simple to learn and produce no side effects.
- Therapeutic massage. Therapeutic massage is often recommended as a complementary treatment to mainstream cancer therapy, but should not be given near the area of any recent surgery.
- Dance therapy. Dance therapy allows patients to release strong emotions as well as exercising their joints and muscles.

Diets and digestive treatments

These forms of treatment are based on the belief that the human digestive tract stores or produces toxic substances and should be cleansed periodically by special foods, fasting, or washing out the lower bowel.

Dietary therapies vary in their usefulness as complementary cancer treatments:

- Vegan diets. Vegan diets are vegetarian diets that omit eggs and dairy products as well as meat. They are thought to offer some protection against cancer, because the milk as well as the tissues of animals

raised for meat may contain carcinogenic (cancer-causing) chemicals. In addition, the high fiber content of vegan diets appears to lower the risk of colon cancer.
- Fasting and juice therapies. These therapies are a major part of naturopathic treatment. Naturopaths maintain that the body can devote more of its energy to healing itself when it does not have to digest high-fat, high-calorie foods. In addition, they regard fasting as a way to help the body rid itself of toxic wastes.
- Macrobiotics. Macrobiotic diets originated in Japan, and classify foods according to the Eastern distinction between yin and yang rather than Western nutritional categories. These diets emphasize brown rice, fruits and vegetables eaten in season, and cooking over a flame rather than using electricity. Although macrobiotic diets have been credited with preventing or curing cancer, no scientific studies have verified these claims.
- Colonic irrigation. This is a treatment method that circulates warm water through the patient's large intestine to remove feces and toxic substances from the walls of the colon. It has been recommended by some alternative therapists for AIDS-related cancers.

Herbal therapies and food supplements

Herbal treatments are historically important because of their role in the development of a number of standard medications. Complementary herbal treatments are presently used to relieve the side effects of mainstream cancer therapy, such as peppermint tea for **nausea** or ginger for **diarrhea**. Patients should, however, consult a health professional before taking any herbal preparation by mouth to make sure that the herb(s) will not interact with prescription medications. Fragrant herbs (rosemary, lemongrass, mint, etc.) can be added to massage oils or bath water for aromatherapy.

Other herbal therapies and dietary supplements have been advertised as cures for cancer:

- Hoxsey formulas. The Hoxsey formulas are herbal remedies for external as well as internal use. The external Hoxsey formula contains bloodroot, which was used by some Native Americans to treat cancer. The internal formula is a mixture of red clover, buckthorn, burdock, licorice root, and several other herbs. The American Cancer Society placed the Hoxsey formulas on its list of unproven methods in 1968.
- Cartilage. Both bovine (cow) and shark cartilage are available in the United States as dietary supplements. Shark cartilage is presently being studied as a cancer

treatment in clinical trials approved by the FDA. It appears to slow down or stop the formation of new blood vessels (angiogenesis) in tumors in animals. As of 2009, however, shark cartilage has not been approved by the FDA as an effective anti-cancer treatment in humans.

- **Coenzyme Q$_{10}$.** Coenzyme Q$_{10}$, also known as vitamin Q$_{10}$, ubiquinone, or ubidecarenone, is a compound that occurs naturally in the human body. It appears to help cells produce energy and to stimulate the immune system. Coenzyme Q$_{10}$ has not been investigated widely as a treatment for cancer in humans, but it has been reported to lengthen the survival of cancer patients. It is sold in the United States as a dietary supplement.

- Mistletoe. Mistletoe (*Viscum album*) is a parasitic plant that has been shown to kill cancer cells in laboratory tests and stimulate the immune system. Although the leaves and berries are toxic to humans, mistletoe extracts are available over the counter in Europe and Asia. There is no clinical evidence that mistletoe is an effective treatment for human cancer, and mistletoe extracts have not been approved for sale in the United States.

- Pau d'arco. Pau d'arco comes from a tree in the South American rainforest. The bark is dried and used to brew a medicinal tea. Pau d'arco was investigated by the NCI for possible anti-tumor effectiveness, but the study concluded in 1974 that a dose strong enough to shrink tumors in humans would have toxic side effects. In small doses, however, pau d'arco tea does appear to stimulate the immune system. It can be purchased in the United States in health food stores.

- Essiac tea. Essiac is a mixture of herbs including burdock, slippery elm inner bark, sheep sorrel, Turkish rhubarb, watercress, red clover, and kelp. Promoters of Essiac claim that the tea strengthens the immune system, relieves pain, increases appetite, reduces tumor size, and extends survival. Some also claim that it cleanses the blood, promotes cell repair, restores energy levels, and detoxifies the body. Despite testimonials, there is no scientific evidence to support the use of this mixture for cancer treatment. NCI studies of Essiac in 1983 found no anti-cancer activity. However, serious side effects from these herbs are rare, and patients may benefit psychologically from the treatment.

External energy therapies

Treatments in this category are based on the belief that there are forms of energy in the universe that can be tapped for purposes of human healing. These energies, which are sometimes called "subtle energies," are thought to be present in mineral formations, plants, the earth's magnetic field, the spectrum of visible light, interpersonal contact, and certain structures or energy fields within the human body itself. Most practitioners of external energy therapies do not ask cancer patients to avoid or give up conventional treatment methods.

The most common forms of external energy therapies include:

- Crystal/gemstone healing. Crystal or gemstone healing is based on the theory that the human body is surrounded by an invisible energy field, or aura, and that the color or crystal structure of a gemstone or mineral can transmit healing energy to the body through the aura.

- Shamanism. Shamanism is the belief that certain persons (shamans) have unusual spiritual powers that can be used for healing. The shaman (who may be a woman in some traditions) acts as an intermediary between the patient and supernatural beings or powers. Native American healers are one type of shaman.

- Bach flower remedies. The 38 Bach flower remedies are tinctures of wildflowers discovered by an English homeopath in the 1920s. They are said to assist physical healing by clearing up negative emotional states or conditions.

- Light/color therapy. Light or color treatment combines the physical effects of the different wavelengths in visible light with the psychological or symbolic meanings attached to specific colors. The practitioner may suggest wearing or visualizing certain colors, or shine colored lights on specific energy points on the patient's body.

- Reiki. Reiki is a holistic approach based on Eastern concepts of universal life energy in which the practitioner holds her or his hands in symbolic patterns over the affected part of the patient's body. It is not a form of massage. Reiki can be used for self-healing as well as treating someone else.

- Therapeutic touch. Therapeutic touch resembles Reiki in that the practitioner is thought to transmit universal energy or "life force" to the patient. Instead of touching the patient directly, however, the practitioner passes his or her hands over the patient's energy field, two to four inches above the body.

Mind- and spirituality-based approaches

Mind-based or spirituality-based approaches draw on the mental and spiritual dimensions of human beings to treat the physical side effects of cancer treatment. They are related to the belief that all dimensions of a person's being should be involved in cancer treatment, and that the mind and spirit can affect or influence physical processes.

These approaches are frequently recommended by health professionals as complementary treatments that allow patients to regain a sense of personal effectiveness and active participation in their lives:

- Prayer. Prayer has been shown in over a hundred reputable double-blind clinical studies to have positive effects on anxiety, high blood pressure, headaches, heart disease, and wounds. The NCCAM considers the act of prayer to be a mind-body therapy.
- Meditation. Meditation is helpful in relieving stress, pain, and other side effects of cancer treatment. There are several different approaches to meditation, such as using a mantra (a sacred word or phrase), chanting, focusing on a visual image, or focusing on one's breath.
- Biofeedback. Biofeedback is a method of learning to modify certain body functions (temperature, heart rate, etc.) related to relaxation with the help of electronic monitors. Eventually, the patient can learn to control his or her relaxation responses without feedback from the machine.
- Hypnosis. Hypnosis is often recommended to lower anxiety and relieve pain. Patients can be hypnotized by a therapist or taught to hypnotize themselves. Hypnosis and biofeedback have both been shown to ease chemotherapy-related nausea and anticipatory nausea (queasiness caused by psychological triggers, such as the sight of the chemotherapy room or smell of treatment chemicals).
- Imagery and visualization. Patients are asked to picture or create an inner image that symbolizes their resistance to cancer. They might visualize their medications as a fire burning up their cancer cells, or their white blood cells as soldiers fighting the enemy.

Sensory-based therapies

Treatments in this category are often used in integrative treatment plans. They are given to help cancer patients cope with the side effects of radiation or **chemotherapy**, to provide positive sensory experiences, and to improve overall quality of life.

Sensory-based treatments include:

- Aromatherapy. Aromatherapy is the use of fragrances—usually the essential oils of flowers and other plant parts—to relax cancer patients or lift their spirits. The fragrant oils are used to scent oil for massage or added to bath water.
- Art therapy. Art therapy allows cancer patients to express their feelings through their creations and to

find satisfaction in learning new skills or techniques. Art therapy may include painting, sculpture, making pottery, quilting, metalwork, print making, photography, or other activities.

- Journaling. Keeping a journal can aid a patient's psychological well being by providing an emotional and creative outlet. Journaling also offers an arena in which patients can sort out thoughts and concerns about their disease.
- Music therapy. Music therapy can be used to help patients relax, release feelings of sadness or anger, or participate in a group activity. It can involve making music as well as listening to it.
- Pet therapy. Pet therapy is the use of trained animals (usually cats, small dogs, birds, or rabbits) in hospital settings to provide comfort and companionship to cancer patients. Petting and talking to the animals has been shown to benefit patients psychologically and physically.

Traditional approaches

Some of the therapies in this category developed outside the European medical tradition, while the last two developed in the West during the eighteenth and nineteenth centuries:

- Native American medicine. Specific beliefs about the causes of disease vary among the five hundred tribes of Native Americans. In general, however, Native American medicine emphasizes the importance of people living in beauty, harmony, and peace with one another and with their environment. Native American healing rituals are most often used as complementary treatments within integrative treatment plans.
- Ayurveda. Ayurveda is the traditional medical system of India. It emphasizes identifying a person's physical and psychological constitution as part of the healing process. Treatments include dietary recommendations and herbal or mineral remedies.
- Traditional Chinese medicine (TCM). TCM includes five major forms of treatment: diet, exercise, acupuncture, massage, and traditional herbal remedies. It regards human health as resulting from balancing the various vital energies within the human body and keeping the body in harmony with its external environment. As of 2009, the NCCAM is funding three studies of Chinese herbal remedies.
- Homeopathy. Homeopathy is a system of treating disease with extremely small doses of substances that would produce symptoms in a healthy person similar to those of the disease being treated. For example, a

homeopathic practitioner might give a feverish patient belladonna, which can cause fever in a healthy person.

- Naturopathy. Naturopathy is an approach to healing that rejects surgery and synthetic drugs. Naturopaths recommend vitamin supplements, natural herbal remedies, diets, and fasting to assist the body's natural healing processes.

Special concerns

Because complementary and alternative therapies vary so widely in their underlying assumptions, their claims to effectiveness, their licensing standards for practitioners, and the materials and equipment involved in their use, patients should talk to their doctor before beginning any complementary or alternative form of treatment. Patients should also investigate said treatments and the practitioner's level of experience in this area.

Surgery

Cancer patients who have had recent surgery should consult their doctor before starting yoga, t'ai chi, or any other form of movement therapy. In addition, Swedish massage and certain forms of deep tissue massage are not suitable for patients who have not fully recovered from surgery.

Clinical trials

Patients who are interested in a specific complementary or alternative therapy may wish to participate in a study of that treatment. Information about CAM trials can be obtained from the NCI's website at http://www.cancernet.nci.nih.gov.

Fraudulent treatments

False claims about a treatment, such as stating that it cures or prevents cancer when it is known to be useless, are sometimes referred to as "quackery." Several groups and organizations can help patients evaluate questionable therapies.

Treatment decisions

Patients considering CAM therapies should ask their doctor:

- What does the treatment claim to do? Cure cancer? Increase the effectiveness of standard treatments? Or relieve symptoms or side effects?
- How is the practitioner licensed or credentialed? For example, there are licensing boards in most states for massage therapists, acupuncturists, practitioners of Chinese medicine, yoga instructors, and homeopaths.

- Is the treatment based on specific theories about the causes of cancer? How are these theories regarded by mainstream health professionals?
- Is the treatment associated with specific types of cancer, such as cancers of the digestive tract or the nervous system?
- Does the treatment have any restrictions or side effects of its own?
- Is the treatment recommended for other diseases or conditions, or only for cancer?
- How is the treatment advertised or promoted? In medical journals, mainstream health publications, the mass media, or only in "New Age" or special-interest magazines?

Patients should look for "red flags" that may indicate that a treatment is fraudulent:

- The treatment is unusually expensive.
- It is based on unproven or discredited theories.
- It claims to be a "secret" offered by only a few providers.
- Patients must go outside the United States or Canada for the treatment.
- Patients are told not to use standard cancer treatments.
- The treatment lacks any connection to reputable licensing bodies, medical schools, research institutions, or cancer organizations.

Resources

BOOKS

American Cancer Society. *The American Cancer Society's Guide to Complementary and Alternative Cancer Methods.* New York: American Cancer Society, 2000.

National Cancer Institute of the National Institutes of Health. *Chemotherapy and You: A Guide to Self-Help During Cancer Treatment.* NIH Publication #99-1136. Can be downloaded from http://cancernet.nci.nih.gov.

OTHER

Cancer Supportive Care Programs. [cited June 21, 2001]. http://www.cancersupportivecare.com. Provides information about pain control, nutrition, and other aspects of supportive care for cancer patients.

The Wellness Community. [cited June 21, 2001]. http://www.wellness-community.org. Offers support groups, stress reduction workshops, exercise programs, social events, and nutritional counseling for cancer patients and their families.

ORGANIZATIONS

American Academy of Medical Acupuncture. (800) 521-2262.

American Association of Naturopathic Physicians. 601 Valley St., Suite 105, Seattle, WA 98109. (206) 298-0126. Fax: (206) 298-0129. http://www.naturopathic.org.

American Botanical Council. http://www.herbalgram.org.

American Cancer Society (ACS). 1599 Clifton Road, NE, Atlanta, GA 30329. (404) 320-3333 or (800) ACS-2345. Fax: (404) 329-7530. http://www.cancer.org.

American Foundation of Traditional Chinese Medicine (AFTCM). 505 Beach Street, San Francisco, CA 94133. (415) 776-0502. Fax: (415) 392-7003. E-mail: aftcm@earth link.net.

American Herbal Products Association. 8484 Georgia Ave., Suite 370, Silver Spring, MD 20910. (301) 588-1174. http://www.ahpa.org.

American Indian Science and Engineering Society (AISES). 5661 Airport Blvd., Boulder, CO 80301-2339. (303) 939-0023. Fax: (303) 939-8150. E-mail: aisehq@spot.color-ado.edu. http://www.colorado.edu/aises.

Consumer Reports Health Letter. P.O. Box 52145, Boulder, CO 80321.

Delta Society (pet therapy). http://www.deltasociety.org.

National Cancer Institute, Office of Cancer Communications. 31 Center Drive, MSC 2580, Bethesda, MD 20892-2580. (800) 4-CANCER. TTY: (800) 332-8615. Email: cancermail@cips.nci.nih.gov. http://www.nci. nih.gov.

National Center for Homeopathy (NCH). 801 North Fairfax St., Suite 306, Alexandria, VA 22314. (703) 548-7790. Fax: (703) 548-7792.

National Certification Board for Therapeutic Massage and Bodywork. 8201 Greensboro Drive, Suite 300, McLean, VA 22102. (703) 610-9015.

National Council Against Health Fraud. P.O. Box 1276, Loma Linda, CA 92354.

NIH National Center for Complementary and Alternative Medicine (NCCAM) Clearinghouse. P. O. Box 8218, Silver Spring, MD 20907-8218. TTY/TDY: (888) 644-6226. Fax: (301) 495-4957. http://www.nccam. nih.gov.

NIH Office of Dietary Supplements. Building 31, Room 1B25, 31 Center Drive, MSC 2086. Bethesda, MD 20892-2086. (301) 435-2920. Fax: (301) 480-1845. Web site: http://odp.od.nih.gov/ods.

Office of Cancer Complementary & Alternative Medicine of the National Cancer Institute (OCCAM). Email: ncioccam1-r @mail.nih.gov. http://www.occam.nci.nih.gov.

Quackwatch. http://www.quackwatch.com.

Rebecca J. Frey, Ph.D.

Computed tomography

Definition

Computed tomography (CT) scanning is a valuable diagnostic tool that provides physicians with views of internal body structures. During a CT scan, multiple **x rays** are passed through the body, producing cross-sectional images, or "slices," on a cathode-ray tube (CRT), a device resembling a television screen. These images can then be preserved on film for examination.

Patient passes into a CT (computed tomography or CAT) scanner. *(Copyright Volker Steger/Science Photo Library, Science Source/Photo Researchers, Inc. Reproduced by permission.)*

CT scan (without color added) of cancer of the rectum. *(Custom Medical Stock Photo. Reproduced by permission.)*

Purpose

CT scans are used to image bone, soft tissues, and air. Since the 1990s, CT equipment has become more affordable and available. CT scans have become the imaging exam of choice for the diagnoses of most solid tumors. Because the computerized image is sharp, focused, and three-dimensional, many structures can be better differentiated than on standard x rays.

Common indications for CT scans include:

• Sinus studies. The CT scan can show details of sinusitis, bone fractures, and the presence of bony tumor involvement. Physicians may order a CT scan of the sinuses to provide an accurate map for surgery.

• Brain studies. Brain CT scans can detect hematomas, tumors, strokes, aneurysms, and degenerative or

A colorized computed tomography (CT) scan, of the human brain. *(Custom Medical Stock Photo. Reproduced by permission.)*

infected brain tissue. The introduction of CT scanning, especially spiral CT, has helped reduce the need for more invasive procedures such as cerebral angiography.

- Body scans. CT scans of the chest, abdomen, spine, and extremities can detect the presence of tumors, enlarged lymph nodes, abnormal collection of fluid, and vertebral disc disease. These scans can also be helpful in evaluating the extent of bone breakdown in osteoporosis.

- Heart and aorta scans. CT scans can focus on the thoracic or abdominal aorta to locate aneurysms and other possible aortic diseases. A newer type of CT scan, called electron beam CT, can be used to detect calcium buildup in arteries. Because it is a new technology, it is not yet widely used and its indications are not yet well-defined.

- Chest scans. CT scans of the chest are useful in distinguishing tumors and in detailing accumulation of fluid in chest infections.

Precautions

Pregnant women or those who could possibly be pregnant should not have a CT scan, particularly a full body or abdominal scan, unless the diagnostic benefits outweigh the risks. If the exam is necessary for obstetric purposes, technologists are instructed not to repeat

films if there are errors. Pregnant patients receiving a CT scan or any x ray exam away from the abdominal area may be protected by a lead apron; most radiation, known as scatter, travels through the body, however, and is not blocked by the apron.

Contrast agents are often used in CT exams, though some types of tumors are better seen without it. Patients should discuss the use of contrast agents with their doctor, and should be asked to sign a consent form prior to the administration of contrast. One of the common contrast agents, iodine, can cause allergic reactions. Patients who are known to be allergic to iodine or shellfish should inform the physician prior to the CT scan; a combination of medications can be given to such patients before the scan to prevent or minimize the reaction. Contrast agents may also put patients with diabetes at risk of kidney failure, particularly those taking the medication glucophage.

Description

Computed tomography, also called CT scan, CAT scan, or computerized axial tomography, is a combination of focused x-ray beams and the computerized production of an image. Introduced in the early 1970s, this radiologic procedure has advanced rapidly and is now widely used, sometimes in the place of standard x rays.

CT equipment

A CT scan may be performed in a hospital or outpatient imaging center. Although the equipment looks large and intimidating, it is very sophisticated and fairly comfortable. The patient is asked to lie on a gantry, or narrow table, that slides into the center of the scanner. The scanner looks like a doughnut and is round in the middle, which allows the x-ray beam to rotate around the patient. The scanner section may also

KEY TERMS

Aneurysm—The bulging of the blood vessel wall. Aortic aneurysms are the most dangerous. Aneurysms can break and cause bleeding.

Contrast (agent, medium)—A substance injected into the body that illuminates certain structures that would otherwise be hard to see on the radiograph (film).

Gantry—A name for the couch or table used in a CT scan. The patient lies on the gantry while it slides into the x-ray scanner.

Hematoma—A collection of blood that has escaped from the vessels. It may clot and harden, causing pain to the patient.

Metastasis—Secondary cancer, or cancer that has spread from one body organ or tissue to another.

Radiologist—A medical doctor specially trained in radiology (x ray) interpretation and its use in the diagnosis of disease and injury.

Spiral CT—Also referred to as helical CT, this method allows for continuous 360-degree x-ray image capture.

Thoracic—Refers to the chest area. The thorax runs between the abdomen and neck and is encased in the ribs.

be tilted slightly to allow for certain cross-sectional angles.

CT procedure

The gantry moves very slightly as the precise adjustments for each sectional image are made. A technologist watches the procedure from a window and views the images on a computer screen. Generally, patients are alone during the procedure, though exceptions are sometimes made for pediatric patients. Communication is possible via an intercom system.

It is essential that the patient lie very still during the procedure to prevent motion blurring. In some studies, such as chest CTs, the patient will be asked to hold his or her breath during image capture.

Following the procedure, films of the images are usually printed for the radiologist and referring physician to review. A radiologist can also interpret CT exams on the computer screen. The procedure time will vary in length depending on the area being imaged. Average study times are from 30 to 60 minutes. Some

patients may be concerned about claustrophobia but the width of the "doughnut" portion of the scanner is such that many patients can be reassured of openness. Doctors may consider giving sedatives to patients who have severe claustrophobia or difficulty lying still.

The CT image

While traditional x-ray machines image organs in two dimensions, often resulting in organs in the front of the body being superimposed over those in the back, CT scans allow for a more three-dimensional effect. CT images can be likened to slices in a loaf of bread. Precise sections of the body can be located and imaged as cross-sectional views. The screen before the technologist shows a computer's analysis of each section detected by the x-ray beam. Thus, various densities of tissue can be easily distinguished.

Contrast agents

Contrast agents are often used in CT exams and in other radiology procedures to illuminate certain details of anatomy more clearly. Some contrasts are natural, such as air or water. A water-based contrast agent is sometimes administered for specific diagnostic purposes. Barium sulfate is commonly used in gastroenterology procedures. The patient may drink this contrast or receive it in an enema. Oral or rectal contrast is usually given when examining the abdomen or cells, but not when scanning the brain or chest. Iodine is the most widely used intravenous contrast agent and is given through an intravenous needle.

If contrast agents are used in the CT exam, these will be administered several minutes before the study begins. Patients undergoing abdominal CT may be asked to drink a contrast medium. Some patients may experience a salty taste, flushing of the face, warmth or slight **nausea**, or hives from an intravenous contrast injection. Technologists and radiologists have the equipment and training to help patients through these minor reactions and to handle more severe reactions. Severe reactions to contrast are rare, but do occur.

Newer types of CT scans

The spiral CT scan, also called a helical CT, is a newer version of CT. This type of scan is continuous in motion and allows for the continuous re-creation of images. For example, traditional CT allows the technologist to take slices at very small and precise intervals one after the other. Spiral CT allows for a continuous flow of images, without stopping the scanner to move to the next image slice. A major advantage of spiral CT is the ability to reconstruct images anywhere along the length of the study area. Because the procedure is faster, patients are required to lie still for shorter periods of time. The ability to image contrast more rapidly after it is injected, when it is at its highest level, is another advantage of spiral CT's high speed.

Electron beam CT scans are another newer type of CT technology that can be used to detect calcium buildup in arteries. These calcium deposits are potential risk factors for coronary artery disease. Electron beam CT scans take pictures much more quickly than conventional CTs, and are therefore better able to produce clear images of the heart as it pumps blood. Because it is a newer and expensive test, electron beam CT scanning is not widely used.

Some facilities will have spiral, electron, and conventional CT available. Although spiral is more advantageous for many applications, conventional CT is still a superior and precise method for imaging many tissues and structures. The physician will evaluate which type of CT works best for the specific exam purpose.

Preparation

If a contrast medium is administered, the patient may be asked to fast for about four to six hours prior to the procedure. Patients will usually be given a gown (like a typical hospital gown) to be worn during the procedure. All metal and jewelry should be removed to avoid artifacts on the film. Depending on the type of study, patients may also be required to remove dentures.

Aftercare

Generally, no aftercare is required following a CT scan. Immediately following the exam, the technologist will continue to watch the patient for possible adverse contrast reactions. Patients are instructed to advise the technologist of any symptoms, particularly respiratory difficulty. The site of contrast injection will be bandaged and may feel tender following the exam.

Risks

Radiation exposure from a CT scan is similar to, though higher than, that of a conventional x ray. Although this is a risk to pregnant women, the risk for other adults is minimal and should produce no effects. Severe contrast reactions are rare, but they are a risk of many CT procedures.

Normal results

Normal findings on a CT exam show bone, the most dense tissue, as white areas. Tissues and fat will show as various shades of gray, and fluids will be gray or black. Air will also look black. Intravenous, oral, and rectal contrast appear as white areas. The radiologist can determine if tissues and organs appear normal by the sensitivity of the gray shadows.

Abnormal results

Abnormal results may show different characteristics of tissues within organs. Accumulations of blood or other fluids where they do not belong may be detected. Radiologists can differentiate among types of tumors throughout the body by viewing details of their makeup.

Sinus studies

The increasing availability and lowered cost of CT scanning has lead to its increased use in sinus studies, either as a replacement for a sinus x ray or as a follow-up to an abnormal sinus radiograph. The sensitivity of CT allows for the location of areas of sinus **infection**, particularly chronic infection. Sinus tumors will show as shades of gray indicating the difference in their density from that of normal tissues in the area.

Brain studies

The precise differences in density allowed by CT scan can clearly show tumors, strokes, or lesions in the brain area as altered densities. These lighter or darker areas on the image may indicate a tumor or hematoma within the brain and skull area. Different types of tumors can be identified by the presence of edema, by the tissue's density, or by studying blood vessel location and activity. The speed and convenience of CT often allows for detection of hemorrhage before symptoms even occur.

Body scans

The body CT scan can identify abnormal body structures and organs. A CT scan may indicate tumors or cysts, enlarged lymph nodes, abnormal collections of fluids, blood or fat, or cancer **metastasis**. Tumors resulting from metastasis are different in makeup than primary (original) tumors.

Chest scans

In addition to those findings that may indicate aortic aneurysms, chest CT studies can show other problems in the heart and lungs, and distinguish between an aortic aneurysm and a tumor adjacent to the aorta. CT will not only show differences between air, water, tissues and bone, but will also assign numerical values to the various densities. Coin-sized lesions in the lungs may be indicative of tuberculosis or tumors. CT will help distinguish among the two. Enlarged lymph nodes in the chest area may indicate **Hodgkin's disease**.

Resources

BOOKS

Abeloff, M. *Clinical Oncology*. 2nd ed. Orlando, Florida: Churchill Livingstone, Inc., 2000.

PERIODICALS

Holbert, J. M. "Role of Spiral Computed Tomography in the Diagnosis of Pulmonary Embolism in the

Emergency Department." *Annals of Emergency Medicine* May 1999: 520-28.

Teresa G. Odle

Computerized axial tomography *see* **Computed tomography**

Cone biopsy

Definition

A cone **biopsy** is a surgical procedure in which a cone-shaped tissue sample from the cervix is removed for examination. Also called cervical conization, a

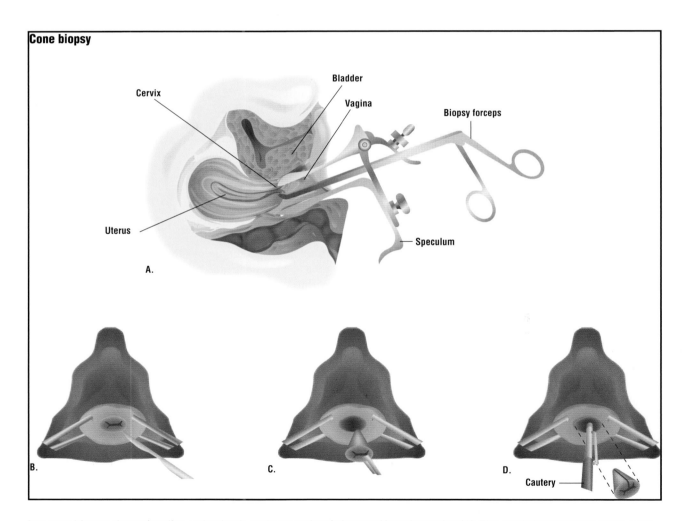

Cone biopsy

In a cone biopsy, the patient lies on her back, and a speculum is inserted into the vagina (A). The cervix is visualized, and a cone-shaped piece of the cervix is removed (B and C). A cauterizing tool is used to stop any bleeding (D). *(Illustration by GGS Information Services. Cengage Learning, Gale.)*

cone biopsy is done to diagnose **cervical cancer** or to remove cancerous or precancerous tissue.

Purpose

The cervix is the neck-shaped opening at the lower part of the uterus. The American Cancer Society estimated that in 2007, approximately 11,150 women would be diagnosed with **cancer** of the cervix, and 3,670 women would die of the disease. When cervical cancer is detected and treated in its early stages, however, the long-term rate of survival is almost 100%.

A cone biopsy is performed to diagnose cancer of the cervix or to detect precancerous changes. The procedure is often recommended if a Pap test indicates the presence of abnormal cells. In some cases, a cone biopsy may be used as a conservative treatment for cervical cancer for women who wish to avoid a hysterectomy (surgical removal of the uterus).

Demographics

The risk of developing cervical cancer increases with age through a woman's 20s and 30s; the risk remains about the same for women over the age of 40. Minority women and women of low socioeconomic status have higher rates of cervical cancer and an increased mortality rate. According to the Centers for Disease Control and Prevention (CDC), African-American, Asian-American, and Hispanic women have a higher-than-average incidence of the disease, while African-American and Hispanic women have a higher rate of cervical cancer-related death.

Description

The procedure is performed with the patient lying on her back with her legs in stirrups. General anesthesia is commonly used, although regional (spinal or epidural) or local anesthesia may also be used. A speculum is inserted into the vagina to hold it open during surgery.

There are several different methods that may be used to perform a cone biopsy. Cold-knife conization is the removal of a cone-shaped wedge of tissue with a scalpel. The tissue may also be removed using a carbon dioxide laser, a procedure called laser conization. A loop electrosurgical excision procedure (LEEP) uses low-voltage, high-frequency radio waves to excise the tissue. Some surgeons choose to cover the open cervical tissue with flaps of tissue stitched into place.

The tissue sample will then be examined under a microscope for the presence of cancerous cells. If abnormal cells are found around the edge of the biopsy, then further surgery will be required to excise any remaining cancer. If there is evidence of invasive cancer (i.e., the cancer has spread to surrounding tissues), then other treatments, such as more extensive surgery, **chemotherapy**, and/or radiation, may be recommended.

Diagnosis/Preparation

A number of tests may be performed prior to cone biopsy to determine if precancerous or cancerous cells exist. A Pap test involves scraping the cervix for a sample of cells and then staining and examining the cells for any abnormalities. Colposcopy is a procedure that allows a physician to examine a woman's cervix and vagina using a special microscope called a colposcope. A cervical biopsy involves the extraction of a smaller tissue sample and is less invasive than a cone biopsy. Based on the results of these tests, a cone biopsy may be indicated if moderate to severe cell abnormalities are found.

As cone biopsy is commonly performed under general anesthesia, the patient is usually instructed to refrain from eating and drinking after midnight on the day of surgery.

Aftercare

After the procedure, the patient may experience some cramping, discomfort, or mild to moderate bleeding. The biopsy site may take up to six weeks to completely heal. The patient will be instructed to avoid intercourse, tampons, and douches for at least three weeks following the procedure.

Risks

Bleeding during and after cone biopsy is the most common complication. Rarely, uncontrolled bleeding during the procedure may result in an emergency hysterectomy. Other potential complications include reaction to the anesthesia, **infection** of the biopsy site, injury to the uterus or other tissues, cervical stenosis (when the cervical canal narrows or becomes closed), and failure to remove all cancerous tissue. If too much tissue is removed during a cone biopsy so that the internal opening of the cervix to the uterus (called the internal os) is affected, a woman may have difficulty carrying a pregnancy to term, increasing her risk of miscarriage or premature birth.

Normal results

Numerous studies have indicated that cone biopsy is successful in excising all cancerous tissue in 90% of patients with cervical cancer.

Morbidity and mortality rates

Between 2% and 8% of women who undergo a cone biopsy will experience bleeding for up to two weeks. One study found that cervical stenosis occurs at a rate of 3–8%, depending on the method of conization.

Alternatives

Cryotherapy (freezing and destroying of abnormal cells) or laser vaporization (using a laser to destroy abnormal cells) may be used to treat early-stage cancer. A hysterectomy may be necessary to remove more invasive cancer. In a subtotal hysterectomy, only the uterus is removed. In a radical hysterectomy, the uterus, cervix, ovaries, fallopian tubes, lymph nodes, and lymph channels are removed. The type of hysterectomy performed depends on how far the cancer has spread. In all cases, menstruation stops and a woman loses the ability to bear children.

Resources

BOOKS

Abeloff, M. D., et al. *Clinical Oncology.* 3rd ed. Philadelphia: Elsevier, 2004.

Gabbe, S. G., et al. *Obstetrics: Normal and Problem Pregnancies.* 5th ed. London: Churchill Livingstone, 2007.

Katz, V. L., et al. *Comprehensive Gynecology.* 5th ed. St. Louis: Mosby, 2007.

PERIODICALS

Brun, J. L., A. Youbi, and C. Hocke. "Complications, Sequellae and Outcome of Cervical Conizations: Evaluation of Three Surgical Techniques." *Journal of Gynecology and Obstetrics and Reproductive Biology* 31, no. 6 (January 10, 2002): 558–64.

OTHER

"All About Cervical Cancer: Overview." *American Cancer Society* 2003 [March 18, 2003]. http://www.cancer.org/docroot/CRI/CRI_2_1x.asp (accessed March 11, 2008).

National Cervical Cancer Coalition May 23, 2002 [cited March 18, 2003]. http://www.nccc-online.org/ (accessed March 11, 2008).

Nyirjesy, Istvan. "Conization of Cervix." *eMedicine* June 28, 2002 [cited March 18, 2003]. http://www.emedicine.com/med/topic3338.htm (accessed March 11, 2008).

Ries, L. A., et al., (eds). "SEER Cancer Statistics Review, 1973–1999." *National Cancer Institute* 2002 [cited March 18, 2003]. http://seer.cancer.gov/csr/1973_1999 (accessed March 11, 2008).

ORGANIZATIONS

American Cancer Society. 1599 Clifton Road NE, Atlanta, GA 30329. (800) ACS-2345. http://www.cancer.org (accessed March 11, 2008).

American College of Obstetricians and Gynecologists. 409 12th St., S.W., PO Box 96920, Washington, D.C. 20090-6920. http://www.acog.org (accessed March 11, 2008).

Stephanie Dionne Sherk
Rosalyn Carson-DeWitt, MD

Corticosteroids

Definition

Corticosteroids are a group of related drugs used in **cancer** treatment to reduce the growth of tumors, stimulate the appetite, and treat skin rashes, **nausea and vomiting**, allergic reactions, inflammation, accumulation of fluid in the brain, and autoimmune disease.

Purpose

Corticosteroids have broad use in cancer treatment. Some are used to treat adult leukemias, adult lymphomas, acute childhood leukemia, **multiple myeloma**, and advanced **prostate cancer**. Others are used in creams to treat skin rashes from **radiation therapy**. Corticosteroids are also used to reduce swelling, especially in the brain and spinal column, reduce **nausea** and **vomiting**, and improve appetite.

Description

Corticosteroids occur naturally in the body. They are produced by the cortex of the adrenal glands, a small, pea-sized pair of glands that are located in the lower back, just above the kidney. Some corticosteroids regulate fluid balance in the body. Others influence fat and sugar (glucose) usage. Corticosteroids are chemically related to the sex hormones estrogen and **testosterone**.

Many different corticosteroids are produced artificially to use as drugs. They are administered as creams, tablets, liquids, or intravenously (or injection directly into a vein). Many people are already familiar with hydrocortisone, a corticosteroid found in low doses in over-the-counter creams.

The most common corticosteroids used in cancer treatment are:

- dexamethasone (Decadron)
- hydrocortisone
- methylprednisolone (Medrol)
- prednisone
- cortisone
- betamethasone
- prednisolone

There are many trade names for drugs containing these corticosteroids.

Recommended dosage

Corticosteroids come in tablets, liquids, intravenous solutions, and creams. Because of their wide variety of uses and forms, there is no standard recommended dose. Dosage is individualized, and depends on the type of cancer, the patient's body weight and general health, the goal of the treatment, the other drugs being given, and the way a patient's cancer responds to the drug. Corticosteroids should be stored away from heat.

Precautions

People taking corticosteroids may want to go on a low-salt, high-potassium diet in order to reduce water retention. They may also want to watch their calorie intake unless corticosteroids are being given to improve appetite. Patients taking large doses of corticosteroids are more susceptible to **infection** and should try to avoid contact with crowds or any individuals that may have an infection. Patients should seek immediate medical advice if they are exposed to chicken pox or measles.

Side effects

Corticosteroids have several side effects. Not every side effect is seen in every patient. The most serious, although rare, side effect is an allergic reaction to corticosteroids when given intravenously (IV). Other side effects can include:

- salt and water retention
- excessive potassium loss
- high blood pressure
- other fluid and electrolyte imbalances
- loss of muscle tissue
- loss of bone strength (osteoporosis)
- easily fractured bones
- heartburn and ulcers
- thin, fragile skin
- slow wound healing
- skin rashes
- masking of infection
- convulsions
- headache
- dizziness
- reproductive irregularities
- strong mood changes
- changes in the functioning of the adrenal gland
- increased pressure in the eye
- glaucoma, cataracts, and blindness (rare)
- nausea
- fatigue
- increased appetite
- weight gain
- increased urination

Interactions

Many drugs interact with nonprescription (over-the-counter) drugs and herbal remedies. Patients should always tell their health care providers about these remedies, as well as any prescription drugs they are taking. Patients should also notify their physician if they are on a special diet.

Corticosteroids can also interact with anticoagulants (blood thinners such as Coumadin), **cyclosporine**, phenobarbitol, and antidepressants.

Tish Davidson, A.M.

Coughing up blood *see* **Hemoptysis**

Craniopharyngioma

Definition

Craniopharyngioma is a **cancer** that arises in the pituitary gland, in tissue originally found in the embryo. One of the most common childhood brain cancers, it is also sometimes called a Rathke's pouch tumor or a suprasellar cyst.

Description

Craniopharyngioma is the second most common type of childhood brain tumor, accounting for almost 10% of all **brain tumors** in children. This cancer has very little tendency to spread to other parts of the body. It readily invades local tissues, however, and since it occurs deep within the brain, invasion of local tissues alone can result in serious illness or even death.

Magnetic resonance image (MRI) of a craniopharyngioma brain tumor. *(Custom Medical Stock Photo. Reproduced by permission.)*

The pituitary gland produces many hormones that play critical roles in the development and regulation of the body. Because this cancer arises in the pituitary gland, it often results in deficiencies of the various hormones that the pituitary gland produces. The tumor can be either solid or cystic or mixed, and most (up to 90%) of craniopharyngiomas contain calcium deposits, an indication of diseased tissue readily observable on **x rays**.

Demographics

The large majority of craniopharyngiomas are childhood tumors. The median age at diagnosis is eight years; peak incidence is between the ages of six and eleven. Almost 70% of all craniopharyngiomas occur before the age of 20, although a small peak occurs after the age of 50. Diagnosis before the age of two is very rare. Girls and boys and all races are affected equally.

Causes and symptoms

The cause of craniopharyngioma is not really understood, although it is believed to be primarily a congenital illness. Nests of embryonic cells exist in a part of the pituitary gland known as Rathke's pouch. In craniopharyngioma, these nests appear to contain cancerous cells which, over time, multiply and become a tumor.

The symptoms of craniopharyngioma can be divided into two categories. Some are nonspecific symptoms which occur because of increased pressure within the skull; some result from deficiencies of the hormones that the pituitary gland normally produces. Any individual patient may have various combinations of symptoms and both the number of symptoms and the severity of the symptoms typically increase over time. Nonspecific symptoms of increased intracranial pressure include:

- headache
- visual disturbances
- irritability
- personality changes
- mental disturbances

Symptoms that can result from hormone deficiencies include:

- diabetes
- growth retardation
- sexual dysfunction (in adults)

Diagnosis

Most patients seek medical attention because of headaches or visual disturbances, failure to match normal growth patterns (due to a deficiency of growth hormone), or symptoms of diabetes. If (after other causes of symptoms are ruled out) a craniopharyngioma is suspected, usually some kind of imaging technique is performed. Traditional x rays reveal an enlargement of the space at the base of the skull where the tumor is typically found, and will also show calcification of cancerous cells. **Computed tomography** (CT scan or CAT scan) may show calcification that does not show up on x rays and also shows whether the tumor is cystic or solid in nature. **Magnetic resonance imaging** (MRI) can show how much the tumor has invaded the surrounding tissues.

Often the amounts of pituitary hormones in the blood are measured as well. Measurements may be made of gonadatropins (hormones which regulate reproduction), thyrotropin (a hormone that regulates the thyroid gland), growth hormones (regulates growth), corticotropin (a hormone that regulates carbohydrate metabolism, vasopressin (a hormone that regulates water retention), or prolactin (a hormone that regulates milk production in mothers of infants).

Treatment team

As the understanding of cancer grows and new treatment approaches are developed, the complexity of cancer treatment also increases. Today, a multidisciplinary approach to cancer treatment is considered necessary for effective patient care. Since craniopharyngioma is a neuroendocrine tumor that occurs deep in the brain and mainly in children, optimal treatment requires a particularly complex and sophisticated team of health professionals. The types of people who may be involved in treating or caring for a patient with craniopharyngioma and their family typically include oncologists (pediatric), pathologists (neuropathologists), radiation oncologists, radiation technicians, psychiatrists, oncology social workers, nutritionists, home health care providers, endocrinologists, rehabilitative specialists, and neurosurgeons. The surgeon, specifically, should be a pediatric neurosurgeon, as these specialists have been shown to provide better long-term outcomes than general neurosurgeons.

Clinical staging, treatments, and prognosis

Standard treatment for craniopharyngioma consists of surgical removal of as much of the tumor as is readily accessible, followed by **radiation therapy**. Although total removal of the tumor yields the best odds of survival, the location in which this cancer occurs (and the fact that these tumors are typically covered by a thick membrane that adheres tightly to surrounding tissues) can make total removal difficult. Attempts to remove the tumor completely, therefore, often result in significant and unacceptable side effects. A better quality of life, and therefore better overall outcome, is obtained through partial removal of the tumor followed by radiation therapy. This is now generally accepted as the best treatment approach.

Chemotherapy is not routinely used for treatment of craniopharyngioma, although some medications are commonly used to treat symptoms. Drugs that decrease inflammation and reduce the probability of convulsions may be given preoperatively to make surgical removal of the tumor safer. Hormone replacement therapy may be necessary if the cancer, occurring in the pituitary gland, causes serious hormone deficiency problems.

Therapies that are not routinely used but have shown some promise include internal placement of radioactive material and improvements in surgical techniques, including **stereotactic surgery**, which utilizes a radioactive "gamma knife" for excision of the tumor.

Since this type of cancer does not demonstrate a tendency to spread to remote areas of the body, staging or grading systems are not usually used. Factors that improve survival are complete removal of the tumor (although this often results in greatly decreased quality of life), the size of the tumor at diagnosis, a cystic rather than solid nature of the tumor, and an age of at least five years old at diagnosis. Unfortunately, most patients who survive have significant remaining illness, and predicting how much function may be lost is as important in this cancer as prognosis of survival. It is important to remember, especially with regards to extent of functional capacity to be expected, that the physician's prognosis is only an educated guess, and that positive thinking can contribute significantly to a better quality of life.

Alternative and complementary therapies

Alternative and complementary therapies are treatments which are not traditional, first-line therapies like surgery, chemotherapy and radiation. Complementary therapies are those that are meant to supplement traditional therapies and usually have the objective of relieving symptoms or helping cancer patients cope with the disease or traditional treatments. Alternative therapies are nontraditional treatments which are chosen instead of traditional treatments in an attempt to cure the disease. Alternative therapies have typically not been proven to be effective in the same way that traditional drugs are evaluated, in studies called **clinical trials**, and are usually not recommended for use with children.

Common complementary therapies that may be employed by cancer patients include aromatherapy, art therapy, massage, meditation, music therapy, prayer, t'ai chi, and yoga or other forms of exercise, which reduce anxiety and can increase a patient's feeling of well-being. Many patients also take high doses of **vitamins** and other nutritional supplements, especially A, C, E, and selenium, which are thought to act as **antioxidants**. Any physical activities or nutritional supplements (especially when treating a child) should be discussed with then patient's physician.

Numerous alternative therapies exist in cancer treatment. Special caution must be used, however, when considering alternative therapies for children's cancers. Although alternative treatments, by definition, have not been proven effective by scientific methods, some brain tumor patients believe that the use of alternative therapies has been beneficial. Some alternate therapies include:

- Laetrile, a product of apricot seeds, contains a form of cyanide that proponents believe may be released by tumor enzymes and act to kill cancerous cells. Laetrile is not approved by the Food and Drug Administration for use in the United States. The National Cancer Institute sponsored two studies of laetrile in the late 1970s and early 1980s, but concluded after the second study that no additional research was necessary.

- Vitamin E, melatonin, aloe vera, and a compound called beta-1,3-glucan are reported to stimulate the immune system. Some practitioners believe that natural substances like garlic, ginger, and shark cartilage shrink tumors, although how they are supposed to work is not really defined.

- Antineoplastons are believed by some to be another alternative approach to a cancer cure. Antineoplastons are small proteins which may act as molecular messengers and which may be absent from the urine and blood of many cancer patients. The therapy is based on the idea that replacing these proteins may have beneficial effects. However, the National Cancer Institute proposed phase II clinical trials, and protocols were developed, but the trials never got underway on a large scale because of lack of patient participation. The National Cancer Institute draws no definitive conclusions about the treatment's effectiveness due to lack of clinical trials.

Coping with cancer treatment

Children have special needs when coping with treatment, depending on their age. Some comprehensive resources are available about how families can cope with cancer diagnoses, but some coping strategies are summarized here. Very young children need affection, soothing, time to play, and reassurances; toddlers have these same needs, but also may need to be taught how to express their anger or frustration, and will need simple explanations about what is happening. School-age children may enjoy a little more involvement in their treatment plan, and will need empathy about missing school and activities. They may benefit from drawing or keeping a journal, communicating with friends, and, if possible, a little physical activity each day. Adolescents have similar needs, but also may want to keep some thoughts and feelings private, and also may have more complex spiritual concerns along with feelings of anger and frustration. The siblings and parents of the child with cancer will have needs and concerns and will need to adopt coping strategies as well. The patient's treatment team can help point the family to helpful resources.

Treatment of craniopharyngioma commonly includes surgery and radiation therapy. Although the use of radiation therapy in addition to surgery has improved the quality of life for craniopharyngioma patients, treatments unavoidably result in damage to some healthy tissues and other undesirable side effects.

Fatigue is a very common side effect of radiation therapy. Patients should expect to be very sleepy and therefore to cut back on activities, allowing plenty of time for resting and letting the body heal. It is also important to try maintain a well-balanced, nutritious diet. Patients should avoid as much extra stress as possible and should limit visitors, if needed, to avoid being overtired.

Another problem for those undergoing radiation therapy is dry, sore skin in the area being treated. (Radiation does not hurt during treatment and does not make the person radioactive.) Skin in the treatment area is essentially "burned" and may blister and peel, becoming painful. Patients with fair skin or those who have undergone previous chemotherapy have a greater risk of more serious reactions. Dry, itchy, or sore skin is temporary, but skin in the treatment area may remain more sensitive to sun exposure, so a good sunscreen should be used whenever affected skin is exposed to sunlight.

Radiation therapy requires a substantial level of commitment from the patient in terms of time and emotional energy. Fear and anxiety are major factors in coping with cancer in general and these cancer treatments specifically. The feelings are completely normal. Some patients find that concentrating on restful, pleasurable activities like hobbies, prayer, or meditation is helpful in decreasing negative emotions. It is also very important that patients have people to whom they can express their fears and other negative emotions. If friends or family members are unable to provide this to patients, support groups may help to provide an environment where fears can be freely expressed and understood.

Clinical trials

Although numerous clinical trials are in progress that evaluate treatments for childhood brain tumors, few of these are specifically concerned with craniopharyngioma. Most clinical trials for childhood brain tumors are evaluating new medications or new chemotherapy combinations. Although some of these may prove effective against craniopharyngiomas, chemotherapy at this time is not considered an appropriate approach to treatment of this disease. Some new therapies with potential value for cranipharyngioma patients include new forms of drug delivery, including liposomes, and immune-based therapies like **monoclonal antibodies**. In addition, new refinements of surgical techniques, including MRI-assisted surgery and stereotactic surgery, including the bloodless "gamma knife" surgery, are being evaluated. A clinical trial evaluating a pharmaceutical therapy for a common side effect of surgical treatment of craniopharygioma, hypothalmic obesity, is ongoing.

Prevention

Craniopharyngioma is believed to be a congenital disease, and there is no known way to prevent this cancer.

Special concerns

This tumor is characterized by various diseases related to hormone deficiencies that may arise as the result of the tumor itself or as the result of either surgical or radiation therapy. The tumor may cause problems related to hormone deficiencies, especially diabetes or growth retardation, and these are often the reason that medical attention is first sought. Craniopharyngioma patients may also experience sleep disorders, changes in personality, and mental disturbances. In addition, treatment for craniopharyngioma can create a condition called hypothalmic obesity, in which a patient steadily gains weight although eating patterns may not have changed. Although many of these problems may significantly improve with time, care of a family member with a brain tumor is a significantly stressful experience for caregivers, which creates a huge strain on normal family life.

As mentioned, **childhood cancers** create unique concerns for the children diagnosed and their families.

Parents and siblings, as well as the cancer patient, all have emotional issues to address, in addition to everyday concerns, such as social development, friends, and school. Hospital staff and social workers can help direct a family to useful resources for support. Support groups for craniopharyngioma patients and for parents of craniopharyngioma patients offer patients and parents a place to discuss their fears and concerns with other people who have been impacted by this disease.

Resources

BOOKS

Abeloff, editor. *Clinical Oncology*. New York: Churchill Livingstone.

Buckman, R. *What You Really Need to Know About Cancer*. Baltimore: Johns Hopkins University Press, 1999.

PERIODICALS

Lafferty, A. R. "Pituitary Tumors in Children and Adolescents." *Journal of Clinical Endocrinology and Metabolism* 84 (December 1999): 4317-4322.

ORGANIZATIONS

American Cancer Society. 1599 Clifton Road, NE, Atlanta, GA 30329-4251. (800)586-4872 http://www.cancer.org.

Candlelighter Childhood Cancer Foundation. 3910 Warner St., Kensington, MD 20895. 1-800-366-2223.http://www.candlelighters.org.

Childhood Brain Tumor Foundation. 20312 Watkins Meadow Drive, Germantown, MD 20867. (301)515-2900. http://www.childhoodbraintumor.org.

National Cancer Institute. 9000 Rockville Pike, Bethesda, Maryland, 20892. (800)422-6237. http:www.nci.nih.gov.

National Children's Cancer Society, Suite 600, 1015 Locust St. St. Louis, MO 63101. 1-800-532-6459. http://www.children-cancer.com.

The Wellness Community. 10921 Reed Harman Highway, Cincinnati, Ohio, 45242 (888)793-9355.

Wendy Wippel, M.Sc.

Craniosynostosis

Definition

Craniosynostosis is a birth defect of the brain in which the cranial sutures (the fibrous joints between the bones of the skull) in the skull of an infant close too early, causing problems with normal brain and skull growth. Premature closure of the sutures may cause the skull or facial bones to change from a normal, symmetrical appearance to an abnormal, asymmetrical

appearance and may also cause the pressure inside of the head to increase.

Description

The skull of an infant is made up of five free-floating bones separated by cranial sutures, which allows the infant to pass through the birth canal. The five bones are: the occipital bone, in the back portion of the skull; the two parietal bones, on either side of the skull; and two frontal bones, on the front portion of the skull. The bones fit together like a puzzle, and the areas where the bones meet one another are called the sutures, which are the fibrous joints. The bones and the sutures serve as a protective shield for the brain.

As the infant's brain grows rapidly during early infancy, the open sutures allow the skull to expand and to develop into a normal shape. However, if one or more of the sutures closes prematurely, either before birth or during the first few months of life, the skull compensates by expanding in the direction of the remaining open sutures, resulting in an abnormal shape. Children with craniosynostosis may also have increased pressure on the brain, resulting in developmental delays, and vision problems as a result of an imbalance in their ocular muscles. Craniosynostosis occurs in one out of 2,000 live births and affects males twice as often as females.

There are several types of craniosynostosis. The sagittal suture, the most common single suture involved in craniosynostosis, runs from a spot at the front of the head to the back of the skull. In sagittal synostosis, the sagittal suture closes, resulting in the infant's head growing long and narrow, rather than expanding in width, in order to accommodate the growth of brain. There may or may not be bulging of both the front and back of the head.

The metopic suture runs from the nose up to the top of the skull, where it meets the sagittal suture. When the metopic suture closes, in metopic synotosis, the infant has a ridge down the forehead that can be seen or felt, and the forehead is narrow and triangular. The eyebrows may appear pinched on either side, and the eyes often seem to be close together. This head shape is referred to as trigonocephaly.

Early closure of one side of the coronal suture, which goes from ear to ear on the top of the head, is referred to as unilateral coronal synotosis (plagiocephaly). The forehead and orbital rim (eyebrow) have a flattened appearance on the affected side of the skull, resulting in a "winking" effect. In bicoronal synotosis, both sides of the coronal suture are fused, and the child may have a flat, recessed forehead. In addition, the head is short and wide, and there may be bulging of the eyes and bulging of the skull around the ears. This type of synotosis is most often found in children with Crouzon's and Apert's syndromes.

Lambdoid synotosis, the most rare form, resulting in bulging over the suture, and the ear on the affected side is pulled up and backwards over the suture, resulting in a flattening of the backside of the skull.

Multiple suture synotosis involves the fusing of all of the skull sutures. This condition requires emergency intervention.

The psychological effects of a noticeably misshapen forehead and face can be devastating to a child, resulting in low self-esteem and behavioral problems. Therefore it is important to correct cosmetic deformities of the skull and face.

Causes and symptoms

Most cases of craniosynostosis have no known causes. Some cases may be attributed to intrauterine restraint or early engagement of the head. Craniosynostosis is also associated with some known genetic chromosomal defects, including Apert, Crouzon, Pfieffer, and Saethre-Chotzen Syndromes.

Most children with craniosynostosis do not have any symptoms, except that the head shape is abnormal, and the face may be malformed. Rarely, the affected child may suffer symptoms such as increased pressure in the head, headaches, decreased appetite, **vomiting**, or even developmental delays or mental retardation.

Diagnosis

An infant with a distorted, misshapen head at birth should be examined by a pediatric neurosurgeon and a craniofacial surgeon to determine if the abnormality is due to abnormal fetal positions and neck tightness or due to craniosynotosis. The physical examination includes feeling the skull for suture ridges, spot spots, and checking the neck position, and taking measurements of the infant's face and head. Computerized tomography, which is a series of photographic images of the brain, is uses to diagnose early suture fusion and to develop surgical correction plans.

Treatment

Treatment of craniosynostosis is used to correct the deformities associated with craniosynostosis and is accomplished by restoring the normal shape and relationship of the forehead and orbital rims through craniofacial surgery. Surgery is less often needed to reduce intracranial pressure. In some cases helmet or band therapy is used after surgery to encourage further correction of the skull and face.

Ideally surgery to correct craniosynotosis should be carried out in an affected child who is less than three months old, when a less-invasive, microscopic procedure can be used that results in smaller incisions, less blood loss, and a shorter hospital stay than the traditional corrective surgery that is used on older children. Also the skull bones of an infant are easier to work with, and the covering of the brain, referred to as the dura, can make bone on its own. The growing brain continues to reshape the skull and face after surgery. However, surgery to correct craniosyntosis can be done at any age. Usually only one surgery is required to correct simple craniosynostosis, but some children may require minor surgery at four to five years of age to correct remaining minor abnormalities. When multiple sutures are involved, usually multiple surgeries are required.

The surgeons make an incision in the skull behind the hairline so that the scar will be covered by hair. The bone in the area of the defect is reshaped or replaced with bone from a different area of the skull.

Surgery for sagittal synostosis involves removing the suture and widening the skull by opening up the coronal and lambdoid sutures, which are found on both sides of the head. In some case bone grafts are used to keep the bones apart.

Surgery for unilateral coronal synotosis involves removing the fused suture, reshaping the forehead and brow, and bringing the forehead and brow forward to match the other side. The cheek is also brought forward to reposition the eye socket. For bicoronal synotosis, both sutures are removed, and the skull is narrowed and lengthened. Both cheekbones are brought forward to reposition the eye socket.

Metopic synotosis is corrected by releasing the metopic suture and expanding and rounding out the upper face, forehead, and skull. Surgery for lambdoid synotosis entails reconstruction of the back portions of the skull.

When all of the sutures are fused, the child must be operated on as soon as possible, with all of the sutures released and repositioned to allow for normal brain growth and to relieve the pressure on the eyes and brain.

Alternative treatment

Conventional surgical treatments should be relied upon for the treatment of craniosynotosis.

Prognosis

The prognosis for craniosynostosis is dependent on whether single or multiple cranial sutures are involved and whether other abnormalities are present. The prognosis is better when there is only single suture involvement and no abnormalities. Surgery is usually successful, and children can lead normal lives with no residual effects from craniosynostosis.

Prevention

Since the causes of craniosynostosis have not been identified, it is unknown as to what measures could be taken that would prevent the condition.

Resources

BOOKS

Parker, James M. and Parker, Philip M., editors. *The Official Parent's Sourcebook on Craniosynostosis.* San Diego, CA: Icon Health Publications, 2003.

OTHER

Craniosynostosis And Positional Plagiocephaly Support, Inc.6905 Xandu Court, Fredericksburg, VA 22407. Telephone: Website: http://www.cappskids.org

ORGANIZATIONS

Children's Craniofacial Association, 13140 Coit Road, Suite 307, Dallas, TX 75240. Telephone: (800) 535-3643; Fax: (214) 570-3643. Website: www.ccakids.com

Craniotomy

Definition

A craniotomy is the surgical removal of part of the skull to expose the brain.

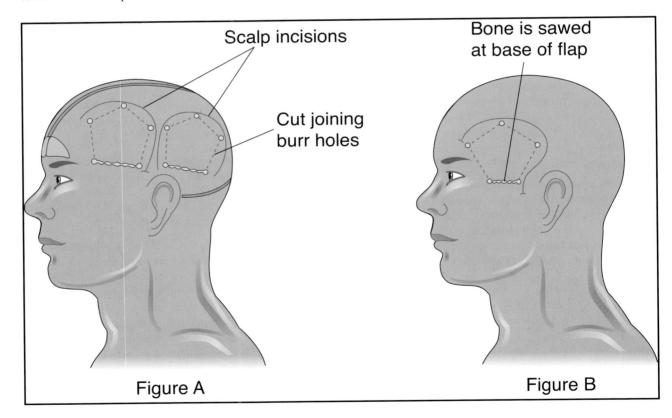

Figure A

Figure B

A craniotomy is the most commonly performed brain surgery for brain tumor removal. There are two basic ways to open the skull: a curving incision from behind the hairline in front of the ear and at the nape of the neck (figure A). To reach the brain, the surgeon uses a hand drill to make holes in the skull, pushing a soft metal guide under the bone. The bone is sawed through until the bone flap can be removed to expose the brain (figure B). *(Illustration by Electronic Illustrators Group. Cengage Learning, Gale.)*

KEY TERMS

Craniotome—A type of surgical drill used to operate on the skull. It has a self-controlled system that stops the drill when the bone is penetrated.

Computed tomography (CT or CAT) scan—Using x rays taken from many angles and computer modeling, CT scans help locate and size tumors and provide information on whether they can be surgically removed.

Magnetic resonance imaging (MRI)—MRI uses magnets and radio waves to create detailed cross-sectional pictures of the interior of the body.

Purpose

A craniotomy is the most commonly performed surgery to remove a brain tumor. It may also be done to remove a blood clot and control hemorrhage, to inspect the brain, to perform a **biopsy**, or to relieve pressure inside the skull.

Precautions

The outcome of surgery will depend on the type and location of the tumor. **Radiation therapy** or **chemotherapy** are sometimes given before surgery to shrink the tumor.

Description

There are two basic ways to open the skull. A curving incision may be made from behind the hairline, in front of the ear, to arch above the eye, or at the nape of the neck around the occipital lobe. The surgeon marks with a felt tip pen a large square flap on the scalp that covers the surgical area. Following this mark, the surgeon makes an incision into the skin as far as the thin membrane covering the skull bone. Because the scalp is well supplied with blood, the surgeon will have to seal many small arteries. The surgeon then folds back a skin flap to expose the bone.

Using a high speed hand drill or an automatic craniotome, the surgeon makes a circle of holes in the skull and pushes a soft metal guide under the bone from one hole to the next. A fine wire saw is then moved along the guide channel under the bone between adjacent holes. The surgeon saws through the bone until the bone flap can be removed to expose the brain.

After the surgery for the underlying cause is completed, the piece of skull is replaced and secured with pieces of fine, soft wire. Finally, the surgeon sutures the membrane, muscle, and skin of the scalp.

Recent advances in computer-assisted technology have enhanced this operation. Image-guided craniotomy uses information from **magnetic resonance imaging** scans (MRIs) or **computed tomography** (CT) scans to produce three-dimensional images of the brain for the surgeon before the operation is begun. This makes it possible for the surgeon to remove less skin and bone, to tell exactly where the tumor stops and the healthy brain begins, and to remove tumors that were previously too deep for surgery.

Preparation

Before the operation, the patient undergoes diagnostic procedures such as CT and MRI scans to determine the underlying problem that requires the craniotomy and to get a better look at the brain's structure. Cerebral **angiography** is a diagnostic procedure that may be used to study the blood supply to the tumor, aneurysm, or other brain lesion.

Before the surgery, patients are given drugs to ease anxiety, and other medications to reduce the risk of swelling, seizures, and **infection** after the operation. Fluids may be restricted, and a diuretic (water pill) may be given before and during surgery if the patient has a tendency to retain water. A urinary catheter is inserted before the patient goes to the operating room. The scalp is shaved in the operating room immediately before surgery; this is done so that any small nicks in the skin won't have a chance to become infected before the operation.

Aftercare

Oxygen, painkillers, and drugs to control swelling and seizures are given after the operation. Codeine may be given to relieve potential headaches caused by the stretching or irritation of the nerves of the scalp. Some type of drainage from the head may be in place, depending on the reason for the surgery.

Patients are usually out of bed within a day and out of the hospital within a week. Headache and pain from the scalp wound can be controlled with medications. Some patients will receive radiation therapy or chemotherapy after surgery.

The bandage on the skull should be changed regularly. Sutures closing the scalp will be removed, but soft wires used to reattach the skull are permanent and require no further attention. The patient should avoid getting the scalp wet until all the sutures have been removed. A clean cap or scarf can be worn until the hair grows back.

Risks

Accessing the area of the brain that needs repair may damage other brain tissue. Therefore, the procedure carries with it risk of brain damage that could leave the patient with some loss of brain function. The surgeon performing the operation can give the patient an assessment of the risk of his or her particular procedure based on the location of the tumor.

Normal results

While every patient's experience is different depending on the reason for the surgery, age, and overall health, recovery from a successful surgery is usually rapid because of the good supply of blood to the area.

Abnormal results

Possible complications after craniotomy include:

- swelling of the brain
- excessive intracranial pressure
- infection
- seizures

See also Brain and central nervous system tumors; Computed tomography; Magnetic resonance imaging.

Resources

ORGANIZATIONS

American Cancer Society. 1599 Clifton Road NE, Atlanta, GA 30329. 800 (ACS)-2345). http://www.cancer.org.

National Cancer Institute. Building 31, Room 10A19, 9000 Rockville Pike, Bethesda, MD 20892. (800) 4-CANCER. http://www.nci.nih.gov.

Carol A. Turkington

Cryoablation

Definition

Cryoablation is the destruction of tissue by controlled freezing.

Purpose

Cryoablation, also called **cryotherapy**, is used primarily to treat male **prostate cancer**, although it can also be used in selective cases to treat abnormal uterine bleeding as an alternative to hysterectomy or to destroy certain localized liver tumors.

Cryotherapy came into use in 1966 with the development of thin probes that could be cooled to very low temperatures with liquid nitrogen. As of 2005, probes cooled with argon have been developed that can reach temperatures of -304°F (-187°C) causing quick and complete freezing of tissues.

Freezing tissue is thought to destroys cells in several ways. The formation of ice crystals inside the cells causes them to burst. Freezing also causes dehydration of certain cells and may destroy blood vessels supplying nutrients to the cells. In addition, freezing may activate an immune system response against the frozen tissue.

The prostate gland lies under the bladder and surrounds the urethra. Its main function is to produce seminal fluid that mixes with sperm prior to ejaculation. Prostate **cancer** is a leading cause of death in men.

Cryoablation of the prostate is not used as often as other therapies for prostate cancer. A survey of by the American Urological Association in 2001 found that fewer than 2% of urologists performed cryoablation; however, the frequency with which these doctors performed the procedure was increasing. Medicare began paying for cryoablation procedures in 1999. Some private insurers will pay for the procedure, but only if the insured individual meets certain conditions with regard to his cancer status.

Advantages of cryoablation are that it is less invasive and less painful than surgery. The recovery period is short. The procedure can be performed again if it is not completely successful or the individual can receive additional therapies such as radiation or **chemotherapy**. The main disadvantages of cryoablation are that it does not destroy cancer cells that have spread beyond the prostate and that it has a high risk of causing impotence.

Precautions

Not all men with prostate cancer are good candidates for cryoablation. Those most likely to benefit

KEY TERMS

Androgens—Male hormones, most commonly testosterone.

Hysterectomy—Surgical removal of the uterus.

Prostate-specific antigen (PSA)—A type of protein made only by the prostate gland. High levels of PSA are a good indication of prostate cancer. Levels can be determined by a simple blood test.

Transrectal ultrasound—A procedure in which a device inserted into the rectum uses the echoes of sound waves to create an image of an organ or gland.

Urethra—The tube which drains urine from the bladder.

from this procedure have low-risk tumors with their cancer limited to the prostate gland. A second group of men who may benefit from this procedure are those whose cancer has not responded to **radiation therapy**, chemotherapy, and androgen withdrawal therapy. Men with very large prostates, those with urinary obstruction, and those who have had certain types of rectal surgery are not good candidates for this procedure.

Description

Cryoablation of the prostate is a minimally invasive procedure that is performed under general or regional anesthesia in a hospital or surgical clinic. An ultrasound device is inserted into the rectum to produce an image of the prostate and guide the placement of probes used to freeze the tissue. This procedure is called a transrectal ultrasound (TRUS). A catheter is inserted into the urethra and filled with warm saline (salt water) in order to avoid freezing the urethra.

Freezing of the prostate takes place one section at a time, with temperatures reaching -40°F (-40°C). The tissue is then allowed to thaw and a second cycle of freezing and thawing is performed after which the probes are removed. Patients may be kept overnight for observation after the procedure or discharged the same day.

Preparation

Prior to cryoablation, tests will be done to determine the size and shape of the prostate and the extent to which the cancer may have spread. Men with large prostates may be put on androgen deprivation therapy to shrink their prostate in order to make freezing more

effective. The day before cryoablation is scheduled, the man will cleanse his bowel by drinking magnesium citrate. On the morning of the procedure, he will be administered an enema.

Aftercare

A catheter remains in the urethra for two to three weeks following the procedure. Because of swelling in of the urethra, the ability to urinate normally does not return for about two weeks. The individual may also be given **antibiotics** for 10–14 days after the procedure. A prostate-specific antigen (PSA) blood test and a prostate **biopsy** may be done three to six months following the procedure. If treatment is unsuccessful, individuals may receive chemotherapy, radiation therapy, or surgery.

Risks

Although technical advances have improved this procedure, significant risks still exist, because freezing is not always limited to cancerous tissue. This procedure results in a high rate (as much as 95%) of erectile dysfunction, although a few men (about 5%) regain function within a year and a half. Another significant risk is the development of a urinary-rectal fistula. This is an abnormal connection between the bladder and the rectum that can result in persistent urinary tract infections as feces leaks into the bladder. Other less common risks include an ongoing inability to empty the bladder, (although this is normal for a few weeks after the procedure), loss of bladder control, pelvic and rectal pain, and permanent numbness of the penis.

Normal results

Individuals with low- and moderate-risk tumors that have not spread beyond the prostate gland have a good likelihood (60–75%) maintaining low PSA levels for five or more years, indicating that they are cancer free. For those with high-risk tumors, the success rate falls to about 40%.

Abnormal results

Failure of this therapy is indicated by rising PSA levels, presence of prostate cancer in post-treatment biopsy, or spread of cancer to other parts of the body.

Resources

RESOURCES
OTHER

American Urological Association. *Cryoablation for Prostate Cancer.* May 2004 [cited 21 February 2005]. http.www.urologyhealth.org/.

Cooperberg, Matthew and Peter Carroll. *Prostate Cancer: Cryotherapy*, 22 July 2004 [3 March 2005]. http://www.emedicine.com/med/topic3539.htm.

ORGANIZATIONS

Prostate Cancer Institute. 10949 Bren Road East, Minnetonka, MN 55343-9613. 952-852-5560.

Tish Davidson, A. M.

Cryotherapy

Definition

Cryotherapy is a technique that uses an extremely cold liquid or instruments to freeze and destroy abnormal or cancerous skin cells that require removal. The prefix *cryo-* comes from the Greek word for frost. The technique has been in use since the turn of the century,

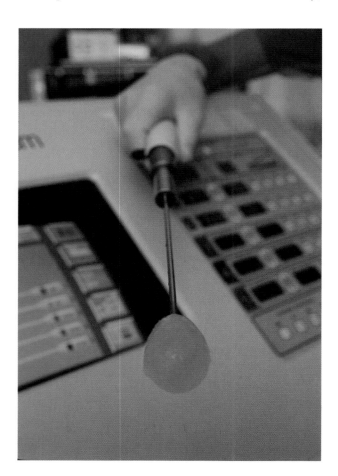

Metal cryoprobe used to treat prostate cancer. *(Copyright Hank Morgan, Science Source/Photo Researchers, Inc. Reproduced by permission.)*

but modern techniques have made it widely available to dermatologists and primary care doctors. Recent advances have also led to more frequent use of cryotherapy in treating internal **cancer**. The technique is also called cryosurgery.

Purpose

Cryotherapy can be employed to destroy a variety of such benign skin growths as warts, precancerous lesions (such as actinic keratoses), **Bowen's disease**, and such malignant lesions as basal cell and squamous cell carcinomas. It has also found new use in treating internal cancers, such as cancers of the prostate gland and the breast. The goal of cryotherapy is to freeze and destroy targeted skin growths or cancers while preserving the surrounding tissue from injury. For this reason cryosurgery appears to be useful in performing lumpectomies for smaller breast cancers.

Internal cancers that are being treated with cryosurgery as of 2009 include cancers of the kidney and liver as well as of the prostate gland.

Precautions

Cryotherapy is not recommended for certain areas of the body because of the danger of destruction of normal tissue or unacceptable scarring. These areas include: skin that overlies nerves, the corners of the eyes, the fold of skin between the nose and lip, the skin surrounding the nostrils, and the border between the lips and the rest of the face. Lesions that are suspected or known to be malignant **melanoma**, an aggressive form of **skin cancer**, should not be treated with cryotherapy, but should instead be removed surgically. Similarly, basal cell or squamous cell skin cancers that have reappeared at the site of a previously treated tumor should also be removed surgically.

If it remains unclear whether a growth is benign or malignant, a sample of tissue should be removed for analysis (**biopsy**) by a pathologist before any attempts to destroy the lesion with cryotherapy. Care should be taken in people with diabetes or certain circulation problems when cryotherapy is considered for growths located on their lower legs, ankles, and feet. In these patients, healing can be poor and the risk of **infection** can be high.

Description

There are three main techniques used to perform cryotherapy. In the simplest technique, usually reserved for warts and other benign skin growths, the physician will dip a cotton swab or other applicator into a cup containing a "cryogen," such as liquid nitrogen, and apply it directly to the skin growth to freeze it. At a temperature of -320°F (-196°C), liquid nitrogen is the coldest cryogen available. The goal is to freeze the skin growth as quickly as possible, and then let it thaw slowly to cause maximum destruction of the skin cells. A second application may be necessary depending on the size of the growth.

In another cryotherapy technique, a device is used to direct a small spray of liquid nitrogen or other cryogen directly onto the skin growth. Freezing may last from 20–30 seconds, depending on the size of the lesion. A second freeze-thaw cycle may be required. In a third option, liquid nitrogen or another cryogen is circulated through a probe to cool it to low temperatures. The probe is then brought into direct contact with the lesion, either on the skin or in the case of internal cancers, inside the patient. The freeze time can take two to three times longer than with the spray technique.

Preparation

Extensive preparation prior to cryotherapy is not required for external lesions. The area to be treated should be clean and dry, but sterile preparation is not necessary. Patients should know that they will experience some pain at the time of the freezing, but local anesthesia is usually not required. The physician may want to reduce the size of certain growths, such as warts, prior to the cryotherapy procedure, and may have patients apply salicylic acid preparations to the growth over several weeks. Sometimes, the physician will pare away some of the tissue using a device called a curette or a scalpel.

Preparation for treating cancers inside the body, such as **prostate cancer**, is slightly more complicated. The areas that are to be cooled are precisely mapped using ultrasound imaging or a specialized x-ray machine known as a computed axial tomography (CAT) scan. Temperature sensors are then placed inside and around the tumor to monitor the temperature. Lastly, cooling probes are then placed in and around the tumor.

Risks

Cryotherapy poses little risk and can be well tolerated by elderly and other patients who are not good candidates for other surgical procedures. As with other surgical procedures, there is some risk of scarring, infection, and damage to underlying skin and tissue. These risks are generally minimal in the hands of experienced users of cryotherapy.

Normal results

Some redness, swelling, blistering, and oozing of fluid are all common results of cryotherapy. Healing time can vary by the site treated and the cryotherapy technique used. When cryogen is applied directly to the growth, healing may occur in three weeks. Growths treated on the head and neck with the spray technique may take four to six weeks to heal; growths treated on other areas of the body may take considerably longer. Cryotherapy boasts high success rates in permanently removing skin growths; even for malignant lesions such as squamous cell and basal cell cancers, studies have shown a cure rate of up to 98%. For certain types of growths, such as some forms of warts, repeat treatments over several weeks are necessary to prevent the growth's return.

In the case of internal tumors, such as cancers of the prostate, cryotherapy has been shown to be at least as effective as other means, such as **radiation therapy**, with fewer side effects and faster recovery time. In addition, cryosurgery appears to have less severe effects on the patients' quality of life than other forms of treatment for prostate cancer.

Abnormal results

Although cryotherapy is a relatively low-risk procedure, some side effects may occur as a result of the treatment. They include:

- Infection. Though uncommon, infection is more likely on the lower legs where healing can take several months.

- Pigmentary changes. Both hypopigmentation (lightening of the skin) and hyperpigmentation (darkening of the skin) are possible after cryotherapy. Both generally last a few months, but can be longer lasting.

- Nerve damage. Though rare, damage to nerves is possible. Reports suggest this will disappear within several months.

Resources

BOOKS

Abeloff, Martin D., James O. Armitage, Allen S. Lichter, and John E. Niederhuber. *Clinical Oncology*. New York: Churchill Livingstone, 2000.

Beers, Mark H., MD, and Robert Berkow, MD, editors. "Principles of Cancer Therapy: Hyperthermia and Cryotherapy." In *The Merck Manual of Diagnosis and Therapy*. Whitehouse Station, NJ: Merck Research Laboratories, 2007.

PERIODICALS

Anastasiadis, A. G., R. Sachdev, L. Salomon, et al. "Comparison of Health-Related Quality of Life and Prostate-Associated Symptoms After Primary and Salvage Cryotherapy for Prostate Cancer." *Journal of Cancer Research and Clinical Oncology* 129 (December 2003): 676–682.

Johnson, D. B., and S. Y. Nakada. "Cryoablation of Renal and Prostate Tumors." *Journal of Endourology* 17 (October 2003): 627–632.

Nadler, R. B., S. C. Kim, J. N. Rubinstein, et al. "Laparoscopic Renal Cryosurgery: The Northwestern Experience." *Journal of Urology* 170 (October 2003): 1121–1125.

Shinohara, K. "Prostate Cancer: Cryotherapy." *Urology Clinics of North America* 30 (November 2003): 725–736.

Subar, D. A., A. J. Sheen, and D. J. Sherlock. " Cryoablation for Liver Tumors—Is There Clinical Utility?" *Medscape General Medicine* 7 (November 2003): 19.

Tafra, L., S. J. Smith, J. E. Woodward, et al. "Pilot Trial of Cryoprobe-Assisted Breast-Conserving Surgery for Small Ultrasound-Visible Cancers." *Annals of Surgical Oncology* 10 (November 2003): 999.

OTHER

National Cancer Institute. http://cis.nci.nih.gov.

ORGANIZATIONS

American Academy of Dermatology. 930 N. Meacham Road, P.O. Box 4014, Schaumburg, IL 60168-4014. (847)330-0230. http://www.aad.org.

Edward R. Rosick, D.O., M.P.H.
Rebecca J. Frey, PhD

CT-guided biopsy

Definition

A CT-guided **biopsy** is a procedure by which the physician uses a very thin needle and a syringe to withdraw a tissue or fluid specimen from an organ or suspected tumor mass. The needle is guided while being viewed by the physician on a **computed tomography** (CT) scan.

Purpose

A definite diagnosis of **cancer** is almost always based on the histological examination of cell or tissue samples. The procedure used to obtain a specimen for this testing is called a biopsy. Biopsies can be performed by surgical removal of the specimen if the suspicious area is located near the surface of the body or during surgery. If, however, the suspected tumor is located deep inside the body and cannot be seen or felt by the physician, he may decide to perform a CT-guided biopsy. The main advantage of a CT-guided biopsy is that it does not require an incision, but the disadvantage is that in some cases, the needle may not be able to remove enough tissue for analysis.

Precautions

CT-guided biopsy can be performed on almost all organs of the body, for example on the lungs, liver, kidneys, adrenal glands, pancreas, and pelvis. The procedure is not indicated for the spleen because there is a high risk of severe post-biopsy hemorrhage. CT-guided biopsy is not indicated for patients with bleeding disorders such as hemophilia, or who are at risk for bleeding as a result of cancer treatments (chemo-radiation) or the cancer itself, as when a patient develops **thrombocytopenia**.

Description

The development of CT technology provided a powerful means to visualize the inner features of the human body which previously could only be seen during surgery or autopsy. Before CT, if a patient had a tumor located in the chest, abdomen, or pelvis, biopsies could only be performed with a surgical procedure. If the patient needed surgery so as to treat the tumor, then biopsy specimens were also collected at the same time for analysis. However, there was no way to obtain samples from patients whose tumors could not be treated with surgery, such as patients with metastatic cancer or with general conditions not

KEY TERMS

Anesthesia—Loss of normal sensation or feeling. Insensitivity to pain.

Autopsy—Postmortem surgical procedure performed to examine body tissues and determine the cause of death.

Hemorrhage—Escape of blood from blood vessels; bleeding.

Histology—The study of tissue with a microscope.

Incision—Cutting through the skin.

Metastasis—The transfer of cancer from one organ to another one not directly connected to it.

Pelvis—Bassin-shaped body cavity containing and protecting the bladder, the rectum, and the reproductive organs.

Pneumothorax—A collapse of the lung due to a sudden change of pressure within the chest cavity.

Sterile—Procedures carried out with instruments that have been sterilized, meaning that they are completely free from microorganisms (germs) that could cause infection.

QUESTIONS TO ASK THE DOCTOR

- Will the CT-guided biopsy procedure be painful?
- How many times will I need to have one?
- What is the normal success rate in obtaining enough tissue to make a diagnosis?
- What kind of complications may I experience at the biopsy site?
- When will I know the results?

allowing surgery. CT-guided needle biopsy has become a welcome alternative to surgical exploration and biopsy.

Preparation

The technique will vary depending on the site of specimen collection and the patient's general condition. In most procedures, the patient lies on the CT table on his back, or on either side, depending on where the needle is to be inserted. Some patients may require intravenous injection of pain killers. A CT scan is first performed, to locate the best site for needle insertion. The skin is then disinfected and anesthetized with its underlying tissue. The needle is inserted through the skin into the body. Another CT scan is perfomed to confirm that the tip of the needle lies at the desired location. When the tip of the needle is seen to be in the proper position, the biopsy specimen is withdrawn through the needle.

Aftercare

After the procedure, the patient is monitored in the hospital or clinic department or in an observation unit for a few hours, and then sent home.

Risks

CT-guided biopsy is a fairly safe procedure. The risks are certainly less than the risks involved with the alternative method, surgical biopsy. In any case, recovering from CT-guided biopsy takes considerably less time than it would if the biopsy were surgically performed.

The risks associated with CT-guided biopsy depend on the site where the biopsy specimen is collected. They include:

- Bleeding: Most patients have had their blood evaluated before the procedure. Although rare, bleeding can occur and may require surgery to control.

- Infection: An infection is possible whenever an object, such as the needle used in CT-guided biopsy, pierces, the skin, even if sterile procedures are always followed during the procedure. This is a very rare complication.

- Pneumothorax: Partial or total collapse of a lung is a reported complication in approximately 25% of lung biopsies. It is also a risk during CT-guided biopsies of the liver and adrenal glands.

Normal results

A preliminary evaluation of the CT-guided biopsy specimen is often performed by the physician. If enough tissue has been obtained for the required tests, the procedure is terminated and the specimen is sent to the histology lab for analysis.

Abnormal results

If the CT-guided biopsy has not been successful, it may be repeated or another biopsy procedure may be selected. Abnormal results indicate that a malignancy or other abnormality is present.

See also Biopsy; Imaging studies.

Resources

BOOKS

Seeram, E. *Computed Tomography: Physical Principles, Clinical Applications and Quality Control.* W. Saunders & Co., 2001.

PERIODICALS

Sklair-Levy, M., Polliack, A., Shaham, D., Applbaum, Y. H., Gillis, S., Ben-Yehuda, D., Sherman, Y., and E. Libson. "CT-guided core-needle biopsy in the diagnosis of mediastinal lymphoma." *European Radiology* 10 (2000): 714-8.

Monique Laberge, Ph.D.

CT scan *see* **Computed tomography**
CUP *see* **Cancer of unknown primary**

▌Cushing's syndrome

Definition

Cushing's syndrome is a relatively rare endocrine (hormonal) disorder resulting from excessive exposure to the hormone cortisol. The disorder, which leads to a variety of symptoms and physical abnormalities, is most commonly caused by taking medications containing the hormone over a long period of time. A more rare form of the disorder occurs when the body itself produces an excessive amount of cortisol.

Description

The adrenals are two glands, each of which is perched on the upper part of the two kidneys. The outer part of the gland is known as the cortex; the inner part is known as the medulla. Each of these parts of the adrenal gland is responsible for producing different types of hormones. Regulation of hormone production and release from the adrenal cortex involves the pituitary gland, a small gland located at the base of the brain. After the hypothalamus (the part of the brain containing secretions important to metabolic activities) sends "releasing hormones" to the pituitary gland, the pituitary secretes a hormone called adrenocorticotropic hormone (ACTH). The ACTH then travels through the bloodstream to the adrenal cortex, where it encourages the production and release of cortisol (sometimes called the "stress" hormone) and other adrenocortical hormones.

Cortisol, a very potent glucocorticoid—a group of adrenocortical hormones that protects the body from stress and affect protein and carbohydrate

Woman exhibiting symptoms of Cushing's syndrome.
(Copyright John Radcliff Hospital/Science Source/Photo Researchers, Inc. Reproduced by permission.)

metabolism— is involved in regulating the functioning of nearly every type of organ and tissue in the body, and is considered to be one of the few hormones absolutely necessary for life. Cortisol is involved in:

- complex processing and utilization of many nutrients, including sugars (carbohydrates), fats, and proteins
- normal functioning of the circulatory system and the heart
- functioning of muscles
- normal kidney function
- production of blood cells
- normal processes involved in maintaining the skeletal system
- proper functioning of the brain and nerves
- normal responses of the immune system

Cushing's syndrome, also called hypercortisolism, has an adverse effect on all of the processes described

KEY TERMS

Adenoma—A type of noncancerous (benign) tumor that often involves the overgrowth of certain cells of the type normally found within glands.

Adrenocorticotropic hormone (ACTH)—A pituitary hormone that stimulates the cortex of the adrenal glands to produce adrenal cortical hormones.

Cortisol—A hormone secreted by the cortex of the adrenal gland. Cortisol regulates the function of nearly every organ and tissue in the body.

Ectopic—In an abnormal position.

Endocrine—Pertaining to a gland that secretes directly into the bloodstream.

Gland—A collection of cells whose function is to release certain chemicals (hormones) that are important to the functioning of other, sometimes distantly located, organs or body systems.

Glucocorticoids—General class of adrenal cortical hormones that are mainly active in protecting against stress and in protein and carbohydrate metabolism.

Hormone—A chemical produced in one part of the body, which travels to another part of the body in order to exert its effect.

Hypothalamus—The part of the brain containing secretions important to metabolic activities.

Pituitary—A gland located at the base of the brain, the pituitary produces a number of hormones, including hormones that regulate growth and reproductive function.

above. The syndrome occurs in approximately 10 to 15 out of every one million people per year, usually striking adults between the ages of 20 and 50.

Causes and symptoms

The most common cause of Cushing's syndrome is the long-term use of glucocorticoid hormones in medications. Medications such as prednisone are used in a number of inflammatory conditions. Such conditions include rheumatoid arthritis, asthma, vasculitis, lupus, and a variety of other autoimmune disorders in which the body's immune cells accidentally attack some part of the body itself. In these disorders, the glucocorticoids are used to dampen the **immune response**, thereby decreasing damage to the body.

Cushing's syndrome can also be caused by three different categories of disease:

- a pituitary tumor producing abnormally large quantities of ACTH
- the abnormal production of ACTH by some source other than the pituitary
- a tumor within the adrenal gland overproducing cortisol

Although it is rare, about two-thirds of endogenous (occurring within the body rather than from a source outside the body, like a medication) Cushing's syndrome is a result of Cushing's disease. The term "Cushing's disease" refers to Cushing's syndrome, which is caused by excessive secretion of ACTH by a pituitary tumor, usually an **adenoma** (noncancerous tumor). The pituitary tumor causes increased growth of the adrenal cortex (hyperplasia) and increased cortisol production. Cushing's disease affects women more often than men.

Tumors in locations other than the pituitary can also produce ACTH. This is called ectopic ACTH syndrome ("ectopic" refers to something existing out of its normal place). Tumors in the lung account for more than half of all cases of ectopic ACTH syndrome. Other types of tumors which may produce ACTH include tumors of the thymus, the pancreas, the thyroid, and the adrenal gland. In each case, the secreting part of the tumor may be in the primary tumor, part of the primary tumor, or may be a small, difficult-to-find, metastatic lesion(s). Nearly all adrenal gland tumors are benign (noncancerous), although in rare instances a tumor may actually be cancerous.

Symptoms of cortisol excess (resulting from medication or from the body's excess production of the hormone) include:

- weight gain
- an abnormal accumulation of fatty pads in the face (creating the distinctive "moon face" of Cushing's syndrome); in the trunk (termed "truncal obesity"); and over the upper back and the back of the neck (giving the individual what has been called a "buffalo hump")
- purple and pink stretch marks across the abdomen and flanks
- high blood pressure
- weak, thinning bones (osteoporosis)
- weak muscles
- low energy
- thin, fragile skin, with a tendency toward both bruising and slow healing

- abnormalities in the processing of sugars (glucose), with occasional development of actual diabetes
- kidney stones
- increased risk of infections
- emotional disturbances, including mood swings, depression, irritability, confusion, or even a complete break with reality (psychosis)
- irregular menstrual periods in women
- decreased sex drive in men and difficulty maintaining an erection
- abormal hair growth in women (in a male pattern, such as in the beard and mustache area), as well as loss of hair from the head (receding hair line)

Diagnosis

Diagnosing Cushing's syndrome can be complex. Diagnosis must not only identify the cortisol excess but also locate its source. Many of the symptoms listed above can be attributed to numerous other diseases. Although a number of these symptoms seen together would certainly suggest Cushing's syndrome, the symptoms are still not specific to Cushing's syndrome. Following a review of the patient's medical history, physical examination, and routine blood tests, a series of more sophisticated tests is available to achieve a diagnosis.

24-hour free cortisol test

This is the most specific diagnostic test for identifying Cushing's syndrome. It involves measuring the amount of cortisol present in the urine over a 24-hour period. When excess cortisol is present in the bloodstream, it is processed by the kidneys and removed as waste in the urine. This 24-hour free cortisol test requires that an individual collect exactly 24-hours' worth of urine in a single container. The urine is then analyzed in a laboratory to determine the quantity of cortisol present. This technique can also be paired with the administration of **dexamethasone**, which in a normal individual would cause urine cortisol to be very low. Once a diagnosis has been made using the 24-hour free cortisol test, other tests are used to find the exact location of the abnormality causing excess cortisol production.

Dexamethasone suppression test

This test is useful in distinguishing individuals with excess ACTH production due to a pituitary adenoma from those with ectopic ACTH-producing tumors. Patients are given dexamethasone (a synthetic glucocorticoid) orally every six hours for four days. Low doses of dexamethasone are given during the first two days; for the last two days, higher doses are administered. Before dexamethasone is administered, as well as on each day of the test, 24-hour urine collections are obtained.

Because cortisol and other glucocorticoids signal the pituitary to decrease ACTH, the normal response after taking dexamethasone is a drop in blood and urine cortisol levels. Thus, the cortisol response to dexamethasone differs depending on whether the cause of Cushing's syndrome is a pituitary adenoma or an ectopic ACTH-producing tumor.

However, the dexamethasone suppression test may produce false-positive results in patients with conditions such as **depression**, alcohol abuse, high estrogen levels, acute illness, and stress. On the other hand, drugs such as **phenytoin** and phenobarbital may produce false-negative results. Thus, patients are usually advised to stop taking these drugs at least one week prior to the test.

Corticotropin-releasing hormone (CRH) stimulation test

The CRH stimulation test is given to help distinguish between patients with pituitary adenomas and those with either ectopic ACTH syndrome or cortisol-secreting **adrenal tumors**. In this test, patients are given an injection of CRH, the corticotropin-releasing hormone that causes the pituitary to secrete ACTH. In patients with pituitary adenomas, blood levels of ACTH and cortisol usually rise. However, in patients with ectopic ACTH syndrome, this rise is rarely seen. In patients with cortisol-secreting adrenal tumors, this rise almost never occurs.

Petrosal sinus sampling

Although this test is not always necessary, it may be used to distinguish between a pituitary adenoma and an ectopic source of ACTH. Petrosal sinus sampling involves drawing blood directly from veins that drain the pituitary. This test, which is usually performed with local anesthesia and mild sedation, requires inserting tiny, flexible tubes (catheters) through a vein in the upper thigh or groin area. The catheters are then threaded up slowly until they reach veins in an area of the skull known as the petrosal sinuses. **X rays** are typically used to confirm the correct position of the catheters. Often CRH is also given during the test to increase the accuracy of results.

When blood tested from the petrosal sinuses reveals a higher ACTH level than blood drawn from a vein in the forearm, the likely diagnosis is a pituitary adenoma. When the two samples show similar levels of ACTH, the diagnosis indicates ectopic ACTH syndrome.

Radiologic imaging tests

Imaging tests such as **computed tomography** scans (CT) and **magnetic resonance imaging** (MRI) are only used to look at the pituitary and adrenal glands after a firm diagnosis has already been made. The presence of a pituitary or adrenal tumor does not necessarily guarantee that it is the source of increased ACTH production. Many healthy people with no symptoms or disease whatsoever have noncancerous tumors in the pituitary and adrenal glands. Thus, CT and MRI is often used to image the pituitary and adrenal glands in preparation for surgery.

Treatment

The choice of a specific treatment depends on the type of problem causing the cortisol excess. Pituitary and adrenal adenomas are usually removed surgically. Malignant adrenal tumors always require surgical removal.

Treatment of ectopic ACTH syndrome also involves removing all of the cancerous cells which are producing ACTH. This may be done through surgery, **chemotherapy** (using combinations of cancer-killing drugs), or **radiation therapy** (using x rays to kill **cancer** cells), depending on the type of cancer and how far it has spread. Radiation therapy may also be used on the pituitary (with or without surgery), for patients who cannot undergo surgery, or for patients whose surgery did not successfully decrease pituitary release of ACTH.

There are a number of drugs that are effective in decreasing adrenal production of cortisol. These medications include **mitotane**, ketoconazole, metyrapone, trilostane, **aminoglutethimide**, and mifepristone. These drugs are sometimes given prior to surgery in an effort to reverse the problems brought on by cortisol excess. However, the drugs may also need to be administered after surgery (sometimes along with radiation treatments) in patients who continue to have excess pituitary production of ACTH.

Because pituitary surgery can cause ACTH levels to drop too low, some patients require short-term treatment with a cortisol-like medication after surgery. Patients who need adrenal surgery may also require glucocorticoid replacement. If the entire adrenal gland has been removed, the patient must take oral glucocorticoids for the rest of his or her life.

Prognosis

Prognosis depends on the source of the problem. When pituitary adenomas are identified as the source of increased ACTH leading to cortisol excess, about 80% of patients are cured by surgery. When cortisol excess is due to some other form of cancer, the prognosis depends on the type of cancer and the extent of its spread.

Resources

PERIODICALS

Boscaro, Marco, Luisa Barzon, and Nicoletta Sonino. "The Diagnosis of Cushing's Syndrome: Atypical Presentations and Laboratory Shortcomings." *Archives of Internal Medicine* 160 (2000): 3045-53.

Boscaro, Marco, Luisa Barzon, Francesco Fallo, and Nicoletta Sonino. "Cushing's Syndrome." *Lancet* 357 (2001): 783-91.

Kirk, Lawrence F., Robert B. Hash, Harold P. Katner, and Tom Jones. "Cushing's Disease: Clinical Manifestations and Diagnostic Evaluation." *American Family Physician* 62, no.5 (September 1, 2001): 1119-27.

Newell-Price J., and A. Grossman. "Diagnosis and Management of Cushing's Syndrome." *Lancet* 353 (1999): 2087-88.

Rosalyn Carson-DeWitt, M.D.

Cutaneous T-cell lymphoma

Definition

Cutaneous T-cell **lymphoma** (CTCL) is a malignancy of the T helper (CD4+) cells of the immune system.

Itchy, crusted plaque on the skin of a patient with cutaneous T-cell lymphoma. *(Custom Medical Stock Photo. Reproduced by permission.)*

KEY TERMS

Alkylating agent—A chemical that alters the composition of the genetic material of rapidly dividing cells, such as cancer cells, causing selective cell death; used as a topical chemotherapeutic agent to treat CTCL.

Erythroderma—An abnormal reddening of the entire skin surface.

Mycosis fungoides—A well-defined subset of CTCL in which mushroom shaped tumors form on the skin.

Retinoids—A group of natural and synthetic compounds that resemble vitamin A in their activity. Retinoids are used in the treatment of CTCL.

Sézary syndrome—A variant of CTCL that is characterized by circulating abnormal T cells and erythroderma.

T-helper cells—A cellular component of the immune system that plays a major role in ridding the body of bacteria and viruses, characterized by the presence of the CD4 protein on its surface; the type of cell that divides uncontrollable with CTCL.

Total-skin Electron Beam Therapy—A method of radiation therapy used to treat CTCL that involves bombarding the entire body surface with high energy electrons.

QUESTIONS TO ASK THE DOCTOR

- What is the stage of the disease at this point and what is the prognosis?
- What are the treatment options and what side effects can be expected?
- Is total-skin electron beam therapy (TSEB) available and is this a treatment that should be considered?
- What are the chances of complete clearance of the disease?

Description

CTCL is a **cancer** of the white blood cells that primarily affects the skin and only secondarily affects other sites. The disease usually develops slowly, advancing from itchy dark patches on the skin to mushroom shaped tumors, a condition known as **mycosis fungoides**. This disease involves the uncontrollable proliferation of T-lymphocytes known as T-helper cells, so named because of their role in the **immune response**. T-helper cells are characterized by the presence of a protein receptor on their surface called CD4. Accordingly, T-helper cells are said to be CD4+.

The proliferation of T-helper cells results in the penetration, or infiltration, of these abnormal cells into the epidermal layer of the skin. The skin reacts with slightly scaling lesions that itch, although the sites of greatest infiltration do not necessarily correspond to the sites of the lesions. The lesions are most often located on the trunk, but can be present on any part of the body. In the most common course of the disease,

the patchy lesions progress to palpable plaques that are deeper red and have more defined edges. As the disease worsens, skin tumors develop that are often mushroom-shaped, hence the name mycosis fungoides (the name was not meant to imply that a fungus is involved in the disease). Finally, the cancer progresses to extracutanous involvement, often in the lymph nodes or the viscera.

The progression of the disease is often not linear, although the probability of spread to the viscera (internal organs in the abdomen) is directly related to the amount of skin involvement. Visceral involvement is almost never seen with minimal skin involvement. About 8% of those with generalized plaques have extracutaneous spread, while 30% with tumors have viscera involved. Overall, visceral involvement occurs with only 15–20% of all patients diagnosed with the disease.

Some patients present with an overall redness of the skin, with or without overlying plaques or tumors. The skin can be atrophic (shrunken) or lichenified (having small, firm bumps, close together), with cold intolerance and intense **itching**. These patients have swollen lymph nodes and large numbers of abnormal cells circulating the blood. This particular manifestation of CTCL is known as **Sézary syndrome**.

Demographics

CTCL is a rare disease, with an annual incidence of about .29 cases per 100,000 persons in the United States. It is about half as common in Eastern Europe. However, this discrepancy may be attributed to a differing physician awareness of the disease rather than a true difference in occurrence. In the United States there are about 500 to 600 new cases a year and about 100 to 200 deaths. Usually seen in older adults, CTCL strikes twice as many men as women and the median age at diagnosis is 55 to 60 years.

Causes and symptoms

The cause of CTCL is unknown. Exposure to chemicals or pesticides has been suggested but the most recent study on the subject failed to show a connection between exposure and development of the disease. The ability to isolate various viruses from cell lines grown from cells of CTCL patients raises the question of a viral cause, but studies have been unable to confirm these suspicions.

The symptoms of CTCL are seen primarily in the skin, with itchy red patches or plaques and, usually over time, mushroom-shaped skin tumors. Any part of the skin can be involved and the extent and distribution of the rash or tumors vary greatly from patient to patient. The only universal symptom of the disease is the itch and this symptom is usually what brings the patient to the doctor for treatment. If the disease spreads outside of the skin, the symptoms include swelling of the lymph nodes, usually most severe in those draining the areas with skin involvement. Spread to the viscera is most often manifested as disorders of the lungs, upper digestive tract, central nervous system, or liver but virtually any organ can be shown to be involved at autopsy.

Diagnosis

Diagnosis of CTCL is often difficult in the early stages because of its slow progression and ability to mimic many other benign skin conditions. The early patches of CTCL resemble closely the rashes of eczema, psoriasis, and contact dermatitis. In a further complication, the early manifestations of the disease can respond favorably to the topical corticosteroid treatments prescribed for these skin disorders. This has the unfortunate result of the disease being missed and the patient remaining untreated for years. CTCL is most likely discovered when a physician maintains a suspicion about the disease, performs multiple skin biopsies, and provides close follow-up after the initial presentation.

Skin biopsies showing penetration of abnormal cells into the epidermal tissue are necessary to make a firm diagnosis of CTCL. Several molecular studies can also help support the diagnosis. The first looks at the cellular proteins seen on the surface of the abnormal cells. Many cases of CTCL show the retention of the CD4+ protein, but the loss of other proteins usually seen on the surface of mature CD4+ cells, such as Leu-8 or Leu-9. The abnormal cells also show unusual rearrangements at the genetic level for the gene that encodes the T-cell receptors. These rearrangements can be identified using Southern blot analysis. The information from the molecular tests, combined with the presence of abnormal cells in the epidermis, strongly supports the CTCL diagnosis.

Treatment team

This disease is treated by a dermatologist, a medical oncologist, and, if **radiation therapy** is used, a radiation oncologist.

Clinical staging, treatments, and prognosis

The current staging of this disease was first presented at the International Consensus Conference on CTCL in 1997. This staging attempts to show the complex interaction between the various outward symptoms of the disease and prognosis. The system has seven clinical stages based on skin involvement (tumor = T), lymph node involvement (LN), and presence of visceral metastases (M).

The first stage, IA, is characterized by plaques covering less than 10% of the body (T1) and no visceral involvement (M0). Lymph node condition at this stage can be uninvolved, reactive to the skin disease, or dermatopathic (biopsies showing CTCL involvement) but not enlarged (LN0-2). The shorthand expression of this stage is therefore T1, LN0-2, M0. Prognosis is very good if the disease has only progressed this far, with an average survival of 20 or more years. Most deaths occurring to persons in this group are unrelated to CTCL.

The next stage, IB, differs from IA in that greater than 10 percent of the body is covered by plaques (T2, LN0-2, M0). Stage IIA occurs with any amount of plaques in addition to the ability to palpate the lymph node and the lymph uninvolved, reactive, or dermatopathic (T1-2, LN0-2, M0). Average survival for patients in stages IB and IIA is about 12 years.

Treatments applied to the skin are preferred for patients having these preliminary stages of the disease. These commonly include topical **chemotherapy** with **mechlorethamine** hydrochloride (nitrogen mustard) or phototherapy of psoralen plus ultraviolet A (PUVA). Topical chemotherapy involves application to the skin of nitrogen mustard, an alkylating agent, in a concentration of 10 to 20 mg/dL in an aqueous or ointment base. Treatment of affected skin is suggested at a minimum and application over the entire skin surface is often recommended. Care needs to be taken that coverage of involved skin is adequate, as patients who self-apply the drug often cannot reach all affected areas. The most common side effect is skin hypersensitivity to the drug. Nearly all patients respond favorably to this treatment, with a 32–61% complete response rate, based on amount of skin involvement. Unfortunately, only 10–15% of patients maintain a complete response rate after discontinuing the treatment.

Phototherapy involves treatment with an orally administered drug, 8-methyloxypsoralen, that renders the skin sensitive to long-wave ultraviolet light (UVA), followed by controlled exposure to the radiation. During the initial treatment period, which may last as long as six months, patients are treated two to three times weekly. This is reduced to about once monthly after initial clearing of the lesions. Redness of the skin and blistering are the most common side effects of the treatment and are much more common in patients presenting with overall skin redness, or erythroderma, so lower intensities of light are usually used in this case. About 50% of all patients experience complete clearance with this treatment. Some patients with very fair skin and limited skin involvement can successfully treat themselves at home with special lamps and no psoralen.

The next stage, IIB, involves one or more cutaneous tumors, in combination with absent or present palpable lymph nodes, lymph uninvolved, reactive, or dermatopathic, and no visceral involvement (T3, LN0-2, M0). Stage III is characterized by erythroderma, an abnormal redness over widespread areas of the skin (T4, LN0-2, M0). The disease in both of these stages involves intermediate risk to the patient.

For more extensive disease, radiation therapy is an effective treatment option. It is generally used after the topical treatments have proven ineffective. Individual plaques or tumors can be treated using electrons, orthovoltage **x rays**, or megavoltage photons with exposure in the range of 15 to 25 Gy. Photon therapy has proven particularly useful once the lymph nodes are involved. Another possibility is total-skin electron beam therapy (TSEB), although the availability of this treatment method is limited. It involves irradiation of the entire body with energized electrons. Side effects of this treatment include loss of finger and toe nails, acute redness of the skin, and inability to sweat for about 6 to 12 months after therapy. Almost all patients respond favorably to radiation treatment and any reoccurrence is usually much less severe.

Combinations of different types of treatments is a very common approach to the management of CTCL. Topical nitrogen mustard or PUVA is often used after completion of radiation treatment to prolong the effects. The addition of genetically engineered interferon to PUVA therapy significantly increases the percentage of patients showing a complete response. Furthermore, although treatments using chemotherapy drugs alone, such as deoxycofomycin or etretinate, have been disappointing for CTCL, combining these drugs with interferon has shown promising results. Interferon has also been combined with retinoid treatments, although the mechanism of action of retinoids (Vitamin A analogues) against CTCL is unknown.

The final two stages of the disease are IVA and IVB. IVA presents as any amount of skin involvement, absent or present palpable lymph nodes, no visceral involvement, and lymph that contains large clusters of convoluted cells or obliterated nodes (T1-4, LN3-4). Patients in stage III and IVA have an average life expectancy of about five years. IVB differs in the addition of palpable lymph nodes and visceral involvement (T1-4, LN3-4, M1). At these stages the disease is high risk, with most deaths occurring by **infection**, due to the depleted immune system of the later stage patient. Once a patient has reached stage IVB, the average life expectancy is one year. All of the treatment methods described above are appropriate for the final two stages of the disease.

Alternative and complementary therapies

Itching of the skin is one of the most troublesome symptoms of CTCL. One alternative treatment for itchiness is the application of a brewed solution of chickweed that is applied to the skin using cloth compresses. Another suggested topical application is a mixture of vitamin E, vitamin A, unflavored yogurt, honey, and zinc oxide. Evening primrose oil applied topically may also reduce itch and promote healing.

Coping with cancer treatment

Topical chemotherapy and radiation treatment of the skin require special care of the areas being exposed to the drug or emission. Use of mild soap and special sensitive formulas for moisturizer and other skin products is suggested. Tight clothing in the area should be avoided. It is important that the treated area is not exposed to the sun during the treatment course. In general, special care to not irritate the area that is being treated will help ease the treatment course.

Clinical trials

Recent **clinical trials** for CTCL have focused on testing molecular treatment approaches. Anti-T-cell **monoclonal antibodies**, which would theoretically target the abnormal T cells for destruction by the patient's own immune system, have been tried. Unfortunately, the responses to this treatment have been brief and limited by the development of an immune reaction against the antibodies themselves (which are made in mouse cells and therefore seen as foreign by the patient's immune system). Studies continue using newly developed, more specific antibodies and radiolabeled antibodies (to target radiation therapy to the T-helper cells).

Genetically engineered fusion proteins that link diphtheria toxin (a protein that kills cells) with interleukin-2 (a protein that binds to T-helper cells through a receptor on its surface) have also been administered intravenously to CTCL patients. The toxin was taken into the abnormal cells and did kill them. Three out of five patients in a phase I trial achieved significant tumor response to this novel therapy.

As of 2009, other experimental treatments for CTCL include CPG 7909, a drug given by injection; vorinostat; and romidep.

Additional new approaches to the treatment of CTCL include vaccine therapy and stem cell transplantation. A group of researchers in Japan is currently testing various peptides introduced through the skin as a possible form of immunization against CTCL, while German and American researchers are investigating the potential of stem cell transplantation in the treatment of CTCL. As of late 2003, bone marrow transplants from unrelated donors offer the best hope of a curative treatment for CTCL.

Prevention

Studies have been unable to link CTCL to any environmental or genetic factors, so prevention is not possible as of the early 2000s.

Special concerns

Because the initial diagnosis of CTCL can be difficult, any dermatitis-like or eczema-like rash that does not respond to treatment or recurs after running the full course of topical **corticosteroids** should be brought to the attention of a doctor. This is particularly important given the good prognosis with early diagnosis and treatment of CTCL but rapidly worsening prognosis with progression of the disease.

See also Non-Hodgkin's lymphoma.

Resources

BOOKS

Beers, Mark H., MD, and Robert Berkow, MD, editors. "Mycosis Fungoides." Section 11, Chapter 139 In *The Merck Manual of Diagnosis and Therapy*. Whitehouse Station, NJ: Merck Research Laboratories, 2002.

Hoppe, Richard, T. "Mycosis Fungoides and Other Cutanous Lymphomas." In *The Lymphomas*, edited by George P. Canellos, et al. Philadephia: W.B. Saunders Co., 1999, pp. 495–406.

Wilson, Lynn D., et al. "Cutaneous T-Cell Lymphomas." In *Cancer Principles & Practice of Oncology*, edited by Vincent T. DeVita, et al. Philadelphia: Lippincott Williams & Wilkins, 2001, pp. 2316–2329.

PERIODICALS

Beyeler, M., and R. Dummer. "Standard and Experimental Therapy of Cutaneous T-cell Lymphoma." [in German] *Hautarzt* 54 (December 2003): 1177–1184.

Dippel, E., C. D. Klemke, and S. Goerdt. "Current Status of Cutaneous T-cell Lymphoma: Molecular Diagnosis, Pathogenesis, Therapy and Future Directions." *Onkologie* 26 (October 2003): 477–483.

Kempf, W., N. Kettelhack, M. Duvic, and G. Burg. " Topical and Systemic Retinoid Therapy for Cutaneous T-cell Lymphoma." *Hematology/Oncology Clinics of North America* 17 (December 2003): 1405–1419.

Oyama, Y., J. Guitart, T. M. Kuzel, et al. "High-Dose Therapy and Bone Marrow Transplantation in Cutaneous T-cell Lymphoma." *Hematology/Oncology Clinics of North America* 17 (December 2003): 1475–1483.

Seo, N., F. Furukawa, Y. Tokura, and M. Takigawa. "Vaccine Therapy for Cutaneous T-cell Lymphoma." *Hematology/Oncology Clinics of North America* 17 (December 2003): 1467–1474.

ORGANIZATIONS

Cutaneous Lymphoma Foundation. PO Box 374, Birmingham, MI 48012. (248) 644-9014. http://www.clfoundation.org.

National Cancer Institute. Building 31 Room 10A31 31 Center Drive MSC 2580 Bethesda, MD 20892-2580. (800)4-CANCER. http://cancernet.nci.nih.gov.

Michelle Johnson, M.S., J.D.
Rebecca J. Frey, PhD

Cyclooxygenase 2 inhibitors

Definition

Cyclooxygenase 2 inhibitors, also known as COX-2 inhibitors, are useful as pain and antiflammatory medications for **cancer** patients. COX-2 inhibitors are not better at stopping pain and inflammation than other non-steroidal anti-inflammatory drugs (NSAIDs), but are less likely to cause stomach ulcers and bleeding.

Purpose

Nonsteroidal anti-inflammatory drugs (NSAIDs) used to treat pain and inflammation are relatively effective in controlling these symptoms but can cause serious side effects. These side effects include stomach

KEY TERMS

Cyclooxygenase—A chemical important for the normal functioning of the human body. The body produces cyclooxygenase 1 (COX 1) and cyclooxygenase 2 (COX 2).

Cyclooxygenase 1 (COX 1) —The cyclooxygenase that helps the stomach, kidneys, and blood function well.

Cyclooxygenase 2 (COX 2)—The cyclooxygenase that helps mediate inflammation and that helps the brain feel pain and regulate fever.

ulcers, kidney problems, and increased likelihood of bleeding. Aspirin is the most serious offender, although other pain medications in the NSAID class of medication present similar problems. COX-2 inhibitors were developed as a type of pain medication less likely to cause stomach and bleeding problems than existing NSAID pain medications.

COX-2 inhibitors may also have future applications in cancer therapy. Recent research suggests that COX-2 is involved in the growth of cancerous tumors; therefore, COX-2 inhibitors may prove to be helpful in preventing or slowing the growth of certain types of cancer. One group of researchers in Taiwan reported in 2003 that celecoxib inhibits the growth of cell lines derived from mouth cancers, while another group in Arizona found that COX-2 inhibitors may be effective in slowing the growth of malignant **melanoma**.

Description

Cyclooxygenase is a chemical important for the normal functioning of the human body. Cyclooxygenase helps the stomach and kidneys to function normally, the platelets in the blood to function normally, and the brain to regulate body temperature and feel pain. Scientists have discovered that there are two distinct types of cyclooxygenase (abbreviated COX). These two types of COX are known as COX-1 and COX-2. COX-1 is needed to maintain the normal body functions of platelet aggregation, the regulation of blood flow in the kidney and stomach, and the regulation of gastric acid secretion in the stomach.

COX-2 is produced only when the body's tissues have been injured. COX-2 mediates inflammation, helps the nerves feel pain, and helps the brain regulate **fever**. A medication that inhibits COX-2 can suppress inflammation, relieve pain, and reduce fever. Inhibition

of COX-1, on the other hand, results in bleeding and kidney and stomach toxicity.

The problem with many older pain medications is that they affect both COX-1 and COX-2, even though they provide benefit only through how they affect COX-2. That is why their long-term use may be associated with such side effects as stomach ulcers, decreased kidney function, and a tendency for excessive bleeding. COX-2 inhibitors inhibit COX-2 while exerting less effect on COX-1.

At the end of 2003, three COX-2 inhibitors were available by prescription in the United States. Celecoxib (brand name Celebrex) was the first to be made available, followed by rofecoxib (brand name Vioxx) and valdecoxib (brand name Bextra), which was approved by the Food and Drug Administration (FDA) in late 2001. In addition, the pharmaceutical company Novartis had hoped to secure FDA approval in 2003 for a fourth COX-2 inhibitor named lumiracoxib, to be sold under the brand name Prexige. The FDA requested more data, however, and as of 2009 lumiracoxib has not yet been approved for use in the United States.

The FDA's reluctance to approve lumiracoxib may have been prophetic, insofar as the agency issued a public health advisory in late September 2004 regarding the safety of rofecoxib. The FDA was concerned about reports that Vioxx increased patients' risks of heart attack or stroke. The manufacturer voluntarily removed the drug from the market on September 30, 2004.

Recommended dosage

Celecoxib comes in 100 mg and 200 mg capsules that are taken orally either once or twice a day.

Valdecoxib is available in 10 and 20 mg tablets.

Precautions

Celecoxib should not be taken by patients with sulfonamide allergy. This medication should not be taken during the last few months of pregnancy.

Valdecoxib should not be taken during the last trimester of pregnancy. In addition, patients taking valdecoxib should tell their doctor if they are pregnant or might become pregnant during treatment with the drug.

Side effects

Celecoxib has few side effects. A small number of patients report stomach upset and even fewer report abdominal pain. Other effects reported rarely with celecoxib include kidney problems, fluid retention, and retention of water in the tissues. The occurrence of ulcers in patients taking celecoxib is less frequent than for many other pain medications. However, the long-term safety of celecoxib has not been well-researched.

Valdecoxib has been reported to cause weight gain, skin rashes, **nausea** and abdominal pain, **itching**, yellowing of the skin, flu-like symptoms, or unusual bruising or bleeding in some patients.

Interactions

Celecoxib may affect the activities of **warfarin**, a medication that limits the ability of blood to clot. Celecoxib may also be involved in interactions with: furosemide, a diuretic; angiotensin-converting enzyme inhibitors (ACE inhibitors), medicines used for high blood pressure and some heart problems; lithium, a medication for bipolar disorder; and fluconazole, an antifungal medication. Celecoxib may be taken with any of the medicines mentioned above; however, the doctor should closely monitor these drug combinations. Because celecoxib is a relatively new medication, more remains to be learned about its potential to interact with other drugs.

Valdecoxib may interact with NSAIDs, aspirin, lithium, steroid medications, ACE inhibitors, blood thinners (anticoagulants), and diuretics. In general, patients should make sure that their doctor has a complete list of all medications that they take on a regular basis—including over-the-counter pain relievers—before taking any COX-2 inhibitor.

Resources

PERIODICALS

Foral, P. A., K. K. Nystrom, A. F. Wilson, and C. M. Christensen. " Gastrointestinal-Related Adverse Effects of COX-2 Inhibitors." *Drugs Today (Barcelona)* 39 (December 2003): 939–948.

Goulet, A. C., J. G. Einsphar, D. S. Alberts, et al. "Analysis of Cyclooxygenase 2 (COX-2) Expression During Malignant Melanoma Progression." *Cancer Biology and Therapy* 2 (November-December 2003): 713–718.

Yang, C. Y., C. L. Meng, C. L. Liao, and P. Y. Wong. "Regulation of Cell Growth by Selective COX-2 Inhibitors in Oral Carcinoma Cell Lines." *Prostaglandins and Other Lipid Mediators* 72 (November 2003): 115–130.

OTHER

FDA press release, September 30, 2004. "FDA Issues Public Health Advisory on Vioxx as its Manufacturer Voluntarily Withdraws the Product." FDA document P04-95. http://www.fda.gov/bbs/topics/news/2004/NEW01122.html.

ORGANIZATIONS

United States Food and Drug Administration (FDA). 5600 Fishers Lane, Rockville, MD 20857-0001. (888) INFO-FDA (463-6332). http://www.fda.gov.

Bob Kirsch
Rebecca J. Frey, PhD

Cyclophosphamide

Definition

Cyclophosphamide is an anticancer (antineoplastic) agent. It also acts as a suppressor of the immune system. It is available under the brand names Cytoxan and Neosar.

Purpose

Cyclophosphamide is approved by the Food and Drug Administration (FDA) to treat several forms of **cancer**. These include:

- breast cancer
- leukemia
- malignant lymphoma
- multiple myeloma
- ovarian cancer
- soft tissue sarcoma
- mycosis fungoides
- nephrotic syndrome
- neuroblastoma
- Wilms' tumor
- retinoblastoma

Cyclophosphamide has activity against a wide variety of other cancers and conditions not specifically approved by the FDA, and patients should be aware that it may be commonly prescribed for these other disease states:

- bone cancer
- cervical cancer
- endometrial cancer
- germ cell tumors
- gestational trophoblastic tumors
- histiocytosis X
- lung cancer
- prostate cancer
- testicular cancer
- Wilms' tumor

Description

Cyclophosphamide chemically interferes with the synthesis of the genetic material (DNA and RNA) of cancer cells by cross-linking DNA strands, preventing these cells from being able to reproduce and continue the growth of the cancer.

Recommended dosage

Cyclophosphamide may be taken either orally (in pill form) or as an injection into the vein. The dosage prescribed may vary widely depending on the patient, the cancer being treated, and whether or not other medications are also being taken.

A typical oral dosage for adults is 1 to 5 mg per kg of body weight per day for initial and maintenance dose, or 400 to 1,000 milligrams per squared meter of body surface area for four to five days every three to four weeks. A typical dosage by injection is 40 to 50 mg per kg, divided in several smaller doses, for two to five days. The dose for patients receiving bone marrow transplant may be as high as 60 mg per kg per day for two days.

Precautions

Cyclophosphamide should be taken on an empty stomach. If stomach irritation occurs, it should be taken with small amounts of food or milk. Cyclophosphamide should always be taken with plenty of fluids.

Cyclophosphamide can cause an allergic reaction in some people. Patients with a prior allergic reaction to cyclophosphamide should not receive this drug.

Cyclophosphamide can cause serious birth defects if either the man or the woman is taking this drug at the time of conception or if the woman is taking this drug during pregnancy. Contraceptive measures should be taken by both men and women while on this drug. Sterility is a common side effect of cyclophosphamide. This sterility is dependent upon the dose, duration of therapy, and state of function of the ovary or testicle at the time of administration of the drug. The sterility may be irreversible in some patients.

Because cyclophosphamide is easily passed from mother to child through breast milk, breast feeding is not recommended while under treatment.

Cyclophosphamide suppresses the immune system and interferes with the normal functioning of certain organs and tissues, and its excretion from the body is dependent on a normal functioning kidney and liver. For these reasons, it is important that the prescribing physician is aware of any of the following pre-existing medical conditions:

- a current case of, or recent exposure to, chicken pox
- herpes zoster (shingles)
- all current infections
- kidney disease
- liver disease
- a prior removal of one, or both, adrenal gland(s)

Also, because cyclophosphamide is such a potent immunosuppressant, patients taking this drug must exercise extreme caution to avoid contracting any new infections.

Side effects

Inflammation and irritation of the bladder, causing blood in the urine, is a common and severe side effect of cyclophosphamide. However, this side effect can be prevented and controlled with the administration of vigorous hydration with intravenous fluids before, during, and after **chemotherapy**. Patients should urinate frequently (at least every two hours) to enhance removal of the drug from the body, and should drink 3 to 4 liters of fluids a day while taking the drug by mouth and for two to three days after discontinuation of the drug unless otherwise instructed by the physician. Patients who are taking cyclophosphamide orally should avoid taking the drug at night so that they can go to the bathroom frequently during the day. The bladder-protectant drug **mesna** is usually administered if the patient is receiving more than 2,000 mg per square meter of body surface area of the cyclophosphamide. Another common side effect of cyclophosphamide is increased susceptibility to **infection** due to decreased production of cells that fight infection. Increased risk of bleeding can occur due to decrease of platelets, which are involved with the clotting process. Decreased production of red blood cells can cause **anemia** and patients may experience **fatigue**, and shortness of breath.

Nausea and vomiting can occur, usually at the higher doses. Taking the appropriate **antiemetics** prescribed by the physician can prevent this side effect. Temporary hair loss (**alopecia**) usually begins three to six weeks after the start of therapy, but hair will regrow (although it may be a different color and/or texture). Sterility can occur in both men and women, and some women may also experience stoppage of menstruation. **Diarrhea** and ulcers of the mouth are also possible side effects of cyclophosphamide treatment.

Less common side effects include:

- nasal stuffiness
- runny eyes
- runny nose
- sinus congestion
- dizziness
- darkening of skin or fingernails
- skin rash
- sneezing (if the drug is given too rapidly by injection into the vein)
- facial flushing

Some patients may also develop a second cancer years later with cyclophosphamide therapy alone or in combination with other anti-cancer drugs. Patients should discuss this side effect with their physicians and determine the risks versus the benefits of this drug for treatment of the immediate cancer.

A doctor should be consulted immediately if the patient experiences any of the following:

- painful or difficult urination
- increase in frequency or feeling of urgency to urinate
- blood in the urine
- shortness of breath
- signs of infection such as cough, sore throat, fever and chills
- pain in the lower back or sides
- unusual bleeding or bruising
- blood in the stool
- tiny red dots on the skin
- delayed healing of any wounds
- skin rash
- yellowing of the skin or eyes

Interactions

Cyclophosphamide should not be taken in combination with any prescription drug, over-the-counter drug, or herbal remedy without prior consultation with a physician.

Paul A. Johnson, Ed.M.

Cyclosporine

Definition

Cylosporine is an immunosuppressant drug used to prevent rejection of kidney, liver, and heart transplants; to prevent graft-versus-host disease in patients receiving allogeneic bone marrow transplants; and for severe autoimmune diseases that are resistant to **corticosteroids** and other therapy. Cyclosporine, also spelled as cyclosporin and ciclosporin, takes several brand names in the United States, including Neoral, Sandimmun, Sandimmune, and Sang Cya. It is also known in slight variant forms, such as cyclosporin A, CsA, and CyA. The Neoral and Sang Cya brand name products are interchangeable, but the Sandimmune brand name product can not be used interchangeably for those other two products.

Purpose

Cyclosporine is best known as a drug used to prevent the rejection of organ transplants and bone grafts.

Description

Discovered in 1972, cyclosporine was first isolated from a fungus. It suppresses (prevents the activity of) the cells in the lymphatic system, known as T cells, that would otherwise mount an **immune response**. This suppression makes cyclosporine useful in conjunction with organ transplants. (In a transplant, the patient receiving a donated organ can react to the organ as though it were a foreign substance, rejecting it.) Cyclosporine is also used to treat severe rheumatoid arthritis, and is being used investigationally as a drug that may help to temper multidrug resistance in **cancer** patients.

The drug is available in several forms, including an intravenous (I.V.) solution, an oral solution, and an oral capsule. Cyclosporine is broken down in the liver.

Recommended dosage

The dosage varies, depending on the reason for use and the patient, and the dosage is also often adjusted by the physician. The dosage is based on the patient's ideal body weight, and the oral dose is approximately three times higher than the intravenous dose. I.V. use is only reserved for patients who cannot take the oral dose, and it is recommended that patients who can be switched to the oral form be switched as soon as possible.

The usual initial oral dose is 14–18 mg/kg per day, beginning 4–12 hours before organ transplantation. After the transplantation, the dose is decreased, and then usually tapered to 3–10 mg/kg per day.

Precautions

Cyclosporine can cause **infection** and possibly **lymphoma**, and is toxic to the kidneys. The use of this drug along with other drugs that are toxic to the kidneys must be closely monitored. It should be ingested and swallowed in its capsule without breaking the capsule. The liquid solution should only be mixed in a glass container. Pregnant or nursing women should not take this drug, and patients taking this drug will be more susceptible to infection. Therefore, crowds of people should be avoided, and no live **vaccines** should be adminstered to the patient without consulting the patient's doctor. Patients should inform their doctor of any hypersensitivities or drug allergies they have before taking this drug. (Cyclosporine in both liquid and capsule form has some castor oil components in it, which could cause an allergic reaction for some.) Some allergic reactions to the I. V. solution may be severe. This drug has not been specifically studied for use with the elderly.

Side effects

More than 10% of patients taking this drug experience the following:

- high blood pressure
- unusual hair growth
- kidney toxicity
- tremors
- thickening of the gums

Other, less common side effects include: seizures, headache, acne, abdominal pain, **nausea and vomiting**, leg cramps, and some endocrine/metabolic conditions known as hypomagnesia, hypokalemia, hyperkalemia, and hyperlipidemia.

Interactions

Cyclosporine interacts with a long list of other drugs. A physician should be informed about each and every drug a person eligible for treatment with cyclosporine is taking. Drugs that may make cyclosporine less effective include: **carbamazepine**, phenobarbital, **phenytoin**, and others. Drugs that may increase cyclopsporine's toxicity include: acyclovir, amphotericin B, corticosteroids, erythromycin, certain **antibiotics**, and some antifungals including fluconazole, itraconazole, and ketaconazole. Cyclosporine should not be taken with grapefruit or related juices because the combination can make it more toxic. Vaccinations should not be given while a person is taking cyclosporine.

Diane M. Calabrese

Cystectomy

Definition

Cystectomy is a surgical procedure that removes all or part of the urinary bladder, the muscular organ that collects urine from the kidneys for excretion at a later time. Partial or segmental cystectomy removes part of the bladder; simple cystectomy removes the entire bladder; and radical cystectomy removes the bladder as well as other pelvic organs or structures.

Purpose

Cystectomy is most commonly performed to treat **cancer** of the bladder. Once a patient has been diagnosed with **bladder cancer**, a staging system is used to indicate how far the cancer has spread and determine appropriate treatments. Superficial tumors isolated to the inner lining of the bladder (stage 0 or I) may be treated with non-surgical therapies such as **chemotherapy** or radiation, or with partial or simple cystectomy. Radical cystectomy is the standard treatment for cancer that has invaded the bladder muscle (Stage II, III, or IV). Muscle-invasive cancer accounts for 90% of all bladder cancers.

Other conditions that may require cystectomy include interstitial cystitis (chronic inflammation of the bladder), endometriosis that has spread to the bladder, severe urinary dysfunction, damage to the bladder from radiation or other treatments, or excessive bleeding from the bladder.

Demographics

Approximately 56,500 cases of urinary bladder cancer are diagnosed in the United States annually, with approximately 12,600 men and women dying of the disease each year. Men are more often diagnosed with bladder cancer (2.6 men for each woman diagnosed), and they also have a higher mortality rate (two men for each woman that dies). The average age that the disease is diagnosed is 65 years.

More cases of bladder cancer are found among white men and women. According to the American Cancer Society, whites are diagnosed with bladder cancer twice as often as African Americans. The mortality rate, however, is similar among white and African-American patients. It is believed that this similarity is due to the cancer being diagonsed at a more advanced stage in African Americans.

Description

Partial cystectomy

During partial or segmental cystectomy, only the area of the bladder where the cancer is found is removed. This allows for most of the bladder to be preserved. Because the cancer must not have spread to the bladder muscle and must be isolated to one area, partial cystectomy is only used infrequently for the patients who meet these select criteria.

The patient is first placed under general anesthesia. After an incision is made into the lower abdomen, the bladder is identified and isolated. The surgeon may choose to perform the operation with the bladder remaining inside the abdominal cavity (transperitoneal approach) or with the bladder lifted outside of the abdominal cavity (extraperitoneal approach). The cancerous area is excised (cut out) with a 0.8 in (2 cm) margin to ensure that all abnormal cells are removed. The bladder is then closed with stitches. The pelvic lymph nodes may also be removed during the procedure. After the cancerous tissue is removed, it is examined by a pathologist to determine if the margins of the tissue are clear of abnormal cells.

Simple or radical cystectomy

While partial cystectomy is considered a bladder-conserving surgery, simple and radical cystectomy involves the removal of the entire bladder. In the case of radical cystectomy, other pelvic organs and structures are also removed because of the tendency of bladder cancer to spread to nearby tissues. After the patient is placed under general anesthesia, an incision is made into the lower abdomen. Blood vessels leading to and from the bladder are ligated (tied off), and the bladder is divided from the urethra, ureters, and other tissues holding it in place. The bladder may then be removed.

The surgical procedure for radical cystectomy differs between male and female patients. In men, the prostate, seminal vesicles, and pelvic lymph nodes are removed with the bladder. In women, the uterus, fallopian tubes, ovaries, anterior (front) part of the vagina, and pelvic lymph nodes are removed with the bladder. If the surgery is being performed as a treatment for cancer, the removed tissues may be examined for the presence of abnormal cells.

Urinary diversion

Once the bladder is removed, a new method for excreting urine must be created. One commonly used approach is the ileal conduit. A piece of the small intestine is removed, cleaned, and tied at one end to form a tube. The other end is used to form a stoma, an opening through the abdominal wall to the outside. The ureters are then connected to the tube. Urine produced by the kidneys flows down the ureters, into the tube, and through the stoma. The patient wears a bag to collect the urine.

For continent cutaneous diversion, a pouch is constructed out of portions of the small and large intestine; the ureters are connected to the pouch and a stoma is created through the abdominal wall. Urine is removed by inserting a thin tube (catheter) into the stoma when the pouch is full. Alternatively, a similar pouch called a neobladder may be created, attached to both the ureters and the urethra, in an attempt to preserve as close to normal bladder function as possible.

Diagnosis/Preparation

The medical team will discuss the procedure and tell the patient where the stoma will appear and what it will look like. The patient will receive instruction on caring for a stoma and bag. A period of fasting and an enema may be required.

Aftercare

After the operation, the patient is given fluid-based nutrition until the intestines begin to function normally again. **Antibiotics** are given to prevent **infection**. The nature of cystectomy means that there will be major lifestyle changes for the person undergoing the operation. Men may become impotent if nerves controlling penile erection are cut during removal of the bladder. Infertility is a consequence for women undergoing radical cystectomy because the ovaries and uterus are removed. Most women who undergo cystectomy, however, are postmenopausal and past their childbearing years.

Patients are fitted with an external bag that connects to the stoma and collects the urine. The bag is generally worn around the waist under the clothing. It takes a period of adjustment to get used to wearing the bag. Because there is no bladder, urine is excreted as it is produced. The stoma must be treated properly to ensure that it does not become infected or blocked. Patients must be trained to care for their stoma. Often, there is a period of psychological adjustment to the major change in lifestyle created by the stoma and bag. Patients should be prepared for this by their physician.

Risks

As with any major surgery, there is a risk of infection; in this case, infection of the intestine is especially dangerous as it can lead to peritonitis (inflammation of the membrane lining the abdomen). In the case of partial cystectomy, there is a risk of urine leakage from the bladder incision site. Other risks include injury to nearby organs, complications associated with general anesthesia (such as respiratory distress), excessive blood loss, sexual dysfunction, or urinary **incontinence** (inadvertent leakage of urine).

Normal results

During a successful partial cystectomy, the cancerous or damaged area of the bladder is removed and the patient retains urinary control. A successful simple or

radical cystectomy results in the removal of the bladder and the creation of a urinary diversion, with little or no effect on sexual function. Intestinal function returns to normal and the patient learns proper care of the stoma and bag. He or she adjusts to lifestyle changes and returns to a normal routine of work and recreation.

Morbidity and mortality rates

The overall rate of complications associated with radical cystectomy may be as high as 25–35%; major complications occur at a rate of 5%. The rate of radical cystectomy-related deaths is 1–3%. Partial cystectomy has a complication rate of 11–29%. Some studies have placed the rate of cancer reoccurrence after partial cystectomy at 40–80%.

Alternatives

Transurethral resection (TUR) is one method that may be used to treat superficial bladder tumors. A cystoscope (a thin, tubular instrument used to visualize the interior of the bladder) is inserted into the bladder through the urethra and used to remove any cancerous tissue. Non-surgical options include chemotherapy and radiation.

Resources

BOOKS

Walsh, Patrick C., et al., eds. *Campbell's Urology,* 8th ed. Philadelphia: Elsevier Science, 2002.

PERIODICALS

"Bladder Cancer, Part III: Treatment Approaches in Current Practice and in Evaluation." *Future Oncology* 6, no. 5 (April 30, 2001): 1322–40.

Carrion, Rafael, and John Seigne. "Surgical Management of Bladder Carcinoma." *Cancer Control: Journal of the Moffitt Cancer Center* 9, no. 4 (October 31, 2002): 284–92.

ORGANIZATIONS

American Cancer Society. 1599 Clifton Road NE, Atlanta, GA 30329. (800) ACS-2345. http://www.cancer.org.

Cancer Information Service, National Cancer Institute. Building 31, Room 10A19, 9000 Rockville Pike, Bethesda, MD 20892. (800) 4-CANCER. http://cis.nci.nih.gov.

OTHER

"All About Bladder Cancer." American Cancer Society, 2003 [cited April 4, 2003]. http://www.cancer.org/docroot/CRI/CRI_2x.asp.

"Cancer Facts and Figures, 2002." American Cancer Society, 2002 [cited April 4, 2003]. http://www.cancer.org/downloads/STT/CancerFacts&Figures2002TM.pdf.

Eggner, Scott, and Steven Campbell. "Cystectomy, Radical." *eMedicine,* August 1, 2001 [cited April 4, 2003]. http://www.emedicine.com/med/topic3061.htm.

Feng, Adrian H. "Cystectomy, Partial." *eMedicine,* February 8, 2002 [cited April 4, 2003]. http://www.emedicine.com/med/topic3043.htm.

Ries, L. A. G., et al., eds. "SEER Cancer Statistics Review." National Cancer Institute, 2002 [cited April 4, 2003]. http://seer.cancer.gov/csr/1973_1999.

John T. Lohr, PhD
Stephanie Dionne Sherk

Cystosarcoma phyllodes

Definition

Cystosarcoma phyllodes (CSP) is a rare type of breast tumor. It is categorized by the National Cancer Institute (NCI) as a tumor subtype that occurs within the breast but is not considered a typical cancer. Its name comes from two Greek words that mean "fleshy tumor" and "leaflike," because its internal structure resembles a leaf when the tumor is cross-sectioned. The term phyllodes tumor is considered preferable to CSP as of the early 2000s because most of these tumors

GALE ENCYCLOPEDIA OF CANCER 3

KEY TERMS

Areola—The darkened ring of skin surrounding the nipple.

Fibroadenoma—A benign tumor derived from glandular tissue that contains fibrous tissue as well. Phyllodes tumors are sometimes referred to as giant fibroadenomas of the breast.

Mitosis—The process of cell division. The rate of mitosis in a tissue sample is one measurement used to determine whether a phyllodes tumor is benign or malignant.

Pathologist—A doctor who examines biopsy specimens and tissues removed during surgery for evidence of changes caused by disease.

Stroma—The supporting connective tissue of the breast or other organ.

---

are benign. Phyllodes tumors are also known as giant fibroadenomas of the breast.

Description

Phyllodes tumors develop only in the breast; they are never found in other parts of the body. They are formed within the stroma (connective tissue) of the breast and contain glandular as well as stromal tissue. Phyllodes tumors can grow noticeably within a matter of weeks, causing the overlying skin to become semitransparent or reddish and warm to the touch. They do not, however, usually involve the nipple or areola.

A phyllodes tumor can be moved freely within the breast when the doctor performs a manual examination. The tumor has a firm, smooth texture, can be easily distinguished from the surrounding tissue, and may grow to be quite large and bulky. The average size of phyllodes tumors is about 2 in (5 cm), although tumors as large as 11.8 in (30 cm) have been reported. These tumors do not cause pain when touched. For reasons that are not yet understood, phyllodes tumors are more likely to develop in the left breast than the right.

There is some disagreement among specialists regarding the number of phyllodes tumors that prove to be malignant. Although figures of 16–30% are commonly given, some doctors think that the actual incidence may be higher, as more cases of malignant tumors have been reported in the early 2000s.

QUESTIONS TO ASK YOUR DOCTOR

- What are the chances that my phyllodes tumor is either borderline or malignant?
- What are the chances of a recurrence?
- Would you recommend a total mastectomy rather than local excision to minimize the risk of recurrence?

Demographics

Phyllodes tumors account for less than 1% of all breast tumors. Almost all occur in women, although a few cases have been reported in men. Phyllodes tumors have been identified in women in all age groups but are uncommon in adolescents. They are most likely to occur in women over 35.

As far as is known, phyllodes tumors occur with the same frequency in women of all races and in all parts of the world.

Causes and symptoms

The cause of phyllodes tumors is not known as of the early 2000s.

The symptoms of a phyllodes tumor include the rapid but painless growth of a smooth, bulky mass within the affected breast. The patient may notice that her entire breast is enlarged and its shape distorted. The skin overlying the tumor may feel warm to the touch and develop a shiny appearance; it may also become translucent.

Patients with metastases from a malignant phyllodes tumor may experience difficulty breathing (dyspnea), **bone pain**, and **fatigue**.

Diagnosis

The diagnosis of a phyllodes tumor may be made when the patient notices a rapidly growing mass in her breast and consults her doctor. After palpating (feeling) the mass and evaluating the appearance of the overlying skin, the doctor will order **imaging studies** and an open breast **biopsy**. Although a mammogram or ultrasound study may be useful in evaluating the size and location of the tumor, these tests are not reliable in distinguishing among benign phyllodes tumors, fibroadenomas, and malignant phyllodes tumors. In addition, fine-needle aspiration does not usually confirm the diagnosis; an open biopsy is considered the definitive diagnostic test as of the early 2000s.

There are no tumor marker or other blood tests that can be used to diagnose phyllodes tumors as of 2005.

Treatment team

The treatment team for a patient with a phyllodes tumor will usually include a diagnostic radiologist, a gynecologist, a general surgeon, and a pathologist.

Clinical staging, treatments, and prognosis

Staging

Phyllodes tumors are not staged in the usual sense; they are classified on the basis of their appearance under the microscope as benign, borderline (or indeterminate), or malignant. The pathologist makes the decision on the basis of the cells' rate of division (mitosis) and the number of irregularly shaped cells in the biopsy sample. In one series of 101 patients with phyllodes tumors, 58% were identified as benign, 12% as borderline, and 30 percent as malignant.

Treatments

Surgical excision (removal) is the usual treatment for phyllodes tumors, whether benign or malignant. In the case of benign tumors, the surgeon will usually try to spare as much breast tissue as possible, generally removing about 1 in (2 cm) of normal breast tissue from the area around the tumor as well as the tumor itself. If the tumor is very large, however, the doctor may remove the entire breast.

In the case of malignant tumors, the surgeon will remove a wider area of normal tissue along with the tumor—a technique known as wide local excision (WLE)—or perform a complete **mastectomy**.

Although **radiation therapy** has been tried as follow-up treatment after surgery, phyllodes tumors do not respond well to either radiotherapy or **chemotherapy** if they recur or metastasize. In addition, malignant phyllodes tumors do not respond to hormone therapy.

Prognosis

The prognosis for benign phyllodes tumors is good following surgical removal, although there is a 20–35% chance of recurrence, particularly in patients over the age of 45. Recurrence is usually treated with further surgery, either another local excision or a complete mastectomy.

The prognosis for patients diagnosed with borderline or malignant phyllodes tumors is more guarded. About 4% of borderline tumors will eventually metastasize. A Mayo Clinic study of 50 patients with malignant tumors found that 32% had a recurrence within two years after surgery; 26% developed metastases, and 32% of the group died from their malignancy. The most common sites for metastases from malignant phyllodes tumors are the lungs, bones, liver, and chest wall, although metastases to the lymph nodes have also been reported. Most patients with metastases from a malignant phyllodes tumor die within three years of their first treatment.

Alternative and complementary therapies

Women who have had surgery for removal of a phyllodes tumor appear to use CAM therapies as often and for the same reasons as women treated for **breast cancer**. According to the Behavioral Research Center of the American Cancer Society, breast cancer survivors are highly likely to use some form of alternative or complementary therapy during cancer treatment or within a year or two of completing conventional treatment. A survey of 608 longer-term (8 years or longer) breast cancer survivors reported in early 2005 that the majority were still using CAM therapies. The survey respondents gave four reasons for using alternative treatments:

- to maintain an active role in recovery from cancer
- to reduce their stress level
- to reduce the risk of recurrence
- to maintain hope

Specific CAM therapies mentioned by the women in the ACS survey included exercise, humor, self-help books (bibliotherapy), prayer or spiritual practice, vitamin treatments, relaxation exercises, and support groups. Dr. Kenneth Pelletier, the former director of the program in complementary and alternative medicine at Stanford University School of Medicine, lists hypnosis, visualization, naturopathy, and journaling as other alternative approaches that breast cancer patients find helpful. Acupuncture is frequently mentioned as a useful method of pain control.

Coping with treatment

Coping with the aftereffects of surgery for a phyllodes tumor is similar to coping with the effects of surgery for breast cancer. Patients who have had a complete mastectomy may experience pain, limited range of motion or weakness in the affected arm, scarring, or swelling. Exercises, outpatient physical therapy, and massage help to relieve these side effects of breast

surgery. In terms of follow-up, most patients treated for phyllodes tumors are scheduled for a postoperative visit with the surgeon one to two weeks after surgery, with periodic checkups thereafter.

Clinical trials

The National Cancer Institute (NCI) is not conducting any **clinical trials** involving phyllodes tumors as of 2009.

Prevention

There is no way to prevent phyllodes tumors as of the early 2000s because their cause is not yet known.

Special concerns

The special concerns of patients with phyllodes tumors are similar to those of patients diagnosed with breast cancer, particularly concern about disfigurement, physical weakness, or recurrence if the entire breast has been removed.

See also Breast cancer; Fibroadenoma.

Resources

BOOKS

"Cystosarcoma Phyllodes." In *The Merck Manual of Diagnosis and Therapy*, edited by Mark H. Beers, MD, and Robert Berkow, MD. Whitehouse Station, NJ: Merck Research Laboratories, 2007.

Pelletier, Kenneth R., MD. *The Best Alternative Medicine.* New York: Simon & Schuster, 2002.

PERIODICALS

Asoglu, O., M. M. Ugurlu, K. Blanchard, et al. "Risk Factors for Recurrence and Death after Primary Surgical Treatment of Malignant Phyllodes Tumors." *Annals of Surgical Oncology* 11 (November 2004): 1011–1017.

Chaney, A. W., A. Pollack, M. D. McNeese, et al. "Primary Treatment of Cystosarcoma Phyllodes of the Breast." *Cancer* 89 (October 1, 2000): 1502–1511.

Hann, D., F. Baker, M. Denniston, and N. Entrekin. "Long-Term Breast Cancer Survivors' Use of Complementary Therapies: Perceived Impact on Recovery and Prevention of Recurrence." *Integrative Cancer Therapies* 4 (March 2005): 14–20.

Konstantakos, Anastasios K., MD, and John H. Raaf, MD. "Cystosarcoma Phyllodes." *eMedicine*, 26 August 2004. http://www.emedicine.com/med/topic500.htm.

Parfitt, J. R., C. Armstrong, F. O'Malley, et al. "In-Situ and Invasive Carcinoma with a Phyllodes Tumor Associated with Lymph Node Metastases." *World Journal of Surgical Oncology* 2 (December 15, 2004): 46.

OTHER

American Cancer Society (ACS), Cancer Reference Information. *Detailed Guide: Breast Cancer: What Is Breast Cancer?*. http://www.cancer.org/docroot/CRI/content/CRI_2_4_1X_What_is_breast_cancer_5.asp.

American Cancer Society (ACS), Cancer Reference Information. *Non-Cancerous Breast Conditions*. http://www.cancer.org/docroot/CRI/content/CRI_2_6X_Non_Cancerous_Breast_Conditions.asp.

National Cancer Institute (NCI). *Breast Cancer (PDQ®): Treatment*. http://www.cancer.gov/cancertopics/pdq/treatment/breast/HealthProfessional/page2.

ORGANIZATIONS

Behavioral Research Center, American Cancer Society. 1599 Clifton Road NE, Atlanta, GA 30329. (800) 758-0227 or (404) 329-7772. http://www.cancer.org.

Norris Cotton Cancer Center, Dartmouth-Hitchcock Medical Center. One Medical Center Drive, Lebanon, NH 03756. (603) 653-9000. http://www.cancer.dartmouth.edu.

Rebecca Frey, PhD

Cystoscopy

Definition

Cystoscopy (cystourethroscopy) is a diagnostic procedure that is used to look at the bladder (lower urinary tract), collect urine samples, and examine the prostate gland. Performed with an optic instrument known as a cystoscope (urethroscope), this instrument uses a lighted tip for guidance to aid in diagnosing urinary tract disease and prostate disease. Performed by a urologist, this surgical test also enables biopsies to be taken or small stones to be removed by way of a hollow channel in the cystoscope.

Purpose

Categorized as an endoscopic procedure, cystoscopy is used by urologists to examine the entire bladder lining and take biopsies of any areas that look questionable. This test is not used on a routine basis but may benefit the urologist who needs further information about a patient who displays the following symptoms or diagnosis:

- blood in the urine (also known as hematuria)
- incontinence, or the inability to control urination
- a urinary tract infection
- a urinary tract that display signs of congenital abnormalities

- tumors located in the bladder
- the presence of bladder or kidney stones
- a stiffness or strained feeling of the urethra or ureters
- symptoms of an enlarged prostate

Blood and urine studies, in addition to **x rays** of the kidneys, ureters, and bladder may all occur before a cystoscopy. At the time of the procedure, a retrograde pyelogram may also be performed. Additional blood studies may be needed immediately following cystoscopy.

Precautions

While the cystoscopy procedure is commonly relied on to gather additional diagnostic information, it is an invasive surgical technique that may involve risks for certain patients. Those who are extremely overweight (obese), smoke, are recovering from a recent illness, or are treating a chronic condition may face additional risks from surgery.

Surgical risk also increases in patients who are currently using certain drugs including antihypertensives, muscle relaxants, tranquilizers, sleep inducers, insulin, sedatives, beta blockers, or cortisone. Those who use mind-altering drugs also put themselves at increased risk of complications during surgery. The following mind-altering drugs should be avoided: narcotics, psychedelics, hallucinogens, marijuana, sedatives, hypnotics, or cocaine.

Description

Depending on the type of information needed from a cystoscopy, the procedure typically takes 10–40 minutes to complete. The patient will be asked to urinate before the procedure, which allows an accurate measurement of the remaining urine in the bladder. A well-lubricated cystoscope is inserted through the urethra into the bladder, where a urine sample is taken. Fluid is then pushed in to inflate the bladder and allow the urologist to examine the entire bladder wall.

During an examination, the urologist may take the following steps: remove either bladder or kidney stones; gather tissue samples; and treat any suspicious lesions. In order to perform the x-ray studies known as a retrograde pyelogram, a harmless dye is injected into the ureters by way of a catheter that is passed through the previously placed cystoscope. After completion of all needed tests, the cystoscope is removed.

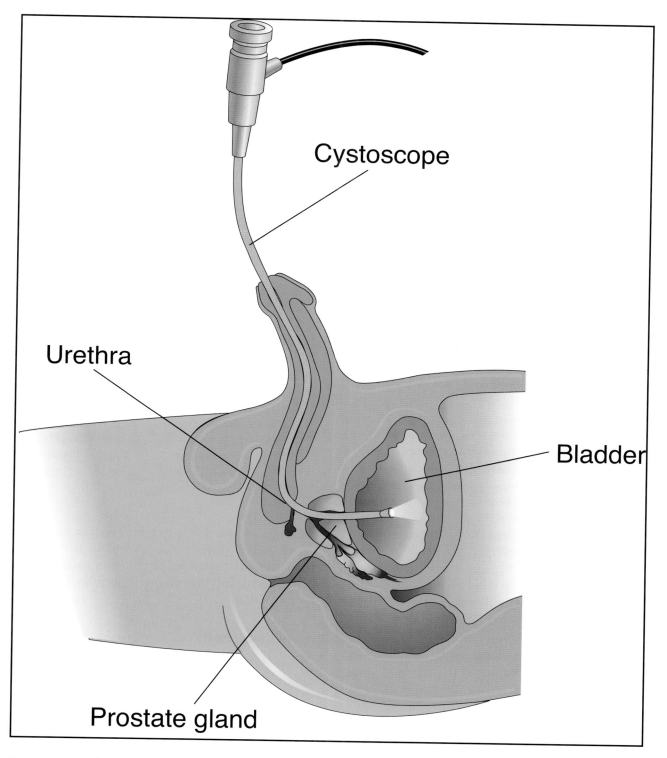

Cystoscope

Urethra

Bladder

Prostate gland

Cystoscopy is a diagnostic procedure which is used to view the bladder, collect urine samples, and examine the prostate gland. This procedure also enables biopsies to be taken. The primary instrument used in cystoscopy is the cystoscope, a tube which is inserted through the penis, into the urethra, and ultimately into the bladder. *(Illustration by Electronic Illustrators Group. Cengage Learning, Gale.)*

Preparation

A cystoscopic procedure can be completed in a hospital, a doctor's office, or an outpatient surgical facility. An injection of spinal or general anesthetic may be used prior to a cystoscopy. Although this test is typically performed on an outpatient basis, a patient may require up to three days' recovery in the hospital.

Aftercare

Patients who have undergone a cystoscopy will be instructed to follow these steps to ensure a quick recovery:

- Because of soreness or discomfort that may occur in the urethra, especially while urinating, several warm baths a day are recommended to relieve any pain.
- Allow four days for recovery.
- Be aware that blood may appear in the urine. This is common and soon clears up in one to two days following the procedure.
- Avoid strenuous exercise for a minimum of two weeks following cystoscopy.
- Sexual relations may continue when the urologist determines that healing is complete.
- Wait at least two days after surgery before driving.

Patients may also be prescribed pain relievers and **antibiotics** following surgery. Minor pain may also be treated with over-the-counter, nonprescription drugs such as acetaminophen.

Risks

As with any surgical procedure, there are some risks involved with a cystoscopy. Complications may include profuse bleeding, a damaged urethra, a perforated bladder, a urinary tract **infection**, or an injured penis.

Patients should also contact their physician if they experience any of the following symptoms following surgery: pain at or redness or swelling around the surgical site; drainage or bleeding from the surgical

site; signs of infection, which may include headache, muscle aches, dizziness, an overall ill feeling, and **fever**; **nausea** or **vomiting**; strenuous or painful urination; or symptoms that may result as side effects from the medication.

Normal results

A successful cystoscopy includes a thorough examination of the bladder and collection of urine samples for cultures. If no abnormalities are seen, the results are indicated as normal.

Abnormal results

Cystoscopy allows the urologist to detect inflammation of the bladder lining, prostatic enlargement, or tumors. If these are seen, further evaluation or biopsies may be needed, in addition to the removal of some tumors.

Resources

PERIODICALS

Chew, Lisa, and Stephan D. Fihn. "Recurrent cystitis in nonpregnant women." *Western Journal of Medicine* 170 (May 1999): 274-277.

Gilmour, D.T., P.L. Dwyer, and M.P. Carey. "Lower urinary tract injury during gynecologic surgery and its detection by intraoperative cystoscopy." *Obstetrics and Gynecology* 5, no. 2 (1999): 883-889.

Neumayer, Leigh, A., Mary K. Mastin, and Douglas M. Hinson. "Performance Standards: Piece of Cake or Pie in the sky?" *Journal of Surgical Research* 88 (2000): 47-50.

ORGANIZATIONS

American Cancer Society. 1599 Clifton Road, NE, Atlanta, GA 30329-4251. (800)ACS-2345. http://www.cancer.org/.The American Cancer Society (ACS) is a nationwide community-based voluntary health organization dedicated to eliminating cancer as a major health problem and is the largest source of private, nonprofit cancer funds. The ACS hopes to prevent cancer, save lives, and diminish suffering from cancer through research, education, advocacy, and service.

Interstitial Cystitis Association (ICA). 51 Monroe Street, Suite 1402, Rockville, MD 20850. 1-800-HELP-ICA. http://www.ichelp.org. Founded in 1984, the ICA is a not-for-profit health organization dedicated to providing patient and physician educational information and programs, patient support, public awareness, and research funding.

National Institute of Diabetes & Digestive & Kidney Disease. Office of Communications and Public Liaison, NIDDK, NIH, 31 Center Drive, MSC 2560, Bethesda, MD 20892-2560. NIDDK_Inquiries@nih.gov. http://www.niddk.nih.gov. Mission to understand, treat, and prevent diseases, such as diabetes and obesity, digestive diseases such as hepatitis and inflammatory bowel disease, kidney and urologic diseases such as kidney failure and prostate enlargement, and blood diseases such as the anemias.

National Kidney and Urologic Diseases Information Clearinghouse. 3 Information Way, Bethesda, MD 20892-3580. 1-800-891-5390. nkudic@info.niddk.nih.gov. http://www.niddk.nih.gov/health/kidney/nkudic.htm. Knowledge and understanding about diseases of the kidneys and urologic system among people with these conditions and their families, health care professionals, and the general public.

Beth A. Kapes

Cytarabine

Definition

Cytarabine (also known as ARA-C, and by the brand name Cytosar) is an anticancer agent that kills **cancer** cells. It is very frequently used with other **anticancer drugs** in the treatment of acute myelocytic

---

KEY TERMS

Cytotoxic drug—A medicine that kills (cancer) cells.

DNA—An acid found in all living cells that contains tiny bits of genetic information.

Lipids—Substances including fats, waxes, and related compounds that (with proteins and carbohydrates) constitute the principal structural components of living cells.

---

leukemia (AML), lymphomas, and for leukemia and **lymphoma** affecting the surrounding membranes of the brain and spinal cord (meninges).

Purpose

There are two formulations of this drug: cytarabine, and cytarabine liposomal, where the drug is encapsulated in a molecule of lipid. Cytarabine is used to treat acute myelogenous leukemia, **acute lymphocytic leukemia** (ALL), **chronic myelocytic leukemia** (CML), central nervous system (CNS) leukemia affecting the membrane surrounding the brain and spinal cord, and Hodgkin's and **non-Hodgkin's lymphoma** (NHL). Cytarabine liposomal (brand name Depocyt) is primarily used to treat lymphoma involving the meninges (the membrane covering the brain and spinal cord).

Description

Cytarabine is a cytotoxic drug. This means that its task is to kill cancer cells. Cytarabine kills cells by interfering with the production of DNA.

Recommended dosage

The dose for cytarabine may be different depending on the protocol used by the physician. An example dose of cytarabine is 100 to 200 mg per square meter of body surface area per day for seven days as an intravenous (IV) medication.

High-dose cytarabine may be 2 to 3 grams per square meter of body surface area twice a day for three days. Cytarabine is also administered directly into the cerebral spinal fluid for lymphoma or leukemia involving the meninges. The dose is 5 to 75 mg per square meter of body surface area every two to seven days. The dose for cytarabine liposomal in the cerebral spinal fluid is usually 50 mg.

Precautions

Liposomal cytarabine not be given to patients with infections of the meninges, allergic reaction to cytarabine, or if the patient is pregnant.

Side effects

Side effects include **fever** in greater than 80% of patients, hair loss (**alopecia**), **nausea and vomiting, diarrhea**, ulcers of the mouth, decreased white blood cells (responsible for fighting infections), decreased platelets (responsible for blood clotting), decreased red blood cells (responsible for oxygenation of tissues), and decrease in liver function. Abdominal pain, loss of appetite, and a metallic taste in the mouth may develop, as may an allergic reaction. Tearing, eye pain, foreign body sensation in the eye, blurred vision, and sensitivity of the eyes to light occurs with high-dose cytarabine and may be prevented or relieved with corticosteroid eyedrops. Patients receiving high-dose cytarabine may also experience skin sloughing, redness and pain of the palms of the hand and soles of the feet, dizziness, headaches, drowsiness, confusion, personality changes, abnormal movements of the eye, loss of coordination, and in severe cases, loss of consciousness.

Although it is uncommon, one of the most serious side effects of cytarabine may involve sudden respiratory distress involving abnormal, shallow, and rapid breathing, which may progress to **pneumonia**.

High doses of cytarabine may trigger what is known as cytarabine syndrome, which consists of fever, muscle ache, **bone pain**, occasional chest pain, rash, inflammation of the membrane that covers the outer surface of the eye. This syndrome occurs 6 to 12 hours after the drug is given. **Corticosteroids** can treat this syndrome or prevent it from occurring.

Interactions

Drugs that decrease the function of the kidneys may increase the toxic side effects of cytarabine. Cytarabine may decrease the effect of digoxin and the **antibiotics** gentamicin and flucytosine. Prior to starting any new medications or herbal remedies, patients should consult with their physician, nurse, or pharmacist to prevent any drug interactions.

Bob Kirsch

Cytogenetic analysis

Definition

Cytogenetics is the analysis of blood or bone marrow cells that reveals the organization of chromosomes. Chromosomes are the physical structures that contain the genetic material DNA.

Purpose

Cytogenetic analyses are essential to the diagnosis and treatment of different forms of **cancer**, especially leukemia, cancers of the blood cell-forming system. The results of cytogenetic tests can help to confirm the diagnosis of a particular form of leukemia, and permit the best treatment to be selected for each patient.

Precautions

This test is performed on tissue or cells that have been removed during the initial surgery or diagnostic procedure used to determine the precise nature of the leukemia or other cancer. It usually does not require any new surgery or blood draw on the patient and, so, does not entail any additional precautions for the patient.

Description

The development of leukemia and other cancers involves alterations, or mutations, in the cellular genetic material. The types of changes seen differ among various forms of cancer, but include changes in the specific sequence of DNA substituent units (termed nucleotides), as well as more dramatic alterations. Some of these more dramatic alterations include loss or duplication of large stretches of DNA sequence, or chromosomal rearrangements that correspond to the movement of genetic sequences from one chromosome to another. These rearrangements can lead to the production of novel, and often characteristic, molecules that are believed to play essential parts in the development of particular cancers.

Cytogenetic analysis focuses upon chromosomal rearrangements. In essence, this type of testing is a hybrid approach that combines genetics, analysis of mutations, with examination of cells. The cells to be tested, usually obtained from circulating blood or bone marrow, are treated in such a way that the chromosomes are made visible. Cells that are about to divide and which have condensed and organized their chromosomes into pairs are most suitable for this type of analysis. Often cells will be treated in the

KEY TERMS

Chromosome—The self-replicating genetic of structure cells that contains the cellular DNA, which includes the genes in a particular order.

DNA sequence—The relative order of nucleotides, the chemical subunits of a DNA molecule.

Gene rearrangement—A change in the structure of a chromosome that changes the order of genes.

Karyotype—A complete set of chromosomes that are examined to look for genetic abnormalities.

QUESTIONS TO ASK THE DOCTOR

- Are the cytogenetic results what you were expecting based upon other diagnostic tests and examinations I have undergone?
- Will you want to repeat this test? At what point in my treatment will you want to do so?
- Do these test results tell you anything about my prospects for a disease-free future?

laboratory to increase the frequency of such cells, in which the chromosomes are visible as what are called mitotic figures. Cells containing such mitotic figures are then chemically stained in a way that makes it possible to identify specific chromosomes. When such stained chromosomes are visualized and enumerated, the resulting pattern is termed the karyotype of that cell.

The karyotypes of many cells are usually scrutinized to establish whether some fraction of cells display a reproducible genetic alteration that can be associated with a specific cancer. Historically, the first such abnormality recognized was the Philadelphia chromosome, which is associated with chronic myelogenous leukemia (also called **chronic myelocytic leukemia**, or CML). In virtually all cases of CML, cytogenetic analyses will reveal a Philadelphia chromosome. The presence of this marker can be used to monitor response to treatment. There are a variety of other genetic abnormalities that are associated with specific forms of cancer. Most of these have been recognized using cytogenetics, and to varying degrees have become useful in diagnosis of leukemia and solid tumors, or in predicting treatment outcome.

Cytogenetics examines microscopically visible chromosomal changes. More recently developed molecular approaches can recognize the same sorts of genetic rearrangements as seen in abnormal karyotypes. In addition, these molecular tests can recognize smaller, more subtle alterations affecting just one or a few of the nucleotide units within a cancer-related gene. These techniques can, in some cases, be more sensitive than cytogenetic approaches, and along with the large body of information derived from the human genome project, hold the promise or providing more accurate tests for diagnosis and treatment of cancer.

Preparation and Aftercare

The only preparation and aftercare would be the preparation and aftercare required for the sample collection—a blood draw or a **bone marrow aspiration and biopsy**. The cytogenetic analysis itself requires no additional preparation or aftercare on the part of the patient.

Risks

This test is performed on tissue or cells that have been removed during the initial surgery or diagnostic procedure used to determine the precise nature of the leukemia or other cancer. It usually does not require any new surgery or blood draw on the patient and, so, does not entail any additional risk to the patient.

Results

Human body cells, exclusive of reproductive cells, have 23 pairs of chromosomes. Any deviation from this is considered abnormal. Cytogenetic analysis directed toward leukemia or other cancer cells is considered to have an abnormal result when a specific, distinctive genetic alteration is seen in the configuration of these chromosomes. The absence of a cytogenetic alteration is not, by any means, a basis to conclude there is an absence of a particular disease or that the prognosis is better than if a genetic abnormality was observed. For example, in **acute lymphocytic leukemia** (ALL) there are several different genetic rearrangements that are each associated with a different outcome. The patients who do the best are not those without any cytogenetic abnormality, but rather those with one specific chromosomal rearrangement. Therefore the potential use of cytogenetics, and similar molecular analyses, is to enable doctors to more accurately determine the diagnosis, treatment, and follow-up of patients with leukemia and other forms of cancer.

See also Chromosome rearrangements.

Resources

PERIODICALS

Nowell P.C., J. D. Rowley, A. D. Knudson, Jr. "Cancer genetics, cytogenetics: defining the enemy within." *Nature Medicine* 4(October 1998):1107-11.

Warren Maltzman, Ph.D.

Cytology

Definition

Cytology is the examination of individual cells and small clusters of cells, and may be used for the diagnosis and screening of diseases, including cancers. Cytology also refers to the study of diseases at the cellular level. For diagnosing diseases such as **cancer**, cytology may be referred to as cytopathology.

Purpose

Diagnostic tests are used to detect a disease in individuals who have signs, symptoms, or some other

Kidney cancer cells for examination by a pathologist. *(Copyright Parviz M. Pour, Science Source/Photo Researchers, Inc. Reproduced by permission.)*

abnormality that indicates a disease. A **screening test** identifies those who might have a certain disease, sometimes before they develop any symptoms, but does not absolutely prove the disease is present. If a screening test is positive, a diagnostic test can be used as follow-up to verify the diagnosis.

Precautions

Procedures to gather cells for cytology are often less invasive than other forms of **biopsy**, and therefore may cause less discomfort, be less likely to result in serious complications, and cost less to perform. In some situations, however, where a piece of tissue is removed rather than individual cells, a different type of biopsy may be required to confirm the cytologic diagnosis.

Description

Samples for cytology can be obtained in more than one way. Fine needle aspiration (FNA) is a type of biopsy in which tumor samples are taken through thin needles.

Scrape or brush cytology is another technique in which cells are scraped or brushed from the organ or tissue being tested. Samples from the esophagus, stomach, bronchi (breathing tubes that lead to the lungs), mouth, and cervix (Pap smear) can be obtained using this type of procedure.

Liquid-based cytology has been introduced in Great Britain as an alternative to the scrape method for collecting cervical cells for Pap smears. It is considered more comfortable and as effective by those who have introduced the method.

Researchers at binocular light microscopes analyze biological samples in a laboratory. The samples have been prepared on glass slides in trays and have been stained with dyes to highlight certain types of cells or tissues. *(Copyright CC Studio, Science Source/Photo Researchers, Inc. Reproduced by permission.)*

How a cytology sample is processed depends on what type of sample it is. A doctor can smear a sample directly on a glass microscope slide. The slide is then stained and viewed by a cytopathologist. In other cases, the fluid is concentrated before being smeared and stained on a slide. This is especially useful for dilute samples such as those from body cavities.

Most routine cytology results are available one or two days after the sample is received in the laboratory. There are many reasons why some results take longer to return, such as if special stains are required to confirm a diagnosis.

Preparation, Aftercare, and Risks

Cytology analysis is performed on cells gathered during diagnostic procedures. The preparation, aftercare, and risks depend on the procedure used to gather the cells.

Normal results

A cytopathologist examines the cells through a microscope and identifies the normal and abnormal cells on the slide using a microscope. Normal results generally indicate no sign of cancer.

Abnormal results

A cytopathologist examines the cells through a microscope. Abnormal cells may show signs that point to a possible diagnosis of cancer.

See also Biopsy; Pap test.

Resources

PERIODICALS

Cooper, Maggie. "Liquid Based Cytology: It's Been Approved as the Modern Replacement to the Conventional Smear Test, But What is Liquid Based Cytology?" *Primary Health Care* March 2004: 22–26.

Dahlstrom, Jane E., Gillian M. Langdale-Smith, and Daniel T. James. "Fine Needle Aspiration Cytology of Pulmonary Lesions: A Reliable Diagnostic Test." *Pathology* 33 (2001): 13-16.

ORGANIZATIONS

American Cancer Society. 1599 Clifton Road NE, Atlanta, GA 30329. (404) 320-3333. http://www.cancer.org.

American Society for Clinical Pathologists (ASCP). 2100 West Harrison Street, Chicago, IL 60612. (312) 738-1336. http://www.ascp.org.

American Society for Cytopathology (ASC). 400 West 9th Street, Suite 201, Wilmington, DE 19801. (302) 429-8802. http://www.cytopathology.org.

College of American Pathologists (CAP). 325 Waukegan Road, Northfield, IL 60093. (800) 323-4040. http://www. cap.org.

International Academy of Cytology (IAC). 1640 East 50th Street, Ste. 20C, Chicago, IL 60615-3161. (773) 955-1406. http://www.cytology-iac.org.

Laura Ruth, Ph.D.

Cytopenias *see* **Neutropenia and Thrombocytopenia**

D

D & C *see* **Dilatation and Curettage**

Dacarbazine

Definition

Dacarbazine, also known as DTIC-Dome or DTIC, is an anticancer agent best known for its long-time use in treating metastatic malignant **melanoma.**

Purpose

Dacarbazine has been approved by the Federal Drug Administration (FDA) for use in the treatment of metastatic malignant melanoma and Hodgkin's **lymphoma,** as well as other neoplasms.

Metastatic malignant melanoma

Dacarbazine used alone produces a response in up to 25% of patients with **metastasis** to the surrounding skin and lymph nodes. Though it has been studied in combination with other drugs, and some three-drug combinations (such as CVD, or **cisplatin, vincristine,** and dacarbazine) have shown promise, evidence thus far does not indicate a clear advantage over traditional single-agent treatment with dacarbazine. Some reserchers have treated patients with a four-drug regimen known as BVLD, for **bleomycin,** vincristine, **lomustine,** and dacarbazine. Again, however, this regimen has not been found to be clearly superior to monotherapy with dacarbazine.

Dacarbazine is sometimes given as palliative therapy for disseminated malignant melanoma. Palliative therapy is treatment that is given to relieve symptoms when a cure is no longer possible.

Hodgkin's disease

In **Hodgkin's disease,** dacarbazine is indicated as a second-line therapy, meaning it is used after initial therapies have failed or if the patient's disease recurs. It is usually used in conjunction with other drugs, most commonly in a regimen called "ABVD," which is comprised of the drugs **doxorubicin** (Adriamycin), bleomycin, **vinblastine** and dacarbazine. ABVD has produced complete remission in up to 70% of cases.

Other neoplasms

Dacarbazine has other, unlabeled uses. It has been used to treat soft tissue sarcomas and malignant metastatic pheochromocytomas. When used with other **chemotherapy** agents, it has also shown to have some activity in the treatment of **non-small cell lung cancer.**

Description

Dacarbazine is a non-classical alkylating agent that causes DNA mispairing and strand breakage, leading to cell death (necrosis). Its exact mechanism is not completely understood. It is a cell cycle non-specific drug, meaning that it causes cell damage and death throughout the life cycle of a cell, and not at any one particular time. When a patient is treated with dacarbazine 50% of the drug is metabolized by the liver, and 50% excreted in urine.

Recommended dosage

Dacarbazine comes in a vial, and must be mixed with sterile water according to manufacturer instructions prior to administration. It may be given directly into a vein, slowly, or by infusion over a time period of 15 minutes to an hour. Safety and effectiveness of this drug have not yet been established in children.

Chemotherapy dosages are usually based on a person's body surface area (BSA), which is calculated in square meters using height and weight measurements. Drug dosages are ordered in milligrams per square meter (mg/m^2). In some cases, chemotherapy may be ordered in milligrams per kilogram body weight. (One kilogram equals 2.2046 pounds.)

There are three regimens that may be considered when prescribing dacarbazine for metastatic malignant melanoma: the ten-day, five-day, and one-day regimen. The dosages recommended are as follows: 2-4.5mg/kg/day for ten days, repeated every four weeks; 250mg/square meter/day every five days, and repeated every three weeks; and 850-1,000mg/square meters for one day, repeated every three weeks. Because of recently developed drugs called 5HT3 **antiemetics** that treat **nausea and vomiting**, the one-day regimen is currently the most commonly used. To date, no studies have indicated that schedule or daily dose affects response rates.

Dacarbazine is usually given in combination with other drugs in the treatment of Hodgkin's lymphoma. The recommended dosage is 150mg/square meter, given once a day for five days. Treatment is repeated every four weeks. Alternatively, the drug may be given on only the first day of treatment, and every 15 days thereafter. For this regimen, the recommended dose is 375mg/square meter.

Precautions

Anaphylaxis is rarely associated with dacarbazine. Dacarbazine should not be used in patients who have demonstrated previous sensitivity to it.

Dacarbazine is classified as an irritant, meaning that the drug has the potential to cause pain and inflammation at the site if it seeps out of the vein and into the surrounding tissue. Should this event, called extravasation, occur, hot packs should be applied. Rarely, extravasation of dacarbazine results in tissue damage or death.

Animal studies have indicated that dacarbazine may be carcinogenic and damaging to an unborn fetus. It should be used only when the need outweighs the risks. There have not been adequate studies to determine whether it does pass to the milk. To be safe, women undergoing treatment with dacarbazine should not breast-feed.

Side effects

Hematopoietic

The most common side effect of dacarbazine is moderate bone marrow suppression. White blood cells and platelets are most affected, though red blood cells may also be decreased. These effects are potentially life threatening, requiring frequent blood level monitoring, and potentially a decrease or complete cessation of the drug. These effects may be delayed from two to four weeks after the drug is administered. Patients should be monitored for symptoms of low white blood cell count. Symptoms may include sore throat, burning during urination, **diarrhea**, or **fever**. Symptoms of low platelet count may include bleeding, increased bleeding with menstruation, and unexplained bruising. Symptoms of **anemia** may include dizziness, **fatigue**, and/or pallor.

Gastrointestinal

Dacarbazine is a highly emetogenic drug, meaning it frequently causes **nausea** and/or **vomiting**. Symptoms begin after one to six hours of administration, and can last up to five days. However, with appropriate supportive care, dacarbazine is usually well tolerated. Preventing nausea and vomiting can usually be accomplished by administering antiemetic medications before dacarbazine is administered, and even up to several days afterwards. There are several regimens available. In addition, restricting food intake for several hours prior to the administration of the drug can help reduce adverse gastrointestinal effects.

Cardiovascular

Dacarbazine has been associated with episodes of low blood pressure that resolve when the drug is stopped. Dacarbazine is prepared in vials with citric acid and the drug mannitol. There is some consideration that these hypotensive episodes may be related to the citric acid, and not the dacarbazine itself.

Dermatological

Although photosensitivity (sensitivity to sunlight) is rare, patients should be instructed to avoid sun exposure after treatment. When outdoors, patients should wear sunscreen and protective clothing. Reactions may include redness, swelling, and/or **itching** of the skin. In more serious cases, blisters may develop.

Dacarbazine may also affect the skin in other ways. For example, it may cause hyperpigmentation of the nails. When used in conjunction with the drugs doxorubicin, bleomycin, and vinblastine, dacarbazine can cause brown streaks to form over the sites of infusion. Dacarbazine may also cause flushing, a temporary redness of the face, neck, and chest area. Dacarbazine can also cause hair loss, although uncommon. Once treatment stops, hair growth nearly always recurs.

Other

Dacarbazine is sometimes associated with a flu-like syndrome that causes fatigue, muscle aches, and sometimes an increased temperature. Reportedly, symptoms begin about a week after therapy, and resolve within one to three weeks. Rarely, dacarbazine causes liver toxicity, symptoms of which may include yellowing of the whites of the eyes or skin, abdominal pain, and nausea.

Interactions

Dacarbazine is best administered in dextrose 5% water or normal saline. It should not be given with the following medications, as they are chemically incompatible: **allopurinol** sodium, cefepime HCl, **Heparin** sodium, or piperacillin sodium. Patients should let their doctors know what medications they are taking, as there may be some adverse reactions. Patients at risk for bone marrow suppression, such as those taking dacarbazine, should avoid aspirin-containing medicines as they may increase the risk of bleeding.

Resources

BOOKS

Beers, Mark H., MD, and Robert Berkow, MD, editors. "Malignant Melanoma." In *The Merck Manual of Diagnosis and Therapy*. Whitehouse Station, NJ: Merck Research Laboratories, 2007.

PERIODICALS

Eigentler, T. K., U. M. Caroli, P. Radny, and C. Garbe. "Palliative Therapy of Disseminated Malignant Melanoma: A Systematic Review of 41 Randomised Clinical Trials." *Lancet Oncology* 4 (December 2003): 748–759.

Lens, M. B., and T. G. Eisen. "Systemic Chemotherapy in the Treatment of Malignant Melanoma." *Expert Opinion on Pharmacotherapy* 4 (December 2003): 2205–2211.

Rapidis, A. D., C. Apostolidis, G. Vilos, and S. Valsamis. "Primary Malignant Melanoma of the Oral Mucosa." *Journal of Oral and Maxillofacial Surgery* 61 (October 2003): 1132–1139.

ORGANIZATIONS

United States Food and Drug Administration (FDA). 5600 Fishers Lane, Rockville, MD 20857-0001. (888) INFO-FDA (463-6332). http://www.fda.gov.

Tamara Brown, R.N.
Rebecca J. Frey, PhD

Daclizumab

Definition

Daclizumab is a humanized monoclonal antibody of the IgG1 type produced by recombinant DNA technology that binds to a specific interleukin-2 (IL-2) receptor known as CD25 or Tac. This receptor is expressed on the surface of cancerous lymphocytes in a number of blood malignancies. Daclizumab has also been known as dacliximab and is marketed in the United States under the Zenapax brand name.

Purpose

When used against **cancer**, this drug is intended to stop the growth of blood cell (hematologic) cancers that express the CD25 protein on the surface of the cancerous cells. Some representative cancers include adult T-cell leukemia/lymphoma (ATL), **hairy cell leukemia (HCL)**, **cutaneous T-cell lymphoma** (CTCL), chronic lymphocytic **lymphoma** (CLL), **Hodgkin's disease**, **non-Hodgkin's lymphoma** (NHL), and other peripheral T-cell or lymphoid leukemias or lymphomas.

Based on the antibody's known ability to block IL-2 binding experimentally, this drug would be expected to work most effectively at the times that the cancerous cells require IL-2 for growth. Generally, this is in the early stages of the disease. However, limited clinical evidence and some experimental evidence support an as of yet uncharacterized alternative method of action that may work during the later, IL-2 independent stages of the cancers.

Description

Daclizumab is a genetically engineered monoclonal antibody that was approved by the FDA in late 1997 as an immunosuppressive drug for use in kidney transplantation. The use of this drug in transplantation is based on the known interaction of activated lymphocytes with IL-2 during the rejection of transplanted tissue. It has not yet been approved for use as a cancer therapy. As of 2009 there were at least six active **clinical trials** to test the ability of daclizumab to treat hematologic cancers. The drug has also been used experimentally to treat IL-2-mediated autoimmune diseases such as uveitis and tropical spastic paraparesis.

Monoclonal antibodies are proteins of the immune system that bind specifically to a particular antigen. Daclizumab was constructed to bind specifically to the alpha subunit of the IL-2 high affinity receptor, a protein also known as CD25 or Tac. By binding to the IL-2 receptor, it is theorized that daclizumab will block the action of IL-2 on the cell, whether it be uncontrolled growth or an uncontrolled immune reaction.

Fusion antibodies related to daclizumab have been developed and are being studied in clinical trials. One fusion antibody links the antibody with radioactive yttrium (Y 90), effectively bringing **radiation therapy** directly to the cancer cells. Another called LMB-2 fuses the antibody binding site with a bacterial exotoxin that is toxic to the cancer cells. This drug is the first recombinant immunotoxin to induce major responses in cancer during a clinical trial.

Most of the daclizumab sequence is derived from human sequences, while about 10% are from mouse sequences. The human sequences were derived from the constant domains of human IgG1 (called "constant" because it is essentially the same for all IgG antibodies) and the variable framework regions of a human antibody against an antigen seen on the surface of **myeloma** cells. These areas do not bind to the IL-2 receptor. Using human sequences in this part of the antibody helps to reduce patient **immune response** to the antibody itself and is called humanization. The actual binding site of daclizumab to the IL-2 receptor is from a mouse anti-Tac antibody.

Recommended dosage

Clinical trials are currently ongoing to determine the most effective dosage and treatment cycles for daclizumab against hematologic cancers.

Precautions

Daclizumab therapy on an outpatient basis requires regular visits to the doctor to check progress. Laboratory tests are needed to make sure daclizumab is working properly and not overly compromising immune function. Because of the possible suppression of the immune system by this drug it is important to maintain good dental hygiene and see a dentist regularly. Also, because the drug would cross the placenta and the effects on an unborn child is unknown, effective contraception is necessary for women of childbearing age while receiving this medicine.

Side effects

Some uncommon side effects of daclizumab needing medical attention include chest pain; coughing; dizziness; **fever**; **nausea**; rapid heart rate; red, tender, oozing skin; shortness of breath; swelling of the feet or lower legs; trembling or shaking of the hands or feet; **vomiting**; weakness; and, rarely, frequent urination.

Some also uncommon and less serious side effects include constipation, **diarrhea**, headache, heartburn, joint pain, muscle pain, slow wound healing, and trouble in sleeping.

Interactions

The following medications have been administered in clinical trials with daclizumab with no increase in adverse reactions: **cyclosporine**, **mycophenolate mofetil**, ganciclovir, acyclovir, **azathioprine**, and **corticosteroids**. Daclizumab has also been used by small numbers of patients without reaction with other immune suppressive drugs such as **tacrolimus, muromonab-CD3**, antithymocyte globulin, and antilymphocyte globulin.

See also Monoclonal antibodies.

Michelle Johnson, M.S., J.D.

Dactinomycin

Definition

Dactinomycin is a chemotherapeutic agent belonging to a family of medicines known as antineoplastic drugs. Alternative trade names or brand names for dactinomycin include Actinomycin-D and Cosmegen.

Description

Dactinomycin is one of the older **chemotherapy** drugs, having gained approval from the Food and Drug Administration (FDA) in 1982. This highly potent and effective cytotoxic agent is a mixture of substances produced by the bacteria *Streptomyces parvullus*. Its toxic properties prevent its use as an antibiotic.

Dactinomycin interferes with the growth of **cancer** cells by complexing with a cell's genetic material (deoxyribonucleic acid, or DNA). This prevents the cell from producing the proteins necessary to function and grow, thereby killing it. Dactinomycin may be used as a single chemotherapeutic agent or in conjunction with other antineoplastics (such as **vincristine** and **cyclophosphamide**) for greater efficacy.

Purpose

Dactinomycin is used in the treatment of **Ewing's sarcoma**, **Wilms' tumor**, **rhabdomyosarcoma**, **gestational trophoblastic tumors**, **Kaposi's sarcoma**, and soft tissue sarcomas. It is less commonly used for cancers of the uterus and testis.

Recommended dosage

The exact schedule and method of dactinomycin administration will be prescribed by an oncologist based on the type and stage of the cancer. An appropriate starting treatment regimen for adult patients is 500 mg/day for five consecutive days at two to four week intervals if the drug is tolerated. For children the dose is 15 mg/day over the same time course as prescribed for adults. Dactinomycin is not recommended for children less than one year of age; little clinical data is available on the use of dactinomycin in the elderly. Administration may be by intravenous (IV) injection, through a running IV infusion, or through a central line inserted under the skin into a vein near the collarbone.

Precautions

To maximize treatment effects, patients receiving dactinomycin should observe the following guidelines, as well as any modifications given by the oncologist:

- The area surrounding the injection site should be monitored.

- Patients should have regular laboratory testing for white blood cell count and kidney, liver, and bone marrow function.

- In order to reduce the possibility of immunosuppression, immunizations not approved or prescribed by the oncologist should be avoided.

- Patients should avoid contact with individuals taking or that have recently taken the oral polio vaccine, or individuals that have an active infection. When necessary a protective facemask should be worn.

- Oral hygiene procedures should be followed to reduce the risk of gum abrasion.

- Patients should not touch eye and nasal areas unless hands have been properly washed immediately prior to contact.

- To reduce bleeding and bruising complications, patients should exercise extreme caution when handling sharp instruments and decline participation in contact sports.

- Prior to treatment, the patient's medical history should be thoroughly reviewed to avoid complications that might arise from previous conditions such as gout, kidney stones, liver disease, chickenpox, shingles, or a history of allergic reactions to various drugs.

- The oncologist should be made aware if the patient is pregnant or if there is the possibility the patient might be pregnant, or if the patient is a breast-feeding mother.

- Only prescribed medications or over the counter (OTC) drugs approved by the oncologist should be taken by a patient receiving dactinomycin.

Side effects

Possible side effects of treatment with dactinomycin should be discussed with the patient prior to initiation of treatment. The patient should be instructed to notify the oncologist of any side effects. Side effects that may not be life threatening but give the patient cause for concern include hair loss (**alopecia**), intermittent **diarrhea**, **nausea and vomiting**, loss of appetite, difficulty swallowing, mouth sores or ulcers, and a general rash or change in skin tone. Side effects that should be reported immediately to the oncologist include unusual bleeding or bruising, black tarry stools, blood in the urine or stool, development of a cough, wheezing or hoarseness, **fever** or chills, lower back or side pain, painful or difficult urination, pinpoint red spots on the skin, and pain at the site of the injection. The oncologist will decide what type of intervention is best suited to control or extinguish the presented side effects, including changing the dosage, changing the treatment schedule, or discontinuing dactinomycin treatment.

Interactions

Certain medications should never be used together, but there are cases in which multiple drug treatment may be advisable even when drug interaction is well documented. Dactinomycin may be used in conjunction with other antineoplastic drugs or **radiation therapy** for increased efficacy of treatment. Under such conditions the oncologist will balance dosage and treatment schedules to maximize the positive effects of all drugs given and minimize any negative interactions.

It is essential that the oncologist be aware of any drugs that the patient is presently taking or has recently taken, or if the patient has recently received radiation therapy. A careful review of drugs that may interact with dactinomycin to lower its efficiency should be covered with the patient prior to treatment. These may include, but are not limited to, amphotericin B, antithyroid agents, **azathioprine**, chloramphenicol,

flucytosine, ganciclovir, interferon, **plicamycin**, zidovudine, probenecid, and sulfinpyrazone.

See also Antineoplastic agents.

Jane Taylor-Jones, Research Associate, M.S.

Dalteparin *see* **Low molecular weight Heparin**

Danazol

Definition

Danazol is a synthetic androgen hormone that the Federal Drug Administration (FDA) approved in 1976. It is also known by its trade name, Danocrine.

Purpose

Danazol is approved for use in the treatment of endometriosis, fibrocystic breast changes, and in the prevention of hereditary angioedema. In addition, it has shown promise in the treatment of certain cytopenias.

Endometriosis

Endometriosis is a condition in which endometrial tissue, normally found in the uterus, implants itself in other areas of the body. The tissue continues to respond to hormones estrogen and progesterone during menstruation as it does in the uterus, but because the tissue cannot exit the body through the vagina during menstruation, it builds up, causing pain and inflammation. Danazol does not cure endometriosis, but renders the endometrial tissue located outside the uterus inactive. In most cases that are amenable to hormonal treatment, the endometrial lesions completely resolve, but can return within six months of stopping treatment.

Fibrocystic breast changes

Many women experience benign lumps or cystic changes in the breast. Most often, supportive bras and over-the-counter pain medication relieves symptoms. However, in some women, pain and discomfort may be so great that medical treatment is warranted. Danazol is the only drug approved by the FDA for fibrocystic breast disease, and in this patient population usually results in complete resolution of nodularity

KEY TERMS

Androgen—A steroid that produces masculine characteristics.

Cytopenia—Deficiencies of certain elements in blood, such as red blood cells, white blood cells and/or platelets.

Menorrhagia —Excessive menstrual bleeding.

and pain. However, symptoms usually return when medication is stopped.

Hereditary angioedema

Hereditary angioedema is a condition in which parts of the body, most dangerously the airway, develop episodic swelling. Danazol is used to prevent these rare, but potentially fatal, attacks.

Other

In addition to the aforementioned indications, there are other, unlabeled uses for danazol. The drug may be used to treat precocious puberty (premature sexual development), menorrhagia (excessively long menstrual periods), and gynecomastia (excess breast development in males).

Because it stimulates erythropoiesis (the production of red blood cells), it is sometimes administered to treat certain types of **anemia**. However, the use of danazol to combat anemia has declined since the recent developments in the synthetic production of erythropoeitin, a hormone naturally produced by the kidney that promotes the formation of red blood cells in bone marrow. In **cancer** patients, danazol may be used for its ability to stimulate erythropoiesis in individuals with types of **thrombocytopenia** (decreased platelets), often associated with HIV, or anemia. Danazol has shown promise in the management of autoimmune **hemolytic anemia**, a group of conditions in which the body produces antibodies that attack red blood cells. **Myelodysplastic syndrome** (MDS), a term that describes a group of hematologic cancers that often develop into acute leukemia, has shown some response to danazol treatment. However, more research is needed to better evaluate its potential in these patient populations.

Description

The pituitary gland produces hormones necessary for reproduction—follicle stimulating hormone (FSH) and luteinizing hormone (LH). Danazol suppresses the production of these and other hormones (estrogen and progesterone), inhibiting ovulation as a result. The effects are usually reversible. Approximately 60 to 90 days after treatment is stopped, ovulation and cyclic bleeding usually return.

Recommended dosage

The lowest therapeutic dose possible should be administered to minimize side effects. In some cases, doctors may periodically stop treatment or decrease dosages. In women, danazol should be started during menstruation or after tests to ensure the woman is not pregnant. Patients should be careful not to miss a dose, and if they do, should not take a double dose.

Endometriosis

Severe cases of endometriosis are initially treated with 800 milligrams (mg) of danazol, given in two divided doses. Gradually, the amount of medication is reduced to a level that is sufficient to suppress menstruation. Mild cases of endometriosis respond to lower doses of danazol. Typically, a doctor will first prescribe 200 to 400 mg a day, in two divided doses. Treatment should continue for three to six months, but in some cases, may last up to nine months.

Fibrocystic breast changes

Treatment for fibrocystic breast changes ranges from 100 to 400 mg given in two divided doses. Up to six months of danazol treatment may be needed to reduce breast nodularity and pain. However, in half of women treated with danazol, symptoms recur within a year. In these cases, treatment can be restarted.

Hereditary angiodema

Treatment for hereditary angioedema usually starts with a 200 mg dose given two or three times a day. Further adjustments are made based on the patient's response. If episodes are prevented, the amount may be decreased by half. If an attack occurs, the dose can be increased by up to 200 mg.

Other

Treatment of anemia in myelodysplastic syndrome usually begins with a dose of 200 mg three times a day.

Precautions

The use of danazol requires that liver and kidney function be routinely tested, as it can cause damage to these organs. In fact, with long-term use, there have been reported incidents of cancerous tumors in the liver.

Breast cancer should be ruled out prior to starting treatment. This may be difficult when there are multiple nodules in the breast. Any lumps that persist once danazol has started warrant consideration for breast cancer. Although danazol is effective in managing dysfunctional uterine bleeding, it should not be used in cases where **endometrial cancer** has not been ruled out.

Danazol should be used cautiously in people with high cholesterol. Danazol may cause a decrease in high-density lipoproteins (HDL; "good cholesterol"), which in high levels remove cholesterol from the arteries. At the same time, danazol can cause an increase in the low density lipoproteins (LDL; "bad cholesterol"), which act to move cholesterol into the arteries.

Danazol can cause androgenic effects on the fetus, and should not be used during pregnancy. Effects on a female fetus can include genital abnormalities such as clitoral enlargement, labia fusion, or vaginal closure. Treatment should not be initiated until pregnancy is ruled out. Throughout therapy, non-hormonal methods of birth control should be used to prevent pregnancy. If pregnancy does occur, the drug should be stopped and a doctor notified immediately.

Danazol is rarely associated with a condition called benign intracranial hypertension, symptoms of which include headache, **nausea**, **vomiting**, and visual disturbances. Should these symptoms occur, patients should stop taking the drug and see a neurologist.

When men, particularly adolescent men, take danazol, semen should be tested for volume, viscosity, sperm-count, and sperm motility every three to four months. Any changes may indicate a need to stop treatment.

Conditions that are worsened by swelling, a possible side effect of danazol, should be carefully monitored. This is particularly relevant in patients with epilepsy or cardiac problems.

Side effects

Long-term effects of danazol are unknown. Androgenic side effects may result, and may be an effect of decreased estrogen. These symptoms may include acne, swelling, abnormal hair growth, decreased breast size, deepening of voice, oily skin or hair, weight gain, enlargement of the clitoris, or reduction in the size of the testicles. Flushing, sweating, vaginitis, nervousness or emotional lability (instability) may also develop. Danazol may cause liver damage. In addition to routine lab testing, patients should be monitored for yellowing of the skin or whites of the eyes due to jaundice.

Interactions

The effects of oral anticoagulants, such as coumadin, may be increased in patients taking danazol, and should be used with caution. Individuals taking insulin for diabetes should carefully monitor their blood sugars. Taken in conjunction with danazol, insulin's effects are reduced. Danazol is also known to increase effects of the medications **carbamazepine** and **cyclosporine**.

Tamara Brown, R.N.

Dasatinib

Definition

Dasatinib (Sprycel) is a second generation BCR-ABL inhibitor drug manufactured by Bristol-Myers Squibb. Under certain conditions it is used to treat chronic myeloid leukemia (CML) and Philadelphia positive acute lymphoblastic leukemia (Ph+ ALL).

Purpose

Dasatinib is used to treat two types of leukemia. Chronic myeloid leukemia (CML), also called chronic myelogenous leukemia, is **cancer** that develops in myeloid cells in the bone marrow and results in the production of abnormal blood cells. These blood cells mature incorrectly or incompletely and live longer than normal so that they slowly build up in the blood, usually over several years, before causing symptoms of CML.

CML accounts for between 10% and 15% of all leukemias, and almost all CML is associated with a specific non-inherited genetic defect. When cells divide, their chromosomes double and also divide in order for each cell to have a complete set of genetic information. Sometimes during this doubling and division process material from one chromosome incorrectly gets attached to or exchanged with material from another chromosome. This process is called translocation. CML starts when part of chromosome 9 is exchanged with part of chromosome 22. The resulting abnormal chromosome 22 is known as the Philadelphia chromosome. People who have it are said to be Philadelphia chromosome positive or Ph+. Although it is not clear what factors cause this translocation, almost everyone with CML is Ph+.

As the result of the formation of the translocation between chromosomes 9 and 22, a new gene called bcr-abl is formed on the Philadelphia chromosome. This gene produces a tyrosine kinase protein called BCR-ABL. BCR-ABL causes myeloid cells to become cancer (malignant) cells. These malignant cells grow and reproduce abnormally. Dasatinib is a tyrosine kinase inhibitor. It interferes with the activities of the BCR-ABL protein and stops the production of cancerous myeloid cells while allowing the production of normal blood cells to continue.

Dasatinib is used only after another tyrosine kinase inhibitor drug, **imatinib mesylate** (Gleevec), has been tried. Imatinib mesylate successfully treats CML in many people. Those people whose cancer does not respond to the drug or who cannot tolerate the side effects of imatinib mesylate may be treated with dasatinib.

Acute lymphoblastic leukemia (ALL), also called **acute lymphocytic leukemia**, is cancer that develops in white blood cells in the bone marrow called lymphocytes. Unlike CML, ALL spreads rapidly through the blood to other organs. Some people who have ALL also carry the Philadelphia chromosome (ALL Ph+). Dasatinib is used to treat people with ALL who are Ph+ and whose cancer has not responded to other treatments.

Description

Dasatinib is sold in the United States and the European Union under the brand name of Sprycel. The drug was first given accelerated approval by the United Sates Food and Drug Administration (FDA) on July 28, 2006. After additional data collection and evaluation, it received full FDA approval for treating CML on May 26, 2009.

Dasatinib is a white to off-white, round tablet. It is supplied in strengths of 20 mg, 50 mg, 70 mg, and 100 mg and should be stored at controlled room temperature. Dasatinib continues to be tested in **clinical trials** in the United States for use against other cancers and in combination with other therapies. A list of clinical trials currently enrolling volunteers can be found at: http://www.clinicaltrials.gov.

Recommended dosage

Dasatinib must be taken exactly as prescribed, and the dosage should not be changed or the drug discontinued except on order of a physician. The usual dose for people in the early (chronic) phase of CML is 100 mg taken once daily either in the morning or evening. The usual dose for people who have advanced CML (accelerated or blast crisis stages) or who have Ph+ ALL is 140 mg taken once daily either in the morning or the evening. Dasatinib tablets must be taken whole; they should never be crushed or divided.

They may be taken with or without food, but grapefruit juice should not be ingested while taking this drug.

There are no special dosage recommendations for use of dasatinib in the elderly or those with kidney (renal) impairment. Although no specific dosage recommendations are made for individuals with liver (hepatic) impairment, caution is urged when prescribing for these individuals. The safety and effectiveness of this drug have not been established in children. Very limited data suggests that overdosage is associated with suppression of normal production of blood cells in the bone marrow (**myelosuppression**) and increased risk of bleeding due to low platelet count.

Precautions

The following precautions should be observed.

- Severe decrease in the number of normal blood cells (myelosuppression) may occur. Decrease in the number of blood platelets (thrombocytopenia) may reduce the ability of the blood to clot and increase the risk of serious bleeding episodes. Decrease in the number of neutrophils (neutropenia) may decrease the ability of the body to fight infection. Decrease in the number of red blood cells (anemia) may reduce the ability of the blood to supply oxygen. Blood count should be monitored frequently. In severe cases, medication may need to be temporarily discontinued.

- Bleeding in the digestive (gastrointestinal) system may occur with such severity as to require blood transfusion. Dasatinib should be used cautiously in patients taking anticoagulant (blood-thinning) drugs such as warfarin (Coumadin).

- Edema (fluid retention) may occur not only in the arms and legs, but also around the heart (pericardial effusion), lungs (pleural effusion), and in the abdomen (ascites). Edema should be monitored and treated as needed.

- Dasatinib can alter heart rhythm, prolonging a phase of heart contraction cycle called the QT interval. Heart monitoring may be necessary.

Pregnant or breastfeeding

Dasatinib is a pregnancy category D drug. Woman who are pregnant or who might become pregnant should not use dasatinib. It is not known whether the drug is excreted in breast milk. Women taking this drug who are or who want to breast feed should discuss the risks and benefits with their doctor and err on the side of caution, as there is the potential for this drug to cause serious adverse effects on nursing infants.

Dasatinib

GALE ENCYCLOPEDIA OF CANCER 3

455

Side effects

Side effects that occurred in more than 20% of individuals given dasatinib during clinical trials included:

- myelosuppression (see precautions)
- fluid retention (see precautions)
- diarrhea
- headache
- difficulty breathing (dyspnea)
- skin rash
- fatigue
- nausea
- bleeding (hemorrhage) events (see precautions)

Interactions

Dasatinib is known to interact with many drugs and some foods. If these drugs cannot be avoided, the dosage of dasatinib may need to be adjusted. All interactions are not known. Patients should provide their doctor and pharmacist with a complete list of all prescription and nonprescription drugs, herbs, and dietary supplements that they are taking.

When taken with dasatinib, these drugs increase the amount of dasatinib circulating in the blood. These drugs include:

- ketoconazole (Nizoral)
- itraconazole (Sporanox)
- ritonavir (Norvir)
- atazanavir sulfate (Reyataz)
- indinavir (Crixivan)
- nelfinavir (Viracept)
- saquinavir (Invirase)
- telithomycin (Ketek)
- erythromycin (E-mycin)
- clarithromycin (Biaxin)

When taken with dasatinib, these drugs decrease the amount of dasatinib circulating in the blood.

- dexamethasone (Decadron)
- phenytoin (Dilantin)
- carbamazepine (Tergretol)
- rifampin (Rimactane)
- phenobarbitol (Luminal)

Drugs that may interfere with the absorption of dasatinib include antacids and proton pump inhibitor such as famotidine (Pepcid) and omeprazole (Prilosec).

Grapefruits and grapefruit juice should be avoided while taking dasatinib.

Dasatinib contains a small amount of lactose as an inactive ingredient. Individuals who are lactose-intolerant should discuss this with their physician.

Drugs whose blood level may be changed when taken with dasatinib include:

- cyclosporine (Sandimmune)
- alfentanil (Alfenta)
- fentanyl
- pimozide (Orap)
- sirolimus (Rapamune)
- tacrolimus (Prograf)
- ergotamine (Ergomar)

Resources

OTHER

Detailed Guide Leukemia, Chronic Myeloid (CML) American Cancer Society. 2009 [October 6, 2009]. http://www.cancer.org/docroot/CRI/CRI_2_3x.asp?rnav=cridg&dt=83

Leukemia, Adult Chronic. MedlinePlus. September 30, 2009 [October 6, 2009]. http://www.nlm.nih.gov/medlineplus/leukemiaadultchronic.html

"Oncolink." Abramson Cancer Center of the University of Pennsylvania. 2009 [October 6, 2009]. http://www.oncolink.upenn.edu

Sprycel (dasatinib) Fact Sheet. Bristol-Myers Squibb [October 6, 2009]. http://www.bms.com/Documents/news/media_kit/sprycel/sprycel_fact.pdf

ORGANIZATIONS

American Cancer Society, 1599 Clifton Rd., NE, Atlanta, GA, 30329, (404) 320-3333, (800) ACS-2345, http://www.cancer.org.

Leukemia & Lymphoma Society, 1311 Mamaroneck Avenue, Suite 310 , White Plains, NY, 10605, (800) 955-4572, http://www.leukemia-lymphoma.org.

National Cancer Institute Public Inquires Office., 6116 Executive Boulevard, Room 3036A, Bethesda, MD, 20892-8322, (800) 4-CANCER. TTY (800) 332-8615, http://www.cancer.gov.

Tish Davidson, A.M.

Daunorubicin

Definition

Daunorubicin is an anti-cancer drug that kills **cancer** cells. The brand names are DaunoXome for the liposomal formulation and Cerubidine for the daunorubicin hydrochloride formulation.

Purpose

Daunorubicin is available in two different formulations, the daunorubicin hydrochloride and daunorubicin citrate liposome. The liposomal daunorubicin formulation places the drug in lipid molecules. This formulation is able to penetrate cancer cells more effectively because of its smaller size, and it remains in the body longer when compared to the daunorubicin hydrochloride formulation. The daunorubicin hydrochloride is approved by the Food and Drug Administration (FDA) to treat acute myelocytic leukemia (AML) and **acute lymphocytic leukemia** (ALL). It is also sometimes used to treat chronic myelogenous leukemia (CML), **non-Hodgkin's lymphoma**, and psoriasis. The liposomal formulation of daunorubicin is used to treat advanced HIV-associated **Kaposi's sarcoma**.

Description

Daunorubicin interferes with the cells' production of DNA and RNA by inserting itself between the molecules that make up DNA and RNA. It also works by inhibiting the enzyme responsible for repairing of DNA (topoisomerase II enzyme). The structure of daunorubicin is very similar to that of **doxorubicin**, and both drugs function in the same way.

Recommended dosage

In the treatment of acute myelocytic leukemia (AML), the dose is 30 to 60 mg of daunorubicin per square meter of body surface area given for three to five days, and the dose is repeated every three to four weeks.

In acute lymphocytic leukemia (ALL), 25 to 45 mg per square meter of body surface area of daunorubicin may be given on day one every week for four cycles, or alternatively may be given at a dose of 30 to 45 mg per square meter of body surface area for three days. The dose for patients receiving daunorubicin citrate liposome is 20 to 40 mg per square meter of body surface area every two weeks, or 100 mg per square meter of body surface area every three weeks.

Patients with decreased liver or kidney function may receive lower doses of the medication than other patients. This medication is usually administered directly into the vein (intravenous, or IV) over the course of three to five minutes. It may also be diluted in a solution to be given over fifteen minutes to one hour.

Precautions

A major problem with the use of daunorubicin is that it may cause a serious heart problem known as heart failure. Some authorities suggest that giving any individual patient more than 900 to 1000 mg of daunorubicin per square meter over the course of their entire life may increase risk of heart injury. Other authorities recommend that the total lifetime cumulative dose not exceed 550 milligrams per square meter. The patient's baseline heart function is obtained prior to starting therapy and is monitored every few cycles of **chemotherapy**. If the heart function is significantly decreased from baseline, the drug is discontinued.

Side effects

There is a risk that heart rhythm problems will occur during daunorubicin therapy. Later, patients may develop heart failure. However, patients receiving daunorubicin are, in fact, less likely to develop such problems than are patients receiving doxorubicin.

In addition, the activity of the bone marrow in producing white blood cells to fight infections, platelets to control bleeding, and red blood cells for oxygenation may be impaired by the drug. This and the development of heart problems are the major side effects that may cause doctors to lower the dose of daunorubicin.

Other side effects associated with daunorubicin therapy are **nausea**, **vomiting**, ulcerations of the mouth, **diarrhea**, and hair loss. In addition, the medication has a harmless side effect about which patients should be forewarned; urine and tears may take on a red color.

Patients receiving daunorubicin in conjunction with certain other **anticancer drugs** may (very rarely) develop a certain type of leukemia. The drug is also an irritant to the skin and tissues of the body. Patients who notice burning or pain with infusion of the drug should notify the nurse immediately to assess if the drug has leaked from the vein into the surrounding tissue. If this occurs, the drug infusion is stopped immediately and appropriate actions are taken to minimize side effects due to tissue damage.

Bob Kirsch

Degarelix

Definition

Degarelix for injection (Firmagon) is a gonadotropin-releasing hormone (GnRH) receptor antagonist manufactured by Ferring Pharmaceuticals. It is used to treat advanced **prostate cancer**.

Purpose

The prostate is a gland found only in men. It is about the size of a walnut and surrounds the neck of the urethra. Almost all prostate cancers arise from prostate gland cells that produce a fluid that is part of semen. Prostate **cancer** can be slowed by eliminating the male hormone **testosterone** from the body. Testosterone is produced in the testicles in response to the hormone gonadotropin, which is released from the pituitary gland. Degarelix is used to treat advanced prostate cancer. It works by binding with gonadotropin-releasing receptors in the pituitary. When degarelix is bound to these receptors, the pituitary no longer releases gonadotropin. Without gonadotropin, the testicles are not stimulated to produce testosterone. This method of eliminating testosterone from the body is referred to as chemical castration. Men retain their testicles, but they no longer produce testosterone. Degarelix is very effective in reducing the amount of testosterone in the body.

Description

Degarelix manufactured by Ferring Pharmaceuticals and is marketed in the United States under the brand name Firmagon. The United States Food and Drug Administration (FDA) approved its use on December 24, 2008. As of October 2009, the drug had not received approval in the European Union or other countries where it was in **clinical trials**. Degarelix is intended only for subcutaneous injection (under the skin, not in a vein). It is supplied as a sterile powder in vials containing either 120 mg or 80 mg of the drug. The powder must be dissolved in sterile water before use. Degarelix continues to be tested in clinical trials in different dosage regimens and in combination with other therapies that treat prostate cancer. A list of clinical trials currently enrolling volunteers can be found at: http://www.clinicaltrials.gov

Recommended dosage

Degarelix is given as a subcutaneous injection in the abdomen at an injection site that will not be irritated by pressure or clothing. The starting dose is 240 mg divided into two injections of 120 mg each at a concentration of 40 mg/mL. This is followed every 28 days by a maintenance dose of 80 mg at a concentration of 20 mg/mL. In clinical trials maintenance doses were continued for one year.

There are no special dosage adjustments needed when using degarelix in the elderly. Because of the limited data available from the clinical trials, caution is urged when using degarelix in people with moderate to severe kidney damage (renal impairment) or liver damage (hepatic impairment). This drug should not be used in females, and its safety and efficacy have not been tested in children.

Degarelix requires special handling when it is dissolved for use. Gloves should be warn to avoid skin contact with the drug. Special procedures are needed to prepare degarelix for injection, and the drug should be used within one hour of being prepared.

Precautions

Long-term use of drugs such as degarelix that deprive the body of testosterone and other androgens (male hormones) can prolong a phase of the heart contraction cycle called the QT interval. This can lead to irregular heartbeat (arrhythmias). Patients who already have a long QT interval, who are taking drugs to treat heart arrhythmia, or who have congestive heart failure should discuss with their physician whether the benefits of degarelix outweigh the risks. Heart monitoring (electrocardiogram) may be necessary.

The effectiveness of degarelix should be monitored by periodically measuring blood concentrations of prostate-specific antigen (PSA), which gives an indication of cancer activity.

Allergies

Degarelix contains mannitol as an inactive ingredient. Individuals who are allergic to mannitol should discuss use of this drug with their physician.

Pregnant or breastfeeding

Degarelix is a pregnancy category X drug. Women who are pregnant should not use or be exposed to degarelix. Fetal abnormalities and fetal death may result. It is not known whether the drug is excreted in breast milk. Women taking this drug should not breast feed. This drug is not FDA-approved for use in women. Female healthcare workers should use care when reconstituting and injecting degarelix.

Side effects

The most serious side effect is prolongation of the QT interval in the heart contraction cycle. Other side effects that may occur include:

- hot flashes
- pain, redness, and swelling at the injection site
- weight gain
- abnormal increases in some liver enzymes
- fatigue
- high blood pressure (hypertension)
- joint pain
- chills
- urinary tract infection
- decreased sex drive and impotence

Interactions

Drug interactions are not known. No formal drug interaction studies have been completed. Before starting and while taking degarelix, patients should provide their doctor and pharmacist with a complete list of all prescription and nonprescription drugs, herbs, and dietary supplements that they are taking.

Resources

OTHER

Degarelix Injection. MedlinePlus. July 1, 2009 [October 9, 2009]. http://www.nlm.nih.gov/medlineplus/druginfo/meds/a609022.html.

Detailed Guide: Prostate Cancer. American Cancer Society. 2009 [October 9, 2009]. http://www.cancer.org/docroot/CRI/CRI_2_3x.asp?dt=36.

Firmagon.com Ferring Pharmaceuticals. 2009 [October 9, 2009]. http://www.firmagon.us/us/us-homeg/pcl-homeg/accessser/0/261/0/default.html.

ORGANIZATIONS

American Cancer Society, 1599 Clifton Rd., NE, Atlanta, GA, 30329, (404) 320-3333, (800) ACS-2345, http://www.cancer.org.

Men's Health Network, P.O. Box 75972, Washington, DC, 20013, (202) 543-MHN-1 (6461, info@menshealthnetwork.org, http://www.menshealthnetwork.org.

National Cancer Institute Public Inquires Office, 6116 Executive Boulevard, Room 3036A, Bethesda, MD, 20892-8322, (800) 4-CANCER. TTY (800) 332-8615, http://www.cancer.gov.

Prostate Cancer Foundation, 1250 Fourth Street, Santa Monica, CA, 90401, (310) 570-4700, (800) 757-CURE (2873), (310) 570-4701, info@pfc.org, http://www.prostatecancerfoundation.org.

Tish Davidson, A.M.

Demeclocycline

Definition

Demeclocycline, more accurately demeclocycline hydrochloride, is a broad-spectrum antibiotic of the tetracycline family. Demeclocycline is marketed under the trade name Declomycin.

Purpose

Demeclocycline is used to treat **cancer** patients who have developed a condition known as **syndrome of inappropriate antidiuretic hormone** (SIADH). A wide variety of malignacies, especially small-cell lung cancer, as well as various other non-cancer conditions, give rise to SIADH, which is caused by overproduction of antidiuretic hormone (ADH). SIADH can also develop as a side effect of the **anticancer drugsvincristine**, **vinblastine**, **cisplatin**, **melphalan**, and **cyclophosphamide**. The increased ADH levels lead to insufficient elimination of water from the kidneys, and the retained water leads to dilution of the serum sodium concentration, a condition called hyponatremia. Symptoms of hyponatremia include weight gain in spite of appetite loss, **fatigue**, headache, and confusion. When the condition is severe or the onset sudden, the symptoms may develop into seizures or coma. Although treating the underlying cancer is the ideal approach, the metabolic imbalances may be alleviated in other ways. The tetracycline derivative demeclocycline has been found to be effective in treating SIADH.

Demeclocycline was originally approved by the Food and Drug Administration (FDA) to treat a wide variety of bacterial infections. It is thought that the tetracyclines work by preventing bacteria from synthesizing protein.

More recently, demeclocycline has been combined with hydrocortisone in a paste used by dentists to control inflammation and prevent **infection** in root canal and other endodontic procedures. The paste is sold under the trade name Ledermix.

Description

This tetracycline derivative is isolated from a mutant strain of the bacterium *Streptomyces aureofaciens*.

Demeclocycline was first investigated as a treatment for SIADH in 1976, and had become established as the treatment regimen of choice by 1986. The drug acts to interfere with the response of the kidneys to ADH and has consistently been found to be effective in treating SIADH with relatively few side effects.

Recommended dosage

Demeclocycline hydrochloride is taken orally. It is supplied as 150 and 300 mg tablets and 150 mg capsules. The usual dosage of demeclocycline for SIADH is from 600 to 1,200 mg/day, and should not exceed 2,400 mg/day. Within five days of beginning the drug, the diuretic action begins, and it generally lasts for two to six days after the drug is discontinued.

Precautions

Absorption of demeclocycline is reduced when taken with food or dairy products, and thus should be given one hour before or two hours after a meal or ingestion of dairy products. The dose should be taken with 8 oz (240 mL) of water, and the last dose of the day should be taken at least one hour before bedtime.

Antacids containing aluminum, calcium, or magnesium interfere with absorption of orally administered tetracyclines and should not used by patients taking demeclocycline.

Photosensitivity reactions are more frequent and more severe with demeclocycline than with other tetracyclines. Patients should be advised that this reaction can occur and be cautioned to avoid exposure to direct sunlight or ultraviolet light.

With renal impairment, even usual doses of demeclocycline may lead to accumulation of the drug and the possibility of liver toxicity. Serum level determinations of the drug may be advisable under such conditions, and the dosage should be lower than usual.

Tetracyclines can cross the placenta and can have toxic effects on the developing fetus, and the drug is found in the milk of lactating women taking tetracyclines. Tetracyclines form a complex with calcium and act to decrease the rate of bone growth in any bone-forming tissue while the drug is being administered.

Side effects

Dermatological

Skin reactions, including redness, swelling, rashes, and flaking or peeling of the skin can result from demeclocycline administration. Demeclocycline should be discontinued if the skin becomes swollen and reddened.

Patients taking demeclocycline are likely to be photosensitive. Phototoxic reactions occur with moderate to large doses and are characterized by severe skin burns resulting from direct exposure to sunlight.

Gastrointestinal

Demeclocycline can cause loss of appetite, **nausea**, **vomiting**, and **diarrhea**. Inflammations of the upper GI tract have also been reported as side effects, involving the tongue and esophagus, with resultant dysphagia, but many of these patients were found to have taken the medication immediately before going to bed. Inflammation of the small and large intestines has also been reported, and, as with all antibiotic therapy, overgrowth in the lower GI tract of other organisms, especially of the *candida* genus of yeast-like fungi, can lead to inflammatory lesions in the anogenital area.

KEY TERMS

Anaphylactoid purpura—A short-term allergic condition of blood vessels, found chiefly in children, that is characterized by wet sores on the skin of the buttocks, legs, and lower abdomen. Joint pain, stomach bleeding, and blood in the urine are also common findings. The disease, also called Henoch-Schonlein (Schonlein-Henoch) purpura, usually lasts for about six weeks and has no long-term effects unless kidney involvement is severe.

Anaphylaxis—A severe allergic reaction to a foreign substance (antigen) that a patient has had previous contact with, characterized by redness and swelling, itching, water build-up, and, in severe cases, extremely low blood pressure, lung spasms, and shock.

Angioedema—A sudden, painless, swelling of short duration that can affect the face, neck, lips, throat, hands, feet, genitals, or abdominal organs; also called angioneurotic edema.

Antidiuretic hormone—A peptide hormone, also called vasopressin, synthesized in the hypothalamus and released by the posterior pituitary gland in response to decreased blood volume, that stimulates capillary muscles and concentrates and reduces the elimination of urine.

Benign intracranial hypertension—Also called pseudotumor cerebri or meningeal hydrops, a condition of swelling of the optic nerve and mild paralysis of the cranial nerves, with headache, nausea, and vomiting.

Dysphagia—Difficulty in swallowing.

Hyponatremia—A condition in which the serum sodium concentration falls to less than 135 milliequivalents per liter (mEq/L), caused by too little excretion of water or by too much water in the bloodstream; in severe cases, hyponatremia leads to water

intoxication, characterized by confusion, lethargy, muscle spasms, convulsions, and coma.

Lupus erythematosus—A long-term disease that affects women four times more often than men, characterized by severe swelling of the blood vessels giving rise to arthritis, kidney disorders, red rash over the nose and cheeks, weakness, fatigue, weight loss, photosensitivity, fever, and skin sores that may spread to the mucous membranes and other tissues of the body; also called systemic or disseminated lupus erythematosus.

Nephrogenic diabetes insipidus—A condition in which the kidneys do not retain urine, resulting in excess urination and thirst, and very watered-down urine.

Pancreatitis—An inflammation of the pancreas diagnosed on the basis of severe pain that begins in the abdomen and moves to the back, fever, loss of appetite, nausea, vomiting, and jaundice.

Pericarditis—An inflammation of the pericardium, the membrane covering the heart, marked by pain that begins in the chest and moves to the shoulder or neck, fever, difficulty breathing, and a dry cough.

Photosensitivity—An abnormal sensitivity of the skin to ultraviolet light, often resulting from use of an oral or topical drug, that leads to accelerated and severe burning and blistering of the skin.

Prothrombin—A plasma protein, produced by the liver and converted to thrombin by activation factors in the plasma, involved in blood coagulation; also called factor II.

Superinfection—An overgrowth, during antimicrobial treatment for another infection, of a microorganism not affected by the treatment.

Tetracycline—A broad-spectrum antibiotic.

Tinnitus—A sensation of ringing or other similar sound in the ears.

Central nervous system

Dizziness, tinnitus, benign intracranial hypertension (pseudotumor cerebri), and visual disturbances have been reported. More rarely, myasthenic (Eaton-Lambert) syndrome and muscle weakness have been reported.

Immune system

Possible allergic reactions to demeclocycline include hives, angioedema, anaphylaxis, anaphylactoid purpura, pericarditis, and worsening of systemic lupus erythematosus.

Other

Superinfection due to overgrowth of nonsusceptible organisms is a common side effect of demeclocycline administration. Renal toxicity has been reported. Acute pancreatitis and nephrogenic diabetes insipidus are possible side effects of demeclocycline treatment. Increases in liver enzymes and hepatic toxicity have been rarely observed. Blood conditions such as **hemolytic anemia**, **thrombocytopenia**, **neutropenia**, and eosinophilia have also been reported. Individuals still undergoing tooth development (infants and children up to eight years old, and in the fetus during the last half of pregnancy) may develop permanent yellowish-grayish-brown discoloration of the teeth and poor enamel development.

Interactions

Tetracyclines including demeclocycline can interfere with the bactericidal action of penicillins, and should not be administered together with penicillin. Tetracyclines coadministered with oral contraceptives can render oral contraceptives less effective. The activity of plasma prothrombin can be depressed by tetracyclines, thus patients on anticoagulant therapy may be required to decrease their anticoagulant dosage.

Resources

BOOKS

Beers, Mark H., MD, and Robert Berkow, MD, editors. "Abnormal Renal Transport Syndromes." In *The Merck Manual of Diagnosis and Therapy*. Whitehouse Station, NJ: Merck Research Laboratories, 2007.

Beers, Mark H., MD, and Robert Berkow, MD, editors. "Antibacterial Drugs: Tetracyclines." In *The Merck Manual of Diagnosis and Therapy*. Whitehouse Station, NJ: Merck Research Laboratories, 2007.

Wilson, Billie Ann, Margaret T. Shannon, and Carolyn L. Stang. *Nurse's Drug Guide 2003*. Upper Saddle River, NJ: Prentice Hall, 2003.

PERIODICALS

Goh, K. P. "Management of Hyponatremia." *American Family Physician* 69 (May 15, 2004): 2387–2394.

Wicht, M. J., R. Haak, H. Schutt-Gerowitt, et al. "Suppression of Caries-Related Microorganisms in Dentine Lesions after Short-Term Chlorhexidine or Antibiotic Treatment." *Caries Research* 38 (September-October 2004): 436–441.

OTHER

Food and Drug Administration (FDA). "Medwatch Safety File, Declomycin Tablets." http://www.fda.gov/med watch/SAFETY/2003/03May_Pl/Declomycin_Pl.pdf.

ORGANIZATIONS

American Society of Health-System Pharmacists (ASHP). 7272 Wisconsin Avenue, Bethesda, MD 20814. (301) 657-3000. www.ashp.org.

United States Food and Drug Administration (FDA). 5600 Fishers Lane, Rockville, MD 20857-0001. (888) INFO-FDA. www.fda.gov.

Patricia L. Bounds, Ph.D.
Rebecca Frey, PhD

Denileukin diftitox

Definition

Denileukin diftitox (Ontak) is a genetically engineered biologic response modifier manufactured by Eisai Medical Research. It is used to treat a specific subtype of **cutaneous T-cell lymphoma** that has failed to respond to other drug treatments.

Purpose

Denileukin diftitox is used to treat a subtype of persistent or recurrent cutaneous T-cell **lymphoma** (CTCL) that carries a high number of interleukin-2 (IL-2) protein receptors on the surface of the malignant (cancerous) cells. CTCL is a rare (about four cases per 1,000,000 population) type of non-Hodgkin's lymphoma that affects the skin, most often in individuals ages 40–60 years.

Description

Denileukin diftitox is sold in the United States and internationally under the brand name Ontak. It belongs to a class of genetically engineered drugs called biologic modifiers. Biologic modifiers are a type of targeted therapy designed to destroy **cancer** cells without harming healthy cells. The drug was first given accelerated approval by the United Sates Food and Drug Administration (FDA) in 1999. After additional data collection and evaluation, it received full FDA approval for treating CTCL on October 15, 2008. Denileukin diftitox continues to be tested in **clinical trials** in the United States for use against other cancers and in combination with other therapies. A list of clinical trials currently enrolling volunteers can be found at: http://www.clinicaltrials.gov.

Denileukin diftitox consists of two components that are united through genetic engineering. The first component is the protein IL-2, which is used to attach the drug to cancer cells. The second component is a diphtheria toxin (poison), which kills the cell. The IL-2 component only attaches to cancer cells with IL-2 receptors; it does not attach to healthy cells that do not have IL-2 receptors. Once attached, the diphtheria toxin enters the cancer cell and stops protein synthesis. This kills the cell. Denileukin diftitox works on both actively dividing and non-dividing (quiescent) cancer cells. Before treatment with denileukin diftitox, the individual's T cells should be analyzed to determine if they carry IL-2 receptors, as the presence of appropriate IL-2 receptors on the surface of the malignant cells is critical to how this drug works.

Recommended dosage

Before receiving denileukin diftitox, the patient is given an antihistamine and acetaminophen (Tylenol) to help reduce the severity of any infusion reaction. The drug is supplied as a frozen solution in single-use vials. It must be stored below 14°F (-10°C). Before use, the drug is thawed and brought to room temperature, after which an appropriate dose is added to an IV infusion bag. The drug is then slowly dripped into a vein over a period of 30–60 minutes. The exact dosage depends on the individual's weight, health status, and other drugs being taken. Generally, a dose of 9 mcg/kg/day or 18 mcg/kg/day is given for 5 consecutive days. This dosage is repeated every 21 days for eight cycles.

Precautions

Denileukin diftitox can cause serious and life-threatening reactions. Deaths have occurred with the administration of denileukin diftitox. The drug carries a boxed warning concerning administration of the drug. The following boxed warnings must be observed:

- Serious and fatal infusion reactions can occur within 24 hours of infusion. In clinical trials, serious infusion reactions occurred in about 8% of patients. They were most common during the first and second infusion cycles. Denileukin diftitox should be given only in a facility where cardiopulmonary resuscitation equipment and staff are present.
- Capillary leak syndrome is a serious condition in which fluid leaks out of the blood vessels and collects in the body. Symptoms include low blood pressure (hypotension), especially when changing position (orthostatic hypotension); fluid retention (edema); and a decrease; in the blood protein called serum albumin. Symptoms may be delayed up to two weeks following infusion.
- Loss of visual acuity (sharpness) and color vision may occur. In some cases this is reversible, but most patients report some permanent vision impairment.

The following additional precautions should be observed:

- Denileukin diftitox is a pregnancy category C drug. Woman who are pregnant or who might become pregnant should not use denileukin diftitox. It is not known whether the drug is excreted in breast milk. Women taking this drug who are or who want to breast feed should discuss the risks and benefits with their doctor and err on the side of caution, as there is the potential for this drug seriously harm nursing infants.
- Certain precautions must be taken by healthcare professionals in handling denileukin diftitox. The drug may be thawed for 24 hours in a refrigerator

or 1–2 hours at room temperature. This drug contains no antibacterial additives, so special care must be taken to ensure that the drug remains sterile when mixed and measured and that it is used promptly.

- Serum albumin levels should be measured before each administration of denileukin diftitox. The drug may not be given if levels are too low.

Side effects

Denileukin diftitox causes many side effects, the most serious of which are listed in the Precautions section. Patients should promptly inform their doctor about any side effects or unusual occurrences after receiving this drug. Common side effects that occurred in more than 30% of patients during clinical trials include:

- capillary leak syndrome (see Precautions)
- fever
- chills
- decrease in the number of lymphocytes (white blood cells) in the blood
- low levels of serum albumin in the blood
- **nausea, vomiting,** and **diarrhea**
- weakness and fatigue
- swelling of the hands and feet (edema)
- infection
- loss of appetite
- low blood pressure
- pain
- skin rash

Other less common side effects include headache, difficulty breathing (dyspnea), chest pain, cough, dizziness, **itching**, **weight loss**, rapid heart rate (tachycardia), anxiety, blood in the urine, and cloudy urine.

Interactions

Drug interactions are not known. No formal drug interaction studies have been completed. Before starting and while taking denileukin diftitox, patients should provide their doctor and pharmacist with a complete list of all prescription and nonprescription drugs, herbs, and dietary supplements that they are taking.

Resources

OTHER

Chemotherapy Drugs: Ontak. Chemocare.com and the Cleveland Clinic Cancer Center [October 8, 2009]. http://www.chemocare.com/bio/ontak.asp.

"Oncolink." Abramson Cancer Center of the University of Pennsylvania 2009 [October 8, 2009]. http://www.oncolink.upenn.edu.

What Is Cutaneous T Cell Lymphoma (CTCL)? Cancer Research UK. December 12, 2008 [October 4, 2009]. http://www.cancerhelp.org.uk/help/default.asp?page=3962.

ORGANIZATIONS

American Cancer Society, 1599 Clifton Rd., NE, Atlanta, GA, 30329, (404) 320-3333, (800) ACS-2345, http://www.cancer.org.

Leukemia & Lymphoma Society, 1311 Mamaroneck Avenue, Suite 310 , White Plains, NY, 10605, (800) 955-4572, http://www.leukemia-lymphoma.org.

National Cancer Institute Public Inquires Office, 6116 Executive Boulevard, Room 3036A, Bethesda, MD, 20892-8322, (800) 4-CANCER. TTY (800) 332-8615, http://www.cancer.gov.National Organization for Rare Diseases (NORD), P. O. Box 1968, Danbury, CT, 06813-1968, (203) 744-0100, (800)999-NORD (6673), orphan@rarediseases.org, http://www.rarediseases.org.

Tish Davidson, A.M.

Depression

Description

Everybody feels sad sometimes, but to be clinically depressed is not just a matter of feeling sad. A patient with **cancer** is diagnosed as having major depression only if certain symptoms, such as loss of pleasure or thoughts of death, are present for at least two weeks. Only a healthcare professional can accurately determine whether a patient is depressed or is simply upset because of the disease.

A note on depression and children with cancer

Few children with cancer experience depression. For many children survivors of cancer, the experience of having had cancer makes them deeper, more understanding human beings later in adulthood and old age. However, some children with cancer do experience depression, sleep problems, and relationship problems. Depression appearing in a child who has cancer should be treated by a healthcare professional.

The symptoms of depression in children are somewhat different from those in adults. The physician should be notified of a sad mood (or, in children less than six years of age, a facial expression that appears to express sadness) that continues for at least two weeks and is accompanied by at least four of the following: (a) appetite changes, (b) sleep problems or excessive sleep, (c) excessive activity or inactivity, (d) loss of pleasure, (e) not caring about anything, (f) **fatigue**, (g) being overly critical of himself or herself, (h) feeling worthless or guilty for no apparent reason, (i) inability to concentrate, and (j) thoughts of death.

Are most people who have cancer depressed?

Most people who have cancer are not depressed. Depression is found in cancer patients about as frequently as in patients hospitalized for major, noncancer illnesses such as heart disease. However, depression is more often present in people who have cancer than in the general population. Approximately one out of eight people with cancer are depressed. Among hospitalized people with cancer, roughly one in four is depressed.

Depression and embarrassment

Doctors and nurses can do a great deal to help a depressed person feel better. Being embarrassed can get in the way of the patient's getting help. While depression is a disease that happens to a minority of cancer patients, it does appear in a sizable number of these patients. Doctors and nurses are trained to deal with depression in cancer patients. If one out of eight people with cancer are depressed, it is no surprise to healthcare professionals that some patients require treatment for depression. It is not "bothering" a good health care professional to let them know that the patient is experiencing some symptoms that may signal depression. Competent doctors and nurses will not think less of a patient who is depressed. Rather, they will respect the patient who acknowledges the willingness to seek and accept treatment for depression. Cooperative patients are not those who hide depression but those who deal with depression when it appears. Dealing honestly and with the aid of doctors and allied healthcare professionals is the right way to address any cancer-related symptom.

How does depression affect someone who has cancer?

Depression is not something that can be pointed to, as one would point to a runny nose or an earache. That does not mean it is not real, nor does it mean the depression does not have a major effect on the cancer patient. The fact is that depression may not only affect what patients can do and how they feel, depression may also affect how well they function and how long they live.

A study of patients with acute leukemia who were receiving **bone marrow transplantation** found that those who were not depressed lived longer. A study of **breast cancer** patients showed that depression can be treated successfully and life extended. In this study, women with metastatic breast cancer who joined a support group lived twice as long as matched patients who did not join a support group. In light of these types of studies it would be incorrect to assume that depressed cancer patients who work with their doctors and nurses to treat their depression do not live as long as patients without depression.

Untreated depression or inadequately treated depression may slow recovery time. A study of depressed colorectal cancer patients found they were not able to function as well six months after surgery as patients who were not depressed. Another study found that breast cancer patients who were more anxious and depressed felt more pain than those who were not. Other studies have also shown that depression affects how people function and cope with illness.

Causes

It is certainly understandable that someone with a serious illness feels sad. Many cancer patients are confronted with difficulties. These may include having to take medications, dealing with the side effects of these medications, undergoing operations, submitting to other medical procedures, and generally taking time away from other things they would prefer to do. In addition, many patients feel a sense of loss. They may feel a loss of good health; there may be a loss of part of the body, such as a segment of a breast; there may be a loss of the ability to do certain tasks. There may also be financial strains. Any such things are difficult for most people to deal with. It takes time and effort, and sometimes medical intervention, for people to deal with such loss and gradually get their lives back on track.

If patients are in pain it is extremely important that the pain be adequately treated. Pain is often under-treated. When pain is not treated appropriately, patients may be more likely to develop depression.

Patients with cancer of the pancreas are particularly likely to become depressed. In addition, patients with breast, colon, gynecologic, oropharyngeal, and **stomach cancer** are more likely to experience depression than patients with other types of cancers. No one knows why depression is more likely to be associated with these cancers.

Approximately one out of every four patients with depression associated with cancer already was depressed at the time of diagnosis. In contrast, approximately three out of four develop the depression after the diagnosis has been made.

Risk factors for depression among cancer patients

Anyone can become depressed, and this includes people with cancer and people who are perfectly healthy. Often, there is no way of predicting who will develop major depression. However, some groups of cancer patients are more likely to develop depression than are others. This include patients who:

- are younger
- have a personal or family history of depression or other mental health problems
- have a personal or family history of substance abuse
- have body image problems
- are hospitalized
- are experiencing unrelieved cancer-related symptoms, such as pain
- have advanced or relapsed cancer, or have experienced a treatment failure
- have been diagnosed with stroke or with Parkinson's disease

In addition, some patients are receiving medicines that may cause depression as a side effect. Among these medicines are certain **anticancer drugs**, antihistamines, blood pressure medicines, anti-Parkinson's disease medicines, medications for convulsions, sedatives, steroids, stimulants, and tranquilizers.

Signs and symptoms

A patient with cancer is diagnosed as having major depression only if certain symptoms are present for at least two weeks. Among these symptoms are: (a) loss of pleasure or interest in activities, (b) major **weight loss** or weight gain not associated with dieting, (c) serious sleep problems, (d) loss of energy, (e) fatigue, (f) feeling worthless, (g) feeling guilty without adequate reason, (h) problems concentrating, (i) indecisiveness, and (j) thoughts of death or suicide. Symptoms such as sleep problems, fatigue, and weight loss may, however, affect cancer patients who are not depressed in the slightest. So, the diagnosis must be made by a healthcare professional.

Often depression appears gradually. At first, the patient seems no more than sad. At times, the person who is in a very early stage of depression brightens up. For many people things never get worse than this and true depression never touches them. However, other people progress to where negative thoughts have a grip upon them.

Gradually, some of the neurotransmitters in the nervous system may stop working in the most healthy way. Neurotransmitters are the chemicals released by nerves to communicate with other nerves. Once a patient's neurotransmitters are affected, the depression is definitely not simply happening in the patient's mind. The way the body uses actual chemicals is being altered by the depressive disease.

Precisely how the depression shows itself may differ from patient to patient. For example, some patients start to respond to little setbacks as though these are catastrophes. Other patients start making big assumptions, usually in negative directions; for example, they may assume their current therapy will not help them, even although there is good medical evidence that it probably will. For yet another example, they may blame themselves for having cancer, or irrationally see the cancer as a punishment visited upon them for something they have done. Patients may try to be too perfect and repeatedly fail. They may think other people have negative feelings about them, or they may focus upon the negative portions of situations. One danger is that the looming depression may encourage patients to push away and alienate those health professionals, friends, and family members who are trying to be helpful. For a final example, a depressed patient may deny the seriousness of the cancer, saying something like, "The tumor is small so I don't really need to be careful about taking my medicines."

Some patients experience a milder form of depression, called dysthymia. Symptoms of dysthymia include annoyance, feelings of sadness, irritability, loss of pleasure, and self-criticism. The patient with dysthymia may develop aches and pains, express excessive guilt, and distance themselves from loved ones. Dysthymia may be almost unnoticeable; however, many patients with dysthymia are unable to function quite as well as they can when they are healthy.

Depression screens

The attending doctor or nurse may request that the patient complete a depression screen. This screen is nothing more than a page or two of questions about how the patient is feeling. The patient's responses give healthcare professionals a picture of whether or not depression may be present.

Prevention

It is important for patients to have an idea of the psychological and social stressors they may have to address because of the cancer. Knowing in advance that something may be a problem is a good way of making sure that it is not quite as stressful once it does appear as it otherwise would be. Patients, their families, and close friends should be able to recognize the most important signs and symptoms of depression and should know which healthcare professional to call should depression appear. However, no one except a professional is capable of accurately diagnosing depression. It is a good idea to try to develop an honest relationship with a healthcare professional you trust. Parents of a child who has cancer may find a parent support group helpful, as there is a great deal to learn from other parents who have been through a similar situation.

Treatments

Most important is that study after study has shown that depression in cancer patients can be successfully treated. It is important to understand that this problem probably can get better. Several different approaches to treatment can be taken, and several of these approaches can be effectively combined with one another

If the patient has a doctor or nurse capable of providing sustained emotional support, that can be helpful. On the other hand, it is important for patients to realize that doctors and nurses are usually extremely busy and that it may be necessary to find someone else to provide sustained emotional support. This other person may be a trained professional, such as a social worker, a psychiatric nurse, a psychologist, or a psychiatrist. The persons who provide support may also be family members or friends. A support group may be helpful. During periods of crisis, it is beneficial to have several people who can provide support. The family member or friend who is trying to provide such support should try to listen well and sympathetically.

Cognitive interventions

Cognitive interventions are also known as cognitive-behavioral treatment (CBT). CBT helps patients' view in a realistic way what is happening to them, where they are, and what they should or should not be doing. This type of intervention can be useful in helping patients give up negative perspectives and replace them with views that rely more upon the facts about what is going on. CBT may be practiced with a healthcare provider, or in a group with other patients and one or more providers.

Among the techniques CBT makes use of are:

- Cognitive distraction: This is the phrase used for techniques that shift the mind-frame of the patient from negative things to more positive thoughts. Music is one of the basic tools of cognitive distraction. Patients should be encouraged to listen to the type of music they like best. Headphones may be helpful if brought to diagnostic and treatment sessions and occasions when waiting is necessary. Imagery is another technique important for cognitive distraction. Imagery can help the mind shift from negative thoughts and difficult situations to helpful images. Each patient should select those images that feel right and good. For one patient this may be swimming at the beach; for another, visiting special friends; for another, walking through the forest.
- Psychoeducation: This CBT technique involves providing information to patients so patients can feel that what is going on is not entirely beyond their control. People often find it difficult to deal with the unknown, and psychoeducation attempts to remove some of what is unknown. Another important psychoeducation technique is having patients make lists of questions to ask their nurse or doctor.
- Image rehearsal: This CBT technique involves working with a healthcare professional. The patient may use image rehearsal to rehearse some activity she or he finds to be stressful. For example, image rehearsal may be used if the patient finds MRI scans or radiation treatments to be stressful.

Other CBT techniques involve relaxation techniques and the conscious decision to participate in activities the patient likes doing.

Psychotherapy

Talking to a psychologist, social worker, psychiatric nurse, psychiatrist, or other health care professional can be helpful. In addition to the cancer and problems associated with therapy, this talk therapy can help the patient address unresolved matters that were already bothersome before cancer was diagnosed.

Group therapy

Studies have shown group therapy to be an effective approach for patients with cancer-related depression. Various approaches to group therapy may be taken. In all, however, it involves communication not only between patient and healthcare professional, but also among and between patients. Group therapy can also be helpful for loved ones of cancer patients.

Important to note is that studies have shown that cancer patients may tend to isolate themselves from friends and family. In other words, the amount of contact and communication between friends and family may be less than it had been before cancer was diagnosed. This is not a helpful trend. Research suggests that social support can have beneficial effects on a person's physical health. Group therapy can provide this type of social support to patients. In addition, group therapy may furnish a place where patients are able to learn about how to maintain contact with family and friends. It can also provide a way for patients to identify which family members and friends are not supportive.

Medication

A variety of antidepressant medications are available. Among those most frequently prescribed are psychostimulants, tricyclic antidepressants (TCAs), selective serotonin reuptake inhibitors (SSRIs), and monoamine oxidase inhibitors (MAOIs). These medications help return the neurotransmitters to a normal, balanced function. There are at least three different psychostimulants, six different TCAs, three different SSRIs, and three different MAOIs that doctors may choose among. In addition, there are various other medications that have proven to be effective as treatment for depression. All of these drugs have been shown to work well in general; however, while one specific type of drug may be appropriate for one patient, another patient may require a completely different type of drug. Use of some of these drugs may be accompanied by side effects. Just as there are different antidepressant drugs, so are there different side effects that may appear. However, many patients have no side effects from antidepressant medications or, at most, exhibit only minor side effects. Other patients find that, although they had side effects from one drug, they experienced no side effects after they switched to another medication. Many patients find they are able to successfully combine medications and other treatment approaches, but honest communication with the physician is essential.

The suicidal patient

If a patient is suicidal it is extremely important to immediately contact a healthcare professional capable of dealing with such a crisis.

Resources

BOOKS

Spiegel, David, and Catherine Classen. *Group Therapy for Cancer Patients: A Research-Based Handbook of Psychosocial Care.* New York: Basic Books, 2000.

Waller, Alexander, and Nancy L. Caroline. *Handbook of Palliative Care in Cancer.* 2nd ed. Boston: Butterworth Heinemann, 2000.

Yarboro, Connie H., Margaret H. Frogge, and Michelle Goodman. *Cancer Symptom Management.* 2nd ed. Boston: Jones and Bartlett Publishers, 1999.

PERIODICALS

Lovejoy, Nancy C., Derek Tabor, Margherite Matteis, and Patricia Lillis. "Cancer-related Depression: Part I— Neurologic Alterations and Cognitive-Behavioral Therapy." *Oncology Nursing Forum* 27 (2000): 667-677.

Sheard, T., and P. Maguire. "The Effect of Psychological Interventions on Anxiety and Depression in Cancer Patients: Results of Two Meta-Analyses." *British Journal of Cancer* 80 (1999): 1770-1780.

Bob Kirsch

Dexamethasone

Definition

Dexamethasone is a synthetic glucocorticoid. Its naturally occuring counterparts are hydrocortisone and cortisone. Although the drug is used in a variety of ways, in general, it reduces inflammation and depresses the immune system. Dexamethasone may also be called by its brand name, Decadron.

Purpose

Dexamethasone is used in the treatment of many disorders. For example, it may be used:

- as replacement therapy in the treatment of Addison's disease
- in the management of various inflammatory disorders, such as rheumatoid arthritis
- to coat drug-eluting stents, which are devices used in treating coronary artery disease to reduce the chance that previously clogged arteries will become blocked again
- in managing such allergic disorders as asthma

- as induction therapy prior to stem cell transplantation

Patients with ulcerative colitis may benefit from dexamethasone therapy, as might those with exacerbations of multiple sclerosis. Such blood disorders as thrombocytopenic purpura or erythroblastopenia, may also be managed with dexamethasone.

Dexamethasone is often prescribed to patients with **cancer**. In some cases, the drug is part of the drug treatment for the disease, and in other cases it is used to manage side effects caused by the treatment or the cancer itself. For example, dexamethasone may be given to treat **nausea and vomiting** associated with **chemotherapy**.

Dexamethasone may be used to decrease abnormally high levels of potassium that develop in association with cancer. In some cases, it may be used as palliation in leukemia or **lymphoma**. Because of its antiinflammatory properties, dexamethasone may help reduce swelling in the brain caused by a brain tumor. It may also help prevent hypersensitivity reactions associated with drugs like paclitaxel. Dexamethasone is also commonly used to treat **nausea** associated with chemotherapy. It is particularly useful with the drug **cisplatin**, which frequently causes nausea and **vomiting**.

In **non-Hodgkin's lymphoma** (NHL), dexamethasone is part of a drug regimen known as DHAP. Here, dexamethasone is given with chemotherapy drugs called cisplatin and **cytarabine**. Also in treating NHL, dexamethasone may be used in a regimen caled "m-BACOD," which also includes the administration of **methotrexate**, **leucovorin**, **bleomycin**, **doxorubicin**, **cyclophosphamide**, and **vincristine**. Dexamethasone may also be helpful in patients with **multiple myeloma**. In the EDAP regimen, dexamethasone is given with **etoposide**, cytosine arabinoside (cytarabine), and cisplatin; in VAD, it is given with vincristine and doxorubicin.

Description

Patients should not stop taking dexamethasone without first consulting their physician. When dexamethasone treatment stops, it must be gradually reduced over time before it can be completely discontinued. Sudden withdrawal of glucocorticoids may result in adrenal insufficiency.

When possible, the drug should be taken before nine A.M. to imitate the time that the body's corticosteroid levels are typically at their highest. A child taking dexamethasone will be carefully monitored to ensure the drug is not affecting his or her growth. Patients taking large doses of dexamethasone should try to take the drug with meals. Antacids may be recommended between meals to reduce gastrointestinal effects and to prevent peptic ulcer.

KEY TERMS

Addison's disease—A potentially life-threatening condition that results when adrenocortical function fails.

Elute—In chemistry, to remove by dissolving or washing. A drug-eluting stent is one that contains a medication to reduce inflammation.

Glucocorticoid—An adrenocortical steroid hormone that is stimulated by the anterior pituitary. The three naturally occuring types are hydrocortisone, corticosterone, and cortisone.

Hyperglycemia—An abnormally increased level of glucose (sugar) in the blood.

Induction therapy—Chemotherapy that is given as the initial treatment for cancer, prior to surgery or transplantation.

Palliation—Therapy aimed at relieving symptoms and promoting comfort, but not producing a cure.

Stent—A small tube inserted surgically into an artery to hold it open. Stents may be coated with dexamethasone to reduce inflammation within the blood vessel.

Recommended dosage

Dexamethasone is available in oral, intravenous (IV), topical, ophthalmic, or inhaled form. In cancer patients, the oral and IV routes are used most frequently. The pill is available in several color-coded dosages [0.25 milligrams (mg), 0.5mg, 0.75mg, 1.5mg, 4mg, and 6mg]. Dexamethasone should be given very slowly by the IV route.

Dosages to treat disease are highly individualized, but generally start at 0.75 to 9.0 mg per day. The lowest therapeutic dose should be given, though amounts given may need to be increased during times of stress. Dosages of medications may be changed based on factors specific to the individual. The following dosages are general guidelines for dexamethasone when it is used in conjunction with chemotherapy agents:

- DHAP. Forty milligrams of dexamethasone is given in pill or IV form per day for the first four days of treatment, followed by cisplatin and cytarabine.

- M-BACOD. Six milligrams per meter square (mg/m2) of dexamethasone is given as a pill on the first five days of treatment.

- EDAP. Forty milligrams of dexamethasone is given in pill form on the first four days of treatment. It is given again on days 9-12, and 17-20.

When used to prevent or manage nausea or vomiting associated with chemotherapy, dexamethasone is given in the following dosages: 4–20 mg IV every four to six hours. Alternatively, a one-time dose of 10–20 mg may be given IV. When pills are preferred, 4–8 mg of dexamethasone may be given four times, every four hours. When used to prevent hypersensitivity reactions in paclitaxel treatment, 20mg should be given orally twelve and six hours before treatment begins.

Precautions

Dexamethasone should be used cautiously in patients with kidney or liver problems, hypothyroidism, high blood pressure, or a history of heart attack. Patients with diabetes mellitus should monitor blood sugar levels carefully, as hyperglycemia may result. If changes occur, patients should notify their doctors immediately. Sudden cessation of dexamethasone therapy is dangerous for patients on therapy for longer than two weeks. The drug should be gradually withdrawn under a physician's guidance.

Side effects

Adverse effects vary widely, and depend on the dosage and route of the drug. Certain drugs may result in decreased blood levels, and therefore render dexamethasone less effective. Patients taking the following drugs should be carefully monitored for decreased levels of dexamethasone: **phenytoin**, phenobarbitol, ephedrine, and rifampin. Conversely, some drugs, such as troleandomycin, may increase blood levels of dexamethasone.

Because of its immunosuppressive properties, dexamethasone may decrease the signs and symptoms of **infection**. Depending on the amount of drug being administered, patients may consider taking measure to prevent infection by avoiding crowded areas and washing their hands frequently. Patients should inform their doctor if they notice a **fever**, sore throat, or cuts or abrasions that don't heal. Laboratory tests may also be affected—false negative results may occur in the nitroblu-tetrazolium test for bacterial infections.

Glucocorticoids, such as hydrocortisone, tend to make the body retain salt. Although dexamethasone's salt-retaining properties are not as severe as hydrocortisone's, salt retention may result in fluid and electrolyte imbalances. Patients at risk may experience high blood pressure or even congestive heart failure.

Weight gain or swelling may indicate salt and fluid retention.

Other adverse effects may include headache, dizziness, insomnia, increased appetite, mood swings, menstrual changes, muscle weakness, acne and/or sweating. **Depression** may be worsened with dexamethasone use. Some men experience changes in the motility and number of their sperm with steroid treatment. Patients should talk to their doctors about any unusual symptoms they experience. In cancer patients, increased appetite may actually be beneficial.

Dexamethasone crosses the placenta and is excreted in breast milk. If a pregnant woman is taking large doses of the drug, her newborn should be monitored for evidence of hypoadrenalism. Optimally, breast-feeding should be avoided. There is some concern that dexamethasone, in large quantities, suppresses growth or disrupts the baby's normal corticosteroid production.

Interactions

Patients should discuss all their medications, prescription and non-prescription, with their doctor. If dexamethasone is administered in amounts that suppress the immune system, live **vaccines**, such as small pox, should not be administered. Dexamethasone may alter the effect of anticoagulant drugs. Frequent laboratory tests should be performed to monitor blood levels. If dexamethasone is given with diuretics, potassium levels may be abnormally low, and should be frequently monotired. Doctors may recommend that patients on long-term therapy follow a potassium-rich diet.

Resources

BOOKS

Wilson, Billie A., Margaret T. Shannon, and Carolyn L. Stang. *Nurses Drug Guide 2000*. Stamford, CT: Appleton & Lange, 2000.

PERIODICALS

Hesketh, P. J. "New Treatment Options for Chemotherapy-Induced Nausea and Vomiting." *Supportive Care in Cancer* 12 (August 2004): 550–554.

Kumar, S., M. Q. Lacy, A. Dispenzieri, et al. "Single-Agent Dexamethasone for Pre-Stem Cell Transplant Induction Therapy for Multiple Myeloma." *Bone Marrow Transplantation* 34 (September 2004): 485–490.

Liu, X., I. de Scheerder, and W. Desmet. "Dexamethasone-Eluting Stent: An Anti-Inflammatory Approach to Inhibit Coronary Restenosis." *Expert Review of Cardiovascular Therapy* 2 (September 2004): 653–660.

ORGANIZATIONS

American Society of Health-System Pharmacists (ASHP). 7272 Wisconsin Avenue, Bethesda, MD 20814. (301) 657-3000. www.ashp.org.

United States Food and Drug Administration (FDA). 5600 Fishers Lane, Rockville, MD 20857-0001. (888) INFO-FDA. www.fda.gov.

Tamara Brown, R.N.
Rebecca J. Frey, PhD

Dexrazoxane

Definition

Dexrazoxane, known by the brand name Zinecard or may be referred to as ADR-529, is a medicine that protects the heart from damage caused by the **chemotherapy** drug **doxorubicin**.

Purpose

Dexrazoxane is approved by the Food and Drug Administration (FDA) as a protectant medicine given to women with metastatic **breast cancer** who are being treated with the chemotherapy drug doxorubicin. In most cases these women already will have received greater than 300 mg per square meter (mg/m^2) of the chemotherapy drug doxorubicin before dexrazoxane is added. Dexrazoxane is given in combination with doxorubicin. Doxorubicin can cause damage to heart muscle and the risk of this damage increases as the total dose increases. The addition of dexrazoxane at the appropriate time in therapy can decrease the extent of damage to the heart muscle.

Description

Dexrazoxane is a clear, colorless solution. It is administered intravenously, into a vein, over a 15-30 minute period. Dexrazoxane is given within 30 minutes prior to receiving the doxorubicin. When doxorubicin gets into cells, it combines with iron to form toxic substances that destroy heart muscle. Dexrazoxane interferes with the doxorubicin binding to the iron compound so that the toxic substance is not formed and the heart muscle is protected.

Recommended dosage

Dexrazoxane doses can be determined using a mathematical calculation that measures a person's body surface area (BSA). This number is dependent

KEY TERMS

Anemia—A lower than normal red blood cell count.

Anthracyclines—A group of chemotherapy medicines that are used to treat cancer. They have similar characteristics and are known for their ability to cause heart damage. The drugs included as anthracyclines are doxorubicin, daunorubicin, idarubicin, and epirubicin.

Antineoplastics—Medicines used to treat cancers.

Chemotherapy—A specific drug used to treat cancer.

Food and Drug Administration—A government agency that oversees public safety in relation to drugs and medical devices. The FDA gives approval to pharmaceutical companies for commercial marketing of their products

Intravenous—To enter the body through a vein.

Metastatic—Cancer that has spread to one or more parts of the body.

Neutropenia—A lower than normal white blood cell count.

Radiation therapy—The use of high-energy beams focused to treat cancerous tumors.

Sterility—Inability to have children.

Toxic—Poisonous.

upon a patient's height and weight. The larger the person, the greater the body surface area. Body surface area is measured in units known as meters squared (m^2). The body surface area is calculated and then multiplied by the drug dosage in mg/m^2. This calculates the actual dose a patient is to receive.

Dexrazoxane is dosed in mg/m^2 as a 10:1 ratio of the doxorubicin dose. For example, if a patient is to receive doxorubicin 50 mg/m^2, then the patient would receive dexrazoxane 500 mg/m^2. Once the dose is determined, the drug is administered either directly into the vein over a few minutes as an intravenous push, or as a quick infusion from an infusion bag. This is then followed by the doxorubicin intravenously.

Precautions

Blood counts will be monitored regularly while on dexrazoxane therapy. During a certain time period after receiving chemotherapy, there is an increased risk of getting infections. Caution should be taken to avoid unnecessary exposure to crowds and people with infections.

Patients should not expect their doctor to use dexrazoxane the first time they receive chemotherapy. It is thought that dexrazoxane may interfere with the chemotherapy drug's ability to destroy **cancer** cells. Dexrazoxane is therefore only used when absolutely necessary.

Patients who may be pregnant or are trying to become pregnant should tell their doctor before receiving dexrazoxane.

Chemotherapy can cause men and women to be sterile (not able to have children). It is unknown if dexrazoxane causes sterility.

Patients should check with their doctors before receiving live virus **vaccines** while on chemotherapy along with dexrazoxane.

Side effects

The most common side effect from receiving the dexrazoxane is pain at the injection site. Another common side effect when dexrazoxane is given with chemotherapy is that the blood counts fall lower than with just chemotherapy alone. However, the time it takes for the blood counts to return to normal is the same with or without the dexrazoxane.

Low blood counts, referred to as **myelosuppression**, are expected due to chemotherapy with dexrazoxane administration. A low white blood cell count is called **neutropenia**, and patients are at an increased risk of developing a **fever** and infections. Platelets are blood cells in the body that allow for the formation of clots. When the platelet count is low, patients are at an increased risk for bruising and bleeding. Low red blood cell counts, referred to as **anemia**, may also occur due to chemotherapy administration. Low red counts cause **fatigue**.

Most other side effects occur due to the administration of the chemotherapy agents that accompany dexrazoxane. Common side effects include **nausea and vomiting**. Patients are given medicines before receiving chemotherapy that can help prevent or decrease these side effects from happening. Other common side effects are hair loss (**alopecia**), fatigue, loss of appetite, mouth sores, fevers, infections, **diarrhea**, and changes in liver function.

Less common side effects are nerve damage, swelling and inflammation of the veins where the chemotherapy is administered, difficulty swallowing, bleeding, **itching**, and skin reactions in areas of previous radiation.

All side effects a patient experiences should be reported to his or her doctor.

Interactions

Dexrazoxane should only be used with chemotherapy combinations that contain doxorubicin or other agents in the anthracycline class of antineoplastics.

Patients should tell their doctors if they have a known allergic reaction to dexrazoxane or any other medications or substances, such as foods and preservatives. Before taking any new medications, including nonprescription medications, **vitamins**, and herbal medications, the patients should notify their doctors.

Nancy J. Beaulieu, RPh., BCOP

Diarrhea

Definition

Diarrhea is the abnormal increase of liquid in stool and increase in the frequency of passing stool (defecation). It is not a specific disease but a condition that occurs as a result of other diseases, medications, toxic substances, or **cancer** therapy. The name *diarrhea* comes from a Greek word that means "to flow through." The person with diarrhea has watery or loose stools more than three times a day. Other symptoms include cramping, pain, feeling the urge to defecate, irritation of the skin around the anus (perianal), and inability to control defecation (fecal **incontinence**). Diarrhea lasting two weeks or less is called acute diarrhea and diarrhea lasting for longer than two months is called chronic diarrhea. Viral and bacterial infections are the most common causes of acute diarrhea.

In addition to frequency of bowel movements, researchers have found that diarrhea best correlates with an increase in stool weight; stool weights above 10oz (300 grams) per day generally indicates diarrhea. This weight is mainly due to excess water, which normally makes up 60–85% of fecal matter. In this way, true diarrhea is distinguished from diseases that cause only an increase in the number of bowel movements (hyperdefecation) or incontinence (involuntary loss of bowel contents).

Doctors also distinguish between osmotic diarrhea, in which water is drawn into the lumen of the intestines because of an unabsorbable substance (such as some artificial sweeteners), and secretory diarrhea, in which an irritant (usually a bacterium) causes the cells lining the intestine to actively secrete fluid into the lumen.

Demographics

Diarrhea caused by infections (including parasites) or food poisoning is very common in all age groups worldwide. Acute infectious diarrhea has a huge impact around the world, causing over five million deaths per year. While most deaths are among children under five years of age in developing nations, the impact is considerable even in developed countries. For example, over 250,000 individuals are admitted to hospitals in the United States each year because of an episode of acute diarrhea.

The World Health Organization (WHO) estimates that at least 30 million adolescents and adults every year get traveler's diarrhea during visits to underdeveloped countries. Diarrhea in children is most commonly caused by rotavirus infections. About 1 child in 80 in the United States and Canada is hospitalized for diarrhea caused by rotavirus by age five. The Centers for Disease Control and Prevention (CDC) estimates that there are about 76 million cases of diarrhea related to food poisoning in the United States each year. Approximately 10% of patients with advanced cancer suffer from diarrhea.

Diarrhea is equally common among both sexes and all races and ethnic groups around the world.

Description

In many cases, acute infectious diarrhea is a mild, limited annoyance. Diarrhea can be, however, a debilitating condition that significantly affects a person's quality of life. Diarrhea can prevent patients from participating in social activities and going to work. Persons with diarrhea fear soiling their clothing or bed linens, a fear that prevents them from leaving home. Loss of sleep due to nighttime diarrhea can cause **fatigue**, which ultimately affects the patient's ability to function normally. Uncontrolled diarrhea can lead to chemical imbalances, loss of fluids (dehydration), and even death. Rapid diagnosis and proper treatment can prevent much of the suffering associated with these devastating illnesses.

Chronic diarrhea also has a considerable effect on health, as well as on social and economic well-being. Patients with celiac disease, inflammatory bowel disease, and other prolonged diarrheal illnesses develop nutritional deficiencies that diminish growth and immunity. They affect social interaction and result in the loss of many working hours.

Risk factors

Risk factors for diarrhea include:

- frequent travel to countries or wilderness areas with poor sanitation
- lack of proper precautions in food purchasing, storage, and preparation
- history of chronic gastrointestinal disorders, including Crohn's disease and irritable bowel syndrome
- taking certain medications, particularly antibiotics
- receiving chemotherapy or radiation therapy for cancer
- exposure to rotavirus infection
- having surgery for gallbladder removal or other surgery in the abdomen
- history of heavy alcohol intake
- lactose intolerance
- heavy consumption of foods containing sorbitol, mannitol, and other artificial sweeteners

Causes and symptoms

Causes

Diarrhea occurs because more fluid passes through the large intestine (colon) than that organ can absorb. As a rule, the colon can absorb several times more fluid than is required on a daily basis. However, when this reserve capacity is overwhelmed, diarrhea occurs.

Diarrhea is caused by infections or illnesses that either lead to excess production of fluids or prevent absorption of fluids. Also, certain substances in the colon, such as fats and bile acids, can interfere with water absorption and cause diarrhea. In addition, rapid passage of material through the colon can also do the same.

Symptoms related to any diarrheal illness are often those associated with any injury to the gastrointestinal tract, such as **fever**, **nausea**, **vomiting**, and abdominal pain. All or none of these may be present depending on the disease causing the diarrhea. The number of bowel movements can vary—up to 20 or more per day. In some patients, blood or pus is present in the stool. Bowel movements may be difficult to flush (because they float) or contain undigested food material.

The most common causes of acute diarrhea are infections (the cause of traveler's diarrhea), food poisoning, and medications. Medications are a frequent and often over/looked cause, especially **antibiotics** and antacids. Less often, various sugar-free foods, which sometimes contain poorly absorbable materials, cause diarrhea.

Chronic diarrhea is frequently due to many of the same things that cause the shorter episodes (infections, medications, etc.) but the symptoms just last longer. Some infections can become chronic. This occurs mainly with parasitic infections (such as *Giardia*) or when patients have altered immunity (AIDS).

The following are the more usual causes of chronic diarrhea:

- AIDS
- colon cancer and other bowel tumors
- endocrine or hormonal abnormalities (thyroid, diabetes mellitus, etc.)
- food allergy
- inflammatory bowel disease (Crohn's disease and ulcerative colitis)
- lactose intolerance
- malabsorption syndromes (celiac and Whipple's disease)
- other (alcoholism, microscopic colitis, radiation, surgery)

CANCER-RELATED DIARRHEA. The most common cause of diarrhea in cancer patients is related to constipation or its treatment. Cancer patients may experience diarrhea as a result of their treatment, or it can be due to dietary changes, infections, hormone imbalances, digestion disorders, or inflammation. Treatment-related diarrhea can be caused by **chemotherapy**, hormone therapy, **radiation therapy**, **biological response modifiers** (drugs that improve the patient's immune system), or surgery. In addition, cancer patients may develop temporary lactose intolerance, which causes diarrhea.

Chemotherapy drugs kill the rapidly growing cancer cells. However, certain normal cells of the body are rapidly growing and they too are affected. Rapidly growing cells are found in the intestines, as well as other parts of the body. Diarrhea occurs as a result of injury to the cells of the intestine. These effects are temporary. Chemotherapy drugs, hormones, and biological response modifiers that frequently cause diarrhea include:

- Dactinomycin
- Daunorubicin
- Diethylstilbestrol diphosphate
- Doxorubicin
- Fluorouracil
- Flutamide
- Hydroxyurea
- Interferon
- Interferon-2 (aldesleukin)

- Irinotecan
- Methotrexate
- Thioguanine

Radiation therapy can cause diarrhea if the intestines are in the treatment field. Diarrhea results from the injury and destruction of the cells lining the intestines, which leads to a decrease in the uptake (absorption) of fluids and an increase in the speed with which stool moves through the intestines. Radiation therapy can cause diarrhea, and other intestinal problems, many months or years after treatment has been completed.

Diarrhea usually develops within one week following pretreatment (chemotherapy and irradiation) for **bone marrow transplantation**. This diarrhea usually disappears within two weeks. Also, bone marrow transplant patients with graft-versus-host disease develop severe diarrhea.

Symptoms and complications

The major effects of diarrhea are dehydration, malnutrition, and **weight loss**. Signs of dehydration can be hard to notice, but increasing thirst, dry mouth, weakness or lightheadedness (particularly if worsening on standing), or a darkening/decrease in urination are suggestive. Severe dehydration leads to changes in the body's chemistry and could become life-threatening. Dehydration from diarrhea can result in kidney failure, neurological symptoms, arthritis, and skin problems.

Diagnosis

Most cases of acute diarrhea never need diagnosis or treatment, as many are mild and produce few problems. But patients with fever over 102 °F (38.9 °C), signs of dehydration, bloody bowel movements, severe abdominal pain, known immune disease, or prior use of antibiotics need prompt medical evaluation. The doctor will take a patient history that includes occupation as well as recent travel to countries with poor sanitation or to wilderness areas. The doctor will ask what the patient has eaten recently and how much; whether the patient has lost weight; whether the patient has felt dizzy or unusually drowsy; when the patient last had a bowel movement and what its appearance was like; whether the patient noticed any blood in or on the stool; when the patient last urinated and the amount of fluid taken in the last 24 hours; and whether the patient presently feels feverish. In some cases the doctor will ask about the patient's customary diet, medications that the patient may be taking, and herbal remedies or alternative therapies that the patient may be using.

Chronic diarrhea is quite different from acute diarrhea, and most patients with this condition will receive some degree of testing. Many exams are the same as for an acute episode, as some infections and parasites cause both types of diarrhea. A careful history to evaluate medication use, dietary changes, family history of illnesses, and other symptoms is necessary. Key points in determining the seriousness of symptoms are weight loss of over 10 lb (4.5 kg), blood in the stool, and nocturnal diarrhea (symptoms that awaken the patient from sleep).

Both prescription and over-the-counter medications can contain such additives as lactose and sorbitol that will produce diarrhea in sensitive individuals. Review of allergies or skin changes may also point to a cause. Social history may indicate whether stress is playing a role or identify activities that may be associated with diarrhea (for example, diarrhea that occurs in runners).

Examination

The doctor will first look for signs of dehydration during an office examination for a patient with diarrhea. A healthcare professional or observant adult can usually tell by looking at someone that they are moderately or severely dehydrated. Such visual signs as sunken eyes and dry skin are often enough to begin treatment. The doctor will typically examine the skin lining the patient's mouth for evidence of dehydration. In addition, the patient's blood pressure may be low, breathing or pulse rate may be rapid, and he or she may have a fever. The doctor will also palpate (gently feel) the patient's abdomen and listen to bowel sounds through a stethoscope. In most cases the doctor will also perform a rectal examination in the office and may take a stool sample.

Tests

When diagnostic studies are needed, the most useful are stool culture and examination for parasites; however these are often negative and a cause cannot be found in a large number of patients. The earlier cultures are performed, the greater the chance of obtaining a positive result. For those with a history of antibiotic use in the preceding two months, stool samples need to be examined for the toxins that cause antibiotic-associated colitis. Tests are also available to check stool samples for microscopic amounts of blood and for cells that indicate severe inflammation of the colon. Tests to check changes in blood chemistry (potassium, magnesium, etc.) and a complete blood count (CBC) are also often performed.

Procedures

Examination with an endoscope is sometimes helpful in determining the severity and extent of inflammation in cases of severe acute diarrhea.

A combination of stool, blood, and urine tests may be needed in the evaluation of chronic diarrhea; in addition a number of endoscopic and x-ray studies are frequently required.

Treatment

Traditional

Treatment is ideally directed toward correcting the cause; however, the first aim should be to prevent or treat dehydration and nutritional deficiencies. The type of fluid and nutrient replacement will depend on whether oral feedings can be taken and the severity of fluid losses. Of the utmost importance in the treatment of diarrhea is the replacement of fluids lost by frequent, watery stools. Patients who can take fluids by mouth should drink six to eight glasses of fluid daily, including clear broth, ginger ale that has been allowed to go flat, water, weak tea, and commercial formulas that contain sugars and minerals (electrolytes). Patients with severe diarrhea may need intravenous fluid replacement either at home or in the hospital. Oral rehydration solution (ORS) or intravenous fluids are the choices; ORS is preferred if possible.

A physician should be notified if the patient is dehydrated, and if oral replacement is suggested then commercial (Pedialyte and others) or homemade preparations can be used. The World Health Organization (WHO) has provided this easy recipe for home preparation, which can be taken in small frequent sips:

- table salt—3/4 tsp
- baking powder—1 tsp
- orange juice—1 cup
- water—1 qt (1 liter)

When feasible, food intake should be continued even in those with acute diarrhea. A physician should be consulted as to what type and how much food is permitted.

Drugs

Anti-motility agents (loperamide, diphenoxylate) are useful for those with chronic symptoms; their use is limited or even contraindicated in most individuals with acute diarrhea, especially in those with high fever or bloody bowel movements. They should not be taken without the advice of a physician.

Other treatments are available, depending on the cause of symptoms. For example, the bulk agent psyllium helps some patients by absorbing excess fluid and solidifying stools; cholestyramine, which binds bile acids, is effective in treating bile salt induced diarrhea. Low fat diets or more easily digestible fat is useful in some patients. New antidiarrheal drugs that decrease excessive secretion of fluid by the intestinal tract offer another approach for some diseases. Avoidance of medications or other products that are known to cause diarrhea (such as lactose) is curative in some, but should be discussed with a physician.

Cancer patients with chronic diarrhea may be given atropine sulfate (Lomotil), codeine phosphate, loperamide (Imodium), or octreotide (Sandostatin); these drugs should not be taken, however, until bacterial **infection** has been eliminated as a cause of the diarrhea. Cancer patients who are experiencing diarrhea due to graft-versus-host disease will continue to take their immunosuppressant drugs. They may also be treated with **corticosteroids** and antidiarrheal medications.

Alternative

It is especially important to find the cause of diarrhea, since stopping diarrhea when it is the body's way of eliminating something foreign is not helpful and can be harmful in the long run.

One effective alternative approach to preventing and treating diarrhea involves oral supplementation of the normal flora in the colon with the yeasts *Lactobacillus acidophilus*, *L. bifidus*, or *Saccharomyces boulardii*. In clinical settings, these "biotherapeutic" agents have repeatedly been helpful in the resolution of diarrhea, especially antibiotic-associated diarrhea.

Nutrient replacement also plays a role in preventing and treating episodes of diarrhea. Zinc especially appears to have an effect on the immune system, and deficiency of this mineral can lead to chronic diarrhea. Also, zinc replacement improves growth in young patients. Plenty of fluids, especially water, should be taken by individuals suffering from diarrhea to prevent dehydration. The BRAT diet also can be useful in helping to resolve diarrhea. This diet limits food intake to bananas, rice, applesauce, and toast. These foods provide soluble and insoluble fiber without irritation. If the toast is slightly burnt, the charcoal can help sequester toxins and pull them from the body.

Acute homeopathic remedies can be very effective for treating diarrhea, especially in infants and young children. A cancer treatment team at Duke University in North Carolina reported in 2009 that relaxation techniques and electroacupuncture are effective in relieving diarrhea in some cancer patients.

Herbal remedies for diarrhea include peppermint tea, chamomile tea, valerian capsules, or aloe vera juice, which may reduce cramping and intestinal spasms. An Ayurvedic physician may recommend taking equal parts of yogurt and water with fresh ginger, or a powder of beleric myrobalan fruit. Other Ayurvedic practitioners recommend as many as 28 different plants for the treatment of diarrhea, including buckthorn, jujube, and several plants related to yams. Ginger capsules may relieve intestinal spasms and pain. **Glutamine** supplements may speed up the healing process and relieve irritated intestines.

Personal care

Diarrhea can cause the perianal skin to become irritated and painful; therefore, it needs to be cleaned thoroughly after each episode of diarrhea. Baby wipes or a mild soap with water can be used to clean the irritated skin. The area should be patted dry and occasionally exposed to air. Taking a sitz bath (sitting in a bathtub of shallow water) with lukewarm water may relieve the discomfort. Petroleum jelly or other type of barrier cream may be used after cleansing the irritated area.

Prognosis

Prognosis is related to the cause of the diarrhea; for most individuals in developed countries, a bout of acute infectious diarrhea is at best uncomfortable. However, in both industrialized and developing areas, serious complications and death can occur. According to WHO, 500,000 children die each year around the world from diarrhea caused by rotavirus infection.

For those with chronic symptoms, an extensive number of tests are usually necessary to make a proper diagnosis and begin treatment; a specific diagnosis is found in 90% of patients. In some, however, no specific cause is found and only treatment with bulk agents or anti-motility agents is indicated.

The prognosis of diarrhea in cancer patients is usually related to the prognosis of the cancer and the therapies used to treat it.

Prevention

Proper hygiene and food-handling techniques will prevent many cases of diarrhea. Rotavirus infections in small children can be prevented by a new oral vaccine introduced in 2006. The most important action is to prevent the complications of dehydration.

QUESTIONS TO ASK YOUR DOCTOR

- What is causing the diarrhea?
- Is the diarrhea acute or chronic?
- Can I take care of fluid intake at home, or will I need professional medical treatment to prevent dehydration?
- What medications, if any, would you recommend?
- Will I need to make changes in my usual diet?

It is difficult to prevent all cases of traveler's diarrhea, although with care, the chances of getting sick can be reduced. Some commonsense preventative measures include the following:

- Avoid tap and well water including ice cubes in drinks.
- Avoid raw unpeeled fruits and raw vegetables.
- Avoid unpasteurized milk, dairy products (e.g., ice cream, yogurt) and unpasteurized fruit juices.
- Do not buy food from street vendors.
- Wash hands often in uncontaminated water.
- Choose hot drinks such as coffee or tea or canned or bottled drinks
- In wilderness situations, travelers should boil water for 3–5 minutes (depending on elevation); filter water with appropriate filters; or use chlorine bleach (2 drops per quart) or tincture of iodine (5 drops per quart) in the water.

For cancer patients, there are some measures that can prevent diarrhea related to anticancer treatments. Patients who are receiving abdominal radiation therapy can be put into certain positions to minimize exposure of healthy intestines to radiation. Diarrhea caused by chemotherapy cannot be prevented; however, the administration of atropine during treatment with **irinotecan** may prevent diarrhea. Patients should stop taking dietary supplements, as these can cause diarrhea. Specific advice about foods to choose and foods to avoid can be found on the American Cancer Society (ACS) website at the link listed below.

Resources

BOOKS

Chiodini, Jane, and Lorna Boyne. *Atlas of Travel Medicine and Health*. Hamilton, Ontario, and Lewiston, NY : BC Decker, 2003.

Goroll, Allan H., and Albert G. Mulley Jr., eds. *Primary Care Medicine: Office Evaluation and Management of the Adult Patient*, 6th ed. Philadelphia : Wolters Kluwer Health/Lippincott Williams and Wilkins, 2009.

Lyman, Gary H., and Jeffrey Crawford, eds. *Cancer Supportive Care: Advances in Therapeutic Strategies*. New York : Informa Healthcare, 2008.

Porter, Robert S., ed. *The Merck Manual of Patient Symptoms: A Concise, Practical Guide to Etiology, Evaluation, and Treatment*. Whitehouse Station, NJ: Merck Laboratories, 2008.

PERIODICALS

Abernethy, A.P., et al. "Detailing of Gastrointestinal Symptoms in Cancer Patients with Advanced Disease: New Methodologies, New Insights, and a Proposed Approach." *Current Opinion in Supportive and Palliative Care* 3 (March 2009): 41–49.

Bishop, R. "Discovery of Rotavirus: Implications for Child Health." *Journal of Gastroenterology and Hepatology* 24 (October 2009): Suppl. 3, S81–S85.

Cabada, M. M., and A. C. White, Jr. "Travelers' Diarrhea: An Update on Susceptibility, Prevention, and Treatment." *Current Gastroenterology Reports* 10 (October 2008): 473–9.

Canavan, A., and B.S. Arant, Jr. "Diagnosis and Management of Dehydration in Children." *American Family Physician* 80 (October 1, 2009): 692–96.

Dupont, H. L. "Bacterial Diarrhea." *New England Journal of Medicine* 361 (October 15, 2009): 1560–69.

Prasad, A. S. "Zinc: Role in Immunity, Oxidative Stress and Chronic Inflammation." *Current Opinion in Clinical Nutrition and Metabolic Care* 12 (November 2009): 646–52.

Tetali, P., et al. "Ethnobotanical Survey of Antidiarrhoeal Plants of Parinche Valley, Pune District, Maharashtra, India." *Journal of Ethnopharmacology* 123 (June 2009): 229–36.

Yarris, J. P., and C.R. Warden. "Gastrointestinal Bleeding in the Cancer Patient." *Emergency Medicine Clinics of North America* 27 (August 2009): 363–79.

Yates, Johnnie. "Travelers' Diarrhea." *American Family Physician* 71 (April 1, 2005): 2107–8.

OTHER

American Cancer Society (ACS). *Diarrhea*. http://www.cancer.org/docroot/MBC/content/MBC_6_2X_Diarrhea.asp?sitearea=MBC.

Guandalini, Stefano, Richard Frye, and M. Akram Tamer. "Diarrhea." *eMedicine*, January 5, 2009. http://emedicine.medscape.com/article/928598-overview.

Mayo Clinic. *Diarrhea*. http://www.mayoclinic.com/health/diarrhea/DS00292.

National Cancer Institute (NCI). *Gastrointestinal Complications: Diarrhea*. http://www.cancer.gov/cancertopics/pdq/supportivecare/gastrointestinalcomplications/Patient/page6.

National Institute of Diabetes and Digestive and Kidney Diseases (NIDDK). *Diarrhea*. http://digestive.niddk.nih.gov/ddiseases/pubs/diarrhea/index.htm.

Surawicz, Christina M., and Blanca Ochoa. "Patient Information: Diarrheal Diseases." http://www.acg.gi.org/patients/gihealth/diarrheal.asp.

ORGANIZATIONS

American Cancer Society (ACS), 250 Williams Street NW, Atlanta, GA, 30303, 800-ACS-2345 (227-2345), www.cancer.org.

American College of Gastroenterology, P.O. Box 342260, Bethesda, MD, 20827-2260, 301-263-9000, http://www.acg.gi.org/.

Centers for Disease Control and Prevention (CDC), 1600 Clifton Road, Atlanta, GA, 30333, 800-232-4636, cdcinfo@cdc.gov, http://www.cdc.gov.

International Society of Travel Medicine (ISTM), 2386 Clower Street, Suite A-102, Snellvile, GA, United States, 30078, + 1 770 736 060, + 1-770 736 0313, istm@istm.org, https://www.istm.org/.

National Cancer Institute (NCI), 6116 Executive Blvd., Room 3036A, Bethesda, MD, 20892-8322, 800-422-6237, cancergovstaff@mail.nih.gov, www.cancer.gov.

National Institute of Diabetes and Digestive and Kidney Diseases (NIDDK), Building 31. Rm 9A06, 31 Center Drive, MSC 2560, Bethesda, MD, 20892-2560, 301-496-3583, http://www2.niddk.nih.gov/Footer/Contact NIDDK.htm, http://www2.niddk.nih.gov/.

Wilderness Medical Society (WMS), 2150 S 1300 E, Suite 500, Salt Lake City, UT, 84106, 801-990-2988, 801-990-2987, wms@wms.org, http://www.wms.org/.

World Health Organization (WHO), Avenue Appia 20, 1211 Geneva 27, Switzerland, + 41 22 791 21 11, + 41 22 791 31 11, info@who.int, http://www.who.int/en/.

David Kamenstein, MD
Belinda Rowland, PhD
Rebecca J. Frey, PhD

Diazepam

Definition

Diazepam is a common mild tranquilizer or anti-anxiety drug. It is a member of a large class of chemically related medications known as **benzodiazepines**, which depress the activity of the central nervous system. Diazepam and other benzodiazepines block the effects of a specific chemical that is involved in the transmission of nerve impulses in the brain, thereby decreasing the excitement level of neurons.

Purpose

Diazepam is prescribed for millions of people on a short-term basis to relieve mild to moderate anxiety. It is also used to control some types of seizures; ease muscle spasms; treat nervous tension, insomnia, and irritable bowel syndrome; and lessen symptoms of panic attacks and agitation caused by alcohol withdrawal.

Description

Diazepam is usually supplied as an oral tablet, as an oral capsule that releases the active drug at a slower rate, or as an oral liquid. It is available as a generic drug. The time-release capsule should be swallowed whole. It is also available as a rectal gel and in an injectable form for use during a serious seizure or severe muscle spasms. Diazepam should be stored at room temperature in a tightly closed container to avoid alteration in the compound due to excessive heat or moisture.

U.S. brand names

- Valium
- Diastat
- Diastat AcuDial
- Diazepam Intensol

Canadian brand names

- Valium
- Diastat
- Apo-Diazepam
- Diazemuls

International brand names

- Apaurin
- Diazemuls
- Diazepam
- Stesolid
- Valium

Recommended dosage

Diazepam dosage is determined by a physician, taking into account the condition being treated, severity of the symptoms, and the patient's weight and response to the drug. It is taken one to four times each day, depending on the strength of the dose. This maintains the concentration of the drug at a therapeutic level, since diazepam is quickly absorbed from the gastrointestinal tract. Peak levels of the drug are reached within a couple of hours after administration, with levels dropping below therapeutic effectiveness within six to eight hours.

A typical dose of diazepam for treating anxiety or seizures in healthy adults ranges from 2–10 milligrams (mg), two to four times per day. Children and elderly adults are typically given 1–2 mg, one to four times

daily. Children generally receive lower doses even if their body weight is equivalent to that of a small adult. For acute treatment of seizures, a higher dose of diazepam is given intravenously (directly into the vein) in a controlled medical setting such as a hospital or emergency room. The typical dose for alcohol withdrawal is a total of 30–40 mg per day, given in three or four doses.

Diazepam can be taken with or without food. The liquid form can be mixed with other fluids or select foods such as applesauce.

Precautions

Diazepam and all benzodiazepines cause sedation, drowsiness, and reduced mental and physical alertness. Patients taking diazepam should not drive, operate dangerous machinery, or engage in hazardous activities that require mental alertness.

The prescribing physician should be consulted regularly if diazepam is taken consistently for more than two weeks. The recommended dosage should not be exceeded, nor should it continue to be taken after the prescribed time. Diazepam and other benzodiazepines can be habit-forming. Diazepam can be abused and should be used with caution in patients with a history of **substance abuse**. If diazepam is stopped abruptly, withdrawal symptoms including shaking, stomach cramps, nervousness, and irritability may occur.

Pediatric

Children under the age of six months should not be given diazepam and all children should be carefully evaluated before being prescribed the drug.

Geriatric

Elderly patients should be carefully evaluated before being prescribed diazepam. The sedative effects of diazepam can last longer in the elderly and accidental falls are common in older adults taking benzodiazepines.

Pregnant or breastfeeding

Pregnant and breastfeeding women should not take diazepam. It is in pregnancy category D, meaning that it can cause birth defects. Women should use effective means of birth control while taking diazepam. It can also pass into breast milk and harm the nursing baby.

Other conditions and allergies

Anyone with significant health conditions should be evaluated carefully before receiving diazepam.

Patients with **myasthenia gravis**, sleep apnea, severe liver disease, narrow-angle glaucoma, severe breathing problems, or allergies to any benzodiazepine should not take diazepam. The drug should be used cautiously in epileptics, since diazepam can trigger an epileptic seizure. Diazepam should be used with caution in patients with a history of liver disease, kidney disease, or low levels of albumen in the blood.

Patients who are allergic to diazepam or other benzodiazepines can be treated with other drugs such as alprazolam (Xanax), chlordiazepoxide (Librium), or triazolam (Halcion).

Side effects

More common side effects of diazepam include:

- drowsiness
- dizziness
- clumsiness
- slurred speech
- blurred vision
- headache
- fatigue
- muscle weakness
- memory loss
- skin rash
- **diarrhea**
- dry mouth
- stomach upset
- decreased sexual drive
- altered appetite

Less common side effects of diazepam include:

- irritability
- insomnia
- muscle spasms
- jaundice
- decreased white blood cell count (leukopenia)

Less common but serious side effects of diazepam include:

- anxiety
- irregular heartbeat
- forgetfulness
- mental **depression**
- confusion
- behavior changes
- hallucinations
- low blood pressure

Common side effects of diazepam withdrawal include:

- sleeping difficulties
- nervousness
- irritability

Less common side effects of withdrawal include:

- abdominal cramps
- sensitivity to light
- nausea
- shaking
- increased sweating
- mental depression
- confusion

Rare but serious withdrawal side effects include:

- seizures
- hallucinations
- paranoia

Diazepam overdoses can be fatal. Symptoms of overdose include:

- extreme drowsiness
- confusion
- limp or weak muscles
- fainting
- shallow breathing
- cessation of breathing

Interactions

Diazepam should not be taken with other central nervous system depressants such as narcotics, other tranquilizers, sedatives, sleeping pills, or alcohol. Such combinations can lower blood pressure and suppress breathing to the point of unconsciousness and death. Diazepam should not be combined with other drugs for treating mental illness, except under the careful supervision and monitoring of a doctor.

Diazepam interacts with a long list of other medications. Anyone starting diazepam should review their other medications with their physician and pharmacist for possible interactions. Patients should always inform all their healthcare providers, including dentists, that they are taking diazepam.

Several drugs reduce the ability of diazepam to be broken down and cleared from the body. This results in higher levels of the drug in the blood and increases the probability of side effects. These medications include several **antibiotics** such as erythromycin, anti-stomach acid drugs such as cimetidine (Tagamet), and antifungal drugs such as fluconazole.

Other common medicines that may interact with diazepam include:

- antihistamines
- disulfiram (Antabuse)
- depression medications including fluoxetine (Prozac)
- pain medications
- medications for Parkinson's disease
- asthma medications
- cold medicines
- muscle relaxants
- antiseizure medications
- oral contraceptives
- some vitamins

Most of these interactions cause increased drowsiness.

Diazepam can produce false results on urine tests using Clinistix and Diastix to monitor blood sugar. Testape should be used instead.

Diazepam may interact with grapefruit juice.

Resources

BOOKS

Corey, E. J., et al. *Molecules and Medicine.* Hoboken, NJ: John Wiley & Sons, 2007.

Hales, Robert E., et al. *What Your Patients Need To Know About Psychiatric Medications.* Washington, DC: American Psychiatric Publishing, 2007.

Toufexis, Donna, and Sayamwong E. Hammac. *Anti-Anxiety Drugs.* New York: Chelsea House Publishers, 2006.

PERIODICALS

de Lusignan, Simon, et al. "New Patient Asking for Benzodiazepine Prescription." *British Medical Journal* 337, no. 7677 (November 1, 2008): 1054.

"Megan's Story." *The Exceptional Parent* 37, no. 7 (July 2007): A10.

Travis, Alan. "Mother's Little Helper is Back: Heroin Shortage Makes Valium the Street Drug of Choice: Survey Reveals Soaring Use of Illicit Diazepam." *The Guardian* (September 3, 2008): 3.

OTHER

American Society of Health-System Pharmacists. "Diazepam." *MedlinePlus.* http://www.nlm.nih.gov/medlineplus/druginfo/meds/a682047.html.

"Diazepam." *Drugs.com.* http://www.drugs.com/diazepam.html.

"Diazepam." *University of Maryland Medical Center.* http://www.umm.edu/altmed/drugs/diazepam-040900.htm.

"Valium Brand of Diazepam Tablets." *FDA.* http://www.accessdata.fda.gov/drugsatfda_docs/label/2008/013263s083lbl.pdf.

ORGANIZATIONS

American Psychiatric Association, 1000 Wilson Blvd., Ste. 1825, Arlington, VA, 22209-3901, (703) 907-7300, apa@psych.org, http://www.psych.org.

National Institute of Mental Health, 6001 Executive Boulevard, Room 8184, MSC 9663, Bethesda, MD, 20892-9663, (301) 443-4513, (866) 615-6464 , (301) 443-4279, nimhinfo@nih.gov, http://www.nimh.nih.gov.

U.S. Food and Drug Administration, 10903 New Hampshire Ave., Silver Spring, MD, 20993-0002, (888) INFO-FDA, http://www.fda.gov.

Mark Mitchell, MD
Emily Jane Willingham, PhD
Brian Douglas Hoyle, PhD
Margaret Alic, PhD

Diethylstilbestrol diphosphate

Definition

Diethylstilbestrol diphosphate is a synthetic (manufactured) form of the female hormone estrogen. Brand names for diethylstilbestrol include Stilphostrol, and is also referred to as Stilbestrol and DES.

Purpose

Diethylstilbestrol is used to relieve symptoms of advanced **breast cancer** that has metastasized, or spread, from the breast to other parts of the body. It is used to treat breast **cancer** in men and in postmenopausal women. Diethylstilbestrol also has been used to relieve symptoms of advanced cancer of the prostate in men.

Description

Diethylstilbestrol was the first form of estrogen made in the laboratory. It was prescribed to millions of women in the 1950s and 1960s to prevent miscarriage and premature birth. This use was discontinued in the 1970s, when abnormalities of the reproductive systems were found in some children of women who

KEY TERMS

Estrogen—Female sex hormone.

Hormone—Substance produced by the body to regulate the activity of a tissue or organ.

Metastasis—Spread of cancer from its point of origin to other parts of the body.

Prostate—Gland in males that surrounds the urine tube (urethra) at the base of the bladder.

Testosterone—Principal male sex hormone.

took the drug during pregnancy. Furthermore, daughters of women who took this drug during pregnancy are at an increased risk for developing certain types of cervical and vaginal cancers.

Diethylstilbestrol is used to relieve some symptoms of advanced breast cancer in certain men and women. The drug can interfere with the spread of cancer cells that require estrogen to grow and divide.

Diethylstilbestrol sometimes is used to relieve symptoms of advanced **prostate cancer** in men. This drug can lower the levels of the male hormone **testosterone**, which is required for the growth and division of these cancer cells. However, diethylstilbestrol can cause severe side effects in men, including breast enlargement and increased risk of heart disease and blood clots. Thus, it is no longer widely used for the treatment of prostate cancer.

Recommended dosage

Diethylstilbestrol usually is given as a pill, which should be taken at the same time each day. The dosage varies depending on body weight and the type of cancer that is being treated. For breast cancer, the dose is 15 mg per day.

For inoperable prostate cancer, the dose is 50 mg three times a day and can be increased up to 200 mg or more three times a day. Maximum dose is 1 gram a day. For the treatment of prostate cancer, diethylstilbestrol can also be injected slowly into a vein. The dosage may be as high as 1 gram per day for five or more days. The dosage then may be lowered to 250-500 mg once or twice per week.

Precautions

Diethylstilbestrol can cause serious birth defects in humans. Children of women who take diethylstilbestrol (DES) during pregnancy may develop reproductive system abnormalities at puberty, and daughters are at an

increased risk for developing **vaginal cancer**. Therefore, this drug should not be taken by pregnant women, or by either the man or the woman at the time of conception. Women should not breast-feed infants while taking this drug, since estrogens pass into the breast milk.

Diethylstilbestrol may not be indicated, or should be used with caution, for individuals whose medical histories include any of the following:

- heart, kidney, or liver damage
- disease of the gallbladder or gallstones
- inflammation of the pancreas
- bone or uterine cancer
- fibroid tumors of the uterus
- unusual vaginal bleeding
- endometriosis (uterine cells in the ovaries or other pelvic organs)
- high cholesterol
- blood clots or circulatory problems in males

Side effects

Diethylstilbestrol affects normal cells as well as cancer cells, so side effects can occur with this medicine. The side effects associated with diethylstilbestrol usually are mild and temporary. Common side effects include:

- enlargement of the breasts
- breast tenderness
- decreased sexual desire
- voice changes
- swelling of the feet and lower legs
- fluid retention
- weight gain

Less common side effects of diethylstilbestrol include:

- nausea and vomiting during the first few weeks of treatment
- changes in vaginal bleeding
- loss of bladder control
- lumps or discharge from the breasts
- stomach, side, or abdominal pain
- yellow skin or eyes

Taking the medicine with food may reduce or prevent **nausea**.

Rarely, diethylstilbestrol results in the formation of blood clots in the legs or in the lungs. This primarily affects men who are receiving high-dosage treatment for breast or prostate cancers. Symptoms of blood clots include:

- pain, redness, or swelling in the calf
- weakness or tingling in an arm or leg

- faintness
- sudden severe headache
- vision changes
- shortness of breath
- chest pain
- coughing up blood (hemoptysis)

Interactions

Medicines that may adversely affect the liver when taken along with diethylstilbestrol include:

- acetaminophen (as in Tylenol; long-term or high-dose usage)
- amiodarone (Cordarone)
- anabolic steroids (such as nandrolone, oxandrolone, oxymetholone, stanozolol)
- androgens (male hormones)
- antithyroid drugs that are used to treat an overactive thyroid
- birth control pills containing estrogen
- carbamazepine (Tegretol)
- carmustine (BiCNU)
- chloroquine (Aralen)
- dantrolene (Dantrium)
- daunorubicin (Cerubidine)
- disulfiram (Antabuse)
- divalproex (Depakote)
- etretinate (Tegison)
- gold salts to treat arthritis
- hydroxychloroquine (Plaquenil)
- isoniazid
- medicines to treat infections
- mercaptopurine (Purinethol)
- methotrexate (Mexate)
- methyldopa (Aldomet)
- naltrexone (Trexan; long-term or high-dose usage)
- phenothiazines
- phenytoin (Dilantin)
- plicamycin (Mithracin)
- valproic acid (Depakene)

In addition, diethylstilbestrol and other estrogens can prevent **cyclosporine** (Sandimmune) from being removed from the body, leading to possible kidney or liver problems. Protease inhibitors such as ritonavir (Norvir) may reduce the activity of diethylstilbestrol.

Margaret Alic, Ph.D.

Digital rectal examination

Definition

The digital rectal examination (DRE) is a routine part of the physical examination and includes manual examination of the rectum, anus, and, in men, the prostate.

Purpose

The purpose of the digital rectal examination is to identify lesions within the rectum and the prostate. It is the most widely used and oldest technique for the detection of **prostate cancer** and is used in screening for **colon cancer** and for the detection of rectal polyps.

Description

Usually the patient is positioned on the left side with the knees close to the chest. Sometimes the patient is asked to stand up and lean over the examination table. For women, sometimes this examination is part of the routine gynecological exam, and it may be done in a different manner than described here.

During the examination, the health care practitioner examines the anus and the surrounding skin for hemorrhoids, tags, fissures, and abscesses. After lubricating the gloved finger and anus, the examiner gently slides the finger into the anus and follows the contours of the rectum. The examiner notes the tone of the anus and feels the walls and the edges for texture, tenderness, and masses as far as the examining finger can reach. The examiner evaluates the prostate for nodules and tenderness. Stool on the finger should be examined for blood, color, and texture, and tested for fecal occult blood.

The examination takes less than two minutes and can be uncomfortable when the patient is not relaxed or is anxious. Occasionally, when the DRE is performed on a man the penis may become erect. A gentle reminder and reassurance helps to relieve the embarrassment associated with the unexpected erection.

Preparation

The patient must be carefully positioned and the doctor should take care to explain the examination to the patient and to explain to the patient what to expect. The digital rectal examination may be uncomfortable and embarrassing. Much of the discomfort can be reduced by an understanding, unhurried, and gentle examiner.

Precautions

When there are infections of the anus and of the rectum, the digital rectal examination should not be performed. Manipulation of the anal and rectal tissues increases the risk of **infection** and of bleeding.

Results

In the normal anus and rectum, there are no hemorrhoids or bleeding about the anus. The anal tone is not loose. The rectum is smooth and non-tender. No masses should be palpated, or felt.

The digital rectal examination is helpful in identifying areas of peritonitis or tender areas that can be felt through the wall of the rectum. It is used to identify perineal disease or deformity, abnormal location of the anus, rectal prolapse, and atrophy of the gluteal muscle. Digital examination can detect a stenosis (or narrowing) of the anal canal, assess the tone and strength of the anal muscles, or detect the presence of a rectal mass or fecal impaction.

Any masses, including hard stool, blood, or tenderness is considered abnormal. **Cancer** masses may be flattened, nodular, cauliflower-like, or ring-shaped. Polyps can be felt, but must be visualized using **anoscopy** or flexible **sigmoidoscopy** to be distinguished from other lesions, such as internal hemorrhoids or malignant growths. Hard masses of feces may be felt and may be removed.

Aftercare

Aftercare of the digital rectal examination is minimal. It requires removal of the lubricating jelly residue from around the anus. The lubricating jelly dissolves easily in water and may be washed off in bathing after the examination. It can be removed with toilet paper immediately after the examination.

See also Rectal cancer.

Resources

BOOKS

DeGowin, R., and D. D. Brown. *DeGowin's Diagnostic Examination.* 7th ed. New York, New York: McGraw-Hill, 2000.

Yamada, Tadatake, editor. *Textbook of Gastroenterology Volumes One and Two.* 3rd ed. Philadelphia: Lippincott, Williams & Wilkins, 1999.

Cheryl L. Branche, M. D.

DiGuglielmo syndrome *see* **Acute erythroblastic leukemia**

Dilatation and curettage

Definition

Dilatation and curettage (D&C) is a gynecological procedure in which the lining of the uterus (endometrium) is scraped away.

Purpose

D&C is commonly used to obtain tissue for microscopic evaluation to rule out **cancer**. The procedure may also be used to diagnose and treat heavy menstrual bleeding and to diagnose endometrial polyps and uterine fibroids. D&C can be used to remove pregnancy tissue after a miscarriage, incomplete abortion, or childbirth, or as an early abortion technique up to 16 weeks. Endometrial polyps may be removed, and sometimes benign uterine tumors (fibroids) may be scraped away.

Description

D&C is usually performed under general anesthesia, although local or epidural anesthesia can also be used. Using local anesthesia reduces risk and costs, but the patient will feel cramping during the procedure. The type of anesthesia used often depends upon the reason for the D&C.

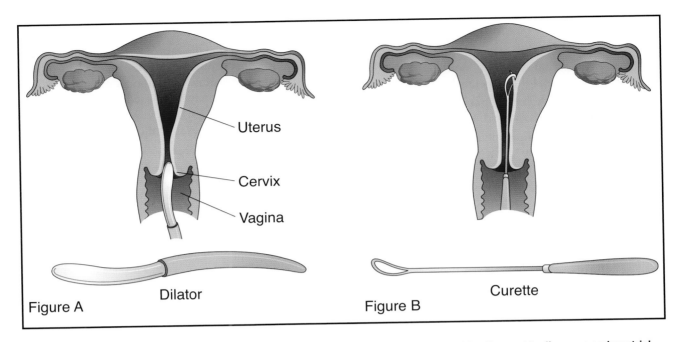

Uterus

Cervix

Vagina

Dilator

Figure A

Curette

Figure B

Dilatation and curettage (D & C) is used primarily to diagnose and treat heavy menstrual bleeding and to diagnose endometrial polyps, uterine fibroids, uterine cancer and cervical cancer. When performing a D & C, the physician inserts a speculum to separate and hold the vaginal walls, then stretches open the cervix with a dilator. Once the cervix is dilated, the physician will insert a curette into the uterus and scrape away small portions of the uterine lining for laboratory analysis. *(Illustration by Electronic Illustrators Group. Cengage Learning, Gale.)*

Dilatation and curettage (D & C) is used primarily to diagnose and treat heavy menstrual bleeding and to diagnose endometrial polyps, uterine fibroids, uterine cancer and **cervical cancer**. When performing a D & C, the physician inserts a speculum to separate and hold the vaginal walls, then stretches open the cervix with a dilator. Once the cervix is dilated, the physician will insert a curette into the uterus and scrape away small portions of the uterine lining for laboratory analysis.

To begin the procedure (which takes only minutes to perform), the doctor inserts an instrument to hold open the vaginal walls, and then stretches the opening of the uterus to the vagina (the cervix). This is done by inserting a series of tapering rods, each thicker than the previous one, or by using other specialized instruments. The process of opening the cervix is called dilation.

Once the cervix is dilated, the physician inserts a spoon-shaped surgical device called a curette into the uterus. The curette is used to scrape away the uterine lining. One or more small tissue samples from the lining of the uterus or the cervical canal are sent for analysis by microscope to check for abnormal cells.

Although simpler, less expensive techniques such as a vacuum aspiration are quickly replacing the D&C as a diagnostic method, it is still often used to diagnose and treat a number of conditions, especially when cancer is suspected.

Preparation

Because opening the cervix can be painful, sedatives may be given before the procedure begins. Deep breathing and other relaxation techniques may help ease cramping during cervical dilation.

Aftercare

A woman who has had a D&C performed in a hospital can usually go home the same day or the next day. Many women experience backache and mild cramps after the procedure, and may pass small blood clots for a day or so. Vaginal staining or bleeding may continue for several weeks.

Most women can resume normal activities almost immediately. Patients should avoid sexual intercourse, douching, and tampon use for at least two weeks to prevent **infection** while the cervix is closing and to allow the endometrium to heal completely.

Risks

The primary risk after the procedure is infection. Signs of infection include:

KEY TERMS

Endometrial hyperplasia—Thickening of the uterine lining. The types of hyperplasia include: simple, complex, and atypical.

Endometrial polyps—A growth in the lining of the uterus (endometrium) that may cause bleeding and can develop into cancer.

Epidural anesthesia—A type of anesthesia that is injected into the epidural space of the spinal cord to numb the nerves leading to the lower half of the body.

Hysteroscopy—A procedure in which the doctor can see the uterine lining with a tube and viewing system. This is sometimes done with a D&C.

Uterine fibroid—A noncancerous tumor of the uterus that can range from the size of a pea to the size of a grapefruit. Small fibroids require no treatment, but those causing serious symptoms may need to be removed.

- fever
- heavy bleeding
- severe cramps
- foul-smelling vaginal discharge

A woman should report any of these symptoms to her doctor, who can treat the infection with **antibiotics** before it becomes serious.

D&C is a surgical operation, which carries certain risks associated with general anesthesia. Rare complications include puncture of the uterus (which usually heals on its own) or puncture of the bowel or bladder (which requires further surgery to repair).

Normal results

Results are considered normal if no unusual thickening, growths, or cancers are found. Removal of the uterine lining causes no side effects, and may be beneficial if the lining has thickened so much that it causes heavy periods. The uterine lining soon grows again normally, as part of the menstrual cycle.

Abnormal results

Some types of uterine thickening, called hyperplasia, are considered abnormal. Simple hyperplasia is a benign condition in which the uterine lining becomes thicker and with more endometrial glands. In complex hyperplasia, another condition where the

QUESTIONS TO ASK THE DOCTOR

- What are you looking for in the D&C?
- Do you recommend any special preparation before the procedure?
- How long will the procedure take?
- What is the risk of finding cancer in my case?
- What action will be taken if cancer is found?
- Will a repeat D&C be necessary?

uterine lining has thickened, the endometrial glands are crowded together. In 80% of cases these conditions will improve, and there is little risk of cancer. Only 1% of simple hyperplasia and 3% of complex hyperplasia will become cancerous.

Atypical hyperplasia is a more serious finding. In this type of endometrial thickening, the cells are abnormal. Twenty-nine percent of women with atypical hyperplasia develop cancer. In fact, in 17% to 25% of women with atypical hyperplasia who have a hysterectomy within one month of diagnosis, a **carcinoma** is found elsewhere in the endometrium.

A D&C is not a fool-proof procedure because only a portion of the uterine lining is sampled. Therefore, it is possible for a cancer to be missed. Because of this, patients with atypical hyperplasia must have another D&C in three or four months. Combining a hysteroscopy (a procedure where a physician can see the lining of the uterus using a special tool) with D&C may increase the accuracy of the diagnosis in some cases. However, this combination is not recommended when endometrial carcinoma is suspected because of the possibility that the hysteroscopy itself can aid in the spread of cancer through the fallopian tubes.

See also Biopsy; Endometrial cancer; Gynecologic cancers.

Resources

BOOKS

Berman, Michael L., and Michael T. McHale. "Uterus." In *Cancer Treatment*, edited by Charles M. Haskell. 5th ed. Philadelphia: W.B. Saunders, 2001, pp. 951-55.

Byers, Lowell J. et al. "Uterus." *Clinical Oncology*, edited by Abeloff, Martin D. et al., 2nd ed. Philadelphia: Churchill Livingstone, 2000, pp. 1987-97.

ORGANIZATIONS

American College of Obstetricians and Gynecologists. 409 12th St. SW, PO Box 96920, Washington, DC 20090-6920. http://www.acog.org.

Carol A. Turkington

Diphenhydramine

Definition

Diphenhydramine is an antihistamine that is used to treat symptoms of conditions varying from the common cold, motion sickness, allergic reactions, and Parkinson's disease to side effects from **cancer** treatments and psychiatric medications.

Purpose

After exposure to an allergen or injury, cells of the immune system release histamines, which have widespread effects throughout the body. Antihistamines such as diphenhydramine compete with histamine for its receptor sites. By preventing histamine from attaching to its receptors, diphenhydramine decreases itchiness, runny nose, hives, and other symptoms of allergic reactions.

Diphenhydramine is a multipurpose antihistamine:

- It is used to relieve red, irritated, itchy, and watery eyes, sneezing, and runny nose caused by colds, hay fever, or allergies.
- It is used to prevent and treat motion sickness.
- Its sedative properties are used for treating insomnia.
- Is is used in cough syrups to relieve coughs and minor throat irritation due to colds or hay fever.
- It is used to control nausea and vomiting.
- It is used to treat stiffness and tremor caused by mild Parkinson's disease, in combination with centrally acting anticholinergic drugs.
- It may be given after a blood transfusion to limit allergic reactions to blood products.
- It may be used prior to imaging studies to limit reactions to radiocontrast media.
- In cancer treatment it is frequently used to control itching and nausea and to minimize the toxic side effects of such drugs as docetaxel.
- It is used to control extrapyramidal neurologic movement symptoms—tremors and abnormal involuntary muscle movements—that are side effects of

drugs called phenothiazines that are used to treat psychotic disorders such as schizophrenia.

Description

Diphenhydramine is an antihistamine that is easily absorbed when taken orally and readily spreads through the body where it induces drying and sedation. Peak action occurs about one hour after ingestion, with effects lasting from four to six hours.

Diphenhydramine comes in many different forms:

- tablets
- rapidly dissolving tablets
- capsules
- liquid-filled capsules
- dissolving strips
- oral liquid or cough syrup
- an injectable form

Diphenhydramine is supplied alone or in combination with pain relievers, **fever** reducers, and decongestants, including over-the-counter (OTC) cough and cold medicines. Some formulations are specifically for children. Diphenhydramine is prescribed in its generic form for treatment of tremors caused by phenothiazines.

U.S. brand names

- AllerMax
- Benadryl
- Benadryl Allergy
- Compoz Nighttime Sleep Aid
- Diphen AF Elixir
- Diphenhist
- Diphenhydramine Hydrochloride Caplets
- Excedrin P.M.
- Genahist
- Goody's PM Powder
- Hydramine Cough Syrup
- Hydramine Elixir
- Miles Nervine Nighttime Sleep-Aid
- Nytol
- Simply Sleep Nighttime Sleep Aid
- Sleepinal Night-time Sleep Aid
- Sominex
- Twilite
- Unisom SleepGels Maximum Strength

Combination products containing diphenhydramine include:

- Alka-Seltzer PM
- Bayer PM Extra Strength Caplets
- Benadryl products
- Doan's P.M. Extra Strength Caplets
- Legatrin PM Caplets
- Percogesic Aspirin-Free Caplets Extra Strength
- Sine-Off Night Time Relief Sinus Cold & Flu Medicine Gel Caplets
- Sominex Pain Relief Formula
- Sudafed Sinus Nighttime Plus Pain Relief Caplets
- Tylenol products

Canadian brand names

- Allerdryl
- Allernix
- Benadryl
- Nytol
- PMS-Diphenhydramine
- Simply Sleep

International brand names

- Benadryl
- Benocten
- Caladryl
- Nytol

Recommended dosage

Diphenhydramine dosages depend on the condition being treated and the patient's response to the medication, but are most often taken as needed. In general, adult oral dosages are 25–50 milligrams (mg), three to four times daily. As a sleep aid, the usual dose is 50 mg 30 minutes before bedtime. For motion sickness, diphenhydramine is taken 30 minutes before departure and, if needed, with meals and at bedtime. The usual dose of injected diphenhydramine is 10–50 mg, administered into a vein or muscle. Some patients may require 100-mg injections. The daily dose of diphenhydramine should not exceed 400 mg. If a dose is missed, the next one should be taken at its regularly scheduled time without doubling up.

Children weighing more than 20 pounds may take 12.5–25 mg, three to four times daily, with a maximum daily dose of 300 mg. The doctor may calculate the dosage based on the child's weight. Parents should not double up on doses if one is missed.

Lotions or creams containing 1–2% diphenhydramine may be applied to the skin three to four times daily to relieve **itching** in adults and children older than two.

Precautions

Because diphenhydramine causes drowsiness, those taking the drug should refrain from driving, operating machinery or appliances, or performing hazardous tasks requiring mental alertness until the medication has worn off.

Topical diphenhydramine should not be applied to large areas of the body, to blistered or oozing skin, to sunburn, or to lesions caused by poison ivy or chickenpox.

Pediatric

It is very important to check all the ingredients on cough and cold medicines given to children, to make sure that they are not taking two medicines that both contain diphenhydramine, since this could cause an overdose. Diphenhydramine should not be used to induce sleepiness in children.

Geriatric

Elderly patients are especially prone to the sedating effects of diphenhydramine. This drug may also cause dizziness and lower blood pressure in older adults. While taking this medication, moving from lying or sitting to a standing position should be performed slowly to prevent dizziness and fainting.

Pregnant or breastfeeding

Pregnant and breastfeeding women should discuss the use of this and all drugs with their physician prior to use. Diphenhydramine enters breast milk and is contraindicated for breastfeeding.

Other conditions and allergies

Patients with the following conditions should use diphenhydramine only under careful medical monitoring:

- angle-closure glaucoma
- peptic ulcer disease
- bowel obstructions
- enlarged prostate
- difficulty urinating due to a blockage in the bladder

Patients with the following conditions should exercise caution and discuss the risks and benefits with their doctor before using diphenhydramine:

- asthma
- heart disease
- high blood pressure

• overactive thyroid

Diphenhydramine should not be used for several days prior to an allergy test, since it will interfere with the results.

Side effects

Drowsiness is the most common side effect of diphenhydramine. Stomach distress—including poor appetite, **nausea**, **vomiting**, **diarrhea**, or constipation—is also a relatively common side effect of diphenhydramine.

Less common side effects of diphenhydramine include:

• dry mouth and nose
• dizziness
• poor coordination
• restlessness
• nervousness
• confusion
• insominia
• blurry or double vision
• ringing in the ears
• headache
• convulsions
• low blood pressure
• palpitations
• rapid or irregular heart beat
• early onset of menstruation
• frequent urination
• difficulty urinating, with urine retention in the bladder
• hives or rash
• sensitivity to the sun

A less common but potentially serious side effect of high doses of diphenhydramine is weakening or deterioration of muscle tissue. Patients should be careful not to take higher-than-recommended doses of the drug.

Pediatric

OTC cough and cold combination medicines containing diphenhydramine can cause serious side effects and even death in young children. These medicines should not be given to children under age four. Children should only be given medicines that are labeled as safe for their age group. Although children also may experience drowsiness with diphenhydramine, in young children the drug sometimes has the opposite effect.

Geriatric

Drowsiness and dizziness may be increased in elderly patients taking diphenhydramine. Thickened lung secretions are also more common in the elderly.

Interactions

Diphenhydramine should not be used in conjuction with hay-fever medicines, sedatives, narcotics, anesthetics, barbiturates, or muscle relaxants. Diphenhydramine should not be used in conjunction with any other preparation containing an antihistamine, unless specifically ordered by a physician. Topical diphenhydramine should not be used with other antihistamine-containing lotions or creams.

Alcohol or other central nervous system depressants, such as pain medications, sleeping pills, or tranquilizers, and antidepressants may increase the drowsiness associated with diphenhydramine. Monoamine oxidase inhibitor (MAOI) antidepressants may increase the drying effects of diphenhydramine and cause their effects to last longer.

Resources

PERIODICALS

Hou, R. H. et al. "Comparison of Diphenhydramine and Modafinil on Arousal and Autonomic Functions in Healthy Volunteers." *Journal of Psychopharmacology* 21, no. 6 (August 2007): 567.

Ryan, Teresa, et al. "Over-the-Counter Cough and Cold Medication Use in Young Children." *Pediatric Nursing* 34, no. 2 (March/April 2008): 174–181.

Scaife, J. C., et al. "Sensitivity of Late-Latency Auditory and Somatosensory Evoked Potentials to Threat of Electric Shock and the Sedative Drugs Diazepam and Diphenhydramine in Human Volunteers." *Journal of Psychopharmacology* 20, no. 4 (July 2006): 485–495.

Thomas, A., et al. "Diphenhydramine Abuse and Detoxification: A Brief Review and Case Report." *Journal of Psychopharmacology* 23, no. 1 (January 2009): 101.

Turner, Claire, Alison D. F. Handford, and Anthony N. Nicholson. "Sedation and Memory: Studies with a Histamine H-1 Receptor Antagonist." *Journal of Psychopharmacology* 20, no. 4 (July 2006): 506–517.

OTHER

American Society of Health-System Pharmacists. "Diphenhydramine." *MedlinePlus.* http://www.nlm.nih.gov/medlineplus/druginfo/meds/a682539.html#skip.
"Diphenhydramine." *University of Maryland Medical Center.* http://www.umm.edu/altmed/drugs/diphenhydramine-043500.htm.

ORGANIZATIONS

American Academy of Family Physicians, 11400 Tomahawk Creek Parkway, Leawood, KS, 66211-2680, (913) 906-6000, (800) 274-6000, (913) 906-6075, http://www.aafp.org/online/en/home.html.
American Society for Pharmacology and Experimental Therapeutics, 9650 Rockville Pike, Bethesda, MD, 20814-3995, (301) 634-7060, info@aspet.org, http://www.aspet.org.
Parkinson's Disease Foundation, 1359 Broadway, Suite 1509, New York, NY, 20814-3995, (212) 923-4700, (800) 457-6676, (212) 923-4778, info@pdf.org, http://www.pdf.org.
U.S. Food and Drug Administration, 10903 New Hampshire Ave., Silver Spring, MD, 20993-0002, (888) INFO-FDA, http://www.fda.gov.

Debra Wood, RN
Rebecca J. Frey, PhD
Fleming L. Fallon, Jr, MD, PhD
Ruth A. Wienclaw, PhD
Margaret Alic, PhD

Diphenoxylate *see* **Antidiarrheal agents**

Disseminated intravascular coagulation

Description

Disseminated intravascular coagulation, or DIC, is a bleeding disorder resulting from the widespread overstimulation of the body's clotting and anticlotting mechanisms in response to illness, stress, or both. Disseminated intravascular coagulation (DIC) occurs mainly within the capillaries or the microcirculation. It is a secondary complication of a diverse group of disorders that activate, in some way, the coagulation system.

Causes

Disseminated intravascular coagulation occurs when the body's clotting mechanisms are activated throughout the body in response to an injury or a disorder, instead of being isolated to the area of initial onset. Platelets circulating throughout the body form small blood clots (thrombi) primarily in the area of the capillaries. This eventually causes the clotting factors to be used up, and none are left to form clots at the site of the injury. The presence of numerous small clots precipitates the release of clot-dissolving mechanisms, and the end result is generalized bleeding throughout the body. It is, in essence, a paradoxical situation—numerous microthrombi are being formed in the capillaries and the body reacts to dissolve these clots. It is sometimes called consumptive coagulopathy to indicate this paradox because the intravascular clotting rapidly consumes the products necessary for clotting: fibrinogen, platelets, prothrombin, and clotting factors V, VIII, and X.

Disseminated intravascular coagulation should be suspected in any individual who has an unexplained tendency toward bleeding and has experienced any clinical condition that introduces coagulation-promoting factors into the circulation. These conditions include placental abruption; retained dead fetus; amniotic fluid embolism; metastatic **cancer** of the pancreas, lung, stomach, or prostate; and acute leukemia. Any condition that also causes decreased blood flow, such as hypotension, can stimulate DIC. Widespread injury to the tissues throughout the body, as in severe burns, trauma, heat stroke, surgery, various types of infections by bacteria and fungus, snake bites, and fat embolism, can precipitate the cascade of factors to produce DIC. Excessive bleeding can appear suddenly and progress rapidly to severe or fatal hemorrhage. Signs and symptoms that appear gradually are prolonged bleeding from a venipuncture site, bleeding gums, nosebleeds, and bruising easily as well as the presence of minute, pinpoint red spots caused by bleeding under the layer of the skin.

Treatments

The objective of treatment is to determine the underlying cause of DIC and treat it, because this underlying cause predicts the probable outcome. The presence of inadequate blood components can be overcome with fresh frozen plasma and blood transfusions. Fibrinogen replacement can also occur by transfusion of blood products. When the primary disease cannot be treated, intravenous injections of **heparin**, a medication used to prevent thrombosis, are sometimes used in combination with replacement therapy. The use of heparin is, however, very controversial because it can cause bleeding itself.

Alternative and complementary therapies

Disseminated intravascular coagulation is an extremely serious condition precipitated by extraordinary events. Because it is an immediate, life-threatening situation, alternative and complementary therapies are not recommended during this phase. As an individual improves, it is important to utilize relaxation, visualization and imagery as well as vitamin and mineral supplements to promote healing.

Linda K. Bennington, C.N.S., M.S.N.

DNA *see* Cancer genetics

DNA flow cytometry

Definition

DNA **flow cytometry** is a method of measuring the amount of deoxyribonucleic acid (DNA, genetic material) in tumor cells and the percentage of cells actively replicating.

Purpose

DNA flow cytometric analysis is sometimes done to assess a patient's prognosis. It is used to help the physician determine how the tumor cells are likely to behave. It may also be used to monitor a patient if the tumor is expected to recur.

Description

DNA flow cytometric analysis may be performed on tissue from a **biopsy** or it may require a sample of blood or body fluid from the patient. If a blood sample is used, it will be separated into its different components and the red blood cells will be removed. If material from a biopsy is used, cells from the solid tissue will be separated from each other. The cells to be analyzed will then be mixed with a dye called propidium iodide that binds tightly to DNA. This dye gives off fluorescent light as the cells pass through the laser beam of the cytometer. The cytometer can also measure other information about the cells, such as their size.

By analyzing the amount of fluorescence that the cells emit, the pathologist can evaluate the DNA content; this is also sometimes referred to as the DNA

index or **ploidy analysis**. It can also determined whether or not the **cancer** cells are dividing; this is called S-phase analysis. The physician sometimes uses this information to determine the patient's prognosis and choose the most effective treatment.

Preparation

If a biopsy is required, the patient should be prepared for the biopsy as suggested by the physician. Alternatively, a routine blood or body fluid sample may be required. Other special preparations are not usually necessary.

Risks

The risks associated with DNA flow cytometry are limited to those associated with blood or biopsy sample collection.

Normal results

Most cells are normally in a resting, or non-proliferating, phase of the cell cycle. During this time the cells are diploid, meaning they have two copies of each chromosome. Cells duplicate their DNA during what is called S-phase so that they can reproduce, resulting in four copies of each chromosome. The cells rest again until a period called mitosis, when they begin to divide.

Normal DNA flow cytometry results will show that most of the cells are resting and have only two copies of each chromosome. Less than 10% of the cells will be in S-phase. DNA flow cytometry results are usually presented in graphical form for easier analysis. A normal graph will show one large peak of resting cells, followed by a flat area and another smaller peak of cells about to divide.

Abnormal results

Abnormal results will show as several peaks of differing sizes. This means that some of the cells in the sample have extra DNA or an irregular number of chromosomes. An increased percentage of cells may be in S-phase replicating their DNA. An abnormal result does not necessarily mean malignancy; DNA flow cytometry results must be combined with other tests to diagnose malignancy. Interpretation of results is also dependent on the type of tumor being examined. In most types of cancers the presence of cells with irregular amounts of DNA is associated with a poor prognosis, but in some types of cancers, it may indicate a good prognosis.

See also Tumor grading.

Resources

BOOKS

Javois, Lorette C., editor. *Immunocytochemical Methods and Protocols.* Totowa, NJ: Humana Press, 1999.

PERIODICALS

Chassevent, A., et al. "S-phase Fraction and DNA Ploidy in 633 t1t2 Breast Cancers: A Standardized Flow Cytometric Study." *Clinical Cancer Research* 7 (April 2001): 909-17.

OTHER

"FACS Laboratory." *Imperial Cancer Research Fund* [cited July 3, 2001]. http://www.icnet.uk/axp/facs/davies/flow.html.

"Flow Cytometry Core Educational Links." *University of Florida.* [cited July 3, 2001]. http://www.biotech.ufl.edu/~fccl/flow_edu.html.

Racquel Baert, M.Sc.

Docetaxel

Definition

Docetaxel is a drug used to treat certain types of **cancer**. Docetaxel is available under the trade name Taxotere.

KEY TERMS

10-deacetyl baccatin III—A naturally occuring compound that can be converted to docetaxel.

Hypersensitivity—An abnormally sensitive reaction to a stimulus; similar to an allergic reaction.

Microtubles—A tubular structure located in cells that helps them to replicate.

Taxoids—A complex molecule that is chemically similar to paclitaxel.

Therapeutic index—A ratio of the maximum tolerated dose of a drug divided by the dose used in treatment.

Purpose

Docetaxel is an antineoplastic agent used to treat **breast cancer** and non-small cell lung **carcinoma**.

Description

Docetaxel was approved by the Food and Drug Administration (FDA) in 1996.

Docetaxel is a synthetic derivative of the naturally occurring compound paclitaxel. Docetaxel is synthesized from the naturally occurring compound, 10-deacetyl baccatin III, which is extracted from the needles of yew plants. Docetaxel belongs to a group of chemicals called taxoids. The chemical structure and biological action of docetaxel is similar to that of paclitaxel.

Docetaxel promotes the formation of microtubules that do not function properly. One of the roles of normal microtubules is to aid in cell duplication. By disrupting this function, docetaxel inhibits cell reproduction.

Docetaxel is used in patients who have breast cancer that has recurred or progressed following treatment with other drugs. It is also used alone to treat non-small cell lung carcinoma, or in combination with platinum-containing drugs such as **cisplatin**. Some increases in survival times have been observed in patients treated with regiments that include docetaxel compared to control populations.

Recommended dosage

There is no known antidote for docetaxel overdose, so patients should be carefully monitored during treatment for toxicity.

Docetaxel is administered intravenously, in a dose that ranges from 60–100 mg/m^2, over one hour, once every three weeks. The initial dose may be adjusted downward depending on patient tolerance to the toxic side effects of the drug. Also, blood tests may be necessary to ensure that the bone marrow is functioning adequately to continue treatment at the recommended interval.

All patients should be pretreated with **corticosteroids** such as **dexamethasone** prior to docetaxel administration, to help prevent adverse side effects. These side effects include severe hypersensitivity to docetaxel treatment and fluid retention. Premedication should start one day prior to docetaxel treatment and continue for three to five days.

Precautions

Docetaxel should only be used under the supervision of a physician experienced in the use of cancer chemotherapeutic agents. Special caution should be taken to monitor the toxic effects of docetaxel, especially suppression of bone marrow function and hypersensitivity reactions. Premedication to prevent hypersensitivity reactions is recommended. Minor to severe hypersensitivity reactions may occur within a few minutes of the start of treatment. Severe hypersensitivity requires treatment. Certain complications will only be possible to manage if the necessary diagnostic and treatment resources are readily available.

Because docetaxel is administered intravenously, the site of infusion should be monitored for signs of inflammation.

Adverse effects of docetaxel treatment in patients with significant liver dysfunction are more likely. High doses of treatment also may increase the likelihood and severity of adverse side effects.

Docetaxel should not be administered to patients who are known to have severe hypersensitivity to polysorbate 80, which is a component of the treatment that helps dissolve the drug.

The safety of docetaxel in children under 16 years of age has not been established.

Docetaxel can cause harm to a fetus when administered to pregnant women. This treatment should be used during pregnancy only in life-threatening situations. Women of childbearing age are advised not to become pregnant during treatment. Women should stop nursing before beginning treatment, due to the potential for serious adverse side effects in nursing infants.

Side effects

Suppression of bone marrow function is the principal adverse side effect associated with docetaxel treatment. Blood tests will allow a doctor to determine if there is adequate bone marrow function to begin or continue treatment. Hypersensitivity and fluid retention may also occur during treatment. Corticosteroids are administered prior to treatment to lessen these side effects. Ulceration of the mouth and surrounding areas is possible. Additional side effects, including **fever**, decrease in blood pressure, **nausea and vomiting**, **diarrhea**, pain, abnormal liver function, skin rash, nerve damage, and hair loss (**alopecia**) may occur.

A 2003 study showed that although docetaxel produced higher toxicities among patients in the short-term, breast cancer patients treated with docetaxel had higher survival and similar quality of life scores than those treated with paclitaxel. Although the women experienced more side effects such as reduction in white blood cells, some loss of strength, **infection**, and mouth ulcers, among others, the effects did not affect their quality of life over time. And the women survived longer.

Interactions

Drugs that may alter the metabolism of docetaxel such as **cyclosporine**, terfenadine, ketoconazole, erythomycin, and troleandomycin should be used with caution due to the potential for interactions. Patients should inform their doctors of all other medications before taking docetaxel.

Resources

PERIODICALS

"Comparison Study Finds Better Overall Response Rate, Survival with Docetaxel." *Drug Week* October 17, 2003: 67.

"Study Shows Improved Survival Rates, Time to Disease Progression with Docetaxel." *Women's Health Weekly* December 25, 2003: 33.

Marc Scanio
Teresa G. Odle

Docusate *see* **Laxatives**

Dolasetron *see* **Antiemetics**

Double contrast barium enema *see* **Barium enema**

Doxorubicin

Definition

Doxorubicin, which kills **cancer** cells, is among the most widely used **chemotherapy** drugs. It is also known by its trade name, Adriamycin.

Purpose

This anticancer drug may be used to fight several different cancers: **breast cancer**, **ovarian cancer**, gastric (stomach) cancer, **thyroid cancer**, lung cancer, **testicular cancer**, and **endometrial cancer**. In addition it may be used against Hodgkin's and non-Hodgkin's **lymphoma**, acute lymphoblastic leukemia (ALL), acute myeloblastic leukemia (AML), sarcomas of the soft tissue, sarcomas of the bone (osteosarcomas), **neuroblastoma**, **Wilms' tumor**, **small cell lung cancer** (SCLC), and **non-small cell lung cancer** (NSCLC).

Because doxorubicin is used to treat so many different cancers, a complete description of how it may be combined with other medications in the treatment of each of the cancers cannot be given here. A few examples follow: In the treatment of Hodgkin's disease, one widely used chemotherapy regimen is the so-called ABVD, which consists of doxorubicin, **bleomycin**, **vinblastine**, and **dacarbazine**. Another is the so-called MOPP/ABV, which consists of **mechlorethamine**, **vincristine** (Oncovin), prednisone, **procarbazine**, doxorubicin, bleomycin, and vinblastine. Yet another is the so-called EVA: **etoposide**, vinblastine, and doxorubicin. Still another is the so-called EPOCH, which consists of etoposide, vincristine, doxorubicin, **cyclophosphamide**, and prednisone.

Doctors may treat stage III and IV non-Hodgkin's lymphoma with the so-called m-BACOD chemotherapy regimen, which consists of **methotrexate**, bleomycin, doxorubicin, cyclophosphamide, vincristine, and **dexamethasone**. Yet another regimen is called the ProMACE-CytaBOM, which consists of cyclophosphamide, doxorubicin, etoposide, prednisone, **cytarabine**, bleomycin, vincristine, methotrexate, and **leucovorin**.

Complete remission (CR) is the total elimination of all diseased cells detectable following therapy. Continuous complete remission is CR that continues indefinitely. In the treatment of **acute lymphocytic leukemia** (ALL), it has been found that the likelihood that continuous complete remission will be achieved is increased if the patient receives at least three drugs. Two of these are usually prednisone and vincristine. The third may be doxorubicin.

Description

Doxorubicin is a DNA-binding anticancer drug and belongs to an anthracycline antibiotic, although doctors do not use this drug to attack microbial infections.

Recommended dosage

Between 60 and 90 milligrams per square meter of doxorubicin are administered via a single intravenous (IV) injection every 21 days. Alternately, between 20 and 30 milligrams per square meter per day may be given via IV for three days every three to four weeks. Alternately, 20 milligrams per square meter may be given via IV weekly. The dose of doxorubicin used depends upon which regimen for cancer is being followed.

For example, in the treatment of acute myelocytic leukemia (AML), 30 milligrams per square meter may be given over a period of three days. When the medication is used in the treatment of breast cancer, one chemotherapy regimen is the so-called AC, which consists of doxorubicin plus cyclophosphamide. A total of 60 milligrams of doxorubicin per square meter are given per day. AC is then repeated every 21 days.

Another chemotherapy regimen used for breast cancer is known as either FAC or CAF: **fluorouracil**, doxorubicin, and cyclophosphamide. In this regimen, 50 milligrams of doxorubicin are given per square meter per day.

Doxorubicin is not given by mouth, as an insufficient amount of the medication would be transported through the stomach wall if this were done. Rather this medication is usually administered through an intravenous (IV) procedure. Patients with liver problems may be given a reduced dose of doxorubicin.

Precautions

Doxorubicin may cause serious heart problems. To prevent these, doctors may limit the amount of doxorubicin given to each patient so that the total amount of doxorubicin a patient receives over her or his entire lifetime is 550 milligrams per square meter, or less. An encouraging recent development is that medication is now available that appears to help protect the patient's heat from the effects of doxorubicin. This new medication is called **dexrazoxane** (Zinecard).

Side effects

Patients may develop problems with heart rhythms while doxorubicin is being taken. In addition, a serious heart illness known as heart failure may develop later. Some patients develop heart failure more than 20 after having received doxorubicin.

Studies have shown that the use of the new medication dexrazoxane (Zinecard) helps protect the patient's heart from the harmful effects of doxorubicin. However, dexrazoxane itself has side effects. For example, it may intensify the reduction of blood cells that may occur with doxorubicin therapy. In addition, it may make doxorubicin less effective in attacking cancer. Dexrazoxane is used only in patients being treated for breast cancer and only in patients who have already been given more than half of the total lifetime amount of doxorubicin they should ever receive.

The activity of the bone marrow in producing blood cells may be harmed by doxorubicin. Side effects affecting the heart and bone marrow may cause doctors to lower the dose of doxorubicin. Other side effects associated with doxorubicin are **nausea and vomiting**, stomach problems, eye problems, loss of appetite (**anorexia**), and hair loss (**alopecia**). Blistering may result if bleeding occurs. In addition, the medication has a harmless side effect about which patients should be forewarned: the urine and tears may have a red color.

Patients receiving doxorubicin in conjunction with certain other **anticancer drugs** may, very rarely, develop a type of leukemia.

Bob Kirsch

Dronabinol *see* **Antiemetics**
Droperidol *see* **Antiemetics**

Drug resistance

Definition

Drug resistance refers to the ability of an organism, such as the HIV virus, the tuberculosis bacillus (TB), or **cancer**, to overcome the effects of a drug prescribed to destroy it. Well-known examples are the resistance of the HIV virus to AZT, or that of TB to **antibiotics**. Resistance has been observed to occur with every anti-HIV drug prescribed. According to the Mayo Clinic in Rochester, Minnesota, drug resistance may have played a role in the 58% rise in infectious disease deaths observed in the United States between 1980 and 1992.

Due to the immunocompromised state of cancer patients caused by the cancer treatment effect, infections with viruses and bacteria are commonplace and infectious disease treatment is paramount.

Causes

A virus like HIV becomes resistant to drugs because it has the ability to mutate. This happens because a typical virus creates billions of new viruses in the body every day—viruses that are replicas of itself. However, these replicas are not always perfect. In this daily production of billions of viruses, several small differences can occur in some of the new viruses. These differences are called *mutations*. When such mutations occur on that part of the virus that the drug is designed to chemically attach to, the drug's action is effectively stopped because it cannot attach. When a drug no longer works against its target, this is called drug resistance and the virus that the drug can no longer destroy is said to be resistant to the drug.

An example of drug resistance is a patient with AIDS. The patient may have a few HIV viruses that mutate in such a way that prevents AZT from working on those mutated viruses. The drug will still work against the HIV that has not mutated, eventually destroying it. However, reproduction of the mutated virus is then unchecked, and the **infection** keeps spreading as the mutated virus makes more copies of itself, which are also resistant to AZT. After some time, this mutated AZT-resistant HIV will be the only type of HIV left, and AZT will no longer work for that patient.

A similar scenario may occur with cancer drug resistance. Since the early 1970s, multiple drug resistance (MDR) has also been known to exist in several types of cancer cells. It now appears that certain cancers have the capacity to resist the cytotoxic (toxic to cells) effects of cancer **chemotherapy**, probably due to genetic abnormalities in the cancer cells. Normal tissues never develop resistance to chemotherapy. Initially, sensitive cancer cells are destroyed by chemotherapy but since mutated cancer cells are allowed to replicate (unlike normal cells that are destroyed when defective) these mutated cancer cells are no longer sensitive to some chemotherapy.

Resistance of cytomegalovirus (CMV) against antiviral drugs is another example showing that drug resistance is becoming an increasingly serious medical problem.

Like viruses, bacteria can also become drug resistant. Every time a patient takes an antibiotic, such as penicillin, to fight a bacterial infection, the antibiotic destroys most of the bacteria. However, a few tough germs may survive—either by mutating like viruses or by obtaining resistance genes from other bacteria. These survivors can then reproduce quickly, creating new drug-resistant bacteria. As is the case with mutated viruses, the presence of these resistant bacterial strains usually means that the next infection will not be cured by the first-choice antibiotic prescribed by the doctor.

Some bacteria that have already become resistant to antibiotic attack include:

- Staphylococcus aureus: This bacterium causes the majority of infections in patients in U.S. hospitals. It spreads and infects cuts, burns, skin, and surgical wounds. Since 1996, at least four patients have been reported to be infected with a strain that was partially resistant to normal doses of the most powerful antibiotic available, vancomycin.

- Streptococcus pneumoniae: This bacterium causes pneumonia, meningitis, and ear infections. According to the Mayo Clinic, it has also become partially resistant to antibiotics of the penicillin family.

- Enterococcus: This bacterium can cause everything from urinary tract to heart valve infections and it is also becoming increasingly antibiotic-resistant, including vancomycin-resistant.

If a virus or bacteria mutates at a specific location that represents the target for the drug to attach to, then modifying the drug so as to have it attach at a different place will succeed in overcoming the drug resistance. In the case of HIV, compiled databases of mutations in HIV genes that confer resistance to anti-HIV drugs are available to assist researchers in the design and production of new drugs.

Treatments

The strategies used to overcome drug resistance depend upon the nature of the organism causing the infection but generally involve the following steps:

- Accurate and rapid diagnosis: Swift identification and treatment—the sooner the infectious organism is detected and correctly identified, the higher the chances that it will not become drug resistant since it will have less time to mutate.

- Drug combination: New combinations of drugs can be very effective. Given a mixture of mutated and unmutated pathogens, a drug "cocktail" is likely to contain a drug that may be effective against a new mutated form of the virus, thus preventing it from making billions of new copies every day. The less virus created, the less chance of further mutations occurring.

- New drugs: There is a problem facing all the strategies used to overcome drug resistance and it is that drugs have to be given at high—and sometimes toxic—doses, and also in combinations that have become quite expensive. Increasingly, they also must be taken on

schedules that are difficult to follow by patients. Even then, new varieties of resistant strains still appear. There is, therefore, an urgent need to understand how drug resistance develops at the molecular level, and to use this understanding to develop more effective drugs.

See also AIDS-related cancers.

Resources

BOOKS
Kaspers, G. J. L., R. Pieters, and A. J. P. Veerman, editors.*Drug Resistance in Leukemia and Lymphoma III (Advances in Experimental Medicine and Biology)*. New York: Plenum Press, 1999.

PERIODICALS
Brenner, B. G., and M. A. Wainberg. "The Role of Antiretrovirals and Drug Resistance in Vertical Transmission of HIV-1 Infection." *Annals of the New York Acadademy of Sciences* 918 (November 2000): 9-15.

Broxterman, H. J., and N. Georgopapadakou. "Cancer Research 2000: Drug Resistance, New Targets and Drugs In Development." *Drug Resistance Updates* 3 (June 2000): 133-138.

Clavel, F., E. Race, and F. Mammano. "HIV Drug Resistance and Viral Fitness." *Advances in Pharmacology* 49 (2000): 41-66.

Durant, J., P. Clevenbergh, P. Halfon, P. Delgiudice, S. Porsin, et al. "Drug-Resistance Genotyping in HIV-1 Therapy." *Lancet* 353 (June 1999): 2195-2199.

Norgaard, J. M., and P. Hokland "Biology of Multiple Drug Resistance in Acute Leukemia." *International Journal of Hematology* 72 (October 2000): 290-297.

Teicher, B. A. "Molecular Targets and Cancer Therapeutics: Discovery, Development and Clinical Validation." *Drug Resistance Updates* 3 (April 2000): 67-73.

OTHER
The AIDS Treatment Data Network. *Factsheet: Trials of drugs for treating HIV* [cited July 1, 2001]. http://www.aidsinfonyc.org/network/trials/hiv.html.

The AIDS Treatment Data Network. *Factsheet: Understanding Drug Resistance* [cited July 1, 2001]. http://www.aidsinfonyc.org/network/simple/resistance.html.

ORGANIZATIONS
HIV Drug Resistance Database. http://204.121.6.64:581/Resist_DB/default.htm.

National Cancer Institute, HIV Drug Resistance Program. NCI-Frederick, Building 535, Room 109, P.O. Box B, Frederick, MD 21702-1201. Phone:(301)846-1168. http://www.ncifcrf.gov/hivdrp.

U. S. Food and Drug Administration. 5600 Fishers Lane, Rockville, MD 20857. Phone:(888)INFO-FDA [(888)463-6332] http://www.fda.gov/default.htm.

Monique Laberge, Ph.D.

Dryness of the mouth, mouth dryness *see* **Xerostomia**

Ductogram

Definition

A ductogram, also called a galactogram, is a special type of mammogram used for imaging the breast ducts. It can aid in diagnosing the cause of abnormal nipple discharges.

Purpose

The purpose of a ductogram is to locate the origin of an abnormal discharge from the nipple of the breast.

Precautions

Women who are pregnant should not undergo a ductogram without adequate protection of the abdomen from the **x rays** that are used in this test.

Description

A ductogram is performed by first cleansing the nipple and areola with an antiseptic. The radiologist performing the test then presses gently on the nipple to determine which duct is leaking fluid. Once the leaking duct has been identified, a small needle (cannula) is inserted into that duct. A dye is then injected into the leaking duct and an x ray similar to a mammogram is performed.

This test is performed in a **mammography** or breast imaging facility, either in a hospital department or an outpatient x-ray center. During this procedure, the patient is in a sitting, standing, or horizontal position depending on the x-ray equipment available at the testing center where the ductogram is to be performed. The x-ray camera may change position during the study, but the patient is usually stationary. The procedure typically takes 30 to 60 minutes. It is important for the patient not to move except when directed to do so by the technologist.

Preparation

There is usually little or no preparation required of the patient for a ductogram. Prior to the test, the patient should not attempt to express a discharge from the affected nipple or nipples. Jewelry or metallic objects that may interfere with the x-ray image should be removed for the duration of the ductogram. No deodorant or powder should be used as this can interfere with the test.

If the nipple drainage suddenly stops on the day of the ductogram, the patient should notify her health care provider prior to undergoing this test.

Aftercare

No special care is required after the test. Fluids are encouraged after the procedure to aid in the excretion of the dye from the body.

Risks

The risks of a ductogram are very low. Most ductograms use the same amount of radiation as a conventional x ray. Side effects or negative reactions are very rare. Possible side effects include pain, **infection**, and bleeding from the nipple where the cannula was inserted.

Normal results

A normal ductogram shows the expected distribution of the dye material within the ducts of the breast and no unusual shape or size of the scanned tissue.

Abnormal results

An abnormal ductogram shows an abnormality within the ducts of the breast that may be causing the pathologic discharge of fluid from that breast. If an abnormality is identified, additional procedures, including surgery, may be necessary.

Resources

OTHER

Breast Cancer Overview [cited May 25, 2001]. http://cancer. mps-group.com/breast_cancer.htm.

ORGANIZATIONS

American Cancer Society. (800) ACS-2345. http://
www.cancer.org.

National Alliance of Breast Cancer Organizations
(NABCO). 9 East 37th St., 10th Floor, New York, NY
10016. (888) 806-2226. http://www.nabco.org.

Paul A. Johnson, Ed.M.

Duplex ultrasound *see* **Ultrasonography**

Dutasteride

Definition

Dutasteride (Avodart) is a 5-alpha reductase
inhibitor used to treat benign prostatic hyperplasia.

Purpose

Benign prostatic hyperplasia (BPH) is a non-cancerous enlargement of the prostate. The prostate is a gland
found only in men. It is about the size of a walnut and
surrounds the neck of the urethra. When the prostate
enlarges, it can press on the urethra making it difficult to
urinate or blocking urine flow completely. Dutasteride
treats these symptoms by shrinking the prostate. This
reduces the risk of needing BPH-related surgery.

As of mid-October 2009, dutasteride has not been
approved anywhere in the world for prevention or treatment of **prostate cancer**. A study was presented in April
2009 at the American Urological Association meeting
that found that dutasteride lowered the risk for prostate
cancer by 23%. Use of dutasteride for prostate **cancer
prevention** is controversial, and the United States Food
and Drug Association (FDA) has not approved this use.
In 2009 **clinical trials** were underway to investigate the
potential role of dutasteride in prostate cancer.

Description

Dutasteride is marketed by GlaxoSmithKline
under the brand name Avodart. It was approved by
the FDA to treat symptoms of BPH in 2002. The drug
is supplied as an oblong, dull yellow soft gelatin capsule containing 0.5 mg of the drug.

Dutasteride reduces the size of the prostate. A
male hormone called dihydrotesterone (DHT) causes
the prostate to enlarge. **Testosterone**, an abundant
male hormone, is converted by the action of an enzyme
(5-alpha reductase) into DHT. Dutasteride blocks this
conversion. When there is less DHT in the body, the

prostate shrinks and pressure on the urethra may be
reduced. Dutasteride continues to be tested in clinical
trials in different dosage regimens and in combination
with other therapies. It is also being tested in the possible prevention or treatment of prostate cancer. A list
of clinical trials currently enrolling volunteers can be
found at: http://www.clinicaltrials.gov.

Recommended dosage

The recommended dosage for dutasteride for treatment of symptoms of BPH is one capsule (0.5 mg) taken
once daily. Capsules should be stored at controlled
room temperature. They should be swallowed whole
and never chewed or crushed. Men who are unable to
swallow capsules should discuss with their doctor how
to take this drug. Dutasteride generally is taken long-
term (two or more years) and its effect is often not felt
for three to six months.

Precautions

Taking dutasteride will reduce the blood level of
prostate-specific antigen (PSA) in the blood. Measuring serum concentrations of PSA gives an indication
of cancer activity. The decrease in PSA levels is predictable, and this test can still be used to detect prostate cancer, but it is important for men to tell their
doctor that they are taking dutasteride and for how
long they have been using the drug so that PSA results
can be accurately interpreted.

Men taking dutasteride may not donate blood for
at least six months after taking the last dose. This is to
prevent a pregnant female transfusion recipient from
accidentally being exposed to dutasteride.

QUESTIONS TO ASK YOUR PHARMACIST

- How long will I need to take this drug before you can tell if it helps me?
- How often do I have to have blood work and other laboratory tests done to check the effect the drug is having?
- Is this drug safe to take with the other drugs that I am currently taking?
- What side effects should I watch for? When should I call the doctor about them?
- Are there any clinical trials of this drug combined with other therapies that might benefit me?

Pregnant or breastfeeding

Dutasteride is a pregnancy category X drug. Women who are pregnant or who may become pregnant should not use, handle, or be exposed to dutasteride. Fetal abnormalities are likely and fetal death may result. It is not known whether the drug is excreted in breast milk. Women who are breast-feeding should avoid exposure to the drug. Dutasteride is not FDA-approved for use in women for any reason. Dutasteride can be absorbed through the skin. Women who are or may become pregnant should avoid handling the drug.

Side effects

Side effects of dutasteride are mainly sexual and include:

- difficulty maintaining an erection
- decreased sex drive
- difficulty ejaculating
- enlarged or tender breasts

Interactions

Among the drugs studied, no clinically significant interactions with dutasteride have been found. However, all interactions are not known. Before starting and while taking dutasteride, patients should provide their doctor and pharmacist with a complete list of all prescription and nonprescription drugs, herbs, and dietary supplements that they are taking.

Resources

OTHER

Avodart. Rxlist.com. July 9, 2008 [October 9, 2009]. http://www.rxlist.com/avodart-drug.htm.

Prostate Diseases. MedlinePlus. October 5, 2009 [October 9, 2009]. http://www.nlm.nih.gov/medlineplus/prostatediseases.html.

ORGANIZATIONS

Men's Health Network, P.O. Box 75972, Washington, DC, 20013, (202) 543-MHN-1 (6461), info@menshealthnetwork.org, http://www.menshealthnetwork.org.

National Kidney and Urologic Disease Information Clearinghouse, 3 Information Way, Bethesda, MD, 20892-3580, http://kidney.niddk.nih.gov/kudiseases/pubs/glomerular/index.htm.

Tish Davidson, A.M.

Dysplastic nevus syndrome *see* **Melanoma**

E

Eaton-Lambert syndrome *see* **Lambert-Eaton myasthenic syndrome**

Edatrexate

Definition

Edatrexate is an investigational (experimental) medicine similar to **methotrexate** used to stop growth of **cancer** and formation of new cancer cells.

Purpose

Edatrexate has been shown to have anticancer activity in research studies in patients with lung cancer, head, and neck cancer, **breast cancer**, and non-Hodgkin's **lymphoma**.

Description

Edatrexate is an anticancer drug that belongs to a family of drugs called antimetabolites. It is an antagonist of **folic acid** closely related to methotrexate in its structure and antitumor activity. However, edatrexate has several potential advantages over methotrexate, including better transport across cancer cell membranes (walls surrounding cancer cells), increased selectivity for tumor cells, and greater antitumor effect. Edatrexate inhibits formation of genetic material and reproduction of cancer cells by inhibiting a certain enzyme needed to make folic acid. Without folic acid, formation of protein and new genetic material in cancer cells cannot occur. Unlike methotrexate, edatrexate has additive activity when used with **cisplatin** (a **chemotherapy** agent often used to treat **non-small cell lung cancer**) in animal studies. It also showed additive anticancer effects with **cyclophosphamide**, paclitaxel and **docetaxel**.

Edatrexate has been used in combination with paclitaxel, cisplatin, clyclophosphamide, mitomycin, or **vinblastine** in research studies. **Leucovorin** has been shown to be effective in reducing edatrexate side effects, but it may also decrease its antitumor effectiveness.

Recommended dosage

Adults

SOLID TUMORS (LUNG, BREAST, HEAD AND NECK CANCER). Doses vary between different chemotherapy protocols. The most commonly used dose in research studies was 40-80 mg per square meter of body surface area given as intravenous infusion once a week. Maximum tolerated dose when edatrexate was used in combination with paclitaxel was 120 mg per meter square per week.

Children

There is no data available on dosing and use of edatrexate in children.

Precautions

To maximize treatment effects, patients receiving edatrexate should observe certain guidelines. Including any modifications given by the oncologist, these guidelines should include regular visits with the oncologist and laboratory testing for white blood cell count, kidney, liver, and bone marrow function. Patients should avoid any immunizations not approved or prescribed by the oncologist, and they should avoid contact with individuals taking or who have recently taken oral polio vaccine, or individuals who have an active **infection**. When necessary, patients should wear a protective facemask, and patients should avoid prolonged or direct exposure to sunlight, as some patients experience an increased sensitivity. Patients should also ask for specific instructions on oral hygiene procedures to reduce the risk of gum abrasion, and avoid touching the eye and nasal areas unless hands have been properly washed immediately prior to contact. To reduce bleeding and bruising complications, patients should exercise extreme caution when handling sharp instruments and decline participation in contact sports. Prior to treatment, the patient's medical history should be thoroughly reviewed to avoid complications that might arise from previous conditions such as gout, kidney stones or kidney disease, liver disease, chickenpox, shingles, intestinal blockage, colitis, suppressed immune system, stomach ulcers, mouth sores, or a history of allergic reactions to various drugs.

The oncologist should also be made aware if the patient is pregnant or if there is the possibility the patient might be pregnant, or if the patient is a breast-feeding mother. Only prescribed medications or over the counter (OTC) drugs approved by the oncologist should be taken by a patient receiving edatrexate.

Side effects

The side effect profile of edatrexate is similar to that of methotrexate, with mouth ulcers as the dose-limiting toxicity. Other side effects include bone marrow suppression and decreased formation of all blood elements, **diarrhea**, skin rash, **nausea**, **vomiting**, inflammation of the lungs (pneumonitis) and mild increase in liver function tests.

Interactions

There is no published information available at this point about any potential drug or food interactions with edatrexate. As a general rule, **vaccines** should be avoided due to the immunosuppressive action of edatrexate, and alcohol should be avoided to reduce the risk of liver complications.

Olga Bessmertny, Pharm.D.

Endocrine system tumors

Definition

The group of tumors that are associated with the hormone-secreting (endocrine) glands of the body.

Description

The glands in the body that make and secrete hormones comprise the endocrine system. All endocrine glands secrete hormones directly into the bloodstream, where they travel to a target organ or cell to trigger a specific reaction. These glands are primarily involved in controlling many of the slow and long-term activities in the body, such as growth, sexual development, and regulation of blood levels for many important proteins and essential chemical elements.

Endocrine glands are found in the head and neck region, the abdominal region, and the pelvic area (the region where the reproductive organs are located). The following are the main endocrine glands of the body:

- Pituitary gland. Found at the base of the brain, this small gland is important because it secretes several hormones that control the activity of other endocrine glands.
- Thyroid gland. Situated in the front of the neck, in the region of the Adam's apple, this gland secretes hormones that regulate body temperature, heart rate, and metabolism.
- Parathyroid glands. These four glands, with a pair on either side of the thyroid gland in the neck region, produce parathyroid hormone, which helps control the level of calcium in the blood.
- Pancreas. Found close to the stomach in the abdominal region, the pancreas contains two groups of cells.

Endocrine system tumors

Pituitary tumors

Thyroid tumors
Parathyroid tumors
Endocrine pancreatic tumors, including gastrinoma, insulinoma, and glucagonoma
Adrenal tumors, including pheochromocytoma and adrenocortical carcinoma
Ovarian tumors
Testicular tumors
Multiple endocrine gland tumors (tumors on several endocrine glands at once)

(Table by GGS Creative Resources. Cengage Learning, Gale.)

KEY TERMS

Endocrine gland—Any gland that makes hormones and secretes them directly into the bloodstream.

Exocrine gland—Any gland that secretes substances outward through a duct into a body cavity or onto a body surface (e.g., sweat glands and salivary glands).

Germ cell—Any cell in the body that eventually produces either a mature egg cell (female) or a mature sperm cell (male).

Inherited disorder—A disease that has a tendency to occur within a family. A disorder may be acquired due to a gene or genes that are passed from parent to child.

One group functions as an exocrine gland, secreting digestive enzymes into the intestines through a duct. The other, known as islets of Langerhans (or islet cells), functions as an endocrine gland and secretes hormones that control blood sugar levels and aid digestion.

- Adrenal glands. These two glands, one located above each kidney, secrete hormones that prevent inflammation and help regulate blood pressure, blood sugar levels, and metabolism.

- Ovary. A woman has two small ovaries in the pelvic area. They contain the egg cells and secrete the hormones progesterone and estrogen. These hormones have many functions, including controlling the onset of puberty, the timing of menstruation, and the changes associated with pregnancy.

- Testis (also called testicle). Men typically have two testes located outside the body in the lower pelvic area. They produce sperm and the hormone testosterone, which signals the onset of puberty, maintains the expression of male characteristics, such as facial hair, and stimulates sperm production.

Endocrine system tumors are rare. Although certain types are likely to be diagnosed as malignant (cancerous), endocrine tumors are often noncancerous (benign). Each year endocrine system cancers account for only around 4% of all new **cancer** cases in the United States.

The most common cancers of the endocrine system are **ovarian cancer** and **thyroid cancer**. Ovarian cancer represents about 44% of all endocrine system cancers and affects eight out of every 100,000

American women. New cases of ovarian cancer in 2009 will likely reach over 21,550, and nearly 14,600 will die from the disease. Roughly six out of every 100,000 Americans develop thyroid cancer, which accounts for 36% of all endocrine system cancers. It is estimated that 37,200 new cases will be diagnosed in 2009 and result in 1,630 deaths. Other malignant endocrine tumors are much rarer. **Testicular cancer** affects about two out of every 100,000 American men, while the remaining cancer types combined affect roughly one out of every 100,000 Americans.

Many benign and malignant endocrine tumors are treatable with a combination of surgery and medication, and the survival rates for many endocrine cancers is good. Two exceptions are ovarian cancer and **adrenocortical carcinoma**, a tumor of the adrenal gland. About 50% of ovarian cancer patients and 40% of those diagnosed with an adrenocortical **carcinoma** will survive five years or more after the initial diagnosis. These cancers have poor survival rates because they are usually first diagnosed after they have spread or reached an advanced stage. Among the different cancers, thyroid cancer and testicular cancer have some of the better 5-year survival rates; both approach 95%.

Symptoms of many endocrine tumors are associated with the excessive secretion of hormones. Hormone-producing tumors are called functional tumors, while those that do not secrete hormones are called nonfunctional tumors. Both types are potentially malignant.

Types of cancers

Proceeding from the head region to the pelvic area, endocrine system tumors include:

- Pituitary tumors. These tumors are classified by the type of hormone they secrete. They are rarely malignant but can cause heath problems, including visual complications. One type of tumor results in Cushing's syndrome.

- Thyroid tumors. Only 5% of the tumors found on the thyroid are malignant. A malignant tumor can indicate one of the four types of thyroid cancer.

- Parathyroid tumors. Around 5% are malignant and result in a diagnosis of parathyroid cancer. Overproduction of parathyroid hormone, a condition known as hyperparathyroidism, is a common condition associated with both benign and malignant tumors. Untreated, hyperparathyroidism can result in osteoporosis (bones become brittle and fracture easily), kidney stones, peptic ulcers, and nervous system problems.

- Endocrine pancreatic tumors. Benign and malignant tumors are often treatable with surgery. Malignant tumors are rare. The most common types of tumors are a gastrinoma, which is associated with Zollinger-Ellison syndrome, insulinoma, and glucagonoma.
- Adrenal tumors. One type of tumor, a pheochromocytoma, is found on the inner part of the adrenal gland (the adrenal medulla). About 10% are malignant. An adrenocortical carcinoma is a malignant tumor on the outer part of the gland (adrenal cortex), and a common symptom is the occurrence of Cushing's syndrome. Both tumors are very rare.
- Ovarian tumors. Tumors can develop in the egg cells inside the ovary (germ cell tumors), but most occur in the cells lining the outside of the ovary, and most of these tumors are benign.
- Testicular tumors. Tumors can occur in one or both of the testes. Over 90% develop in the germ cells and only 4% involve the endocrine cells of the testes.
- Multiple endocrine gland tumors. Some disorders result in the simultaneous occurrence of tumors on several endocrine glands. Many of these are inherited disorders, including multiple endocrine neoplasia syndromes, von Hippel-Lindau syndrome, and von Recklinghausen's neurofibromatosis.

See also Adenoma; Craniopharyngioma; Neuroendocrine carcinomas; Pancreatic cancer, exocrine.

Resources

PERIODICALS

Monson, J. C. "The Epidemiology of Endocrine Tumours." *Endocrine-Related Cancer* 7 (2000): 29–36.

OTHER

EndocrineWeb.com. [cited July 3, 2001]. http://www.endocrineweb.com.

ORGANIZATIONS

American Association of Clinical Endocrinologists. 1000 Riverside Ave., Suite 205, Jacksonville, FL 32204. (904) 353-7878. http://www.aace.com.

Monica McGee, M.S.

Endometrial cancer

Definition

Endometrial **cancer** develops when the cells that make up the inner lining of the uterus (the endometrium) become abnormal and grow uncontrollably.

Demographics

Endometrial cancer (also called uterine cancer) is the fourth most common type of cancer among women and the most common gynecologic cancer. Approximately 42,160 women are diagnosed with endometrial cancer each year. In 2009, the American Cancer Society predicted that approximately 7,780 women would die from this cancer that year. More than half of all endometrial cancer diagnoses occur in women who are between ages 55 and 74. The average age at diagnosis is 60 years old.

The highest incidence of endometrial cancer in the United States is in Caucasians, Hawaiians, Japanese, and African Americans. American Indians, Koreans, and Vietnamese have the lowest incidence. African American and Hawaiian women are more likely to be diagnosed with advanced cancer and, therefore, have a higher risk of dying from the disease.

Description

The uterus, or womb, is the hollow female organ that supports the development of the unborn baby during pregnancy. The uterus has a thick muscular wall and an inner lining called the endometrium. The endometrium is very sensitive to hormones and it changes daily during the menstrual cycle. The endometrium is designed to provide an ideal environment for the fertilized egg to implant and begin to grow. If pregnancy does not occur, the endometrium is shed causing the menstrual period.

More than 95% of uterine cancers arise in the endometrium. The most common type of uterine cancer is **adenocarcinoma**. It arises from an abnormal multiplication of endometrial cells (atypical adenomatous hyperplasia) and is made up of mature, specialized cells (well-differentiated). Less commonly, endometrial cancer arises without a preceding hyperplasia and is made up of poorly differentiated cells. The more common of these types are the papillary serous and clear cell carcinomas. Poorly differentiated endometrial cancers are often associated with a less promising prognosis.

Causes and symptoms

Although the exact cause of endometrial cancer is unknown, it is clear that high levels of estrogen, when not balanced by progesterone, can lead to abnormal growth of the endometrium. Factors that increase a woman's risk of developing endometrial cancer are:

- Age. The risk is considerably higher in women who are over the age of 50 and have gone through menopause.
- Obesity. Being overweight is a very strong risk factor for this cancer. Fatty tissue can change other normal

502

Cancer located in the uterus. *(Illustration by Argosy Publishing, Inc. Cengage Learning, Gale.)*

body chemicals into estrogen, which can promote endometrial cancer.

- Estrogen replacement therapy. Women receiving estrogen supplements after menopause have a 12 times higher risk of getting endometrial cancer if progesterone is not taken simultaneously.

- Diabetes. Diabetics have twice the risk of getting this cancer as nondiabetic women. It is not clear if this risk is due to the fact that many diabetics are also obese and hypertensive. One 1998 study found that women who were obese and diabetic were three times more likely to develop endometrial cancer than women who were obese but nondiabetic. This study also found that nonobese diabetics were not at risk of developing endometrial cancer.

- Hypertension. High blood pressure (or hypertension) is also considered a risk factor for uterine cancer.

- Irregular menstrual periods. During the menstrual cycle, there is interaction between the hormones estrogen and progesterone. Women who do not ovulate regularly are exposed to high estrogen levels for longer periods of time. If a woman does not ovulate regularly, this delicate balance is upset and may increase her chances of getting uterine cancer.

- Early first menstruation or late menopause. Having the first period at a young age (the mean age of menses is 12.16 years in African American girls and 12.88 years in caucasian girls) or going through menopause at a late age (over age 51) seem to put women at a slightly higher risk for developing endometrial cancer.

- Tamoxifen. This drug, which is used to treat or prevent breast cancer, increases a woman's chance of developing endometrial cancer. Tamoxifen users tend to have more advanced endometrial cancer with an associated poorer survival rate than those who do not take the drug. In many cases, however, the value of tamoxifen for treating breast cancer and for preventing the cancer from spreading far outweighs the small risk (one in 500) of getting endometrial cancer.

Colored scanning electron micrograph of adenocarcinoma cancer in the endometrium, the lining of the uterus. Here, surface epithelial cells are seen (yellow), with cavities forming the openings of glands. Adenocarcinoma cells are large (green) and proliferative, invading the surface and glands. *(Copyright Professors P.M. Motta and S. Makabe, Science Source/Photo Researchers, Inc. Reproduced by permission.)*

- Family history. Some studies suggest that endometrial cancer runs in certain families. Women with inherited mutations in the BRCA1 and BRCA2 genes are at a higher risk of developing breast, ovarian, and other gynecologic cancers. Those with the hereditary nonpolyposis colorectal cancer gene have a higher risk of developing endometrial cancer.

- Breast, ovarian, or colon cancer. Women who have a history of these other types of cancer are at an increased risk of developing endometrial cancer.

- Low parity or nulliparity. Endometrial cancer is more common in women who have born few (low parity) or no (nulliparity) children. The high levels of progesterone produced during pregnancy has a protective effect against endometrial cancer. The results of one study suggest that nulliparity is associated with a lower survival rate.

- Infertility. Risk is increased due to nulliparity or the use of fertility drugs.

- Polycystic ovary syndrome. The increased level of estrogen associated with this abnormality raises the risk of cancers of the breast and endometrium.

The most common symptom of endometrial cancer is unusual vaginal spotting, bleeding, or discharge. In women who are near menopause (perimenopausal), symptoms of endometrial cancer could include bleeding between periods (intermenstrual bleeding), heavy bleeding that lasts for more than seven days, or short menstrual cycles (fewer than 21 days). For women who have gone through menopause, any vaginal bleeding or abnormal discharge is suspect. Pain in the pelvic region and the presence of a lump (mass) are symptoms that occur late in the disease.

Diagnosis

If endometrial cancer is suspected, a series of tests will be conducted to confirm the diagnosis. The first step will involve taking a complete personal and family medical history. A physical examination, which will include a thorough pelvic examination, will also be done.

The doctor may order an endometrial **biopsy**. This is generally performed in the doctor's office and does not require anesthesia. A thin, flexible tube is inserted through the cervix and into the uterus. A small piece of endometrial tissue is removed. The patient may experience some discomfort, which can be minimized by taking an anti-inflammatory medication (like Advil or Motrin) an hour before the procedure.

If an adequate amount of tissue was not obtained by the endometrial biopsy, or if the biopsy tissue looks abnormal but confirmation is needed, the doctor may perform a **dilatation and curettage** (D & C). This procedure is done in the outpatient surgery department of a hospital and takes about an hour. The patient may be given general anesthesia. The doctor dilates the cervix and uses a special instrument to scrape tissue from inside the uterus.

The tissue that is obtained from the biopsy or the D & C is sent to a laboratory for examination. If cancer is found, then the type of cancer will be determined. The treatment and prognosis depends on the type and stage of the cancer.

Transvaginal ultrasound may be used to measure the thickness of the endometrium. For this painless procedure, a wand-like ultrasound transducer is inserted into the vagina to enable visualization and measurement of the uterus, the thickness of the uterine lining, and other pelvic organs.

Other possible diagnostic procedures include sonohysterography and hysteroscopy. For sonohysteroscopy, a small tube is passed through the cervix and into the uterus. A small amount of a salt water (saline) solution is injected through the tube to open the space within the uterus and allow ultrasound visualization of the endometrium. For hysteroscopy, a wand-like camera is passed through the cervix to allow direct visualization of the endometrium. Both of these procedures cause discomfort, which may be reduced by taking an anti-inflammatory medication prior to the procedure.

Treatment

Clinical staging

The International Federation of Gynecology and Obstetrics (FIGO) has adopted a staging system for endometrial cancer. The stage of cancer is determined after surgery. Endometrial cancer is categorized into four stages (I, II, III, and IV) that are subdivided (A, B, and possibly C) based on the depth or spread of cancerous tissue. Seventy percent of all uterine cancers are stage I, 10–15% are stage II, and the remainder are stages III and IV. The cancer is also graded (G1, G2, and G3) based upon microscopic analysis of the aggressiveness of the cancer cells.

The FIGO stages for endometrial cancer are:

- Stage I. Cancer is limited to the uterus.
- Stage II. Cancer involves the uterus and cervix.
- Stage III. Cancer has spread out of the uterus but is restricted to the pelvic region.
- Stage IV. Cancer has spread to the bladder, bowel, or other distant locations.

The mainstay of treatment for most stages of endometrial cancer is surgery. **Radiation therapy**, hormonal therapy, and **chemotherapy** are additional treatments (called adjuvant therapy). The necessity of adjuvant therapy is a controversial topic which should be discussed with the patient's treatment team.

Surgery

Most women with endometrial cancer, except those with stage IV disease, are treated with a hysterectomy. A simple hysterectomy involves the removal of the uterus. In a bilateral salpingo-oophorectomy with total hysterectomy, the ovaries, fallopian tubes, and uterus are removed. This may be necessary because endometrial cancer often spreads to the ovaries first. The lymph nodes in the pelvic region may also be biopsied or removed to check for **metastasis**. Hysterectomy is traditionally performed through an incision in the abdomen (laparotomy), however, endoscopic surgery (**laparoscopy**) with vaginal hysterectomy is also being used. Women with stage I disease may require no

further treatment. However, those with higher grade disease will receive adjuvant therapy.

Radiation therapy

The decision to use radiation therapy depends on the stage of the disease. Radiation therapy may be used before surgery (preoperatively) and/or after surgery (postoperatively). Radiation given from a machine that is outside the body is called external radiation therapy. Sometimes applicators containing radioactive compounds are placed inside the vagina or uterus. This is called internal radiation therapy or brachytherapy and requires hospitalization.

Side effects are common with radiation therapy. The skin in the treated area may become red and dry. **Fatigue**, upset stomach, **diarrhea**, and **nausea** are also common complaints. Radiation therapy in the pelvic area may cause the vagina to become narrow (vaginal stenosis), making intercourse painful. Premature menopause and some problems with urination may also occur.

Chemotherapy

Chemotherapy is usually reserved for women with stage IV or recurrent disease because this therapy is not a very effective treatment for endometrial cancer. The **anticancer drugs** are given by mouth or intravenously. Side effects include stomach upset, **vomiting**, appetite loss, hair loss, mouth or vaginal sores, fatigue, menstrual cycle changes, and premature menopause. There is also an increased chance of infections.

Hormonal therapy

Hormonal therapy uses drugs like progesterone to slow the growth of endometrial cells. These drugs are usually available as pills. This therapy is usually reserved for women with advanced or recurrent disease. Side effects include fatigue, fluid retention, and appetite and weight changes.

Alternative treatment

Although alternative and complementary therapies are used by many cancer patients, very few controlled studies on the effectiveness of such therapies exist. Mind-body techniques, such as prayer, biofeedback, visualization, meditation, and yoga, have not shown any effect in reducing cancer, but they can reduce stress and lessen some of the side effects of cancer treatments. Clinical studies of hydrazine sulfate found that it had no effect on cancer and even worsened the health and well-being of the study subjects. One clinical study of the drug amygdalin (Laetrile) found that it had no effect on cancer. Laetrile can be

QUESTIONS TO ASK YOUR DOCTOR

- What kinds of diagnostic studies will be required to ascertain the type and spread of this cancer?
- Could there be a genetic component to this tumor? Should other family member be tested?
- What types of treatments are available?
- What types of side effects from treatments can I expect? What are your recommendations to help me deal with those side effects?
- Am I eligible for any clinical trials? Would these be helpful to consider?
- Are there any lifestyle changes that I should make?
- What type of diet should I follow? Are there foods I should avoid?
- Should I avoid any medications?
- How often should I be checked after treatment has ended?
- Is there a support group that I can join to hear about other people's experiences with this disorder?

toxic and has caused deaths. Shark cartilage, although highly touted as an effective cancer treatment, is an improbable therapy that has not been the subject of clinical study.

The American Cancer Society has found that the "metabolic diets" pose serious risk to the patient. The effectiveness of the macrobiotic, Gerson, and Kelley diets and the Manner metabolic therapy has not been scientifically proven. The FDA was unable to substantiate the anticancer claims made about the popular Cancell treatment.

There is no evidence for the effectiveness of most over-the-counter herbal cancer remedies. Some herbals have shown an anticancer effect. As shown in clinical studies, Polysaccharide krestin, from the mushroom *Coriolus versicolor*, has significant effectiveness against cancer. In a small study, the green alga *Chlorella pyrenoidosa* has been shown to have anticancer activity. In a few small studies, evening primrose oil has shown some benefit in the treatment of cancer.

Prognosis

Because it is possible to detect endometrial cancer early, the chances of curing it are excellent. The overall five year survival rate for endometrial cancer (accounting for all stages of this disease) is about 83%. The five year survival rates for endometrial cancer by stage are: 92-99%, stage I; 80%, stage II; 60%, stage III; and 30%, stage IV. Endometrial cancer most often spreads to the lungs, liver, bones, brain, vagina, and certain lymph nodes.

Prevention

Women (especially postmenopausal women) should report any abnormal vaginal bleeding or discharge to the doctor. Controlling obesity, blood pressure, and diabetes can help to reduce the risk of this disease. Women on estrogen replacement therapy have a substantially reduced risk of endometrial cancer if progestins are taken simultaneously. Long term use of birth control pills has been shown to reduce the risk of this cancer. Women who have irregular periods may be prescribed birth control pills to help prevent endometrial cancer. Women who are taking **tamoxifen** and those who carry the hereditary nonpolyposis colorectal cancer gene should be screened regularly, receiving annual pelvic examinations.

Resources

BOOKS

Abeloff, MD et al. *Clinical Oncology*. 3rd ed. Philadelphia: Elsevier, 2004.

Gabbe, SG et al. *Obstetrics: Normal and Problem Pregnancies*. 5th ed. London: Churchill Livingstone, 2007.

Katz VL et al. *Comprehensive Gynecology*. 5th ed. St. Louis: Mosby, 2007.

OTHER

"Cancer of the Uterus." *Cancernet*. December 2000. [cited March 13, 2001]. <http://cancernet.nci.nih.gov/wyntk_pubs/uterus.htm.>

ORGANIZATIONS

American Cancer Society. 1599 Clifton Rd. NE, Atlanta, GA 30329. (800) 227-2345. <http://www.cancer.org/.>

Cancer Research Institute, National Headquarters. 681 Fifth Ave., New York, NY 10022. (800) 992-2623. <http://www.cancerresearch.org.>

Gynecologic Cancer Foundation. 401 North Michigan Ave., Chicago, IL 60611. (800) 444-4441. <http://www.wcn.org.>

National Cancer Institute, National Institutes of Health. 9000 Rockville Pike, Bethesda, MD 20892. (800) 422-6237. <http://cancernet.nci.nih.gov/.>

Lata Cherath, PhD
Belinda Rowland, PhD

Endorectal ultrasound

Definition

Ultrasound is a type of imaging technique that painlessly uses sound waves to produce an image of internal structures, organs, and masses. Endorectal ultrasound, also called transrectal ultrasound, is a special ultrasound technique in which the transducer is directly inserted through the anus and into the patient's rectum. The sound wave echoes detected by the transducer are converted by a computer into an image.

Purpose

Ultrasound technology has been used in medicine since World War II and is recognized as a non-invasive, non-radiative, real-time and inexpensive imaging capacity. It has become standard medical practice to produce fetal images and to identify and assess various anatomical features of the body.

Endorectal ultrasound is a specialized ultrasound application and it represents one of the most useful diagnostic tools for diseases of the anal and rectal regions of the body, especially for rectal, anal, and prostrate **cancer** screening and staging.

For **rectal cancer**, endorectal ultrasound is the most preferred method for staging both depth of tumor penetration and local lymph node metastatic status. Endorectal ultrasound:

- differentiates areas of invasion within large rectal adenomas that seem benign
- determines the depth of tumor penetration into the rectal wall
- determines the extent of regional lymph node invasion
- can be combined with other tests (chest x rays and computed tomography scans, or CT scans) to determine the extent of cancer spread to distant organs, such as the lungs or liver The resulting rectal cancer staging allows physicians to determine the need for—and order of— radiation, surgery, and **chemotherapy**.

For patients diagnosed with **anal cancer**, endorectal ultrasound may help to stage the lesion and may be used as follow-up care to check for recurrence of cancer after treatment.

In the diagnosis of prostrate cancer, endorectal ultrasound has become a companion technique to **digital rectal examination** (DRE). It is also the most frequent method used to guide **biopsy** needle insertion. If surgery is indicated, endorectal ultrasound can also assist the preoperative evaluation of the depth of

cancer penetration and of the presence of metastases, as required to design appropriate surgical procedures.

Endorectal ultrasounds can also be used to check the overall treatment results.

Precautions

This is a very easy procedure. Unlike other imaging techniques, it uses no radiation and thus requires no special precautions.

Description

The instrumentation used for endorectal ultrasound consists of a hand-held probe, the transrectal transducer, a scanner, and an imaging screen. During the procedure, high-frequency acoustical (sound) waves are sent out by the small microphone-like transducer, which is inserted into the rectum. The waves bounce off the organ being examined and produce echoes sent by the transducer to a computer so as to generate a picture called a sonogram. Doctors examine the sonogram for echoes that may represent abnormal areas.

Usually, the patient lies on his side during the test. An endorectal probe is covered with a protective covering and inserted into the patient. The probe looks like a small enema tip and there is a minimal amount of discomfort associated with the procedure itself. Once inserted, the sonographer or radiologist gently moves the probe forward and backward to best evaluate the organ being examined. An endorectal ultrasound generally takes five to ten minutes. After the procedure, the radiologist interprets the results and sends a report to the referring physician.

Preparation

The patient requires no anesthetic or sedation, but needs an enema about two hours before the test in order to provide a clean rectal wall through which to scan. The evening before the procedure, it is recommended that the patient eat a small dinner, drinking only clear liquids and avoiding coffee, tea, or soft drinks after dinner.

Aftercare

The patient should enjoy a good meal and remember to keep a follow-up appointment if scheduled. In some cases, there may be some bleeding from the rectum, though this usually settles within a few days. **Antibiotics** may be prescribed in some cases.

Risks

Multiple studies have shown that the sound waves used with ultrasound imaging are harmless and may be directed at patients with complete safety. However, some patients may develop infections following the procedure, which could require further treatment. These may cause shivering and **fever**. Any manifestation of such symptoms should be immediately reported to the treating physician. Generally speaking, the entire procedure is well tolerated and there is usually minimal bleeding afterwards.

Normal results

Normal sonograms produce images that have the correct shape of the organ or tissue examined by the procedure, meaning that it corresponds to the true anatomy.

Abnormal results

Abnormal sonograms produce images which highlight abnormal features of the organ being scanned. In a tumor is present, it will show up as a distinct contrast feature on the sonogram.

See also Imaging studies.

Resources

BOOKS

Bankman, I. *Handbook of Medical Imaging.* Academic Press, 2000.

Bushong, S. C. *Diagnostic Ultrasound.* New York: McGraw-Hill & Co., 1999.

Edelstein, Peter, M.D. *Colon and Rectal Cancer.* New York: Wiley-Liss, 2000.

PERIODICALS

Gavioli, M., A. Bagni, I. Piccagli, S. Fundaro, and G. Natalini. "Usefulness of endorectal ultrasound after preoperative radiotherapy in rectal cancer: comparison between sonographic and histopathologic changes." *Diseases of the Colon and Rectum* 43 (August 2000): 1075-83.

Hsieh, J.-S., C.-J. Huang, J.-Y. Wang, and T.-J. Huang. "Benefits of Endorectal Ultrasound for Management of Smooth-Muscle Tumor of the Rectum." *Diseases of the Colon and Rectum* 42 (August 1999): 322-8

Sudhanshu, G., et al. "Staging of prostate cancer using 3-dimensional transrectal ultrasound images: a pilot study." *Journal of Urology* 162 (1999): 1318-1321.

van den Berg, J. C., J. P. van Heesewijk, and H. W. van Es. "Malignant stromal tumour of the rectum: findings at endorectal ultrasound and MRI." *British Journal of Radiology* 73 (September 2000): 1010-12.

Monique Laberge, Ph.D.

Endoscopic retrograde cholangiopancreatography

Definition

Endoscopic retrograde cholangiopancreatography (ERCP) is a technique in which a hollow tube called an endoscope is passed through the mouth and stomach to the duodenum (the first part of the small intestine). This procedure was developed to examine abnormalities of the bile ducts, pancreas, and gallbladder. It was developed during the late 1960s and is used today to diagnose and treat blockages of the bile and pancreatic ducts.

The term has three parts to its definition:

- "Endoscopic" refers to the use of an endoscope.
- "Retrograde" refers to the injection of dye up into the bile ducts in a direction opposing, or against, the normal flow of bile down the ducts.
- Cholangiopancreatography means visualization of the bile ducts (cholangio) and pancreas (pancreato).

Purpose

Until the 1970s, methods to visualize the bile ducts produced images that were of relatively poor quality and often misleading; in addition, the pancreatic duct could not be examined at all. Patients with symptoms related to the bile ducts or pancreatic ducts frequently needed surgery to diagnose and treat their conditions.

Using ERCP, physicians can obtain high-quality **x rays** of these structures and identify areas of narrowing (strictures), cancers, and gallstones. This procedure can help determine whether bile or pancreatic ducts are blocked; it also identifies where they are blocked along with the cause of the blockage. ERCP may then be used to relieve the blockage. For patients requiring surgery or additional procedures for treatment, ERCP outlines the anatomical changes for the surgeon.

Precautions

The most important precaution is that the examination should be performed by an experienced physician. The procedure is much more technically difficult than many other gastrointestinal endoscopic studies. Patients should seek physicians with experience performing ERCP. Patients should inform the physician about any allergies (including allergies to contrast

dyes, iodine, or shellfish), medication use, and medical problems. Occasionally, patients may need to be admitted to the hospital after the procedure.

Description

After sedation, a specially adapted endoscope is passed through the mouth, through the stomach, then into the duodenum. The opening to ducts that empty from the liver and pancreas is identified, and a plastic tube or catheter is placed into the orifice (opening). Contrast dye is then injected into the ducts, and with the assistance of a radiologist, pictures are taken.

Preparation

The upper intestinal tract must be empty for the procedure, so patients should NOT eat or drink for at least 6 to 12 hours before the exam. Patients should ask the physician about taking their medications before the procedure.

Aftercare

Someone should be available to take the person home after the procedure and stay with them for a while; patients will not be able to drive themselves because they undergo sedation during this test. Pain or any other unusual symptoms should be reported to the physician.

Risks

ERCP-related complications can be broken down into those related to medications used during the procedure, the diagnostic part of the procedure, and those related to endoscopic therapy. The overall complication rate is 5% to 10%; most of those occur when diagnostic ERCP is combined with a therapeutic procedure. During the exam, the endoscopist can cut or stretch structures (such as the muscle leading to the bile duct) to treat the cause of the patient's symptoms. Although the use of sedatives carries a risk of decreasing cardiac and respiratory function, it is very difficult to perform these procedures without these drugs.

The major complications related to diagnostic ERCP are pancreatitis (inflammation of the pancreas) and cholangitis (inflammation of the bile ducts). Bacteremia (the passage of bacteria into the blood stream) and perforation (hole in the intestinal tract) are additional risks.

Normal results

Because certain standards have been set for the normal diameter or width of the pancreatic duct and bile ducts, measurements using x rays are taken to determine if the ducts are too large (dilated) or too narrow (strictured). The ducts and gallbladder should be free of stones or tumors.

Abnormal results

When areas in the pancreatic or bile ducts (including those in the liver) are too wide or too narrow compared with the standard, the test is considered abnormal. Once these findings are demonstrated using ERCP, symptoms are usually present; they generally do not change without treatment. Stones, identified as opaque or solid structures within the ducts, are also considered abnormal. Masses or tumors may also be seen, but sometimes the diagnosis is made not by direct visualization of the tumor, but by indirect signs, such as a single narrowing of one of the ducts. Overall, ERCP has an excellent record in diagnosing these abnormalities.

Resources

PERIODICALS

"Guidelines:The role of ERCP in diseases of the biliary tract and pancreas." *Gastrointestinal Endoscopy* 50, no. 6 (1999): 915-920.

OTHER

Endoscopic Retrograde Cholangiopancreatography. [cited June 21, 2001]. http://www.asge.org.
Measuring Procedural Skills.[cited June 21, 2001]. http://www.acponline.org/journals/annals/15dec96/procskil.htm.
Treatment of Acute Biliary Pancreatitis. [cited June 21, 2001]. <http://content.nejm.org>.

David S. Kaminstein, M.D.

Enoxaparin *see* **Low molecular weight Heparin**

Enteritis

Description

Enteritis is an inflammation of the intestine; the term applies chiefly to the small intestine. In the context of **cancer**, enteritis is a functional disorder of the large and small bowel that occurs as a result of **radiation therapy** applied to the abdomen, pelvis, or rectum. It occurs at the onset of radiation therapy (acute radiation enteritis) and may also reappear after completion of the radiation treatment (chronic enteritis).

Enteritis also occurs in connection with such disorders as Crohn's disease and **infection** by such pathogens as *Helicobacter pylori*. Patients who receive hemodialysis for kidney disorders as well as cancer patients have an increased risk of enteritis.

Causes

Radiation enteritis occurs because the large and small intestines are sensitive to all forms of ionizing radiation. Some areas of the gastrointestinal tract are more sensitive to radiation than others; the colon is more sensitive to the effects of radiation than the small intestine, for example. Although the probability of tumor control increases with the radiation therapy dose, so does the probability of damage to normal healthy tissues. Since the doses required to destroy many tumors are very high, acute side effects to the intestines also occur, chief among which is enteritis. Thus, the majority of patients undergoing radiation to the abdomen, pelvis, or rectum will show signs of acute enteritis.

Symptoms of the disorder are observed during the first course of radiation treatment and take about eight weeks to become acute. Chronic radiation enteritis may also occur months to years after a patient has undergone a course of radiation therapy. The symptoms include colicky abdominal pain, bloody **diarrhea**, tenesmus, **weight loss**, **nausea and vomiting**, bowel obstruction and rectal bleeding, sometimes very severe.

Several factors influencing the occurrence and extent of radiation enteritis have been identified. They include the dose of radiation given to the patient, the size of the tumor being treated, the concomitant prescription of **chemotherapy** and the general state of the patient's health. For example, enteritis will be more severe in patients with a history of hypertension, diabetes or inadequate nutrition.

Treatments

Some symptoms of radiation enteritis are caused by an overgrowth of bacteria. In these cases, **antibiotics** may be prescribed. Patients who develop acute enteritis report **nausea**, **vomiting**, abdominal cramping, and diarrhea. Diarrhea impairs the digestive and absorptive functions of the gastrointestinal tract, resulting in malabsorption of fat, lactose, bile salts, and vitamin B12. Patients also complain about rectal pain and bleeding. Treatment of acute enteritis accordingly includes treating diarrhea, dehydration and abdominal and rectal pain or discomfort. Antidiarrheal drugs are usually prescribed, such as Kaopectate, Lomotil, Paregoric or Imodium. Additionally, bile salt–retaining drugs may also be indicated, such as cholestyramine. Bowel cramps may be alleviated with antispasmodic drugs, such as Donnatal.

Some patients with radiation enteritis can be fed through a tube leading into the stomach provided the small intestine is functioning normally. Otherwise, they may require parenteral alimentation, which means that a nutrient solution is given intravenously.

Approximately 5–10% of patients having received radiation therapy for abdominal or pelvic cancers develop chronic enteritis. In some cases, surgery may be indicated. There is at present no agreement as to the proper timing and choice of surgical intervention in such cases. Surgery is thus only undertaken after careful assessment of individual patient conditions and health status.

Surgery may also be indicated for patients who have developed radiation enteritis–induced strictures. (Strictures are narrowing of passages or canals.)

Alternative and complementary therapies

An important complementary therapy is nutrition management. Another side effect of radiation is to destroy the intestinal villi, which impairs the body's capacity to absorb nutrients and also destroys enzymes required for digestion, such as lactase, required to digest milk and dairy products. Thus a lactose-free diet is often recommended.

Besides milk and dairy products, it is often recommended to avoid foods such as whole bran bread and cereals, nuts, seeds and coconuts, fried and greasy foods, fruit and some fruit juices (prune juice especially), uncooked vegetables, potato chips, pretzels, strong spices and herbs, chocolate, coffee, tea, alcohol and tobacco.

Recommended foods include fish, poultry, and cooked, broiled, or roasted meat, bananas, apple sauce, peeled apples, apple and grape juices, white bread, noodles, baked, boiled, or mashed potatoes, cooked vegetables such as asparagus tips, green and waxed beans, carrots, spinach, mild processed cheese, eggs, smooth peanut butter, buttermilk, yogurt and nutmeg.

Additionally, patients with radiation enteritis may be helped by eating their food at room temperature and by drinking plenty of water every day. Carbonated sodas should be allowed to lose their carbonation prior to drinking.

Resources

BOOKS

Beers, Mark H., MD, and Robert Berkow, MD, editors. "Principles of Cancer Therapy: Management of Adverse Effects." In *The Merck Manual of Diagnosis and Therapy*. Whitehouse Station, NJ: Merck Research Laboratories, 2007.

PERIODICALS

Gore, J. I., and C. Surawicz. "Severe Acute Diarrhea." *Gastroenterology Clinics of North America* 32 (December 2003): 1249–1267.

Koffeman, G. I., W. G. van Gemert, E. K. George, and R. A. Veenendaal. "Intestinal Failure: Classification, Epidemiology and Aetiology." *Best Practice and Research: Clinical Gastroenterology* 17 (December 2003): 879–893.

Tsukada, K., T. Miyazaki, H. Katoh, et al. "*Helicobacter pylori* Infection in Hemodialysis Patients." *Hepatogastroenterology* 50 (November-December 2003): 2255–2258.

Monique Laberge, Ph.D.
Rebecca J. Frey, PhD

Environmental factors in cancer development

Definition

Environment as a cause of **cancer** is a complex and often misunderstood topic. The term environment has several different meanings when referring to causation of cancer. Originally, the term "environmental cause of cancer" was used to refer to all cancers that were not caused by hereditary or inherited factors. This definition included all cancers caused by lifestyle practices such as diet and tobacco use, viruses, and many other causes. For purposes of clarification, the term "environment" has been further defined by adding the labels "personal environment" and "external environment" when referring to causes of cancer.

By this definition, causes of cancer related to an individual's personal environment includes lifestyle choices such as diet, use of tobacco, and other factors that may place the individual at high risk for the development of cancer. External environmental causes of cancer refer to factors in the environment such as environmental pollutants that increase risk for cancer. Up to 85% of cancer is due to lifestyle choices made by individuals, which places them at higher risk for the development of cancer. For example, tobacco is directly related to more than 30% of cancer deaths. Considering more than 500,000 deaths per year are caused by tobacco alone, risk for cancer development due to external environmental factors pales in comparison.

Epidemiologists are scientists who research and identify factors that are common to cancer patients' histories and lifestyles, and then evaluate those factors within the context of current biological and disease causation theories. Eventually, evidence may persuade epidemiologists to conclude that one or more factors or characteristics shared by a study group "caused" a disease such as a type of cancer. The science of epidemiology enables researchers to determine causes of diseases such as specific types of cancer, and also to estimate or project numbers of deaths that can be attributed to the cause on an annual basis.

Personal environment/lifestyle choices

Tobacco use

Tobacco is known as one of the most potent carcinogens in humans. Tobacco causes more than 148,000 deaths each year in the form of various cancers such as lung, trachea, bronchus, larynx, pharynx, oral cavity, and esophagus. Other cancers linked to tobacco use include cancers of the pancreas, kidney, bladder, and cervix. Smoking's effects on cancer continue to be shown. Research in 2004 linked a mother's smoking to increased risk of **testicular cancer** in their children. Cigarette smoking is more common among men; however, because of the increase in the number of women who smoke, more women die from lung cancer each year than from **breast cancer**. The life span of an individual who smokes is shortened by an average of 12 years.

Diet and nutrition

According to the American Cancer Society, the single most important dietary intervention to lower risk for cancer is eating five or more servings of fruits and vegetables daily. Consuming a diet rich in plant sources provides phytochemicals—non-nutritive substances in plants that possess health protective benefits. A diet rich in foods from plant sources reduces the risk for development of cancers of the gastrointestinal tract, respiratory tract, and colon. Increased consumption of fruits and vegetables is also associated with decreased risk for lung cancer.

Diets high in fat have been associated with increased risk for colon, rectal, prostate, and endometrial cancers. The association between high-fat diets and the development of breast cancer is much weaker. Specific recommendations are to replace high-fat foods with fruits and vegetables, eat smaller portions of high-fat foods, and limit consumption of meats—especially those that are considered high fat. Foods from animal sources remain a staple in American diets. Consumption of meat, especially red meats such as beef, pork, and lamb, have been associated with increased risk of colon and **prostate cancer**.

Obesity is often the result of meat-based, high-fat diets. Obesity has been linked to cancers at several sites including colon and rectum, prostate, kidney, and endometrium. Weight gain in early adulthood seems to increase risk for breast cancer, especially if the gain occurred in the third decade of life. The highest risk related to obesity and the development of breast cancer is in postmenopausal women.

Alcohol use

Drinking alcohol increases the risk of developing cancers of the mouth, esophagus, pharynx, larynx, and liver in men and women; and increases the risk of breast cancer in women. Cancer risk increases as the amount of alcohol consumed increases. An individual who both smokes and drinks alcohol greatly increases the risk of developing cancer when compared to either smoking or drinking alone.

Physical activity

Recommendations related to physical exercise have included engaging in moderate levels of activity for at least 30 minutes on most days of the week. Many physicians have encouraged even more exercise to decrease obesity and increase overall health. Studies have revealed an association between physical activity and a reduced risk of the development of certain types of cancers, including colon, breast, and prostate cancer.

Radiation exposure

Only high frequency radiation such as ultraviolet (UV) radiation and ionizing radiation (IR) has been proven to cause cancer in humans. A source of UV radiation is sunlight. Prolonged exposure to UV radiation is the major cause of basal and squamous cell skin cancers. UV radiation is also a major cause of **melanoma**.

IR has cancer-causing capability, as proven by studies on atomic bomb survivors and other groups. Virtually any part of the body can by affected by IR, but the areas most affected are the bone marrow and the thyroid gland. IR is released in very low levels from diagnostic equipment such as medical and dental X-ray equipment. Much higher levels of IR are released from machines delivering **radiation therapy** to patients. Great precautions are taken not to expose patients or staff unnecessarily to the effects of IR.

Exposure to radon, a form of IR, can increase risk for lung cancer, especially among smokers. Radon is a naturally occurring radioactive gas formed by the decay of uranium in rocks and soil. The gas is odorless, colorless, tasteless, and cannot be detected by sight. Radon seeps up through the ground and is released into the air. Radon gas exists at harmless levels outdoors. In areas where there is poor ventilation, such as underground mines, radon can accumulate to levels that pose a risk for the development of lung cancer. Radon causes cancer by emitting radioactive particles as it decays. These particles damage the lining of the lung when the radon is inhaled. Individuals at highest risk for the development of cancer from radon exposure include uranium miners and those individuals who live in well-insulated, tightly sealed homes built on uranium-rich soil. Testing for radon is the only way to determine if a home has elevated radon levels.

Reproductive and gynecologic factors

Lifestyle choices linked to breast cancer include diet, **alcohol consumption**, oral contraceptives, estrogen replacement therapy, postmenopausal obesity, and nulliparity (a woman who has never had a child). The relationship between dietary fats and breast cancer continues to be studied. Women who consume more than two alcoholic drinks per day are at higher risk. Oral contraceptive use has been linked to the development of breast cancer. Nulliparous women who began using oral contraceptives prior to the age of 18 years and continued uninterrupted use for more than eight years have a minimally increased risk. In 2002, a large study of hormone replacement therapy for postmenopausal women was halted because of the large risk of breast cancer (and heart disease) the therapy produced in women. In early 2004, researchers also found increased risk of breast cancer recurrence in women who used the hormone therapy for postmenopausal symptoms.

Full-term pregnancy seems to exert a deterrent effect on the development of breast cancer. Women who become pregnant after the age of 30 years, or who never become pregnant, are at higher risk. Historically, lactation and breast-feeding have been recognized as protective mechanisms for breast cancer development. A correlation between the development of breast cancer and abortion has been documented in United States studies. A large study conducted in Denmark to investigate the correlation found no increased risk of breast cancer among women who had undergone abortions.

Precancerous and cancerous lesions of the cervix are associated with many personal risk factors, including a higher incidence in women who become sexually active prior to age 17, have many sex partners, and are multiparous (have borne at least one living child). An association has also been described between type of employment and increased **cervical cancer** mortality. Women with higher mortality rates include women once employed in farm work, manufacturing, personal services, or who worked as nurses' aides. Women who are infected with the human immunodeficiency virus (HIV) are at higher risk for the development of squamous intraepithelial lesions of the cervix. Cervical cancer is not often diagnosed in women who are nulliparous, those who are lifetime celibates, or who are lifetime monogamous (having sex with only one person).

Psychological stress

Stress is known to activate the body's endocrine or hormonal system which in turn causes changes in the immune system. There is no specific evidence that changes in the immune system caused by stress directly cause cancer. However, some studies report significantly higher rates of breast cancer in women who experienced stressful life events and losses in the years immediately preceding the diagnosis of breast cancer. Other studies do not support the association between stress and breast cancer development.

Cellular phone use

Studies in the United States and Denmark in 2000 and 2001 revealed there is no link between cellular telephone use and tumors of the brain, salivary gland, leukemia, or other cancers. The type of telephone, the duration of the cell phone use, or age of the phone user had no effect on cancer risk.

External environment

Chemicals and other substances

Exposure to certain chemicals, pesticides, and metals can increase an individual's risk for cancer. Carcinogens in this category include nickel, cadmium, vinyl chloride, and benzene. These carcinogens may act alone or in combination with another carcinogen, such as cigarette smoke, to increase risk for cancer.

Environmental tobacco smoke (secondhand smoke)

Environmental tobacco smoke (ETS) is a combination of two forms of smoke from tobacco products—sidestream smoke and mainstream smoke. Sidestream smoke is smoke released between puffs of a burning cigarette, cigar, or pipe. Mainstream smoke is the smoke that is exhaled by the smoker. Sidestream smoke contains essentially the same compounds as those in the mainstream smoke inhaled by the smoker. Tobacco smoke is known to contain at least 60 different carcinogens. Nonsmokers who are exposed to ETS absorb nicotine and other harmful compounds from the smoke. ETS can cause lung cancer in healthy adults who are nonsmokers and there is a 20% increased risk of lung cancer in nonsmokers exposed to ETS. ETS has been linked to other cancers, including cancers of the nasal cavity, cervix, breast, and bladder. In 1992, the U.S. Environmental Protection Agency classified ETS as a Group A carcinogen. Group A is reserved by the EPA to categorize only the most dangerous cancer-causing agents to humans.

Asbestos exposure

Asbestos is a group of minerals that occur naturally as strong, flexible fibers that can be separated into threads and then woven. Asbestos fibers cannot conduct electricity and are not affected by heat or chemicals. Because of these properties there have been many industrial applications of asbestos. Some of the applications include insulation, fireproofing, and absorption of sound. Serious health risks related to asbestos occur as a result of exposure to the dust that is formed when the fibers break into tiny particles. These asbestos particles can then be inhaled or swallowed. Exposure to asbestos can lead to lung, larynx, and gastrointestinal tract cancers, as well as to the rare cancer—mesothelioma. Individuals at highest risk include those with the combination of asbestos exposure and smoking. Smoking increases risk for lung cancer by 10 times more than for the nonsmoker also exposed to asbestos. Due to government regulations and public concerns about the health hazards from asbestos exposure, the use of asbestos in the United States has declined significantly. Workplace practices involving asbestos are highly regulated by industry and government to minimize worker exposure.

Electric and magnetic field (EMF) exposure

EMFs are emitted from devices that produce, transmit, or use electric power and arise from the motion of electrical charges. Examples of these devices include power lines, transmitters, and household products such as microwave ovens, electric blankets, televisions, and computers. EMFs are considered forms of nonionizing radiation. According to the National Cancer Institute (NCI), public concern has increased over the health effects of EMFs, particularly in relation to the risk of developing cancer in both children and adults exposed to EMFs. Numerous studies have been conducted in the past 15 years to evaluate risk of cancer from exposure to EMFs. As of 2001, the results have been inconsistent according to the NCI. One large NCI/Children's Cancer Group study sought to determine whether exposure to magnetic fields contributed to the development of acute lymphoblastic leukemia (ALL) in children under the age of 15 years. The results of this study revealed little evidence of a relationship between risk for ALL in children and exposure to magnetic fields.

Other studies focused on determining links between magnetic fields and central nervous system (CNS) tumors such as brain cancers continue to be actively researched. To date, expert panels that have reviewed the existing data have concluded that data are insufficient to support the conclusion that magnetic fields cause cancer.

Nuclear facility exposure

An NCI study published in 1991 concluded there was no general increased risk of death from cancer for people living in more than 100 U.S. counties containing, or closely adjacent to, nuclear facilities. A British survey of cancer mortality in areas around nuclear facilities in the United Kingdom reported an increase in deaths from childhood leukemia near some of the facilities. Other smaller surveys of cancer deaths around nuclear facilities in both countries yielded conflicting results.

See also Cigarettes; Occupational exposures and cancer; Cancer prevention.

Resources

BOOKS

Yarbro, J. W. "Carcinogenesis" In *Cancer Nursing Principles and Practice,* edited by C. H. Yarbro, M. H. Frogge, M. Goodman, and S. L. Groenwald. Boston: Jones and Bartlett, 2000, pp.48-59.

PERIODICALS

Ballard-Barbash, R., M. R. Forman, and V. Kipnis. "Dietary Fat, Serum Estrogen Levels, and Breast Cancer Risk." *Journal of the National Cancer Institute* 91 (1999): 492-494.

Franco, E. L., T. E. Rohan, and L. L. Villa. "Epidemiologic Evidence and Human Papillomavirus Infection as a Necessary Cause of Cervical Cancer." *Journal of the National Cancer Institute* 91 (1999): 506-511.

"HRT Trail Terminated Over Risk of Breast Cancer." *GP* February 9, 2004: 8.

"Maternal Smoking May Play Etiologic Role in Testicular Cancer." *Cancer Weekly* June 22, 2000: 232.

"Top 10 Health Stories of 2003." *Harvard Health Letter* December 2003.

OTHER

"Cancer." *CancerNet.* 2000, National Cancer Institute. [cited April 22, 2001 and July 1, 2001]. http://www.cancernet.nci.nih.gov/wyntk_pubs/cancer.htm.

"Environmental Factors and Cancer." *OncoLink* 1994-2001, The Trustees of the University of Pennsylvania. [cited April 3, 2001 and July 1, 2001]. http://www.oncolink.upenn.edu/causeprevent/environment.

"Lifestyle and Environmental Risk Factors for Breast Cancer." *The Komen Foundation.* 2000, Breast Health. [cited April 22, 2001 and July 1, 2001]. http://www.breastcancerinfo.com/bhealth/html/environmental_risk_factors.html.

Melinda Granger Oberleitner, R.N., D.N.S.

A brain surgery in progress. When possible, surgery is the first form of treatment for ependymoma. *(Custom Medical Stock Photo. Reproduced by permission.)*

Ependymoma

Definition

An ependymoma is a rare type of primary brain tumor that develops from the ependymal cells lining the ventricles of the brain and the central canal of the spinal cord. It is classified as a glioma because it arises from glial (supportive) cells in the brain. Ependymomas can be found anywhere in the brain or spine but are usually located in the main part of the brain, the cerebrum, and may spread from the brain to the spinal cord via the cerebrospinal fluid (CSF). They were first identified as a distinctive type of central nervous system **cancer** in 1924.

Demographics

Ependymomas are infrequent tumors, representing 2–3% of all primary **brain tumors**. However, ependymomas are the third most common brain tumor in children (5–10%) and are diagnosed in about 75 to 150 children each year in the United States. More than 50% of all ependymomas are diagnosed during childhood, 30% in children below the age of three years. Ependymomas of the spine in adults account for over half of all spinal tumors. In adults, 60% of all ependymomas occur along the spine, whereas in children, 90% of these tumors are in the brain. In children, ependymomas are more likely to occur in boys than

in girls, although the reason for the difference is not known as of 2009.

The occurrence of ependymomas is equal for male and female adults and among all races, although a few subtypes of ependymomas are more common in African Americans than in members of other races in North America. The frequency of ependymomas is thought to be the same around the world.

Description

Most brain tumors are named after the cells in which they are found, thus the name ependymoma for a tumor of ependymal cells. Ependymomas are located with respect to the tentorium, a thick membrane that separates the upper two-thirds of the brain from the lower third. Ependymomas are thus classified as either supratentorial (above the tentorium, located in the top part of the head) or infratentorial (below the tentorium, located in the back of the head). In children, most ependymomas are of the infratentorial type and occur in or close to the fourth ventricle of the brain. Ependymomas are soft tumors, greyish or reddish in color and may contain cysts.

Ependymomas may block the flow of cerebrospinal fluid out of the ventricles causing them to enlarge—a condition called hydrocephalus. Unlike other types of brain tumors, ependymomas as a rule do not spread into healthy brain tissue or outside the brain or spinal cord. As a result, it is often the case that they can be removed and cured by surgery, especially spinal cord ependymomas.

Causes and symptoms

Causes

As is the case for most brain tumors, the cause of ependymomas is unknown. Ependymal cells usually grow in an orderly and controlled way, but if for some reason this process is disrupted, the cells continue to divide and form a tumor. Research is being carried out to identify possible contributing factors. Little is known, but researchers have begun to make progress in the areas of genetic and hereditary causes. As of 2009, researchers are looking at glial cells known as radial glia as the possible point of origin of ependymomas. Chromosomes that have been implicated include chromosomes 6, 9, 16, 17, and 22. No toxic chemicals or other environmental factors have been identified as possible causes of ependymomas.

Symptoms

The first symptoms of any type of brain tumor are usually due to increased pressure within the skull. This may be the result of a blockage in the ventricles of the brain causing a buildup of CSF or may be induced by swelling around the tumor itself. The increased pressure can cause headaches, **vomiting** and visual problems in older children and adults. In younger children, the earliest symptoms of an ependymoma may include swelling of the head, irritability, and unusual sleepiness. Other symptoms specific to ependymomas include swelling of the optic nerve, rapid and jerky eye movements, and neck pain. Seizures, fits and personality changes are also general symptoms associated with a brain tumor. About 25% of children with ependymomas have seizures.

Other ependymoma symptoms depend on which area of the brain is affected:

- If located in the frontal lobe of the brain, ependymomas may cause mood swings, personality changes, and paralysis on one side of the body.
- If occurring on the temporal lobe of the brain, coordination, speech, and memory problems may result.
- If located on the parietal lobe of the brain, the condition may affect writing and related tasks.
- If located in the cerebellum, ependymomas may cause unsteady gait and problems with coordination and balance.

Adults with ependymomas of the spine may experience tingling, electric shock-like sensations, numbness, or weakness in the arms and legs. They may also have problems with bowel or bladder control (**incontinence**).

Diagnosis

The diagnosis of an ependymoma is usually made within 3 to 6 months of the onset of symptoms. To plan treatment, doctors need to find out as much as they can about the type, location, and size of the ependymoma. A number of diagnostic tests and examinations are scheduled. The first test is a neurological examination to evaluate any effect the tumor may have had on the nervous system. Every patient with ependymoma is usually subjected to diagnostic imaging of the spinal cord and brain. The most sensitive method available for evaluating spinal cord **metastasis** is spinal **magnetic resonance imaging** (MRI) performed with gadolinium, a contrast agent injected into the patient before the procedure.

Other imaging studies—such as a CT scan—may also be performed to find the exact location and size of the ependymoma. To confirm the diagnosis, a **biopsy** will be perfomed and an ependymoma specimen will be examined under a microscope. About 10% to 15% of ependymomas spread from their original location through the CSF; infratentorial ependymomas are more likely to spread to the spinal cord than supratentorial tumors. An additional test called a myelogram may be done to check for this condition and to see whether the tumor has spread to the spinal cord.

Tests

There are no laboratory tests that are useful in diagnosing ependymomas. Spinal taps are potentially dangerous for the patient because of the increased fluid pressure inside the skull.

Treatment

Traditional

CLINICAL STAGING AND TREATMENTS. There is no formal staging system for ependymomas. They are divided into supratentorial and infratentorial tumors and treated accordingly. Treatment will proceed depending on a number of factors such as the patient's general health and age, the size and location of the ependymoma, and whether it has spread. Before any treatment is given for ependymoma, it will be important to reduce the pressure in the skull if this has occurred. If it is due to a buildup of CSF, a shunt may be inserted to drain off the excess fluid. Steroid drugs may also be prescribed to reduce swelling around the ependymoma.

When possible, surgery is the first form of treatment for ependymoma. The purpose of surgery is to remove as much of the tumor as possible without damaging the healthy brain tissue. However, it may not be possible to remove it entirely and follow-up treatment may be required. One approach is to prescribe repeated surgery in patients who still have ependymoma remaining after a first surgery and **radiation therapy**.

Radiation therapy, or the use of high-energy rays to destroy the cancer cells, is often used after surgery to destroy any remaining cancer cells. It may also be used alone to treat ependymomas that cannot be reached by surgery. Since ependymomas may spread to the spinal cord, radiation therapy is sometimes given to both the brain and spinal cord. Radiation oncologists are also using focal radiation techniques, meaning that they give a single large dose of radiation so as to kill residual cancer cells after regular radiation therapy in patients who have significant tumor tissue remaining after surgery.

TREATMENT TEAM. The primary physician will recommend one or more types of treatment based on the ependymoma diagnosis (size, location, type) and on the patient's medical history, age, and overall health. As a rule, the treatment team includes a neurosurgeon, a neurologist, a radiation oncologist and a medical oncologist.

Drugs

Chemotherapy, or the use of anti-cancer drugs to destroy cancer cells, is another form of treatment indicated for ependymomas. It may be given alone or in conjunction with surgery and radiation therapy. Newer and improved chemotherapeutic drugs are now being used after surgery, with the goal of shrinking the ependymoma before radiation therapy.

Patients who are having seizures are usually given levetiracetam (Keppra), **phenytoin** (Dilantin), or **carbamazepine** (Tegretol). Those with swelling or inflammation of the brain tissue may be treated with **corticosteroids**, usually **dexamethasone** (Decadron).

Alternative

In a search for less toxic therapies and improved quality of life, patients with primary brain tumors are increasingly considering complementary and alternative treatments. The American Brain Tumor Association provides a list of therapies such as acupuncture, antioxidant therapy, acupressure, meditation, and others. The association does not officially endorse any of them, however. The treatment team will be able to offer the best advice as to whether alternative and/or complementary treatments are indicated.

Coping with cancer treatment

Learning to live with ependymoma can be difficult for both patient and family. Several national associations exist to educate, support and advocate for families of children with cancer, survivors of childhood cancer, and the health professionals who care for

QUESTIONS TO ASK YOUR DOCTOR

- Where is the ependymoma located?
- What is the next step? Are more tests necessary
- What kinds of specialists should I seek out for treatment?
- What medication is necessary, and what is it for? What are the side-effects?
- Considering age and the extent of the ependymoma, what is the current prognosis?

them. These organizations offer contacts with peer-support groups and distribute a wealth of cancer-related brochures and publications.

Clinical trials

In 2009, the National Cancer Institute (NCI) supported over 183 ependymoma-related **clinical trials** to evaluate a variety of new treatments. The NCI monitors clinical trials and should be contacted at http://www.cancer.gov/for up-to-date information.

Prognosis

Postoperative radiation therapy has definitely been shown to improve chances of recovery from an ependymoma but results of chemotherapy are considered somewhat disappointing. Age is also a factor in recovery; usually the younger the patient, the less favorable the prognosis. As of 2009, the 10-year survival rate for ependymomas in people of all age groups is 45–55%. The five-year survival rate is 76% in adults and 14% in children. The most rapid recoveries usually occur in patients who have no visible tumor after surgery.

Prevention

A large coordinated investigation recently carried out in Europe, Israel, and North America studied the factors that might affect the occurrence of primary brain tumors in infants and children under the age of 20. The study concluded that women taking vitamin supplements containing C, A, E, and/or folate during the entire period of their pregnancy were half as likely to have their child develop a brain tumor before age 5 compared to those who did not take **vitamins**.

Special concerns

Recurrence of an ependymoma is very dependent upon the extent of surgical removal as well as on the success of the treatment course following the initial diagnosis. Most recurrent ependymomas occur in the vicinity of the cavity from which the original tumor was surgically removed. Treatment options for an individual with a recurrent ependymoma usually include more surgery, chemotherapy, and further radiotherapy. An ependymoma can also metastasize into adjacent areas of the brain or, less commonly, to distant parts of the central nervous system. Approximately 12% of patients will have evidence of metastasis at the time of diagnosis. In these situations, more extensive treatment is used to treat the disease.

Children diagnosed with ependymomas are the object of special concern because of their vulnerability to radiation therapy. The organs in children are, generally speaking, significantly more sensitive to radiation than those of adults. Thus, radiation doses delivered to a child may have devastating side effects and must therefore be designed to address the issues of toxicity as well as that of treatment effectiveness.

When the ependymoma causes blockage of CSF flow and leads to hydrocephalus, a special tubing called a ventriculo-peritoneal shunt (VP shunt) can be surgically implanted in the brain ventricles to drain the excess CSF into the abdomen. This procedure allows the fluid to bypass the tumor blockage and relieves the pain and symptoms of hydrocephalus.

Resources

BOOKS

Estlin, Eddy, Richard J. Gilbertson, and Robert Wynn, eds. *Pediatric Hematology and Oncology: Scientific Principles and Clinical Practice.* Hoboken, NJ: Wiley-Blackwell, 2010.

Estlin, Eddy, and Stephen Lowis, eds. *Central Nervous System Tumours of Childhood.* London: Mac Keith Press, 2005.

PERIODICALS

Boop, F. A., and S. Sqouros. "Intracranial Ependymoma in Children: Current Status and Future Trends on Diagnosis and Management." *Child's Nervous System* 25 (October 2009): 1163–65.

Kilday, J. P., et al. "Pediatric Ependymoma: Biological Perspectives." *Molecular Cancer Research* 7 (June 2009): 765–86.

Lopez-Gines, C., et al. "Metastasizing Anaplastic Ependymoma in an Adult. Chromosomal Imbalances, Metabolic and Gene Expression Profiles." *Histopathology* 54 (Match 2009): 500–504.

Mack, S. C., and M.D. Taylor. "The Genetic and Epigenetic Basis of Ependymoma." *Child's Nervous System* 25 (October 2009): 1195–1201.

Massimino, M., et al. "Intracranial Ependymoma: Factors Affecting Outcome." *Future Oncology* 5 (March 2009): 207–16.

McGuire, C. S., et al. "Incidence Patterns for Ependymoma: A Surveillance, Epidemiology, and End Results Study." *Journal of Neurosurgery* 110 (April 2009): 725–29.

Mueller, S., and S. Chang. "Pediatric Brain Tumors: Current Treatment Strategies and Future Therapeutic Approaches." *Neurotherapeutics* 6 (July 2009): 570–86.

OTHER

American Brain Tumor Association (ABTA). *Ependymoma.* http://www.abta.org/sitefiles/pdflibrary/Ependymoma_Pamphlet_F.pdf

Bruce, Jeffrey N., and David J. Fusco. "Ependymoma." *eMedicine,* January 26, 2009. http://emedicine.medscape.com/article/277621-overview

National Cancer Institute (NCI). *Childhood Ependymoma Treatment.* http://www.cancer.gov/cancertopics/pdq/treatment/childependymoma/healthprofessional/allpages

National Institute of Neurological Disorders and Stroke (NINDS). *Brain and Spinal Tumors: Hope through Research.* http://www.ninds.nih.gov/disorders/brainandspinaltumors/detail_brainandspinaltumors.htm

ORGANIZATIONS

American Brain Tumor Association (ABTA), 2720 River Road, Des Plaines, IL, 60018, 847-827-9910, 800-886-2282, 847-827-9918, info@abta.org, http://www.abta.org/.

American Cancer Society, 250 Williams Street NW, Atlanta, GA, 30303, 800-ACS-2345 (227-2345), www.cancer.org.

American Society of Clinical Oncology (ASCO), 2318 Mill Road, Suite 800, Alexandria, VA, 22314, 571-483-1300, 888-282-2552, membermail@asco.org, http://www.asco.org/ASCOv2?edition = default.

The Childhood Brain Tumor Foundation (CBTF), 20312 Watkins Meadow Drive, Germantown, MD, 20876, 301-515-2900, 877-217-4166, cbtf@childhoodbraintumor.org, http://www.childhoodbraintumor.org/.

National Cancer Institute, 6116 Executive Blvd., Room 3036A, Bethesda, MD, 20892-8322, 800-422-6237, cancergovstaff@mail.nih.gov, www.cancer.gov.

National Institute of Neurological Disorders and Stroke (NINDS), P.O. Box 5801, Bethesda, MD, 20824, 800-352-9424, 301-496-5751, http://www.ninds.nih.gov/index.htm.

Monique Laberge, PhD
Rebecca J. Frey, PhD

Epidermal growth factor receptor agonists

Definition

Epidermal growth factors receptors are proteins found in cell membranes that help to regulate cell growth and cell division. Epidermal growth factor receptor antagonists are **chemotherapy** drugs that interfere with the action of epidermal growth factor receptors.

Purpose

Many different types of normal and **cancer** (malignant) cells have epidermal growth factor receptors in their cell membranes. When epidermal growth factor (a protein) binds to an epidermal growth factor receptor, new proteins are produced inside the cell that stimulate the cell to grow and divide. Some cells, when they become malignant, develop too many or overactive epidermal growth factor receptors. This stimulates the overproduction of growth-regulating proteins in the cell, with the result that malignant cells grow and divide wildly and form a tumor.

Epidermal growth factor also plays a role in the sequence of metabolic events that leads to the formation of new blood vessels, a process called angiogenesis. As tumors grow larger, they need more oxygen and nutrients. To meet these needs, new blood vessels must grow into the tumor. Epidermal growth factor receptor antagonist drugs bind with the epidermal growth factor receptors and stop or slow the production of the proteins that stimulate the formation of new blood vessels. Therefore, epidermal growth factor receptor antagonists fight cancer in two ways. They directly inhibit tumor growth, and they also limit tumor size by stopping or slowing the development of new blood vessels necessary to feed the tumor.

As of 2009, at least four different subtypes of epidermal growth factor receptors had been discovered. Different subtypes are present (expressed) on different kinds of cancer cells. As a result, specific epidermal growth factor receptor antagonists drugs are used to target different types of cancer including **pancreatic cancer**, metastic **breast cancer**, **non-small cell lung cancer**, squamous cell **carcinoma** of the head and neck, and colorectal cancer. Generally, epidermal growth factor receptor antagonists are used as second-line treatment after treatment with other drugs has failed to control the cancer. Occasionally they are used as first-line treatment in combination with other cancer therapies.

Description

There are two distinctly different types of epidermal growth factor receptor antagonist drugs: small-molecule epidermal growth factor receptor antagonists and **monoclonal antibodies**. These work in different ways, although both interfere with the production of proteins that cause cells to grow and divide. Since epidermal growth factor receptors are also found on normal cells, these drugs kill both normal and malignant cells.

Small-molecule epidermal growth factor receptor antagonists are drugs that block the actions of an enzyme called tyrosine kinase. Tyrosine kinase is a signaling molecule that is involved in cell growth and division. By interfering with tyrosine kinase, small-molecule epidermal growth factor receptor antagonists disrupt cell division. Small-molecule epidermal growth factor antagonist drugs include:

- erlotinib (Tarceva) used to treat pancreatic cancer and non-small cell lung cancer
- lapatinib (Tyverb, Tykerb) approved in 74 countries for the treatment of breast cancer that has metastasized (spread to other organs)
- gefitinib (Iressa) used to treat non-small cell lung cancer but available in the United States only through a special access program since 2005.

Monoclonal antibodies are identical antibodies that are produced in great numbers in the laboratory from a single cell. These antibodies can be genetically engineered to target particular receptors on cells. The epithelial growth factor receptor antagonist drugs that are monoclonal antibodies include **cetuximab** (Erbitux), used to treat squamous cell carcinoma of the head and neck and colorectal cancer, and **panitumumab** (Vectibix) used to treat metastic colorectal cancer. These drugs bind with epidermal growth factor receptors in the cell membrane and disrupt their activity.

All approved epithelial growth factor antagonists continue to be tested in **clinical trials** for use against other cancers and in combination with other therapies. A list of clinical trials currently enrolling volunteers can be found at http://www.clinicaltrials.gov.

Recommended dosage

The recommended dosage varies with the specific epithelial growth factor antagonist prescribed. Dosage also varies depending on the health status of the patient, the type of cancer being treated, and other drugs the patient is taking. Small-molecule drugs are tablets while monoclonal antibodies are given as injections. All epithelial growth factor antagonists have strict requirements about when and how they must be taken. See individual drug entries and consult a physician or pharmacist for additional information.

Precautions

Epithelial growth factor antagonists have potentially severe, possibly life-threatening side effects. For example, cetuximab carries a boxed warning stating that serious infusion reactions may occur and that cardiopulmonary arrest and sudden death occurred in some patients during clinical trials. Precautions and warnings vary somewhat with each drug. See individual drug entries and consult a physician or pharmacist for additional information about specific drugs.

Pediatric

The safety and effectiveness of this drug have not been established in children.

Pregnant or breastfeeding

Epithelial growth factor antagonists described in this entry are either pregnancy category C or pregnancy category D drugs. Woman who are pregnant or who might become pregnant should not use these drugs. It is not known whether these drugs are excreted in breast milk. Women taking these drug should avoid breastfeeding, as there is the potential for these drugs to cause serious harm to nursing infants. Women should discuss with their doctor how long after stopping the drug they should wait before becoming pregnant or beginning to breast feed. Some drugs require that the woman wait at least six months after stopping the drug before becoming pregnant and wait at two months before beginning to breast feed.

Side effects

All epithelial growth factor antagonists have the potential to cause serious or live-threatening side effects. They almost universally also cause common side effects of chemotherapy such as **nausea, vomiting**, headache, pain, and abnormalities in blood count and liver function. Side effects and their frequency vary somewhat with each drug. See individual drug entries and consult a physician or pharmacist for additional information about specific drugs.

Interactions

Epithelial growth factor antagonists interact in a variety of ways with many drugs. A pharmacist or physician must be consulted for the most up-to-date information about interactions for the specific drug being taken. All interactions are not known. Patients should provide their doctor and pharmacist with a complete list of all prescription and nonprescription drugs, herbs, and dietary supplements that they are taking.

Resources

OTHER

Angiogenesis Inhibitors Therapy. National Cancer Institute November 6, 2008 [October 11, 2009]. http://www.cancer.gov/cancertopics/factsheet/therapy/angiogenesis-inhibitors

ORGANIZATIONS

American Cancer Society, 1599 Clifton Rd., NE, Atlanta, GA, 30329, (404) 320-3333, (800) ACS-2345, http://www.cancer.org.
National Cancer Institute Public Inquires Office., 6116 Executive Boulevard, Room 3036A, Bethesda, MD, 20892-8322, (800) 4-CANCER. TTY (800) 332-8615, http://www.cancer.gov.

Tish Davidson, A.M.

Epirubicin

Definition

Epirubicin is a semi-synthetic anthracycline-based anticancer (or antineoplastic) drug derived from **doxorubicin**. It is also known by its trade name Ellence.

Purpose

Epirubicin is used as the **chemotherapy** agent for adjuvant therapy in patients diagnosed with **breast cancer**, and, as determined by the attending oncologist, epirubicin may be used in the treatment of lung, gastric, and pancreatic cancers.

Description

Epirubicin has been used extensively since the mid-1980s for both early stage and metastatic breast **cancer**. Epirubicin received Federal Drug Administration approval in the fall of 1999 for adjuvant therapy in patients with node-positive breast cancer. Like other DNA-interactive antineoplastic family members,

KEY TERMS

Adjuvant therapy—Treatment that is prescribed to increase the effectiveness of a primary treatment.

Anthracycline—Drugs that have a characteristic four-ring structure that are linked, via a glycosidic bond, to daunosamine, an amino sugar, which are used in leukemia therapy to prevent cell division by disrupting the structure of the DNA.

Antineoplastic—Agents that inhibit or prevent the maturation and proliferation of malignant cells.

Cytotoxic—A term that refers to chemicals that are directly toxic to a cell, preventing the growth or reproduction of the cell.

Doxorubicin—An extremely effective anticancer drug isolated from the *Streptomyces peucetius* bacteria.

Free radicals—Highly reactive molecules that act as agents of tissue damage.

Oncologist—A physician who specializes in the diagnosis and treatment of cancer patients.

epirubicin binds to DNA to inhibit DNA, RNA, and protein synthesis resulting in cell death. It has been demonstrated that epirubicin also acts to block cell growth and to increase the production of cytotoxic free radicals. For breast cancer treatment, epirubicin has proven highly effective when administered as a single agent in a sequential regimen. Epirubicin may be given in combination with **cyclophosphamide**, and 5-fluorouracil; however, currently there is no clinical evidence to suggest that long-term survival is greater in the combination regimen than with epirubicin alone. The lower toxicity associated with epirubicin treatment promotes better quality of life for the patient.

Recent research has examined the role of epirubicin in treating **prostate cancer**. Study of its effects in helping to relieve pain, quality of life, and survival are preliminary, but it appears that eprirubicin is not effective alone in treating metastatic prostate cancer. A study in 2003 reported that epirubicin, used in combination with cancer drugs **cisplatin** and **irinotecan**, might have promising broad antitumor activity. In the future, epirubicin might be used in combination therapies to treat many types of tumors.

Recommended dosage

Epirubicin is administered as a red fluid via intravenous injection (IV) into a cannula placed into the vein or through a central line inserted under the skin into a vein near the collarbone. The dose of epirubicin prescribed will vary among patients, correlated with patient body size, the purpose of the dose, whether the epirubicin will be used as a single agent or in combination, and the stage and aggressiveness of the cancer type. A starting dose of 50 mg/m^2 of body surface per dose cycle of epirubicin is an appropriate regimen. Treatment cycles may be given weekly. With higher doses, cycles may be reduced to only two to three times per month. The maximum cumulative dose for anthracyclines is defined by cardiotoxicity. Studies on epirubicin have only been conducted on adult patients; therefore, with the associated risk of cardiotoxicity there are no recommendations for dosage on young children or the elderly.

Precautions

To maximize treatment effects, patients receiving epirubicin should observe certain guidelines. Along with any specific modifications given by the oncologist, these guidelines should include monitoring the area surrounding the injection site, and regular laboratory testing for white blood cell count, and kidney, liver, and bone marrow function. In order to reduce the possibility of immunosupression, immunizations not approved or prescribed by the oncologist should be avoided. Those receiving epirubicin should avoid contact with individuals taking, or that have recently taken, oral polio vaccine or individuals that have an active **infection**. When necessary, a protective facemask can be worn. Specific instructions on oral hygiene procedures to reduce the risk of gum abrasion should be received. Avoiding touching the eye and nasal areas unless hands have been properly washed immediately prior to contact is advised. To reduce bleeding and bruising complications, patients should exercise extreme caution when handling sharp instruments and decline participation in contact sports. The oncologist may suggest increased fluid intake to prevent kidney problems and to ensure proper kidney function.

Prior to treatment, the patient's medical history should be thoroughly reviewed to avoid complications that might arise from previous conditions such as bone marrow depression; viral, fungal, or bacterial infection; heart, kidney disease, or liver disease; or tumor cell infiltration of bone marrow. The oncologist should also be made aware if the patient is pregnant, if there is the possibility the patient might be pregnant, or if the patient is a breast-feeding mother. Only prescribed medications or over the counter (OTC) drugs approved by the oncologist should be taken by a patient receiving epirubicin

Side effects

Along with the desired anticancer effects from epirubicin treatment, less desirable side effects are to be anticipated. All presenting side effects should be discussed with the oncologist. Some side effects may occur that do not require medical attention, but nonetheless concern the patient. These commonly include hair loss (**alopecia**), lack of menstrual periods, discolored urine, **nausea and vomiting**, occasional **diarrhea**, hot flashes, and temporary decrease of bone marrow function. Less frequently, the patient also may experience loss of appetite with accompanying **weight loss**, darkening of the soles of the feet, palms, or nails, and cardiotoxicity. Most of these side effects disappear with the end of treatment or may be eased during treatment with prescribed intervention from the oncologist.

Other side effects from epirubicin treatment require immediate attention from a healthcare professional. These indicators of potentially life-threatening conditions or medical overdose frequently include bleeding and bruising; the presence of ulcers, sores, or redness in the mouth, throat, or on the lips; a cough or hoarseness; pain or difficulty in urination; **fever** or chills; lower back or side pain; black tarry stools; redness or drainage from the eyes or eye area; pinpoint red spots on the skin; and red streaks around the injected vein. More rare, but no less critical side effects may include wheezing or shortness of breath; joint pain; fast or irregular heartbeat; skin rash or **itching**; discoloration, redness, or warmth at the site of the injection; swelling in feet, legs, and abdomen; and tenderness of the abdomen or lymph nodes.

Interactions

More than 70 regularly prescribed drugs are known to have interactive effects with epirubicin. A complete and exhaustive list should be documented in the patient's history prior to treatment. In particular, the patient should be made aware of specific drugs that, when given concurrently with epirubicin, produce increased problems and risks in the following areas:

- liver problems
- blood disorders
- risk of infection
- risk of heart damage and heart failure
- extended clearance time of epirubicin from the body
- risk of secondary leukemia

Resources

PERIODICALS

"Cisplatin, Irinotecan, and Epirubicin Have Promising Broad Antitumor Activity." *Cancer Weekly* October 14, 2003: 12.
"Epirubicin Alone Should Not be Used to Treat Hormone-Resistant Prostate Cancer." *Drug Week* October 31, 2003: 333.

Jane Taylor-Jones, M.S.

Epoietin alfa *see* **Erythropoietin**

Epstein-Barr virus

Definition

Epstein-Barr virus, or EBV, is the name given to a member of the herpesvirus family that is associated with a variety of illnesses—from infectious mononucleosis (IM) and multiple sclerosis to **nasopharyngeal cancer** and **Burkitt's lymphoma**. EBV is also known as human herpesvirus 4 or HHV-4. It is named for Anthony Epstein and Yvonne Barr, who identified the virus in 1964 in tissue samples sent to them from Uganda by Denis Burkitt (1911–1993), for whom Burkitt's **lymphoma** was named.

Demographics

EBV occurs in nearly all regions of the world, and is considered among the most common infectious viruses known to humankind. It is likely as of 2009 that its genetic diversity is greater than was thought when it was first identified. In the United States, the

Epstein-Barr virus in situ. *(Custom Medical Stock Photo. Reproduced by permission.)*

Center for Disease Control (CDC) estimates that 95% of adult Americans between the ages of 35 and 40 years have been infected with EBV, but it is less prevalent in children and teenagers. This pattern of infecting adults more than children persists throughout other prosperous Western countries, but does not hold true in underdeveloped regions such as Africa and Asia. In Africa, most children have been infected by EBV by the age of three years.

About 10% of cancers of the stomach are associated with EBV. The reason for this association is not known as of 2009.

Nasopharyngeal **cancer** is uncommon in the West but more prevalent in the Far East. It affects three times as many men as women, and usually occurs in adults between the ages of 40 and 50 years. This type of cancer is diagnosed in fewer than 1 in every 100,000 Caucasians but in 10–53 persons per 100,000 in mainland China, Taiwan, Hong Kong, and Malaysia. It also occurs more frequently in Eskimos in Greenland and Alaska, and in Tunisians, with about 20 cases per 100,000 people per year. The prevalence rate for adults of Asian descent in the United States is 3–4.2 cases per 100,000 persons per year. Nasopharyngeal cancer accounts for less than 1% of malignancies in children. It affects 1 in every 100,000 children in North America and Europe each year, but between 8 and 25 of every 100,000 children in Asia.

Description

Herpesviruses have long been known. The name actually comes from the Greek adjective *herpestes*, which means creeping. Many herpesvirus species appear to establish a lifelong presence in the human body, remaining dormant for long periods and becoming active for some, often inexplicable, reason. EBV is only one of several members of the Herpesvirus family that have similar traits. Others include varicella zoster virus—the cause of both chickenpox and shingles—, and the **herpes simplex** virus responsible for both cold sores and genital herpes. EBV is usually transmitted through saliva but not blood, and is not normally an airborne **infection**.

Individuals with EBV infections typically show some elevation in the white blood cell count and a noticeable increase in lymphocytes—white blood cells associated with the **immune response** of the body. IM is a time-limited infection that usually lasts from one to two months. Symptoms include **fever**, malaise, sore throat, swollen glands and (sometimes) swollen spleen and/or liver.

EBV infections that lead to Burkitt's lymphoma in Africa typically affect the jaw and mouth area, while the (very rare) incidences of Burkitt's lymphoma found in developed countries are more apt to manifest tumors in the abdominal region, most commonly in the intestines, kidneys, or ovaries.

Causes and symptoms

EBV and mononucleosis

EBV is normally transmitted by contact with the saliva of an infected person; it is not ordinarily transmitted through the air. The virus takes about 4 to 6 weeks to incubate, and thus infected persons can spread the disease to others over a period of several weeks. After entering the patient's mouth and upper throat, the virus infects B cells, which are a certain type of white blood cell produced in the bone marrow. The infected B cells are then carried into the lymphatic system, where they affect the liver and spleen and cause the lymph nodes to swell and enlarge. The infected B cells are also responsible for the fever, swelling of the tonsils, and sore throat that characterize mononucleosis.

Most people who become infected with EBV do not have any symptoms, however. In children, EBV infection is usually asymptomatic; when it does cause symptoms, they are difficult to distinguish from routine mild childhood infections. Teenagers who were not exposed to EBV in childhood have a 35–50% chance of developing infectious mononucleosis (IM) from EBV. The most common symptoms of IM in teenagers are fever, sore throat, and swollen lymph glands. The patient may also have an enlarged spleen and liver.

After the symptoms of mononucleosis go away, the EBV virus remains in a few cells in the patient's throat tissues or blood for the rest of the person's life. The virus occasionally reactivates and may appear in samples of the person's saliva, but it does not cause new symptoms of illness. EBV infection does not cause any problems during pregnancy, such as miscarriages or birth defects.

EBV and cancer

EBV has been linked to IM in the Western world for decades. It has also become associated consistently with nasopharyngeal cancers in Asia (especially China) and Burkitt's lymphoma in Africa and Papua New Guinea. According to the CDC, EBV is not the sole cause of these two malignancies, but does play an important role in the development of both cancers. The mechanism that allows Epstein-Barr virus to at least help in producing such diverse illnesses in diverse regions of the world has been the subject of increasing research and scrutiny. One theory regarding the higher rate of nasopharyngeal cancer in Asia is that EBV interacts with chemicals called nitrosamines, used in the preparation of salted fish and other preserved foods popular in the region, to trigger changes in cells that lead to cancer.

It is known that EBV is one of the herpesviruses that remain in the human body for life. Under certain, still not-understood conditions, it alters white blood cells normally associated with the immune system, changing the B cells (white blood cells normally associated with making antibodies), and causing them to reproduce uncontrollably. EBV can bind to these white blood cells to produce a solid mass made up of B cells—called Burkitt's lymphoma—or to the mucous membranes of the mouth and nose and cause nasopharyngeal cancer. Since Burkitt's lymphoma typically occurs in people living in moist, tropical climates, the same regions where people usually contract malaria, some doctors speculate that the immune system is altered by its response to malaria. When EBV infection occurs, the altered immune system reacts by producing a tumor.

Special concerns

Though studies about the hereditary tendency of abnormal cell development after EBV infection are incomplete, researchers have found it to be associated with abnormalities on multiple human chromosomes, including chromosomes 1, 2, 3, 4, 5, 6, 8, 9, 11, 13, 14, 15, 16, 17, 22, and the X chromosome.

Diagnosis

The diagnosis of mononucleosis caused by EBV is usually based on the results of blood tests combined with the doctor's examination of the patient's throat and neck. The doctor will also tap on or feel the patient's abdomen to see whether the liver and spleen have become enlarged.

A patient infected by EBV will have an increased number of white blood cells in the blood sample, an increased number of abnormal white blood cells, and antibodies to the Epstein-Barr virus. These antibodies can be detected by a test called the monospot test, which gives results within a day but may not be accurate during the first week of the patient's illness. Another type of blood test for EBV antibodies takes longer to perform but gives more accurate results within the first week of symptoms.

Treatment

Traditional

Drugs

Because EBV infections are viral in origin, **antibiotics** are ineffective against them. Much research is geared toward the development of a **vaccines** effective against both the virus and cancer.

Treatment for mononucleosis caused by EBV consists of self-care at home until the symptoms go away. Patients should rest in bed if possible and drink plenty of fluids. Nonaspirin pain relievers like Advil or Tylenol can be taken to bring down the fever and relieve muscle aches and pains. Throat lozenges or gargling with warm salt water may help ease the discomfort of a sore throat.

Because mononucleosis can affect the spleen, patients should avoid vigorous exercise or contact sports for at least one month after the onset of symptoms or until the spleen returns to its normal size. This precaution will lower the risk of rupture of the spleen.

With regard to cancers associated with EBV, such **anticancer drugs** as **cyclophosphamide** or **radiation therapy** have been shown to be effective against Burkitt's lymphoma in four out of five cases.

Alternative

The goal of alternative treatment is to lower the white blood cell count to normal levels. Treatment often includes such nutritional supplements as flaxseed oil or shark cartilage, vitamins—including **vitamins** C and K, and mineral supplements containing magnesium and potassium. Well-conducted randomized **clinical trials** have not yet been conducted to prove the efficacy of these therapies.

Prognosis

Mononucleosis caused by EBV rarely leads to serious complications. In most patients, the fever goes down in about 10 days but **fatigue** may last for several weeks or months. Some people do not feel normal again for about three months. A patient who feels sick longer than four months, however, should go back to the doctor to see whether they have another disease or disorder in addition to mononucleosis. In some cases the patient is diagnosed with chronic fatigue syndrome or CFS. The Epstein-Barr virus does not cause CFS; however, it appears to make some patients with mononucleosis more susceptible to developing chronic fatigue syndrome.

QUESTIONS TO ASK YOUR DOCTOR

- Should I be concerned about EBV infection?
- How can I tell whether I have been exposed to EBV?
- Does having mononucleosis increase a person's risk of cancer?

The prognosis for nasopharyngeal cancer associated with EBV in adults is poor, because about 60% of these cancers have already metastasized to other regions of the head and neck by the time diagnosis is made. The prognosis for this type of cancer in children is also relatively poor. The survival rates for children treated only with radiation therapy are about 45%. When **chemotherapy** and radiation therapy are used together, long-term survival rates range from 55–80%.

Prevention

As of 2009 there is no vaccine that can prevent mononucleosis caused by EBV. In addition, the fact that many people can be infected with the virus and transmit it to others without having symptoms of the disease means that mononucleosis is almost impossible to prevent. The best precautionary measure is for patients who have been diagnosed with mono to avoid kissing or other close personal contact with others, and to wash their drinking glasses, food dishes, and eating utensils separately from those of other family members or friends for several days after the fever goes down. It is not necessary for people with mono to be completely isolated from other people, however.

Because the Epstein-Barr virus remains in the body after the symptoms of mononucleosis go away, people who have had IM should not donate blood for at least 6 months after their symptoms started.

Resources

BOOKS

Gluckman, Toma R. *Herpesviridae Viral Structure, Life Cycle, and Infections.* New York: Nova Science Publishers, 2009.

Krueger, Hans, et al. *HPV and Other Infectious Agents in Cancer: Opportunities for Prevention and Public Health.* New York: Oxford University Press, 2010.

Tao, H. E., ed. *DNA Tumor Viruses.* New York: Nova Science Publishers, 2009.

PERIODICALS

Bagert, B.A. "Epstein-Barr Virus in Multiple Sclerosis." *Current Neurology and Neuroscience Reports* 9 (September 2009): 405–410.

Boysen, T., et al. " EBV-associated Gastric Carcinoma in High- and Low-incidence Areas for Nasopharyngeal Carcinoma." *British Journal of Cancer* 101 (August 4, 2009): 530–33.

Chang, C.M., et al. "The Extent of Genetic Diversity of Epstein-Barr Virus and its Geographic and Disease Patterns: A Need for Reappraisal." *Virus Research* 143 (August 2009): 209–21.

Morris, M. A., et al. "Role of the Epstein-Barr Virus-encoded Latent Membrane Protein-1, LMP1, in the Pathogenesis of Nasopharyngeal Carcinoma." *Future Oncology* 5 (August 2009): 811–25.

Oluwadara, O., and F. Chiappelli. "Biomarkers for Early Detection of High Risk Cancers: From Gliomas to Nasopharyngeal Carcinoma." *Bioinformation* 3 (April 21, 2009): 332–39.

Shinozaki, A., et al. "Epstein-Barr Virus-associated Gastric Carcinoma: A Distinct Carcinoma of Gastric Phenotype by Claudin Expression Profiling." *Journal of Histochemistry and Cytochemistry* 57 (August 2009): 775–85.

OTHER

Centers for Disease Control and Prevention (CDC). *Epstein-Barr Virus and Infectious Mononucleosis.* http://www.cdc.gov/ncidod/diseases/ebv.htm

Lin, Ho-Sheng, and Willard E. Fee, Jr. "Malignant Nasopharyngeal Tumors." *eMedicine*, December 21, 2007. http://emedicine.medscape.com/article/848163-overview

Paulino, Arnold C., and Stephan A. Grupp. "Nasopharyngeal Cancer." *eMedicine*, October 17, 2008. http://emedicine.medscape.com/article/988165-overview

National Library of Medicine Tutorial. . http://www.nlm.nih.gov/medlineplus/tutorials/epsteinbarrvirusmono/htm/index.ht

Virology Down Under. *Epstein-Barr Virus.* http://www.uq.edu.au/vdu/VDUEBV.htm

ORGANIZATIONS

American Society for Virology (ASV), asv@asv.org, http://www.asv.org/.

Centers for Disease Control and Prevention (CDC), 1600 Clifton Road, Atlanta, GA, 30333, 800-232-4636, cdcinfo@cdc.gov, http://www.cdc.gov.

International Association for Research on Epstein-Barr Virus and Related Diseases, [site hosted at Baylor College of Medicine, Houston, TX], ebv-webmaster@bcm.edu, http://www.bcm.edu/ebvassociation/index.htm.

Joan Schonbeck, RN
Rebecca J. Frey, PhD

ERCP *see* **Endoscopic retrograde cholangiopancreatography**

ERCP stenting *see* **Stenting**

Erlotinib

Definition

Erlotinib is a type of anti-cancer medication that targets part of the chemical pathway responsible for **cancer** growth. Erlotinib specifically targets a chemical receptor expressed by some cancer cells known as the epidermal growth factor receptor (EGFR).

Purpose

Erlotinib is an anti-cancer drug that is used to treat multiple types of cancer. Specifically erlotinib treats a type of lung cancer known as **non-small cell lung cancer** and **pancreatic cancer**. Erlotinib is used in non-small cell lung cancer when it has failed treatment with another agent. Erlotinib is therefore considered a second line agent in the treatment of non-small cell lung cancer. Erlotinib is a first line agent in the treatment of pancreatic cancer. Erlotinib may be used in combination with other agents to treat cancer that is locally advanced, located in a place not amenable to surgery, or metastatic. Metastatic cancer is cancer that has traveled from another part of the body and settled in a new location.

Description

Erlotinib is produced by multiple pharmaceutical companies. Both Genentech and OSI Pharmaceuticals make erlotinib in the United States. Roche produces erlotinib under the trade name Tarceva. Erlotinib specifically targets the EGFR expressed by cancer cells to prevent cancer cell growth and replication. The EGFR is a type of chemical receptor that sits on the outer membrane of both normal cells and cancer cells. Chemical receptors in the body activate a sequence of cellular events known as a chemical cascade or signaling pathway. It is these signaling pathways that are responsible for many normal body functions. Drugs or natural chemicals that bind to and activate the receptor signaling pathway are known as receptor agonists. Drugs or natural chemicals that bind to the receptor and block them from creating a signaling pathway are known as receptor antagonists, because they antagonize the effects of that receptor. EGFR are receptors bind growth factors to create signaling cascades that are a natural part of cell development and necessary for normal cell growth. The agonist that normally binds to the EGFR is epidermal growth factor. When EGF binds to the EGFR, it initiates chemical signals that tell the cell how to grow and replicate. Some cancer cells have a mutated form of

the EGFR that can be targeted by drugs that differentiate between the normal and mutated EGFR. Erlotinib antagonizes the mutant EGFR by binding and prevent the signaling pathway for growth from happening. Erlotinib mainly acts on cancer cells instead of normal cells because it targets the mutated form of the EGFR.

Studies have shown that use of erlotinib increases median survival time and progression-free survival compared to placebo in non-small cell lung cancer and compared to placebo or other agents tested in pancreatic cancer. Median survival time is a term used to describe the time from either diagnosis or treatment at which half of the patients with a given disease are expected to still be alive. The term progression-free survival describes the length of time during and after treatment in which a patient is living with a disease that does not get worse. In a clinical trial designed to test out a cancer drug in humans, both median survival time and progression-free survival are ways to measure how effective a treatment is.

Recommended dosage

Erlotinib is taken as an oral drug in pill form. Erlotinib is manufactured in 25, 100, and 150 mg tablets. The minimum effective dose is 100 mg and the maximum dose used is 150 mg per day. Erlotinib is administered once a day at least 1 hour before or 2 hours after ingestion of food. Treatment of cancer with erlotinib is continued until the cancer is shown to be progressing and nonresponsive to treatment, or until unacceptable toxicity occurs. For the second-line treatment of locally advanced or metastatic non-small cell lung cancer, the usual adult dosage is 150 mg taken once daily. In initial studies done on the effectiveness of erlotinib as a treatment for this type of cancer, therapy was given for an average of 9 to 10 weeks. For the first-line treatment of locally advanced or metastatic pancreatic cancer, the usual adult dosage is 100 mg taken once a week in combination with another chemotherapeutic called **gemcitabine**. When toxicity makes dosage adjustment necessary, erlotinib is reduced in 50 mg decrements.

Cigarette smoking reduces the exposure of the body to erlotinib therapy. Patients who medically require erlotinib treatment are advised to stop smoking. In patients who need to continue to smoke for a brief time as they address **smoking cessation**, a cautious increase in the dose level of erlotinib may be considered not exceeding 300 mg. Very careful monitoring by a specialist physician is required. The effectiveness and long-term (greater than 14 days) safety for use of this dose level have not been established in smoking patients and may be toxic in non-smoking patients.

Precautions

Erlotinib is a category D pregnancy drug. Category D pregnancy drugs are drugs for which there is evidence of human fetal risk based on data from marketing experience or studies in done in humans, but for which the potential medical benefit is great enough that it may warrant use of the drug in pregnant women despite the risks. Erlotinib use during pregnancy may result in death to the fetus. Erlotinib is only used in pregnancy if medically necessary for survival of the mother, and is not recommended for use in breastfeeding. The safety and effectiveness of erlotinib

have not been established in children younger than 18 years of age.

Erlotinib is not contraindicated for use with any disease, but may be more likely to cause toxicity in patients with certain medical conditions. Toxicity developing in certain medical conditions has proven fatal. Caution should be used if administered to patients with lung disease, liver or kidney disease, heart disease, history of stroke, or **hemolytic anemia**.

Side effects

Common side effects seen with erlotinib use include an acne-like rash, loss of appetite, **diarrhea**, **fatigue**, **nausea**, **vomiting**, infections, and abdominal pain. Erlotinib has been associated with the development of some serious side effects. Toxicity to the lungs, heart, liver, and kidney may occur. Serious or fatal exfoliative skin conditions and gastrointestinal tract conditions have occurred. Erlotinib has also been associated with serious eye inflammation, stroke, hemolytic **anemia**, severely tender or burning rash, **itching**, hair loss, and brittle loose fingernails.

Interactions

Erlotinib is metabolized by a set of liver enzymes known as cytochrome P450 (CYP-450) subtype 3A4. Drugs that induce, or activate these enzymes increase the metabolism of erlotinib. This results in lower levels of therapeutic erlotinib, thereby negatively affecting treatment of cancer. For this reason drugs that induce CYP-450 subtype 3A4 may not be used with erlotinib. This includes some anti-epileptic drugs such as **carbamazepine**, some anti-inflammatory drugs such as dexamethasone, anti-tuberculosis drugs such as rifampin, and the herb St. John's Wort.

Drugs that act to inhibit the action of CYP-450 subtype 3A4 may cause undesired increased levels of erlotinib in the body. This could lead to toxic doses. Some examples are **antibiotics** such as clarithromycin, antifungal drugs such as ketoconazole, antiviral drugs such as indinavir, antidepressants such as fluoxetine, and some cardiac agents such as verapamil. Grapefruit juice may also increase the amount of erlotinib in the body. Patients should avoid drinking grapefruit juice or eating grapefruit while taking erlotinib.

Resources

BOOKS

Goodman and Gilman's The Pharmacological Basis of Therapeutics, Eleventh Edition: McGraw Hill Medical Publishing Division, 2006.
Tarascon Pharmacopoeia Library Edition: Jones and Bartlett Publishers, 2009.

OTHER

Medscape*Erlotinib*. http://www.medscape.com.
RxList*Tarceva*. http://www.rxlist.com.

ORGANIZATIONS

National Cancer Institute. 6116 Executive Boulevard, Room 3036A, Bethesda, MD 20892-8322. (800)4-CANCER http://www.cancer.gov.
FDA U.S. Food and Drug Administration. 10903 New Hampshire Ave, Silver Spring, MD 20993. (888)INFO-FDA. http://www.fda.gov.

Maria Basile, Ph.D.

Erythropoietin

Definition

Erythropoietin, which is also referred to by the names Epogen, Procrit, epoetin alfa, and EPO, is a medicine used to treat a low red blood cell count.

Purpose

Erythropoietin is a drug approved by the Food and Drug Administration (FDA) to treat low red blood cell counts called **anemia**. This anemia can be caused by **cancerchemotherapy** treatment, kidney failure, or a drug used to treat AIDs. Erythropoietin has also been used to increase the red blood cell count in patients who are anemic and scheduled to have surgery. This can decrease the risk of needing blood transfusions.

Description

Erythropoietin is a natural substance made by the kidneys in the body. Sometimes the body cannot make enough erythropoietin to cause red blood cells to be produced. The synthetic drug erythropoietin can be given to act like the natural erythropoietin and increase red blood cells.

Chemotherapy drugs destroy cancer cells, but they also destroy normal cells in the bone marrow. Oxygen, which is needed by the body to make energy, is carried to cells by the red blood cells. The destruction of the red blood cells causes anemia, which can make patients feel tired or dizzy.

Erythropoietin acts to stimulate the bone marrow to make more red blood cells. Patients need an adequate supply of iron in the body for erythropoietin to work best. If a patient's iron is low, the doctor may recommend oral iron tablets to keep the level of iron up. The increase in red blood cell levels should be seen in two to six weeks after beginning therapy in cancer-related anemia patients. When the red blood cell count rises, patients generally feel better.

Recommended dosage

Erythropoietin is a clear, colorless liquid that must be kept refrigerated. It is administered as an intravenous injection or an injection directly underneath the skin, referred to as a subcutaneous injection. There are several dosing schedules used to treat patients with anemia.

To treat cancer-related anemia

Erythropoietin is dosed in units per kilogram of body weight, starting at 150 units per kilograms of body weight administered three times per week. This dosage can be increased to 300 units per kilogram of body weight three times per week.

Manufacturers continue to improve the effectiveness of the drug and physicians select dosage amount and frequency based on the drug type, brand, method of administration, and the individual patient's situation. Erythropoietin may be administered at a physician office or at home subcutaneously. Typically, it has been administered once a week, though in 2004, a study revealed that a form of the drug could safely be dosed every two weeks for some cancer patients, making it more convenient.

To treat patients with renal failure

Erythropoietin starting dose is 50-100 units per kilogram of body weight three times a week. This would be adjusted based on blood work and patient response.

To treat AIDS patients on the drug zidovudine

Erythropoietin starting dose is 100 units per kilogram of body weight three times per week for 8 weeks. This would be adjusted based on blood counts and patient response.

To treat patients prior to surgery

Erythropoietin starting dose is 300 units per kilogram of body weight per day for 10 days prior to surgery, the day of surgery, and four days after surgery.

An alternate schedule is erythropoietin 600 units per kilogram of body weight administered once weekly beginning three weeks before surgery, then a fourth dose on the day of surgery.

Surgery patients need to take iron replacement with the start of erythropoietin injections.

Precautions

Blood counts will be monitored before receiving erythropoietin and regularly while on the drug erythropoietin. This allows the doctor to determine if patients are candidates for this treatment and if the dose the patient is receiving needs to be increased or decreased.

Blood pressure should also be monitored regularly while on erythropoietin. Patients who have high blood pressure that is not under control should not use erythropoietin.

Patients may be instructed to take oral iron tablets while on erythropoietin to increase the drug's effectiveness.

It is not recommended to give erythropoietin to patients who have cancer, such as leukemias, arising from their bone marrow.

Patients with a known previous allergic reaction to erythropoietin or the drug albumin should tell their doctor.

Patients who may be pregnant or trying to become pregnant should tell their doctor before receiving erythropoietin.

Side effects

A common side effect due to erythropoietin administration is pain or burning at the site of the injection. This can be decreased by making sure that the erythropoietin is at room temperature before giving the **infection**. Ice can be placed in the area of injection to numb it before receiving the shot, and the site of injection should be changed with each shot.

Common side effects of patients who receive erythropoietin include **diarrhea** and swelling.

Less common side effects in cancer patients include **fever**, **nausea and vomiting**, **fatigue**, shortness of breath, and weakness.

Seizures have been reported in patients with kidney failure who are taking erythropoietin.

Erythropoietin can cause an increase in blood pressure, but this is uncommon in cancer patients. Blood pressure should be monitored while on this medicine.

Interactions

In clinical studies erythropoietin did not have any drug interactions.

In addition to taking oral iron replacement, patients should increase their intake of iron in their diet. This would include eating foods such as red meats, green vegetables, and eggs.

Patients should tell their doctors if they have a known allergic reaction to erythropoietin or any other medications or substances, such as foods and preservatives. Before taking any new medications, including nonprescription medications, **vitamins**, and herbal medications, the patients should notify their doctors.

Resources

PERIODICALS

"Studies: Aranesp Dosed Semiweekly Is Comparable to Epoetin Alfa Once a Week." *Obesity, Fitness & Wellness Week* July 10, 2004: 59.

Nancy J. Beaulieu, RPh.,BCOP
Teresa G. Odle

Esophageal cancer

Definition

Esophageal **cancer** is a malignancy that develops in tissues of the hollow, muscular canal (esophagus) along which food and liquid travel from the throat to the stomach.

Description

Esophageal cancer usually originates in the inner layers of the lining of the esophagus and grows outward. In time, the tumor can obstruct the passage of food and liquid, making swallowing painful and difficult. Since most patients are not diagnosed until the late stages of the disease, esophageal cancer is associated with poor quality of life and low survival rates.

Squamous cell **carcinoma** is the most common type of esophageal cancer, accounting for 95% of all esophageal cancers worldwide. The esophagus is normally lined with thin, flat squamous cells that resemble tiny roof shingles. Squamous cell carcinoma can develop at any point along the esophagus but is most common in the middle portion.

Adenocarcinoma has been increasing, and, among white males in the United States incidence of adenocarcinoma is almost equal to that of squamous cell carcinoma. Adenocarcinoma originates in glandular tissue not normally present in the lining of the esophagus. Before adenocarcinoma can develop, glandular cells must replace a section of squamous cells. This occurs in **Barrett's esophagus**, a precancerous condition in which chronic acid reflux from the

A close-up view of a cancerous esophageal tumor. *(Copyright S. Benjamin. Custom Medical Stock Photo. Reproduced by permission.)*

stomach stimulates a transformation in cell type in the lower portion of the esophagus.

A very small fraction of esophageal cancers are melanomas, sarcomas, or lymphomas.

Demographics

There is great variability in the incidence of esophageal cancer with regard to geography, ethnicity, and gender. The overall incidence is increasing. About 16,000 new cases of esophageal cancer are diagnosed in the United States each year. During the same 12-month period, 14,000 people die of this disease. It strikes between five and ten North Americans per 100,000. In some areas of China the cancer is endemic.

Squamous cell carcinoma usually occurs in the sixth or seventh decade of life, with a greater incidence in African-Americans than in others. Adenocarcinoma develops earlier and is much more common in white patients. In general, esophageal cancer occurs more frequently in men than in women.

Causes and symptoms

Causes

The exact cause of esophageal cancer is unknown, although many investigators believe that chronic irritation of the esophagus is a major culprit. Most of the identified risk factors represent a form of chronic irritation. However, the wide variance in the distribution of esophageal cancer among different demographic groups raises the possibility that genetic factors also play a role.

Several risk factors are associated with esophageal cancer.

- Tobacco and alcohol consumption are the major risk factors, especially for squamous cell carcinoma. Smoking and alcohol abuse each increase the risk of squamous cell carcinoma by five-fold. The effects of the two are synergistic, in that the combination of smoking and alchohol increases the risk by 25- to 100-fold. It is estimated that drinking about 13 ounces of alcohol every day for an extended period of time raises the risk of developing esophageal cancer by 18%. That likelihood increases to 44% in individuals who also smoke one or two packs of cigarettes a day. Smokeless tobacco also increases the risk for esophageal cancer.

- Gastroesophageal reflux is a condition in which acid from the stomach refluxes backwards into the lower portion of the esophagus, sometimes causing symptoms of heartburn. In some cases of gastroesophageal reflux, the chronic exposure to acid causes the inner lining of the lower esophagus to change from squamous cells to glandular cells. This is called Barrett's esophagus. Patients with Barrett's esophagus are roughly 30 to 40 times more likely than the general population to develop adenocarcinoma of the esophagus.

- A diet low in fruits, vegetables, zinc, riboflavin, and other vitamins can increase risk of developing to esophageal cancer.

- Caustic injury to the esophagus inflicted by swallowing lye or other substances that damage esophageal cells can lead to the development of squamous cell esophageal cancer in later life.

- Achalasia is a condition in which the lower esophageal sphincter (muscle) cannot relax enough to let food pass into the stomach. Squamous cell esophageal cancer develops in about 6% of patients with achalasia.

- Tylosis is a rare inherited disease characterized by excess skin on the palms and soles. Affected patients have a much higher probability of developing esophageal cancer than the general population. They should have regular screenings to detect the disease in its early, most curable stages.

- Esophageal webs, which are protrusions of tissue into the esophagus, and diverticula, which are outpouchings of the wall of the esophagus, are associated with a higher incidence of esophageal cancer.

Symptoms

Unfortunately, symptoms generally don't appear until the tumor has grown so large that the patient cannot be cured. Dysphagia (trouble swallowing or a sensation of having food stuck in the throat or chest) is the most common symptom. Swallowing problems may occur occasionally at first, and patients often react by eating more slowly and chewing their food more carefully and, as the tumor grows, switching to soft foods or a liquid diet. Without treatment, the tumor will eventually prevent even liquid from passing into the stomach. A sensation of burning or slight mid-chest pressure is a rare, often-disregarded symptom of esophageal cancer. Painful swallowing is usually a symptom of a large tumor obstructing the opening of the esophagus. It can lead to regurgitation of food, **weight loss**, physical wasting, and malnutrition. Anyone who has trouble swallowing, loses a significant amount of weight without dieting, or cannot eat solid food because it is too painful to swallow should see a doctor.

Diagnosis

A barium swallow is usually the first test performed on a patient whose symptoms suggest esophageal cancer. After the patient swallows a small amount of barium, a series of **x rays** can highlight any bumps or flat raised areas on the normally smooth surface of the esophageal wall. It can also detect large, irregular areas that narrow the esophagus in patients with advanced cancer, but it cannot provide information about disease that has spread beyond the esophagus. A double contrast study is a barium swallow with air blown into the esophagus to improve the way the barium coats the esophageal lining. Endoscopy is a diagnostic procedure in which a thin lighted tube (endoscope) is passed through the mouth, down the throat, and into the esophagus. Cells that appear abnormal are removed for **biopsy**. Once a diagnosis of esophageal cancer has been confirmed through biopsy, staging tests are performed to determine whether the disease has spread (metastasized) to tissues or organs near the original tumor or in other parts of the body. These tests may include **computed tomography**, endoscopic ultrasound, **thoracoscopy**, **laparoscopy**, and **positron emission tomography**.

Treatment team

The treatment team includes the surgeon, radiologist, radiation therapist, and oncologist. Nutrition therapists are also vital in optimizing a diet that the patient can swallow easily.

Clinical staging, treatments, and prognosis

Staging

Stage 0 is the earliest stage of the disease. Cancer cells are confined to the innermost lining of the esophagus. Stage I esophageal cancer has spread slightly deeper, but still has not extended to nearby tissues, lymph nodes, or other organs. In Stage IIA, cancer has invaded the thick, muscular layer of the esophagus that propels food into the stomach and may involve connective tissue covering the outside of the esophagus. In Stage IIB, cancer has spread to lymph nodes near the esophagus and may have invaded deeper layers of esophageal tissue. Stage III esophageal cancer has spread to tissues or lymph nodes near the esophagus or to the trachea (windpipe) or other organs near the esophagus. Stage IV cancer has spread to distant organs like the liver, bones, and brain. Recurrent esophageal cancer is disease that develops in the esophagus or another part of the body after initial treatment.

Treatment

Treatment for esophageal cancer is determined by the stage of the disease and the patient's general health. The most important distinction to make is whether the cancer is curable. If the cancer is in the early stages, cure may be possible. If the cancer is advanced or if the patient will not tolerate major surgery, treatment is usually directed at palliation (relief of symptoms only) instead of cure.

SURGERY. The most common operations for the treatment of esophageal cancer are esophagectomy and **esophagogastrectomy**. Esophagectomy is the removal of the cancerous part of the esophagus and nearby lymph nodes. This procedure is performed only on patients with very early cancer that has not spread to the stomach. Esophagogastrectomy is the removal of the cancerous part of the esophagus, nearby lymph nodes, and the upper part of the stomach. The resected esophagus is replaced with the stomach or parts of intestine so the patient can swallow. These procedures can significantly relieve symptoms and improve the nutritional status of more than 80% of patients with dysphagia. Although surgery can cure some patients whose disease has not spread beyond the esophagus, but more than 75% of esophageal cancers have spread to other organs before being diagnosed. Less extensive surgical procedures can be used for palliation.

CHEMOTHERAPY. Oral or intravenous **chemotherapy** alone will not cure esophageal cancer, but pre-operative treatments can shrink tumors and increase the probability that cancer can be surgically eradicated. Palliative chemotherapy can relieve symptoms of advanced cancer but will not alter the outcome of the disease.

RADIATION. External beam or internal radiation, delivered by machine or implanted near cancer cells inside the body, is only rarely used as the primary form of treatment. Post-operative radiation is sometimes used to kill cancer cells that couldn't be surgically removed. Palliative radiation is effective in relieving dysphagia in patients who cannot be cured. However, radiation is most useful when combined with chemotherapy as either the definitive treatment or preoperative treatment.

Palliation

In addition to surgery, chemotherapy, and radiation, other palliative measures can provide symptomatic relief. Dilatation of the narrowed portion of the esophagus with soft tubes can provide short-term relief of dysphagia. Placement of a flexible, self-expanding stent within the narrowed portion is also useful in allowing more food intake.

Follow-up treatments

Regular barium swallows and other **imaging studies** are necessary to detect recurrence or spread of disease or new tumor development.

Prognosis

Since most patients are diagnosed when the cancer has spread to lymph nodes or other structures, the prognosis for esophageal cancer is poor. Generally, no more than half of all patients are candidates for curative treatment. Even if cure is attempted, the cancer can recur.

Alternative and complementary therapies

Photodynamic therapy (PDT) involves intravenously injecting a drug that is absorbed by cancer cells and kills them after they are exposed to specific laser beams. PDT can be used for palliation, but it also cured some early esophageal cancers during preliminary studies. Researchers are comparing its benefits with those of more established therapies.

Endoscopic laser therapy involves delivering short, powerful laser treatments to the tumor through an endoscope. It can improve dysphagia, but multiple treatments are required, and the benefit is seldom long-lasting.

Coping with cancer treatment

Many cancer patients have found it helpful to discuss cancer and treatment with other cancer patients and survivors in support groups. Guidance from a nutritionist may be helpful to maintain a balanced diet and to ensure that the patient is receiving adequate **nutritional support**. The hospital staff and treatment team may be valuable resources for locating support groups and other community resources.

Clinical trials

Researchers are searching more effective chemotherapeutic agents and radiation treatment regimens. Many studies are aimed at defining the most beneficial combination of surgery, chemotherapy, and radiation in the treatment of esophageal cancer.

Prevention

There is no known way to prevent esophageal cancer.

Resources

BOOKS

Heitmiller, Richard F., Arlene A. Forastiere, and Lawrence R. Kleinberg. "Esophagus." In *Clinical Oncology*, edited by Martin D. Abeloff, 2nd ed. New York: Churchill Livingstone, 2000, pp.1517–1539.
Zwischenberger, Joseph B., Scott K. Alpard, and Mark B. Orringer. "Esophageal Cancer." In *Sabiston Textbook of Surgery*, edited by Courtney Townsend Jr. 16th ed. Philadelphia: W.B. Saunders Company, 2001, pp.731–749.

ORGANIZATIONS

American Cancer Society. "Esophageal Cancer.". [cited July 6, 2001]. http://www3.cancer.org.
National Coalition for Cancer Survivorship. 1010 Wayne Avenue, 5th Floor, Suite 300, Silver Spring, MD 20910. Telephone: 1-888-650-9127.

Maureen Haggerty
Kevin O. Hwang, M.D.

Esophageal resection

Definition

An esophageal resection is the surgical removal of the esophagus, nearby lymph nodes, and sometimes a portion of the stomach. The esophagus is a hollow muscular tube that passes through the chest from the mouth to the stomach—a "foodpipe" that carries food and liquids to the stomach for digestion and nutrition. Removal of the esophagus requires reconnecting the remaining part of the esophagus to the stomach to allow swallowing and the continuing passage of food. Part of the stomach or intestine may be used to make this connection. Several surgical techniques and approaches (ways to enter the body) are used, depending on how much or which part of the esophagus needs to be removed; whether or not part of the stomach will be removed; the patient's overall condition; and the surgeon's preference.

There are two basic esophageal resection surgeries. Esophagectomy is the surgical removal of the esophagus or a cancerous (malignant) portion of the esophagus and nearby lymph nodes. **Esophagogastrectomy** is the surgical removal of the lower esophagus and the upper part of the stomach that connects to the esophagus, performed when **cancer** has been found in both organs. Lymph nodes in the surrounding area are also removed.

An esophageal resection may be performed in combination with pre- and postoperative radiation and **chemotherapy** (chemoradiation).

Purpose

An esophagectomy is most often performed to treat early-stage cancer of the esophagus before the cancer has spread (metastasized) to the stomach or other organs. Esophagectomy is also a treatment for esophageal dysplasia (Barrett's esophagus), which is a precancerous condition of the cells in the lining of the esophagus. Lymph nodes are removed to be tested for the presence of cancer cells, which helps to determine if the cancer is spreading. Esophagectomy is also recommended when irreversible damage has occurred as a result of traumatic injury to the esophagus; swallowing of caustic (cell-damaging) agents; chronic inflammation; and complex motility (muscle movement) disorders that interfere with the passage of food to the stomach.

An esophagogastrectomy is performed when cancer of the esophagus has been shown to be spreading to nearby lymph nodes and to the stomach, creating new tumors. When cancer invades other tissues in this way, it is said to be metastatic. The goal of esophagogastrectomy is to relieve difficult or painful swallowing (dysphagia) in patients with advanced **esophageal cancer**, and to prevent or slow the spread of metastases to more distant organs such as the liver or the brain.

Demographics

The candidates for esophageal resection parallel those at high risk for esophageal cancer. Esophageal

KEY TERMS

Achalasia—Failure to relax. The term is often applied to sphincter muscles.

Adenocarcinoma—A type of cancer that develops in the esophagus near the opening into the stomach.

Anastomosis—A surgically created joining or opening between two organs or body spaces that are normally separate.

Barrett's esophagus—A potentially precancerous change in the type of cells that line the esophagus, caused by acid reflux disease.

Carcinoma—The common medical term for cancer.

Dysphagia—Difficulty and pain in swallowing.

Dysplasia—The presence of precancerous cells in body tissue.

Endoscopic ultrasound—An imaging procedure that uses high-frequency sound waves to visualize the esophagus via a lighted telescopic instrument (endoscope) and a monitor.

Esophagus—The upper portion of the digestive system, a tube that carries food and liquids from the mouth to the stomach.

Gastroesophageal reflux disease (GERD)—A condition of excess stomach acidity in which stomach acid and partially digested food flow back into the esophagus during or after eating.

Malignancy—The presence of tumor-causing cancer cells in organ tissue.

Metastasis (plural, metastases)—The spread of cancer cells from a cancerous growth or tumor into other organs of the body.

Resection—The surgical cutting and removing of a body organ, portion of an organ, or other body part.

Sphincter—A circular band of muscle fibers that constricts or closes a passageway in the body. The esophagus has sphincters at its upper and lower ends.

Squamous cell carcinoma—A type of cancer that develops in the cells in the top layer of tissue.

Thoracotomy—An open surgical procedure performed through an incision in the chest.

Thorascopy—Examination of the chest through a tiny incision using a thin, lighted tube-like instrument (thorascope).

cancer is found among middle-aged and older adults, with the average age at diagnosis between 55 and 60. Esophageal cancer and esophageal dysplasia occur far more often in men than in women. One type of esophageal cancer (squamous cell **carcinoma**) occurs more frequently in African Americans; another type (**adenocarcinoma**) is more common in Caucasian males. Caucasian and Hispanic men with a history of gastroesophageal reflux disease (GERD) are also at increased risk, because GERD has been shown to cause changes in the cells of the esophagus that may lead to cancer. Higher risks are also associated with smoking (45%), alcohol abuse (20%), and lung disorders (23%).

Description

Esophageal cancer is diagnosed in about 16,000 people annually in the United States; it is responsible for approximately 14,000 deaths each year. Although it is not as prevalent as breast and **colon cancer**, its rate of occurrence is increasing. This rise is thought to be related to an increase in gastroesophageal reflux disease, or GERD.

The esophagus has a muscular opening, or sphincter, at the entrance to the stomach, which usually keeps acid from passing upward. In people with GERD, the esophageal sphincter allows partially digested food and excess stomach acid to flow back into the esophagus. This occurrence is known as regurgitation. Regurgitation continually exposes the lining of the esophagus to large amounts of acid, causing repetitive damage to the cells of the esophageal lining. The result is Barrett's esophagus, a condition in which the normal cells (squamous cells) of the esophageal lining are replaced by the glandular type of cells that normally line the stomach. Glandular cells are more resistant to acid damage but at the same time, they can more readily develop into cancer cells. Studies at New York's Memorial Sloan-Kettering Hospital have shown that only 30% of people diagnosed with Barrett's esophagus will later be diagnosed with cancer; the other 70% will not develop dysplasia, the precancerous condition. Effective medical treatment of acid reflux is thought to be a factor in the low incidence of cancer in people with Barrett's esophagus. Other types of cancer can also occur in the esophagus, including **melanoma**, **sarcoma**, and **lymphoma**.

The risk factors for esophageal cancer include:

- Use of tobacco. The highest risk for esophageal cancer is the combination of smoking and heavy alcohol use.

- Abuse of alcohol.
- Barrett's esophagus as a result of long-term acid reflux disease.
- A low-fiber diet; that is, a diet that is low in fruits and vegetables, and whole grains that retain their outer bran layer. Other dietary risk factors include vitamin and mineral deficiencies, such as low levels of zinc and riboflavin.
- Accidental swallowing of cleaning liquids or other caustic substances in childhood.
- Achalasia. Achalasia is an impaired functioning of the sphincter muscle between the esophagus and the stomach.
- Esophageal webs. These are bands of abnormal tissue in the esophagus that make it difficult to swallow.
- A rare inherited disease called tylosis, in which excess layers of skin grow on the hands and the soles of the feet. People with this condition are almost certain to develop esophageal cancer.

Cancer of the esophagus begins in the inner layers of the tissue that lines the passageway and grows outward. Cancer of the top layer of the esophageal lining is called squamous cell carcinoma; it can occur anywhere along the esophagus, but appears most often in the middle and upper portions. It can spread extensively within the esophagus, requiring the surgical removal of large parts of the esophagus. Adenocarcinoma is the type of cancer that develops in the lower end of the esophagus near the stomach. Both types of cancer may develop in people with Barrett's esophagus. Prior to 1985, squamous cell carcinoma was the most common type of esophageal cancer, but adenocarcinoma of the esophagus and the upper part of the stomach is increasing more rapidly than any other type of cancer in the United States. Up to 83% of patients undergoing esophagectomy have been shown to have adenocarcinoma. This development may be related to such changes in risk factors as decreased smoking and alcohol use as well as increased reflux disease. People at high risk for esophageal cancer should be examined and tested regularly for changes in cell types.

Esophageal cancer is classified in six stages determined by laboratory examination of tissue cells from the esophagus, nearby lymph nodes, and stomach. The six stages are:

- Stage 0. This is the earliest stage of esophageal cancer, in which cancer cells are present only in the innermost lining of the esophagus.
- Stage I. The cancer has spread to deeper layers of cells but has not spread into nearby lymph nodes or organs.
- Stage IIA. The cancer has invaded the muscular layer of the esophageal walls, sometimes as far as the outer wall.
- Stage IIB. The cancer has invaded the lymph nodes near the esophagus and has probably spread into deeper layers of tissue.
- Stage III. Cancer is present in the tissues or lymph nodes near the esophagus, especially in the trachea (windpipe) or stomach.
- Stage IV. The cancer has spread to more distant organs, such as the liver or brain.

Unfortunately, the symptoms of esophageal cancer usually don't appear until the disease has progressed beyond the early stages and is already metastatic. Without early diagnostic screening, patients may wait to consult a doctor only when there is little opportunity for cure. The symptoms of esophageal cancer may include difficulty swallowing or painful swallowing; unexplained **weight loss**; hiccups; pressure or burning in the chest; hoarseness; lung disorders; or **pneumonia**.

The decision to perform an esophageal resection will be made when staging tests have confirmed the presence of cancer and its stage. Two-thirds of people who undergo endoscopy, a close examination of the inside lining of the esophagus, and biopsies (testing esophageal tissue cells) will already have cancer, which can progress rapidly. Some will be treated with surgery and others with medical therapy, depending on the stage of the cancer, the patient's general health status, and the degree of risk. Removing the esophagus or the affected portion is the most common treatment for esophageal cancer; it can cure the disease if the cancer is in the early stages and the patient is healthy enough to undergo the stressful surgery. Esophagectomy will be recommended if early-stage cancer or a precancerous condition has been confirmed through extensive diagnostic testing and staging. Esophagectomy is not an option if the cancer has already spread to the stomach. In this case an esophagogastrectomy will usually be performed to remove the cancerous part of the esophagus and the upper part of the stomach.

Esophagectomy

An esophagectomy takes about six hours to perform. The patient will be given general anesthesia, keeping him or her unconscious and free of pain during surgery. One of several approaches or incisional strategies will be used, chosen by the surgeon to gain adequate access to the upper abdomen and remove the esophagus or the tumor and the nearby lymph nodes. The four common incisional approaches are: transthoracic, which involves a chest incision; Ivor-Lewis, a side entry through the fifth rib; three-hole esophagectomy, which uses small incisions in the chest and abdomen to accommodate the use of instruments; and transhiatal, which involves a mid-abdominal incision. The approach chosen depends on the extent of the cancer, the location of the tumor or obstruction, and the overall condition of the patient.

In a minimum-access laparoscopic and thorascopic procedure, the surgeon makes several small incisions on the chest and abdomen through which he or she can insert thin telescopic instruments with light sources. The abdomen will be inflated with gas to enlarge the abdominal cavity and give the surgeon a better view of the procedure. First, the camera-tipped laparoscope will be inserted through one small incision, allowing images of the organs in the abdominal area to be displayed on a video monitor in the operating room. If the surgeon is going to use a portion of the stomach to replace the resected esophagus, he or she will first locate the fundus, or upper portion of the stomach. The fundus will be manipulated, stapled off, and removed laparoscopically, to be sutured in place (gastroplasty) as a replacement esophagus.

Next, the surgeon will pass thorascopic instruments into the chest through another incision. The esophagus or cancerous portion of the esophagus will be visualized, manipulated, cut and removed. Lymph nodes in the area will also be removed. Then the surgeon will either pull up a portion of the stomach and connect it to the remaining portion of the esophagus (anastomosis), or use a piece of the stomach or intestine, usually the colon, to reconstruct the esophagus. Either procedure will allow the patient to swallow and pass food and liquid to the stomach after recovery. As discussed above, other approaches may be used to gain access to the affected portion of the esophagus.

There are several variations of an esophagectomy, including:

- Standard open esophagectomy. This technique requires larger incisions to be made in the chest (thoracotomy) and in the abdomen so that the surgeon can dissect the esophagus or cancerous portion and remove it along with the nearby lymph nodes. The esophagus can then be reconnected to the stomach using a portion of either the stomach or the colon.

- Laparoscopic esophagectomy. This is a less invasive technique performed through several small incisions on the chest and abdomen with the camera-tipped laparoscope and a video monitor to guide removal of

the esophagus or tumor along with nearby lymph glands.

- Vagal-sparing esophagectomy. This procedure preserves the branches of the vagus nerve that supply the stomach, with only minimal alteration of the size of the stomach and the nerves that control acid production and digestive functions.

Esophagogastrectomy

An esophagogastrectomy is also major surgery performed with the patient under general anesthesia. The surgeon will choose the incisional approach that allows the best possible access for resecting the lower portion of the esophagus and the upper portion of the stomach. The surgeon's decision will depend on the extent of the cancer, the amount of the esophagus that must be removed, and the patient's overall health status. An esophagogastrectomy can be performed as an open procedure through large incisions, or as a laparoscopic procedure through small incisions.

In a minimum-access laparoscopic procedure, several small incisions are made in the patient's abdomen. A laparoscope will be inserted through one small incision, allowing images of the abdominal organs to be displayed on a video monitor. As in an esophagectomy, gas may be used to inflate the abdominal cavity for better viewing and space for the surgeon to maneuver. The cancerous upper portion of the stomach will first be stapled off and resected. The cancerous portion of the esophagus will then be cut and removed along with nearby lymph nodes. Finally, a portion of the stomach will be pulled upward and connected to the remaining portion of the esophagus (anastomosis); or, if most of the esophagus has been removed, a piece of the colon will be used to construct a new esophagus. Sometimes the surgeon must make an incision in the neck in order to gain access to and resect the upper portion of the esophagus, followed by making an anastomosis between the esophagus and a portion of the stomach.

Diagnosis/Preparation

Diagnosis

The diagnosis of esophageal cancer begins with a careful history and a review of symptoms, and involves a number of different diagnostic examinations. An esophagoscopy may be performed in the doctor's office, allowing the doctor to examine the inside of the esophagus with a lighted telescopic tube (esophagoscope). A barium swallow is another common **screening test**, performed in the radiology (x-ray) department of the hospital or in a private radiology office. In a barium swallow, the patient drinks a small amount of radiopaque (visible on x ray) barium that will highlight any raised areas on the wall of the esophagus when chest **x rays** are taken. The x-ray studies will reveal irregular patches that may be early cancer or larger irregular areas that may narrow the esophagus and could represent a more advanced stage of cancer. If either of these conditions is present, the doctors will want to confirm the diagnosis of esophageal cancer; determine how far it has invaded the walls of the esophagus; and whether it has spread to nearby lymph nodes or organs. This staging process is essential in order to determine the best treatment for the patient.

One staging technique is a diagnostic procedure called endoscopic ultrasound. The doctor will thread an endoscope, which is a tiny lighted tube with a small ultrasound probe at its tip, into the patient's mouth and down into the esophagus. This procedure allows the inside of the esophagus to be viewed on a monitor to show how far a tumor has invaded the walls of the esophagus. At the same time, the doctor can perform biopsies of esophageal tissue by cutting and removing small pieces for microscopic examination of the cells for cancer staging. Staging tests may also include **computed tomography** (CT scans); thorascopic and laparoscopic examinations of the chest and abdomen; and **positron emission tomography** (PET).

Preparation

The patient will be admitted to the hospital on the day of the operation or the day before, and will be taken to a preoperative nursing unit. The surgeon and anesthesiologist will visit the patient to describe the resection procedure and answer any questions that the patient may have. The standard preoperative blood and urine tests will be performed. Intravenous lines (IV) will be inserted in the patient's vein for the administration of fluids and pain medications during and after the surgery. Sedatives may be given before the patient is taken to the operating room.

Aftercare

Immediately after surgery the patient will be taken to a recovery area where the pulse, body temperature, and heart, lung, and kidney function will be monitored. Several hours later, the patient will be transferred to a concentrated care area. Surgical wound dressings will be kept clean and dry. Pain medication will be given as needed. A chest tube inserted during surgery will be checked for drainage and removed when the drainage stops. A nasogastric (nose to stomach) tube, also placed during surgery, will be used to drain stomach secretions. Nurses will check it

regularly and rinse it out. It will eventually be removed by the surgeon. Until the patient is able to swallow soft foods, he or she will be fed intravenously or through a feeding tube that was placed in the small intestine during surgery. Patients will be encouraged to cough and to breathe deeply after surgery to fully expand the lungs and help prevent **infection** and collapse of the lungs. Walking and movement will also be encouraged to promote a quicker recovery.

About 10–14 days after the surgery, the patient will be given another barium swallow so that the doctor can examine the esophagus for any areas of leaking fluid. If none are seen, the nasogastric tube can be removed. The patient can then begin to sip clear liquids, followed gradually by small amounts of soft foods. Patients being treated for esophageal cancer may begin chemotherapy (cytotoxic or cell-killing medications), **radiation therapy**, or both, before or soon after discharge from the hospital. Patients typically remain in the hospital as long as two weeks after surgery if no complications have occurred.

When the patient goes home, any remaining bandages must be kept clean and dry. Frequent walking and gentle exercise are encouraged. Because laparoscopic and thorascopic surgery is less invasive and uses only small incisions, there is less trauma to the body and activity can be resumed more quickly than with open procedures that require larger incisions. The patient should report any **fever** or chills, persistent pain, or incision drainage to the surgeon. The patient's diet will typically be restricted for a while to soft foods and small portions; a normal diet can be resumed in about a month, but with smaller quantities. Patients are advised not to drive if they are still taking prescribed narcotic pain medications. Daily care and assistance at home is recommended during the recuperation period. Regular medical care and periodic diagnostic testing, such as endoscopic ultrasound, is essential to monitor the condition of the esophagus and to detect recurrence of the cancer or the development of new tumors.

Risks

One of the primary risks associated with esophageal resection surgeries is leakage at the site of the anastomosis, where a new feeding tube was sutured (stitched) to the remaining esophagus. As many as 9% of all patients have been reported to develop leaks, most occurring when a portion of the stomach rather than the colon was used to construct the new section of the esophagus.

Other risks include:

- formation of blood clots that can travel to the heart, lungs, or brain

- nerve injury, which can cause defective emptying of the stomach
- infection
- breathing difficulties and pneumonia
- adverse reactions to anesthesia
- narrowing of the remaining esophagus (strictures), which may cause swallowing problems
- increased acid reflux and heartburn as a result of injury to or removal of the esophageal sphincter

Normal results

Esophageal resection, especially esophagectomy, can be curative if cancer has not spread beyond the esophagus. About 75% of patients undergoing esophagectomy will be found to have metastatic disease that has already spread to other organs. Esophagectomy will reduce symptoms in most patients, especially swallowing difficulties, which will improve the patient's nutritional status as well. Patients whose esophagectomy is preceded and followed by a combination of chemotherapy and radiation treatments have longer periods of survival.

The typical result of an esophagogastrectomy is palliation, which is the relief of symptoms without a cure. Because esophagogastrecomy is always performed when metastases have already been found elsewhere in the body, the procedure may relieve pain and difficulty in swallowing, and may delay the spread of the cancer to the liver and brain. Cure of the disease, however, is not an expectation.

Patients having less invasive laparoscopic and thorascopic resection procedures will experience less pain and fewer complications than patients undergoing open procedures.

Morbidity and mortality rates

Because 75% of all esophagectomy patients and 100% of all esophagogastrectomy patients will have metastatic disease, morbidity and mortality rates for these procedures are high. Thirty-day mortality for esophagectomy ranges from 6–12%; it is 10% or higher for esophagogastrectomy. Survival of early-stage cancer patients after esophagectomy ranges from 17 to 34 months if surgery alone is the treatment. The mortality rate for early-stage cancer patients having esophagectomy alone is higher than when surgery is combined with pre- and postoperative chemoradiation. The three-year survival rate for early-stage cancer patients who received pre- and post-esophagectomy chemoradiation is about 63%. Better staging techniques, more careful selection of patients, and improved surgical techniques

WHO PERFORMS THE SURGERY AND WHERE IS IT PERFORMED?

Esophageal resection surgeries are performed in a hospital or medical center operating room by a general surgeon or a thoracic surgeon.

QUESTIONS TO ASK THE DOCTOR

- Why do I need this surgery?
- How will the surgery be performed? How long will it take?
- How many times have you performed this procedure? How often is it performed in this hospital?
- How much discomfort can I expect in the short term? Over the long term?
- Will this surgery cure my cancer? Will it allow me to live longer?
- What are the chances that the cancer will come back?
- What are my options if I don't have the surgery?
- What are the risks involved in having this surgery?
- What kind of care will I need at home afterward?
- How quickly will I recover?

are also believed to be responsible for the increase in postoperative survival rates. Recurrence of cancer in esophagectomy patients has been shown to be about 43%. A higher percentage of patients undergoing esophageal resections survive beyond the 30-day postoperative period in hospitals where the surgeons perform these procedures on a regular basis.

Alternatives

People with Barrett's esophagus can be treated with medicine and dietary changes to reduce acid reflux disease. These nonsurgical approaches are effective in relieving heartburn, calming inflamed tissues, and preventing further cell changes.

Fundoplication, or anti-reflux surgery, can strengthen the barrier to acid regurgitation when the lower esophageal sphincter does not work properly, curing GERD and reducing the exposure of the esophagus to excessive amounts of acid.

Photodynamic therapy (PDT) is the injection of a cytotoxic (cell killing) drug in conjunction with laser treatments, delivering benefits comparable to more established treatments. Endoscopic laser treatments that deliver short, powerful laser beams to the tumor through an endoscope can improve swallowing difficulties; however, multiple treatments are required and the benefits are neither long-lasting nor shown to prevent cancer.

Resources

BOOKS

American Cancer Society. *The American Cancer Society's Complementary and Alternative Cancer Methods Handbook.* Atlanta, GA: American Cancer Society, 2002.

Harpham, Wendy S., MD. *Diagnosis Cancer: Your Guide Through the First Few Months.* New York: W. W. Norton, Inc., 1998.

Heitmiller, R. F., et al. "Esophagus," in Martin D. Abeloff, ed., *Clinical Oncology*, 2nd ed. New York: Churchill Livingstone, 2000.

ORGANIZATIONS

American Cancer Society. 1599 Clifton Road NE, Atlanta, GA 30329. (800)ACS-2345. www.cancer.org.

American Gastroenterological Association. 4930 Del Ray Avenue, Bethesda, MD 20814. (301) 654-2055. www.gastro.org.

OTHER

Ferguson, Mark, MD. *Esophageal Cancer.* Society of Thoracic Surgeons. www.sts.org/doc4121.

National Cancer Institute (NCI). *General Information About Esophageal Cancer.* Bethesda, MD: NCI, 2003.

L. Lee Culvert

Esophagogastrectomy

Definition

Esophagogastrectomy is a surgical procedure in which a section of diseased esophagus is removed, along with part of the stomach and neighboring lymph nodes. The remaining piece of the esophagus is then reattached to the remaining stomach.

Purpose

Esophagogastrectomy is performed to treat **cancer** of the esophagus. There are two types of **esophageal cancer**: squamous cell and **adenocarcinoma**. Squamous

cell cancer of the esophagus used to be the most common type, but now is only responsible for fewer than 50% of cases of esophageal cancer. Squamous cell cancer occurs when the cells of the esophageal lining convert into malignant cells. This type of esophageal cancer is more common in white patients. Adenocarcinoma of the esophagus often follows a condition called Barrett's esophagus, in which the lower cells of the esophagus convert into cells resembling the glandular cells of the stomach. Over time, these abnormal Barrett's cells have the potential of converting into truly malignant cells. Adenocarcinoma of the esophagus is the more common type of esophageal cancer in African-American patients.

Men are three to four times more likely to develop esophageal cancer than are women, and African-Americans are about 50% more likely to develop the condition. According to the American Cancer Society, about 16,470 new cases of esophageal cancer will be diagnosed in the United States in 2009, and the disease will be responsible for about 14,530 deaths. The disease is much more common in other countries, such as Iran, northern China, India, and southern Africa, where rates are between ten and 100 times as high as they are in the United States. Still, esophageal cancer rates among white men in Western countries are increasing steadily, at a rate of about 2% per year; the rate has held steady among white women. Among patients diagnosed at all stages of esophageal cancer, five-year survival rates are about 18% in white patients and 11% in African-American patients.

Precautions

Patients who are taking blood thinners, aspirin, or nonsteroidal anti-inflammatory medications may need to discontinue their use in advance of the test, to avoid increasing the risk of bleeding.

Description

Patients undergoing esophagogastrectomy require general anesthesia. This will be administered in the form of intravenous medications as well as anesthetic gasses that are inhaled. The patient will be intubated for the duration of the surgery, and a ventilator will breathe for them.

Esophagogastrectomy can be achived through a traditional upper abdominal incision, or through multiple very small laparoscopic incision. Traditional open abdominal esophagogastrectomy exposes the entire upper abdomen in order to allow careful visual inspection of all the structures and lymph nodes surrounding the stomach an esophagus. Laparoscopic esophagogastrectomy involves the introduction of a scope through one of the keyhole incisions, and the use of other tiny incisions for introducing the miniature surgical instruments necessary for the operation. The exact technique utilized in the surgery will depend on where in the esophagus the cancerous segment is located, and how much of the stomach is involved. Surgical preference is to be able to preserve part of the esophagus, in order to allow it to be reconnected to the remaining stomach. In some cases, however, so much esophagus must be removed that there is not enough left to reattach to the stomach. When this occurs, a piece of intestine can be removed and used to connect the throat to the stomach. Requiring this step considerably increases the complexity and risks of the operation.

Preparations

Patients will need to stop eating and drinking for about 12-16 hours prior to their operation. The evening before the operation, a series of enemas and/or **laxatives** are used to empty the GI tract of feces. An intravenous line will be placed in order to provide the patient with fluids, general anesthesia agents, sedatives, and pain medicines during the operation. A urinary catheter will be placed in the patient's bladder. The patient will be attached to a variety of monitors to keep track of blood pressure, heart rate, and blood oxygen level throughout the procedure.

Aftercare

Esophagogastrectomy is major surgery, and often requires that the patient remain hospitalized for recuperation for as much as two weeks after the operation. Over this time, the patient's diet will slowly be reinstated, progressing gradually from liquids to soft foods to solids. Because esophageal cancer often causes symptoms of dysphagia (difficulty swallowing), a therapist specializing in re-teaching swallowing may be needed to help design a rehabilitative program.

Risks

Esophagogastrectomy carries a number of significant risks, including the general risks accompanying major surgery, such as blood clots, bleeding, heart attack, and **infection**. Specific complications that can occur with esophagogastrectomy include:

- Leakage of the new esophageal-stomach connection
- Slow stomach emptying due to surgical effects on the nerves controlling this function, sometimes resulting in chronic nausea and vomiting
- Severe heartburn if the lower part of the esophagus and upper part of the stomach are weakened by the surgery, allowing stomach contents to reflux back up into the esophagus
- Strictures or narrowing of the esophagus due to scarring from the surgery

The risk of fatal complications from esophagogastrectomy may range from about three to about seventeen percent. In general, studies have shown that hospital and surgeon experience with esophagogastrectomy reduces the risk of morbidity and mortality for patients.

Normal results

Normal results occur when the cancerous tissue is completely removed, and a patent, functional connection is created between the remaining esophageal and stomach tissue.

Abnormal results

Abnormal results range from remaining malignant tissue, to those complications detailed above, such as a leaky esophageal-stomach connection, chronic **nausea** secondary to nerve damage and slow stomach emptying, dysphagia due to strictures, etc.

Resources

BOOKS

Abeloff, M. D., et al. *Clinical Oncology,* 3rd ed. Philadelphia: Elsevier, 2004.

Goldman, L., D. Ausiello, eds. *Cecil Textbook of Internal Medicine,* 23rd ed. Philadelphia: Saunders, 2008.

Khatri, VP and JA Asensio. *Operative Surgery Manual,* 1st ed. Philadelphia: Saunders, 2003.

Rosalyn Carson-DeWitt, MD

Essiac

Definition

Essiac is a medically untested and unproven alternative treatment for **cancer**, AIDS, and other diseases. It consists of a blend of four herbs: burdock root (arctium lappa), Indian rhubarb root (rheum palmatum, sometimes known as Turkish rhubarb), sheep sorrel (rumex acetosella), and the inner bark of slippery elm (ulmus fulva or ulmus rubra).

Purpose

Essiac tea is generally used by alternative healthcare practitioners to treat various forms of cancer and

KEY TERMS

Chemotherapy—The use of chemical agents to treat or control diseases, especially cancer.

Cholesterol—A steroid alcohol found in human cells and body fluids, implicated in the onset of heart disease.

Degenerative diseases—Diseases characterized by progressive degenerative changes in tissue, including arteriosclerosis, diabetes mellitus, and osteoarthritis.

Diabetes—A degenerative disease characterized by inadequate production or absorption of insulin, excessive urine production, and excessive amounts of sugar in the blood and urine.

the side effects of conventional cancer therapy. It is also used to treat AIDS. It is used to a lesser extent to treat a variety of other medical conditions, including diabetes, skin inflammation, liver and thyroid problems, **diarrhea**, ulcers, and some other degenerative diseases. Other uses include treating pain, purifying the blood, healing wounds, lowering cholesterol, and increasing energy levels. Essiac tea is more commonly used in Canada than the United States.

Although each of the four main ingredients in essiac tea are used to treat other conditions, only the sorrel is used separately to treat cancer. Only when the four are combined do they effect anticancer properties. Alternative healthcare practitioners do not claim to know how or why the ingredients work in combination, but one idea is that they work synergistically to stimulate production of antibodies. Rene Caisse (pronounced "Reen Case", d. 1978), a Canadian nurse who ran her own clinic from 1934 to 1942, was convinced that this tea could cure cancer. She believed essiac tea purified the blood and carried away damaged tissue and **infection** related to the cancer. She also believed the tea strengthened the immune system, allowing healthy cells to destroy cancerous cells.

Caisse maintained that tumors not destroyed by essiac tea would be shrunk and could be surgically removed after six to eight weeks of treatment. To insure any malignant cells that remained after treatment and surgery were destroyed, Caisse recommended at least three months of additional weekly essiac treatments.

One of Caisse's patients was her mother, Friseide Caisse, who was diagnosed with **liver cancer** at the age of 72. Her mother's physician reportedly said she had only days to live. Rene Caisse began giving her mother

daily intramuscular injections of the tea. Friseide began recovering within a few days and after a few months, with less frequent doses of essiac, her cancer was gone. She lived to be 90, finally succumbing to heart disease.

Description

Essiac tea is based on a Canadian Ojibwa Indian formula containing primarily burdock root, Turkish rhubarb root, sheep sorrel, and the inner bark of the slippery elm. It is used in alternative medicine mainly as a treatment for cancer.

The formula, said to have been first developed by an Ojibwa healer, was intended to purify the body and balance the spirit. In 1922, the formula came to the attention of Rene Caisse (essiac is Caisse spelled backwards), a nurse in Ontario, Canada, after hearing firsthand accounts of its curative effects on cancer. She began administering the tea to cancer patients and found it to have remarkable healing abilities. Despite considerable objection from the medical profession, Caisse continued treating cancer patients with the tea until she died in 1978. In 1977, Caisse sold the essiac tea formula to the Resperin Corp. of Ontario, Canada. It is now produced generically by at least 35 companies and sold mainly in health food stores and on the Internet. It is sold as a dry mix and as a brewed liquid.

Caisse reported that hundreds of her patients had been cured of their cancers through the use of her tea, sometimes used as intramuscular injections. Most of the patients came to her after conventional cancer treatments (surgery, **chemotherapy**, and **radiation therapy**) failed. Several alternative healthcare practitioners report essiac tea seems to work best in patients who have had the least amount of radiation therapy or chemotherapy.

The mainstream medical community does not embrace essiac tea. Critics contend that a certain number of cancers deemed incurable spontaneously go into remission without adequate medical explanation. Others chalk up the successes to the so-called placebo effect, in which the belief that the treatment is working effects a cure rather than the treatment itself. The treatment is not approved by the American Medical Association or the American Cancer Society. In 2000, the U.S. Federal Trade Commission (FTC) began a crackdown on Internet distributors of essiac tea. The FTC said claims by the distributors that essiac tea cured or was an effective treatment for cancer, AIDS, and other diseases were misleading and illegal.

In 1938, a bill in the Canadian Parliament to legalize essiac tea failed by three votes. As of 2009 the tea still is not approved for marketing in the United States or Canada. However, the Canadian Health and Welfare Department permits compassionate use of essiac tea on an emergency basis.

In 1975 and again in 1982, the Memorial Sloan-Kettering Cancer Center in New York tested only the sorrel component in the tea. They boiled it, which may have neutralized any beneficial compounds in the leftover tea, and administered it to mice with cancerous tumors. It determined the formula had no anticancer effects. The National Cancer Institute and Canadian Bureau of Prescription Drugs reached the same conclusion in the 1980s.

Recommended dosage

The four main ingredients of essiac tea are sold separately and can be combined at home. Essiac tea is also marketed as tea bags and in bottles of the prepared formula. The formula is ready to use immediately. When ready, the bottle is shaken to mix the sediments. Four tsp of the essiac formula are blended with 4 tsp of warm spring water. The usual daily dosage is 2–4 oz of tea for persons weighing 100–150 pounds and 2 oz for every 50 pounds over 150 pounds. Some alternative health practitioners recommend regular doses of essiac to strengthen the immune system and as a preventative for certain diseases, including cancer. The frequency ranges from daily to weekly.

Precautions

Essiac tea is not recommended for pregnant or lactating women. The formula should not be prepared or stored in plastic or aluminum containers. Sunlight and freezing temperatures are believed to destroy the formula's effectiveness. It is generally recommended that persons consult with their physician before treating any condition with essiac. It is important to remember that essiac is often used in combination with traditional cancer treatments, such as chemotherapy, radiation, and surgery.

Side effects

No major adverse side effect have been associated with essiac tea.

Interactions

Essiac is not known to adversely interact with other medications or nutritional supplements.

Ken R. Wells

Estramustine

Definition

Estramustine is a combination of two drugs, estradiol and **mechlorethamine**, that is used to slow the growth of and kill malignant cells in **prostate cancer**. It is also known by the brand names Emcyt and Estracyte.

Purpose

Estramustine is used in the palliative treatment of metastatic or progressive **cancer** of the prostate. Palliative treatment helps to relieve symptoms, but does not cure the cancer.

In the early 2000s, estramustine was also being investigated in several **clinical trials** evaluating its usefulness in managing asymptomatic prostate cancer patients; its effectiveness in combination with **docetaxel** as an alternative to radical **prostatectomy**; and its usefulness in increasing the effectiveness of a microtubule drug in treating prostate cancer. These studies suggest that estramustine may have beneficial applications outside the field of palliative care.

Description

Estramustine is classified as an antineoplastic drug. Estramustine is a combination of two drugs: estradiol, a potent female hormone (estrogen), and mechlorethamine, a nitrogen mustard. Its action is to decrease **testosterone**, increase estrogen level, and suppress cell growth. Estramustine is approved by the United States Food and Drug Administration (FDA) for the palliative treatment of metastatic or progressive cancer of the prostate.

Recommended dosage

As with many cancer-fighting drugs, the dose of estramustine a patient receives is individualized and depends on the patient's body weight and general health, as well as what other **chemotherapy** drugs are being used. A standard dose of estramustine is 14 mg per kg of body weight per day, divided into three or four doses. This is equivalent to one 140 mg capsule for each 22 lb (10 kg) of body weight. It takes one to three months for estramustine to start to work. The therapy is continued as long as the patient has a favorable response. Some patients have successfully taken this drug for as long as three years.

Precautions

Estramustine should not be used by men who have a history of problems with blood clots, a blood clotting

KEY TERMS

Malignant—Cancerous. Cells tend to reproduce without normal controls on growth and form tumors or invade other tissues.

Metastatic—Spreading of cells from the original site of the cancer to other parts of the body where secondary tumors are formed.

Palliative—Serving to relieve or alleviate the symptoms of a disease or disorder without curing the disease.

disorder, or allergic reactions to estrogen or nitrogen mustard.

Estramustine must be taken more than one hour before or more than two hours after meals. It should not be taken with dairy products, calcium supplements, of any food that is high in calcium.

Patients taking estramustine should avoid having any vaccinations while taking the drug, and should consult their doctor immediately if exposed to chicken pox or measles, as this drug may make them more susceptible to these diseases.

Side effects

Nausea and vomiting can occur within 2 hours of taking estramustine. This side effect is mild and patients will respond to **antiemetics** to control the **nausea** and **vomiting**. **Diarrhea** and flatulence can occur while taking this drug. Patients taking estramustine also have an increased risk of developing blood clots, congestive heart failure, and heart attacks, although these side effects are rare. Therefore, men with a history of blood clots and heart disease require frequent monitoring while receiving this drug. Estramustine also decreases the glucose (sugar) tolerance in people with diabetes, and frequent blood sugar monitoring is recommended in this patient population. Blood pressure may also be increased with estramustine, and monitoring of blood pressure is recommended, especially in patients with a history of high blood pressure. Men receiving estramustine may also experience enlargement of their breasts due to the estrogen component in the drug combination. Patients may also experience decreased sexual drive, although this side effect is reversible. If sexually active, the patient should use a contraceptive method (even if he is impotent) prior to initiating therapy, because estramustine may reverse impotency while on the drug. Estramustine may also cause genetic mutations. Therefore, use of

contraceptive measures is advisable. Other side effects include lethargy, rash, **itching**, dry skin, easy bruising, flushing, and thinning hair. If any of the above side effects occur, patients should alert their physician to these side effects immdediately.

Serious side effects that require immediate medical attention include:

- sudden or severe headaches
- sudden shortness of breath or difficulty breathing
- increased weight gain or swelling of the feet or legs
- pain in the chest
- sudden pain or cramping in the legs or calves
- weakness or numbness in the legs or arms

Interactions

Dairy products and other foods containing calcium interfere with the absorption of estramustine. Prior to treatment, patients should notify their physician about any medications they are taking and of any known allergies.

Patients taking estramustine should not use tobacco products, as smoking causes the blood vessels to narrow and may increase the risk of circulation problems during treatment with estramustine..

Estramustine intensifies the effects of **vinblastine**, another anticancer drug.

Resources

PERIODICALS

Eastham, J. A., W. K. Kelly, G. D. Grossfeld, et al. "Cancer and Leukemia Group B (CALGB) 90203: A Randomized Phase 3 Study of Radical Prostatectomy Alone Versus Estramustine and Docetaxel Before Radical Prostatectomy for Patients with High-Risk Localized Disease." *Urology* 62, Supplement 1 (December 29, 2003): 55–62.

Gulley, J., and W. L. Dahut. "Novel Approaches to Treating the Asymptomatic Hormone-Refractory Prostate Cancer Patient." *Urology* 62, Supplement 1 (December 29, 2003): 147–154.

Oh, W. K. "The Evolving Role of Chemotherapy and Other Systemic Therapies for Managing Localized Prostate Cancer." *Journal of Urology* 170, 6 Part 2 (December 2003): S28–S32.

Smaletz, O., M. Galsky, H. I. Scher, et al. "Pilot Study of Epothilone B Analog (BMS-247550) and Estramustine Phosphate in Patients with Progressive Metastatic Prostate Cancer Following Castration." *Annals of Oncology* 14 (October 2003): 1518–1524.

ORGANIZATIONS

United States Food and Drug Administration (FDA). 5600 Fishers Lane, Rockville, MD 20857-0001. (888) INFO-FDA (463-6332). http://www.fda.gov.

Tish Davidson, A.M.
Rebecca J. Frey, PhD

Etidronate *see* **Bisphosphonates**

Etoposide

Definition

Etoposide is a **chemotherapy** medicine used to treat **cancer** by destroying cancerous cells. Etoposide is also sold under the brand name VePesid.

Purpose

Etoposide is approved by the Food and Drug Administration (FDA) to treat refractory **testicular cancer** and **small cell lung cancer**. It has also been useful for other types of cancer, including non-small cell cancer, leukemia (acute myeloocytic leukemia), Hodgkin's and **non-Hodgkin's lymphoma**, muscle, **brain tumors**, bladder, stomach, **Kaposi's sarcoma**, **Ewing's sarcoma**, **Wilms' tumor**, **multiple myeloma**, hepatoma, uterine **carcinoma**, myeloblastoma, **mycosis fungoides**, **neuroblastoma**, and **prostate cancer**. It is presently being studied as a treatment for lung cancer that hsa metastasized to the central nervous system.

Description

Etoposide is formulated as a clear liquid for infusion into a vein and it is also available as a pink capsule form to be taken by mouth. It may also be referred to as VP-16, VP-16-213, and epipodophyllotoxin. Etopophos is a different formulation of the intravenous form of etoposide. Etoposide was originally derived from a plant and has been made for longer than 20 years. Etoposide is a member of the group of chemotherapy drugs known as topoisomerase II inhibitors. Topoisomerase II inhibitors cause breaks in the genetic material (DNA) inside the cancer cells and prevent them from further dividing and multiplying. Then the cells die.

The oral form of etoposide is preferred for longer cycles of treatment, while the intravenous form is used primarily for short-term infusion. Studies indicate that lower doses of oral etoposide are utilized by the body more efficiently than higher doses.

Recommended dosage

An etoposide dose can be determined using a mathematical calculation that measures a person's body surface area (BSA). This number is dependent upon a patient's height and weight. The larger the person, the greater the body surface area. BSA is measured in the units known as square meter (m^2). The body surface area is calculated and then multiplied by the drug dosage in milligrams per square meter (mg/m^2). This formula is used to calculate the actual dose a patient is to receive.

To treat refractory testicular cancer

Etoposide injection dosed at the range of 50–100 mg per square meter per day given into a vein over 30–60 minutes daily for 5 consecutive days, every 3–4 weeks. This is done in combination with other chemotherapy drugs, **cisplatin** and **bleomycin**.

Etoposide can also be dosed at 100 mg per square meter per day injected into a vein over 30–60 minutes on day 1, day 3, and day 5.

To treat lung cancer

Etoposide injection dosed at the range of 35 mg per square meter per day is given into a vein infused over 30–60 minutes for 4 consecutive days. It is dosed up to 50 mg per square meter per day given into a vein infused over 30–60 minutes for 5 days in a row. This is usually in combination with other chemotherapy drugs such as cisplatin or **carboplatin**.

Etoposide phosphate formulation is dosed the same as etoposide, but administered over a shorter period of time. The formulation is often used in transplant patients because it does not need to be mixed in large amounts of intravenous fluid and can be administered over less than 30 minutes, unlike regular etoposide.

Oral etoposide 50 mg capsules for lung cancer are dosed by doubling the intravenous dose and rounding the number to the nearest 50 mg.

Patients with kidney problems may receive smaller doses of etoposide than patients with normal kidneys. The doctor will monitor a patient's kidney function prior to therapy by checking certain blood counts. Patients with liver abnormalities may also need dose adjustments of the etoposide.

Precautions

Blood counts will be monitored regularly while on etoposide therapy. During a certain time period after receiving etoposide, there is an increased risk of getting infections. Caution should be taken to avoid unnecessary exposure to crowds and people with infections.

Patients with a known previous allergic reaction to chemotherapy drugs should tell their doctor.

Patients who may be pregnant or are trying to become pregnant should tell their doctor before receiving etoposide. Chemotherapy can cause men and women to be sterile, or unable to have children.

Patients should check with their doctors before receiving live virus **vaccines** while on chemotherapy.

Patients who develop mouth sores from etoposide treatment should discontinue smoking, drinking alcohol, and eating highly acidic or spicy foods.

Side effects

The most common side effect from etoposide is low blood counts (**myelosuppression**). When the white blood cell count is low (**neutropenia**), patients are at an increased risk for developing a **fever** and infections. Etoposide also causes the platelet count to fall. Platelets are blood cells in the body that allow for the formation of clots. When the platelet count is low, patients are at an increased risk for bruising and bleeding. Low red blood cell counts (**anemia**), may also occur due to etoposide administration. Low red counts may make patients feel tired, dizzy, and lacking in energy.

Etoposide infusions, if given too quickly into the vein, can cause a significant drop in blood pressure. This can usually be avoided by administering the etoposide over a time period of at least 30–60 minutes. A patient's blood pressure may be taken when receiving an etoposide infusion. To minimize dizziness from a drop in blood pressure, the patient should sit up slowly following an etoposide infusion.

Etoposide can cause mild to moderate **nausea and vomiting**. This is more common in patients taking the oral capsules. Patients will be given **antiemetics** before receiving etoposide to help prevent or decrease this side effect. Hair loss (**alopecia**) is common with etoposide administration. **Diarrhea**, loss of appetite (**anorexia**), and mouth sores are less common but have been reported to occur.

Liver problems may occur due to etoposide administration, though they are mild. The liver returns to normal when the drug is stopped. This side effect is more common with higher etoposide doses.

Males receiving etoposide for testicular cancer typically have a lowered sperm count during chemotherapy. As with liver function, however, testicular function gradually returns to normal after etoposide treatment is stopped. In one group of 38 patients treated for testicular cancer, 13 fathered a total of 16 children within two years after the end of etoposide treatment. None of the children had any birth defects.

Less common neurological side effects caused by etoposide include tingling and numbness of the fingers and toes, dizziness, headache, sleepiness, visual disturbances, and confusion.

Other less common side effects caused by etoposide include rash, **itching**, sores in the mouth, darkening skin, fever, development of another type of cancer or leukemia, redness and pain at the site of injection into the vein, chest pain, and irregular heart rate.

Rare side effects from using etoposide are allergic, or anaphylactic-type, reactions, which include fever, chills, tongue swelling, shortness of breath, low blood pressure, and increased heart rate.

Interactions

Etoposide, if given with the oral drug **warfarin** (also known as coumadin), can increase bleeding.

Resources

BOOKS

Beers, Mark H., MD, and Robert Berkow, MD, editors. "Acute Leukemia." In *The Merck Manual of Diagnosis and Therapy*. Whitehouse Station, NJ: Merck Research Laboratories, 2007.

Everolimus

Beers, Mark H., MD, and Robert Berkow, MD, editors. "Kaposi's Sarcoma." In *The Merck Manual of Diagnosis and Therapy*. Whitehouse Station, NJ: Merck Research Laboratories, 2007.

Karch, A. M. *Lippincott's Nursing Drug Guide*. Springhouse, PA: Lippincott Williams & Wilkins, 2003.

PERIODICALS

Marsh, J. W., M. Donovan, D. R. Burholt, et al. "Metastatic Lung Disease to the Central Nervous System: In vitro Response to Chemotherapeutic Agents." *Journal of Neurooncology* 66 (January 2004): 81–90.

Pectasides, D., M. Pectasides, D. Farmakis, et al. "Testicular Function in Patients with Testicular Cancer Treated with Bleomycin-Etoposide-Carboplatin (BEC(90)) Combination Chemotherapy." *European Urology* 45 (February 2004): 187–193.

Toffoli, G., G. Corona, B. Basso, and M. Boiocchi. "Pharmacokinetic Optimisation of Treatment with Oral Etoposide." *Clinical Pharmacokinetics* 43 (March 2004): 441–466.

ORGANIZATIONS

American Society of Health-System Pharmacists (ASHP). 7272 Wisconsin Avenue, Bethesda, MD 20814. (301) 657-3000. www.ashp.org.

United States Food and Drug Administration (FDA). 5600 Fishers Lane, Rockville, MD 20857-0001. (888) INFO-FDA. www.fda.gov.

Nancy J. Beaulieu, R.Ph., B.C.O.P.
Rebecca J. Frey, PhD

Everolimus

Definition

Everolimus (Afinitor) is a kinase that interferes with the protein called mammalian target of rapamycin (mTOR), a protein that regulates tumor cell reproduction and blood vessel growth. Everolimus is used to treat advanced **kidney cancer** (renal cell **carcinoma** [RCC]) after treatment with **sunitinib** (Sutent) or **sorafenib** (Nexavar) has failed.

Purpose

Everolimus is a second-line treatment for RCC, the most common type of kidney **cancer**. It is used only after another drug treatment has failed. Tumors formed in RCC begin in the lining of the kidney tubules and spread to nearby lymph nodes and other organs. In these cancerous (malignant) cells, the protein mTOR is inappropriately "switched on." mTOR controls cell division, and when too much of it is present, malignant cells can reproduce wildly, forming

a tumor. mTOR also plays a role in the sequence of metabolic events that lead to the formation of new blood vessels (a process called angiogenesis). As tumors grow, they need more oxygen and nutrients. To meet these needs, new blood vessels must grow into the tumor. Everolimus inhibits the activity of mTOR. In doing this, it stops or slows cell division and also stops or slows the development of new blood vessels necessary to feed the tumor. In some cases tumors shrink in size after treatment with everolimus.

Description

Everolimus is manufactured by Novartis Pharmaceuticals and sold in the United States and the European Union under the brand name Afinitor. The United States Food and Drug Administration (FDA) first approved everolimus for the treatment of RCC following failure of treatment with sunitinib (Sutent) or sorafenib (Nexavar) on March 30, 2009. Everolimus is also approved for sale in the EU. As of October 2009 approval of everolimus is pending in Japan and Switzerland. Everolimus comes as a white to yellowish elongated tablet.

Abnormal production of mTOR occurs in many types of cancer. Everolimus is being tested in **clinical trials** for use against other kinds of cancer and in combination with other therapies. A list of clinical trials currently enrolling volunteers can be found at http://www.clinicaltrials.gov.

Recommended dosage

Everolimus comes in tablets with strengths of 5 mg or 10 mg. The recommended dosage is 10 mg taken once daily at the same time every day. Tablets should be swallowed whole with water and may be taken with or without food. Tablets should never be crushed, divided, or chewed. Individuals who cannot swallow tablets should consult their doctor about how to take this drug. Everolimus should be stored at room temperature and kept dry and out of direct light.

For individuals with moderate liver damage (hepatic impairment), the recommended dose is 5 mg daily. This drug has not been evaluated in individuals with severe liver damage. If the individual is taking certain drugs that interact with everolimus, dosage also may be adjusted (see Interactions below). In the event of serious side effects, the dosage may be reduced, generally to 5 mg, or the drug may be halted temporarily.

Precautions

Patients and their physicians should be alert to the following precautions.

- Non-infectious (cannot be passed to other people) pneumonitis can cause low blood levels of oxygen (hypoxia), fluid build-up around the lungs (pleural effusion), shortness of breath (dyspnea), and cough. Non-infectious pneumonitis has been fatal in some patients. Patients should tell their doctor immediately about any worsening of respiratory symptoms so that the drug regimen can be modified and the condition treated.

- Infections, including and bacterial and fungal systemic infections (sepsis), may occur and be serious enough to require hospitalization. Sepsis has resulted in patient deaths during clinical trials. Patients should immediately report any signs of infection (e.g., fever, chills) to their physician.

- Elevated serum creatinine, elevated blood sugar (hyperglycemia), elevated lipids and fats in the blood (hyperlipidemia and hyper triglyceridemia) all occurred during clinical trials. Kidney function and blood chemistries should be monitored.

- A decrease in the number of blood platelets (thrombocytopenia) may reduce the ability of the blood to clot and increase the risk of serious bleeding episodes. Decrease in the number of neutrophils (neutropenia) may decrease the ability of the body to fight infection. Decrease in the number of red blood cells (anemia) may reduce the ability of the blood to supply oxygen. Blood count should be monitored frequently.

- Patients taking everolimus should not receive any live vaccines (e.g., intranasal influenza, measles, mumps, rubella [German measles], oral polio, BCG [tuberculosis], yellow fever, varicella [chickenpox], typhoid). They also should avoid people who have recently been vaccinated with a live vaccine.

Allergies

Individuals who are allergic to **sirolimus** (Rapamune, rapamycin), or temsirlimus (Torisel) should avoid everolimus.

This drug contains lactose as an inactive ingredient. People who are highly lactose-intolerant should discuss use of this drug with their physician.

Pregnant or breastfeeding

Everolimus is a pregnancy category D drug. Woman who are pregnant or who might become pregnant should not use everolimus. It is not known whether the drug is excreted in breast milk. Women taking this drug should not breastfeed, as there is the potential for this drug to cause serious harm to the nursing infant.

Side effects

Everolimus has many potential side effects, the most serious of which are listed above in Precautions. In addition, the following side effects may occur:

- Mouth sores, mouth ulcers, and inflammation of the mucous membrane lining the mouth
- fatigue
- cough, difficulty breathing (see Precautions)
- diarrhea
- skin rash and itching
- nausea and vomiting
- fever (see Precautions)
- loss of appetite
- fluid retention (edema)
- distorted sense of taste
- headache
- nose bleeds
- inflammation of the digestive system
- pain in the arms or legs

Interactions

Everolimus is known to interact with certain drugs. If these drugs cannot be avoided, the dosage of everolimus may need to be adjusted. All interactions are not known. Patients should provide their doctor and pharmacist with a complete list of all prescription and nonprescription drugs, herbs, and dietary supplements that they are taking.

When taken with everolimus, these are examples of drugs that are likely to increase the amount of everolimus circulating in the blood.

- ketoconazole (Nizoral)
- erythromycin (E-mycin)
- verpamil (Calan, Isoptin, Verlan)

When taken with everolimus, these are examples of drugs are likely to decrease the amount of everolimus circulating in the blood.

- dexamethasone (Decadron)
- phenytoin (Dilantin)
- carbamazepine (Tergretol)
- rifampin (Rimactane)
- phenobarbitol (Luminal)

Patients should tell their doctor if they are taking St. John's wort (*Hypericum perforatum*).

Resources

OTHER

Afinitor (everolimus) Tablets. Novartis Pharmaceuticals. 2009 [October 9, 2009]. http://www.afinitor.com/index.jsp

Detailed Guide: Kidney Cancer. American Cancer Society 2009 [October 9, 2009]. http://www.cancer.org/docroot/CRI/CRI_2_3x.asp?dt=22

Kidney Cancer. MedlinePlus September 30, 2009 [October 9, 2009]. http://www.nlm.nih.gov/medlineplus/kidneycancer.html

ORGANIZATIONS

American Cancer Society, 1599 Clifton Rd., NE, Atlanta, GA, 30329, (404) 320-3333, (800) ACS-2345, http://www.cancer.org.

Kidney Cancer Association, P.O. Box 96503, Washington, DC, 20090, (800) 850-9132, (312) 327-7002, kidney.cancer@hotmail.com, http://www.kidneycancer.org.

National Cancer Institute Public Inquires Office., 6116 Executive Boulevard, Room 3036A, Bethesda, MD, 20892-8322, (800) 4-CANCER. TTY (800) 332-8615, http://www.cancer.gov.

Tish Davidson, A.M.

Ewing's sarcoma

Definition

Ewing's **sarcoma** is a **cancer** that affects children, teens, and less often, young adults. It begins in developing bone cells. Ewing's sarcoma cells grow uncontrollably and form masses or lumps called tumors. They can start in any bone in the body but about half of all cases involve flat bones such as the pelvic bones and the long bones in the leg—the tibia, fibula, and femur.

A femur of a patient diagnosed with Ewing's sarcoma. Ewing's sarcoma is the second most common bone tumor among children and teens, and half of all cases involve flat or long bones, such as the femur. *(Custom Medical Stock Photo. Reproduced by permission.)*

Description

Ewing's sarcoma is the second most common bone tumor among children and teens. It accounts for about 1% of all **childhood cancers**. This cancer is named for James Ewing, the researcher who first described the tumor in 1921. There are some rare cases of Ewing's sarcoma that do not begin in bones. These tumors are thought to start in nerve or other soft tissues.

Demographics

Ewing's sarcoma occurs most frequently in children ages 11 to 15 years old. Slightly more males than females develop Ewing's sarcomas, and like **osteosarcoma**, the most common bone cancer found in children, it is more often diagnosed in taller teens. The disease is rarely diagnosed in children younger than 5

KEY TERMS

Biopsy—The surgical removal and microscopic examination of living tissue for diagnostic purposes.

Chemotherapy—Treatment of cancer with synthetic drugs that destroy the tumor either by inhibiting the growth of cancerous cells or by killing them.

Metastasize—The spread of cancer cells from a primary site to distant parts of the body.

Oncologist—A doctor who specializes in cancer medicine.

Pathologist—A doctor who specializes in the diagnosis of disease by studying cells and tissues under a microscope.

Radiation therapy—Treatment using high energy radiation from x–ray machines, cobalt, radium, or other sources.

Stage—A term used to describe the size and extent of spread of cancer.

QUESTIONS TO ASK THE DOCTOR

- How big is the tumor?
- Has the Ewing's sarcoma spread?
- What are the recommended treatments?
- What are the side effects of the recommended treatments?
- Is treatment expected to cure the disease or only to prolong life?

or adults older than 30. It affects primarily Caucasians, and rarely occurs in African Americans and native Chinese.

Causes and symptoms

The causes of Ewing's sarcoma are not known. It is possible that certain inherited conditions increase the risk of developing this cancer.

About two-thirds of patients with Ewing's sarcoma have a painful swelling or lump that can be felt in the affected bone. Along with tenderness, the area of swelling may be hot. The symptoms depend on the site of the tumor and whether it has spread. For example, a tumor on a rib may cause painful breathing. When Ewing's sarcoma has spread, patients may have other symptoms such as **fatigue**, **weight loss**, and **fever**.

Diagnosis

Most patients who have Ewing's sarcomas go to the doctor because they have discovered a lump or mass or swelling on or near a bone. Others have symptoms related to the part of the body that is affected by the tumor, such as pressure on the bladder from a tumor on a pelvic bone.

The patient's doctor will take a detailed medical history to find out about the symptoms. The history is followed by a complete physical examination with special attention to the suspicious symptom or body part.

Depending on the location of the tumor (mass or lump), the doctor will order **imaging studies** such as x ray, **computed tomography** (CT) scans and **magnetic resonance imaging** (MRI) to help determine the size, shape and exact location of the tumor. The doctor will also order a chest x ray to find out if the tumor has spread to the lungs, and bone scans to determine if the tumor has spread to bones. Blood tests will be done and an examination of the bone marrow will be performed to see if the marrow is involved.

A **biopsy** of the tumor is necessary to make a diagnosis of Ewing's sarcoma. During a biopsy, some tissue from the tumor is removed. The tissue sample is examined by a pathologist, a doctor who specializes in the study of diseased tissue.

Types of biopsy

The type of biopsy done depends on the location of the tumor. For some small tumors, such as those on the arm or leg, the doctor may perform an excisional biopsy, removing the entire tumor and a margin of surrounding normal tissue. Most often, the doctor will perform an incisional biopsy, a procedure that involves cutting out only a piece of the tumor. This biopsy provides a core of tissue from the tumor that is used to confirm the diagnosis of Ewing's sarcoma.

Treatment team

Like other cancer patients, teens and young adults with Ewing's sarcoma are usually cared for by a multidisciplinary team of health professionals. The patient's pediatrician, family physician, or primary care doctor may refer the patient to other physician specialists, such as surgeons and oncologists (doctors who specialize in cancer medicine). Radiologic technicians perform x ray, CT and MRI scans and nurses and laboratory technicians may obtain samples of blood, urine and other laboratory tests.

Before and after any surgical procedures, including biopsies, specially trained nurses will explain the procedures and help to prepare patients and families. Depending on the tumor location and treatment plan, patients may also benefit from rehabilitation therapy with physical therapists and nutritional counseling from dieticians.

Clinical staging, treatments, and prognosis

Staging

The purpose of staging a tumor is to determine how far it has advanced. This is important because treatment varies depending on the stage. Generally, stage is determined by the size of the tumor, whether the tumor has spread to nearby lymph nodes, whether the tumor has spread elsewhere in the body, and what the cells look like under the microscope.

There is no commonly accepted system for staging Ewing's sarcomas. As is the case with other cancers, patients with metastases (spread) tend to have worse outlooks than patients whose tumors have not spread.

Between one quarter to one third of patients with Ewing's sarcoma have metastases when they are first diagnosed. Patients with tumors closer to the trunk of the body or in the pelvic bones are more likely to have metastases than patients with tumors located on the lower leg or foot. The most common sites for spread of Ewing's sarcoma are to the lungs or bones.

Treatment

Treatment for Ewing's sarcoma varies depending on the location of the tumor, its size and grade, and the extent of its spread. For most patients, the goals of treatment are to remove or control the tumor and combat the spread of the cancer.

Generally, when removing the tumor will not sharply reduce function, Ewing's sarcoma tumors are surgically removed. The goal of removing as much tumor as possible is to reduce the amount of radiation needed after surgery. The part of the body where the tumor was removed is treated with radiation to destroy remaining tumor cells. Most patients also receive **chemotherapy**, powerful anti-cancer drugs to destroy remaining cancer cells.

When the disease has spread throughout the body, there may be no benefit from surgical removal of the tumor. These patients, who have widespread metastases, are treated with radiation and chemotherapy.

SIDE EFFECTS. The surgical treatment of Ewing's sarcoma carries risks related to the surgical site, such as loss of function resulting from loss of a long bone in the leg. There also are the medical risks associated with any surgical procedure, such as reactions to general anesthesia or **infection** after surgery.

The side effects of **radiation therapy** depend on the site being radiated. Radiation therapy can produce side effects such as fatigue, skin rashes, **nausea** and **diarrhea**. Most of the side effects lessen or disappear completely after the radiation therapy has been completed.

The side effects of chemotherapy vary depending on the medication, or combination of **anticancer drugs**, used. Chemotherapy drugs often given to combat Ewing's sarcoma are **cyclophosphamide, doxorubicin, vincristine,** and **dactinomycin**.

For patients with widespread disease, chemotherapy may be given along with bone marrow transplant and radiation to the entire body. **Nausea and vomiting**, **anemia**, lower resistance to infection, and hair loss (**alopecia**) are common side effects of chemotherapy. Medication may be given to reduce the unpleasant side effects of chemotherapy.

Alternative and complementary therapies

Many patients find that alternative and complementary therapies help to reduce the stress associated with illness, improve immune function and feel better. While there is no evidence that these therapies specifically combat disease, activities such as biofeedback, relaxation, therapeutic touch, massage therapy and guided imagery have been reported to enhance well–being.

Prognosis

The outlook for patients with Ewing's sarcoma varies, depending on the size and volume of the tumor, its stage, and the extent of its spread. Patients with large tumors do not fare as well as those with smaller tumors. Patients with tumors in certain sites, such as the bones of the pelvis and spinal column also seem to have poor outlooks because by the time these tumors are discovered they have already spread.

Ewing's sarcoma may spread locally to areas near the tumor and it can spread to nearby lymph glands. To spread to distant parts of the body, the cancer cells travel in the blood, bone marrow or through the lymph glands. In general, tumors that have spread widely throughout the body are not associated with favorable survival rates.

Nearly three quarters of patients diagnosed before the cancer has spread are disease free for five years after treatment. Patients with tumors that do not respond to treatment and those who suffer recurrences have poor outlooks for long–term survival.

Coping with cancer treatment

Teens undergoing cancer treatment have special needs. The diagnosis of a life–threatening illness, surgery and radiation or chemotherapy may cause fear, anxiety, **depression** and loss of self–esteem. Disruption of normal routines and discomfort from diagnostic tests and treatment may also cause anxiety. There are additional social problems including making up missed school work, explaining the illness and treatment to friends, and coping with physical limitations or disability.

Teens with serious illnesses and disabilities face emotional conflicts and psychological challenges. One conflict is between the teen's growing desire for independence and the reality of dependence on others for the activities of daily living. It is important for teens to be fully informed about their disease and treatment plan and involved in treatment decision making. Many teens benefit from continuing contact with friends, classmates, teachers, and family during hospital stays and recovery at home.

Depression, emotional distress, and anxiety associated with the disease and its treatment may respond to counseling from a mental health professional. Individual and group therapy often help teens and young adults to reveal and express their feelings about illness and treatment. Many cancer patients and their families find participation in mutual aid and group support programs help to relieve feelings of isolation and loneliness. By sharing problems with others who have lived through similar difficulties patients and families can exchange ideas and coping strategies.

Clinical trials

More than 25 clinical studies were underway during 2001. For example, at John Hopkins Oncology Center and other cancer centers across the United States, patients with recurring or widespread Ewing's sarcoma were being given chemotherapy to stop tumor cells from dividing as well as stem cells (**bone marrow transplantation**) to replace immune cells killed by chemotherapy.

Other **clinical trials** compare different combinations of drugs used for chemotherapy or combinations of chemotherapy and radiation to find out which combination is more effective. For example, in one study, patients with Ewing's sarcoma were randomly assigned to two different treatment groups. One group received chemotherapy followed by surgery and radiation therapy. The other group received radiation therapy during chemotherapy.

Other types of clinical research study individuals and families at high risk of cancer to help identify cancer genes. To learn more about clinical trials visit the National Cancer Institute (NCI) web site at http://cancertrials.nci.nih.gov or the Pediatric Oncology Branch of the National Cancer Institute web site at http://www–dcs.nci.nih.gov/pedonc/

Prevention

Since the causes of Ewing's sarcoma are not known, there are no recommendations about how to prevent its development. Among families with an inherited tendency to develop soft tissue sarcomas, careful monitoring may help to ensure early diagnosis and treatment of the disease.

Special concerns

Ewing's sarcoma, like other cancer diagnoses, may produce a range of emotional reactions in patients and families. Education, counseling and participation in group support programs can help to reduce feelings of guilt, fear, anxiety and hopelessness. For many parents suffering from spiritual distress, visits with clergy members and participation in organized prayer may offer comfort.

Resources

BOOKS

Pelletier, Kenneth R. *The Best of Alternative Medicine.* New York: Simon & Schuster, 2000.

PERIODICALS

Arndt, Carola A.R., and William M. Crist. "Medical Progress: Common Musculoskeletal Tumors of Childhood and Adolescence." *New England Journal of Medicine* 29 (July 1999): 342–352.

ORGANIZATIONS

American Cancer Society. 1599 Clifton Road, N.E., Atlanta, GA 30329. (800)227–2345.

Cancer Research Institute. 681 Fifth Avenue, New York, NY 10022. (800)992–2623.

National Cancer Institute Clinical Cancer Trials. <http://cancertrials.nci.nih.gov>.

National Cancer Institute (National Institutes of Health). 9000 Rockville Pike, Bethesda, MD 20892. (800)422–6237.

The Pediatric Oncology Branch of the National Cancer Institute. (877) 624–4878 or (301)496–4256. <http://www–dcs.nci.nih.gov/pedonc/>.

Barbara Wexler, M.P.H.

Exemestane *see* **Aromatase inhibitors**

Exenteration

Definition

An exenteration is a major operation during which all the contents of a body cavity are removed. Pelvic exenteration refers to the removal of all the organs and adjacent structures of the pelvis, and orbital exenteration refers to the removal of the entire contents of the ocular orbit, sometimes including the eyelids as well.

Purpose

The pelvis is the basin-shaped cavity that contains the bladder, rectum and reproductive organs. (The reproductive organs include the ovaries, uterus and cervix for women and the prostate for men.) Pelvic exenteration is performed to surgically remove **cancer** that involves these organs and that has not responded well to other types of treatment. For example, pelvic exenteration might be performed for primary **rectal cancer** because 5–10% of primary rectal cancers spread to nearby pelvic organs. Pelvic exenteration is also indicated when cancer returns after an earlier treatment, as rectal cancer does in some 20% of cases. In women, the operation is additionally performed mostly for advanced and invasive cases of endometrial, ovarian, vulvar, vaginal and **cervical cancer**, and in men for aggressive **prostate cancer**.

Similarly, orbital exenteration is performed to remove the eye and surrounding tissues when cancer of the orbital contents cannot be controlled by simple removal or irradiation. It is often the only course of treatment for advanced **basal cell carcinoma** of the eyelids, for cancers that have spread to the optic nerve, or retinoblastomas larger than 1/4 inch (0.6 cm), as well as for large tumors of the eyeball.

Exenteration is not only a major operation for a patient to undergo, it is also technically very challenging, because it involves elaborate **reconstructive surgery**. It is a radical surgical procedure, but it often provides the only opportunity available for patients to eliminate the cancer and to prevent cancer from recurring.

Precautions

Pelvic exenterations should not be performed on patients diagnosed with inflammation of the roots of spinal nerves, sciatica, lymphedema, **liver cancer**, extrapelvic disease, and obstructions of the urinary tract.

All precautions applying to major surgery apply to exenterations, whether pelvic or ocular.

After pelvic exenteration, sexual intercourse should be avoided as directed by the surgeon. This is to allow the wound to heal properly.

Description

Pelvic exenteration

There are three types of pelvic exenterations.

ANTERIOR EXENTERATION. This operation usually removes in women the uterus, bladder, vagina, and entire urethra. Patients selected for this operation have cancers that are located so as to allow the rectum to be spared. Vaginal reconstruction is performed afterwards if required. It is called anterior because it removes organs toward the front or in front of the pelvis.

POSTERIOR EXENTERATION. This operation removes in women the uterus, ovaries, Fallopian tubes, anus, supporting muscles and ligaments, and all the vagina except a portion of the wall that supports the urethra. In men, the bladder is also removed. It is called posterior because it removes organs located in the back part of the pelvis.

TOTAL PELVIC EXENTERATION. This operation removes the bladder, rectum and anus, supporting muscles and ligaments, together with either the prostate in men or the gynecologic (reproductive) organs in women. Total pelvic exenteration is performed when there is no opportunity to perform a less extensive operation, because of the location and size of the cancer. For women, vaginal reconstruction is performed, which also helps reconstruction of the pelvic area. In both anterior and total pelvic exenteration, a urinary tract can be constructed.

The exact surgical procedure followed depends on the type of exenteration, but generally, all pelvic exenterations start with an incision in the lower abdomen. Blood vessels are clamped and the organs specified by the procedure are removed. The site of incision is then stitched up.

Orbital exenteration

This operation removes the eyeball and surrounding tissues of the orbit. The eye is surrounded by bone, so orbital exenteration is easier to tolerate than pelvic exenteration and patients may even undergo the operation as outpatients. Orbital exenteration with partial preservation of eyelids and conjunctiva can sometimes be achieved. Within two weeks of surgery, patients are usually fitted with a temporary ocular prothesis (plastic eye). Later, facial prostheses are also attached to the facial skeleton.

Both pelvic and orbital exenterations are performed using general anesthesia.

Preparation

The evaluation of patients before pelvic exenteration includes a thorough physical exam with rectal and pelvic examination. **Endorectal ultrasound** and **imaging studies**, such as **computed tomography** scans (CT

scans) and **magnetic resonance imaging** (MRI), are routinely used to obtain pictures of the abdominal and pelvic areas and evaluate the spread of the cancer.

Ocular ultrasound examination, CT scan and **angiography** evaluation is usually performed to prepare for ocular exenteration.

Preparing for the operation usually depends on the type of exenteration procedure selected. Most patients receive a combination of **radiation therapy** and **chemotherapy** before the operation. Surgery is typically performed approximately six weeks later.

In the case of pelvic exenteration, patients are required to clean as much waste as possible out of the large intestine, using various **laxatives** or enemas. This cleaning of the colon and rectum is required so as to eliminate stool and lower the level of bacteria, thus preventing infections after surgery. **Antibiotics** are also typically given to help sterilize the colon.

Aftercare

Pelvic exenteration

After a pelvic exenteration, a drainage tube is inserted at the site of the incision. There usually is some bleeding, discharge and considerable tenderness and pain for a few days. This is a major operation that requires at least a three- to five-day hospital stay. Side effects depend on the type of pelvic exenteration performed, but always include urination difficulty, especially if adjustment to a catheter is required, and a very painful lower abdomen.

Some exenterations require a temporary or permanent **colostomy**, meaning the creation of an opening (stoma) in the abdomen to allow solid waste to leave the body. Permanent colostomy may be needed, for example, if the rectum is removed. In such cases, the patient needs time to adjust and be taught how to irrigate, empty, clean and wear the colostomy bags.

Stitches are usually removed from the skin on the third day or before the patient is sent home. A prescription for pain medication is usually given as well as instructions for follow up care.

Ocular exenteration

After ocular exenteration, most patients have a headache for several days that goes away using medication such as tylenol. An eye ointment is also prescribed that contains antibiotics and steroids to help the healing process.

Risks

No surgical procedure is risk-free. Complications are always possible, especially if the operation is major. As with any operation, possible exenteration risks include possible complications due to the anesthetic and wound **infection**.

In the case of pelvic exenteration, the following complications are also possible:

- hemorrhage that may require a blood transfusion
- injury to the bowel
- urinary tract infection
- urinary retention requiring permanent use of a catheter
- bowel obstruction
- urinary tract infection

The following considerations also apply: after removal of the reproductive organs, women will no longer have monthly periods nor will they be able to become pregnant. For men, surgery involving the prostate and the nerves around the rectum may also result in the inability to produce sperm or to have an erection.

In the case of orbital exenteration, the following complications have been known to occur:

- growth of an orbital cyst (rare)
- chronic throbbing orbital pain
- sinusitis (nasal stuffiness)
- ear problems

See also Adenocarcinoma; Cervical cancer; Endometrial cancer; Melanoma; Ovarian cancer; Vaginal cancer; Vulvar cancer.

Resources

PERIODICALS

Petros, J. G., P. Augustinos, M. Lopez, J. S. Spratt, W. J. Temple, E. B. Saettler, R. E. Hautmann, and D. Turns. "Pelvic exenteration for carcinoma of the colon and rectum." *Seminars in Surgical Oncology* 17 (October-November 1999): 206-212.

Turns, D. "Psychosocial issues: pelvic exenterative surgery." *Journal of Surgical Oncology* 76 (March 2001): 224-236.

OTHER

Information on eye cancer: Websites: http://www.EyeCancer Book.com/ and http://eyecancerinfo.com/.

Women's Health Matters. http://www.womenshealthmatters.ca/centres/cancer/cervical/treatment/index.html.

Monique Laberge, Ph.D.

Extracranial germ cell tumors

Definition

Extracranial **germ cell tumors** are reproductive cells that have developed into a rare form of malignancy within the reproductive system or within another part of the body, outside of the brain.

Description

Germ cells are cells that develop into the reproductive organs (gonads) during a child's embryonic stage; the testicles in males, the ovaries in females. Germ, meaning "seed," refers to directly to these cells' role in production of the sperm and the ovums. On rare occasions, these calls can experience an abnormal transformation and growth, and develop into a germ cell tumor.

After normal embryonic development, germ cells travel down through the midline path of the body and enter the pelvis to form the gonads. For this reason, most germ cells tumors develop in the testes or ovaries and are referred to as gonadal germ cell tumors. However, germ cells can also migrate during the embryonic development and travel to other regions of the body. Also known as **extragonadal germ cell tumors**, these tumors can develop inside the chest, coccyx, abdomen, and pelvis. Because they grow outside the cranium (another location of possible germ cell tumor growth), these types of germ cells are commonly referred to as extracranial germ cell tumors.

Malignant extracranial germ cell tumors can also spread (metastasize) to other parts of the body. The liver, lungs, and the lymph nodes can be commonly affected by **metastasis**, but in rare cases the central nervous system and skeletal structure (bones and marrow) can also be affected. Benign extracranial germ cell tumors do not metastasize, but the increased pressure caused by their growth can damage and/or hinder the function of nearby organs and structures.

Extracranial germ cell tumors are divided into certain types, depending on their characteristics. The four most common forms of extracranial germ cell tumors include:

- Mature teratoma—The most common subtype of extracranical germ cell tumor and generally benign in nature. Mature teratomas are cysts that contain germ cell layers from the ectoderm (skin and nervous tissue), mesoderm (muscle, bone, cartilage, and connective tissue), and endoderm (the lining of the digestive and respiratory systems). As such, any type of tissue can grow within these cysts, usually of a type far different from the surrounding tissue; i.e. hair and

KEY TERMS

Cryptorchidism—A developmental defect marked by the failure of the testes to descend into the scrotum.

Chemotherapy—The treatment of cancer using specific chemical agents and/or drugs, which are selectively destructive to malignant cells and tissues.

Hematologist—A physician specializing in the treatment of blood diseases.

Germ Cell—An ovum or a sperm cell or one of their developmental precursors.

Gonads—The male and female reproductive organs, which produce sperm (testes) and ovum (ovaries).

Oncologist—A physician specializing in the study and treatment of tumors.

Teratoma—A tumor consisting of different types of tissue, as of skin, hair, and muscle, caused by the development of independent germ cells.

Yolk sac—A membranous sac attached to an embryo, which functions as the circulatory system of the human embryo before internal circulation begins.

teeth growing in the testes. Some mature tertomas can even secrete enzymes and hormones, such as insulin, androgens, and growth hormones.

- Immature teratoma—Similar to mature tertomas, but the tissues are more immature. Immature teratomas may also contain neuroepithelium tissues (associated with the development of the nevrous system). Germ cell tumors of this classification are more likely to be malignant in nature.

- Yolk Sac tumor—The most common malignant extracranial germ cell tumor in young children. Yolk sac tumors are also the most common germ cell tumor, benign or malignant, to develop in the testes of infants and young boys. Tumors are soft and brittle with a yellow and/or grayish cystic exterior. Necrosis and extensive hemorrhaging are common experienced with yolk sac tumors.

- Germinoma—Depending on the location of tumor, germinomas are known as dysgerminoas (ovaries) and seminomas (testes). They are most common malignancy to affect the central nervous system of children.

Demographics

Approximately half of all extracranial germ cell tumors are benign in nature. Of these tumors, almost 50% of them will develop in the gonads, 25% in the

QUESTIONS TO ASK YOUR DOCTOR

- Is the tumor benign or malignant, and where is it located? How will that affect the prognosis?
- What risks and side effects my child could face undergoing the different treatments for this type of cancer?
- Has the malignancy spread any further than the original tumor and, if so, what parts of the body are affected?
- WHat is the likelihood the tumor will return?
- Do you know of any support groups my child and I can contact?

coccyx, and roughly 5% in miscellaneous extragonadal locations, such as chest, stomach, liver, and central nervous system.

Extracranial germ cells tumors are particularly rare amongst young children, only accounting for approximately 3% of **cancer** cases for children 15 years of age and younger. However, this incidence rate rises dramatically in adolescents (aged 15 to 19 years of age) accounting for approximately 14% of cancer cases. However, in both categories, the incidence rate of extracranial germ cell tumors has been rising over the last few decades.

Causes and symptoms

The underlying cause behind the development of extracranial germ cell tumors is not fully understood. However, a number of inherited defects of the central nervous system, spine, and genitourinary (genital and urinary organs) tract have been associated with an increased risk of development. Cryptorchidism, for example, has been identified as a possible risk factor for the development of testicular germ cell tumors. Patients with Klinefelter's syndrome (a chromosomal anomaly in males) and Swyer's syndrome (a developmental problem of the gonads) are also at risk of developing extragonadal germ cell tumors in the chest and central nervous system, respectively.

Symptoms

Symptoms of extracranial germ cell tumors will great depend on the type and location of the tumor, as well as the age and gender of the patient. However, general symptoms will include:

- a growth, swelling, or mass that can be felt and/or seen
- constipation and/or urinary retention
- incontinence
- leg weakness
- abnormal testicular shape or size, sometimes painful, in boys
- abdominal pain in girls
- abnormal shortness of breath
- chest pain

Diagnosis

Patients presenting with the various symptoms of extracranial germ cell tumors should be given a thorough history and careful physical examination. This examination should include blood testing and complete blood count. Germ cell tumors often produce proteins in the blood that can be used as markers. In particular, elevated levels of alpha-fetoprotein and human chorionic gonadotropin may indicate the presence of extracranial germ cell tumors. If indicated, this examination should be followed by either a **computed tomography** (CT) scan or **magnetic resonance imaging** (MRI) scan. This will provide the physician with a better picture of where the tumor is located. Chest x-rays can determine if there is tumor growth in the lungs.

If this initial examination indicated the presence of a tumor, a **biopsy** must be conducted to confirm whether or not the tumor is malignant. If the cancer cells are malignant, a pathologist can determine what grade the tumor is and estimate its growth rate. There are three grades of cell malignancy: Low (almost normal appearance, slow growth, unlikely to spread), Intermediate (average appearance and growth, may spread), and High (highly abnormal in appearance, quick growth rate, and likely to spread).

Treatment team

Children and adolescents are the most common patients to be afftected by extracranial germ cell tumors. Unlike adults, they may not always understand what is happening to them and are likely to become upset and scared by both their disease and the various stages of the diagnostic and therapeutic process. As such, children with cancer should always be treated by a multidisciplinary team of cancer specialists. In addition to their family health provider, primary care should be provided by specialists trained in treating children and adolescents, including surgical subspecialists, oncologists, hematologists, and nursing specialists. In addition, social workers and therapists, as well as rehabilitation specialists, can provide the young patient with the effective supportive care they will require during and after treatment. Quality of life should be the focus of any therapeutic regimen for child patients.

Clinical staging, treatments, and prognosis

Initial diagnosis of the germ cell tumor will help determine whether or not it is malignant or benign in nature. If a malignancy is detected, further diagnostic studies will be required to determine if the tumor has spread to other areas of the body. Staging of the tumor depends on its size and whether it has metastasized. There are four stages commonly associated with all extracranial germ cell tumors:

- Stage 1—Cancer has not spread to surrounding tissues and lymph nodes. Surgical removal of tumor will eliminate all cancer cells.
- Stage 2—Cancer has metastasized to surrounding tissues and/or lymph nodes. Surgical removal of tumor cannot eliminate all cancer cells.
- Stage 3—Cancer has metastasized to surrounding tissue, to several lymph nodes, and is present in the fluid of the abdomen. Surgical removal of tumor cannot eliminate all cancer cells.
- Stage 4—The cancer has spread to other organs of the bodTumor has spread to other areas

Treatment

Treatment will depend greatly on the stage, grade, and position of the extracranial germ cell tumor. Other factors will include the child's age, general health, medical history, and their tolerance for specific procedures and medications. Generally, treatment will involve the surgical removal of the tumor and, if required, the surrounding tissue. This is followed by either **chemotherapy** (drugs used to kill the tumor cells) and/or radiotherapy (killing the cancerous cells with radiation). To what lengths these procedures will be employed will depend on the size of the tumor and to what extent it has spread throughout the body.

Effective treatment of extracranial germ cell tumors may require the use of other modalities, including **bone marrow transplantation**, hormonal replacement, **antibiotics** and supportive and follow-up care.

Prognosis

Recent advances in treatment modalities, such as the use of Cisplatin-based chemotherapy, have provided a high five-year survival rate; between 75% and 90%. However, some types of germ cells tumors may respond differently to treatment, thus increasing or worsening the patient's prognosis. For example, germ cell tumors in the lower back have a very low survival rate (approximately 28%) even if the malignancy is localized. Extracranial germ cell tumors can also be recurrent in nature, returning after surgical removal. The tumor may occur in the original location or another area of the body. These can occur in 20% to 30% of all high risk patients. Unfortunately, the presence of recurrent extracranial germ cell tumors offers a poor prognosis. It is important to ask the physician regarding the prognosis of each type of germ cell tumor.

Coping with cancer treatment

Special considerations should be taken with coping with the treatment of extracranial germ cell tumors, as the majority of patients will be adolescents and young children. Some adolescents may find discussing these tumors to be embarrassing. Even so, if possible, older children should be involved in all the details of their treatment. The patient will rely heavily upon family and friends for support during this difficult time. Counselors, therapists, and local support groups may also be of assistance. The goal must be to prevent fear and confusion, as well as to maintain the child's quality of life as much as possible.

Clinical trials

Due to the rarity of **childhood cancers**, all child patients should be considered for entrance into **clinical trials**. New treatments are being researched constantly. Details of current and future clinical trials can be found at the National Cancer Institute's website: http://cancer.gov/clinicaltrials.

Prevention

As these cancerous cells begin very early during pregnancy, there are no known preventive measures against extracranial germ cell tumors.

Resources

BOOKS

Barrett A. "Gene Cell Tumors." In *Cancer in Children: Clinical Management.*, edited by P.A. Voute, C. Kalifa, and A. Barrett. New York, NY: Oxford University Press, 1998, pp. 292-307.

Cushing B, E Perlman, N Marina, and R Castleberry. "Gene Cell Tumors." In *Principles and Practice of Pediatric Oncology (4th ed).*, edited by Phillip Pizzo and David Poplack. Philadelphia, PA: Lippincott Wliams & Wilkins, 2002, pp. 1091-1113.

PERIODICALS

Hawkins E. "Germ Cell Tumors." *American Journal of Clinical Pathology* 109(#4, Suppl 1998): S82-S88.

OTHER

"Childhood Extracranial Germ Cell Tumors." *National Cancer Institute* http://www.cancer.gov/cancerinfo/types/extracranial-germ-cell.

Javeed M. "Gern Cell Tumors." *eMedicine Journal* http://www.emedicine.com/med/topic863.htm.

Jason Fryer

Extragonadal germ cell tumors

Definition

Germ cells are primitive cells within the body that normally mature into ova (egg) or sperm cells. More than 90% of all **germ cell tumors** are gonadal; that is, they develop in the ovaries or the testes (the gonads). The remaining 5–10% of germ cell tumors arise outside of the gonads: these are the extragonadal germ cell tumors. These tumors occur mostly in the chest, lower back, and head.

Description

Extragonadal germ cell tumors are related to developmental problems that occur prior to birth. In the growing embryo, germ cells migrate to the immature ovaries or testes. In some instances, these cells fail to move to the gonads and end up in the midchest area between the lungs (mediastinum), the lowest part of the back (presacral area), or near the pea-sized gland between the two hemispheres of the brain (pineal gland). When these germ cells grow in these extragonadal sites, they sometimes develop into tumors. These tumors can be benign (noncancerous) or malignant (cancerous).

Benign extragonadal germ cell tumors are called benign teratomas. Malignant extragonadal germ cell tumors are subdivided into seminoma and nonseminoma. The nonseminoma germ cell tumors include: embryonal **carcinoma**, malignant teratoma, endodermal sinus tumor, choriocarcinoma, and mixed germ cell tumors. The specific category of extragonadal germ cell tumor that is present has a major influence on both treatment and prognosis.

Demographics

Extragonadal germ cell tumors are quite rare. One new case is diagnosed annually for every 1 million people in the United States.

In young children, extragonadal germ cell tumors tend to occur primarily in the presacral area. The majority of these tumors are benign.

KEY TERMS

Germ cells—Cells that are involved in reproduction. These cells are usually located in the gonads. Sometimes they fail to move to the gonads during embryonic development and cause tumors in other parts of the body.

Gonads—The reproductive organs: the testes and ovaries.

Mediastinum—The mid-chest area between the lungs.

Pineal gland—A pea-sized gland just below the brain.

Presacral area—The lowest part of the back.

In adults, extragonadal germ cell tumors tend to be in the mediastinum. Of these, approximately 40% are malignant.

Malignant extragonadal germ cell tumors occur with equal frequency in boys and girls. But, they are approximately nine times more likely to occur in men than in women.

Extragonadal germ cell tumors occur with equal frequency in members of all races and ethnic groups. There does not appear to be any relationship of extragonadal germ cell tumors to any geographic region.

Causes and symptoms

The cause, or causes, of extragonadal germ cell tumors are not known.

The symptoms of an extragonadal germ cell tumor depend on the type and location of the tumor.

Mediastinum

Germ cell tumors of the mediastinum are primarily diagnosed in men between the ages of 20 and 30. Symptoms include:

- chest pain
- breathing problems
- cough
- fever

Presacral area

Presacral germ cell tumors are primarily diagnosed in children under the age of six. These are generally seen as a mass in the lower abdomen or buttocks. Because of the size and location of the tumor, the patient may have difficulty passing urine or having a bowel movement. Tumors detected in children under the age of six

months are benign in 98% of cases. Tumors detected in children over the age of six months are malignant in approximately 65% of cases.

Pineal area

Almost all pineal germ cell tumors occur in people under the age of 40. Symptoms include:

- headache
- nausea
- vomiting
- lethargy
- difficulty walking
- memory loss
- an inability to look upward
- uncontrolled eye movement
- double vision

In some cases, a pineal germ cell tumor can begin to produce hormones that can cause a child to enter puberty at an abnormally young age (precocious puberty).

Diagnosis

The diagnosis of an extragonadal germ cell tumor usually begins with a thorough physical examination. In cases where a presacral tumor is suspected, this will include a rectal examination and a pelvic examination in women. In cases where a germ cell tumor of the pineal area is suspected, a complete neurological examination will be performed.

Mediastinum

The first test for a tumor of the mediastinum is a standard chest x ray. This will detect the tumor and show its location in 95% of cases. This will be followed by a **computed tomography** (CT) scan of the chest to determine the size of the tumor and by a CT scan of the abdomen to see if there has been a spread (**metastasis**) to the liver or other abdominal sites.

Diagnosis is generally confirmed by taking a needle **biopsy** of the tumor. In this procedure, a needle is injected directly into the tumor and a sample is removed.

Certain types of nonseminomas can be detected via blood tests for levels of alpha-fetoprotein (AFP) and beta-human chorionic gonadotropin (beta-hCG).

Presacral area

Germ cell tumors of the presacral area are diagnosed by either **magnetic resonance imaging** (MRI) or ultrasound imaging techniques. These techniques allow for the determination of both the location and the precise size of the tumor. To check for metastases, a bone scan, chest **x rays**, and a CT scan of the lungs should be performed. Sometimes a **bone marrow biopsy** is also ordered.

Diagnosis of a presacral germ cell tumor is confirmed by a direct biopsy of the tumor. This may be either an excisional biopsy, in which the tumor is first removed, then examined; or, a needle biopsy, in which only a sample of the tumor is removed for examination.

Pineal area

A CT scan of the head will usually show a pineal tumor. An MRI scan, using gadolinium as a tracer chemical, may also be ordered.

Blood tests for AFP and beta-hCG may help to diagnose pineal area germ cell tumors. Tests for these chemicals on the cerebrospinal fluid (spinal tap or **lumbar puncture**) may also be ordered.

The diagnosis of a pineal area germ cell tumor is usually confirmed upon biopsy of the tumor after it has been removed from the patient.

Treatment team

Treatment of an extragonadal germ cell tumor depends on the location of the tumor. Most tumors are treated with a combination of surgery, **chemotherapy**, and radiation treatments.

Germ cell tumors of the mediastinum are generally not surgically removed. They are treated with high-dose radiation and sometimes with chemotherapy. Germ cell tumors of the presacral area are treated with chemotherapy to shrink the tumor, then surgery to remove the tumor. This surgery is generally performed by a physician who specializes in tumor removal surgery of the lower abdomen and pelvis. Germ cell tumors of the pineal area are generally

removed by a brain surgeon and then the patient is treated with radiation and/or chemotherapy.

Chemotherapy is administered under the direction of a physician who specializes in **cancer** (oncologist). Radiation therapies are generally administered by radiological technicians under the direction of an oncologist, a radiologist, a health physicist, and/or a medical radiation dosimetrist.

Clinical staging, treatments, and prognosis

The prognosis for patients with benign extragonadal germ cell tumors is excellent after surgery to remove the tumor is completed.

In the cases of malignant extragonadal germ cell tumors, the prognosis depends on the type and size of the tumor that is found.

Fifty-six percent of nonseminomas and 90% of seminomas have a good prognosis. Another 28% of nonseminomas and the remaining 10% of seminomas have an intermediate prognosis. While 16% of nonseminomas have a poor prognosis. A good prognosis is defined as a five-year survival rate above 85%. An intermediate prognosis is defined as a five-year survival rate between 50% and 85%. A poor prognosis is defined as a five year survival rate lower than 50%.

For both seminomas and nonseminomas, the prognosis is better if the tumors have not metastasized to other tissues. This is particularly true in the case of **mediastinal tumors**: those that have metastasized outside the general region of the lungs lead to particularly poor prognoses.

The prognosis for nonseminomas is based primarily on AFP and hCG concentrations found in the blood. The lower the levels of these two chemicals in the blood, the better the prognosis.

Alternative and complementary therapies

There are no effective alternative treatments for extragonadal germ cell tumors other than surgery, chemotherapy, and radiation.

Coping with cancer treatment

Most patients who undergo surgery to remove their tumors can resume their normal activities within a few days of the operation.

In some cases of presacral area germ cell tumors, it is difficult to remove the entire tumor in a single operation. In these cases, it is necessary for the patient to undergo a second course of chemotherapy prior to a second surgery to remove the remaining tumor.

When extensive chemotherapy is necessary, the patient may require counseling to help cope with the side effects of these treatments, such as loss of head and body hair, **weight loss**, **nausea**, **fatigue**, and changes in psychological well-being.

Clinical trials

There were 12 **clinical trials** underway, in early 2001, aimed at the treatment of extragonadal germ cell tumors. More information on these trials, including contact information, may be found by conducting a clinical trial search at the web site of the National Cancer Institute, CancerNet (http://cancernet.nci. nih.gov).

Prevention

Because the causes of extragonadal germ cell tumors are not known, there are no known preventions.

Special concerns

Repeat surgery may be necessary for extragonadal germ cell tumors, particularly those of the presacral area because these tumors are often difficult to remove completely. Careful monitoring by the medical team will be required.

See also Bone marrow aspiration and biopsy; Nuclear medicine scan; Testicular cancer.

Resources

OTHER

Extragonadal Germ Cell Cancer Articles and Links. 15 April 2001. [cited July 2, 2001]. http://www.acor.org/TCRC/egc_links.html.

ORGANIZATIONS

National Cancer Institute. Building 31, Room 10A03, 31 Center Dr., MSC 2580, Bethesda, MD 20892-2590. (800) 4-CANCER. http://www.nci.nih.gov.

Paul A. Johnson, Ed.M.

Famciclovir *see* **Antiviral therapy**

Familial cancer syndromes

Definition

Familial **cancer** syndromes are genetic conditions associated with an increased risk of specific types of cancers; for this reason they are sometimes called familial cancer susceptibility syndromes since they are not themselves types of cancer as such. Familial cancer syndromes account for only 5–10% of all cancers.

Demographics

Familial cancer syndromes are very rare in the general population; some affect only 1 person in every 30,000 to 100,000. As of 2009, researchers have identified about 55 different familial cancer syndromes.

Description

Most cancers are not inherited. Cancer itself is common; in 2008, more than 1.44 million new cancer cases were diagnosed in the United States. Many people have relatives who have had cancer, but most of the time these cancers are due to chance or environmental factors. In a familial cancer syndrome, however, an inherited or new genetic mutation causes a person to be at increased risk for cancer and other physical symptoms.

There are many different familial cancer syndromes, and each one has a specific set of characteristic cancers and physical symptoms associated with it. For example, **BRCA1** and **BRCA2** gene mutations are associated with an increased risk of breast and **ovarian cancer**. Examples of other familial cancer syndromes include von Hippel-Lindau syndrome, **Peutz-Jeghers syndrome**, Wilms tumor, and **Li-Fraumeni syndrome**.

Risk factors

Below is a list of "clues" in a family tree that make a familial cancer syndrome more suspicious:

- Two or more close relatives with the same type of cancer (on the same side of the family).
- Cancer diagnosed at an earlier age than usual.
- Cancer diagnosed more than once in the same person (more than one primary cancer, not a cancer recurrence).
- Cluster of cancers associated with a known familial cancer syndrome (such as breast and ovarian).
- Many cases of cancer in a family, more than can be accounted for by chance.
- Cancer in a person who also has birth defects.
- Evidence of autosomal dominant inheritance, which occurs when a gene from one parent overrides that of the other parent. When one parent has a dominant abnormal gene, the offspring each have a 50% chance of inheriting that gene.

Different familial cancer syndromes have different risks for cancer and associated symptoms. In general, a person who inherits the syndrome has a higher risk of developing the cancer associated with the syndrome than the general population, but this is not a guarantee that cancer will ever develop. On the other hand, someone who does not inherit the syndrome is not at increased risk for cancer above that of the general population, but this fact is no guarantee that cancer will not develop, and the person should follow screening guidelines for the general population.

Causes and symptoms

The causes of familial cancer syndromes are mutations in individual genes or damage to one or more sections of specific chromosomes. The specific symptoms of these syndromes vary depending on the organ or organ system affected, the inheritance pattern, the number of genes involved, the number of mutations

Gene	Consequence of gene loss
Rb	Retinoblastoma and osteosarcoma
TP53	Li-Fraumeni syndrome
Wt1	Wilms' tumor
VHL	von Hippel-Lindau syndrome; renal cell carcinoma
NF1	von Recklinghausen's disease; neurofibromatosis type 1; schwannoma and glioma
NF2	Neurofibromatosis type 2; acoustic neuroma and meningiomas
APC	Familial adenomatous polyposis; colorectal tumors
MMR	Hereditary nonpolyposis-colorectal cancer

Suppressor genes that, when deleted, predispose families to cancers

(Table by GGS Creative Resources. Cengage Learning, Gale.)

discovered that affect a particular gene, and other factors. As of 2009, the most recent source for brief descriptions of the 55 known familial cancer syndromes is the *Concise Handbook of Familial Cancer Susceptibility Syndromes*, second edition, which can be downloaded from http://jncimono.oxfordjournals.org/cgi/reprint/2008/38/3. It is about 93 pages long and includes information about cancer risk management for each of these syndromes as well as symptom descriptions and genetic information.

Diagnosis

The most important step in determining whether a family has a familial cancer syndrome is gathering an accurate family history. The family history should include children, brothers and sisters, parents, aunts, uncles, grandparents, nieces, nephews, and cousins on both sides of the family. For a person who has had cancer, the type of cancer and age at diagnosis should be listed for each cancer. It may be necessary to obtain medical records to confirm what type of cancer a person had since family members may not always be aware of specific information. Birth defects, unusual skin findings, benign tumors, and special screening tests (such as **colonoscopy** to look for colon polyps) should also be noted. When this type of family information is unavailable, it may be possible to look for clues in one or a small number of family members. A website with instructions for compiling a family health history is ldquo;My Family Health Portrait," at https://familyhistory.hhs.gov/fhh-web/home.action.

Many hospitals have a "familial cancer clinic," which is a team of health professionals with expertise in familial cancer syndromes. Geneticists, genetic counselors, oncologists, and social workers assist individuals and families by providing risk assessment, support, screening and prevention recommendations, and **genetic testing** options (if available).

Inheritance patterns

Some familial cancer syndromes show autosomal dominant inheritance, which means that an affected person has a 50% chance of passing on the genetic mutation to each of his or her children. Other familial cancer syndromes show autosomal recessive inheritance, which means that both parents are usually not affected, but are carriers of a mutation for the condition. In autosomal recessive inheritance, each child born to parents who are carriers has a 25% chance of having the condition. When a person is diagnosed with a familial cancer syndrome, relatives should be examined for signs of the syndrome. Sometimes a person identified as having a familial cancer syndrome is the first person in the family to be affected. That person is able to pass the condition on to his or her children, but the parents and siblings are not affected. Depending on the syndrome, genetics professionals can determine who in the family is at risk.

Tests

Although genetic testing is available for many familial cancer syndromes, there are genes that have yet to be discovered. Each syndrome has special issues surrounding genetic testing; for example, what age should the test be done? How would the results change medical management? Does insurance cover the test? How will the information affect the family? Health professionals familiar with familial cancer syndromes keep up to date with advances in **cancer genetics**, and work with families to discuss the risks, benefits and limitations of genetic testing.

Prevention

Since mid-2002, when the first complete draft of the Human Genome Project was completed, rapid advances have been made in the discovery of specific locations of cancer genes. For example, late in 2003, scientists tracked down the exact chromosome that carries certain familial forms of colorectal cancer. By mapping every normal gene in the human body, scientists can compare abnormal DNA sequences that lead to cancer. For example, the BRAF mutation has been linked to several cancers. Data from the Human Genome Project will help identify cancer genes, develop better genetic tests for cancer, and lead to improved preventive and therapeutic interventions.

The work of the Human Genome Project is continued at the National Human Genome Research Institute (NHGRI). The NHGRI website contains links to many resources for information about specific familial cancer syndromes. One is the Genetics and Rare Diseases (GARD) Information Center at http://rarediseases.info.nih.gov/GARD/Default.aspx?PageID=4. GARD also has information specialists who can be contacted by telephone at 888-205-2311.

Another online resource is the National Library of Medicine's Genetics Home Reference at http://ghr.nlm.nih.gov/. The site includes information about inheritance patterns, genetic testing, and genetic counseling as well as specific information about more than 400 genetically transmitted diseases.

Resources

BOOKS

Lalloo, Fiona, et al, eds. *Risk Assessment and Management in Cancer Genetics*. New York: Oxford University Press, 2005.

PERIODICALS

Castells, A., et al. "Concepts in Familial Colorectal Cancer: Where Do We Stand and What Is the Future?" *Gastroenterology* 137 (August 2009): 404–09.

Goldin, L. R., et al. "Highly Increased Familial Risks for Specific Lymphoma Subtypes." *British Journal of Haematology* 146 (June 2009): 91–94.

Lobb, E. A., et al. "Attendance of Men at the Familial Cancer Clinic: What They Value from the Consultation." *Genetics in Medicine* 11 (June 2009): 443–440.

Oliveira, C., et al. "Hereditary Gastric Cancer." *Best Practice and Research: Clinical Gastroenterology* 23 (February 2009): 147–57.

Reis, M. M., et al. "Evaluation of a Surveillance Programme for Women with a Family History of Breast Cancer." *Journal of Medical Genetics* 46 (May 2009): 319–23.

OTHER

Lindor, Noralane, et al. *Concise Handbook of Familial Cancer Susceptibility Syndromes*, 2nd ed. http://jncimono.oxfordjournals.org/cgi/reprint/2008/38/3.

National Cancer Institute (NCI). *Understanding Gene Testing*. (slide show with text) http://www.cancer.gov/cancertopics/understandingcancer/genetesting/allpages.

Riegert-Johnson, Douglas, ed. *Familial Cancer Syndromes*. This is an online resource provided by the National Center for Biotechnology Information (NCBI). As of September 2009 three chapters have been posted, with six more planned. http://www.ncbi.nlm.nih.gov/bookshelf/br.fcgi?book=famcan.

ORGANIZATIONS

American Cancer Society, 250 Williams Street NW, Atlanta, GA, 30303, 800-ACS-2345 (227-2345), www.cancer.org.

National Cancer Institute, 6116 Executive Blvd., Room 3036A, Bethesda, MD, 20892-8322, 800-422-6237, cancergovstaff@mail.nih.gov, www.cancer.gov.

National Human Genome Research Institute (NHGRI), Building 31, Room 4B09, 31 Center Drive, MSC 2152, 9000 Rockville Pike, Bethesda, MD, 20892-2152, 301-402-0911, 301-402-2218, http://www.genome.gov/.

University of Chicago Comer Children's Hospital Familial Cancer Clinic, 5721 S. Maryland Avenue, Chicago, IL, 60637, 773-702-1000, 888-UCH-0200, http://www.uchicagokidshospital.org/specialties/cancer/familial-cancer.html.

Laura L. Stein, M.S., C.G.C.
Teresa G. Odle
Rebecca J. Frey, PhD

Famotidine *see* **Histamine 2 antagonists**

Fanconi anemia

Definition

Fanconi **anemia** is an inherited form of aplastic anemia characterized by an abnormally low number of cellular components in the blood due to failing bone marrow.

Description

Fanconi anemia (FA) is a rare genetic disease caused by mutations or alterations in one of seven different genes. The disease is an autosomal recessive condition, meaning that the genes are not located on the sex chromosomes and a mutated gene copy must be inherited from both parents in order for a person to be affected. Test results of cells from FA patients suggest that the genetic defects of FA reduce the cell's

KEY TERMS

Aplastic anemia—A disease in which the bone marrow stops producing all three types of cells of the blood: red blood cells, white blood cells, and platelets.

Fludarabine—A drug that inhibits a blood cell's ability to produce DNA, eliminating native cells from FA patients so they can undergo BMT.

Myelodysplastic syndrome—A disease where the bone marrow stops producing healthy blood cells and the cells that are produced function poorly. This syndrome sometimes develops into leukemia.

Neutrophil—A type of white blood cells important in the defense of the body against infection.

QUESTIONS TO ASK THE DOCTOR

- Which FA gene is responsible for my child's illness?
- Are growth factor or gene therapies appropriate for my child?
- When should bone marrow transplantation be considered as an appropriate treatment?

ability to repair damaged deoxyribonucleic acid (DNA), the primary chemical component of chromosomes. Five of the seven genes associated with FA have been isolated.

Demographics

With only approximately 1,000 cases documented in the literature, FA is a rare disease with varied frequency in different ethnic groups. It is particularly prevalent in the Ashkenazi Jewish population, where carriers are 1 in 89 persons, compared to an overall carrier frequency of 1 in 100 to 600. A carrier is a person unaffected by the disease who has one mutated and one normal gene in their genome. Both parents must be carriers in order to produce a child with FA.

Causes and symptoms

FA is caused by inheriting two abnormal copies of one of seven different genes, all thought to be involved in DNA repair. About 67% of children with FA are born with some sort of congenital defect. The problems seen include:

- short stature
- abnormalities of the thumb or arm
- other skeletal abnormalities such as of the hip or ribs
- kidney malformations
- skin discoloration
- small eyes or head
- mental retardation
- low birth weight and failure to thrive
- abnormalities of the digestive system
- heart defects

The defining characteristic of FA is progressive pancytopenia, a gradual reduction of the cellular components of the blood. A reduction in red blood cells is typically noted first, then white blood cells, and finally, platelets. Complete bone marrow failure in FA patients is usually seen between the ages of three and twelve, with a median of seven.

Later in life, FA patients have delayed sexual maturity and an increased probability of developing **cancer**. For FA patients surviving into adulthood, 50% develop leukemia (a malignancy of the white blood cells) and/or **myelodysplastic syndrome** (MDS, a pre-leukemic state). Persons with FA also have an elevated chance of developing squamous cell cancers (originating in the outer layer of the skin), particularly gynecological cancers (for females); head, neck and throat cancers; **gastrointestinal cancers**; and liver cancers.

Diagnosis

Diagnosis can be made upon the appearance of the characteristic congenital defects, but is more common upon development of aplastic anemia (when the bone marrow fails to produce normal numbers of blood cells). Definitive diagnosis involves a showing of an unusual level of chromosome breakage when cells are exposed to DNA damaging agents. Additionally, with five of the seven genes associated with FA isolated, genetic engineering techniques can often be used to determine exactly what gene mutation is responsible for the disease. An estimated 90% of FA patients have mutations within the FANCA, FANCC and FANCG genes, all of which have been isolated.

Treatment team

FA is usually treated by pediatricians, hematologists, and, if a bone marrow transplant (BMT) is performed, a specialized teams of physicians, nurses, and medical assistants who are experienced in BMT.

Clinical staging, treatments, and prognosis

There is no clinical staging system for FA.

BMT and androgen therapy are two long-term non-experimental treatments for FA. BMT involves the suppression of the patient's own marrow and replacement with stem cells of the donor. The effectiveness of BMT is highly dependent on the existence of a donor that is closely matched to the patient. For sibling match (full match) transplants, the two-year survival rate is about 80%, compared to about 37% for less than a full match. The difference is due the prevalence of graft versus host disease (GVHD), where the recipient's body rejects the donor cells. The use of T-cell (a type of immune cell) depletion before transplantation and the drug **fludarabine** have significantly reduced the occurrence of GVHD. BMT does not alter the tendency of FA patients to develop other malignancies later in life, however.

Androgen therapy involves the administration of male hormones to stimulate the production of blood cells. Most FA patients respond for at least a time to this therapy. The cell increase lasts a few years at most, however, and the hormones have serious side effects, including masculinization of female patients and liver disease.

Clinical trials

Growth factor therapy and gene therapy are two treatments being tested in **clinical trials**. Two growth factors—granulocyte/macrophage colony stimulating factor (GM-CSF) and granulocyte colony stimulating factor (G-CSF)—were shown to increase blood cell production. Patients with low neutrophil counts particularly benefit from this treatment.

A clinical trial for gene therapy of FA patients is ongoing. The normal copy of the mutated gene is introduced into the patient's own bone marrow stem cells using a viral vector. When the virus infects the stem cells, the normal FANC gene is integrated into the stem cell's DNA. This therapy will, theoretically, correct the defect in the stem cells and prevent their premature death, curing the aplastic anemia seen in FA patients. As with BMT, however, this gene therapy will not reduce the development of other cancers in FA patients.

Prevention

The only known method of prevention of this disease is prenatal diagnosis and termination of pregnancies for affected embryos. Preimplantation genetic diagnosis, where one or two cells are tested from *in*

vitro fertilized embryos, is also available. This method avoids the need for abortion, but carries more risk.

Special concerns

Because FA can be present without any outward symptoms, it is essential that any potential sibling donor for BMT be carefully tested for the disease using white blood cell exposure to DNA damaging agents or direct examination of their FANC gene copies before the transplant.

See also Bone marrow transplantation; Genetic testing.

Resources

BOOKS

Frohnmeyer, Lynn, and Dave Frohnmeyer. *Fanconi Anemia: A Handbook for Families and Their Physicians.* Eugene, Oregon: Fanconi Anemia Research Fund, Inc., 2000.

PERIODICALS

de Winter, J.P., et al. "The Fanconi anemia protein FANCF forms a nuclear complex with FANCA, FANCC and FANCG." *Human Molecular Genetics* 9 (November 2000): 2665-74.
Garcia-Higuera, I., et al. "Interaction of the Fanconi anemia proteins and BRCA1 in a common pathway." *Molecular Cell* 7 (February 2001): 249-62.

OTHER

Online Mendelian Inheritance in Man (OMIM). John Hopkins University, Baltimore, MD. MIM Nos. 602956, 603467, 227645, 227646, 227650. April 2001. 25 June 2001 http://www.ncbi.nlm.nih.gov/omim/.

ORGANIZATIONS

Fanconi Anemia Research Fund, Inc. 1801 Willamette St., Suite 200, Eugene, OR 97401. (800) 828-4891. www.fanconi.org.

Michelle Johnson, M.S., J.D.

Fatigue

Description

Fatigue is a feeling of exhaustion or loss of strength. The duration of fatigue for a patient with **cancer** has been found to last from one to two times the length of time between diagnosis and completion of treatment, so it is common for fatigue to persist beyond a patient's treatment regimen.

Causes

Many people experience fatigue as a side effect of cancer treatment. Both **chemotherapy** and **radiation therapy** are associated with fatigue. Scientists believe fatigue also occurs because the body is devoting so much of its energy fighting the cancer that it has little left over for daily life. Often the feelings of exhaustion are more intense immediately following a cancer treatment, but they gradually ease over time as the body gains strength.

During chemotherapy, anti-cancer drugs kill both cancer cells and healthy cells, including red blood cells. This can lead to **anemia**, or low red blood cell counts, which causes fatigue. Chemotherapy agents also attack white blood cells, weakening the immune system.

Medications, pain, **depression**, and the stress of the diagnosis and treatment are other factors that result in fatigue.

Treatments

If anemia is a problem, physicians may prescribe iron supplements or drugs, such as **erythropoietin**, to stimulate blood cell growth. In some cases, blood transfusions may be necessary.

Many people with cancer find that they must pace themselves, alternating periods of activity with small naps. Going to bed earlier also seems to help.

Research has shown that people who exercise experience less cancer-related fatigue. Walking or using an exercise bicycle are good choices. For those who have severe weakness, even a few minutes of gentle stretching in bed can make a difference.

Eating nutritious food is another way to get an energy boost to better fight cancer. Include a variety of fruits and vegetables, whole grains and plenty of protein, if **nausea and vomiting** are not a problem. High-calorie liquid meals can help offset severe **weight loss** for those who cannot tolerate solid foods. Drinking plenty of water also helps prevent **diarrhea** and dehydration, which add to fatigue.

Alternative and complementary therapies

Yoga has proven to be highly effective in reducing stress, thereby increasing energy and helping people to relax and sleep better.

Marijuana has been used to help ease **nausea** in cancer patients. Since a loss of appetite can cause weakness and fatigue, marijuana may help indirectly. Most states do not permit the use of marijuana for medical reasons. Physicians will be aware of these regulations.

Other complementary therapies, such as massage, aromatherapy, meditation, or prayer, help people with cancer relax, easing their worries and ultimately combatting fatigue.

See also Complementary cancer therapies.

Resources

BOOKS

Clegg, Holly B., and Gerald Miletello, MD. *Eating Well Through Cancer.* Baton Rouge: Holly B. Clegg Inc., 2001.

Hassett Dahm, Nancy, and Robert Schirmer. *Mind, Body and Soul: A Guide to Living with Cancer.* New York: Taylor Hill Publishing, 2000.

PERIODICALS

Dimeo, F. C., et al. "Effects of Physical Activity on the Fatigue and Psychologic Status of Cancer Patients During Chemotherapy." *Cancer* 85, no. 10 (May 15, 1999): 2273–7.

OTHER

"Fatigue." *American Cancer Society* June 2001. [cited June 28, 2001]. <http://www3.cancer.org/cancerinfo/>.

ORGANIZATIONS

American Cancer Society. 1599 Clifton Road, Atlanta, GA 30329. (800) ACS-2345. http://www.cancer.org.

CancerFatigue.org. Oncology Nursing Society, 501 Holiday Dr., Pittsburgh, PA 15220. (412) 921-7373. http://www.cancerfatigue.org.

Melissa Knopper, M.S.

Fecal occult blood test

Definition

The fecal occult blood test (FOBT) is performed as part of the routine physical examination during the examination of the rectum. It is used to detect microscopic blood in the stool and is a screening tool for colorectal **cancer**.

Purpose

FOBT uses chemical indicators on stool samples to detect the presence of blood not otherwise visible. (The word "occult" in the test's name means that the blood is hidden from view.) Blood originating from or passing through the gastrointestinal tract can signal many conditions requiring further diagnostic procedures and, possibly, medical treatment. These conditions may be benign or malignant and some of them include:

• colon, rectal, and gastric (stomach) cancers
• ulcers

- hemorrhoids
- polyps
- inflammatory bowel disease
- irritations or lesions of the gastrointestinal tract caused by medications (such as nonsteroidal anti-inflammatory drugs, also called NSAIDs)
- irritations or lesions of the gastrointestinal tract caused by stomach acid disorders, such as reflux esophagitis

The FOBT is used routinely (in conjunction with a rectal examination performed by a physician) to screen for colorectal cancer, particularly after age 50. The ordering of this test should not be taken as an indication that cancer is suspected. The FOBT must be combined with regular screening endoscopy (such as a **sigmoidoscopy**) to detect cancers at an early stage.

Precautions

Certain foods and medicines can influence the test results. Some fruits contain chemicals that prevent the guaiac, the chemical in which the test paper is soaked, from reacting with the blood. Aspirin and some NSAIDs irritate the stomach, resulting in bleeding, and should be avoided prior to the examination. Red meat and many vegetables and fruits containing vitamin C also should be avoided for a specified period of time prior to the test. All of these factors could result in a false-positive result.

Description

Feces for the stool samples is obtained either by the physician at the rectal examination or by the patient at home, using a small spatula or a collection device. In most cases, the collection of stool samples can easily be done at home, using a kit supplied by the physician. The standard kit contains a specially prepared card on which a small sample of stool will be spread, using a stick provided in the kit. The sample is placed in a special envelope and either mailed or

brought in for analysis. When the physician applies hydrogen peroxide to the back of the sample, the paper will turn blue if an abnormal amount of blood is present.

Types of fecal occult blood tests

Hemoccult is the most commonly used fecal occult blood test. The Hemoccult test takes less than five minutes to perform and may be performed in the physician's office or in the laboratory. The Hemoccult blood test can detect bleeding from the colon as low as 0.5 mg per day.

Tests that use anti-hemoglobin antibodies (or immunochemical tests) to detect blood in the stool are also used. Immunochemical tests can detect up to 0.7 mg of hemoglobin in the stool and do not require dietary restrictions. Immunochemical tests

- are not accurate for screening for stomach cancer
- are more sensitive than Hemoccult tests in detecting colorectal cancer
- are more expensive than Hemoccult tests

Hemoquant, another fecal occult blood test, is used to detect as much as 500 mg/g of blood in the stool. Like the Hemoccult, the Hemoquant test is affected by red meat. It is not affected by chemicals in vegetables.

Fecal blood may also be measured by the amount of chromium in the red blood cells in the feces. The stool is collected for three to ten days. The test is used in cases where the exact amount of blood loss is required. It is the only test that can exclude blood loss from the gastrointestinal area with accuracy.

Medicare coverage began on January 1, 2004, for a newer fecal occult blood test based on immunoassay. This technique does not rely on guaiac, so it is not influenced by diet or medications used prior to the test. The immunoassay test also requires fewer specimen collections. At a conference of gastroenterologists (physicians who specialize in diseases of the stomach and related digestive systems), a company announced a new fecal occult blood test that was based on DNA and appeared more sensitive than traditional tests. Widespread use of these new tests remains to be seen; the traditional guiaic test has been in place for about 30 years.

Preparation

For 72 hours prior to collecting samples, patients should avoid red meats, NSAIDs (including aspirin), antacids, steroids, iron supplements, and vitamin C, including citrus fruits and other foods containing large amounts of vitamin C. Foods like uncooked broccoli, uncooked turnips, cauliflower, uncooked cantaloupe, uncooked radish and horseradish and parsnips should be avoided and not eaten during the 72 hours prior to the examination. Fish, chicken, pork, fruits (other than melons) and many cooked vegetables are permitted in the diet.

Results

Many factors can result in false-positive and false-negative findings.

Positive results

It is important to note that a true-positive finding only signifies the presence of blood—it is not an indication of cancer. The National Cancer Institute states that, in its experience, less than 10% of all positive results were caused by cancer. The FOBT is positive in 1%–5% of the unscreened population and 2%–10% of those are found to have cancer. The physician will want to follow up on a positive result with further tests, as indicated by other factors in the patient's history or condition.

Negative results

Alternatively, a negative result (meaning no blood was detected) does not guarantee the absence of **colon cancer**, which may bleed only occasionally or not at all. (Only 50% of colon cancers are FOBT-positive.)

Conclusions

Screening using the FOBT has been demonstrated to reduce colorectal cancer. However, because only half of colorectal cancers are FOBT-positive, FOBT must be combined with regular screening endoscopy to increase the detection of pre-malignant colorectal polyps and cancers.

Resources

BOOKS

DeVita, Vincent, Samuel Hellman, and Steven Rosenburg. *Cancer:Principles and Practices of Oncology.* Philadelphia:Lippincott Williams & Wilkins, 2001.

Yamada, Tadetaka, editor. *Textbook of Gastroenterology Volumes One and Two.* Philadelphia:Lippincott Williams & Wilkins, 2001.

PERIODICALS

"DNA-based Stool Test More Sensitive than Fecal Occult Blood Test in Study." *Health & Medicine Week* November 10, 2003: 194.

From the Centers for Disease Control and Prevention. "Trends in screening for colorectal cancer—United States, 1997 and 1999." *Journal of the American Medical Association* 28 (March 2001): 12.

Silverman, Jennifer. "Colorectal Screning Option." *Family Practice News* 33 (December 15, 2003): 49–51.

OTHER

"Colon and Rectum Cancer." *American Cancer Society.* Copyright 2000. [cited July 10, 2001]. http://www.cancer.org.

"ColorectalCancer Screening." *WebMD.* <http://my.webmd.com/content/article/2955.291>.

"Fecal Occult Bood Test." *Virtual Health Fair.* Copyright 1997-2000. [cited July 10, 2001]. <http://vfair.com/resources/lab/fecal.htm>.

ORGANIZATIONS

American Cancer Society. Phone: 1-800-ACS-2345. Web site: http://www.cancer.org.

National Cancer Institute (NCI). 1-800-4-CANCER (1-800-422-6237), TTY: 1-800-332-8615. Web site: <http://rex.nci.nih.gov>.

Jill S. Lasker
Cheryl Branche, M.D.

Fentanyl *see* **Opioids**

Fentanyl transdermal *see* **Fentanyl**

Fertility issues

Overview

Any procedure or medication that interferes with the functioning of the testes or ovaries affects fertility. The choices made before **cancer** treatment begins can determine whether the patient will remain fertile after treatment. Prior to deciding on a treatment plan, it is important for the patient to discuss the issue of fertility with the treatment team so that all options, with their associated risks, can be considered.

Conventional cancer treatments and their effects on fertility

Cancer is usually treated with surgery, **chemotherapy**, and/or radiation, with the type and stage of the cancer dictating the treatment regimen recommended. While some physicians may routinely take into consideration alternatives to spare a patient's fertility, others may not, feeling that to differ from the treatment norm may compromise the patient's best chances for survival. Patients for whom fertility preservation is important, or for whom fertility-sparing measures could compromise treatment outcome, must discuss this issue fully with their treatment team.

Surgery

Surgery for cancer usually involves removal of the cancerous area, with some sampling of the adjacent area and lymph nodes to check for **metastasis**. If surgery must involve the removal of both of the testes or ovaries, the man will not be able to provide his own sperm, and the woman her own egg, towards the development of a biologic child. (A couple may be able to use donated sperm or egg when attempting a future pregnancy, however.) Fertility-sparing surgery may be an option for some individuals, depending on the type and stage of their cancer. For example, a woman with **ovarian cancer** contained to one ovary may be able to have just that one removed. The same is true for a man with **testicular cancer** contained to one testicle. In the case of testicular cancer, removal of retroperitoneal lymph nodes during surgery may damage the nerves affecting ejaculation. Men may wish to discuss nerve-sparing surgery and their concerns for fertility with their surgeon prior to surgery.

Chemotherapy

Chemotherapy affects the whole body, but certain drugs are less harmful to the reproductive tract than others. The drugs used in chemotherapy are highly toxic, in order to kill any cancer cell. However, they are not very selective, meaning that in addition to cancerous cells, normal cells are killed as well. It may take a few years after chemotherapy has finished to understand its temporary or permanent effect on fertility. It is generally recommended that women wait about two years after chemotherapy before attempting to become pregnant, to avoid the risk of a pregnancy that may end in miscarriage or a fetal malformation. Men who have had chemotherapy can have their sperm analyzed after treatment has finished to check sperm counts and motility.

There is a concern that individuals may delay treatment in order to undergo various fertility-preserving measures, such as sperm banking or egg retrieval and cryopreservation, and that this delay could result in a poorer treatment outcome. Some women undergo attempts at egg retrieval and embryo cryopreservation after an initial dose of chemotherapy. Some treatment centers offer the option of doing the chemotherapy in stages. The first stage of chemotherapy uses

medications that are considered less toxic. Then the more intensive treatment follows after the harvesting of egg or sperm. However, it is still not yet clear what kind of damage may have been endured by tissue harvested right after some chemotherapy.

Radiation

Radiation is known to damage the highly sensitive sperm and eggs. Just as chemotherapy attacks healthy cells, so does radiation. However, radiation technology is able to focus very tightly on the cancerous area, which decreases risk to healthy tissue. When radiation for cancer does not involve the pelvic area, it may be possible to successfully shield the reproductive organs to preserve fertility. If the area needing irradiation is the pelvis, the reproductive organs are at great risk of damage.

When radiation is done to the pelvic area, women often experience a pause in menstruation, along with other symptoms of menopause. There may also be vaginal dryness, **itching**, and burning. Radiation may affect sexual desire as well. Men may experience a decrease in sperm count and motility, and difficulty in having or maintaining an erection. These changes may be temporary or permanent, and it may take up to a few years to determine if the effects were temporary or permanent. Sperm banking or cryopreservation of eggs may allow the individual reproductive success in the future.

Since radiation can be harmful to the fetus, pregnancy during **radiation therapy** is contraindicated, and because the full effect of the radiation on fertility cannot be predicted, individuals should use contraception during sexual relations while receiving radiation therapy.

Bone marrow transplant

A bone marrow transplant (BMT) may be part of the suggested treatment regimen. If so, patients need to understand its potential impact on future fertility. While the actual BMT does not jeopardize fertility, chemotherapy or radiation done prior to the BMT in preparation for the body's receiving of the new marrow can damage fertility. This pretreatment can destroy cells in the reproductive organs, rendering the individual infertile. While each case is unique, patients may wish to discuss the impact of their treatment on their reproductive future, and consider sperm banking or egg cryopreservation.

Children's cancers and future fertility

In the case of children, chemotherapy and radiation for childhood cancer can cause permanent damage to the ovaries or testes. In boys who have become sexually mature, sperm banking may provide future reproductive options. Options such as sperm aspiration, and cryopreservation of female ova are still considered experimental in children. While they may be effective, researchers are concerned that parents and their children may be unrealistic in their hopes for future fertility, and that the reintroduction of the harvested tissue may return latent cancer cells into the body. While research may bring new options, obtaining true informed consent involving children and their parents is an issue of moral and practical concern.

Alternative and complementary therapies

Individuals undergoing cancer treatment may turn to alternative therapies for a number of reasons. Techniques such as meditation, therapeutic touch, yoga, t'ai chi, and guided imagery can be very helpful in reducing stress and its effects on the body. Acupuncture has been shown through research studies to be effective in reducing the **nausea and vomiting** associated with chemotherapy. However, a study reported in the March 1999 issue of the medical journal *Fertility and Sterility* investigated several herbal remedies and their effect on sperm and ova. While this study was involved in animal research, the finding that high concentrations of St. John's wort, an herbal supplement used for mild to moderate **depression**, Echinacea, and ginkgo biloba damaged reproductive cells raises concern for its effect on humans. In particular, St. John's wort was found to be mutagenic to sperm cells.

Special concerns

Some cancers, such as testicular cancer, affect primarily young men. Most men diagnosed with testicular cancer are between the ages of 15 and 40. Sperm banking is highly recommended for these men. The method intracytoplasmic sperm injection uses just one sperm to fertilize one egg, by injecting the sperm directly into the egg. This can result in a fertilized egg for insemination, even when the sperm has decreased motility. It has a success rate of 30%.

Fertility issues and the development of cancer

Fertility issues can also play a role in the development of cancer. For example, women having their first child after 30 are at slightly higher risk of developing ovarian cancer than those having their first child before age 30. The number of ovulatory cycles a woman experiences also appears to affect her risk for ovarian cancer. A longer reproductive period (early menarche and late menopause) appears to raise the risk, while having children (there is no ovulation during pregnancy), breastfeeding (there is some suppression of ovulation during breastfeeding), and the use of oral contraceptives for at least five years decreases the risk.

Women who used the infertility medication clomiphene citrate without becoming pregnant were found in some studies to have a greater risk of developing a low malignancy potential ovarian cancer. In a November 1999 issue of the medical journal *Lancet*, researchers reported that women whose infertility remained unexplained were found to have more ovarian and uterine cancers, irrespective of whether or not they had been treated for the infertility. Also, more breast cancers were detected in the first year after treatment for infertility terminated than was expected. The lead author of the study speculated that these cancer diagnoses may be due to closer medical supervision that resulted in early detection. In some cases it was believed that the infertility was a symptom of the undiagnosed cancer.

Resources

BOOKS

Runowicz, Carolyn D., Jeanne A. Petrek, and Ted S. Gansler. *The American Cancer Society: Women and Cancer.* New York: Villard Book, 1999.

Teeley, Peter, and Philip Bashe. *The Complete Cancer Survival Guide.* New York: Doubleday, 2000.

PERIODICALS

Venn, Alison, et al. "Risk of cancer after use of fertility drugs with in-vitro fertilization." *The Lancet* November 6, 1999: 190.

ORGANIZATIONS

American Cancer Society. (800) ACS-2345. http://www.cancer.org.

Esther Csapo Rastegari, R.N., B.S.N., Ed.M.

Fever

Definition

Fever is a condition in which the body's temperature rises above its normal thermoregulatory set point, usually by about 1.8°F to 3.6°F (1°C to 2°C). It is also known as pyrexia. Fever is sometimes categorized as a form of **hyperthermia** (any elevation of body temperature above normal) but it is distinguished from hyperthermia caused by exposure to heat from the environment. The latter condition represents a failure of thermoregulation; that is, the body absorbs or produces more heat than it can dissipate. Fever, on the other hand, represents the immune system's response to an internal threat, usually a disease organism. The role of fever in the body's response to disease was first understood and described by a German physician named Carl Wunderlich (1815–1877) in a report published in 1868.

Demographics

Fever is an extremely common condition worldwide. Almost all children have at least one febrile illness during childhood, and many adults have low-grade fevers with such widespread illnesses as the common cold. According to one estimate, as many as 11% of adults who travel abroad return home with a febrile illness, usually an upper respiratory **infection** or community-acquired **pneumonia**.

Description

A healthy person's body temperature fluctuates between 97 °F (36.1 °C) and 100 °F (37.8 °C), with the average being 98.6 °F (37 °C). The body maintains stability within this range by balancing the heat produced by the metabolism with the heat lost to the environment. Body temperature in humans also varies according to the time of day as well as from individual to individual. Early-morning body temperature may be as low as 97°F, and as high as 99.3°F in the afternoon hours, yet still be considered normal.

It is also important to note that normal human body temperature varies somewhat in different locations in the body. Depending on where a thermometer is inserted, fever can be defined as:

- Rectal: a temperature above 100°F (37.8°C).
- Oral: a temperature above 99.5°F (37.5°C).
- Armpit: a temperature at or above 99°F (37.2°C).
- Ear: a temperature at or above 99°F (37.2°C).

The set point or "thermostat" that controls this process is located in the hypothalamus, a small structure located deep within the brain just above the brain stem. The nervous system constantly relays information about the body's temperature to the thermostat, which in turn activates different physical responses designed to cool or warm the body, depending on the circumstances. These responses include: decreasing or increasing the flow of blood from the body's core, where it is warmed, to the surface, where it is cooled; slowing down or speeding up the rate at which the body turns food into energy (metabolic rate); inducing shivering, which generates heat through muscle contraction; and inducing sweating, which cools the body through evaporation.

A fever occurs when the thermostat resets at a higher temperature, primarily in response to an infection. To reach the higher temperature, the body moves blood to the warmer interior, increases the metabolic rate, and induces shivering. The chills that often accompany a fever are caused by the movement of blood to the body's core, leaving the surface and extremities cold. Once the higher temperature is achieved, the shivering and chills stop. When the infection has been overcome or such drugs as aspirin or acetaminophen (Tylenol) have been taken, the thermostat resets to normal and the body's cooling mechanisms switch on: the blood moves to the surface and sweating occurs.

Fever is an important component of the **immune response**, though its role is not completely understood. Physicians believe that an elevated body temperature has several effects. The immune system chemicals that react with the fever-inducing agent and trigger the resetting of the thermostat also increase the production of cells that fight off the invading bacteria or viruses. Higher temperatures also inhibit the growth of some bacteria, while at the same time speeding up the chemical reactions that help the body's cells repair themselves. In addition, the increased heart rate that may accompany the changes in blood circulation also speeds the arrival of white blood cells to the sites of infection.

How long a fever lasts and how high it may go depends on several factors, including its cause, the age of the patient, and his or her overall health. Most fevers caused by infections are acute, appearing suddenly and then resolving as the immune system defeats the infectious agent. An infectious fever may also rise and fall throughout the day, reaching its peak in the late afternoon or early evening. A low-grade fever that lasts for several weeks is associated with such autoimmune diseases as lupus or rheumatoid arthritis, or with some cancers, particularly leukemia and **lymphoma**.

It is important to note that the degree of a fever in an adolescent or adult does not necessarily reflect the seriousness of the underlying cause. It is possible for relatively minor illnesses to produce high fevers and for serious conditions to produce relatively low fevers.

Risk factors

Risk factors for fever include:

- Living or working in close contact with others with febrile illnesses, particularly small children.
- Having a weakened immune system.
- Frequent travel abroad, particularly to countries with poor sanitation, high rates of malaria, and high rates of other febrile illnesses.
- Being treated for cancer.
- Being hospitalized for any illness or injury. Many people contract pneumonia or other febrile illnesses during a hospital stay.
- Having an autoimmune disorder.
- Having Parkinson's disease or other severe neurological disorder.

Causes and symptoms

Causes

Fevers in the general population are primarily caused by viral or bacterial infections, such as pneumonia or influenza. However, other conditions can induce a fever, including allergic reactions; autoimmune diseases; trauma, such as breaking a bone; **cancer**; excessive exposure to the sun; intense exercise; hormonal imbalances; certain drugs; and damage to the hypothalamus. When an infection occurs, fever-inducing agents called pyrogens are released, either by the body's immune system or by the invading cells themselves, that trigger the resetting of the thermostat. In other circumstances, the immune system may overreact (allergic reactions) or become damaged (autoimmune diseases), causing the uncontrolled release of pyrogens. A stroke or tumor can damage the hypothalamus, causing the body's thermostat to malfunction. Malignant hyperthermia is a rare inherited condition in which a person develops a very high fever when given certain anesthetics or muscle relaxants in preparation for surgery.

Fever associated with cancer can generally be categorized into four major causal groups: infection, tumors, allergic reactions to a drug, or allergic reaction to blood components in transfusion therapies. For cancer patients, fever should be considered a result of infection until an alternative cause is diagnosed. When a fever develops in a cancer patient, the individual must be thoroughly examined to determine the cause. A comprehensive physical examination should be administered by the physician and blood drawn for laboratory analysis.

Symptoms

The most common symptoms of fever in addition to a high temperature include:

- sweating
- shivering
- headache
- muscle cramps or aches
- loss of appetite
- thirst/dehydration
- general feeling of tiredness and weakness

Symptoms that may appear with high fevers (103°F to 106°F; 39.4°C to 41.1°C):

- mental confusion
- hallucinations
- irritability
- seizures or convulsions

SYMPTOMS REQUIRING EMERGENCY TREATMENT. A fever requires emergency treatment under the following circumstances:

- newborn (three months or younger) with a fever over 100.5 °F (38 °C)
- infant or child with a fever over 103 °F (39.4 °C)

- fever accompanied by severe headache, neck stiffness, mental confusion, or severe swelling of the throat
- hyperpyrexia: fever at or over 105°F (41°C) in anyone
- the fever has lasted three days or longer
- unusual skin rash
- inability to swallow or take liquids by mouth
- unusual sensitivity to bright light
- persistent vomiting
- difficulty breathing or chest pain
- abdominal pain or pain when urinating

A very high fever in a small child can trigger seizures (febrile seizures) and therefore should be treated immediately. A fever accompanied by the above symptoms can indicate the presence of a serious infection, such as meningitis, and should be brought to the immediate attention of a physician.

FEVER IN CHILDREN. Children's temperatures are generally higher than those of adults and fluctuate more widely. They may vary depending on the time of day, the child's emotional state or level of physical activity, the amount of clothing worn, or the surrounding room temperature. In general, temperatures under 100°F (37.7°C) are considered subfebrile (i.e., not indicating fever). Rectal temperatures of up to 100.4°F (38°C) may be considered normal.

A child's temperature can be taken in several ways. Rectal temperatures are about one-half a degree higher than oral ones. A rectal reading is considered more accurate than an oral one, which may be affected by previously eaten hot or cold foods or by a child's breathing. Underarm temperatures are considered reliable for young infants, and electronic thermometers can measure temperature through the ear. Although fever is generally a cause for concern among parents, high fevers are not necessarily a sign of serious illness. A mild cold may produce a fever as high as 105°F (40.5°C), while the fever accompanying pneumonia may only be 100°F (37.7°C). The temperatures of newborn infants are particularly unreliable because the baby's temperature control mechanism is not yet adequately developed.

Diagnosis

A fever is usually diagnosed using a thermometer. A variety of different thermometers are available, including traditional glass and mercury ones used for oral or rectal temperature readings and more sophisticated electronic ones that can be inserted in the ear to quickly register the body's temperature. For adults and older children, temperature readings are usually taken orally. Younger children who cannot or will not hold a thermometer in their mouths can have their temperature taken by placing an oral thermometer under their armpit. Infants generally have their temperature taken rectally using a rectal thermometer.

Examination

The cause of fever in adults or adolescents is generally diagnosed during an office visit by a careful patient history (including recent travel, a history of autoimmune disorders, recent immunizations, or exposure to persons with contagious illnesses) and taking the patient's vital signs (temperature, pulse, breathing rate, and blood pressure). The doctor will examine the inside of the patient's mouth and throat for signs of an infectious illness, and may swab the patient's throat to obtain a sample for culture.

In terms of office visits for children, most experts agree that a doctor should be notified immediately when fever appears in an infant under the age of eight weeks. Children at this age are susceptible to serious, even life-threatening, infections that can come on suddenly and need immediate attention. For children up to the age of three years, a doctor should be notified of any fever over 103°F (39.4°C). In older children, a fever of 105°F (40.5°C) or over requires prompt medical attention, as does any fever that lasts longer than four or five days. Medical attention should also be sought for any fever accompanied by unusual irritability or sleepiness, listlessness, pain, a stiff neck, difficulty breathing, reduced urination, or any other symptoms that arouse suspicion.

Tests

Blood tests can aid in identifying an infectious agent by detecting the presence of antibodies against it or providing samples for growth of the organism in a culture. Blood tests can also provide the doctor with white blood cell counts. A urine sample may be collected for testing if the patient's fever is related to a urinary tract infection. A stool sample may be taken if the doctor suspects intestinal parasites or gastrointestinal bleeding. Ultrasound tests, **magnetic resonance imaging** (MRI) tests, or **computed tomography** (CT) scans may be ordered if the doctor cannot readily determine the cause of a fever.

Treatment

Traditional

Most cases of fever are treated with medications of one type or another, at least initially.

Drugs

Physicians agree that the most effective treatment for a fever is to address its underlying cause, such as through the administration of **antibiotics**. Antibiotics are usually given to treat fevers related to ear infections, urinary tract infections, and other illnesses caused by bacteria. Because a fever helps the immune system fight infection, it usually should be allowed to run its course.

Drugs to lower fever (antipyretics) can be given if a patient (particularly a child) is uncomfortable. These include aspirin, acetaminophen (Tylenol), and ibuprofen (Advil). Bathing a patient in cool water can also help alleviate a high fever.

DRUGS IN CHILDREN. Although fevers in children are generally not dangerous, they are treated because they cause discomfort and can prevent children from getting the sleep and nourishment they need in order to get well. Aspirin was the medication most commonly used to lower fevers until 1980, when researchers found that the use of aspirin to treat children's fevers caused by influenza and chicken pox was associated with Reye's syndrome, a dangerous condition that causes liver impairment and brain damage and can result in coma and eventual death. Since then, acetaminophens (sold under such brand names as Tylenol) have become the most widely recommended drugs for treating fever in children. Acetaminophens, which are available in liquid form, tablets and capsules for oral use, and as suppositories, are effective in treating fever but do not share aspirin's inflammation-reducing properties.

Ibuprofen (Advil, Motrin, etc.) is an effective fever reducer that is also an anti-inflammatory agent. However, it has been known to produce allergic and gastrointestinal side effects. Studies have shown that ibuprofen can be more effective than acetaminophen in reducing fever in children, but it does have more potential side effects. This fact has led some physicians to recommend alternating the two drugs for the best effect. Parents can give the drugs every four to six hours over three days; this dosage pattern has been shown to be more effective in lowering fever in infants and children than using either drug alone. Doctors caution, however, that parents may become confused when alternating the medicines and accidentally miss a dose or give the child an extra dose.

Children's fever can also be reduced one or two degrees by sponging the child with room-temperature water (about 70°F [21°C]) while he or she sits in a tub filled with water up to waist level.

FEVER IN CANCER PATIENTS. Once a diagnosis has been made and treatment initiated, it is important to address problems created by the fever itself. It may be necessary to increase fluids and nutritional supplements. Because fever places increased demands on the body, this can be critical in restoring normal health for patients who may already be nutritionally compromised. Fever in a patient with **neutropenia** (low white blood cell count) represents the potential for a critical, life-threatening situation, and treatment should begin as quickly as the patient can reach the emergency room.

Physicians do not fully understand how tumors can cause fever, but certain correlations are well documented. Fever spikes may indicate that a tumor has grown or spread to other areas of the body, or that the tumor has produced some type of blockage. The fever associated with a tumor tends to be cyclic, and subsides with tumor treatment and recurs when the tumor returns or increases in size. In the case of drug-associated fever, the fever is an allergic-type reaction to a particular medication or combination of medications. Similarly, an immune response to donor blood cells is the typical cause of fever associated with blood components.

Each of the major causes for fever associated with cancer has recommended conventional treatment procedures. For infection-related fever, broad-spectrum antibiotics, given orally, rectally, or intravenously, are the principle method of control. Some antibiotics may be started before a definitive diagnosis is made to retard additional complications caused by the infection. Treatment typically is administered for five to seven days as long as the fever and infection show a positive response.

Fever from a tumor is best treated by treating the tumor itself. Supplemental treatment for the fever may include the use of **nonsteroidal anti-inflammatory drugs** (NSAIDs) and acetaminophen. Aspirin should only be used in patients with no risk of bleeding problems. The allergic responses manifesting in drug- or blood-associated fever may be treated by various methods: antihistamines and acetaminophen may be administered prior to drug therapy or blood **transfusion therapy**; discontinuing the present drug and choosing alternate medication may be required; blood may require irradiation or removal of white blood cells from the donor blood.

Alternative

There are several different types of alternative approaches to fever:

- Herbal remedies: Western herbalists commonly recommend teas or tinctures made from catnip, yarrow, feverfew, sage, wormwood, and chamomile. These herbs and preparations made from them are sometimes referred to as febrifuges, from two Latin words that mean "to drive away fever."

- Homeopathy: Homeopathic practitioners usually recommend *Aconite* or *Belladonna* for fevers that come on suddenly; *Pulsatilla* for patients with symptoms of a cold or ear infection related to the fever; *Ferrum phos.* for fever accompanied by a severe cough; and *Nux vomica* for fevers associated with gastrointestinal symptoms, heavy drinking, or the use of recreational drugs.

- Naturopathy: Naturopaths generally regard fever as one of the body's self-regulatory mechanisms. They usually prescribe treatment of the underlying cause of the fever along with self-care at home and extra vitamin or mineral supplements to support the body's immune system, rather than drugs or medications intended to suppress the fever.

- Traditional Chinese medicine (TCM): Practitioners of TCM distinguish between fever caused by disease organisms, fever related to menstruation in women, and fever caused by disorders of the blood or the internal organs (including cancer). There are a number of different herbal remedies prescribed according to the type of condition and its severity. Unlike Western herbal formulations, which tend to be based on a single herb, traditional Chinese medicines typically contain five or more ingredients. In addition to a traditional medicine, the practitioner of TCM will also usually recommend acupuncture, changes in the patient's diet, and in some cases a form of massage known as *tui na*.

- Ayurveda: Practitioners of Ayurveda, the traditional medical system of India, typically regard fever as caused by external infections, disorders of the internal organs, or an imbalance in the three energetic principles within humans known as doshas. To treat fever, an Ayurvedic practitioner may recommend herbal remedies (cumin seeds, coriander, turmeric, or ginger), abstention from sexual activity as well as heavy meals or exercise, and mild sweating. Sweating in Ayurvedic practice is done by covering the patient with a light blanket for 10–20 minutes and giving him or her a hot beverage to drink made from a mixture of raisins and ginger.

- Native American: traditional Native American healers typically boiled fever wort, dogwood, or willow tree bark in water and gave the resulting liquid to the patient to drink. Willow was most commonly used by tribes living in the southern or western

parts of North America, while dogwood was used in the Northeast.

Some cancer patients are investigating and adhering to the use of alternative treatments and complementary therapies. These choices may include holistic healing and therapy utilizing biofeedback, relaxation therapy, prayer and meditation, and imagery techniques. Still other complementary therapies include pet therapy, humor therapy, art therapy, and journaling. Patients maintain that these alternative and complementary therapies add a sense of control to their life during a period when they have little control over anything. No conclusive data exists on the effectiveness of the therapies used alone; however, in conjunction with conventional methods of fever management, they do not appear to hinder mainstream therapy and may provide the patient increased goodwill and a positive outlook.

Prognosis

Most fevers caused by infection end as soon as the immune system rids the body of the pathogen and do not produce any lasting effects. The prognosis for fevers associated with such chronic conditions as autoimmune disease depends upon the overall outcome of the disorder. Hyperpyrexia caused by **sepsis** or other severe infections has a guarded prognosis.

Prevention

The most effective way to prevent fever is to avoid exposure to infectious diseases, follow proper techniques for food storage and preparation, maintain good personal hygiene, and wash the hands frequently.

Resources

BOOKS

Chiodini, Jane, and Lorna Boyne. *Atlas of Travel Medicine and Health.* Hamilton, Ontario, and Lewiston, NY : BC Decker, 2003.

Goroll, Allan H., and Albert G. Mulley Jr., eds. *Primary Care Medicine: Office Evaluation and Management of the Adult Patient*, 6th ed. Philadelphia : Wolters Kluwer Health/Lippincott Williams and Wilkins, 2009.

Landau, Elaine. *Fever*. New York: Marshall Cavendish Benchmark, 2010.

Porter, Robert S., ed. *The Merck Manual of Patient Symptoms: A Concise, Practical Guide to Etiology, Evaluation, and Treatment*. Whitehouse Station, NJ: Merck Laboratories, 2008.

PERIODICALS

Axelrod, Y.K., and M.N. Diringer. "Temperature Regulation in Acute Neurologic Disorders." *Neurologic Clinics* 26 (May 2008): 585–603.

Barone, J.E. "Fever: Fact and Fiction." *Journal of Trauma* 67 (August 2009): 406–409.

Fumagalli, R., et al. "Which Drugs for the Control of Fever in Critical Patients?" *Current Drug Targets* 10 (September 2009): 881–86.

Laupland, K.B. "Fever in the Critically Ill Medical Patient." *Critical Care Medicine* 37 (July 2009): S273–S278.

Marano, C., and D.O. Freedman. "Global Health Surveillance and Travelers' Health." *Current Opinion in Infectious Diseases* 22 (October 2009): 423–29.

Meckler, G., and S. Lindemulder. "Fever and Neutropenia in Pediatric Patients with Cancer." *Emergency Medicine Clinics of North America* 27 (August 2009): 525–44.

St. Clair, M., et al. "Legionella as a Cause of Hyperpyrexia." *Clinical Infectious Diseases* 49 (August 15, 2009): 646–47.

Swischuk, L.E. "Fever, Cough, and Abdominal Pain." *Pediatric Emergency Care* 25 (October 2009): 696–97.

OTHER

American Academy of Pediatrics (AAP). "Fever without Fear." *Healthy Children* (Winter 2008): 20–21. http://www.aap.org/healthychildren/08winter/HC-winter08-fever.pdf

American Academy of Pediatrics (AAP). *Parenting Corner Questions and Answers: Fever: What's the Best Way to Take a Child's Temperature?*. http://www.aap.org/publiced/BR_Fever.htm

American Cancer Society (ACS). *Fever*. http://www.cancer.org/docroot/MBC/content/MBC_2_3X_Fever.asp?sitearea = MBC

Lo Re, Vincent, III, and Stephen J. Glucken. "Fever in the Returned Traveler." *American Family Physician* 68 (October 1, 2003): 1434–50. http://www.aafp.org/afp/20031001/1343.html

Mayo Clinic. *Fever*. http://www.mayoclinic.com/health/fever/DS00077

National Cancer Institute (NCI). *Cancer Supportive Care: Fever*. http://www.cancer.gov/cancertopics/pdq/supportivecare/fever/Patient/page2

ORGANIZATIONS

American Academy of Pediatrics (AAP), 141 Northwest Point Boulevard, Elk Grove Village, IL, 60007-1098, 847-434-4000, 847-434-8000, kidsdocs@aap.org, http://www.aap.org/.

American Cancer Society (ACS), 250 Williams Street NW, Atlanta, GA, 30303, 800-ACS-2345 (227-2345), www.cancer.org.

Centers for Disease Control and Prevention (CDC), 1600 Clifton Road, Atlanta, GA, 30333, 800-232-4636, cdcinfo@cdc.gov, http://www.cdc.gov.

National Cancer Institute (NCI), 6116 Executive Blvd., Room 3036A, Bethesda, MD, 20892-8322, 800-422-6237, cancergovstaff@mail.nih.gov, www.cancer.gov.

National Center for Complementary and Alternative Medicine (NCCAM), 9000 Rockville Pike, Bethesda, MD, 20892, 888-644-6226, info@nccam.nih.gov, http://nccam.nih.gov/.

International Society of Travel Medicine (ISTM), 2386 Clower Street, Suite A-102, Snellvile, GA, United States, 30078, + 1 770 736 060, + 1-770 736 0313, istm@istm.org, https://www.istm.org/.

World Health Organization (WHO), Avenue Appia 20, 1211 Geneva 27, Switzerland, + 41 22 791 21 11, + 41 22 791 31 11, info@who.int, http://www.who.int/en/.

Rebecca J. Frey, Ph.D.

Fibrocystic breast disease *see* **Fibrocystic condition of the breast**

Fibrocystic condition of the breast

Definition

Fibrocystic condition of the breast is a term that may refer to a variety of symptoms: breast lumpiness or tenderness, microscopic breast tissue, and/or the x-ray or ultrasound picture of the breast. It has been called a "wastebasket" diagnosis because a wide range of vaguely defined benign breast conditions may be labeled as fibrocystic condition. It is not a **cancer**, and the majority of types of fibrocystic conditions do not increase the risk of **breast cancer**.

Description

There is no such thing as a normal or typical female breast. Breasts come in all shapes and sizes, with varying textures from smooth to extremely lumpy. The tissues of the female breast change in response to hormone levels, normal aging, nursing (lactation), weight fluctuations, and injury. To further complicate matters, the breast has several types of tissue; each of these tissue types may respond differently to changes in body chemistry.

A mammogram of a female breast indicating multiple cysts.
(Custom Medical Stock Photo. Reproduced by permission.)

Fibrocystic breast condition may be called fibrocystic disease, although it is clearly not a single, specific disease process. Variations or changes in the way the breast feels or looks on x ray may cause the condition to be called "fibrocystic change." Other names have been used to refer to this imprecise and ill-defined term: mammary dysplasia, mastopathy, chronic cystic mastitis, indurative mastopathy, mastalgia, lumpy breasts, or physiologic nodularity.

Estimates vary, but 40–90% of all women have some evidence of "fibrocystic" condition, change, or disease. It is most common among women between the ages 30 and 50, but may be seen at other ages.

Causes and symptoms

Fibrocystic condition of the breast refers to technical findings on diagnostic testing (signs); however, this discussion focuses on symptoms that may fall under the general category of the fibrocystic condition. First, a brief review of the structure and function of the breast may be useful.

The breast is not supposed to be a soft, smooth organ. It is actually a type of sweat gland. Milk, the breasts' version of sweat, is secreted when the breast receives appropriate hormonal and environmental stimulation.

The normal breast contains milk glands, with their accompanying ducts, or pipelines, for transporting the milk. These complex structures may not only alter in size, but can increase or decrease in number as needed. Fibrous connective tissue, fatty tissue, nerves, blood and lymph vessels, and lymph nodes, with their different shapes and textures, lie among the ever-changing milk glands. It is no wonder that a woman's breasts may not feel uniform in texture and that the "lumpiness" may wax and wane.

The fibrocystic condition refers to the tenderness, enlargement, and/or changing "lumpiness" that many women encounter just before or during their menstrual periods. At this time, female hormones are preparing the breasts for pregnancy, by stimulating the milk-producing cells, and storing fluid. Each breast may contain as much as three to six teaspoons of excess fluid. Swelling, with increased sensitivity or pain, may result. If pregnancy does not occur, the body reabsorbs the fluid, and the engorgement and discomfort are relieved.

Symptoms of fibrocystic breast condition range from mildly annoying in some women to extremely painful in others. The severity of discomfort may vary from month to month in the same woman. Although sometimes distressing, this experience is the body's normal response to routine hormonal changes.

This cycle of breast sensitivity, pain and/or enlargement, can also result from medications. Some hormone replacement therapies (estrogen and progesterone) used for postmenopausal women can produce these effects. Other medications, primarily, but not exclusively those with hormones may also provoke these symptoms.

Breast pain unrelated to hormone shifts is called "noncyclic" pain. "Trigger-zone breast pain" is a term that may also be used to describe this area-specific pain. This type of pain may be continuous, or it may be felt intermittently. Trauma, such as a blow to the chest area, a prior breast **biopsy**, or sensitivity to certain medications may also underlie this type of pain. Fibrocystic condition of the breast may be cited as the cause of otherwise unexplained breast pain.

Lumps, apart from those clearly associated with hormone cycles, may also be placed under the heading of fibrocystic condition. These lumps stand out from enlarged general breast tissue. Although noncancerous lumps may occur, the obvious concern with such lumps is cancer.

Noncancerous breast lumps include:

- Adenosis. This condition refers to the enlargement of breast lobules, which contain a greater number of glands than usual. If a group of lobules are found near each other, the affected area may be large enough to be felt.
- Cysts. These are fluid-filled sacs in the breast and probably develop as ducts that become clogged with old cells in the process of normal emptying and filling. Cysts usually feel soft and round or oval. However a cyst deep within the breast may feel hard, as it pushes up against firmer breast tissue. A woman with a cyst may experience pain, especially if it increases in size before her menstrual cycle, as is often the case. Women between the age of 30 and 50 are most likely to develop cysts.
- Epithelial hyperplasia. Also called proliferative breast disease, this condition refers to an overgrowth of cells lining either the ducts or the lobules.
- Fibroadenomas. These are tumors that form in the tissues outside the milk ducts. The cause of fibroadenomas is unknown. They generally feel smooth and firm, with a somewhat rubber-like texture. Typically a fibroadenoma is not attached to surrounding tissue and moves slightly when touched. They are most commonly found in adolescents and women in their early twenties but can occur at any age.
- Fibrosis. Sometimes one area of breast tissue persistently feels thicker or more prominent than the rest of the breast. This feeling may be caused by old hardened scar tissue and/or dead fat tissue as a result of surgery or trauma. Often the cause of this type of breast tissue is unknown.
- Miscellaneous disorders. A number of other benign (noncancerous) breast problems may be placed under the heading of "fibrocystic condition." These problems include disorders that may lead to breast inflammation (mastitis), infection, and/or nipple discharge.

Atypical ductal hyperplasia

The condition known as atypical ductal hyperplasia (ADH) is a condition in which the cells lining the milk ducts of the breast are growing abnormally. This condition may appear as spots of calcium, or calcifications, on the mammogram. A biopsy removed from the breast would confirm the diagnosis. Atypical ductal hyperplasia is not a cancer. In most women, this condition will cause no problems. However, for some women, especially women with family histories of breast cancer, the risk of developing breast cancer is increased. (One study with over 3,000 female participants indicated that about 20% of the participants with atypical hyperplasia and a family history of breast cancer developed breast cancer, as compared to the 8% of participants who developed the disease with atypical hyperplasia and no family history of breast cancer.) For women with ADH and a family history of breast cancer, more frequent mammograms and closer monitoring may be required.

Diagnosis

Breast cancer is the most common concern of women who feel a breast lump or experience an abnormal breast symptom. For peace of mind, and to rule out any possibility of cancer, any newly discovered breast lumps should be brought to the attention of a family physician or an obstetrician-gynecologist. He or she will obtain a history and conduct thorough physical examination of the area. Depending on the findings on physical examination, the patient is usually referred for tests. The most common of these tests include:

- Mammography. A mammogram is an x-ray examination of the breasts. The two major types of abnormalities doctors look for are masses and calcifications; either abnormality may be benign or malignant. The size, shape, and edges of these masses help doctors determine whether or not cancer is present. Sometimes, however, this test may be difficult to interpret, however, due to dense breast tissue.

- Ultrasonography. If a suspicious lump is detected during mammography, an ultrasound (the use of high-frequency sound waves to outline the shape of various organs and tissues in the body) is useful (although not definitive) in distinguishing benign from cancerous growths.

- Ductography. A ductogram (also called a galactogram) is a test that is sometimes useful in evaluating nipple discharge. A very fine tube is threaded into the opening of the duct onto the nipple. A small amount of dye is injected, outlining the shape of the duct on an x ray, and indicates whether or not there is a mass in the duct.

- Biopsy. If a lump cannot be proven benign by mammography and ultrasound, a breast biopsy may be considered. Usually a tissue sample is removed through a needle (fine-needle aspiration biopsy, or FNAB) to obtain a sample of the lump. The sample is examined under the microscope by a pathologist, and a detailed diagnosis regarding the type of benign lesion or cancer is established. In some cases, however, FNAB may not provide a clear diagnosis, and another type of biopsy (such as a surgical biopsy, core-needle biopsy, or other stereotactic biopsy methods—such as the Mammotome or Advanced Breast Biopsy Instrument) may be required.

Other breast conditions such as inflammation or **infection** are usually recognized on the basis of suspicious history, breastfeeding, or characteristic symptoms such as pain, redness, and swelling. A positive response to appropriate therapies often confirms the diagnosis.

Treatment

Once a specific disorder within the broad category of fibrocystic condition is identified, treatment can be prescribed. There are a number of treatment options for women with a lump that has been diagnosed as benign. If it is not causing a great deal of pain, the growth may be left in the breast. However, some women may choose to have a lump such as a fibroadenoma surgically removed, especially if it is large. Another option to relieve the discomfort of a painful benign lump is to have the cyst suctioned, or drained. If there is any uncertainty regarding diagnosis, the fluid may be sent to the lab for analysis.

Symptoms of cycle breast sensitivity and engorgement may also be treated with diet, medication, and/or physical modifications. For example,

- Although there is no scientific data to support this claim, many women have reported relief of symptoms when caffeine was reduced or eliminated from their diets. Decreasing salt before and during the period when breasts are most sensitive may also ease swelling and discomfort. Low-fat diets and elimination of dairy products also appear to decrease soreness for some women. However, it may take several months to realize the effects of these various treatments.

- Over-the-counter analgesics such as acetaminophen (Tylenol) or ibuprofen (Advil) may be recommended. In some cases, treatment with prescription drugs such as hormones or hormone blockers may prove successful. Oral contraceptives may also be prescribed.

- Warm soaks or ice packs may provide comfort. A well-fitted support bra can minimize physical movement and do much to relieve breast discomfort. Breast massage may promote removal of excess fluid from tissues and alleviate symptoms. Massaging the breast with castor oil, straight or infused with herbs or essential oils, can help reduce and dissipate fibroadenomas as well as keep women in touch with changes in their breast tissue.

- Infections are often treated with warm compresses and antibiotics. Lactating women are encouraged to continue breastfeeding because it promotes drainage and healing. However, a serious infection may progress to form an abscess that may need surgical drainage.

- Some studies of alternative or complementary treatments, although controversial, have indicated that vitamins A, B complex and E, and mineral supplements may reduce the risk of developing fibrocystic condition of the breast. Evening primrose oil (*Oenothera biennis*), flaxseed oil, and fish oils have been reported to be effective in relieving cyclic breast pain for some women.

Prognosis

Most benign breast conditions carry no increased risk for the development of breast cancer. However, a small percentage of biopsies uncover overgrowth of tissue in a particular pattern in some women; this pattern indicates a 15–20% increased risk of breast cancer over the next 20 years. Strict attention to early detection measures, such as annual mammograms, is especially important for these women.

Prevention

There is no proven method of preventing the various manifestations of fibrocystic condition from occurring. Some alternative health care practitioners believe that eliminating foods high in methyl xanthines (primarily coffee and chocolate) can decrease or reverse fibrocystic breast changes.

Resources

BOOKS

Goldmann, David R., and David A. Horowitz, editors. *The American College of Physicians Home Medical Guide: Breast Problems*. New York: Dorling Kindersley, 2000.

Love, Susan M., with Karen Lindsey. *Dr. Susan Love's Breast Book*. 3rd rev. ed. Reading, MA.: Addison-Wesley, 2000.

Singer, Sydney Ross. *Get It Off! Understanding the Cause of Breast Pain, Cysts, and Cancer*. Pahoa, HI: ISCD Press, 2000.

PERIODICALS

Horner, N.K., and J.W. Lampe. "Potential Mechanisms of Diet Therapy for Fibrocystic Breast Conditions Show Inadequate Evidence of Effectiveness." *Journal of the American Dietetic Association* 100 (November 2000): 1368-1380.

Mannello, F., M. Malatesta, and G. Gazzanelli. "Breast Cancer in Women With Palpable Breast Cysts." *Lancet* 354 (August 1999): 677- 678.

Morrow, Monica. "The Evaluation of Common Breast Problems." *American Family Physician* 61 (April 15, 2000): 2371-2378, 2385.

OTHER

National Cancer Institute. "Understanding Breast Changes: A Health Guide for All Women." [cited July 10, 2001]. http://rex.nci.nih.gov/MAMMOG_WEB/PUBS_POSTERS/UNDRSTNDNG/UNDER_STANDING_CHANGE.html.

ORGANIZATIONS

American Cancer Society. 1599 Clifton Rd. NE, Atlanta, GA 30329. 1-800-ACS-2345 http://www.cancer.org.

American College of Obstetricians and Gynecologists. 409 12th St., S.W., P.O. Box 96920, Washington, DC 20090-6920. http://www.acog.org.

Cancer Information Service (CIS). 9000 Rockville Pike, Building 31, Suite 10A18, Bethesda, MD 20892. Phone: 1-800-4-CANCER. Free telephone service provided by the National Cancer Institute.

Ellen S. Weber, M.S.N.
Genevieve Slomski, Ph.D.

Fibrosarcoma

Definition

A fibrosarcoma is a malignant tumor that arises from fibroblasts (cells that produce connective tissue). This is a type of **sarcoma** that is predominantly found in the area around bones or in soft tissue.

Excised specimen of a skin tumor known as a fibrosarcoma, sliced open (white). *(Photo Researchers, Inc. Reproduced by permission.)*

Demographics

In general, fibrosarcomas are an uncommon type of **cancer** in humans; they are relatively more common in dogs and cats. Soft-tissue fibrosarcomas are extremely rare in people, with approximately 500 new cases reported in the United States each year. Sarcomas of the bone are also rare and represent about 0.2 percent of all new cancer cases each year.

Fibrosarcomas typically develop in people between the ages of 25–79. The peak age of occurrence is the fourth decade of life. Generally, fibrosarcomas develop equally in men and women, though they are rare in children. They occur with equal frequency in all races and ethnic groups.

Infantile fibrosarcoma, also known as congenital fibrosarcoma or juvenile fibrosarcoma, is unique. Under microscopic examination, it is similar to fibrosarcomas seen in adults. However, infantile fibrosarcomas have a more positive prognosis with a post-treatment, five-year survival rate of 83% to 94%.

Description

Fibrosarcomas develop from fibroblasts, cells that produce such connective tissues as collagen. Fibrosarcoma tumors are consequently rich in collagen fibers. The immature proliferating fibroblasts take on an interlacing or herringbone pattern.

Fibrosarcomas can form from fibroblasts in such soft tissue as muscles, connective tissues, blood vessels, joints, and fat. Soft-tissue fibrosarcoma normally occurs in fibrous tissue of the body's trunk and the extremities (arms and legs). About 43% of fibrosarcomas are found on the arms and legs.

Fibrosarcomas can also occur in bones. While a bone is made up of such inorganic substances as calcium phosphate, it also has an organic element made up of 95% collagen, similar to the collagen found in the skin. Fibrosarcomas of the bone usually occur in the long bones in the bone marrow cavity where collagen is formed. The bones that predominantly yield fibrosarcomas are those in the legs, arms, pelvis, and hip.

The two most common forms of bone cancer are **osteosarcoma** and **Ewing's sarcoma**. Among the less common are **chondrosarcoma**, fibrosarcoma, and **malignant fibrous histiocytoma**, all of which arise from spindle cell neoplasms.

Risk factors

Risk factors for fibrosarcoma include:

- Genetic factors.
- Exposure to radiation therapy for an area of bone or soft tissue.
- Age. Fibrosarcomas are most common in adults between 35 and 45.
- Paget disease and other preexisting diseases of the bone.
- Having metallic implants for joint fixation or reconstruction.

Causes and symptoms

The cause(s) of fibrosarcomas is still unknown as of 2009, although it is known that many sarcomas are associated with genetic mutations, particularly **chromosome rearrangements**. Fibrosarcomas of the bone are sometimes connected with underlying benign bone tumors. Both fibrosarcomas of soft tissue and of the bone can develop as a result of exposure to radiation. This may represent a side effect from previous **radiation therapy** for unrelated primary cancer treatment. Individuals with such other bone diseases as Paget's disease and osteomyelitis are at a higher risk for developing fibrosarcomas.

There are many symptoms associated with the onset of fibrosarcomas. The following is a list of the main symptoms that may be present:

- pain (more common in fibrosarcomas of bone; soft-tissue fibrosarcomas are typically painless)
- swelling
- a firm lump just under the skin or on a bone
- broken bone
- loss of normal range of motion

- limping or other difficulties in walking or using the arms or legs normally
- neurologic symptoms
- gastrointestinal bleeding (seen in soft tissue abdominal fibrosarcomas)
- urinary frequency (seen in pelvic fibrosarcomas)
- urinary obstruction (seen in pelvic fibrosarcomas)

Diagnosis

In order to diagnose fibrosarcoma, a doctor will take the patient's medical history and will conduct a thorough physical exam. Blood tests will be performed to rule out other conditions and to identify cancer markers.

The most revealing initial exam is an x ray. It can show the location, size, and shape of the tumor. If a malignant tumor is present, the x ray will expose a soft tissue mass with ill-defined edges. This procedure takes less than an hour and can be performed in the doctor's office.

Once there is evidence of a tumor, one or more of several other procedures may be performed, including **computed tomography** (CT) scans, **magnetic resonance imaging** (MRI), angiograms, and biopsies.

Treatment

Treatment team

The patient's primary care physician may perform the initial diagnostic tests. However, in order to comprehensively diagnose and treat fibrosarcomas, the primary care physician will refer the patient to an oncologist (cancer specialist). Radiologists, pathologists, and orthopedic surgeons will also be involved to read **x rays**, examine tissue samples, and, if needed, remove the tumor.

Other individuals might be involved with the treatment of fibrosarcoma, including nurses, dieticians, and physical or vocational therapists.

Staging

After the physician makes the diagnosis, it is important to determine the stage of the cancer. Staging will help reveal how far the cancer has progressed and how much tissue has been affected.

The American Joint Committee on Cancer developed the most widely used staging system for fibrosarcomas. The foremost categories of this system include grade (G), size of the tumor (T), lymph node involvement (N), and presence of metastases (M). Low grade and high grade are designated G1 and G3, respectively. The size of the tumor can be less than 5 centimeters (2 inches), designated as T1, or greater than 5 centimeters, designated as T2. If the lymph nodes are involved, N1 is designated, while no lymph involvement is designated N0. Finally, there may be a presence of distant metastases (M1), or no metastases (M0). The following is a list of stages and their indications:

- Stage IA: (G1, T1, N0, M0)
- Stage IB: (G1, T2, N0, M0)
- Stage IIA: (G2, T1, N0, M0)
- Stage IIB: (G2, T2, N0, M0)
- Stage IIIA: (G3, T1, N0, M0)
- Stage IIIB: (G3, T2, N0, M0)
- Stage IVA: (Any G, any T, N1, M0)
- Stage IVB: (Any G, any T, N1, M1)

Tumors with lower stage numbers, such as IA and IB, contain cells that look very similar to normal cells, while tumors with higher stage designations are composed of cells that appear very different from normal cells. In higher staged tumors, the cells appear undifferentiated.

Traditional

Physicians can employ several courses of treatment to remove fibrosarcomas. The most effective treatment is surgical removal; this is used as a primary treatment for all stages of fibrosarcoma. When performing the surgery, the surgeon will remove the tumor and some healthy soft tissue or bone around it to ensure that the tumor does not recur near the original site.

Prior to surgery, large tumors (greater than 5 centimeters, or 2 inches) may be treated with **chemotherapy** or radiation in order to shrink them, thus rendering the surgical procedure more effective. Chemotherapy is particularly effective in shrinking fibrosarcomas in children.

Even individuals with low-grade fibrosarcoma who have undergone surgery experience a 60% risk of local recurrence. To combat recurrence, **adjuvant chemotherapy** (the use of one or more cancer-killing drugs) and radiation therapy (the use of high-energy rays), such as irradiation and brachytherapy, are also used to complement surgery. Employing chemotherapy or radiation therapy individually without surgery is much less effective.

After therapy, low-stage fibrosarcomas (stages IA and IB) have greater five-year survival rates than high stages (Stages IVA and IVB). Because high-grade tumors are more aggressive and more highly metastatic than lower grade tumors, patients with high-grade tumors have a lower survival rate. Not only is the grade of the tumor (the estimate of its aggressiveness) important in determining prognosis, the age of the patient is also crucial. Generally, fibrosarcomas that occur in childhood and infancy have a lower mortality rate than those that occur in adults. Additionally, patients with fibrosarcomas that occur in the extremities have a better survival rate than those with fibrosarcomas in the visceral region.

Metastases appear later in the development of fibrosarcomas. The lungs are the primary sites of **metastasis** for fibrosarcomas that develop in the extremities. Once metastasis to the lungs has occurred, the chances of survival are significantly decreased.

Patients treated for fibrosarcomas are monitored for at least 5 years after treatment.

Alternative

Many individuals choose to supplement traditional therapy with complementary methods. Often, these methods improve the patient's tolerance of side effects and symptoms, as well as enrich their quality of life. The American Cancer Society recommends that patients talk to their doctor to ensure that the methods they choose are safely supplementing their traditional therapy. Some **complementary cancer therapies** include the following:

- yoga
- meditation
- religious practices and prayer
- music therapy
- art therapy
- pet therapy
- massage therapy
- aromatherapy

Coping with cancer treatment

Chemotherapy often results in several side effects, depending on the drug used and the patient's individual tolerance. Patients may have to deal with **nausea**, **vomiting**, loss of appetite (**anorexia**), and hair loss (**alopecia**). Many times, chemotherapy as well as radiation therapy are better handled if patients are eating well. Nurses and dieticians can aid patients in choosing healthful foods to incorporate into their diet.

If the fibrosarcoma necessitated a limb **amputation**, then patients will need to learn how to cope with a prosthetic device. Both physical and vocational therapists can effectively help patients adjust and learn how to use the prosthetic device to perform their daily activities.

Clinical trials

Fibrosarcomas are rare, but advances are being made in both diagnostic and curative procedures. Although surgery is the most effective treatment, both pre- and post-operative adjuvant therapies are being researched to complement surgery. There are 53 **clinical trials** for fibrosarcoma treatment in progress as of 2009.

Exploring the results of chemotherapy trials uncovers a trend of improved results with more intense regimens—meaning higher and more prolonged doses of drug therapy. Drugs that are being studied in 2009 include **cyclophosphamide, ifosfamide, doxorubicin, epirubicin, temozolomide, methotrexate, vincristine, dacarbazine, dactinomycin,** soblidotin, exatecan mesylate, or a combination of two or three of these.

Patients should consult with their physicians or contact the American Cancer Society to learn what procedures are currently being investigated in clinical trials. In some cases, insurance companies will not cover procedures that are part of clinical trials. Patients should talk with their doctor and insurance company to determine which procedures are covered.

Prognosis

The prognosis of a fibrosarcoma depends on its location, stage, and whether it has metastasized.

Prevention

The prevention of cancer can be assisted by avoiding such known chemical carcinogens as alpha-naphthylamine, carbon tetrachloride, and benzene. Another way to avoid developing cancer is to minimize exposure to penetrating radiation such as x rays and radioactive elements. Medical x rays revolutionized the field of medicine and are used to detect and treat many diseases. In most cases, the benefits of medical x rays outweigh the risks.

Special concerns

Treatment, especially surgical amputation, can take a physical and psychological toll on cancer patients and their families. To deal with the psychological impact, there are many different support groups and psychotherapists that can help. Some therapists will consider amputation a posttraumatic stress disorder, and treat it accordingly. To deal with

---

QUESTIONS TO ASK YOUR DOCTOR

- What diagnostic procedures are best for the location and type of tumor suspected?
- What treatments are best for the location and type of tumor suspected?
- What kinds of side effects will this course of treatment cause?
- Are there support services available?
- What treatments are currently in clinical trials?
- What treatments will my health care insurance cover?
- What alternative treatments are safe?

---

their condition, relying on faith practices can also be beneficial for cancer patients. Patients should discuss all options with their physician to determine what is available.

For patients whose fibrosarcoma affected their face or head, Look Good...Feel Better is a free public service program approved by the American Cancer Society. It helps patients with any kind of cancer cope with changes in their looks related to cancer treatment. It began in 1987 when a doctor asked the president of the Personal Care Products Council to help a patient who was so depressed by her appearance during chemotherapy that she refused to leave her hospital room. The president sent a makeup artist to visit the patient, who was so delighted with her makeover that she began to respond better to her cancer treatment. Look Good...Feel Better has expanded to include programs for teens, men, and Spanish-speaking patients; groups are available in all 50 states, the District of Columbia, and Puerto Rico. The main website is http://www.lookgoodfeel better.org/.

Once the cancer has been treated, patients should make sure to schedule follow-up appointments with their physicians. Physicians will want to monitor the patient for side effects or possible recurrence that may develop years after treatment.

Resources

BOOKS

Hasegawa, Sota, ed. *Soft Tissue Cancers: Etiology, Pathogenesis and Interventions.* New York: Nova Science Publishers, 2008.

PERIODICALS

Collini, P., et al. "Sarcomas with Spindle Cell Morphology." *Seminars in Oncology* 36 (August 2009): 324–37.

Russell, H., et al. "Infantile Fibrosarcoma: Clinical and Histologic Responses to Cytotoxic Chemotherapy." *Pediatric Blood and Cancer* 53 (July 2009): 23–27.

Stein-Wexler, R. "MR Imaging of Soft Tissue Masses in Children." *Magnetic Resonance Imaging Clinics of North America* 17 (August 2009): 489–507.

OTHER

Children's Hospital Boston. *My Child Has Fibrosarcoma.* http://www.childrenshospital.org/az/Site897/mainpage S897P0.html.

Dickey, Ian, and James Floyd. "Fibrosarcoma." *eMedicine*, March 2, 2007. http://emedicine.medscape.com/article/1257520-overview.

National Cancer Institute (NCI). *Soft Tissue Sarcomas: Questions and Answers.* http://www.cancer.gov/cancer-topics/factsheet/Sites-Types/soft-tissue-sarcoma.

ORGANIZATIONS

American Academy of Orthopaedic Surgeons (AAOS), 6300 North River Road, Rosemont, IL, 60018, 847-823-7186, 847-823-8125, orthoinfo@aaos.org, http://www.aaos.org/.

American Cancer Society, 250 Williams Street NW, Atlanta, GA, 30303, 800-ACS-2345 (227-2345), www.cancer.org.

National Cancer Institute, 6116 Executive Blvd., Room 3036A, Bethesda, MD, 20892-8322, 800-422-6237, cancergovstaff@mail.nih.gov, www.cancer.gov.

Sally C. McFarlane-Parrott
Rebecca J. Frey, PhD

Filgrastim

Definition

Filgrastim is a medicine used to increase the white blood cell count in the body, which will help prevent **infection**. Filgrastim is known by the brand name Neupogen.

Purpose

Filgrastim is a drug approved by the Food and Drug Administration (FDA) to increase white blood cell counts. If a patient has a lower than normal white blood cell count it is referred to as **neutropenia**.

Filgrastim can be used to treat neutropenia caused by **cancerchemotherapy** treatment. In these patients the filgrastim increases the recovery of white blood cells after chemotherapy. Filgrastim can also be used to treat patients who have a neutropenia not related to chemotherapy. In both cases, the filgrastim decreases the risk of **fever** and infection.

Filgrastim is not usually used in leukemia patients. However, in patients with the disease known as acute myelocytic leukemia, it is approved for use after chemotherapy. Filgrastim can increase the recovery of the white blood cell count thereby decreasing the length of time a patient may have a fever associated with a low white count.

Filgrastim can also be used after **bone marrow transplantation**. Once the new healthy bone marrow has been given back to a patient, filgrastim can be administered to help increase the white blood cell count and decrease the risk of fever and infection.

Filgrastim can be used for patients who will receive a peripheral blood stem cell transplant. Patients will receive the filgrastim before the transplant. The filgrastim in these patients causes young, non-developed blood cells, known as stem or progenitor cells, to move from the bone marrow to the blood where they will then be removed from a patient by the process of apheresis. These blood cells are stored until after the patient receives larges doses of chemotherapy that destroy the bone marrow and the cancer. The patient then receives these stored cells back by an intravenous infusion. The stored cells repopulate the bone marrow and develop into the many types of functioning blood cells.

Description

Filgrastim has been available to cancer patients since the 1990s, and is highly effective at decreasing neutropenia. Filgrastim may be referred to as G-CSF, granulocyte colony stimulating factor, colony stimulating factor. This compound is manufactured by recombinant DNA methods using E. coli as the host organism. Chemotherapy destroys white blood cells temporarily. These white blood cells will grow again, but during the time that the levels are low, patients are at an increased risk of developing fevers and infection. Filgrastim acts to stimulate the bone marrow to make more white blood cells, which can either prevent the white count from dropping below normal or decrease the time that the level is low. By effectively avoiding fevers and infections, patients are able to receive their next doses of chemotherapy without delay.

Recommended dosage

Filgrastim is a clear colorless liquid that is dosed on body weight in kilograms. It is kept refrigerated until ready to use, and it is administered to patients as

KEY TERMS

Food and Drug Administration (FDA)—A government agency that oversees public safety in relation to drugs and medical devices. The FDA gives the approval to pharmaceutical companies for commercial marketing of their products.

Chemotherapy—Specific drugs used to treat cancer.

Subcutaneous—Underneath the initial layer of skin.

Intravenous—To enter the body through a vein.

Reinfusion—The transfer through a vein of healthy stem cells or bone marrow to a patient that had received larges doses of chemotherapy used to destroy cancer cells.

Neutropenia—Low white blood cell count.

Recovery—Blood counts that are returning back to normal levels.

Apheresis—The process of removing and collecting specific cells from the blood through a machine.

Peripheral blood stem cell transplant—A procedure that collects and stores healthy young and non-developed blood stem cells. These are then given back to a patient to help them recovery from high doses of chemotherapy that they received to destroy their cancer.

Bone marrow transplant—A procedure that destroys all of a patients' diseased bone marrow and replaces it with healthy bone marrow.

a subcutaneous injection (directly underneath the skin) It is usually administered in the back of the arms, upper legs, or stomach area. Filgrastim can also be given to patients as a short intravenous infusion into a vein over 15 to 30 minutes.

Chemotherapy-caused neutropenia

The starting dose for patients who have just finished chemotherapy is 5 micrograms per kilogram of body weight per day. This is given as a subcutaneous injection under the skin daily for up to 14 consecutive days, and sometimes longer. The doctor will inform the patient when it is time to stop the filgrastim.

Bone marrow transplants

The recommended dose is 10 micrograms per kilogram per day. This can be administered as a 4- to 24-hour infusion intravenously, or as a 24-hour subcutaneous infusion.

Peripheral blood stem cell transplant

The recommended dose is 10 micrograms per kilogram per day. This can be given either as a under the skin injection, intravenously, or as a continuous infusion over 24 hours. This dosing should begin four days before the first apheresis collection process and continue until the last day of collection.

Other neutropenia

The dose recommendation is variable based on the reason for neutropenia. The range of filgrastim doses has been from 5 micrograms per kilogram per day up to 100 microgram per kilogram per day. Doctors may increase the filgrastim dose based on how the white blood cell count responds to the treatment. Other factors that play a role in filgrastim dosing include how low the white blood cell count is and the length of time the white blood cell count remains low.

Precautions

Filgrastim should not be received by a patient in the 24-hour time frame before or after receiving chemotherapy or reinfusion of bone marrow or stem cells.

Blood counts will be monitored while on the drug filgrastim. This allows the doctor to determine if the drug is working and when to stop the drug.

It is not recommended to give filgrastim to patients who have certain types of leukemias.

Patients with a known previous allergic reaction to filgrastim or to any other substance derived from the bacteria *E. coli* should not take filgrastim.

Patients who may be pregnant, or trying to become pregnant, should tell their doctor before receiving filgrastim.

Side effects

The most common side effect from filgrastim is **bone pain**. The filgrastim causes the bone marrow to produce more white blood cells, and, as a result, patients may experience pain in their bones. Tylenol, an over-the-counter pain reliever, can usually control mild to moderate pain that occurs with standard dosed filgrastim. Larger doses of filgrastim, like those given for bone marrow transplant patients, can cause severe bone pain that may need a prescription pain reliever to ease the pain.

Another common side effect due to filgrastim administration is pain or burning at the site of the injection. This can be decreased by bringing the filgrastim to room temperature before administering the injection, icing the area of injection to numb it before receiving the injection, and moving the site of the injection with each dose.

Patients who have received filgrastim after cancer chemotherapy have reported fever, **nausea and vomiting**, muscle pain, **diarrhea**, hair loss (**alopecia**), mouth sores, **fatigue**, shortness of breath, weakness, headache, cough, rash, constipation, and pain. These side effects may be due to the chemotherapy administration.

Interactions

Filgrastim should not be given at the same time as chemotherapy or **radiation therapy**. Dosing should begin at least 24 hours after the last dose of treatment.

Patients on the drug lithium should tell their doctor before starting filgrastim therapy.

Filgrastim use for delayed **myelosuppression** has not been studied after the use of the chemotherapy agents **mitomycin-C**, and nitrosoureas, or after the drug **fluorouracil**.

Nancy J. Beaulieu, RPh., BCOP

Flow cytometry

Definition

Flow cytometry, is a method of sorting and measuring types of cells by fluorescent labeling of markers on the surface of the cells. It is sometimes referred to as FACS (Fluorescent Activated Cell Sorting) analysis.

Purpose

Flow cytometric analysis is most often clinically used to help determine the type of leukemia or **lymphoma** a patient has and to assess the prognosis. Flow cytometry is quite sensitive; it is able to detect rare cell types and residual levels of disease.

Precautions

Drugs, such as steroids, that suppress the immune system will affect the number of white blood cells in the patient's sample.

Description

The physician will select a sample based on the type of **cancer** the patient is thought to have. In the

case of lymphoma, the sample may be collected by fine needle aspiration **biopsy**, then the tissue sample will be separated into single cells. Analysis of leukemia will require a patient to give a blood sample. The patient's blood sample will be separated and the red blood cells removed. The sample will be mixed with a variety of different antibodies that can interact with markers on the surface of the cells. Different types of cells have characteristic markers on their cell surfaces, so a particular cell type can be identified by the antibodies that bind to it. The antibodies are labeled so that they will give off fluorescent light (glow) as they pass through the laser beam in the cytometer. The cytometer also measures the size of the cell and some information about the interior of the cell. The physician uses this information to determine the specific type of leukemia, such as myelogenous or lymphocytic, which in turn, helps to determine the type of treatment that will be best suited to the patient.

Sample analysis may also be performed using a more complex type of flow cytometer combined with a microscope, called a laser-scanning cytometer. This instrument is similar to a regular flow cytometer, but is better able to analyze solid tumor samples.

Preparation

Flow cytometry is usually performed on blood, body fluids, or bone marrow. In most cases, no special preparation is required. If **bone marrow aspiration** is necessary or a biopsy is required from a solid tumor, the patient should be appropriately prepared for these procedures. However, the flow cytometry itself does not require any additional preparation on the part of the patient.

Aftercare and risks

The only aftercare and risks associated with flow cytometric analysis are those associated with the sample collection procedure. The cell analysis itself requires no effort or risk from the patient.

Normal results

A normal result will indicate that there is no increase in the number of any particular type of immune cell. The pathologist will see several different types of cells, but no one type will be present in increased numbers.

Abnormal results

If the results are abnormal, the pathologist will observe an unusually large number of one particular cell type. The types of marker present on the cell will give further information about the type of leukemia or lymphoma and may indicate the patient's prognosis. For example, leukemic cells that have markers that are normally found on less mature cell types may suggest a poorer prognosis, and therefore more aggressive therapy may be recommended.

See also Tumor grading.

Resources

BOOKS

Javois, Lorette C.*Immunocytochemical Methods and Protocols*. Totowa, NJ: Humana Press, 1999.

PERIODICALS

Rew, David A., et al. "Laser-scanning Cytometry." *The Lancet* 353 (January 23, 1999): 255–56.

OTHER

"FACS Laboratory."*Imperial Cancer Research Fund.* [cited July 5, 2001]. http://www.icnet.uk.

"Flow Cytometry Core Educational Links."*University of Florida.* [cited July 6, 2001]. http://www.biotech.ufl.edu/~fccl/flow_edu.html.

Racquel Baert, M.S.

Floxuridine

Definition

Floxuridine is an anti-cancer drug that is injected directly into the artery that carries blood to the liver or the abdominal cavity. The brand names of floxuridine are Fluorodeoxyuridine, FUDR, and Floxuridine For Injection USP. The generic name product may be available in the United States.

Purpose

Floxuridine is used to treat **gastrointestinal cancers** that have metastasized, or spread, to the liver. These cancers include **rectal cancer** and Stage IV **colon cancer**. Floxuridine also has been used to treat cancerous gastrointestinal tumors; however the response rate is poor and usually the drug is used only to relieve symptoms.

Description

Floxuridine is approved by the United States Food and Drug Administration.

Floxuridine is a type of medicine called an antimetabolite because it interferes with the metabolism and growth of cells. Floxuridine prevents the production of DNA in cells. The cells cannot reproduce and eventually they die.

Floxuridine sometimes is used in conjunction with the drugs **fluorouracil** (5-FU), **cisplatin**, and/or **leucovorin**. Leucovorin increases the activity of floxuridine. In general, floxuridine is more effective than other chemotherapies against liver metastases, but its use does not improve overall survival rates. Ongoing studies are comparing floxuridine with other chemotherapies. The drug may be used in conjunction with surgery. Its use in conjunction with **radiation therapy** is being evaluated.

Recommended dosage

Floxuridine is injected directly into the liver. This is called hepatic intra-arterial infusion, or **hepatic arterial infusion**. A special pump delivers the drug through an implanted infusion port or catheter into an artery that goes to the liver. Injection of floxuridine into a vein is being evaluated. Floxuridine also may be injected into the abdominal cavity (intraperitoneal therapy). The dosage of floxuridine depends on a number of factors including body weight, type of **cancer**, and any other medicines that are being used.

Precautions

Floxuridine may lower the number of white blood cells and, therefore, reduce the body's ability to fight **infection**. Immunizations (vaccinations) should be avoided during or after treatment with floxuridine because of the risk of infection. It also is important to avoid contact with individuals who have recently taken an oral polio vaccine. Treatment with floxuridine may cause chicken pox or shingles (**Herpes zoster**) to become very severe and spread to other parts of the body.

Kidney or liver diseases may increase the effects of floxuridine, since the drug may be removed from the body at a slower rate. Floxuridine also may put an individual at an increased risk for hepatitis.

Floxuridine can cause birth defects in animals. Therefore this drug should not be taken by pregnant women or by either the man or the woman at the time of conception. Women usually are advised against breast-feeding while receiving this drug.

Side effects

Since floxuridine may affect the growth of normal cells as well as cancer cells, side effects may occur during or after drug treatment. Some effects may occur months or even years after the drug is administered. Floxuridine increases the risk of later developing certain types of cancer, such as leukemia.

The more common side effects of floxuridine include:

- **diarrhea**
- loss of appetite (anorexia)
- sores in the mouth or on the lips
- stomach pain or cramps
- numbness or tingling in the hands and feet

Less common side effects of floxuridine include:

- **nausea and vomiting**
- black, tar-like stools

- heartburn
- redness or scaling of the hands or feet
- sore, swollen tongue
- skin rash or itching
- temporary thinning of hair (alopecia)
- bleeding at the site of the catheter
- infection from the catheter
- closing off of the catheter

Other, rare side effects of floxuridine include:

- blood in urine or stools
- hiccups
- hoarseness or coughing
- fever or chills
- sore throat
- difficulty swallowing
- blurred vision
- lower back or side pain
- painful or difficult urination
- small red skin spots
- difficulty walking
- bleeding or bruising
- yellow eyes or skin
- seizures
- depression

In addition to lowering the white blood cell count, increasing the risk of infection, floxuridine may reduce the level of blood platelets that are necessary for normal blood clotting. This can increase the risk of bleeding. The drug also may lead to abnormalities in liver function. Intraperitoneal floxuridine therapy has been associated with the development of fibrous masses in the abdomen.

Interactions

Previous treatment with radiation or other anticancer drugs can increase the effects of floxuridine on the blood.

Drugs that may interact with floxuridine include:

- amphotericin B (Fungizone)
- antithyroid drugs that are used to treat an overactive thyroid
- azathioprine (Imuran)
- chloramphenicol (Chloromycetin)
- colchicine
- flucytosine (Ancobon)
- ganciclovir (Cytovene)

- interferon (Intron A, Roferon-A)
- plicamycin (Mithracin)
- zidovudine (AZT, Retrovir)

Margaret Alic, Ph.D.

Fluconazole *see* **Antifungal therapy**

Fludarabine

Definition

Fludarabine is a **chemotherapy** medicine used to treat certain types of **cancer** by destroying cancerous cells. It is known as the brand name Fludara. Fludarabine may also be referred to as Fludarabine phosphate, 2-fluoroadenine aribinoside 5-phosphate, and FAMP.

Purpose

Fludarabine is approved by the Food and Drug Administration (FDA) to treat refractory **chronic lymphocytic leukemia** (CLL). Patients must have a disease that did not respond to other treatment or a disease that became worse during other treatment. Fludarabine has also been used to treat Hodgkin's and **non-Hodgkin's lymphoma, cutaneous T-cell lymphoma**, macroglobulinemic **lymphoma, mycosis fungoides**, and **hairy cell leukemia**.

Description

Fludarabine has been available for use since the early 1990s, and is a member of the group of chemotherapy drugs known as antimetabolites. Antimetabolites interfere with the genetic material (DNA) inside the cancer cells and prevent them from further dividing and growing more cancer cells.

Recommended dosage

Fludarabine is a clear solution that is administered through a vein.

A fludarabine dose can be determined using a mathematical calculation that measures a person's body surface area (BSA). This number is dependent upon a patient's height and weight. The larger the person, the greater the body surface area. BSA is measured in the units known as square meter (m^2). The body surface area is calculated and then

multiplied by the drug dosage in milligrams per square meter (mg/m^2). This calculates the actual dose a patient is to receive.

The approved dose for chronic lymphocytic leukemia is 25 milligrams per square meter per day for 5 days in a row. The fludarabine is given intravenously into a vein over a 30-minute to 2-hour time period. This 5-day cycle is repeated every 4 weeks.

The dose of fludarabine may need to be decreased in patients who have kidney problems.

Precautions

Blood counts will be monitored regularly while on fludarabine therapy. During a certain time period after receiving fludarabine, there is an increased risk of getting infections. Caution should be taken to avoid unnecessary exposure to crowds and people with infections.

Patients with a known previous allergic reaction to chemotherapy drugs should tell their doctor.

Patients who may be pregnant or are trying to become pregnant should tell their doctor before receiving fludarabine. Chemotherapy can cause men and women to be sterile, or unable to have children. It is unknown if fludarabine has this effect on humans.

Patients should check with their doctors before receiving live virus **vaccines** while on chemotherapy.

Side effects

The most common side effect expected from taking fludarabine is low blood counts (**myelosuppression**). When the white blood cell count is lower than normal (**neutropenia**), patients are at an increased risk of developing a **fever** and infections. Patients may need to be treated with **antibiotics** at this point. The platelet blood count can also be decreased due to fludarabine administration, but generally returns to normal within 2 weeks after the end of the infusion. Platelets are blood cells that cause clots to form to stop bleeding. When the platelet count is low, patients are at an increased risk for bruising and bleeding. Fludarabine causes low red blood cell counts (**anemia**). Low red counts make people feel tired and dizzy.

Fludarabine can cause the development of autoimmune **hemolytic anemia**, which occurs when the body begins to destroy its own red blood cells. It is an uncommon side effect, but very serious when it occurs.

Common side effects from fludarabine include **nausea and vomiting**. If **nausea** and **vomiting** are a problem, patients can be given **antiemetics** before receiving fludarabine. This medication helps prevent or decrease these side effects. Other common side effects include fever, chills, joint pain, fluid gain, **fatigue**, sleepiness, pain, muscle ache, weakness, and **infection**. Other less common side effects include loss of appetite (**anorexia**), **diarrhea**, abnormal touch sensation, cough, **pneumonia**, and shortness of breath.

Damage to the nerves and nervous system tissues can occur with fludarabine. Side effects due to this nerve damage include sleepiness, confusion, weakness, fatigue, irritability, numbness or tingling in the hands and feet, visual changes, and difficulty walking.

Infrequent side effects of fludarabine are skin rashes, pain, **itching**, fever, lung problems, insomnia, headache, muscle and joint aches, swelling, and decreased blood pressure.

Rare side effects of fludarabine include mouth sores, constipation and abdominal cramping, bleeding from the bladder, hair loss, hearing problems, and liver and kidney problems.

Fludarabine can cause the rapid breakdown of cancer cells. Patients who have large numbers of cancer cells in their bloodstream can develop a problem known as **tumor lysis syndrome**. The symptoms of this syndrome include pain in the lower back and blood in the urine. A patient can develop high or low levels of electrolytes and high levels of uric acid, which can lead to gout and kidney damage. The drug **allopurinol** may be given to patients prior to fludarabine treatment to prevent this from occurring. Drinking an increased amount of liquids also may help prevent the kidney damage.

All side effects a patient experiences should be reported to the doctor.

Interactions

Fludarabine should not be used in combination with the drug **pentostatin**. The combination causes severe lung damage.

Nancy J. Beaulieu, R.Ph., B.C.O.P.

Fluorouracil

Definition

Fluorouracil is a medication that kills **cancer** cells. It is also known as 5-FU or 5-fluourouracil, and as the brand name Adrucil.

Purpose

5-FU may be used in combination with other **chemotherapy** agents to treat cancers of the breast, stomach, colon, rectum, and pancreas.

Description

5-FU is a cytotoxic drug. This means that it kills cancer cells. 5-FU kills cells by interfering with the activities of DNA and RNA, which are molecules in the cells important in expressing genetic material.

Recommended dosage

Most frequently, 5-FU is given as an injection into the vein (intravaneous injection or IV). Many different doses and regimens are used depending on the cancer diagnosis, and patients should discuss with their physician the dose based on the individual protocol used. A sample dose is 500 to 1,000 mg per square meter of

KEY TERMS

Cytotoxic drug—A medicine that kills (cancer) cells.

DNA—A molecule found in all living cells that contains tiny bits of genetic information.

Infusion therapy—Administration of a medication as a liquid through an intravenous (IV) device.

RNA—A molecule found in all living cells that plays a role in transmitting information from the DNA to the protein-forming system of the cell.

body surface area given as a 24-hour infusion for four to five days every three weeks. A dose of 425 mg per square meter of body surface area per day for five days given along with the drug **leucovorin** is also common.

Precautions

Patients with allergic reaction to 5-FU should not be administered this drug. It is also inadvisable for pregnant women. 5-FU should be administered with caution to patients with impaired liver or kidney function, or in patients with a history of heart problems.

Side effects

The amount of drug given and the duration of which it is given during a single session greatly influences the side effects seen. For example, when given as a 24-hour continuous infusion, the most common side effects are **diarrhea** and mouth ulcers. If 5-FU is given as a bolus infusion (a high quantity of the drug all at once), the most common side effect is bone marrow suppression; this results in a decrease of the white blood cells responsible for fighting infections, the platelets responsible for blood clotting, and the red blood cells responsible for providing oxygen to the cells of the body.

The severity of the side effects is increased when 5-FU is given with the drug leucovorin. **Vomiting**, diarrhea, **nausea**, and loss of appetite (**anorexia**) may occur regardless of how 5-FU is administered. The diarrhea side effect may be severe in some patients, and it is important for them to alert their doctor immediately so that appropriate medications for the diarrhea can be prescribed.

5-FU may cause rashes, increased sensitivity to sunlight, changes in skin color, changes to the fingernails, and redness and swelling in the palms of the hands and soles of the feet. Patients who have had

heart disease before starting therapy with 5-FU may have problems with blood flow to the heart. Rarely, 5-FU may cause an allergic reaction, dry eyes, sleepiness, confusion, headache, changes in walking gait, involuntary rapid movement of the eyes, and difficulty speaking. When 5-FU is applied directly on the skin, there are usually no side effects except for those to the skin itself. These may include burning sensations, pain, and darkening of the skin color.

Some authorities recommend discontinuation of 5-FU therapy as soon as mild side effects are observed as a way of reducing the extent of injury to the digestive tract. Administration may then be restarted at a lower dose after the side effects have stopped.

Interactions

People taking fluorouracil should consult their doctor before taking any other prescription drug, over-the-counter drug, or herbal remedy.

Bob Kirsch

Fluoxymesterone

Definition

Fluoxymesterone is a synthetic male hormone used to treat women with hormone-dependent **breast cancer**, and may also be used as a **testosterone** replacement for men. Fluoxymesterone is sold as Halotestin, Android-F, and Ora-Testryl.

Purpose

Fluoxymesterone is used to manage metastatic breast **cancer** in menopausal women who have hormone receptor–positive tumors. It may also be used as a supplement to **chemotherapy** for metastatic breast cancer, or as a hormone replacement for men. Additionally, it is sometimes used to treat **anemia**.

Description

Fluoxymesterone is a synthetic androgen, or male hormone, similar in action to testosterone. Fluoxymesterone works by attaching itself to androgen receptors; this causes it to interact with the parts of the cell involved in the making of proteins. It may cause an increase in the synthesis of some proteins or a decrease in the synthesis of others. These proteins have a variety of effects, including blocking the growth of some types of breast cancer cells, stimulating cells that cause male sexual characteristics, and stimulating the production of red blood cells.

When used as a breast cancer treatment, this drug blocks the growth of tumor cells that are dependent on female hormones to grow. It can only be used on female breast cancer patients who have reached menopause one to five years earlier, or as a result of surgery. It may be used in addition to other chemotherapeutic drugs, such as **tamoxifen** or **cyclophosphamide**, **doxorubicin**, and **fluorouracil**.

Fluoxymesterone may be used to treat men; it replaces male hormones which are not being released in the body as a result of tumors, radiation, or surgery affecting the pituitary or hypothalamus.

Recommended dosage

The recommended dosage will depend on the age, sex, and diagnosis of the patient, as well as the response to treatment and occurrence of side effects. Treatment is usually with a full therapeutic dose initially, then adjusted to the individual needs of the patient.

Women being treated for breast cancer usually take 10–40 mg per day orally, divided into several doses. Up to three months may be required for a response to treatment.

Androgen replacement therapy for men is usually started at 5–20 mg per day, taken orally in divided doses.

If a dose is missed, it should be taken as soon as it is remembered, unless it is more than two hours late. If it is more than two hours late, the patient should skip that dose and continue to follow the normal dosing schedule.

Precautions

Fluoxymesterone may be taken with food if it causes stomach upset. Patients taking this medication should ensure that they see their physician regularly during treatment and receive appropriate laboratory tests. Liver function should be monitored and cholesterol and red blood cell levels may need to be examined during treatment. Female breast cancer patients should have their serum and urine calcium levels checked. Prepubescent males will require **x rays** to determine the rate of their bone maturation. Diabetics should be aware that this medication may affect blood sugar levels.

Fluoxymesterone should not be taken by pregnant women as it will affect the sexual development of the fetus. The hormone may also pass into the milk of nursing mothers, affecting sexual development of the infant. Fluoxymesterone should not be taken by people with liver, kidney, heart or blood vessel disease, prostate problems, or sensitivity to the dye tartrazine. Patients with migraines or epilepsy should discuss these conditions with their physician before using the drug. Senior male patients using fluoxymesterone have an increased risk of prostate enlargement.

Patients should consult their physician before discontinuing the drug.

Side effects

Patients who use fluoxymesterone have an increased risk of developing liver disease, and should report symptoms such as yellowing of the eyes and skin to their physicians immediately. Women being treated for breast cancer and patients who are immobilized may develop **hypercalcemia**. Other side effects which may occur include the following:

- fluid retention
- nausea and vomiting
- diarrhea
- anxiety
- depression
- changes in sex drive
- dizziness
- suppression of blood clotting factors II, V, VII, and X
- headache
- itching
- reduction in number of white blood cells
- increase in number of red blood cells

Women who take this medication may also experience menstrual irregularities, acne, enlarged clitoris, and masculine characteristics such as deepening of the voice, increased hair growth, and male pattern baldness. Some of these changes may go away if the medication is stopped, while others may remain.

Men taking fluoxymesterone may experience breast growth, erections of excessive frequency and duration, impotence, decreased ejaculatory volume, and bladder irritation.

Interactions

A large number of medications may cause interactions with fluoxymesterone, including acetaminophen, anabolic steroids, anticoagulants, antidiabetic agents, and many others. Patients should notify their physicians of any medications they are taking before using fluoxymesterone.

Racquel Baert, M.Sc.

Flutamide *see* **Antiandrogens**

Folic acid

Definition

Folic acid is a water-soluble B vitamin essential in the human diet. It is an important cofactor in the synthesis of DNA and RNA of dividing cells, particularly during pregnancy and infancy when there is an increase in cell division and growth.

Purpose

Folic acid is important to the field of oncology in two ways. First, prior to neoplasm formation, folic acid is important in the synthesis of DNA and RNA and the repair of damaged DNA. Second, after a tumor develops, a form of folic acid is used to counter the side effects of **methotrexate** and 5-fluorouracil (also called **fluorouracil** or 5-FU).

Description

Prior to tumor formation

Since folic acid is a cofactor in DNA replication and biosynthesis of purines and also in DNA repair, there is an increasing amount of research (epidemiological, clinical, and experimental) that suggests a folic acid deficiency might be a factor that predisposes the formation of tumors in normal epithelial tissue. There is an inverse relationship associated with low folate diets and an increase in DNA breakage and mutation that is unable to be effectively repaired. The preventative influence of dietary folic acid on the formation of **colon cancer** is currently under heavy research. Although a correlation is observed, it has not yet been proven to show cause and effect. However,

there is enough evidence to encourage consuming minimal daily dietary requirements of folic acid to potentially reduce the risk. When choosing supplements, other names for folic acid that may be encountered are folate and folacin.

After tumors form

Once a neoplasm forms, folic acid levels need to be decreased. In neoplasms, DNA replication and cell division are both occurring in an uncontrolled manner. Folate, which assists in this process, needs to be inhibited, causing an interruption in DNA synthesis and slowing the growth of the tumor. Chemotherapeutic agents called antimetabolites, or folic acid antagonists, such as methotrexate and 5-fluorouracil (5-FU), inhibit the enzymatic pathways for biosynthesis of nucleic acids by substituting for folic acid and sabotaging the reaction. Unfortunately, drugs that inhibit the biosynthesis of **cancer** cells also inhibit the biosynthesis of normal cells, resulting in extremely toxic side effects. To counter the side effects, a drug called **leucovorin** (a form of folate also known as Wellcovorin, Citrovorum and folinic acid) opposes the toxic effects of methotrexate on normal tissue. Leucovorin also increases the anticancer effect of 5-FU.

Recommended dosage

Non-cancer individuals supplementing their diet with folic acid may reduce the risk of cancer. Supplemental folic acid can be purchased over the counter and is also fortified in breakfast cereals and whole grain products produced in the United States. The recommended intake for adults is 400 micrograms (mcg) each day. While the risk of upper limit toxicity is low, adult men and women should not exceed the advised upper limit of 1,000 mcg per day. It is especially important that individuals diagnosed with cancer seek the advice of medical professionals before commencing or continuing supplemental folic acid use because it may interact with **chemotherapy**.

Cancer patients treated with methotrexate may be given leucovorin as a "rescue" treatment approximately 24 hours later to counteract the toxic side effects on normal tissues of the gastrointestinal system and bone marrow. Leucovorin is only available by prescription. It is a systemic drug available in oral form (tablets) or via injections. The dosage varies from person to person and is based on body size.

Precautions

Patients should inform their physician of the following conditions before they begin to take leucovorin:

- Pregnancy or breast-feeding.
- Pernicious anemia.
- Allergies to leucovorin or any other drugs.
- Vitamin B_{12} deficiency. Folic acid may mask hematologic signs of B_{12} deficiency while neurologic damage progresses.

Side effects

Folic acid in general and specifically leucovorin are usually well-tolerated. However, there are some uncommon side effects that include skin rashes, **itching**, **vomiting**, **nausea**, **diarrhea**, and difficulty breathing. Although extremely rare, seizures have occurred in some patients taking leucovorin. Since leucovorin is taken with chemotherapeutic drugs, some side effects may be due to drug interaction.

Interactions

Supplemental folic acid can interact with anticonvulsant medications such as dilantin, **phenytoin**, and primidone. It also complicates the effects of metformin (used in individuals with type 2 diabetes), sulfasalazine (used in individuals with Crohn's disease), and triamterene (a diuretic).

Leucovorin enhances the effects of 5-FU and antagonizes the effects of methotrexate. It additionally interacts with barbiturate medications that may be taken by people with sleep disorders.

Sally C. McFarlane-Parrott

Foscarnet *see* **Antiviral therapy**

Gabapentin

Definition

Gabapentin is an antiseizure or anticonvulsant medication that is used to help manage epilepsy and to treat certain types of nerve pain as well as some other conditions.

Purpose

The U.S. Food and Drug Administration (FDA) first approved gabapentin in 1993 as an antiepileptic to help prevent and manage partial seizures, with or without generalization, in combination with other antiseizure drugs in adults and children over age 12. Partial seizures are caused by brief abnormal electrical activity in localized areas of the brain. They usually do not result in loss of consciousness, but may cause rhythmic contractions in one area of the body or abnormal numbness or tingling sensations. When gabapentin is used along with other drug therapies for managing epileptic partial seizures, improvements are usually observed within 12 weeks. A liquid formulation and its use in children aged three to 12 was approved by the FDA in 2000.

The FDA has also approved gabapentin for the treatment of nerve pain that sometimes accompanies herpes infections (post-herpetic neuralgia from shingles). Gabapentin is used off-label (without specific FDA approval) to treat severe chronic nerve pain due to nerve damage, diabetic **neuropathy**, multiple sclerosis, **cancer**, and trigeminal neuralgia. It is also used as an acute treatment for bipolar mood disorder (manic-depressive disorder), to treat tremors associated with multiple sclerosis, and to prevent migraine headaches. Gabapentin is sometimes prescribed off-label for other mood disorders and for post-menopausal hot flashes.

Gabapentin has begun to replace tricyclic antidepressants (TCAs)—such as **amitriptyline**, nortriptyline, and desipramine—as a first-line treatment for neuropathic pain. Although both gabapentin and TCAs take from one to three weeks to provide pain relief, gabapentin appears to be the safer drug, especially in the elderly and those taking multiple medications. However gabapentin is more expensive than TCAs.

Description

Gabapentin is structurally similar to gamma-aminobutyric acid (GABA), a neurotransmitter in the central nervous system (brain and spinal cord) that decreases the firing of neurons and prevents excitatory electrical impulses from spreading to neighboring cells. Although this could theoretically lead to a decrease in seizure activity, gabapentin does not interact with GABA receptors and its exact mechanism of action for controlling seizures and reducing pain is not known. However gabapentin does appear to alter the activity of nerve cells.

Gabapentin is available as 100-, 300-, and 400-milligram (mg) capsules, as 600- and 800-mg tablets, and as a 250 mg per 5 ml liquid solution.

U.S. brand names

- Gabarone
- Neurontin

Canadian brand names

- Apo-Gabapentin
- Neurontin
- Novo-Gabapentin
- Nu-Gabapentin
- PMS-Gabapentin

International brand names

- Gabapentin
- Neurontin

Recommended dosage

For seizure control in those over age 12, the initial gabapentin dose may be 300 mg three times daily. This may be gradually increased as necessary, usually to no more than a total of 1,800 mg daily in three doses. However some patients may need even higher doses to control their seizures. Doses up to 3,600 mg per day have been well-tolerated in research studies. For children ages three to 12, the dosage is based on body weight, initially 10–15 mg per kilogram (kg; 2.2 lb) per day in three equal doses, increased as necessary until an effective dosage is reached, typically 25–40 mg per kg per day. For children under the age of three, use and dosage of gabapentin is determined by the physician.

To treat neuropathic pain, gabapentin is usually gradually increased from an initial dose of 300 mg on the first day, two 300-mg doses on the second day, and three 300-mg on the third day, up to a maximum daily dose of 1,800 mg. Research studies have found effective doses to range from 300 to 3,600 mg per day. The optimal dosage appears to be 1,200–2,400 mg per day in three doses.

The optimal dosage for treatment of bipolar disorder is not well-established. Doses up to 4,800 mg per day have been used.

To minimize side effects the first dose should be taken at bedtime and doses should be taken at even intervals. If a dose is missed, it should be taken as soon as remembered. However double dosing can be hazardous and should be avoided. Capsules should not be chewed or crushed.

Precautions

- Gabapentin should be taken only as prescribed.
- Gabapentin should not be used alone for the treatment of seizures unless the patient cannot tolerate other anticonvulsant drugs.
- Patients should avoid driving, operating dangerous machinery, or participating in hazardous activities until they learn how gabapentin affects their alertness, reaction time, and judgment.
- Gabapentin should not be discontinued suddenly, since this can increase the risk of seizures; rather, the dosage should be gradually decreased over at least one week.
- Gabapentin has caused the development of tumors in experimental animals, although it is not known whether this occurs in humans.
- In 2008, the FDA issued a warning that gabapentin and other antiepileptic drugs posed an increased risk for suicidal thoughts and behaviors.

Pediatric

Gabapentin should be used with caution in children under 12 years-of-age, due to the lack of safety and efficacy studies in this population.

Pregnant or breastfeeding

Gabapentin has caused fetal abnormalities in mice, rats, and rabbits. Although it has not been studied in pregnant women, it should only be used by women who are pregnant or may become pregnant if its potential benefits outweigh the risks. Breastfeeding mothers should discuss the risks and benefits of gabapentin with their physicians.

Other conditions and allergies

Gabapentin should be used with caution in patients with severe kidney disease and the dosage should be reduced.

Side effects

Gabapentin is usually well-tolerated. The most common side effects are nervous system symptoms including:

- drowsiness
- dizziness
- fatigue
- trembling or shaking
- unsteadiness
- clumsiness
- uncontrollable back-and-forth eye movements or eye rolling
- double or blurred vision
- swelling of the hands, feet, or legs
- muscle weakness or pain

These side effects appear to be dose-related and usually disappear after the first several weeks.

Less common side effects that may occur when first taking gabapentin include:

- dry mouth and eyes
- runny nose
- frequent urination
- indigestion
- nausea and/or vomiting
- constipation or diarrhea
- low blood pressure
- back pain
- decreased sexual drive
- ringing in the ears

- slurred speech
- difficulty concentrating
- insomnia
- weight gain
- twitching

Other less common side effects of gabapentin include:

- irritability
- mood changes
- memory loss
- impotence
- depression
- changes in thinking

Rare side effects of gabapentin include:

- pain in the lower back or side
- difficulty urinating
- fever and/or chills
- cough
- hoarseness

A patient experiencing any of the following should contact their physician or pharmacist immediately:

- mental or mood changes
- tingling or numbness in the hands or feet
- swelling of ankles
- vision problems
- fever or unusual bleeding

Signs of gabapentin overdose may include:

- double vision
- slurred speech
- drowsiness
- diarrhea

Pediatric

Gabapentin can cause behavioral and emotional disorders in children, including hostility and hyperactivity. Children under age 12 who experience the following more common side effects should see a doctor immediately:

- aggressive behavior
- irritability
- anxiety
- difficulty concentrating or paying attention
- crying
- depression
- mood swings
- increased emotionality

- hyperactivity
- suspiciousness or distrust

Geriatric

Elderly patients may be more sensitive to the side effects of gabapentin.

Interactions

Among the advantages of gabapentin are that it is not broken down in the body and, unlike many other drugs that are used to treat epilepsy, it has few interactions with other drugs. In particular, gabapentin does not interfere with other commonly used anticonvulsants such as **phenytoin**, **carbamazepine**, valproic acid, and phenobarbital. However antacids such as Mylanta and Maalox can interfere with the absorption of gabapentin, lowering its level in the blood, and should be taken at least two hours after taking gabapentin to avoid compromising its effectiveness.

Alcohol should be limited or avoided while taking gabapentin since it can intensify drowsiness and dizziness caused by the drug. Foods do not appear to affect the absorption of gabapentin.

The following herbs should be avoided when taking gabapentin:

- evening primrose
- valerian
- St. John's wort
- kava kava
- gotu kola

Resources

BOOKS

Corey, E. J., et al. *Molecules and Medicine*. Hoboken, NJ: John Wiley & Sons, 2007.
Hales, Robert E., et al. *What Your Patients Need To Know About Psychiatric Medications*. Washington, DC: American Psychiatric Publishing, 2007.

Schatzberg, Alan F., and Charles B. Nemeroff. *Essentials of Clinical Psychopharmacology*, 2nd ed. Washington, DC: American Psychiatric Publishing, 2006.

PERIODICALS

Kirkey, Sharon. "Off-Label Drug Use Can Have Painful Consequences; Many Drugs Are Used to Treat Illnesses They Were Not Intended For." *Vancouver Sun* (January 2, 2009): B3.

O'Connor, Alec B., et al. "A Cost-Effectiveness Comparison of Desipramine, Gabapentin, and Pregabalin for Treating Postherpetic Neuralgia." *Journal of the American Geriatric Society* 55, no. 8 (August 2007): 1176.

Steinman, Michael A., et al. "Narrative Review: The Promotion of Gabapentin: An Analysis of Internal Industry Documents." *Annals of Internal Medicine* 145, no. 4 (August 15, 2006): 284–293.

Vieta, Eduard, et al. "A Double-Blind, Randomized Placebo-Controlled, Prophylaxis Study of Adjunctive Gabapentin for Bipolar Disorder." *Journal of Clinical Psychiatry* 67 (2006): 473–477.

OTHER

"ACPA Medications & Chronic Pain." *American Chronic Pain Association*. http://www.theacpa.org/documents/ACPA%20Meds%202007%20Final.pdf.

American Society of Health-System Pharmacists. "Gabapentin." *MedlinePlus*. http://www.nlm.nih.gov/medlineplus/druginfo/meds/a694007.html.

Center for Drug Evaluation and Research. "Drug Details: Neurontin." *U.S. Food and Drug Administration*. http://www.accessdata.fda.gov/scripts/cder/drugsatfda/index.cfm?fuseaction=Search.DrugDetails.

"Gabapentin." *University of Maryland Medical Center*. http://www.umm.edu/altmed/drugs/gabapentin-056540.htm.

"Suicidal Behavior and Ideation and Antiepileptic Drugs." *U.S. Food and Drug Administration*. http://www.fda.gov/Drugs/DrugSafety/PostmarketDrugSafetyInformationforPatientsandProviders/UCM100190.

ORGANIZATIONS

American Chronic Pain Association, PO Box 850, Rocklin, CA, 95677, (800) 533-3231, (916) 632-3208, ACPA@pacbell.net, http://www.theacpa.org.

American Pain Foundation, 201 North Charles Street, Suite 710, Baltimore, MD, 21201-4111, (888) 615-PAIN (7246), info@painfoundation.org, http://www.painfoundation.org.

National Institute of Neurological Disorders and Stroke (NINDS), NIH Neurological Institute, PO Box 5801, Bethesda, MD, 20824, (301) 496-5751, (800) 352-9424, http://www.ninds.nih.gov/index.htm.

U.S. Food and Drug Administration, 10903 New Hampshire Ave., Silver Spring, MD, 20993-0002, (888) INFO-FDA, http://www.fda.gov.

Rosalyn Carson-DeWitt, MD
Emily Jane Willingham, PhD
Margaret Alic, PhD

Gallbladder cancer

Definition

Cancer of the gallbladder is cancer of the pear-shaped organ that lies on the undersurface of the liver.

Description

Bile from the liver is funneled into the gallbladder by way of the cystic duct. Between meals, the gallbladder stores a large amount of bile. To do this, it must absorb much of the water and electrolytes from the bile. In fact, the inner surface of the gallbladder is the most absorptive surface in the body. After a meal, the gallbladder's muscular walls contract to deliver the bile back through the cystic duct and eventually into the small intestine, where the bile can help digest food.

Demographics

About 6,000 people are diagnosed with gallbladder cancer each year in the United States, making it the fifth most common gastrointestinal cancer. It is more common in females than males and most patients are elderly. Southwest American Indians have a particularly high incidence—six times that of the general population.

Causes and symptoms

Gallstones are the most significant risk factor for the development of gallbladder cancer. Roughly 75 to 90 percent of patients with gallbladder cancer also have gallstones. Larger gallstones are associated with a higher chance of developing gallbladder cancer. Chronic inflammation of the gallbladder from **infection** also increases the risk for gallbladder cancer.

Unfortunately, sometimes cancer of the gallbladder does not produce symptoms until late in the disease. When symptoms are evident, the most common is pain in the upper right portion of the abdomen, underneath the right ribcage. Patients with gallbladder cancer may also report symptoms such as **nausea**, **vomiting**, weakness, jaundice, skin **itching**, **fever**, chills, poor appetite, and **weight loss**.

Diagnosis

Gallbladder cancer is often misdiagnosed because it mimics other more common conditions, such as gallstones, cholecystitis, and pancreatitis. But the imaging tests that are utilized to evaluate these other conditions can also detect gallbladder cancer. For example, ultrasound is a quick, noninvasive imaging test that reliably diagnoses gallstones and cholecystitis. It can also detect

KEY TERMS

Cholangiography—Radiographic examination of the bile ducts after injection with a special dye

Cholecystitis—Inflammation of the gallbladder, usually due to infection

Computed tomography—A radiology test by which images of cross-sectional planes of the body are obtained

Jaundice—Yellowish staining of the skin and eyes due to excess bilirubin in the bloodstream

Metastasis—The spread of tumor cells from one part of the body to another through blood vessels or lymphatic vessels

Pancreatitis—Inflammation of the pancreas

Stent—Slender hollow catheter or rod placed within a vessel or duct to provide support or maintain patency

Ultrasound—A radiology test utilizing high frequency sound waves

the presence of gallbladder cancer as well as show how far the cancer has spread. If cancer is suspected, a **computed tomography** scan is useful in confirming the presence of an abnormal mass and further demonstrating the size and extent of the tumor. Cholangiography, usually performed to evaluate a patient with jaundice, can also detect gallbladder cancer.

There are no specific laboratory tests for gallbladder cancer. Tumors can obstruct the normal flow of bile from the liver to the small intestine. Bilirubin, a component of bile, builds up within the liver and is absorbed into the bloodstream in excess amounts. This can be detected in a blood test, but it can also manifest clinically as jaundice. Elevated bilirubin levels and clinical jaundice can also occur with other conditions, such as gallstones.

On occasion, gallbladder cancer is diagnosed incidentally. About one percent of all patients who have their gallbladder removed for symptomatic gallstones are found to have gallbladder cancer. The cancer is found either by the surgeon or by the pathologist who inspects the gallbladder with a microscope.

Treatment team

The main member of the treatment team is the surgeon, since surgical removal of the cancer is the only measure that offers a significant chance of cure.

Sometimes the cancer is too advanced such that surgery would be of no benefit. But the patient might suffer from jaundice or blockage of the stomach. In this case, the gastroenterologist or interventional radiologist may be able to provide non-surgical alternatives to address these complications. In limited scenarios, the oncologist or radiation therapist may treat the patient with **chemotherapy** or **radiation therapy**.

Clinical staging, treatments, and prognosis

Staging of gallbladder cancer is determined by the how far the cancer has spread. The effectiveness of treatment declines as the stage progresses. Stage I cancer is confined to the wall of the gallbladder. Approximately 25% of cancers are at this stage at the time of diagnosis. Stage II cancer has penetrated the full thickness of the wall, but has not spread to nearby lymph nodes or invaded adjacent organs. Stage III cancer has spread to nearby lymph nodes or has invaded the liver, stomach, colon, small intestine, or large intestine. Stage IV disease has invaded very deeply into two or more adjacent organs or has spread to distant lymph nodes or organs by way of **metastasis**.

Early Stage I cancers involving only the innermost layer of the gallbladder wall can be cured by simple removal of the gallbladder. Cancers at this stage are sometimes found incidentally when the gallbladder is removed in the treatment of gallstones or cholecystitis. The majority of patients have good survival rates. Late Stage I cancers, which involve the outer muscular layers of the gallbladder wall, are generally treated in the same way as Stage II or III cancers. Removal of the gallbladder is not sufficient for these stages. The surgeon also removes nearby lymph nodes as well as a portion of the adjacent liver (radical surgery). Survival rates for these patients are considerably worse than for those with early Stage I disease. Patients with early Stage IV disease may benefit from radical surgery, but the issue is controversial. Late Stage IV cancer has spread too extensively to allow complete excision. Surgery is not an option for these patients.

Other therapies

When long-term survival is not likely, the focus of therapy shifts to improving quality of life. Jaundice and blockage of the stomach are two problems faced by patients with advanced cancer of the gallbladder. These can be treated with surgery, or alternatively, by special interventional techniques employed by the gastroenterologist or radiologist. A stent can be placed across the bile ducts in order to re-establish the flow of bile and relieve jaundice. A small feeding tube can be placed in the small intestine to allow feeding when the stomach is blocked. Pain may be treated with conventional pain medicines or a celiac ganglion nerve block.

Current chemotherapy or radiation therapy cannot cure gallbladder cancer, but they may offer some benefit in certain patients. For cancer that is too advanced for surgical cure, treatment with chemotherapeutic agents such as **fluorouracil** (5-FU) may lengthen survival for a few months. The limited benefit of chemotherapy must be weighed carefully against its side effects. Radiation therapy is sometimes used after attempted surgical resection of the cancer to extend survival for a few months or relieve jaundice.

Coping with cancer treatment

After cancer treatment, many patients find that good nutrition, and a strong support system (which may include a support group) improve their quality of life. Treatment team members or hospital social workers can often recommend local resources that can be of assistance to the patient.

Clinical trials

More **clinical trials** are needed to define the role of chemotherapy and radiation therapy after attempted surgical resection of Stage II and III cancer. Some investigators are conducting trials to assess whether extremely radical surgery is beneficial in early Stage IV disease.

Special concerns

After the removal of the gallbladder, patients may experience a temporary change in bowel habits. The bowel movements may be more frequent or more liquid than before surgery. This situation usually resolves within about six months.

Resources

BOOKS

Abeloff, Martin D., editor. "Gallbladder Carcinoma." In *Clinical Oncology*. 2nd ed. New York: Churchill Livingstone, 2000, pp.1730-1737.

Ahrendt, Steven A., and Henry A. Pitt. "Biliary Tract." In *Sabiston Textbook of Surgery*, edited by Courtney Townsend Jr., 16th ed. Philadelphia: W.B. Saunders Company, 2001, pp. 1076-1111.

OTHER

National Cancer Institute Cancer Trials website. http://cancertrials.nci.nih.gov/system.

Kevin O. Hwang, M.D.

Gallium nitrate

Definition

Gallium nitrate is a drug that is used to treat **hypercalcemia**, or too much calcium in the blood. This condition may occur when individuals develop various types of **cancer**. Gallium nitrate is also known by the common brand name Ganite.

Purpose

The purpose of gallium nitrate is to reduce the level of calcium in a patient's blood. It is a liquid medication that is injected into a person's vein.

Description

Due to the fact that hypercalcemia is a serious condition that can be fatal, it is very important that it is effectively treated. Hypercalcemia is a common complication of cancer, affecting approximately 10–20% of all cancer patients. This condition can affect many systems of the body and has various signs and symptoms. Sometimes, these symptoms may be thought to be associated with the cancer, and therefore the hypercalcemia itself may go undiagnosed.

Symptoms of hypercalcemia include frequent urination, thirst, dizziness, constipation, **nausea**, **vomiting**, and disruptions in cardiac rhythm. If severe, this complication can lead to seizure, cardiac arrest, coma, or death.

Hypercalcemia should first be treated with fluids. Doctors should make sure that their patients are properly hydrated, meaning that they have enough fluid in their body. However, fluid treatment alone is usually not effective to treat this condition. Therefore, some physicians may recommend that their patients take gallium nitrate to establish a normal balance of calcium in the blood.

Recommended dosage

The recommended dosage of gallium nitrate differs depending on the patient, and should be determined by a physician. For adults and teenagers, the dosage of this medication is based on body weight/size, and must be calculated by a doctor. The medication is injected into a patient's vein at a slow pace for 24 hours over a period of five days. If a patient's calcium level is still too high, this process can be repeated in two to four weeks. For younger children, up to the age of 12, there are no specific studies to determine the effects of gallium nitrate. Therefore, use and dosage of this medication

KEY TERMS

Cancer—One cell that grows out of control in the body and subsequently invades nearby cells and tissue.

Ganite—The commonly used brand name for gallium nitrate.

Hypercalcemia—Excessive or increased calcium in the blood. Often a complication of cancer.

must be determined by the young cancer patient's personal physician.

While undergoing treatment with gallium nitrate, patients' doctors should check calcium levels at regular intervals. Even if a patient's condition has improved, he or she may still need to be followed closely to make sure that they do not develop hypercalcemia again.

Precautions

Before taking gallium nitrate, there are specific precautions that should be taken to avoid potential complications. Patients should let their physician know if they are allergic to any foods, preservatives or dyes. In addition, patients with certain medical problems, specifically kidney disease, should make sure that their prescribing physician is aware of this, as use of gallium nitrate can exacerbate this condition. Adequate hydration may minimize toxic effects on the kidney.

In addition, use of gallium nitrate has not been studied in pregnant animals or humans. It is not recommended for women who are pregnant or breast-feeding, as it may cause negative side effects.

With regard to children, as stated, there are no studies of gallium nitrate in younger populations. There are also no studies of this medication in the elderly. However, it is not thought that the use of gallium nitrate would cause very different side effects in older people versus younger adults.

Side effects

Individuals who are considering taking gallium nitrate should discuss its use in detail with their physician. This includes talking about the potential benefits versus any potential side effects. Some individuals may experience all, some, or none of these side effects. Some of these side effects may lessen as a person's body gets used to the medication. However, it is important to be aware of these potential side effects because some of them may require medical interventions.

More common side effects:

- blood in the urine
- pain in the bones
- change in urination frequency
- feeling thirsty
- loss of appetite (anorexia)
- weakness of muscles
- feeling nauseous
- diarrhea
- metallic taste in the mouth
- nausea and vomiting
- decrease of phosphate levels in the blood

Less common side effects:

- cramps in the abdomen
- a feeling of confusion
- muscle spasms

Rare side effects:

- excessive fatigue or weakness

Interactions

Patients should tell their physician if they are taking any other medications on a regular basis, especially the ones listed below, as they could cause a negative interaction if taken with gallium nitrate.

- certain medications taken for infections
- cisplatin
- medications for pain that contain acetaminophen or aspirin
- cyclosporine
- deferoxamine
- some medications for treatment of arthritis
- lithium
- methotrexate
- pencillamine
- gentamicin
- amphotericin B
- "nephrotoxic agents"

Tiffani A. DeMarco, MS

Gallium scan

Definition

A gallium scan of the body is a nuclear medicine test that is conducted using a camera that detects gallium, a form of radionuclide, or radioactive chemical substance.

Purpose

Most gallium scans are ordered to detect cancerous tumors, infections, or areas of inflammation in the body. Gallium is known to accumulate in inflamed, infected, or cancerous tissues. The scans are used to determine whether a patient with an unexplained **fever** has an **infection** and the site of the infection, if present. Gallium scans also may be used to evaluate **cancer** following **chemotherapy** or **radiation therapy**.

Precautions

Children and women who are pregnant or breast-feeding are only given gallium scans if the potential diagnostic benefits will outweigh the risks.

Description

The patient will usually be asked to come to the testing facility 24–48 hours before the procedure to receive the injection of gallium. Sometimes, the injection will be given only four to six hours before the study or as long as 72 hours before the procedure. The timeframe is based on the area or organs of the body being studied.

For the study itself, the patient lies very still for approximately 30–60 minutes. A camera is moved across the patient's body to detect and capture images of concentrations of the gallium. The camera picks up signals from any accumulated areas of the radionuclide. In most cases, the patient is lying down throughout the procedure. Back (posterior) and front (anterior) views will usually be taken, and sometimes a side (lateral) view is used. The camera may occasionally touch the patient's skin, but will not cause any discomfort. A clicking noise may be heard throughout the procedure; this is only the sound of the scanner registering radiation.

Preparation

The intravenous injection of gallium is done in a separate appointment prior to the procedure. Generally, no special dietary requirements are necessary. Sometimes the physician will ask that the patient have light or clear meals within a day or less of the procedure. Many patients will be given **laxatives** or an

Nuclear medicine scan of the skeleton. A radioisotope, like gallium, is used to produce this image. This scan reveals that lung cancer has spread to ribs and there is osteomyelitis in ankle. *(Copyright Scott Camazine and Sue Trainor, Science Source/Photo Researchers, Inc. Reproduced by permission.)*

enema prior to the scan to eliminate any residual gallium from the bowels.

Aftercare

There is generally no aftercare required following a gallium scan. However, women who are breastfeeding who have a scan will be cautioned against breastfeeding for four weeks following the exam.

Risks

There is a minimal risk of exposure to radiation from the gallium injection, but the exposure from one gallium scan is generally less than exposure from **x rays**.

Normal results

A radiologist trained in nuclear medicine or a nuclear medicine specialist will interpret the exam

KEY TERMS

Benign—Not cancerous. Benign tumors are not considered immediate threats, but may still require some form of treatment.

Gallium—A form of radionuclide that is used to help locate tumors and inflammation (specifically referred to as GA67 citrate).

Malignant—This term, usually used to describe a tumor, means cancerous, becoming worse and possibly growing.

Nuclear medicine—A subspecialty of radiology used to show the function and anatomy of body organs. Very small amounts of radioactive substances, or tracers, are detected with a special camera as they accumulate in certain organs and tissues.

Radionuclide—A chemical substance, called an isotope, that exhibits radioactivity. A gamma camera, used in nuclear medicine procedures, will pick up the radioactive signals as the substance gathers in an organ or tissue. They are sometimes referred to as tracers.

results and compare them to other diagnostic tests. It is normal for gallium to accumulate in the liver, spleen, bones, breast tissue, and large bowel.

Abnormal results

An abnormal concentration of gallium in areas other than those where it normally concentrates may indicate the presence of disease. Concentrations may be due to inflammation, infection, or the presence of tumor tissue. Often, additional tests are required to determine if the tumors are malignant (cancerous) or benign.

Even though gallium normally concentrates in organs such as the liver or spleen, abnormally high concentrations will suggest certain diseases and conditions. For example, Hodgkin's or **non-Hodgkin's lymphoma** may be diagnosed or staged if there is abnormal gallium activity in the lymph nodes. After a patient receives cancer treatment, such as radiation therapy or chemotherapy, a gallium scan may help to find new or recurring tumors or to record regression of a treated tumor. Physicians can narrow causes of liver problems by noting abnormal gallium activity in the liver. Gallium scans also may be used to diagnose lung diseases or a disease called sarcoidosis, in the chest.

Resources

OTHER

"A Patient's Guide to Nuclear Medicine." *University of Iowa Virtual Hospital.* [cited July 2, 2001].http://www.vh.org/ Patients/IHB/Rad/NucMed/PatGuideNucMed/ PatGuideNucMed.html.

ORGANIZATIONS

American Cancer Society. 1599 Clifton Road NE, Atlanta, GA 30329. (404) 320-3333. http://www.cancer.org.
American College of Nuclear Medicine. PO Box 175, Landisville, PA 31906. (717) 898-6006.
American Liver Foundation. 1425 Pompton Avenue, Cedar Grove NJ 07009. (800) GO LIVER (465-4837). http://www.liverfoundation.org.
Society of Nuclear Medicine. 1850 Samuel Morse Drive, Reston, VA 10016. (703) 708-9000. http://www.snm.org.

Teresa G. Odle

Ganciclovir *see* **Antiviral therapy**

Gastrectomy

Definition

Gastrectomy is the surgical removal of all or part of the stomach.

Purpose

Gastrectomy is performed most often to treat the following conditions:

- stomach (gastric) cancer
- bleeding gastric ulcer
- perforation of the stomach wall
- noncancerous tumors

Demographics

According to the World Health Organization (WHO), **stomach cancer** is the second leading cause of **cancer** deaths in the world, accounting for about 8.8% of all deaths from cancer. (Lung cancer accounts for 17.8% of cancer deaths). Although stomach cancer is a worldwide problem, the incidence rates vary considerably in different countries. The highest death rates from stomach cancer are found in Japan, Korean, South America, especially Chile, and parts of the former Soviet Union. In the United States, the American Cancer Society expected about 21,130 new cases of stomach cancer to be diagnosed and 10,620 deaths to be attributed to the disease. Since gastrectomy is most often

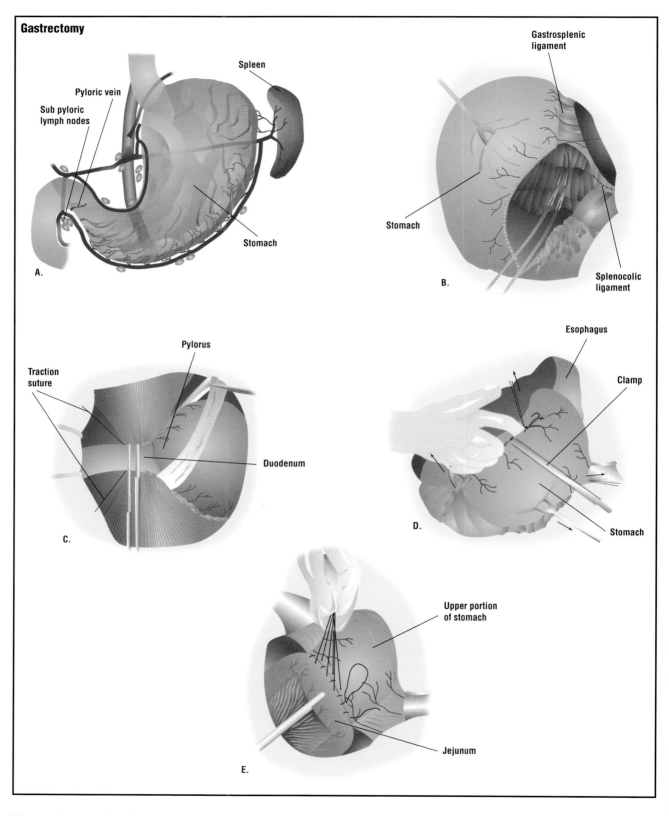

Gastrectomy

A. Sub pyloric lymph nodes / Pyloric vein / Spleen / Stomach

B. Gastrosplenic ligament / Stomach / Splenocolic ligament

C. Traction suture / Pylorus / Duodenum

D. Esophagus / Clamp / Stomach

E. Upper portion of stomach / Jejunum

Ligaments connecting the stomach to the spleen and colon are severed (B). The duodenum is clamped and separated from the the stomach, or pylorus (C). The stomach is clamped, and the portion to be removed is severed (D). The remaining stomach is attached to the jejunum (E). *(Illustration by GGS Information Services. Cengage Learning, Gale.)*

done to treat stomach cancer, gastrectomy rates should mirror stomach cancer rates.

Description

Gastrectomy for cancer

Surgery is the only curative treatment for gastric (stomach) cancer. If the cancer is diagnosed early and limited to one part of the stomach, The tumor and only part of the stomach may be removed (partial or sub-total gastrectomy.) More often, the entire stomach is removed (total gastrectomy) along with the surrounding lymph nodes. When the entire stomach is removed, the esophagus is attached directly to the small intestine.

A gastrectomy is performed under general anesthesia. Once the patient is anesthetized, a urinary catheter is usually inserted to monitor urine output. A thin nasogastric tube is inserted into the nose, through the esophagus, and into the stomach. The abdomen is cleansed with an antiseptic solution. The surgeon makes a large incision from just below the breastbone down to the navel. The surgeon then removes all or part of the stomach and attaches connects either the remaining piece of stomach or the esophagus to the small intestine.

Gastrectomy for gastric cancer is almost always done using the traditional open surgery technique, which requires a wide incision to open the abdomen. However, some surgeons use a laparoscopic technique that requires only a small incision. The laparoscope is connected to a tiny video camera that relays a picture of the abdomen to a monitor to guide the surgeon who then operates through this incision.

The potential benefits of laparoscopic surgery include less postoperative pain, decreased hospitalization, and earlier return to normal activities. The use of laparoscopic gastrectomy is limited, however. Only patients with early-stage gastric cancers or those whose surgery is intended only as palliative treatment (pain and symptomatic relief rather than cure) are considered for this minimally invasive technique.

Gastrectomy for ulcers

Gastrectomy is also used occasionally in the treatment of severe peptic ulcer disease or its complications. While the vast majority of peptic ulcers (gastric ulcers in the stomach or duodenal ulcers in the duodenum) are managed with medication, partial gastrectomy is sometimes required for peptic ulcer patients who have complications. These include patients who do not respond satisfactorily to medical therapy, those who develop a bleeding or perforated ulcer, and those

who develop pyloric obstruction (a blockage to the exit from the stomach). The surgical procedure for severe ulcer disease is also called an antrectomy. An antrectomy is a limited form of gastrectomy in which the antrum, or lower portion of the stomach that produces digestive juices, is removed.

Diagnosis/Preparation

Before undergoing gastrectomy, patients require a variety of tests such as **x rays**, **computed tomography** (CT) scans, **ultrasonography**, or endoscopic biopsies (microscopic examination of tissue) to confirm the diagnosis and localize the tumor or ulcer. **Laparoscopy** and tissue **biopsy** may be used to diagnose a malignancy or to determine the extent of a tumor that is already diagnosed. When a tumor is strongly suspected, laparoscopy is often performed immediately before the surgery to remove the tumor. This avoids the need to anesthetize the patient twice, and sometimes avoids the need for surgery completely if the tumor found through laparoscopy is deemed inoperable.

Aftercare

After gastrectomy surgery, patients are taken to the recovery unit and vital signs are closely monitored by the nursing staff until the anesthesia wears off. Patients commonly feel pain from the incision, and pain medication is prescribed to provide relief and is usually delivered intravenously (IV, directly into a vein). Upon waking from anesthesia, patients have an intravenous line, a urinary catheter, and a nasogastric tube in place. They cannot eat or drink immediately following surgery. In some cases, oxygen is delivered through a mask that fits over the mouth and nose. The nasogastric tube is attached to intermittent suction to keep what remains of the stomach empty.

If the whole stomach has been removed, the tube goes directly to the small intestine and remains in place until bowel function returns. This can take two to three days and is monitored by listening with a stethoscope for bowel sounds. When bowel sounds return, the patient can drink clear liquids. If the liquids are tolerated, the nasogastric tube is removed and the diet is gradually changed from liquids to soft foods, and then to more solid foods. Dietary adjustments may be necessary, as certain foods may now be difficult to digest. Overall, gastrectomy surgery usually requires a stay of 7–10 days in the hospital and recuperation time of at least several weeks.

Risks

Surgery for peptic ulcer is effective, but it may result in a variety of postoperative complications. Following gastrectomy surgery, as many as 30% of patients have significant symptoms. An operation called highly selective vagotomy, in which a nerve that stimulates the stomach is cut, is now preferred for ulcer management, as it is safer than gastrectomy.

After a gastrectomy, several abnormalities may develop that produce symptoms related to food intake. They happen largely because the stomach, which serves as a food reservoir, has been reduced in its capacity by the surgery. Other surgical procedures that often accompany gastrectomy for ulcer disease can also contribute to later symptoms. These other surgical procedures include vagotomy, which lessens acid production and slows stomach emptying, and pyloroplasty, which enlarges the opening between the stomach and small intestine to facilitate emptying of the stomach.

Some patients experience lightheadedness, heart palpitations (racing heart), sweating, **nausea**, and **vomiting** after a meal. These may be symptoms of dumping syndrome, as food is rapidly moved into the small intestine from the remaining stomach or directly from the esophagus. Dumping syndrome is treated by adjusting the diet and pattern of eating, for example, eating smaller, more frequent meals, and limiting liquids.

Patients who have abdominal bloating and pain after eating, followed frequently by **nausea and vomiting**, may have afferent loop syndrome, a serious condition that must be corrected surgically. Patients who have early satiety (feeling of fullness after eating), abdominal discomfort, and vomiting may have bile reflux gastritis (also called bilious vomiting), which is also surgically correctable. Many patients experience **weight loss** after gastrectomy.

Reactive hypoglycemia is a condition that results when blood sugar levels become too high after a meal, stimulating the release of insulin, occurring about two hours after eating. Should this occur after gastrectomy, changing to a high-protein diet and smaller meals is advised.

Ulcers recur in a small percentage of patients after partial gastrectomy for peptic ulcer. Recurrence is usually within the first few years after surgery. Further surgery is usually necessary.

Vitamin and mineral supplementation is necessary after gastrectomy to correct certain deficiencies, especially vitamin B_{12}, iron, and folate. Vitamin D and calcium are also needed to prevent and treat the bone problems that often occur. These include softening

---

WHO PERFORMS THE PROCEDURE AND WHERE IS IT PERFORMED?

A gastrectomy is performed by a board-certified surgeon trained in gastroenterology, the branch of medicine that deals with the diseases of the digestive tract. An anesthesiologist is responsible for administering anesthesia The operation is always performed in a hospital setting.

QUESTIONS TO ASK THE DOCTOR

- What happens on the day of surgery?
- What type of anesthesia will be used?
- How long will it take to recover from the surgery?
- When can I expect to return to work and/or resume normal activities?
- What are the risks associated with a gastrectomy?
- How many gastrectomies do you perform in a year?
- What is the rate of postsurgical complications among your patients?
- Will there be a scar?

---

and bending of the bones, which can produce pain and osteoporosis, which is a loss of bone mass. According to one study, the risk for spinal fracture after gastrectomy may be as high as 50%.

Normal results

Overall, survival after gastrectomy for gastric cancer varies greatly by the stage of disease at the time of surgery. For early gastric cancer, the five-year survival rate is as high as 77%. For late-stage disease, the five-year survival rate is only 3%. The five-year survival rate for cancers in the lower stomach is better than for those found in the upper stomach, and the survival rate for gastric **lymphoma** is better than for gastric adenocarcinomas.

Most studies have shown that patients can have an acceptable quality of life after gastrectomy for a potentially curable gastric cancer. Many patients maintain a healthy appetite and eat a normal diet. Others lose weight and do not enjoy meals as much as before gastrectomy. Some studies show that patients who have total gastrectomies have more disease-related or treatment-related symptoms after surgery and poorer physical function than patients who have subtotal gastrectomies. There does not appear to be much difference, however, in emotional status or social activity level between patients who have undergone total versus subtotal gastrectomies.

Morbidity and mortality rates

Depending on the extent of surgery, the risk for postoperative death after gastrectomy for gastric cancer has been reported as 1–3%, and the risk of non-fatal complications as 9–18%.

Resources

BOOKS

Beers, Mark H., Robert S. Porter, and Thomas V. Jones, eds. "Disorders of the Stomach and Duodenum." In *The Merck Manual*, 18th ed. Whitehouse Station, NJ: Merck, 2007.
Feldman, Mark, et al., eds. "Stomach and Duodenum: Complications of Surgery for Peptic Ulcer Disease." In *Sleisenger's and Fordtran's Gastrointestinal and Liver Disease*, 8th ed. Philadelphia: W. B. Saunders Co., 2006.

ORGANIZATIONS

American College of Gastroenterology. P.O. Box 342260 Bethesda, MD 20827-2260. (301) 263-9000. http://www.acg.gi.org (accessed March 23, 2008).
American Gastroenterological Association (AGA). 4930 Del Ray Avenue, Bethesda, MD 20814. (301) 654-2055. http://www.gastro.org (accessed March 23, 2008).

Caroline A. Helwick
Monique Laberge, PhD
Tish Davidson, AM

Gastric cancer *see* **Stomach cancer**
Gastrinoma *see* **Zollinger-Ellison syndrome**

Gastrointestinal complications

Description

Constipation, fecal impaction, bowel obstruction, and **diarrhea** are common gastrointestinal complications faced by **cancer** patients due to either their cancer or the treatment of it. The seriousness of these complications varies from mildly uncomfortable to life threatening.

Constipation is the slow and infrequent passage of small, dry bowel movements through the large intestine. Unpleasant and sometimes painful, constipation often causes people to strain while trying to have a bowel movement. However, constipation itself is generally not life threatening; however, fecal impaction can be.

Fecal impaction is the collection of hard, dry stool in the colon or rectum that can't be excreted. Patients with fecal impaction may or may not experience the typical gastrointestinal symptoms usually associated with constipation, such as cramping and pressure. For example, if the impaction is pressing on a nerve, there may be back pain. If the impaction is pressing on the urethra or bladder, there may be an increase or decrease in urination. There may be **nausea** and abdominal pain, as well as stool that leaks out when the patient coughs and explosive diarrhea, which is the result of stool moving around the impaction. When movement of the diaphragm is restricted due to abdominal distention (swelling of the abdomen), the patient may not be getting enough oxygen. Breathing, heart, and circulation problems may develop, such as dizziness, hypotension (low blood pressure), hypoxia (a lack of oxygen to the brain), and angina. If left untreated, fecal impaction can cause death.

Bowel obstruction, as defined by the National Cancer Institute, is "a partial or complete blockage of the small or large intestine by a process other than fecal impaction. Classified by type, cause, and location, bowel obstructions can be caused by tumors inside or outside of the bowel, as well as the development of scar tissue after surgery. Patients with colostomies have an increased risk of becoming constipated. Therefore, they need to be especially proactive and report any signs of constipation to their physicians in order to avoid developing bowel obstruction.

Diarrhea is loose, watery stool, which results in abdominal cramps and frequent trips to the bathroom. For cancer patients, diarrhea tends to be especially bothersome. It can affect their eating patterns, as well as cause them to become dehydrated and lose weight. Although it can usually be managed, it sometimes leads to life threatening problems.

Causes

Constipation and fecal impaction

Constipation can have many causes. It can be a symptom of cancer or the result of a growing tumor. It can be linked to certain cancer treatments as well. Sometimes the medications given to cancer patients, such as **opioids** for pain, diuretics, or **chemotherapy** drugs, can cause constipation. Medications prescribed for anxiety and **depression**, not to mention the depression itself, can be the culprits, too. Patients may find it difficult or painful to move and may put off going to the bathroom. Physical illness, exacerbated by depression, can also alter eating habits, resulting in dietary changes that aren't healthy, such as drinking too little water or not eating enough. In addition, certain muscle and nerve damage, such as **spinal cord compression** from a tumor, can lead to a loss of muscle tone in the bowel, making it difficult for a patient to complete a bowel movement. Environmental factors can worsen constipation. For example, patients who are in unfamiliar surroundings, or need assistance getting to the bathroom, or use a bedpan may have difficulty relaxing and this may affect their ability to defecate. Treating cancer patients with dignity and allowing them as much privacy as possible can be very helpful in these situations.

The National Cancer Institute has identified five major factors that can lead to fecal impaction:

- opioid pain medications
- inactivity over a long period of time
- changes in diet
- mental illness
- long-term use of laxatives

Oddly enough, using **laxatives** over a long period of time actually contributes to the development of constipation and fecal impaction, because the higher doses necessary to do the job "make the colon less able to signal the need to have a bowel movement," according to the National Cancer Institute. It may be difficult for cancer patients to avoid repeated bouts of constipation during their cancer treatment, especially if they are taking opioids for pain. However, patients should talk with their physicians about the specific preventative measures that would be the most suitable for them. Every effort should be made to avoid fecal impaction.

Bowel obstruction

According to the National Cancer Institute, "a bowel obstruction may be caused by a narrowing of the intestine from inflammation or damage of the bowel, tumors, scar tissue, hernias, twisting of the bowel, or pressure on the bowel from outside the intestinal tract." Most bowel obstructions, usually due to scar tissue and hernias, occur in the small intestine. Tumors, volvulus (twisting of the bowel), or diverticulitis account for most of the bowel obstructions in the large intestine. Cancers of the colon, stomach, and ovary are the ones that most frequently cause bowel obstructions. When lung and breast cancers spread to the abdomen, they too can cause bowel obstructions. Ripamonti and colleagues reported in the *Annals of Oncology* in 1993 that having abdominal surgery or abdominal radiation puts patients at a greater risk of developing a bowel obstruction.

Diarrhea

Most often when cancer patients have diarrhea, the cause is related to their cancer therapy (i.e., chemotherapy drugs, especially fluoropyrimidines or **irinotecan**, **radiation therapy**, or surgery). Intestinal surgery, for example, can cause diarrhea by negatively affecting the way the bowel functions. Chemotherapy drugs, which can alter the way food is broken down and absorbed in the small intestine, can cause indigestion and diarrhea. According to Tuchmann and Engelkind, the stress and anxiety associated with cancer diagnosis and treatment can also cause diarrhea. Unfortunately, antibiotic therapy to treat **infection**, as the National Cancer Institute points out, "can cause inflammation of the lining of the bowel, resulting in diarrhea that often does not respond to treatment." In other cases, the cause can be directly tied to the patient's diet or use of laxatives. Severe diarrhea may result from concurrent chemotherapy and radiation therapy.

Treatments

Constipation and fecal impaction

A physician can diagnose the causes of constipation by performing a physical examination and reviewing a patient's medical history. The patient's stool can be tested for the presence of blood, which is done by asking the patient to provide a sample. In some cases, the physician might suspect that constipation has progressed to fecal impaction. In that case, an examination might include x-rays of the abdomen or chest, blood tests, and an electrocardiogram, which is a painless test that shows the activity of the heart. Another way to check for fecal impaction is to perform a rectal examination, which involves the physician inserting a lubricated, gloved finger into the rectum. If there is an impaction, there may be some discomfort; however, in general, the worst part of this examination is the embarrassment some people might feel.

A **colonoscopy** might be scheduled to see if cancer is present or to simply rule it out. A colonoscopy takes about thirty minutes to complete and is performed in a clinic or hospital setting. It is relatively painless, because patients are given a sedative and/or pain medicine. By inserting a flexible lighted tube into the patient's anus, the physician is able to see the entire large intestine all the way to the lower end of the small intestine.

Treatments options for patients with constipation may include a combination of preventative measures. Patients will probably be advised to keep track of their bowel movements in a journal. If they are too ill to do so, their caregivers may be asked to perform the task on their behalf. When the patient is trying to defecate, caregivers should be careful to respect their privacy, allowing them enough time and space to encourage success. Some patients find it helpful to run water in the sink or tub; the sound relaxes them and creates a sound barrier. If it is not contraindicated, patients may be advised to add fiber to their diets. Patients may be referred to nutritionists who are familiar with addressing the needs of cancer patients and can create individualized meal plans based on a patient's medical profile.

Adequate fluid intake is critical for patients prone to developing constipation, as well as fecal impaction. Patients may be asked to reduce their use of laxatives. In addition, patients should seek the approval of their physicians before they take any over-the-counter medications. According to the National Institute of Cancer, "impactions are usually treated by moistening and softening the stool with an enema." However, a physician needs to be consulted before an enema is given, because too many enemas can damage the bowel. Nonstimulating bowel softeners may be needed. In some cases, it may be necessary for the fecal material to be manually removed by a physician, although it is understandable that many patients may dislike the thought of it.

Bowel obstruction

To make a diagnosis of bowel obstruction, the physician will need to perform a physical exam to determine if the patient has abdominal pain, gas, or stool in the bowel. The physician will most likely want to draw blood in order to check for infection and body chemistry imbalances. If an obstruction is diagnosed, a **barium enema** may need to be performed to ascertain its location.

Bowel obstruction can be classified into two categories: acute (short term) and chronic (long term). Patients with acute bowel obstruction must be monitored carefully. If their condition cannot be stabilized, it may necessary to insert a lubricated nasogastric tube through the patient's nose and esophagus until it reaches the stomach. Many patients find this procedure initially unpleasant, which is understandable. It is a brief procedure, but it causes many patients to gag and, in some cases, vomit. Some patients may respond better to a tube inserted in their rectum to relieve the pressure. The purpose of inserting the tube is to reduce the patient's swelling, gas, and excess fluid; however, surgery may be unavoidable, if the obstruction worsens and completely blocks the bowel. The insertion of a stent may be required in patients with advanced cancer, if the obstruction cannot be removed through surgical means.

A chronically ill patient may need to have a gastrostomy tube (or feeding tube) inserted through the wall of the abdomen into the stomach. This is done to help the patient eat and to alleviate painful symptoms. A gastroenterologist performs the procedure while the patient is under general anesthesia; therefore, it is completely painless. The tube may need to be temporary or permanent, depending on the patient's condition.

Diarrhea

Many factors can play a part in causing diarrhea, making its treatment challenging. Because severe diarrhea can be very upsetting and even life threatening, physicians will try to establish the cause of the problem as quickly as possible. Patients can expect to be asked a series of questions and to be physically examined. Their vital signs, such as blood pressure and pulse, will be taken and compared to previous readings. The patient may need to provide a stool sample so that it can be tested for the presence of blood or bacteria.

Dietary changes are likely to be suggested. The patient may be given a list of foods to avoid and a list of foods that are acceptable in small quantities. Patients with severe diarrhea may need to monitored closely by their caretakers or admitted to the hospital where intravenous fluids will be administered.

Alternative and complementary therapies

Relaxation therapy

Some patients find that relaxation therapy helps them cope with the anxiety associated with cancer treatments and their side effects. A well-established psychogenic modality, relaxation therapy has been said to help cancer patients alleviate pain. When patients are in pain, they tend to tense up. This increases the pain, which causes even more stress. Learning relaxation techniques can help reverse this negative cycle. For example, some patients have found that by utilizing progressive muscle relaxation techniques, they are better able to handle physical and emotional pain, such as constipation and anxiety.

Comfort measures

Utilizing comfort measures to help patients heal is grounded in the belief that a patient should be seen as a whole person, not just someone with a disease and symptoms. Those who practice Eastern medicine have traditionally embraced this holistic approach, which considers the patient's mind, body, and spirit. Indeed, many Eastern philosophies have begun to greatly influence Western society. Some physicians have begun to change their personal philosophies to incorporate holistic concepts in their therapeutic handling of pain. For example, some cancer patients suffer not only from physical pain, but they also feel anxious and show signs of depression. In an article published by the *New England Journal of Medicine*, Dr. Campion promotes comfort measures as a way to help alleviate depression, recognizing that a person's state of mind affects his or her physical health. Comfort measures that embrace dignity, such as showing the patient kindness and respect, go a long way to promote healing. Patients with diarrhea, for example, can benefit from comfort measures that include a bedside commode, frequently changed sheets, and adjustable beds.

Acupuncture

Over 10,000 acupuncture and Oriental medicine practitioners currently practice in the United States. In a 1997 consensus statement issued by the National Institutes of Health, acupuncture was recognized as being an effective treatment for pain and nausea. It has also been used successfully to treat bowel obstructions. Developed by the Chinese as far back as 3000 B.C., acupuncture is thought to correct an imbalance of energy flow in the body. The technique involves inserting fine, sterile needles into a person's energy points, sometimes referred to as meridians. Some people fear acupuncture because they think the procedure will be painful, but in actuality it is not painful and tends to relax many people. Some people even fall asleep during the procedure.

Not everyone agrees on how acupuncture works, but research has shown that acupuncture increases the body's electromagnetic flow, which could cause the release of endorphins, the body's natural painkillers. Acupuncture is performed in a clinical setting. Patients interested in receiving acupuncture treatments should talk with their doctors to obtain suitable referrals to reputable, well-trained medical practitioners.

Resources

BOOKS

Jacobson, E. *Progressive Relaxation.* Chicago, IL: Chicago University Press, 1938.
Tuchmann L., Engelking, C. Cancer-related diarrhea. In *Oncology Nursing Secrets, edited by R. A. Gates and R. M. Fink.* Philadelphia, PA: Hanley and Belfus, 2001, pp.310–322.

PERIODICALS

Campion, E. W. "Why unconventional medicine?" *New England Journal of Medicine* 328 (1993): 282–283.
Ripamonti, C., De Conno, F., Ventafridda, V., et al. "Management of bowel obstruction in advanced and terminal cancer patients." *Annals of Oncology* 4 (1993): 15–21.

OTHER

National Cancer Institute "Gastrointestinal Complications (PDQ^R). " *National Cancer Institute.* February 2003. National Cancer Institute. 26 Feb. 2005. http://www.nci.nih.gov/.
National Institutes of Health "107 Acupuncture: National Institutes of Health Consensus Development Conference Statement." *National Cancer Institute.* November 1997. National Institutes of Health. 4 April 2005. http://odp.od.nih.gov/consensus/cons/107/107_statement.htm.

Lee Ann Paradise

Gastroduodenostomy

Definition

A gastroduodenostomy is a surgical reconstruction procedure by which a new connection between the stomach and the first portion of the small intestine (duodenum) is created.

Purpose

A gastroduodenostomy is a gastrointestinal reconstruction technique. It may be performed in cases of **stomach cancer**, a malfunctioning pyloric valve, gastric obstruction, and peptic ulcers.

As a gastrointestinal reconstruction technique, it is usually performed after a total or partial **gastrectomy** (stomach removal) procedure. The procedure is also referred to as a Billroth I procedure. For benign diseases, a gastroduodenostomy is the preferred type of reconstruction because of the restoration of normal gastrointestinal physiology. Several studies have confirmed the advantages of the procedure, because it preserves the duodenal passage. Compared to a gastrojejunostomy (Billroth II) procedure, meaning the surgical connection of the stomach to the jejunum, gastroduodenostomies have been shown to result in less modification of pancreatic and biliary functions, as well as in a decreased incidence of ulceration and inflammation of the stomach (gastritis). However, gastroduodenostomies performed after gastrectomies for **cancer** have been the subject of controversy.

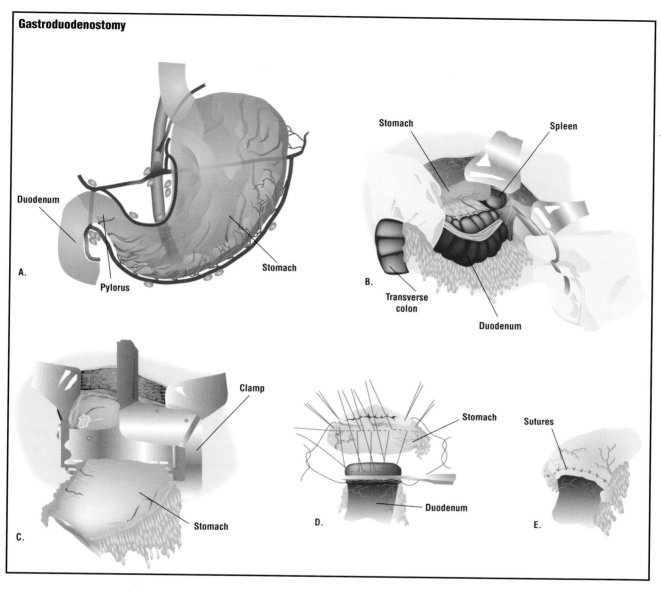

Gastroduodenostomy

A. Duodenum / Pylorus / Stomach

B. Stomach / Spleen / Transverse colon / Duodenum

C. Clamp / Stomach

D. Stomach / Duodenum

E. Sutures

A gastroduodenostomy usually follows a gastrectomy procedure in the treatment of stomach cancer. An abdominal incision exposes the stomach and duodenum (small intestine) (A). The duodenum is freed from connecting materials (B), and is clamped and severed. The stomach is also clamped and severed (C). The remaining stomach is then connected to the duodenum with sutures (D and E). *(Illustration by GGS Information Services. Cengage Learning, Gale.)*

Although there seems to be a definite advantage of performing gastroduodenostomies over gastrojejunostomies, surgeons have become reluctant to perform gastroduodenostomies because of possible obstruction at the site of the surgical connection due to tumor recurrence.

As for gastroduodenostomies specifically performed for the surgical treatment of malignant gastric tumors, they follow the general principles of oncological surgery, aiming for at least 0.8 in (2 cm) of margins around the tumor. However, because gastric adenocarcinomas tend to metastasize quickly and are locally invasive, it is rare to find good surgical candidates. Gastric tumors of such patients are thus only occasionally excised via a gastroduodenostomy procedure.

Gastric ulcers are often treated with a distal gastrectomy, followed by gastroduodenostomy or gastrojejunostomy, which are the preferred procedures because they remove both the ulcer (mostly on the lesser curvature) and the diseased antrum.

KEY TERMS

Adenocarcinoma—The most common form of gastric cancer.

Anastomosis—An opening created by surgical, traumatic, or pathological means between two normally separate spaces or organs.

Barium swallow—An upper gastrointestinal series (barium swallow) is an x-ray test used to define the anatomy of the upper digestive tract; the test involves filling the esophagus, stomach, and small intestines with a white liquid material (barium).

Computed tomography (CT) scan—An imaging technique that creates a series of pictures of areas inside the body, taken from different angles. The pictures are created by a computer linked to an x-ray machine.

Duodenum—The first part of the small intestine that connects the stomach above and the jejunum below.

Endoscopy—The visual inspection of any cavity of the body by means of an endoscope.

Gastrectomy—A surgical procedure in which all or a portion of the stomach is removed.

Gastroduodenostomy—A surgical procedure in which the doctor creates a new connection between the stomach and the duodenum.

Gastrointestinal—Pertaining to or communicating with the stomach and intestine.

Gastrojejunostomy—A surgical procedure where the stomach is surgically connected to the jejunum.

Laparoscopy—The examination of the inside of the abdomen through a lighted tube, sometimes accompanied by surgery.

Lumen—The cavity or channel within a tube or tubular organ.

Small intestine—The small intestine consists of three sections: duodenum, jejunum, and ileum. All are involved in the absorption of nutrients.

Demographics

Stomach cancer was the most common form of cancer in the world in the 1970s and early 1980s. The incidence rates show substantial variations worldwide. Rates are currently highest in Japan and eastern Asia, but other areas of the world have high incidence rates, including eastern Europesan countries and parts of Latin America. Incidence rates are generally lower in western

European countries and the United States. Stomach cancer incidence and mortality rates have been declining for several decades in most areas of the world.

Description

After removing a piece of the stomach, the surgeon reattaches the remainder to the rest of the bowel. The Billroth I gastroduodenostomy specifically joins the upper stomach back to the duodenum.

Typically, the procedure requires ligation (tying) of the right gastric veins and arteries as well as of the blood supply to the duodenum (pancreatico-duodenal vein and artery). The lumen of the duodenum and stomach is occluded at the proposed site of resection (removal). After resection of the diseased tissues, the stomach is closed in two layers, starting at the level of the lesser curvature, leaving an opening close to the diameter of the duodenum. The gastroduodenostomy is performed in a similar fashion as small intestinal end-to-end anastomosis, meaning an opening created between two normally separate spaces or organs. Alternatively, the Billroth I procedure may be performed with stapling equipment (ligation and thoraco-abdominal staplers).

Diagnosis/Preparation

If a gastroduodenostomy is performed for gastric cancer, diagnosis is usually established using the following tests:

- Endoscopy and barium x rays. The advantage of endoscopy is that it allows for direct visualization of abnormalities and directed biopsies. Barium x rays do not facilitate biopsies, but are less invasive and may give information regarding motility.
- Computed tomagraphy (CT) scan. A CT scan of the chest, abdomen, and pelvis is usually obtained to help assess tumor extent, nodal involvement, and metastatic disease.
- Endoscopic ultrasound (EUS). EUS complements information gained by CT. Specifically, the depth of tumor invasion, including invasion of nearby organs, can be assessed more accurately by EUS than by CT.
- Laparoscopy. This technique allows examination of the inside of the abdomen through a lighted tube.

The diagnosis of gastric ulcer is usually made based on a characteristic clinical history. Routine laboratory tests such as a complete blood cell count and iron studies can help detect **anemia**, which is indicative of the condition. By performing high-precision endoscopy and by obtaining multiple mucosal **biopsy** specimens, the diagnosis of gastric ulcer can be confirmed.

Additionally, upper gastrointestinal tract radiography tests are usually performed.

Preparations for the surgery include nasogastric decompression prior to the administration of anesthesia, intravenous or intramuscular administration of **antibiotics**, insertion of intravenous lines for administration of electrolytes, and a supply of compatible blood. Suction provided by placement of a nasogastric tube is necessary if there is any evidence of obstruction. Thorough medical evaluation, including hematological studies, may indicate the need for preoperative transfusions. All patients should be prepared with systemic antibiotics, and there may be some advantage in washing out the abdominal cavity with tetracycline prior to surgery.

Aftercare

After surgery, the patient is brought to the recovery room where vital signs are monitored. Intravenous fluid and electrolyte therapy is continued until oral intake resumes. Small meals of a highly digestible diet are offered every six hours, starting 24 hours after surgery. After a few days, the usual diet is gradually introduced. Medical treatment of associated gastritis may be continued in the immediate postoperative period.

Risks

A gastroduodenostomy has many of the same risks associated with any other major abdominal operation performed under general anesthesia, such as wound problems, difficulty swallowing, infections, **nausea**, and blood clotting.

More specific risks are also associated with a gastroduodenostomy, including:

- Duodenogastric reflux, resulting in persistent vomiting.
- Dumping syndrome, occurring after a meal and characterized by sweating, abdominal pain, vomiting, lightheadedness, and diarrhea.
- Low blood sugar levels (hypoglycemia) after a meal.
- Alkaline reflux gastritis marked by abdominal pain, vomiting of bile, diminished appetite, and iron-deficiency anemia.
- Malabsorption of necessary nutrients, especially iron, in patients who have had all or part of the stomach removed.

Normal results

Results of a gastroduodenostomy are considered normal when the continuity of the gastrointestinal tract is reestablished.

WHO PERFORMS THE PROCEDURE AND WHERE IS IT PERFORMED?

A gastroduodenostomy is performed by a surgeon trained in gastroenterology, the branch of medicine that deals with the diseases of the digestive tract. An anesthesiologist is responsible for administering anesthesia, and the operation is performed in a hospital setting.

QUESTIONS TO ASK THE DOCTOR

- What happens on the day of surgery?
- What type of anesthesia will be used?
- How long will it take to recover from the surgery?
- When can I expect to return to work and/or resume normal activities?
- What are the risks associated with a gastroduodenostomy?
- How many gastroduodenostomies do you perform in a year?
- Will there be a scar?

Morbidity and mortality rates

For gastric obstruction, a gastroduodenostomy is considered the most radical procedure. It is recommended in the most severe cases and has been shown to provide good results in relieving gastric obstruction in most patients. Overall, good to excellent gastroduodenostomy results are reported in 85% of cases of gastric obstruction. In cases of cancer, a median survival time of 72 days has been reported after gastroduodenostomy following the removal of gastric **carcinoma**, although a few patients had extended survival times of three to four years.

Alternatives

In the case of ulcer treatment, the need for a gastroduodenostomy procedure has diminished greatly over the past 20 to 30 years due to the discovery of two new classes of drugs and the presence of the responsible germ (*Helicobacter pylori*) in the stomach. The drugs are the H_2 blockers such as cimetidine and ranitidine and the proton pump inhibitors such as omeprazole; these effectively stop acid production. *H. pylori* can be eliminated from most patients with combination therapy that includes antibiotics and bismuth.

If an individual requires gastrointestinal reconstruction, there is no alternative to a gastroduodenostomy.

Resources

BOOKS

Benirschke, R. *Great Comebacks from Ostomy Surgery.* Rancho Santa Fe, CA: Rolf Benirschke Enterprises Inc, 2002.

Magnusson, B. E. O. *Iron Absorption after Antrectomy with Gastroduodenostomy: Studies on the Absorption from Food and from Iron Salt Using a Double Radio-iron Isotope Technique and Whole-Body Counting.* Copenhagen: Blackwell-Munksgaard, 2000.

PERIODICALS

Kanaya, S., et al. "Delta-shaped Anastomosis in Totally Laparoscopic Billroth I Gastrectomy: New Technique of Intra-Abdominal Gastroduodenostomy." *Journal of the American College of Surgeons* 195 (August 2002): 284–287.

Kim, B. J., and T. O'Connell T. "Gastroduodenostomy after Gastric Resection for Cancer." *American Surgery* 65 (October 1999): 905–907.

Millat, B., A. Fingerhut, and F. Borie. "Surgical Treatment of Complicated Duodenal Ulcers: Controlled Trials." *World Journal of Surgery* 24 (March 2000): 299–306.

Tanigawa, H., H. Uesugi, H. Mitomi, K. Saigenji, and I. Okayasu. "Possible Association of Active Gastritis, Featuring Accelerated Cell Turnover and p53 Overexpression, with Cancer Development at Anastomoses after Gastrojejunostomy. Comparison with Gastroduodenostomy." *American Journal of Clinical Pathology* 114 (September 2000): 354–363.

ORGANIZATIONS

American College of Gastroenterology. 4900-B South 31st St., Arlington, VA 22206. (703) 820-7400. www.acg.gi.org.

American Gastroenterological Association (AGA). 4930 Del Ray Avenue, Bethesda, MD 20814. (301) 654-2055. www.gastro.org.

United Ostomy Association, Inc. (UOA). 19772 MacArthur Blvd., Suite 200, Irvine, CA 92612-2405. (800) 826-0826. http://www.uoa.org.

OTHER

"Gastroduodenostomy After Gastric Resection for Cancer." *Nursing Hands* [cited June 2003] www.nursinghands.com/news/newsstories/1004031.asp.

Monique Laberge, PhD

Gastrointestinal cancers

Definition

Gastrointestinal (GI) cancers include **cancer** of the esophagus, stomach, small intestine, colon, rectum, and anus as well as cancers of the liver, pancreas, gallbladder, and biliary system.

Description

The GI tract, or digestive tract, starts from the oral cavity (mouth) and proceeds to the esophagus, the stomach, the duodenum, the small intestine, the large intestine (colon and rectum), and the anus. It processes all the food consumed. Along the way through the tract, food is digested, nutrients and water are extracted, and waste is eliminated from the body in the form of stool and urine. Cancer can affect any of the gastrointestinal organs. The National Cancer Institute estimates that 25% of all cancers are gastrointestinal, with the majority of these occurring in the colon and rectum (colorectal cancers). The next sites most commonly affected by GI cancers are the

Gastrointestinal cancers

Cancer	Types
Esophageal cancer	Squamous cell carcinoma
	Adenocarcinoma
Stomach cancer	Adenocarcinoma
Liver cancer	Angiosarcoma
	Hepatoblastoma
	Cholangiocarcinoma
	Hepatocellular carcinoma (hepatoma)
Gallbladder cancer	Adenocarcinoma
	Squamous cell carcinoma
	Carcinosarcoma
	Small cell (oat cell) carcinoma
Pancreatic cancer	Adenocarcinoma
	Insulinoma
	Gastrinoma
	Glucagonoma
	Vipoma
	Somatostinoma
	Acinar cell carcinoma
	Cystic tumors
	Papillary tumors
	Pancreatoblastoma
Colorectal cancer	Adenocarcinoma
	Carcinoid tumors
	Gastroinstestinal stromal tumors
	Lymphomas
Anal cancer	Squamous cell carcinoma
	Basal cell carcinoma
	Melanoma
	Adenocarcinoma

(Table by GGS Creative Resources. Cengage Learning, Gale.)

KEY TERMS

Abdomen—A part of the body which lies between the thorax and the pelvis. It contains a cavity (abdominal cavity) which holds organs such as the pancreas, stomach, intestines, liver, gallbladder. It is enclosed by the abdominal muscles and the vertebral column (backbone).

Bile—A greenish-yellow fluid produced by the liver and stored in the gallbladder.

Bile ducts—Passages external to the liver for the transport of bile.

Digestion—The conversion of food in the stomach and in the intestines into substances capable of being absorbed by the blood.

Digestive system—Organs and paths responsible for processing food in the body. These are the mouth, the esophagus, the stomach, the liver, the gallbladder, the pancreas, the small intestine, the colon, and the rectum.

Gastric juice—An acidic secretion of the stomach that breaks down the proteins contained in the ingested food, prior to digestion.

Gland—An organ that produces and releases substances for use in the body, such as fluids or hormones.

Lymph nodes—Small, bean-shaped organs surrounded by a capsule of connective tissue. Also called lymph glands. Lymph nodes are spread out along lymphatic vessels and store special cells (lymphocytes), which filter the lymphatic fluid (lymph).

Lymphatic system—The tissues and organs that produce, store, and carry white blood cells that fight infection. It includes the bone marrow, spleen, thymus, and lymph nodes as well as a network of thin vessels (lymphatic vessels) that carry lymph and white blood cells into all the tissues of the body.

Metastasis—The transfer of cancer from one location or organ to another one not directly related to it.

Ovary—One of two small oval-shaped organs located on either side of the uterus. They are female reproductive glands in which the ova (eggs) are formed.

Small intestine—The part of the digestive tract located between the stomach and the large intestine.

Squamous cells—Flat, thin cells, such as found on the outer layer of the skin.

Stage—The extent to which a cancer has spread from its original site to other parts of the body. A Stage 1 cancer is less advanced than a Stage 4 cancer.

---

pancreas, stomach, liver, and esophagus. A brief overview of GI cancers follows; the reader should refer to other specific encyclopedia entries shown in bold for more comprehensive information on these cancers and their treatment. The reader should also note that the overview below does not discuss oral cavity cancers. Those cancers are also discussed in individual entries.

Types of cancers

Esophageal cancer

The esophagus is a muscular, hollow tube that carries food from the oropharynx (area behind mouth and soft palate) to the stomach. It consists of several layers. **Esophageal cancer** usually develops in the inner layer cells and grows outward. There are two major types of esophageal cancer. The first occurs in the cells found in the lining of the esophagus (squamous cells), and the cancer is called squamous cell **carcinoma**. It can develop anywhere along the entire length of the esophagus and represents approximately half of all reported esophageal cancers. The second type of cancer known to occur in the esophagus is an

adenocarcinoma, which is cancer of the glandular cells that line the inside of organs. Adenocarcinoma occurs near the stomach entrance and may be associated with a condition known as **Barrett's esophagus**. This is a disorder in which the lining of the esophagus undergoes cellular changes as a result of chronic irritation and inflammation resulting from a backwash of acidic stomach gastric juices. Esophageal adenocarcinomas cannot develop unless squamous cells have been transformed by the acid reflux of the stomach juices. The American Cancer Society (ACS) predicted the occurrence of approximately 16,470 new cases of esophageal cancer in 2009 that will result in some 4,530 deaths in the United States.

Stomach cancer

Stomach cancer is also called gastric cancer. The stomach is located in the upper abdomen under the ribs. It is the most expandable organ of the digestive system. Food reaches the stomach from the esophagus and is broken down by gastric juices secreted by the stomach. After leaving the stomach, partially broken down food passes into the small intestine and afterwards into the colon (first part of the large intestine). In cancer of the stomach, cancerous cells are found in the tissues of the stomach and this cancer can develop anywhere in the organ. It may grow along the stomach wall into other organs such as the esophagus or small intestine. Or it may go through the stomach wall and invade the nearby lymph nodes or organs such as the liver, pancreas, and colon. And it may also spread to more distant organs, such as the lungs, the lymph nodes located above the collar bone, and the ovaries. The major type of stomach cancer is adenocarcinoma (90%). Approximately 1,130 new cases of stomach cancer will be diagnosed in the United States in 2009. The number of cases, as well as the death rate, have declined significantly over the past several decades, but it is still the seventh leading cause of cancer deaths. A cure is possible if the cancer is found before spreading to other organs. Unfortunately, the early symptoms are not very noticeable, and by the time stomach cancer is diagnosed, it has in many cases already metastasized.

Liver cancer

The liver is one of the largest organs in the body. In normal adults, it weighs about three pounds and is located in the upper right side of the abdomen, under the right lung and rib cage. It plays a major role in digestion, in the transformation of food into energy and in filtering and storing blood. It is also responsible for processing nutrients and drugs, producing bile, controlling the level of glucose (sugar) in the blood, detoxifying blood, and regulating blood clotting. In cancer of the liver, cancerous cells are found in the tissues of the liver. Primary **liver cancer** is cancer that starts in the liver. As such, it is different from cancer that starts somewhere else and spreads to the liver. Liver cancer is a rare form of GI cancer in the United States with only about 22,620 new cases diagnosed in 2009. Primary cancers of the liver and of the bile ducts are far more common in Africa and Asia than in America, where they only represent 1.5% of all cancer cases. The highest occurrence rate is in Vietnamese men (41.8 per 100,000), probably a result of the high incidence of viral hepatitis infections in their country. Asian-American groups also have higher liver cancer incidence rates than the Caucasian population. Liver cancer mortality rates calculated for populations for which statistics are available are highest in China.

There are four main types of liver cancer: angiosarcoma, a rare type of cancer that starts in the blood vessels of the liver; hepatoblastoma, another rare type of liver cancer occurring chiefly in young children; cholangiocarcinoma, which starts in the bile ducts

and accounts for approximately 13% of liver cancers; and finally, hepatocellular carcinoma, also known as hepatoma. The most common liver cancer is hepatocellular carcinoma which accounts for approximately 84% of liver cancers. As is the case with stomach cancer, liver cancer is hard to diagnose early because there are seldom any clear-cut symptoms.

However, some diseases have been identified as liable to increase a person's risk of getting liver cancer. They include: hepatitis B, hepatitis C, cirrhosis of the liver, exposure to certain chemicals such as aflatoxin (a substance made by a fungus in tropical regions and that can infect wheat, peanuts, soybeans, corn, and rice), vinyl chloride, thorium dioxide, anabolic steroids, arsenic, and birth control pills (of a type no longer prescribed).

Gallbladder cancer

The gallbladder is a pear-shaped organ located just under the liver in the upper abdomen. Its role in digestion is to store and release the bile produced by the liver into the stomach to help break down fat. In **gallbladder cancer**, the cancer cells develop in the tissues of the gallbladder. Several types of cancer can occur, such as adenocarcinoma, squamous cell carcinoma, carcinosarcoma and small cell (oat cell) carcinoma, all of them uncommon. Approximately 6,000 to 7,000 new cases are diagnosed per year in the U. S., affecting women twice as often as men and occurring mostly in the elderly.

Pancreatic cancer

The pancreas is a tongue-shaped glandular organ lying below and behind the stomach. It consists of two areas, the exocrine and endocrine regions. The endocrine pancreas secretes the hormones insulin and glucagon, which regulate blood sugar. The exocrine pancreas secretes pancreatic juice into the small intestine. The juice contains enzymes that break down fats and proteins so that the body can use them. In **pancreatic cancer**, the cancer can develop either in the cells that secrete the pancreatic juice (**exocrine pancreatic cancer**) or in the cells that release the hormones (**endocrine pancreatic cancer**). Exocrine pancreatic cancer is much more common than endocrine. Several types can develop, the majority being various types of carcinomas. The American Cancer Society predicted that, in 2009, about 42,470 people in the U. S. will be diagnosed with pancreatic cancer. Pancreatic cancer is the fourth leading cause of cancer death in men and women. Because the pancreas is located deep inside the body, it cannot be felt during a routine physical exam, and no tests are presently available to allow early detection.

Colorectal cancers

The colon, the first part of the large intestine, extends from the end of the small intestine to the rectum. The colon has four major divisions. The first is called the ascending colon, it starts where the small intestine attaches and extends upward on the right side of the abdomen. The second part is the transverse colon and it extends across the body to the left side where it joins the third section, called the descending colon, which continues downward on the left side. The fourth part of the colon is the sigmoid colon, which joins the rectum. The rectum joins the anus, where stool passes out of the body.

Each of the divisions of the colon and rectum has several layers of tissue. Colorectal cancers usually start in the innermost layer and can grow through some or all of the other layers. Colorectal cancers are common, and occur more frequently in people over the age of 50. The ACS estimated that in 2001 in the U. S., about 46,000 new cases of **colon cancer** will be diagnosed in men, and about 52,000 cases in women. For rectal cancers, the ACS estimates that about 21,000 men and 16,000 women will be diagnosed in 2001. The number of new colorectal cancer cases and reported deaths have declined in recent years due to improved screening and diagnostic methods. Colorectal cancers are highly treatable when detected early, but the symptoms are often not obvious in early stages.

Over 95% of colorectal cancers are adenocarcinomas. Other, less common types of colorectal cancers are: carcinoid tumors, which develop from the hormone-producing cells of the intestine, gastrointestinal stromal tumors, which start in the connective tissue and muscle layers located in the wall of the colon and rectum, and lymphomas, which are cancers of the immune system cells that usually occur in the lymph nodes but may also start in the colon.

Anal cancer

The anus has several types of tissues. Each type of tissue also contains several types of cells and cancer can develop in each of these kinds of tissues. Approximately half are squamous cell carcinomas. This type of cancer is found in the surface cells that line the anus and most of the anal canal. Another 15% of anal cancers consist of adenocarcinomas and usually start in glands found in the anus area. The remaining anal cancers are accounted for by basal cell carcinomas and malignant melanomas. **Anal cancer** is usually diagnosed in people

over 50. People who have the human papillomavirus (HPV) also have a greater chance of developing anal cancer as well as men who practice anal sex. How treatable the cancer is depends partly on where it starts.

See also Bile duct cancer; Carcinoid tumors, gastrointestinal; Human papilloma virus; Laryngeal cancer; Liver cancer, primary; Melanoma; Pancreatic cancer, endocrine; Pancreatic cancer, exocrine; Small intestinal cancer; Upper gastrointestinal endoscopy.

Resources

BOOKS

Daly, J. *Management of Upper Gastrointestinal Cancer.* St. Louis: W. B. Saunders, 1999.

Feczko, P. *Gastrointestinal Imaging: Case Review.* New York: Mosby-Yearbook Inc., 2000.

PERIODICALS

Catalano, V., A. M. Baldelli, P. Giordani, and S. Cascinu. "Molecular markers predictive of response to chemotherapy in gastrointestinal tumors." *Critical Reviews of Oncology and Hematology* 38 (May 2001): 93-104.

Lunn, J. A., and W. M. Weinstein. "Gastric biopsy." *Gastrointestinal Endoscopic Clinicology of North America* 10 (October 2000): 723-38.

Nishida, T., and S. Hirota. "Biological and Clinical Review of Stromal Tumors in the Gastrointestinal Tract." *Histology and Histopathology* 15 (October 2000): 1293-301.

Royce, M. E., P. M. Hoff, and R. Pazdur. "Progress in Colorectal Cancer Chemotherapy: How Far Have We Come, How Far to Go?" *Drugs and Aging* 17 (September 2000): 201-16.

Zock, P. L. "Dietary fats and cancer." *Current Opinions in Lipidology* 12 (February 2001): 5-10.

OTHER

University of Michigan Gastrointestinal Cancer Clinic Website: http://www.cancer.med.umich.edu/clinic/giclinic.htm.

ORGANIZATIONS

American Cancer Society (National Headquarters). 1599 Clifton Road, N.E., Atlanta, GA 30329.(800) 227-2345. Website: http://www.cancer.org.

Cancer Research Institute (National Headquarters). 681 Fifth Avenue, New York, NY 10022. (800)992-2623. Website: http:://www.cancerresearch.org.

National Cancer Institute's Cancer Information Service: 1-800-4-CANCER.

Monique Laberge, Ph.D.

G-CSF *see* **Filgrastim**

Gefitinib

Definition

Gefitinib, which is also known as Iressa, is an anticancer drug used to inhibit the growth of lung **cancer** cells and reduce the size of a cancerous tumor.

Purpose

Gefitinib is used as a single agent for the treatment of advanced **non-small cell lung cancer** that has advanced or failed to respond to other kinds of treatment. It is not suitable for use as an initial treatment, but may help to shrink tumors by as much as 10% when used as a third-line therapy in patients with advanced non-small lung cancer.

Description

In May 2003, gefitinib was approved for use in the United States under the U. S. Food and Drug Administration's (FDA) accelerated approval program. Generally speaking, before the FDA approves a drug for use, a great deal of data regarding the safety, efficacy, and quality of the drug is usually compiled. In fact, it is typical for the FDA to review thousands of pages of data about a medicine under consideration for approval. One of the reasons for this is the FDA's extremely strict approval process, an approval process that is, in fact, among the strictest in the world. FDA approval means that the regulators have decided that the new drug's potential benefits outweigh its risks. When a drug is approved under the accelerated program it is done so because, as Mark B. McClellan, M.D. and FDA Commissioner states, the "FDA believes it is critical for patients to have many safe and effective treatment options available to them in their battles against disease."

In a 2004 article published in the *Pfizer Journal* entitled, "Enhancing Pharmaceutical Safety," Dr. Stephanie Crawford, a member of the FDA's Drug Safety and Risk Management Advisory Committee, said the following: "Approval of a drug as safe is not a blanket statement that it is without risk. It means that the risk is acceptable." Drawing on information provided by the FDA, it was further stated in the article that "the decision to approval a medicine involves consideration of the disease: a product to treat a life threatening condition may be approved even if it presents more of a certain risk, because its potential benefits are so great." In other words, the approval of a valuable cancer drug associated with an adverse side effect might be seen as more acceptable than the approval

of an allergy medicine with the same side effect. As was further stated in the article, "The value of the medicine has to be seen in the context of its benefits, its known adverse effects, the severity and reversibility of these effects, and the availability of other medications for that person."

As the FDA cautiously stated in 2003, "The mechanism by which Iressa [gefitinib] exerts its clinical benefit is not fully understood. However, Iressa was developed to block growth stimulatory signals in cancer cells. These signals are mediated in part by enzymes called tyrosine kinases. Iressa blocks several of these tyrosine kinases, including the one associated with the Epidermal Growth Factor Receptor (EGFR)." Research has shown that the EGFR is sometimes found in abundance on the surface of cancer cells, causing them to divide excessively. Therefore, by blocking EGFR, it is thought that tumor growth can be thwarted.

However, gefitinib was approved by the FDA, as all drugs approved under the accelerated program, with the condition that further studies would be conducted to measure the drug's clinical benefit. According to the FDA, the drug's sponsor would be required to conduct three studies. One would evaluate gefitinib as a third-line therapy drug and evaluate if it prolonged survival as compared to the best supportive care available. Another study would compare gefitinib to **docetaxel**, which is another approved **chemotherapy** drug. And the third trial would analysis whether gefitinib is effective in reducing cancer symptoms in patients with lung cancer that are resistant to all available chemotherapy treatments. As Dr. McClellan indicated, "the studies are needed to confirm the clinical benefit, understand better which patients benefit, and evaluate long-term safety."

However, on March 4, 2005, Public Citizen in a letter to the FDA petitioned for gefitinib's removal from the market, stating that the study conducted to prove gefitinib's efficacy had failed and that the drug had already been removed from the market in Europe. Furthermore, the use of the drug has been tied to deaths in Japan. Therefore, it is possible that before long the FDA will reclassify gefitinib as an experimental drug.

Recommended dosage

Gefitinib is available in 250 mg tablets. Dosage levels may vary, depending on the needs of the patient. However, patients generally take one 250 mg tablet a day. The tablets should not be crushed or broken and the patient should be certain to drink plenty of fluids throughout the day.

Precautions

Women who are pregnant or may become pregnant should not use gefitinib. Patients receiving gefitinib should not breast-feed their babies during the treatment cycle and for a substantial time after the treatment.

Side effects

This drug has been associated with high toxicity in Japan. There have been reports indicating that using gefitinib caused severe side effects, such as inflammation of the lungs (interstitial **pneumonia**) and difficulty in breathing. Therefore, patients should report any side effects, whether they seem severe or not, to their physician. The most common side effects associated with taking 250 mg a day were:

- skin rash
- diarrhea
- acne
- dry skin
- nausea and vomiting

As reported in *Applied Therapeutics: The Clinical Use of Drugs* the most common side effects were skin related, which went away after the drug was discontinued. The symptoms were managed through the use of steroid creams, antihistamines, or topical or systemic **antibiotics**.

Interactions

Gefitinib increases the effect of metoprolol and may increase the risk of bleeding in patients taking **warfarin**. The following drugs may decrease gefitinib's effectiveness:

- cimetidine
- phenytoin
- rifampin
- ranitidine
- sodium bicarbonate

Resources

BOOKS

Hodgson, B. B., Kizior, R. J., Foley, M., et al. *Mosby's 2005 Drug Consultant for Nurses.* St. Louis, MO: Mosby, 2005.

Koda-Kimbl, M. A., Young, L. Y., Kradjan, W. A., Guglielmo, B. J., editors. *Applied Therapeutics: The Clinical Use of Drugs.* 10th ed. Baltimore, MD: Lippencott Williams & Wilkins, 2005.

PERIODICALS

Giorgianni, S. J., editor. "Enhancing pharmaceutical safety." *The Pfizer Journal* 8 (2004): 4–13.

OTHER

Public Citizen "Cancer Drug Should Not Be Approved, Public Citizen Tells FDA." *Public Citizen* 1 May 2003 Public Citizen. 15 April. 2005 http://www.citizen.org/pressroom/.

U.S. Food and Drug Administration "Approvals of FDA-regulated products." *U.S. Food and Drug Administration* Mar. 2004. U.S. Food and Drug Administration. 25 Mar. 2005 http://www.fda.gov/.

U.S. Food and Drug Administration " FDA approves new type of drug for lung cancer." *U.S. Food and Drug Administration* May 2003. U.S. Food and Drug Administration. 25 Mar. 2005 http://www.fda.gov/.

ORGANIZATIONS

Public Citizen. 1600 20th Street, NW, Washington, DC 20009. 1-202-588-1000. http://www.citizen.org/about/.

Lee Ann Paradise

Gemcitabine

Definition

Gemcitabine is a drug that is used to treat advanced stages of pancreatic, lung, and other cancers. Its brand name is Gemzar.

Purpose

Gemcitabine is used to treat **pancreatic cancer**, particularly when it has metastasized, or spread to other parts of the body (Stage IVB). In combination with the drug **cisplatin**, gemcitabine is the first-line treatment for inoperable, metastasized **non-small cell lung cancer**. Sometimes it is used to treat cancers of the bladder or breast, or epithelial **ovarian cancer**.

Description

Gemcitabine is a relatively new anticancer drug. It is a type of medicine called a pyrimidine antimetabolite

KEY TERMS

Deoxycytidine—Component of DNA, the genetic material of a cell, that is similar in structure to gemcitabine.

Metastasis—Spread of cancer from its point of origin to other parts of the body.

Platelet—Blood component that aids in clotting.

Pyrimidine—Class of molecules that includes gemcitabine and deoxycytidine.

Vasculitis—Inflammation of a blood or lymph vessel.

because it interferes with the metabolism and growth of cells. It does this by replacing the pyrimidine deoxycytidine in DNA, thereby preventing the DNA from being manufactured or repaired. As a result, cells cannot reproduce and eventually die.

Gemcitabine was approved by the U.S. Food and Drug Administration (FDA) to treat pancreatic **cancer** in 1998 and non-small cell lung cancer in 2002. Gemzar may relieve pain and other symptoms of advanced pancreatic cancer and increase survival time by several weeks to two months. Clinical studies of pancreatic cancer are comparing the effectiveness of combination treatments using gemcitabine with **fluorouracil** (5-FU), cisplatin, **streptozocin**, or **radiation therapy**. Gemcitabine has activity against metastatic **bladder cancer** and recurrent ovarian cancer, and further **clinical trials** are underway. Gemcitabine is being evaluated for its effectiveness in the treatment of uterine, stomach, laryngeal and hypopharyngeal, and colon and rectal cancers.

Recommended dosage

Gemcitabine is administered by injection over a period of 30 minutes. The dosage and number of administrations depend on a variety of factors, including the type of cancer, body size, the patient's sex, and other concurrent treatments.

Precautions

Gemcitabine may temporarily reduce the number of white blood cells, particularly during the first 10–14 days after administration. A low white blood cell count reduces the body's ability to fight **infection**. Thus, it is very important to avoid exposure to infections and to receive prompt medical treatment. Immunizations (vaccinations) should be avoided during or after treatment with gemcitabine. It also is important to avoid contact with individuals who have recently taken an oral polio vaccine. Treatment with gemcitabine may cause chicken pox or shingles (**herpes zoster**) to become very severe and spread to other parts of the body.

Gemcitabine also may lower the blood platelet count. Platelets are necessary for normal blood clotting. The risk of bleeding may be reduced by using caution when cleaning teeth, avoiding dental work, and avoiding cuts, bruises, or other injuries.

Gemcitabine can cause birth defects and fetal death in animals. Therefore, this drug should not be taken by pregnant women or by either the man or woman at the time of conception. Women usually are advised against breastfeeding while taking this drug.

Side effects

Gemcitabine affects normal cells as well as cancer cells, resulting in various side effects. The most common side effects are related to reduction in red and white blood cells and blood platelets. These side effects may include symptoms of infection or unusual bleeding or bruising. Older patients are more likely to suffer from low blood cell counts after treatment.

Flu-like symptoms are common following the first treatment with gemcitabine. Other common side effects of gemcitabine may include:

- nausea
- vomiting
- chills and fever
- constipation
- diarrhea
- loss of appetite (anorexia)
- headache
- muscle pain
- weakness or fatigue
- shortness of breath
- blood in urine or stools
- skin rash
- swelling of the hands, feet, legs, or face
- insomnia

Less common side effects of gemcitabine may include:

- cough or hoarseness
- lower back or side pain
- painful or difficult urination
- chest, arm, or back pain
- difficulty with speech
- fast or irregular heartbeat

- high blood pressure
- pain or redness at the site of injection
- numbness or tingling in hands or feet
- sores or white spots on lips and in mouth
- hair loss (alopecia)
- itching

Some of these side effects may occur or continue after treatment with gemcitabine has ended. **Itching**, hives, swelling, or a skin rash, particularly if accompanied by breathing problems, may indicate an allergic reaction to gemcitabine. Some researchers have coined the term gemcitabine-induced severe pulmonary toxicity, or GISPT, to describe an inflammatory reaction in the lungs following treatment with gemcitabine. The incidence of GISPT is estimated to range between 0.5% and 5% of patients receiving the drug.

Additional side effects of gemcitabine may be symptoms associated with liver or kidney malfunction. Furthermore, kidney or liver disease may cause gemcitabine to be removed from the body at a slower rate, thus increasing the effects of the drug.

Another potentially fatal side effect of gemcitabine is vasculitis, or inflammation of blood or lymph vessels. A group of physicians in Iowa reported on two cases of women who died of necrotizing enterocolitis resulting from vasculitis associated with gemcitabine treatment for ovarian cancer. A case of vasculitis in a male patient treated with gemcitabine for bladder cancer was reported in Turkey.

Interactions

Previous treatment with radiation or other anti-cancer drugs can increase the risk of very low blood counts with gemcitabine. Serious problems may develop in areas previously treated with radiation.

Drugs that may interact with gemcitabine, or that may increase the risk of infections while being treated with gemcitabine, include live **vaccines** and **warfarin**. Because some other medications have a tendency to interact with gemcitabine, patients should alert their doctor to any drugs they are taking.

It is also important not to take any medicines containing aspirin during treatment with gemcitabine, since aspirin can increase the chances of excessive bleeding.

Resources

BOOKS

Beers, Mark H., MD, and Robert Berkow, MD, editors. "Pancreatic Tumors." Section 3, Chapter 34 In *The Merck Manual of Diagnosis and Therapy*. Whitehouse Station, NJ: Merck Research Laboratories, 2007.

Karch, A. M. *Lippincott's Nursing Drug Guide*. Springhouse, PA: Lippincott Williams & Wilkins, 2003.

PERIODICALS

Barlesi, F., P. Villani, C. Doddoli, et al. "Gemcitabine-Induced Severe Pulmonary Toxicity." *Fundamental and Clinical Pharmacology* 18 (February 2004): 85–91.

Birlik, M., S. Akar, E. Tuzel, et al. "Gemcitabine-Induced Vasculitis in Advanced Transitional Cell Carcinoma of the Bladder." *Journal of Cancer Research and Clinical Oncology* 130 (February 2004): 122–125.

Geisler, J. P., D. F. Schraith, K. J. Manahan, and J. I. Sorosky. "Gemcitabine Associated Vasculitis Leading to Necrotizing Enterocolitis and Death in Women Undergoing Primary Treatment for Epithelial Ovarian/Peritoneal Cancer." *Gynecologic Oncology* 92 (February 2004): 705–707.

Li, D., K. Xie, R. Wolff, and J. L. Abbruzzese. "Pancreatic Cancer." *Lancet* 363 (March 27, 2004): 1049–1057.

ORGANIZATIONS

American Society of Health-System Pharmacists (ASHP). 7272 Wisconsin Avenue, Bethesda, MD 20814. (301) 657-3000. www.ashp.org.

United States Food and Drug Administration (FDA). 5600 Fishers Lane, Rockville, MD 20857-0001. (888) INFO-FDA. www.fda.gov.

Margaret Alic, Ph.D.
Rebecca J. Frey, PhD

Gemtuzumab

Definition

Gemtuzumab ozogamicin is a humanized monoclonal antibody produced by recombinant DNA technology that binds specifically to CD33, a protein that is found on the cell surface of most leukemic blasts, the abnormal, cancerous cells in acute myeloid leukemia (also known as acute myelocytic leukemia, or AML). It is marketed in the United States under the brand name Mylotarg.

Purpose

Gemtuzumab is a monoclonal antibody used to treat AML that is characterized by expression of the CD33 protein on the cancerous cells, called leukemic blasts. The CD33 protein is found on the surface of the leukemic blasts of about 80% of AML patients. After the gemtuzumab antibody is produced in the laboratory, a chemical reaction is used to link it to an antitumor drug called calicheamicin. About half of the antibody succeeds in acquiring the antitumor drug.

Gemtuzumab

KEY TERMS

Antibody—A protective protein made by the immune system in response to an antigen, also called an immunoglobulin.

Blasts—A type of immature cell that lacks some of the outward characteristics of the mature cell. In AML, the cancerous cells are leukemic blasts.

Calicheamicin—An anti-tumor drug that binds to DNA within the tumor cells, causing breaks in the strands and killing the cell.

IgG—Immunoglobulin type gamma, the most common type found in the blood and tissue fluids.

Humanization—Fusing the constant and variable framework region of one or more human immunoglobulins with the binding region of an animal immunoglobulin, done to reduce human reaction against the fusion antibody.

Monoclonal—Genetically engineered antibodies specific for one antigen.

Myelosuppression—Reduction in the number of the cells of the bone marrow, which leads to reduction of many other circulating blood cells that are produced by the marrow.

When the antibody-calicheamicin molecule binds to the cancerous cells, both the antibody and the drug are taken into the cell. There the drug binds to the cell's genetic material (deoxyribose nucleic acid or DNA) inducing breaks in the molecule and killing it. Because the antibody carries and delivers the toxic drug to the leukemic blasts targets, gemtuzumab treatment is called antibody-targeted **chemotherapy**.

Gemtuzumab can also be used to induce remission (remove cancerous cells) in AML patients to prepare them for stem-cell transplantation. It is indicated for refractory AML (AML that does not readily yield to treatment). The use of antibody-targeted chemotherapy has been shown to have fewer side effects than traditional chemotherapy courses and does improve the disease-free survival time after transplantation.

Description

Gemtuzumab is a genetically engineered monoclonal antibody linked to an antitumor antibiotic. It was approved by the FDA in 2000 as a method of treating relapsed AML in older patients (over 60 years of age) that are not candidates for other cytotoxic chemotherapy. About 75% of all patients with

AML experience a relapse after initial treatment. In **clinical trials** focusing on the treatment of older patients with relapsed AML, gemtuzumab had an overall response rate of 30%, with 16% having a complete response.

Most of the gemtuzumab sequence is derived from human sequences, while about 2% are from mice. The human sequences were derived from the constant domains of human IgG4 (called "constant" because it is essentially the same for all IgG antibodies) and the variable framework regions of a human antibody. These areas do not bind to the CD33 protein. Using human sequences in this part of the antibody helps to reduce patient **immune response** to the antibody itself and is called humanization. The actual binding site of gemtuzumab to the CD33 protein is from a mouse anti-CD33 antibody. The antibiotic antitumor drug calcheamicin is linked to the antibody in a way that does not interfere with the ability of the antibody to bind CD33.

Gemtuzumab is not currently approved for use in combination with other chemotherapy drugs or treatments. However, clinical trials that combine the drug with **cytarabine**, **fludarabine**, total-body irradiation, as well as other **cancer** treatments, are ongoing.

Recommended dosage

Gemtuzumab is administered intravenously. In the pivotal clinical trial, the drug was given at a dose of 9 mg/m^2 for two doses that were fourteen days apart.

Precautions

Extreme caution should be used when using gemtuzumab to treat patients with existent liver problems. Animal studies showed that the drug can cause significant harm to the development of a fetus, so it is likely the drug should not be used during pregnancy, and women of childbearing age should avoid pregnancy while on the drug. Because of the adverse effects of calcheamicin on DNA, the drug greatly reduced fertility in animal studies for males, but not females.

Side effects

A severe side effect of gemtuzumab treatment is a depletion of various types of cells in the bone marrow, including those that make white and red blood cells, a condition known as **myelosuppression**. Because CD33 is expressed on a patient's normal bone marrow cells, as well as on the surface of the abnormal leukemic blasts, the treatment eliminates both normal and cancerous cells. This results in severe reduction of the circulating blood cells normally produced by the bone marrow, including red blood cells (**anemia**), white blood cells (**neutropenia**), and clotting cells (**thrombocytopenia**). These conditions are treated with blood transfusions. However, the population of all these cells will rebound after clearance of gemtuzumab because the precursor to cells of the bone marrow, called pluripotent hematopoietic stem cells, do not express CD33 and will restore the various cell populations.

Gemtuzumab can produce a postinfusion symptom complex of **fever** and chills, and less commonly, low blood pressure and labored breathing during the first 24 hours after administration. Some patients developed severe liver function abnormalities, which were generally transient and reversible. The most common side effects were fever, chills, **nausea**, **vomiting**, thrombocytopenia, neutropenia, asthenia (loss of strength or energy), **diarrhea**, abdominal pain, headache, and **stomatitis** (inflammation of the lining of the mouth).

Interactions

There have been no formal drug interaction studies done for gemtuzumab.

See also Monoclonal antibodies.

Michelle Johnson, M.S., J.D.

Genetics of cancer *see* **Cancer genetics**

Genetic testing

Definition

Genetic testing is a process which involves examining individuals' genetic material for the presence of a change that indicates why they may have developed a disease or disorder. Genetic testing may also tell patients if they are at increased risk for developing a disease such as **cancer** in the future, but currently do not have any symptoms of that particular disease.

Description

Genetic testing is usually done by taking a sample of a person's blood. The changes in the genetic material that can be detected by this testing vary in size. Sometimes parts or even entire chromosomes may be altered or missing completely. Other times, a mutation is present on a gene that causes it to malfunction. One type of mutation is known as a hereditary mutation. Hereditary mutations may also be called germline mutations

Researcher examining the genetic code of a sequenced sample of neuroblastoma DNA. *(Copyright Colin Cuthbert, Science Source, Photo Researchers, Inc. Reproduced by permission.)*

because they are found in all the cells of a person's body, including the reproductive or germ cells, the sperm for a male and the egg for a female. This is why hereditary mutations can be inherited, or passed from a parent to a child. Genetic testing often looks for the presence or absence of these types of mutations in genes.

Genes and cancer

Cancer is defined as one cell that grows out of control and subsequently invades nearby cells and tissue. There are several steps involved in the process that causes a normal cell to become malignant (cancerous). It is believed that different genes play a role in this specialized process. Oncogenes typically promote or encourage cell growth. However, if they are overexpressed or mutated, they may cause cancer to arise. Tumor-suppressor genes, when working properly, prevent cells from growing too quickly or out of control. They are often compared to brakes in a car. If these genes cannot perform their function because of the presence of a mutation, cells may grow out of control and become cancerous. Finally, cancer may also be caused by faulty DNA repair genes. These genes usually correct the common mistakes that are made by the body as the DNA copies itself, a normally occurring process. However, if these genes can't correct mistakes, the mistakes may accumulate and lead to cancer.

KEY TERMS

Cancer—The process by which cells grow out of control and subsequently invade nearby cells and tissue.

Cancer susceptibility gene—The type of genes involved in cancer. If a mutation is identified in this type of gene it does not reveal whether or not a person has cancer, but rather whether an individual has an increased risk (is susceptible) to develop cancer (or develop cancer again) in the future.

Colonoscopy—A screening test performed with a tube called a colonoscope that allows a doctor to view a patient's entire colon and rectum.

Chromosome—Structures found in the center of a human cell on which genes are located.

DNA repair genes—A type of gene that usually corrects the common mistakes that are made by the body as DNA copies itself. If these genes are mutated and cannot correct these mistakes they may accumulate and lead to cancer.

Gene—Packages of DNA that control the growth, development and normal function of the body.

Genetic counselor—A specially trained health care provider who helps individuals understand if a disease (such as cancer)is running in their family and their risk for inheriting this disease. Genetic counselors also discuss the benefits, risks and limitations of genetic testing with patients.

Hepatoblastoma—A cancerous tumor of the liver. Individuals with FAP have an increased risk for developing this type of tumor at a young age.

Mammogram—A screening test that uses X-rays to look at a woman's breasts for any abnormalities, such as cancer.

Mutation—An alteration in the number or order of the DNA sequence of a gene.

Oncogene—Genes that typically promote cell growth. If mutated, they may encourage cancer to develop.

Pedigree—A family tree. Often used by a genetic counselor to determine if a disease may be passed from a parent to a child.

Penetrance—The likelihood that a person will develop a disease (such as cancer), if they have a mutation in a gene that increases their risk for developing that disorder.

Polyp—A growth that may develop in the colon. These growths may be benign or cancerous.

Prophylactic surgery—The preventive removal of an organ or tissue before a disease such as cancer develops.

Sequencing—A method of performing genetic testing where the chemical order of a patient's DNA is compared to that of normal DNA.

Sigmoidoscopy—A screening test performed with a flexible scope called a sigmoidoscope, that allows a doctor to view a limited portion of a patient's colon or rectum for the presence of polyps.

Tumor suppressor gene—Genes that typically prevent cells from growing out of control and forming tumors that may be cancerous.

It is very important to remember that while all cancer is genetic, or caused by changes in genes, just a small amount of cancer is hereditary, or passed from parent to child. It is thought that only about 5-10% of cancer falls into this category. Therefore, the majority of cancer is not hereditary. Most cancer is due to other causes, such as environmental exposures. Usually it is very difficult to determine the exact cause of cancer that is not known to be the result of an altered gene.

Identifying at-risk individuals and families for hereditary cancer

Although scientists have identified genetic tests for common cancers, like breast and **colon cancer**, genetic testing is not an option that should be offered to all people with cancer, or even to those who may have cancer in their family. This is primarily due to the fact that most cancer does not run in families. Therefore, genetic testing will not be helpful for many people. In order to determine those who may benefit from undergoing genetic testing for cancer, health care providers need to be aware of certain aspects of an individual's personal and family history of cancer.

A person who is thinking about having a genetic test for cancer often meets with a genetic counselor, a specially trained health care provider. When a patient meets with a genetic counselor, the counselor will ask the patient about their personal and family history of cancer. The counselor will also draw a very detailed family tree, also known as a pedigree. The counselor

QUESTIONS TO ASK THE DOCTOR OR A GENETIC COUNSELOR

- What is the likelihood that the cancer in my family is due to a mutation in a cancer susceptibility gene?
- If the cancer in my family is hereditary, what is the chance that I carry a mutation in a cancer susceptibility gene?
- What are the benefits, limitations and risks of undergoing genetic testing?
- What is the cost of genetic testing and how long will it take to obtain results?
- If I undergo genetic testing, will my insurance company pay for testing? If so, will I want to share my results with them?
- What does a positive test result mean for me?
- What does a negative test result mean for me?
- If I test positive for a mutation in a cancer susceptibility gene, what are the best options available for screening and prevention? What research studies may I be eligible to participate in?
- What legislation is in effect to protect me against discrimination by my insurer or employer?

will then examine the family tree to determine if there are certain "clues" that the cancer may be hereditary.

The clues that may be observed in a family tree are listed below, with **breast cancer** used as an example.

- Multiple relatives in more than one generation with the same type of cancer, or related cancers. For example, a grandmother, mother and daughter with breast cancer. Or, relatives with both breast and ovarian cancer.
- Cancer occurring in the family at younger ages than is typically observed in the general population. For example, breast cancer usually occurs in women as they get older, most commonly in their 60's to 70's. However, in families that may have an alteration in a gene increasing their risk for developing breast cancer, the disease may occur in women at much younger ages.
- Cancer that occurs in paired organs. For example, breast cancer that occurs in both of a woman's breasts. This is also called bilateral breast cancer.
- Development of more than one type of related cancer in the same person within a family. For example, a female relative with both breast and ovarian cancer diagnosed at young ages.

- Specific ethnic background. Mutations in certain cancer susceptibility genes may be more likely to occur in individuals of specific ethnic backgrounds. For this reason, it is very important that a complete family tree includes the country where a person's relatives originally lived.

If a genetic counselor or other health care provider observes one or more of the above features in an individual's family tree, he or she may talk about the option of genetic testing with the patient. In the case of cancer genetic testing, it is only offered to a patient if there are options available to screen for the certain cancer and detect it early, or to possibly prevent it from occurring at all.

The process of genetic testing

The process of genetic testing for genes that may increase risk for cancer is different from other medical tests. Genes involved in cancer are called cancer susceptibility genes. If a mutation is identified in one of these genes, it does not reveal that a person has cancer, but rather whether an individual has an increased risk to develop cancer in the future. In addition, if the person undergoing genetic testing has already had cancer, genetic testing may tell them whether they are at increased risk for developing cancer again. However, the risk for developing cancer is not 100%. The likelihood that a person will develop cancer if they carry an altered gene is called penetrance. Penetrance may differ even among relatives in the same family, and the reasons are not well understood. For example, a mother with a mutation in a cancer susceptibility gene may never develop cancer, but may pass this mutation on to her daughter, who is then diagnosed with cancer at a young age.

For a family in which an inherited mutation has not been previously identified, it is best to begin genetic testing by obtaining a blood sample from a person who has had cancer at a young age. From this blood sample, scientists will be able to extract some DNA. There are a number of different ways that they can then look at the DNA to determine if a mutation is present. The most common is known as sequencing, whereby the chemical sequence of a patient's DNA is compared to DNA that is known to be normal. Scientists will look for any differences, such as missing or extra pieces of DNA in the patient's gene.

Testing can be very expensive and it may take several weeks or months to obtain results. Also, insurance companies will sometimes not cover the cost of testing. Some families are able to participate in research studies where genetic counseling and testing is offered at a lower cost or free of charge.

Categories of results

A positive result indicates the presence of a genetic mutation that is known to be associated with an increased risk for developing cancer. Once this kind of mutation has been found in an individual, it is possible to test this person's relatives, like their children, for the presence or absence of that particular mutation. This testing can be done in a relatively short period of time and provides results that are clearly positive or negative for a particular mutation.

If a relative in a family is tested for a mutation in a cancer susceptibility gene that was previously identified in their family, and they are not found to have this mutation, this type of test result is called a true negative. This means that they did not inherit the mutation in the gene that is the reason why their relative(s)developed cancer. If a person receives a true negative test result, their risk for developing cancer is generally considered to be reduced to that of someone in the general population. Also, because they did not inherit the mutation, they cannot pass it down to any of their children. The term true negative is used to distinguish this test result from a negative or indeterminate result, which is described below.

If the first person tested within a family is not found to have an alteration in a cancer susceptibility gene, this result is negative. However, this result is often called indeterminate. This is because a negative test result cannot completely rule out the possibility of hereditary cancer still being present within a family. The interpretation of this type of result can be very complex. For example, a negative result may mean that the method used to detect mutations may not be sensitive enough to identify all mutations in the gene, or perhaps the mutation is in a part of the gene that is difficult to analyze. It may also mean that a person has a mutation in another cancer susceptibility gene that has not yet been discovered or is very rare. Finally, a negative result could mean that the person tested does not have an increased risk for developing cancer because of a mutation in a single cancer susceptibility gene.

Finally, sometimes mutations are identified in cancer genes and scientists do not know what they mean. They do not know if these types of mutations affect the functioning of the gene and thereby increase a person's risk for cancer, or if they are normal changes in the DNA that just make one person's gene a little bit different from another person's. When this occurs, the genetic counselor may work with the laboratory to determine if future research can be done to find out the meaning of the patient's test result.

In general, a genetic counselor will help a patient to understand the meaning of his or her genetic test result, whether positive, negative, or indeterminate.

Benefits and limitations of undergoing genetic testing for cancer susceptibility genes

There are potential benefits for patients who undergo genetic testing, but there are also possible limitations and risks regarding the information that is obtained. A genetic counselor will discuss these issues in detail with a patient. Before undergoing genetic testing, a patient will also sign a consent form. This is a written agreement indicating that the patient understands the benefits and risks of genetic testing and has made an independent decision to undergo the testing. The informed consent process is a very important part of genetic counseling and testing. With the exception of FAP, where polyps and subsequently colon cancer can occur at young ages or in the teens, the cancers associated with carrying an altered breast or colon cancer susceptibility gene do not typically occur at very young ages. Therefore, genetic testing for mutations in these genes is usually only offered to those men and women who are 18 years of age or older. In addition, individuals who are 18 or older are considered legally able to provide informed consent.

Benefits of participating in genetic testing for alterations in cancer susceptibility genes:

- Results of genetic testing may provide additional information about the increased risk for developing cancer in the future. It may also provide relief from anxiety if a person learns that they do not carry an altered gene.

- If a person finds out that they are at increased risk for developing cancer, they may choose to be screened for this cancer at a younger age and more often than someone without an altered cancer susceptibility gene. Results may also help men and women decide about prophylactic surgery.

- Testing may provide information about cancer risks for children, brothers and sisters, and other relatives.

- Genetic testing may help a person understand why they and/or their family members developed cancer. This may relieve a person from the emotional burden surrounding their cancer diagnosis.

Limitations and risks of participating in genetic testing for cancer susceptibility genes:

- It is possible that the results of genetic testing may be difficult to interpret. Even if a patient receives a positive test result, this does not mean that he/she will definitely develop cancer.
- During the process of undergoing genetic testing, a person may learn information about themselves or their family members. For example, they may learn about an adoption or that an individual is not the biological father of a child. This kind of information may cause strained relationships among relatives.
- Some patients may become sad, angry or anxious if they learn that they have a mutation in a cancer susceptibility gene. If these feelings are very intense, psychological counseling may be helpful.
- Results of genetic testing may place a person at risk for discrimination by health or life insurers, or their employer. There are some laws in effect that provide limited protection to people who undergo genetic testing. The completion of the Human Genome Project, which has mapped all the genes in the human body, will increase the number of genetic tests that are available. Therefore, additional laws need to be passed to completely protect all people who undergo genetic testing from any type of discrimination.

Genes and cancer types

Genes have been discovered that are associated with or responsible for several types of cancer, including **Chronic myelocytic leukemia**, **Burkitt's lymphoma**, **retinoblastoma**, **Wilms' tumor**, and breast and colon cancers. The remainder of this entry will focus only on genetic testing for two of the most common cancers, breast and colon cancer.

Breast cancer genetic testing

Breast and ovarian cancer statistics

All women have a risk for developing breast and **ovarian cancer** during their lifetime. While breast cancer is a common cancer among women in the United States, ovarian cancer is not. Most women are diagnosed with breast or ovarian cancer after the age of 50, and the great majority of cases are not hereditary. But, of the 5-10% of breast and ovarian cancer that does run in families, most is due to mutations in two genes, the BReast CAncer–1 gene (BRCA1) and the BReast CAncer–2 gene (BRCA2). The **BRCA1** gene is located on chromosome 17, and was discovered in 1994. The **BRCA2** gene is on chromosome 13, and was discovered in 1995.

BRCA1 and BRCA2 genes

BRCA1 and BRCA2 genes are tumor suppressor genes and are inherited in a dominant fashion. This means that children of a parent with a mutation in one of the breast cancer genes have a 50% chance to inherit this mutation. These mutations can be passed from either mother or father, and can be inherited by both males and females. The mutations may be detected by performing genetic testing on a patient's blood sample.

Mutations in these genes are more common in people who are Ashkenazi (Eastern or Central European) Jewish. While these mutations may be more common in this specific population, they can be identified in a person of any ethnic background.

Cancer risks

Females who inherit a mutation in the BRCA1 or the BRCA2 gene have an increased risk for developing breast and/or ovarian cancer over their lifetime. The lifetime risk for breast cancer may be as high as 85%, as compared to about 13% in the general population. The lifetime risk for developing ovarian cancer may be as high as 60%, as compared to 1.5% in the general population. Males who inherit a mutation in one of these genes are also at increased risk for developing certain cancers, including prostate, colon and breast cancer.

Men and women who inherit an alteration in the BRCA2 gene also have an increased risk to develop more rare cancers, such as pancreatic and **stomach cancer**. However, these risks are much lower than those observed for breast, ovarian, and **prostate cancer**.

Screening and prevention options

It is recommended that individuals who are at increased risk for developing breast cancer undergo increased surveillance. This means that they may choose to see their physicians for medical screening tests at an earlier age and more often than they would if they did not have an altered gene. For example, it is recommended that women with an altered BRCA1 or BRCA2 gene undergo mammograms at a younger age than is recommended in the general population. It is also recommended that these women see their doctors more often to do a breast exam and also perform breast self-exams regularly. Because women who have a mutation in BRCA1 or BRCA2 are also at increased risk for developing ovarian cancer, they may also choose to be screened closely for this cancer. This screening involves undergoing a test, called a CA-125, which looks for protein levels in a woman's blood. Women may also undergo a pelvic ultrasound to look at the size and shape of the ovaries to determine if cancer may be growing in that area. It is important to mention that ovarian cancer is a difficult cancer to detect, and these screening methods may not be able to find the cancer at an early stage when a woman can undergo successful treatment.

Men with an altered BRCA1 or BRCA2 gene may also choose to be screened earlier and more frequently for the cancers they are at increased risk to develop. Prostate screening consists of a test called prostate specific antigen (PSA) that looks for protein levels in a man's blood. Men may also undergo an examination by a physician. There are no standard screening recommendations for males who are at increased risk for breast cancer. It is usually recommended that they learn to do breast self-exams and talk with their doctors if they find any changes in their breast tissue.

Some women at increased risk for developing breast or ovarian cancer may decide to have prophylactic or preventive surgery. This means that they may choose to have their healthy breasts or ovaries removed before cancer develops. However, even the very best surgeon cannot remove all of the breast or ovarian tissue. Therefore, even if a woman has her breasts or ovaries removed preventively, she may still develop cancer in the remaining tissue, but this risk is believed to be small.

Finally, some healthy women who are at increased risk for breast or ovarian cancer may decide to take certain medications that have been shown to reduce risk. As some of these medications have been studied only in the general population, further research is underway to find out how effective these medications are for women with an inherited risk for developing cancer.

Colon cancer genetic testing

Colon cancer statistics

Males and females in the general population have a 6% risk for developing colon cancer over their lifetime, and the average individual is diagnosed in their 60s to 70s. Similar to breast and ovarian cancer, most colon cancer does not run in families. However, some colon cancer is hereditary, and may be due to a mutation in a colon cancer susceptibility gene. Three of the more common hereditary colon cancer syndromes are described below.

Familial Adenomatous Polyposis (FAP)

FAP is a syndrome in which individuals develop numerous polyps (growths) in their colon or rectum. This disorder may also be called familial polyposis or Gardner's syndrome. Males or females with FAP often

have hundreds of precancerous polyps at young ages, such as when they are teenagers or young adults.

FAP is due to a mutation in a gene called APC. Mutations in this gene are dominantly inherited. In about 80% of families genetic testing performed on a blood sample can find the alteration in the APC gene that is causing this disorder. It is believed that 2/3 of the people with FAP have inherited a mutated gene from their parent. The other 1/3 of individuals with FAP are believed to be new (sporadic) mutations, meaning that the alteration in the APC gene was not inherited from a parent. Individuals with sporadic mutations can pass the mutation on to their children.

Cancer risks

Due to the fact that individuals with FAP develop so many polyps in their colon, there is a very high risk that these polyps, if not removed, will develop into colon cancer. Individuals with FAP may also develop precancerous polyps in other organs, such as their stomach or small intestine. Young people with FAP may also be at increased risk for developing a tumor in the liver, known as a hepatoblastoma. They are also at increased risk for developing tumors in other parts of the body, such as the thyroid gland or pancreas. Males or females with FAP may also have other manifestations of the disease. For example, they may have cysts or bumps on their skin or on the bones of their legs or arms, or freckle-like spots in their eyes.

APC I1307K mutation

In 1997 scientists identified another mutation on the APC gene, known as I1307K. This mutation is found only in individuals who are of Ashkenazi Jewish descent. It is estimated that about 6% of individuals who are Jewish have this particular mutation. The I1307K mutation itself does not cause an increased risk for colon cancer, but rather makes the APC gene more likely to undergo other genetic changes. These other genetic changes increase a person's risk for developing colon cancer. Genetic testing can be performed on a blood sample to determine if an individual carries the I1307K mutation. A person with this mutation has a 50% chance of passing it on to his or her children.

Cancer risks

Individuals who carry the I1307K mutation have an 18-30% risk for developing colon cancer over their lifetime. Research is ongoing to determine if individuals with this mutation may also be at risk for developing other types of cancer, such as breast cancer.

Hereditary Non-Polyposis Colorectal Cancer (HNPCC)

HNPCC, also known as Lynch Syndrome, is a condition in which individuals have an increased risk for developing colon cancer, even if there are very few or no polyps present in the colon. It is believed that mutations in one of five cancer susceptibility genes are associated with most cases of HNPCC. These genes are known as hMSH2, hPMS1, MSH6 (all on chromosome 2), hMLH1 (chromosome 1) and hPMS2 (chromosome 7). It is possible that other genes may be found which are also associated with HNPCC. Mutations in these genes are dominantly inherited, and may be able to be detected through genetic testing performed on a patient's blood sample.

Cancer risks

Individuals with an altered HNPCC gene have a much higher risk for developing colon cancer, often at a younger age (less than 50) than people in the general population. Those with an HNPCC mutation are at increased risk for developing other types of cancer, including stomach, urinary tract, bile duct, uterine and ovarian cancer. It is recommended that men and women also be screened closely for these cancers.

Screening and prevention options

It is recommended that all individuals who are at increased risk for developing colon cancer undergo screening for this cancer. Screening for colon cancer consists of two main types of tests. The first test is called a **sigmoidoscopy**. It is performed by inserting a flexible tube, called a sigmoidoscope into the anus to look at the rectum and the lower colon. The doctor can use the scope to see whether polyps may be present, but these growths can not be removed with this test. The second test is known as a **colonoscopy**. While it is very similar to a sigmoidoscopy, it allows a doctor to see the entire colon. Also, with the use of a colonoscope a polyp can be easily removed at the same time a person is undergoing the test. However, because a colonoscopy is a more invasive test, patients have to be sedated. For patients who are at increased risk for developing colon cancer, it is recommended that they undergo this screening at younger ages and more often then individuals in the general population. For example, because cancer can occur at such young ages for individuals with FAP, it is recommended that they have a sigmoidoscopy beginning at age 11.

Finally, men and women with a mutation in a colon cancer susceptibility gene may take certain medications that have been approved for use in individuals with an increased risk for developing colon cancer.

The only way to prevent colon cancer from developing is to remove the colon entirely. If a person with FAP, HNPCC or the I1307K mutation develops colon cancer he/she may choose to have the colon removed. In addition, if an individual is very anxious about developing colon cancer he or she may choose to have the colon removed before cancer develops. There are several different procedures for removing the colon that allow a person to function normally. Women with an HNPCC mutation may also consider prophylactic removal of their ovaries and uterus.

See also Cancer genetics; Familial cancer syndromes.

Resources

OTHER

Genetic Health. [cited March 27, 2001]. http://www.genetichealth.com/.
Johns Hopkins Hereditary Colorectal Cancer Resources. [cited March 23, 2001]. http://www.hopkins-coloncancer.org/.

ORGANIZATIONS

American Cancer Society. 1599 Clifton Road, NE, Atlanta, GA 30329. (800)ACS-2345.http://www.cancer.org.
National Cancer Institute. 31 Center Drive, MSC 2580 Bethesda, MD 20892-2580. (800)4-CANCER.http://www.nci.nih.gov .
National Society of Genetic Counselors. 233 Canterbury Drive, Wallingford, PA 19086-6617. (610) 872-7608. http://www.nsgc.og.

Tiffani A. DeMarco, M.S.

Gentamicin *see* **Antibiotics**

Germ cell tumors

Definition

Germ cell tumors are a diverse group of tumors that originate in the developing embryo or fetus from cells that would normally become the cells of the gonads—testes—including sperm—in males and ovaries—including eggs (ova)—in females. Germ cell tumors can occur in many parts of the body and can be either benign (non-cancerous) or malignant (cancerous).

Demographics

Germ cell tumors are rare. The incidence of germ cell tumors in the United States and worldwide is about 2.4 children in one million per year. The peak occurrences of germ cell tumors are during infancy and adolescence. They account for about 4% of all cancers in children and adolescents under age 20. Germ cell tumors outside of the brain account for about 16% of all cancers in teenagers aged 15–19. The most common type of germ cell tumors are benign and malignant teratomas in the region of the tailbone during the first few years of life. These are about four times more common in girls than in boys. The second peak incidence reflects testicular cancers in teenage and young adult males. Other relatively common childhood germ cell tumors are abdominal, vaginal, and testicular tumors in infants, **brain tumors** in children, and ovarian tumors in young adolescent girls. Adult germ cell tumors usually occur in the testes or ovaries.

Description

Germ cells are specialized cells in an embryo or fetus that develop into the testes and ovaries. Although most ovarian and testicular tumors are germ cell tumors, most germ cell ovarian tumors are benign. Less than 2% of ovarian cancers are germ cell tumors. In contrast more than 90% of testicular cancers are germ cell tumors.

During embryonic development germ cells can move along the midline to other parts of the body, including the brain, where they may eventually form tumors. These are called **extragonadal germ cell tumors** because they are outside of the gonads (testes and ovaries). More than 60% of germ cell tumors in children are extragonadal. Germ cell tumors that occur outside of the brain are called **extracranial germ cell tumors**. In addition to the gonads and brain germ cell tumors can occur in other parts of the body's midline:

- other reproductive organs such as the cervix, uterus, vagina, or prostate
- middle of the chest
- center back wall of the abdominal cavity
- center of the pelvis
- oral or nasal cavities
- lips

Germ cell tumors are usually discovered either during the first few years of life or shortly after puberty when they grow in response to increasing hormone levels. Extragonadal, extracranial germ cell tumors in early childhood usually originate in the sacrum and coccyx at the lower end of the spinal cord. Extragonadal, extracranial germ cell tumors in teenagers and young adults often originate in the chest. Some germ cell tumors are almost always malignant and others are almost always benign, depending on where in the body they occur.

There are two major types of germ cell tumors: germinomas, which contain only immature germ cells, and embryonic germ cell tumors, which contain both germ cells and some cells that have begun to develop into other tissues, as they normally would in a fetus. Germinomas—also called dysgerminoma if located in the ovaries and seminoma if located in the testes—are malignant tumors. Most embryonic germ cell tumors are a mixture of tissue types:

- Teratomas contain each of the three layers of the developing embryo—the endoderm (inner layer), mesoderm (middle layer), and ectoderm (outer layer). Mature teratomas are usually benign and immature teratomas are usually cancerous
- Endodermal sinus or yolk sac tumors, also called infantile embryonal carcinomas or orchidoblastomas, have cells that resemble the yolk sac of an early embryo and are usually malignant, often aggressively so.
- Embryonal carcinomas look like the tissue of very early embryos and are usually malignant and mixed with other types of germ cell tumors.
- Choriocarcinomas are very rare but often malignant tumors that arise from the chorion layer of the placenta during pregnancy and can spread to the mother and infant. They also occasionally develop in the ovaries or testes of young children.
- Gonadoblastomas and polyembryomas are rare types of embryonic germ cell tumors.

In general any type of germ cell tumor can develop at any germ cell tumor site; however some germ cell tumor types are much more common at some locations:

- About 40% of all germ cell tumors are teratomas in the area of the tailbone and are typically diagnosed in the first month or two of life.
- Teratomas are also the most common type of ovarian germ cell tumor.
- Germinomas and endodermal sinus tumors are most common in the ovaries. Endodermal sinus tumors are also common in the testes.
- Embryonal carcinomas are most common in the testes, usually mixed with endodermal sinus tumors or choriocarcinomas.

Diagnosis, treatment, and prognosis for germ cell tumors depend on the major cell type in the tumor and the most malignant type of cell in the tumor. Malignant germ cell tumors can spread or metastasize to other parts of the body, most often to the lungs, liver, lymph nodes, and central nervous system. Rarely they metastasize to the bone, bone marrow, and other organs.

Risk factors

The known risk factors for germ cell tumors include a number of inherited conditions, especially malformations of the central nervous system and genitourinary tract. Some types of germ cell tumors tend to run in families. Conditions involving extra or missing sex chromosomes can result in abnormal or incomplete reproductive system development, increasing the risk of germ cell tumors. Males with cryptorchidism—failure of the testes to descend into the scrotal sac—are at increased risk for testicular germ cell tumors.

Causes and symptoms

The causes of germ cell tumors are not well understood. Since germ cell tumors usually consist of several different types of **cancer** cells, there are probably multiple causes. Increases in hormone levels at puberty are thought to play a role in the development of ovarian and testicular tumors in adolescents. Some germ cell tumors have a high frequency of certain genetic sequences or abnormal chromosome numbers that may lead to cancer. Testicular germ cell tumors can have structural abnormalities involving chromosome 12, which may play a role in tumor development.

Symptoms of germ cell tumors vary greatly depending on the size and location of the tumor. The most common symptom of germ cell tumors is a mass somewhere along the midline of the body, possibly accompanied by abdominal pain or bloating. Other possible symptoms include:

- constipation, incontinence, and leg weakness if the tumor is located in the sacrum and is compressing structures
- abnormally shaped or irregularly sized testes
- early entry into puberty
- vaginal bleeding
- late onset of menstruation
- menstrual problems
- excessive hair growth
- shortness of breath or other breathing problems
- diabetes
- hormonal abnormalities
- stunted growth
- headaches or vision problems

Diagnosis

Examination

Most germ cell tumors are initially identified by a lump in the testicles or somewhere else along the midline of the body. Childhood teratomas of the tailbone are often externally visible. A complete medical history and physical examination will be performed.

Tests

There are two **tumor markers** that are suggestive of germ cell tumors. Tumor markers are proteins that are produced by tumor cells and are often found at elevated levels in the blood. Teratomas and endodermal sinus tumors produce high levels of alpha-fetoprotein (AFP). Germ cell tumors containing embryonal **carcinoma** or choriocarcinoma are associated with elevated levels beta-human chorionic gonadotropin (beta-HCG). These markers are also used to monitor the effectiveness of surgery or other therapies and to monitor patients for a recurrence of the tumor.

Other blood tests may include:

- complete blood count (CBC)
- blood chemistries
- liver and kidney function
- genetic tests

Procedures

Procedures to identify germ cell tumors often include a **biopsy** of an identified lump. A small piece of the lump is removed and cut into thin sections. A specialist examines these sections under a microscope for the presence of abnormal cells. The degree to which the biopsied tissue differs from healthy tissue is an indication of the probable severity of the disease. Biopsy results are used to grade tumors and provide a prognosis.

Imaging procedures for diagnosing germ cell tumors include **x rays**, **computed tomography** (CT or CAT) scans, **magnetic resonance imaging** (MRI), ultrasound, and bone scans. X rays can reveal calcium deposits in normally soft tissues. CT scans and ultrasound can provide details about the tumor, such as its site of origin, whether it is solid or cystic, and whether its borders are well-defined. Tumors with well-defined borders have a better chance of complete surgical removal.

Staging

Grading and staging of malignant tumors determine treatment and prognosis. Tumor grades are based on the types of tissues present in the tumor.

Staging indicates the spread of the cancer. Separate staging systems exist for childhood and adult ovarian and testicular cancers, which are treated by pediatric and adult oncologists, respectively.

Pediatric testicular cancers are typically staged as follows:

- Stage I tumors are limited to the testes. Postoperative tumor marker levels are within the normal range.
- Stage II tumors have spread to the abdominal lymph nodes and tumor markers are elevated.
- Stage III tumors have greater involvement of the abdominal lymph nodes.
- Stage IV tumors have spread to other organs such as the lungs.

Adult testicular cancers are commonly staged according to a simplified TNM system:

- Stage T, with several sub-levels, is a localized tumor.
- Stage N is a cancer that has spread to local lymph nodes.
- Stage M is a cancer that has spread to distant lymph nodes and organs.

Treatment

Traditional

The treatment and prognosis of germ cell tumors depend on the types of tissues in the tumor, the tumor's location, and the stage of the cancer. The age of the patient, overall health and medical history, prognosis, and the issue of future childbearing also affect treatment choice. Most germ cell tumors require surgical removal of the tumor. More advanced cancers are treated with additional radiation or **chemotherapy**. Sometimes it is possible to completely remove all cancerous tissue with surgery. In other cases debulking surgery is performed to reduce the size of the tumor to be treated with chemotherapy or radiation. Sometimes a **second-look surgery** is performed after **radiation therapy** or chemotherapy to confirm that cancerous tissues have been eradicated.

Germinomas are especially sensitive to radiation and this may be the primary treatment for these types of tumors. However germinomas in the brain are the only type of childhood germ cell tumors that are routinely treated with radiation.

Drugs

Chemotherapy is administered with pills taken by mouth, by injection, or intravenously (IV). Chemotherapy kills cancerous cells, including those that have moved from the initial site. In more advanced stages of disease chemotherapy is sometimes the primary treatment. It usually involves a platinum-based drug such as **cisplatin** in combination with one or two other anti-cancer medications. Using a combination of drugs reduces the risk of serious side effects from high doses of a single drug, since each drug has different side effects. Drug combinations also decrease the risk of the cancer developing resistance to a particular drug. Different combinations of drugs are used to treat different types of tumors.

Clinical trials for germ cell cancer treatment are evaluating a therapy called "peripheral stem cell rescue," in which the patient's red blood cells are removed before high-dose chemotherapy and replaced after the chemotherapy is complete. This decreases the side effects of the medications and improves the patient's chances of successful treatment. **Bone marrow transplantation** also allows the administration of higher-dose chemotherapy. Other clinical trials for germ cell cancer treatments are evaluating different combinations of chemotherapy drugs and new types of drug treatments.

Some of the more common side effects of chemotherapy include:

- hair loss (alopecia)
- fatigue and weakness
- nausea and vomiting
- bedwetting

Hair loss can be especially difficult for teenage patients. Other sources of hair damage—such as curling, blow-drying, or chemical treatments—should be avoided to slow the rate of hair loss. Children should be allowed to choose how to cope with hair loss and their choices should be supported. They may choose to remain bald or to wear hats or scarves. Schools may need to be persuaded to allow a child to wear a head covering. If a wig is chosen, a sample of pretreatment hair can be used to match color and texture. It is important to assure the child that the hair loss is temporary and a sign that the medication is working. Children should be prepared for the possibility that their hair may grow back a different color or texture.

Drugs may be prescribed to combat **nausea and vomiting** from chemotherapy. Desensitization, hypnosis, guided imagery, and relaxation techniques can also help treat **nausea** and **vomiting**. Video games are often an effective means of distracting children who are undergoing treatment.

Bedwetting can be especially distressing for older children. The child should be assured that this is insignificant and temporary. Extra linens and towels should be kept by the bed. Limiting fluids for a few hours before bedtime or waking the child in the night can help prevent bedwetting.

Alternative and complementary therapies

Common complementary therapies in the treatment of germ cell tumors involve reducing anxiety and increasing feelings of well-being. They may include:

- aromatherapy
- art therapy
- massage
- meditation
- music therapy
- prayer
- t'ai chi
- yoga
- other forms of exercise

There are numerous alternative therapies for cancer:

- Vitamins A, C, and E and selenium are believed to act as antioxidants.
- Vitamin E, melatonin, aloe vera, and beta-1,3-glucan may stimulate the immune system.
- Some practitioners believe that substances such as garlic and ginger can shrink tumors. Any supplements should be discussed with the attending physician.

Home remedies

Home treatment of children with germ cell tumors includes:

- a well-balanced diet
- small frequent meals with light nourishing food such as soup to combat nausea and vomiting
- plenty of rest
- avoidance of stress
- allowing the child to pursue normal activities to the extent possible, including choosing activities that are most important to the child and providing backup activities or alternative mobility (such as a stroller or wheelchair) if the child become too fatigued

Prognosis

The prognosis for germ cell tumors depends on the type of tumor, its size and location, and whether a cancerous tumor has metastasized. The overall prognosis for germ cell tumors has improved dramatically in recent decades. About 90% of patients diagnosed with localized tumors are cured and the cure rate for metastasized germ cell cancers is approaching 80%:

- Childhood teratomas of the tailbone are usually diagnosed and treated very early and have a very favorable prognosis.
- Mature teratomas of the ovaries—by far the most common type of ovarian tumor—are almost always benign, unless mixed with other more malignant germ cell tumor types.
- Malignant germ cell ovarian tumors are usually diagnosed at a late stage and have the worst prognosis of all germ cell tumors.
- Embryonal carcinomas and choriocarcinomas are particularly malignant. Without treatment, the average survival time is only a few months.

Since most germ cell tumor patients are children or young adults, future fertility is a major concern. Radiation, in particular, destroys fertility and therefore is not usually used to treat children except in cases of brain germinomas. The surgical removal of reproductive organs to treat germ cell tumors can have major psychological consequences and cause altered feelings of **sexuality**.

Prevention

There are no methods for preventing germ cell tumors. Patients who have been successfully treated for germ cell cancers require frequent follow-ups to check for recurrences. Males who have had **testicular cancer** can improve their chances of detecting a recurrence at an early stage by performing regular self-examinations.

Health care team roles

The treatment a germ cell cancer typically involves the referring physician (often a pediatrician or gynecologist), an oncologist, a pathologist, and nurses. Radiation therapy involves a radiation oncologist, radiation therapist, radiation nurse, radiation physicist, and a dosimetrist. Treatment may also include a psychologist, nutritionist, social worker, and chaplain.

Resources

BOOKS

Bellenir, Karen. *Cancer Sourcebook,* 5th ed. Detroit: Omnigraphics, 2007.

Raghavan, Derek, et al., eds. *Textbook of Uncommon Cancer,* 3rd ed. Hoboken, NJ: Wiley, 2006.

Sutton, Amy L. *Cancer Sourcebook for Women,* 3rd ed. Detroit: Omnigraphics, 2006.

PERIODICALS

Feldman, Darren R., and Robert J. Motzer. "Good-Risk-Advanced Germ Cell Tumors: Historical Perspectives and Current Standards of Care." *World Journal of Urology* 27, no. 4 (August 2009): 463-470.

Schrader, Mark, et al. "Germ Cell Tumors of the Gonads: A Selective Review Emphasizing Problems in Drug Resistance and Current Therapy Options." *Oncology* 76, no. 2 (February 2009): 77-84.

Westermann, Dirk H., and Urs E. Studer. "High-Risk Clinical Stage I Nonseminomatous Germ Cell Tumors: The Case for Chemotherapy." *World Journal of Urology* 27, no. 4 (August 2009): 455-461.

OTHER

"Childhood Extracranial Germ Cell Tumors Treatment." *National Cancer Institute.*http://www.cancer.gov/cancertopics/pdq/treatment/extracranial-germ-cell/patient/.

"Extragonadal Germ Cell Tumors Treatment." *National Cancer Institute.*http://www.cancer.gov/cancertopics/pdq/treatment/extragonadal-germ-cell/patient/.

"Germ Cell Tumors." *Lucile Packard Children's Hospital.*http://www.lpch.org/DiseaseHealthInfo/HealthLibrary/oncology/gct.html.

"Germ Cell Tumors—Childhood.;" *Cancer.Net.* http://www.cancer.net/patient/Cancer + Types/Germ + Cell + Tumor + - + Childhood?sectionTitle = Overview.

"Ovarian Germ Cell Tumors Treatment." *National Cancer Institute.*http://www.cancer.gov/cancertopics/pdq/treatment/ovarian-germ-cell/patient/.

"Testicular Cancer." *MedlinePlus.*http://www.nlm.nih.gov/medlineplus/ency/article/001288.htm.

ORGANIZATIONS

American Cancer Society, 1599 Clifton Road NE, Atlanta, GA, 30329-4251, (800) ACS-2345, http://www.cancer.org.

National Cancer Institute, NCI Public Inquiries Office, 6116 Executive Boulevard, Room 3036A, Bethesda, MD, 20006, (800) 4-CANCER, http://www.cancer.gov.

The National Children's Cancer Society, One South Memorial Drive, Suite 800, St. Louis, MO, 63102, (314) 241-1600, (314) 241-1996, pbeck@children-cancer.org, http://www.nationalchildrenscancersociety.org.

The Wellness Community, 919 18th St. NW, Washington, DC, 20006, (202) 659-9709, (888) 793-well, (202) 659-9703, help@thewellnesscommunity.org, www.thewellnesscommunity.org.

Wendy Wippel, MS
Margaret Alic, PhD

Gestational trophoblastic tumors

Definition

A gestational trophoblastic tumor (GTT)—also called gestational trophoblastic disease (GTD) or gestational trophoblastic neoplasm (GTN)—is a rare **cancer** that develops in the trophoblastic cells that help attach the embryo to the uterus and form the placenta.

Demographics

GTTs account for less than 1% of all **gynecologic cancers**. GTTs are significantly more common in some African and Asian countries than in Europe and North America. In the United States and Europe:

- Hydatidiform moles—the most common type of GTT—occur in about one out of every 1,000 pregnancies.
- About 15% of hydatidiform moles become invasive moles.
- Choriocarcinoma, a malignant form of GTT, occurs in 4% of women who have had a hydatidiform mole that was surgically removed or treated with radiation therapy.
- The overall incidence of choriocarcinoma is about one in 40,000 pregnancies.

GTTs occur only in women of childbearing age, almost always following a failed pregnancy. They are most common in women who:

- are under age 20
- are over age 40
- have had a previous GTT
- have had difficulty becoming pregnant or have had prior miscarriage
- have type A or AB blood
- have taken birth control pills
- have a family history of GTT
- are of lower socioeconomic status

Description

GTTs are highly curable malignancies that originate inside the uterus in cells called trophoblasts that make up one layer of the placenta. The most common types of GTTs are hydatidiform moles, also called molar pregnancies, and choriocarcinomas. A placental-site trophoblastic tumor is an extremely rare type of GTT that originates at the site where the placenta was attached to the wall of the uterus.

A hydatidiform mole can form when a sperm and egg cell unite but a fetus does not develop. If all of the tissue is not expelled, the cells that form the placenta can continue to grow until they look something like a cluster of grapes. Hydatidiform moles are classified as partial or complete. A hydatidiform mole does not spread beyond the uterus, but it can develop into an invasive mole in the uterine muscle or into a choriocarcinoma. Between 2% and 4% of hydatidiform moles progress to choriocarcinomas.

A choriocarcinoma is a malignancy of the trophoblastic cells. It usually originates in a hydatidiform mole. However it can also develop in tissue that remains in the uterus following normal pregnancy and delivery, miscarriage, abortion, or an ectopic pregnancy. A choriocarcinoma is an aggressive, invasive tumor characterized by rapid growth and heavy bleeding. It can spread (metastasize) to any part of the body. **Metastasis** begins at an early stage of the disease and usually involves the lungs, vagina, pelvis, brain, and/or liver. Less frequently a choriocarcinoma spreads to the kidneys, spleen, and/or gastrointestinal tract.

Risk factors

Although the exact cause of GTTs is unknown, the risk of a GTT is higher than normal if a woman's blood group is A and her partner's is O. A woman's risk of a second GTT is twice that of a first GTT, although the risk is still very low.

Causes and symptoms

A partial hydatidiform mole can develop when two sperm fertilize a normal egg cell. Although fetal development may be initiated, the extra genetic material from the second sperm results in early miscarriage.

A complete hydatidiform mole most often develops when one or two sperm fertilize an empty egg cell that has no internal genetic material. Since all of the genetic material is from the father's sperm, no fetal tissue forms.

Choriocarcinomas develop from tissue that remains behind following pregnancy:

- About 50% develop after molar pregnancies.
- About 25% develop following a miscarriage, abortion, or tubal pregnancy (an ectopic pregnancy in a fallopian tube).
- The remaining 25% of choriocarcinomas develop after normal pregnancy and birth.

Although molar pregnancy is almost always diagnosed during the first trimester, it is often difficult to distinguish it from the early stages of a normal pregnancy. The most common symptoms of a hydatidiform mole are vaginal bleeding and severe morning sickness. Other symptoms may include:

- an unusually large uterus for the pregnancy stage
- a uterus that is enlarged on only one side
- absence of a fetal heartbeat
- absence of a visible fetus on a sonogram
- absence of fetal movement at the appropriate stage of pregnancy
- passage of clots with the color and consistency of prune juice or of finger-like structures (villi) containing fetal blood cells
- toxemia
- ovarian cysts
- hyperthyroidism
- iron-deficiency anemia from recurrent bleeding

Choriocarcinomas most often occur following a molar pregnancy. However persistent vaginal bleeding after giving birth can be a symptom of a choriocarcinoma. Irregular, abnormal bleeding can indicate that the choriocarcinoma has invaded the vagina. Other symptoms include lesions that can be seen on a chest x ray but do not cause shortness of breath or other symptoms. Symptoms of lung metastasis include severe shortness of breath (respiratory insufficiency) and coughing up blood. The central nervous system (CNS) is rarely affected by choriocarcinoma unless the disease has spread to one or both lungs. Metastasis to the brain may cause headaches, seizures, and stroke-like symptoms.

Diagnosis

Examination

An internal pelvic examination is performed to detect lumps or abnormalities in the size or shape of the uterus.

Tests

Blood and urine tests measure levels of beta-human chorionic gonadotropin (beta-HCG). This hormone—which is normally produced by the placenta during pregnancy and is the basis for pregnancy tests—is abnormally elevated in the blood and urine of women with a GTT. The presence of beta-HCG in the blood of a woman who is not pregnant is indicative of a GTT. Beta-HCG is a sensitive marker for the presence of a GTT before, during, and after treatment.

Procedures

Imaging studies such as chest **x rays**, **computed tomography** (CT) scans, **magnetic resonance imaging** (MRI), ultrasound, and **positron emission tomography** (PET) scans may be used to locate tumors.

Staging

Cancer centers commonly use the following system to describe the stage or extent of a GTT:

- Hydatidiform mole: Cancer is found only in the space inside the uterus.
- Invasive mole or choriocarcinoma destruens: Cancer is in the muscle of the uterus.
- Placental-site gestational trophoblastic tumor: Cancer is found in the muscle of the uterus and at the site where the placenta was attached.
- Nonmetastatic: Cancer is derived from cells remaining after treatment of a hydatidiform mole or following an abortion or delivery of a baby. Cancer has not spread beyond the uterus.
- Metastatic, good prognosis: Cancer cells have grown inside the uterus from tissue remaining after treatment of a hydatidiform mole or following an abortion or delivery and have invaded tissues outside of the uterus, but have not spread to the liver or brain; blood levels of beta-HCG are low; less than four months have passed since the last pregnancy; the patient has not received previous chemotherapy.
- Metastatic, poor prognosis: Cancer cells have invaded tissues outside of the uterus, including the liver or brain; blood levels of beta-HCG are high; more than four months have passed since the last pregnancy; previous chemotherapy has not eradicated the disease; or the tumor developed after the completion of a normal pregnancy.
- Recurrent: The cancer came back after treatment, in the uterus or elsewhere in the body.

Treatment

Traditional

The choice of treatment for a GTT is determined by the following factors:

- the woman's age and general health

- tumor type
- stage of the disease
- areas of the body where the cancer has spread
- blood levels of beta-HCG
- length of time between conception and initiation of treatment
- prior pregnancy-related problems and their treatments
- whether the woman plans to become pregnant in the future

A GTT is usually treated with surgery to remove the tumor. If the woman does not wish to become pregnant in the future, a hysterectomy may be performed to remove the uterus. If she does wants to become pregnant in the future, a **dilatation and curettage** (D&C) with suction evacuation is performed. This is used only for molar pregnancies. It involves:

- stretching the cervix—the opening of the uterus
- using a small vacuum-like device to remove material from inside the uterus
- gently scraping the walls of the uterus to remove any remaining material.

Radiation therapy is sometimes used to treat a GTT that has spread to other parts of the body. The radiation is either from a machine outside of the body (external beam) or from radiation-producing pellets (radioisotopes) inserted into the area of the body where cancer cells have been found.

In the case of a recurrent GTT that has spread to the liver, radiation does not improve survival and may make **chemotherapy** less effective. The prognosis is even worse if both the liver and brain are affected.

Following diagnosis and treatment of a GTT, blood tests are performed weekly, pelvic exams every other week, and chest x rays every four–six weeks until the blood level of beta-HCG has returned to normal. Once beta-HCG levels have normalized, monthly blood tests are continued for the next year and medical monitoring, including blood tests, with decreasing frequency for the next three years. Women who have been treated for a GTT should wait at least a year before becoming pregnant and should see a doctor as soon as they think they may be pregnant.

Drugs

Following D&C or hysterectomy for a hydatidiform mole, the blood levels of beta-HCG are carefully monitored. Chemotherapy is initiated if:

- Beta-HCG levels continue to rise for two weeks or remain constant for three weeks.

- Beta-HCG levels become elevated after having fallen to normal values.
- Analysis of tissue removed during surgery indicates the presence of invasive disease (choriocarcinoma).
- Heavy, unexplained bleeding occurs.

Chemotherapy may be in oral pill form or administered intravenously to kill any cancer cells remaining after surgery. Chemotherapy is started as early in the course of the disease as possible and administered every 14–21 days until beta-HCG blood levels drop to normal:

- Nonmetastatic disease, the most common form of choriocarcinoma, is usually treated with single-agent chemotherapy.
- Metastatic disease with good prognosis may be treated with chemotherapy alone, hysterectomy followed by chemotherapy, or chemotherapy followed by hysterectomy. Patients are carefully monitored because 40–50% of the cancers will become resistant to the first chemotherapy drug used.
- Metastatic disease with poor prognosis is usually treated with combination chemotherapy.

Metastatic GTT may be further classified as low-risk, medium-risk, or high-risk. High-risk patients are treated with combination chemotherapy regardless of the stage of their disease. Factors used to determine risk include:

- age
- prior pregnancy experiences
- time elapsed between conception and initiation of treatment
- blood beta-HGC levels
- the size of the largest tumor
- the locations of metastasized cancer
- previous chemotherapy

A woman who develops one or more new GTTs after chemotherapy is considered high risk with a poor prognosis and is treated with aggressive chemotherapy, as well as possible surgery. If recurrent disease has spread to the central nervous system, whole brain radiation and systemic chemotherapy are administered simultaneously.

Research into GTT treatment is addressing the following questions:

- How effective are certain chemotherapy drugs for treating a GTT that has not responded to other therapies or that has recurred after treatment?
- At what dosages do specific chemotherapy drugs become toxic?

QUESTIONS TO ASK YOUR DOCTOR

- What are the indications that my pregnancy may not be proceeding normally?
- What stage is my GTT?
- What treatment do you recommend?
- Will my GTT affect my ability to have children in the future?
- How long must I wait before becoming pregnant again?

- How does the frequency of chemotherapy treatments affect a patient's prognosis?
- What is the relationship between the start of chemotherapy and an immediate drop in a woman's beta-HCG levels?

Prognosis

A GTT is one of the most curable cancers of the female reproductive system. This is because GTT cells respond well to chemotherapy and beta-HCG blood tests are a reliable means of determining whether cancer cells are still present and whether therapy should continue. Although it can be life-threatening, with early specialized treatment a GTT is highly curable even when it has spread far beyond the uterus:

- A hydatidiform mole is 100% curable by surgery. Partial hydatidiform moles are usually completely removed by the initial surgery. With about 20% of complete hydatidiform moles, some persistant molar material remains after surgery, usually as an invasive mole and rarely as choriocarcinoma, both of which require further treatment.
- Placental-site GTTs do not generally spread to other parts of the body; however they do not respond well to chemotherapy and can be fatal.
- Nonmetastatic GTT has a cure rate of almost 100%.
- About 80% of patients with widely metastasized disease are cured by prompt, aggressive chemotherapy, sometimes combined with surgery and radiation.

About 70% of patients with high-risk disease go into remission:

- Combination chemotherapy is effective in 74% of patients who have not responded to other forms of treatment and in 76% of those who have not been treated previously with chemotherapy.

- The survival rate for patients treated with combination chemotherapy is 84%.
- When recurrent GTT has spread to the central nervous system, simultaneous whole-brain radiation and systemic chemotherapy result in sustained remission in 50–60% of cases.

About 85% of GTT recurrences are within 18 months of remission and almost all are within 36 months of remission. A GTT recurs in about:

- 2.5% of women treated for nonmetastatic disease
- 3.7% of women treated for metastatic disease, good prognosis
- 13% of women treated for metastatic disease, poor prognosis

Prevention

There are no known preventions for a GTT, other than never becoming pregnant. Women who have had previous molar pregnancies should speak to their doctors about future risks.

Health care team roles

A GTT is typically treated by a team of gynecologists, gynecologic oncologists, medical oncologists, and surgeons. Women with poor prognoses should be treated at a specialized trophoblastic disease center by a physician experienced in caring for high-risk GTT patients.

Resources

BOOKS

Bellenir, Karen. *Cancer Sourcebook*, 5th ed. Detroit: Omnigraphics, 2007.

Johnson, Tara, and Meredith Celene Schwartz. *Gestational Trophoblastic Neophasia: A Guide for Women Dealing with Tumors of the Placenta, such as Choriocarcinoma, Molar Pregnancy and Other Forms of GTN.* Victoria, BC: Trafford, 2007.

Sutton, Amy L. *Cancer Sourcebook for Women*, 3rd ed. Detroit: Omnigraphics, 2006.

PERIODICALS

El-Helw, L. M., and B. W. Hancock. "Treatment of Metastatic Gestational Trophoblastic Neoplasia." *Lancet Oncology* 8 (2007): 715-724.

Shih, I. M. "Gestational Trophoblastic Neoplasia—Pathogenesis and Potential Therapeutic Targets." *Lancet Oncology* 8 (2007): 642-650.

OTHER

"Gestational Trophoblastic Tumor" *National Cancer Institute*.http://cancernet.nci.nih.gov/templates/doc.aspx?viewid = 35DE7EC3-67AD-4A98-921C-6D5BA4D2675C.

Rich, William M. "Gestational Trophoblastic Disease." *OBGYN.net*.http://www.obgyn.net/women/women.asp?page = /women/articles/rich/gest.

"What is Gestational Trophoblastic Disease?" *American Cancer Society*.http://www.cancer.org/docroot/CRI/content/CRI_2_4_1X_What_are_gestational_trophoblastic_disease_49.asp?sitearea = .

ORGANIZATIONS

American Cancer Society, 1599 Clifton Road NE, Atlanta, GA, 30329-4251, (800) ACS-2345, http://www.cancer.org.

American College of Obstetricians and Gynecologists, PO Box 96920, Washington, DC, 20090-6920, (202) 638-5577, resources@acog.org, http://www.acog.org.

National Cancer Institute, NCI Public Inquiries Office, 6116 Executive Boulevard, Room 3036A, Bethesda, MD, 20006, (800) 4-CANCER, http://www.cancer.gov.

Maureen Haggerty
Margaret Alic, PhD

Giant cell tumors

Definition

Giant cell tumor generally refers to a bone tumor and is typically found in the end of arm and leg bones.

Description

Giant cell tumor of the bone is also referred to as an osteoclastoma as it contains a large number of giant cells resembling a type of bone cells called osteoclasts. Half of all giant cell tumors occurs in the knee, at the lower end of femur (thigh bone) or upper tibia (one of the bones of the lower leg). The tumor is usually located eccentrically and often causes expansion of the bone end. The tumor destroys the bony structure and thus could lead to fractures, even in the absence of stress. Other giant cell tumors can occur in virtually any other bone, including the sacrum, pelvis, and small bones of hands and feet. The growth of this tumor is variable and unpredictable. It is considered to be benign, but can recur following surgical removal. It can also have pulmonary metastases that are mostly curable. Some of the giant cell tumors may change into malignant sarcomas, especially when they recur after high-dose radiation treatment.

Giant cell tumor of tendon sheath

Giant cell tumor of tendon sheath is also referred to a localized nodular tenosynovitis. It usually occurs as single, painless mass that grows slowly. It is mainly found in the wrist and fingers. These are benign

Giant cell tumor of a tendon in a woman's finger. *(Custom Medical Stock Photo. Reproduced by permission.)*

growths that can be easily excised (surgically removed). This type is not discussed further in this entry.

Demographics

Giant cell tumor of bone is mostly seen in adults between the ages of 20 and 40 years. It is slightly more common among women than men and is seen in Asians more than other ethnic groups. It is very uncommon in children.

Causes and symptoms

The cause of giant cell tumors of bone is unknown.

The following symptoms may be seen in patients with giant cell tumors:

- Pain: As this tumors mainly occurs in the joints, arthritic pain is usually the first symptom.
- Swelling: Giant cell tumor causes enlargement of the bone and, as it grows, the patient may find a swelling at the site of the tumor.
- Fracture: Giant cell tumors destroy the surrounding bone and, unlike other bone cancers, fractures are common as the tumor grows. Initially the patient may have a sore or painful joint and the fracture could make it suddenly, severely painful.

Diagnosis

Typically the patient with giant cell tumor will go to the doctor because of pain. The doctor will perform routine physical tests and test the affected area for tenderness, swelling, warmth, redness, and mobility. An x ray of the affected area will be obtained. Certain other imaging tests could be done, including **magnetic**

resonance imaging (MRI) and **computed tomography** (CT scan) to see extent of growth. CT scan of the chest will also be done to test for **metastasis** to the lungs. An isotope scan may be also done to test for extent of damage. These techniques are noninvasive and can be performed within a day. A surgical **biopsy** is always done either before or during surgical removal of the tumor. The biopsy determines whether the tumor is malignant and identifies the stage of the tumor. This may done under either local or general anesthesia, depending upon the location of the tumor and the condition and age of the patient.

Treatment team

The treatment team will consist primarily of radiation oncologist, orthopedic oncologist, and oncology nurse. Following surgical removal of the tumor, recovery may be aided by physical therapists.

Clinical staging, treatments, and prognosis

Most giant cell tumors are initially classified as benign (grade 0). The tumor may progress in three stages. Stage 1, or latent stage, consists of a very slow growing tumor. It is well demarcated and there is little destruction of the outer surface of the bone. Stage 2, or the active stage, is the most commonly found stage. In this stage the tumor grows more steadily and the cortex (or outer layer of the bone) is lost. Stage 3 is the aggressive stage and accounts for about 20% of all giant cell tumors. In this stage the tumor grows rapidly and extends beyond the bone into the soft tissue. This stage is also associated more frequently with fractures.

Treatment of giant cell tumors is mainly surgical. Most stage 1 and 2 and some stage 3 tumors are treated by aggressive curettage, and the bone may be treated chemically and filled with cement. In some stage 2 and most stage 3 lesions the affected section of the bone may have to be removed (en bloc resection). In very rare cases the tumor may be so expanded that **amputation** may be necessary. Radiation is used to treat giant cell tumors in a location difficult to treat surgically. **Chemotherapy** has not been shown to be effective against giant cell tumors.

Prognosis following resection is excellent, with less than 5% chance of recurrence. When the tumor is removed by curettage followed by aggressive chemical treatment, there is a 5-10% chance of local recurrence. When the tumors recur locally it is usually within three years of surgical removal and the patient needs to be monitored closely during this time. A small percentage of giant cell tumors can metastasize to the lungs. The metastases can be removed surgically and most can be cured.

When a rare case of malignant **sarcoma** develops from a giant cell tumor, it is treated aggressively by surgery. In these cases, prognosis is poor and long-term survival rate is as low as 20–30%.

Alternative and complementary therapies

There are no alternative or complementary therapies available for giant cell tumors.

Coping with cancer treatment

As the treatment for giant cell tumors is mainly surgical, physical therapy with strengthening exercises to restore range of motion is extremely important. If amputation is required resulting psychological effects will also have to be addressed, especially as this disease occurs in adults who are physically and sexually active.

Clinical trials

As of 2001 there were no ongoing **clinical trials** by any major agencies specifically for treatment of giant cell tumors.

Prevention

As the cause of giant cell tumors is not known, there is no known method for prevention. When adults in the age group of 20 to 40 years notice pain and swelling in the joints, prompt radiological evaluation could identify giant cell tumors in early stages and lead to a complete cure.

Special concerns

Whenever a giant cell tumor is suspected, a chest CT scan should also be performed to check for metastasis to the lungs. During pregnancy the tumor can grow more rapidly, in which case it may be better to wait to perform surgery until the baby can be safely delivered by induction. If a patient with giant cell tumor suffers a fracture at the affected area, it may be best to wait until the fracture is healed before performing the surgery.

Resources

BOOKS

Campanacci, Mario. *Bone and soft tissue tumors.* New York:Springer-Verlag Wien Publishing, 1999.

PERIODICALS

Blackley, H. R., et al. "Treatment of giant cell tumors with curettage and bone grafting." *Journal of Bone and Joint Surgery* American, 81, no. 6 (1999): 811-20.

ORGANIZATIONS

The American Academy of Orthopaedic Surgeons. 6300 N. River Road, Suite 200, Rosemont, IL 60018. (847) 823-8125. http://www.aaos.org.

Malini Vashishtha, Ph.D.

Gliomas *see* Brain/Central nervous system tumors

Glossectomy

Definition

A glossectomy is the surgical removal of all or part of the tongue.

Purpose

A glossectomy is performed to treat **cancer** of the tongue. Removing the tongue is indicated if the patient has a cancer that does not respond to other forms of treatment. In most cases, however, only part of the tongue is removed (partial glossectomy). Cancer of the tongue is considered very dangerous due to the fact that it can easily spread to nearby lymph glands. Most cancer specialists recommend surgical removal of the cancerous tissue.

Demographics

According to the Oral Cancer Foundation, 30,000 Americans will be diagnosed with oral or pharyngeal cancer in 2003, or about 1.1 persons per 100,000. Of these 30,000 newly diagnosed individuals, only half will be alive in five years. This percentage has shown little improvement for decades. The problem is much greater in the rest of the world, with over 350,000 to 400,000 new cases of oral cancer appearing each year.

The most important risk factors for cancer of the tongue are **alcohol consumption** and smoking. The risk is significantly higher in patients who use both alcohol and tobacco than in those who consume only one.

Description

Glossectomies are always performed under general anesthesia. A partial glossectomy is a relatively simple operation. If the "hole" left by the excision of the cancer is small, it is commonly repaired by sewing up the tongue immediately or by using a small graft of skin. If the glossectomy is more extensive, care is taken to repair the tongue so as to maintain its mobility. A common approach is to use a piece of skin taken from the wrist together with the blood vessels that supply it. This type of graft is called a radial forearm free flap. The flap is inserted into the hole in the tongue. This procedure requires a highly skilled surgeon who is able to connect very small arteries. Complete removal of the tongue, called a total glossectomy, is rarely performed.

Diagnosis/Preparation

If an area of abnormal tissue has been found in the mouth, either by the patient or by a dentist or doctor, a **biopsy** is the only way to confirm a diagnosis of cancer. A pathologist, who is a physician who specializes in the study of disease, examines the tissue sample under a microscope to check for cancer cells.

If the biopsy indicates that cancer is present, a comprehensive physical examination of the patient's head and neck is performed prior to surgery. The

patient will meet with the treatment team before admission to the hospital so that they can answer questions and explain the treatment plan.

Aftercare

Patients usually remain in the hospital for seven to 10 days after a glossectomy. They often require oxygen in the first 24–48 hours after the operation. Oxygen is administered through a face mask or through two small tubes placed in the nostrils. The patient is given fluids through a tube that goes from the nose to the stomach until he or she can tolerate taking food by mouth. Radiation treatment is often scheduled after the surgery to destroy any remaining cancer cells. As patients regain the ability to eat and swallow, they also begin speech therapy.

Risks

Risks associated with a glossectomy include:

- Bleeding from the tongue. This is an early complication of surgery; it can result in severe swelling leading to blockage of the airway.
- Poor speech and difficulty swallowing. This complication depends on how much of the tongue is removed.
- Fistula formation. Incomplete healing may result in the formation of a passage between the skin and the mouth cavity within the first two weeks following a glossectomy. This complication often occurs after feeding has resumed. Patients who have had radiotherapy are at greater risk of developing a fistula.
- Flap failure. This complication is often due to problems with the flap's blood supply.

Normal results

A successful glossectomy results in complete removal of the cancer, improved ability to swallow food, and restored speech. The quality of the patient's

QUESTIONS TO ASK THE DOCTOR

- Will the glossectomy prevent the cancer from coming back?
- What are the possible complications of this procedure?
- How long will it take to recover from the surgery?
- How will the glossectomy affect my speech?
- What specific techniques do you use?
- How many new cancers of the head and neck do you treat every year?

speech is usually very good if at least one-third of the tongue remains and an experienced surgeon has performed the repair.

Total glossectomy results in severe disability because the "new tongue" (a prosthesis) is incapable of movement. This lack of mobility creates enormous difficulty in eating and talking.

Morbidity and mortality rates

Even in the case of a successful glossectomy, the long-term outcome depends on the stage of the cancer and the involvement of lymph glands in the neck. Five-year survival data reveal overall survival rates of less than 60%, although the patients who do survive often endure major functional, cosmetic, and psychological burdens as a result of their difficulties in speaking and eating.

Alternatives

An alternative to glossectomy is the insertion of radioactive wires into the cancerous tissue. This is an effective treatment but requires specialized surgical skills and facilities.

Resources

BOOKS

"Disorders of the Oral Region: Neoplasms." in *The Merck Manual of Diagnosis and Therapy*, edited by Mark H. Beers, MD, and Robert Berkow, MD. Whitehouse Station, NJ: Merck Research Laboratories, 2007.

Johnson, J. T., ed. *Reconstruction of the Oral Cavity.* Alexandria, VA: American Academy of Otolaryngology, 1994.

Shah, J. P., J. G. Batsakis, and J. Shah. *Oral Cancer.* Oxford, UK: Isis Medical Media, 2003.

PERIODICALS

Barry, B., B. Baujat, S. Albert, et al. "Total Glossectomy Without Laryngectomy as First-Line or Salvage Therapy." *Laryngoscope* 113 (February 2003): 373-376.

Chuanjun, C., Z. Zhiyuan, G. Shaopu, et al. "Speech After Partial Glossectomy: A Comparison Between Reconstruction and Nonreconstruction Patients." *Journal of Oral and Maxillofacial Surgery* 60 (April 2002): 404-407.

Furia, C. L., L. P. Kowalski, M. R. Latorre, et al. "Speech Intelligibility After Glossectomy and Speech Rehabilitation." *Archives of Otolaryngology - Head & Neck Surgery* 127 (July 2001): 877-883.

Kimata, Y., K. Uchiyama, S. Ebihara, et al. "Postoperative Complications and Functional Results After Total Glossectomy with Microvascular Reconstruction." *Plastic Reconstructive Surgery* 106 (October 2000): 1028-1035.

OTHER

"Oral Cavity Cancer." *Cancer Information Network*.www.ontumor.com/oral/.

"Tongue Base and Tonsil Cancer." *CancerAnswers.com*.www.canceranswers.com/Tongue.Base.Tonsil.html.

ORGANIZATIONS

American Academy of Otolaryngology - Head and Neck Surgery. One Prince Street, Alexandria, VA 22314. (703) 806-4444. www.entnet.org.

American Cancer Society. National Headquarters, 1599 Clifton Road NE, Atlanta, GA 30329. (800) ACS -2345. www.cancer.org

Oral Cancer Foundation. 3419 Via Lido, #205, Newport Beach, CA 92663. (949) 646-8000. www.oralcancer.org

Monique Laberge, Ph.D.

Glutamine

Definition

Glutamine is an amino acid that is used as a nutritional supplement in the treatment of a variety of diseases, including **cancer**.

Purpose

Glutamine is the most abundant free amino acid in the human body and, in addition to its role as a component of protein, serves a variety of functions in the body. It is a non-essential amino acid because it is made by body cells. In addition most dietary protein contains ample amounts of glutamine and healthy people usually obtain all the additional glutamine that they need in their diet.

KEY TERMS

Arginine—An essential amino acid derived from dietary protein; sometimes used in combination with glutamine to boost the immune system.

Beta-hydroxy-beta-methylbutyrate, HMB—A nutritional supplement used to buildup muscles and to treat muscle-wasting caused by disease.

Bone marrow transplant, BMT—The destruction of bone marrow by high-dose chemotherapy or radiation and its replacement with healthy bone marrow taken from the patient prior to chemotherapy or from a donor.

Cachexia—Severe malnutrition, weakness, and muscle-wasting caused by disease.

Gluconeogenesis—The formation of glucose from non-carbohydrates such as protein or fat.

Glutaminase—The enzyme that breaks down glutamine; high glutaminase activity may be correlated with the proliferation of cancer cells.

Glutathione (GSH)—A three-amino-acid tripeptide that reduces harmful oxygen radicals and activates some proteins, including natural killer cells.

Hepatic veno-occlusive disease—Liver failure caused by chemotherapy that may benefit from glutamine supplementation.

Lymphocyte—A white blood cell of the immune system, making up 25–33% of all adult white blood cells.

Mucositis—A common, painful inflammation of the membranes of the mouth caused by chemotherapy.

Natural killer cell—A type of lymphocyte that kills cancer cells and certain microorganisms.

Parenteral nutrition (PN)—Intravenous feeding.

Short bowel syndrome—A condition that occurs after a large segment of the small intestine has been removed; it is treated with glutamine.

Tryptophan—An essential amino acid that is sometimes used in combination with glutamine supplementation.

Cancer and other diseases and injuries induce a state of physiologic stress that is characterized by glutamine deficiency. This deficiency is aggravated by **chemotherapy** and **radiation therapy** used to treat cancer. Therefore, glutamine is sometimes described as a conditionally essential amino acid that needs to be supplemented when the body is stressed.

Cancer-related glutamine deficiency can reduce the tolerance of normal tissues to cancer treatment, necessitating reduced doses and possibly diminishing the effects of treatment. Glutamine supplementation may help protect normal tissues from chemotherapy and radiation while sensitizing tumor cells to these agents.

Increasingly in the early 2000s, glutamine is considered an important component of both oral and parenteral (intravenous) nutrition (PN) therapy during high-dose chemotherapy and radiation treatment. It also is used as a nutritional supplement for bone marrow transplant (BMT) patients, particularly those with leukemia or **lymphoma** whose bone marrow has been destroyed with high-dose chemotherapy.

Glutamine supplementation appears to do the following:

- improve nitrogen retention
- decrease the incidence of infection
- decrease the length of hospitalization, saving thousands of dollars

Glutamine supplementation also appears to reduce the incidence of gastrointestinal, nervous system, and heart complications arising from cancer therapy. Oral glutamine may reduce **diarrhea** and the duration and severity of other gastrointestinal side effects of chemotherapy. In particular it appears to help prevent the intestinal toxicity of the cancer drug **fluorouracil**. Glutamine may reduce the incidence and severity of **mucositis**, a common, painful inflammation of the membranes of the oral cavity that can result from chemotherapy. Rinsing with a glutamine-containing mouthwash can help reduce mouth sores from radiation and chemotherapy treatments. Glutamine also appears to reduce the need for antifungal agents during chemotherapy.

Description

Glutamine (Gln) or L-glutamine is available by prescription as a powder called NutreStore. It is taken as an oral suspension for treating short bowel syndrome. It also is available in nutritional formulas and as an individual nutritional supplement. As an intravenous supplement it may be supplied in the form of alanyl-glutamine dipeptide or glycyl-glutamine dipeptide.

Metabolic effects

There is much speculation about why glutamine appears to be a beneficial adjunct for cancer treatment. Glutamine is required for numerous metabolic processes, including the following:

- Regulation of cell growth and function.

- Synthesis of proteins and nucleic acids (DNA and RNA).

- Movement of nitrogen in the body. Glutamine is the body's primary means of transferring ammonia in a nontoxic form.

- Gluconeogenesis—the formation of glucose from protein and fat.

- Maintenance of acid-base equilibrium in the body.

- As a major fuel for intestinal mucosal cells.

- Improved kidney cell function.

Tumors cause major disruptions in nitrogen and glutamine metabolism. The high rate of protein synthesis in rapidly growing tumors requires a continuous supply of amino acids. Tumors are referred to as nitrogen traps because they actively compete with normal tissues for nitrogen-containing compounds such as glutamine. Tumors also are referred to as glutamine traps because glutamine moves from normal tissues to tumors. Some evidence suggests that glutamine supplementation may diminish tumor growth, in part by improving overall protein metabolism.

Cancer cells generally move glutamine across their cell membranes at a faster rate than normal cells. Glutaminase—the enzyme that breaks down glutamine—has increased activity in cancerous cells, and there is evidence that glutaminase activity correlates with the proliferation of malignant cells.

Immunological effects

Glutamine and arginine may be referred to as immunonutrients because of their important roles in the functioning of the immune system that protects the body from foreign entities, including cancer cells. Glutamine helps to regulate the immune system and is a major fuel for lymphocytes (a type of white blood cell) and other immune system cells. In cancer patients undergoing chemotherapy and total body irradiation, glutamine has been shown to boost the immune system by increasing the levels of circulating lymphocytes and other cells of the immune system.

In patients undergoing chemotherapy with radioactive drugs for advanced **esophageal cancer**, oral glutamine supplementation helped to protect immune system function by causing lymphocytes to divide and multiply. Glutamine supplementation also reduced the permeability of the gastrointestinal tract in these patients.

Antioxidative effects

Glutamine appears to be the rate-limiting factor for the production of liver and intestinal glutathione (GSH), a chemical that protects cells against the damaging effects of oxidation. As cancer cells deplete the glutamine in normal cells, the levels of GSH drop. It has been suggested that PN without added glutamine may itself decrease GSH levels and increase oxidative damage. By increasing GSH levels, oral glutamine supplementation also may increase the selectivity of **anticancer drugs** by protecting normal cells from oxidative damage caused by the drugs. Glutamine supplementation also appears to protect normal cells from radiation-induced oxidative damage. Since GSH depletion reduces the activity of natural killer cells (immune system cells that destroy cancer cells) glutamine supplementation may increase GSH levels and restore natural-killer-cell activity. Some evidence suggests that this may diminish tumor growth.

Effectiveness

Glutamine supplementation during cancer therapy and bone marrow or stem cell transplantation remains under investigation. Although some studies have demonstrated specific benefits in at least some types of cancer, numerous animal and human studies have shown no clear benefit or any effect on tumor response or on the side effects of chemotherapy. However, one study suggested that glutamine supplementation could increase the likelihood of long-term survival in patients with cancers of the blood.

Other studies have found that glutamine supplementation in cancer patients receiving high-dose chemotherapy and BMT decreases the incidence and/or severity of the following:

- chemotherapy-associated mucositis
- diarrhea associated with irinotecan, a drug used to treat colon and rectal cancers
- nervous system damage caused by the anticancer drug paclitaxel
- cardiac toxicity caused by the drug anthracycline

Combination supplements

Cancer-related cachexia (severe malnutrition, weakness, and muscle-wasting) is caused by the increased breakdown of proteins and reduced protein synthesis in patients with advanced cancer. One study demonstrated that supplementation with specific nutrients, including a combination of glutamine, beta-hydroxy-beta-methylbutyrate (HMB), and arginine, could reverse these processes. Patients with stage

IV cancer who received this combination gained significant fat-free body mass in four weeks and continuing over a period of 24 weeks, as compared to control patients who lost body mass.

Case studies have reported that the administration of glutamine orally and intravenously, in combination with oral vitamin E, decreases the signs and symptoms of hepatic veno-occlusive disease. This is an often-fatal type of liver failure that occurs in patients treated with high-dose chemotherapy in preparation for BMT.

Recommended dosage

Glutamine supplementation generally is started three to five days before chemotherapy. The glutamine dosage used to treat short bowel syndrome is 5 g, six times per day for up to 16 weeks. It is taken with food, every two to three hours while awake. Nutritional guidelines for cancer patients generally recommend 2–4 g of glutamine per day to protect against radiation-induced **enteritis** (intestinal inflammation).

Dosages used in clinical studies of glutamine supplementation in cancer patients vary:

- 18–30 g per day, orally
- 10 g three times per day, orally
- 0.57 g per kg (2.2 lb.) of body weight per day
- 50 g per day of dipeptide glycyl-glutamine, intravenously
- 0.4 g per kg (2.2 lb.) of body weight per day of dipeptide glycyl-glutamine, intravenously
- 14 g of glutamine per day in combination with arginine and HMB for up to 24 weeks

Precautions

Glutamine, taken orally or by injection, appears to be safe; however, precautions include the following:

- Excess amino acids may be excreted in the urine without being absorbed by the body.
- Excess amino acids can harm the kidneys.
- Glutamine, like any drug, can potentially cause an allergic reaction.
- It is not known whether glutamine supplementation is safe during pregnancy or while breastfeeding.
- Elderly patients may be more sensitive to glutamine supplementation, requiring lower doses.
- Glutamine can worsen liver disease.

Since glutamine is essential for the growth of both healthy and cancerous cells, it is theoretically possible that glutamine could fuel tumor cells, leading to more rapid growth. However, there is no evidence to suggest this, nor is there evidence that glutamine supplementation adversely affects treatment or clinical outcomes.

Side effects

Glutamine supplementation in cancer patients does not appear to cause side effects or adversely affect quality of life.

Interactions

Glutamine supplementation is not known to negatively interact with other medications.

Margaret Alic, Ph.D.

GM-CSF *see* **Sargramostim**

Gonadal dysfunction *see* **Fertility issues**

Goserelin acetate

Definition

Goserelin acetate is a synthetic (man-made) hormone that acts similarly to the naturally occurring gonadotropin-releasing hormone (GnRH). It is available in the United States under the tradename Zoladex.

Purpose

Goserelin acetate is used primarily to counter the symptoms of late-stage **prostate cancer** in men or is offered as an alternative to treat prostate **cancer** when surgery to remove the testes or estrogen therapy is not an option or is unacceptable for the patient. Goserelin is also given as combination therapy with the drug flutamide to manage prostate cancer that is locally confined and not widespread. It is often used to ease the pain and discomfort of women suffering from endometrosis and to relieve symptoms in women with advanced **breast cancer**.

Description

Goserelin acetate is a man-made protein that mimics many of the actions of gonadotropin-releasing hormone (GnRH). In men, this results in decreased blood levels of the male hormone **testosterone**. In women, it decreases blood levels of the female hormone estrogen.

Recommended dosage

Goserelin acetate is given in the form of an implant containing 3.6 mg of the medication. This implant is placed just under the skin of the upper abdominal wall. The drug lasts for 28 days, after which a new implant has to be placed. Goserelin is also available in a dose of 10.8 mg, in which case the drugs lasts for three months.

Precautions

If a woman becomes pregnant while taking this drug, goserelin acetate may cause birth defects or the loss of the pregnancy. It is not known if goserelin is passed into breast milk; therefore, it is not recommended to breast feed while on this drug.

Goserelin acetate will also interfere with the chemical actions of birth control pills. For this reason, sexually active women who do not wish to become pregnant should use some form of birth control other than birth control pills during treatment with goserelin acetate and for at least 12 weeks after the completion of treatment.

Goserelin acetate will cause sterility in men, at least for the duration of the treatment.

Side effects

In patients of both sexes, common side effects of goserelin acetate include:

- sweating accompanied by feelings of warmth (hot flashes)
- a decrease in sex drive
- depression or other mood changes
- headache
- tumor flare, which is exhibited as bone pain (this is due to a temporary initial increase in testosterone/estrogen before its production is finally decreased)

Other common side effects in men include:

- impotence (erectile dysfunction)
- sterility
- breast enlargement

Other common side effects in women include:

- light, irregular, vaginal bleeding
- no menstrual period
- vaginal dryness and/or itching
- emotional instability
- depression
- change in breast size
- an increase in facial or body hair
- deepening of the voice

Less common side effects, in patients of either sex, include:

- nausea and vomiting
- insomnia
- weight gain
- swollen feet or lower legs
- acne or other skin rashes
- abdominal pain
- increased appetite

A doctor should be consulted immediately if the patient experiences any of the above symptoms.

Interactions

There are no known interactions of goserelin acetate with any food or beverage.

Patients taking goserelin acetate should consult their physician before taking any other prescription, over-the-counter, or herbal medication. Patients taking any other hormone or steroid-based medications should not take goserelin acetate without first consulting their physician.

See also Endometrial cancer; Ovarian cancer.

Paul A. Johnson, Ed.M.

Graft-vs.-host disease

Description

Graft-vs.-host disease is a response by the immune system that occurs when cells from a blood or bone marrow donor attack those of the recipient. The only transplanted tissues that contain enough immune cells to cause graft-vs.-host disease are the blood and the bone marrow. Blood transfusions are used every day in hospitals for many reasons. Bone marrow transplants are used to replace blood-forming cells and immune cells in **cancer** patients whose own bone marrow has been destroyed by **radiation therapy** or **chemotherapy**.

Blood transfusion graft-vs.-host disease affects mostly the blood. Blood cells perform three functions: carrying oxygen, fighting infections, and clotting. All of these functions are decreased in a transfusion graft-vs.-host reaction, leading to **anemia** (lack of red blood cells in the blood), reduced resistance to infections, and increased bleeding. The reaction occurs 4–30 days after the transfusion.

The tissues most affected by bone marrow graft-vs.-host disease are the skin, the liver, and the intestines. One of these forms of tissue is affected in nearly half of the patients who receive bone marrow transplants.

Bone marrow graft-vs.-host disease comes in both an acute and a chronic form. The acute form appears within two months of the transplant, while the chronic form usually appears within three months. The acute disease produces a skin rash, liver abnormalities, and **diarrhea** that can be bloody. The skin rash is primarily a patchy thickening of the skin. Chronic disease can produce a similar skin rash, a tightening or an inflammation of the skin, lesions in the mouth, drying of the eyes and mouth, hair loss (**alopecia**), liver damage, lung damage, and indigestion. The symptoms are similar to an autoimmune disease called scleroderma.

Both forms of graft-vs.-host disease bring with them an increased risk of infections, either because of the process itself or its treatment with cortisone-like drugs and immunosuppressives that inhibit the **immune response**. Patients can die of liver failure, **infection**, or other severe disturbances of their system.

Causes

Cells from the donor who has an active immune system may be transplanted along with the organ or tissue into the host who has a suppressed immune system. These transplanted cells attack the host's body, causing graft-vs.-host disease. Substances made in the body called cytokines are thought to play a role in the development of this reaction. Cytokines are protein substances made by cells that affect other cells.

Even if the donor and recipient are well matched, graft-vs.-host disease can still occur. There are many different components involved in generating immune reactions, and all people (except identical twins) are different. Testing can often find donors who match all the major components, but there are many minor ones that will always be different. Making a match between a donor and recipient depends upon the urgency of the need for a transplant and the chance that a suitable donor will be found.

Treatments

Both the acute and the chronic diseases are treated with cortisone-like drugs, immunosuppressive agents, or with **antibiotics** and immune chemicals from donated blood (gamma globulin). **Cyclosporine** and prednisone are two immunosuppressive drugs that are often used, and **methotrexate** may enhance efficacy. Another way to prevent graft-vs.-host disease is, before transplantation, rid donor bone marrow of the immune cells (T cells) that would attack the recipient's body. Another possibility to avoid complications in **bone marrow transplantation** is to cleanse the bone marrow of cancer cells and use the patient's own cells to grow more bone marrow. Cancer cells that reside in the bone marrow may be removed, leaving behind only those cells that are needed to grow new blood cells (stem cells). These stem cells from the patient can be grown and returned back to the patient.

For recipients of blood transfusions who are especially likely to have graft-vs.-host reactions, the red blood cells can safely be irradiated (using **x rays**) to kill all the immune cells. The red blood cells are less sensitive to radiation and are not harmed by this treatment.

New directions in research may help to solve the problem of graft-vs.-host disease. A potential source for new stem cells is the umbilical cord. Cells from this area do not give such strong immune reactions and may be useful for re-establishing cell populations. Another potential is to use genetically engineered cells to correct genetic defects in stem cells within the marrow.

Alternative and complementary therapies

Alternative and complementary therapies range from herbal remedies, vitamin supplements, and special diets to spiritual practices, acupuncture, massage, and similar treatments. When these therapies are used in addition to conventional medicine, they are called complementary therapies. When they are used instead of conventional medicine, they are called alternative therapies.

Complementary or alternative therapies are widely used by people suffering with illness. Good nutrition and activities, such as yoga, meditation, and massage, that reduce stress and promote a positive view of life have no unwanted side effects and appear to be beneficial. Alternative and experimental treatments are normally not covered by insurance.

Special concerns

If graft-vs.-host disease is suspected as a complication to a cancer treatment, a skin punch **biopsy** may be performed to confirm this diagnosis. This is a relatively minor procedure in which the skin is anesthetized in a local area and a small piece is removed for testing in the laboratory.

Infection with one particular virus, called cytomegalovirus (CMV), is so likely a complication of graft-vs.-host disease that some experts recommend treating it in advance, using ganciclovir or valacyclovir.

It is an interesting observation that patients with leukemia who develop graft-vs.-host disease are less likely to have a recurrence of the leukemia that was being treated. This phenomenon is called graft-vs.-leukemia.

Bone marrow transplant patients who do not have a graft-vs.-host reaction gradually return to normal immune function in a year. A graft-vs.-host reaction may prolong the diminished immune capacity indefinitely, requiring supplemental treatment with immunoglobulins (gamma globulin). The grafted cells develop a tolerance to the recipient's body after 6–12 months, and the medications can be gradually withdrawn.

Graft-vs.-host disease is not the only complication of blood transfusion or bone marrow transplantation. Host-vs.-graft disease, or rejection, occurs when the recipient's immune system is strong enough to attack the transplant. This is also a common occurrence and may require a repeat transplant with another donor organ. Infections are a constant threat in bone marrow transplant because of the disease being treated, the prior radiation or chemotherapy and the medications used to treat the transplant.

See also Bone marrow transplantation; Transfusion therapy.

Resources

BOOKS

Anderson, William L. *Immunology*. Madison, CT: Fence Creek Publishing, 1999.

Janeway, Charles A., et al. *Immunobiology: The Immune System in Health and Disease*. New York, NY: Current Biology Publications; London, England: Elsevier Science London/Garland Publishing, 1999.

Roitt, Ivan and Arthur Rabson. *Really Essential Medical Immunology*. Malden, MA: Blackwell Science, 2000.

OTHER

Complementary and Alternative Medicine Website for the American Cancer Society. http:cancer.org/alt_therapy/index.html.

University of Michigan Patient Education Resource Center (PERC). http://www.cancer.med.umich.edu htm.

University of Michigan Transplant Center. http://www.med.umich.edu/trans/public/.

J. Ricker Polsdorfer, M.D.
Jill Granger, M.S.

Granisetron *see* **Antiemetics**

Gynecologic cancers

Definition

Gynecologic cancers are malignant tumors within the female reproductive organs. Gynecologic cancers include cervical, endometrial (uterine), ovarian, vaginal, and vulvar cancers

Demographics

In the United States the most commonly diagnosed **cancer** of the female reproductive organs is **endometrial cancer** with approximately 42, 160 new cases expected to be diagnosed in 2009. About 50% of the new cases of endometrial cancer occur in women between the ages of 55 and 74 years. The incidence of this type of cancer is higher in white women but more black women die from endometrial cancer than white women. Almost 8,000 women are expected to die from endometrial cancer in the United States in 2009.

The estimated number of new cases of **ovarian cancer** (cancer of the ovaries) in the U.S. in 2009 is 21,550. Ovarian cancers account for about 5% of all cancers in women. Ovarian cancer is the eighth most common cancer in females and the fifth leading cause of death from cancer in women with about 14,600 deaths expected in 2009. Older women (over the age of 60) are most often diagnosed with this type of cancer. Incidence rates for ovarian cancers have been decreasing in recent years.

Over 11,000 new cases of invasive cancers of the cervix (**cervical cancer**) are expected to be diagnosed in 2009 with approximately 4,000 deaths attributed to this type of cancer. The death rate from cervical cancer has declined by almost 75% since the mid-1950s due to implementation of PAP screening for cervical cancer detection. Most women are diagnosed with cervical

Gynecologic cancers

Cancer type	Occurs in	Tumor types
Endometrial cancer	Uterus	Endometrioid tumors Clear-cell carcinomas Papillary serous Sarcomas Mixed tumors
Fallopian tube cancer	Fallopian tubes, but frequently spreads	Serous carcinomas Mucinous tumors Endometrioid tumors
Cervical cancer	Cervix	Squamous cell carcinomas Adenocarcinomas Clear-cell carcinoma Serous carcinoma Glassy-cell carcinoma
Ovarian cancer	Ovaries	Serous carcinomas Mucinous tumors Endometrioid tumors
Vaginal cancer	Vagina	Squamous cell carcinoma Adenocarcinoma Melanoma Sarcoma
Vulvar cancer	Vulva	Squamous cell carcinomas Melanoma Basal cell carcinoma Paget's disease Adenocarcinomas

(Table by GGS Creative Resources. Cengage Learning, Gale.)

cancer prior to the age of 50 but 20% of cases are diagnosed in women over the age of 65 years. Hispanic and African American women are considered high risk groups for the development of cervical cancer.

Cancers of the vulva and vagina account for 4% and 1% of all female reproductive tract cancers respectively. In 2009, the American Cancer Society estimates the diagnosis of 3,580 new cases of vulvar cancers and 2,160 new cases of vaginal cancers. Approximately 900 women will die from **vulvar cancer** and about 800 women will die from **vaginal cancer** in the United States in 2009.

Description

The female reproductive tract is comprised of the ovaries, fallopian tubes, uterus, cervix, vagina, and vulva. Together, these organs allow a woman to become pregnant, protect and nourish an unborn baby, and give birth. An understanding of each organ and its role in reproduction may help the patient to understand her particular gynecologic cancer. There are two ovaries, which are the internal organs dedicated to producing eggs. Released eggs are captured by the fallopian tubes, through which the egg (or fertilized egg) travels to the womb (uterus). The lining of the uterus (endometrium) responds to female hormones, such as estrogen, and becomes thickened to allow for implantation of a fertilized egg. The cervix is the opening of the uterus which opens (dilates) during labor to allow for passage of the baby. The vagina is a short tube that extends from the outer female genitalia (vulva) to the cervix.

Gynecologic cancers are defined not solely by the organ affected but also by the type of cancerous cells in the tumor. The type of cancer depends on the cell types that make up an organ. Adenocarcinomas are cancers that contain primarily cells originating from glands or ducts. Squamous cell carcinomas are tumors that arose from squamous cells, the main cell type found in skin. Sarcomas are cancers that originated from cells of basic connective tissue (mesenchymal cells). Sarcomas are comprised of cells that have become specialized (differentiated) and are named according to the predominant cell type. Endometreoid tumors are those that originated from the endometrium. Clear-cell **carcinoma** is a rare gynecologic tumor that contains cells from the mullerian duct, which gives rise to the uterus, vagina, and fallopian tubes during development.

Because the reproductive organs are interconnected, spread of cancer from one organ to another (direct extension) is not uncommon. Gynecologic cancer carries the name of the organ where the cancer originated (primary cancer site). For example, a tumor restricted to the vagina would be "primary vaginal cancer," whereas one that has extended from the cervix to the vagina would be "primary cervical cancer."

Risk factors

Risk factors for the different kinds of gynecologic cancer vary by type of cancer.

Risk factors related to the development of cervical cancer include:

- history of HPV infection
- history of smoking
- infection with human immunodeficiency virus (HIV)
- chlamydial infection
- diet low in fruits and vegetables
- long-term use of oral contraceptives
- history of multiple pregnancies
- women whose mothers used the drug di-ethylstilbesterol (DES) during pregnancy
- family history of cervical cancer

Risk factors related to the development of endometrial cancer include:

- use of estrogen replacement therapy

- history of early menarche (before age 12) and late menopause (after age 55)
- women who have never been pregnant
- obesity
- small risk (1 in 500) for women taking the drug tamoxifen
- history of polycystic ovarian syndrome
- increasing age
- diet high in animal fat
- history of diabetes
- family history of endometrial cancer
- family history of hereditary nonpolyposis colon cancer
- personal history of breast or ovarian cancer
- prior radiation therapy to the pelvic area of the body
- history of endometrial hyperplasia

Risk factors associated with the development of ovarian cancer include:

- increasing age
- obesity
- history of never being pregnant
- use of androgen drugs
- post-menopausal estrogen use
- family history of ovarian, breast or colorectal cancer
- personal history of breast cancer

Risk factors related to the development of vaginal cancer include:

- increasing age
- women whose mothers took DES in pregnancy have a small risk (1 in 1000)
- personal history of vaginal adenosis
- HPV infection
- HIV infection
- history of cervical cancer
- smoking and alcohol use

Risk factors related to the development of vulvar cancer include:

- increasing age
- HPV infection especially in younger women
- smoking
- HIV infection
- presence of a pre-cancerous condition called vulvar intraepithelial neoplasia (VIN) which is a precursor to squamous cell carcinoma of the vulva
- presence of a dermatologic condition of the vulva called lichen sclerosus
- history of cervical cancer
- personal or family history of melanoma

Types of cancers

Uterine cancer, also called endometrial cancer, is the most common gynecologic cancer. Endometrial cancer primarily affects postmenopausal women, however, 25% of cases are in premenopausal women. There are two types of endometrial cancer: estrogen-dependent and non-estrogen-dependent. Estrogen-dependent cancers are usually comprised of well-differentiated cells and are associated with a good outcome and a long survival time. Non-estrogen-dependent cancers are usually made up of poorly differentiated cells and are invasive and associated with a poor prognosis. Uterine tumors are most frequently endometrioid tumors, usually adenocarcinomas. Clear-cell carcinomas, papillary serous, sarcomas, and mixed tumors also occur.

Ovarian cancer is the second most common cancer of the female reproductive organs. It accounts for 30% of all gynecologic cancers and 53% of the deaths in this group. The high death rate associated with ovarian cancer is due to the fact that most women are not diagnosed until the cancer has progressed to an advanced stage. The average age at diagnosis is 63 years. Serous carcinomas are the most common type of ovarian cancer. Other common types of ovarian cancer include mucinous tumors and endometrioid tumors.

Fallopian tube cancers, as primary cancers, are very rare. They frequently spread widely within the abdominal cavity. Although often diagnosed earlier than ovarian cancer, fallopian tube cancer produces similar symptoms and originates from similar cell types as ovarian cancer.

Cervical cancer is the third most common cancer of the female reproductive tract. Although cervical cancer can affect any adult woman, there are peaks of occurrence around the ages of 37 years and 62 years. Although cervical cancer used to be one of the most common causes of death among American women, in the past 50 years there has been a 75% decrease in mortality from cervical cancer. This primarily due to routine screening with Pap tests to identify pre-cancerous and early-stage invasive stages of cervical cancer. Between 60% and 80% of the cases of cervical cancer are squamous cell carcinomas with the remainder being adenocarcinomas. Clear-cell carcinoma, serous carcinoma, and glassy-cell carcinoma are less frequent cervical cancers.

Cervical cancer is very strongly associated with the **human papilloma virus** (HPV). HPV **infection** accounts for the cause of approximately 90% of all cervical cancer cases. A vaccine, which was introduced in 2006, protects against the two HPV strains that cause 70% of all cervical cancers. The vaccine is known to protect against HPV for at least five years. However, it does not protect or treat women who are already infected with HPV. The vaccine is recommended for females ages 9 through 26 years.

Vulvar cancer is rare and accounts for 4% of the gynecologic cancers. It most often strikes women in their sixties. Squamous cell carcinoma is the most common type and **melanoma** is the second most common type of vulvar cancer. Other types of vulvar cancer include **basal cell carcinoma**, Paget's disease, and adenocarcinomas (arising from the Bartholin's, Skene's, or sweat glands). There is an association between vulvar cancer and human papilloma virus.

Vaginal cancer is also a rare type of cancer and accounts for just 1% of the gynecologic cancers. It most often strikes women in their sixties. Greater than 90% of the vaginal cancers are squamous cell carcinomas. **Adenocarcinoma**, melanoma, and **sarcoma** account for the remaining cases. There is an association between vaginal cancer and human papilloma virus.

Causes and symptoms

The exact cause of most cases of gynecologic cancers remain unknown at this time although several risk factors which place women at higher risk for specific types of gynecologic cancers have been identified.

Symptoms associated with cervical cancer include abnormal vaginal bleeding especially after sexual intercourse. Other symptoms include bleeding between periods or after menopause. Unusual vaginal discharge and pain after intercourse are also symptoms of cervical cancer.

Episodes of unusual bleeding such as bleeding between periods and after menopause are also symptoms of endometrial cancer as is unusual vaginal discharge. Other symptoms, which may be indicative of advanced disease, include pain in the pelvic area and **weight loss**.

Symptoms of vaginal cancer are similar to the symptoms associated with other gynecological cancers including abnormal bleeding and vaginal discharge. Other symptoms include pain during intercourse, pain upon urination, constipation and pain the pelvic area.

Women with ovarian cancer may not experience any symptoms or may experience only vague symptoms until the cancer spreads beyond the ovaries. Symptoms of ovarian cancer include bloating, pain in the abdomen or pelvis, early satiety or the sensation of feeling full after eating very little. Other symptoms include back pain, pain during intercourse, constipation and menstrual changes.

Symptoms associated with cancer of the vulva are somewhat different from that of the other gynecologic cancers. Symptoms associated with VIN include vulvar skin that is often lighter or thicker. There may also be lumps and/or bumps as well as other skin changes including the appearance of cauliflower- or wart-like growths on the vulva. Other non-dermatologic symptoms include persistent **itching**, pain, burning, bleeding, discharge, and/or painful urination.

Diagnosis

Examination

When a gynecologic cancer is suspected, a physical examination, often including an abdominal/pelvic examination will be conducted. The patient may be referred to a gynecologic oncologist for further examination and evaluation.

Tests

Blood tests which may be ordered include a complete blood count (CBC) with platelet count and blood chemistry profile with liver function tests. Other specialized blood tests such as testing for **tumor markers** may be done depending on the type of cancer. For example, CA-125 is considered a tumor marker for ovarian cancer. Levels of CA-125 may be elevated in some women with ovarian cancer.

Other tests may be done specific to a particular cancer including cervical **cytology** tests (such as a Pap test or smear) to determine presence of cervical or uterine cancers. Evaluation of the gastrointestinal system may be clinically indicated as well.

Imaging tests which may be ordered include chest imaging, ultrasound, and/or computerized axial tomography (CT scans) of the abdomen and/or pelvis. **Positron emission tomography** scans (PET scans) may also be included in the workup for gynecologic cancers.

Procedures

Procedures which may be included in the work-up related to the diagnosis of gynecologic cancers include endometrial **biopsy** of uterine tumors, cervical and cone biopsies for cervical cancer and cytoscopy/proctoscopy if there is suspicion of bladder and/or bowel involvement of tumor.

Treatment

Treatment of gynecologic cancers is dependent on several factors including: type of cancer, the extent of tumor involvement or stage of the cancer at time of diagnosis, and patient characteristics such as age and presence of other concurrent medical conditions.

Modalities used in the treatment of an endometrial tumor which considered to be operable include surgical removal of the uterus, cervix, fallopian tubes and ovaries. Adjuvant treatment options which may be employed following surgery include vaginal brachytherapy with or without **radiation therapy** directed to the pelvis and may also include treatment with **chemotherapy**. Women who are less than 60 years old and who are diagnosed with minimal-sized tumors that have not invaded the lymph nodes may be observed prior to being offered further adjuvant treatment.

Primary treatment for ovarian cancer includes laparotomy with total abdominal hysterectomy and bilateral or unilateral salpingo-oophorectomy (performed in select patients to preserve fertility options). All suspicious and/or enlarged lymph nodes should be removed during surgery. Some patients may require surgical removal of the appendix, the spleen and/or parts of the bowel. Chemotherapy may be used prior to surgery to reduce the size of the tumor. Chemotherapy administered after surgery for ovarian cancer includes the drugs **cisplatin**, paclitaxel, **docetaxel** and **carboplatin**.

Treatment options for cervical cancer depend on tumor stage and include observation (for early Stage 1 tumors), hysterectomy, pelvic radiation/brachytherapy, and cisplatin-containing chemotherapy regimens.

The preferred modality for the treatment of most vaginal cancers is radiation therapy. Radiation therapy for vaginal cancer can be delivered via external beam radiation, intracavitary brachytherapy, or by interstitial radiation. Surgery to treat this type of cancer is used only if the cancer is not cured by radiation. Surgery may be an option to remove small Stage 1 tumors. Chemotherapy has not proven to be an effective option in the treatment of vaginal cancers. However, chemotherapy may be used prior to surgery to shrink the tumor size and may be administered concurrently with radiation therapy to enhance the effects of the radiation. Laser surgery and topical drugs such as imiquimod and the chemotherapy drug 5-FU are used to treat cases of non-invasive vaginal cancer.

Surgical treatment options for vulvar cancer include laser surgery, surgical excision of the cancer and surrounding tissue margins, vulvectomy (removal of all or part of the vulva), and pelvic **exenteration**, a procedure which entails removal of the vulva, the pelvic lymph nodes, and possibly the lower colon, rectum, bladder, uterus, cervix, and vagina. Extent of the exenteration depends on the extent of cancer involvement. Radiation therapy

QUESTIONS TO ASK YOUR DOCTOR

- What type of gynecological cancer do I have?
- What are my treatment options?
- Will I require surgery? How extensive will my surgery be?
- Will I still be able to have children after my surgery?
- What side effects can I expect after my cancer treatments?
- How long will my treatments last?
- What is my overall prognosis?

may be given directed to lymph nodes in the groin and pelvis. Chemotherapy, utilizing drugs such as cisplatin, mitomycin, and 5-FU, has been used in the treatment of advanced vulvar cancer but with minimal positive results to date.

Prognosis

Prognosis related to the gynecologic cancers varies by cancer type and is determined by stage of diagnosis. Detection of the cancer in earlier stages is related to better overall survival. The overall 5-year survival rate by specific gynecologic cancer type is as follows:

- cervical cancer – 71%
- endometrial cancer – 73%
- ovarian cancer – 46%
- vaginal cancer -50%

Prevention

The exact cause of most gynecologic cancers is not currently known. However, certain risk factors have been identified which can place women at higher risk for the development of certain types of gynecologic cancers. When possible, steps should be taken to minimize the possibility for developing these cancers. Girls and young women between the ages of 9 and 26 years should be vaccinated with the cervical cancer vaccine. In addition, women should adhere to recommended annual screening guidelines and practices related to the early detection of specific gynecologic cancers as recommended by the American Cancer Society and other national organizations.

Resources

BOOKS

Ozols, R.F., Rubin, S.C., Thomas, G., etal"Epithelial Ovarian Cancer." In*Principles and Practice of Gynecologic Oncology, 4th Edition*,edited by Hoskins, W.J., Perez, C.A., Young, R.C. Philadelphia: Lippincott, Williams, and Wilkins, 2005.

PERIODICALS

Andersen, M.R., Goff, B.A., Lowe, K.A., et al."Combining a Symptoms Index with CA125 to Improve Detection of Ovarian Cancer."*Cancer*113(2008):184–9.

FUTURE II Study Group."Quadrivalent Vaccine Against Human Papillomavirus to Prevent High-grade Cervical Lesions."*N Engl J Med*356(2007):1915–27.

Monk, B.J., Tewari, K.S., Koh, W-J."Multimodality Treatment for Locally Advanced Cerivcal Carcinoma: State of the Art and Future Directions."*J Clin Oncol.*25(2007):2952–65.

Ueda, S.M., Kapp, D.S., Cheung, M.K., et al."Trends in Demographic and Clinical Characteristics in Women Diagnosed with Corpus Cancer and Their Potential Impact on the Increasing Number of Deaths."*Am J Obstet Gynecol.*198(2008):198, e1-6.

OTHER

National Comprehensive Cancer Network. "NCCN Clinical Practice Guidelines in Oncology, Cervical Cancer." vol.1. 2009. http://www.nccn.org/professionals/ physician_gls/PDF/cervical.pdf[cited September 23,2009].

National Comprehensive Cancer Network. "NCCN Clinical Practice Guidelines in Oncology, Ovarian Cancer." vol.2. 2009. http://www.nccn.org/professionals/ physician_gls/PDF/ovarian.pdf[cited September 23, 2009].

National Comprehensive Cancer Network. "NCCN Clinical Practice Guidelines in Oncology, Uterine Neoplasms." vol. 2. 2009. http://www.nccn.org/professionals/ physician_gls/PDF/uterine.pdf[cited September 23, 2009].

ORGANIZATIONS

American Cancer Society. 1599 Clifton Rd. NE, Atlanta, GA 30329. (800) ACS-2345. http://www.cancer.org.

Cancer Research Institute, National Headquarters. 681 Fifth Ave., New York, NY 10022. (800) 992-2623. http://www.cancerresearch.org.

Gynecologic Cancer Foundation. 230 W. Monroe, Suite 2528 Chicago, IL 60606. (312) 578-1439. http:// www.wcn.org/gcf.

National Institutes of Health. National Cancer Institute. 9000 Rockville Pike, Bethesda, MD 20982. (800) 4-CANCER. <http://cancer.gov>.

Belinda Rowland, Ph.D.
Melinda Granger Oberleitner, R.N., D.N.S., A.P.R.N., C.N.S.

Hair loss *see* **Alopecia**

Hairy cell leukemia

Definition

Hairy cell leukemia is a disease in which a type of white blood cell called the lymphocyte, present in the blood and bone marrow, becomes malignant and proliferates. It is called hairy cell leukemia because the cells have tiny hair-like projections when viewed under the microscope.

Description

Hairy cell leukemia (HCL) is a rare **cancer**. It was first described in 1958 as *leukemic reticuloendotheliosis*, erroneously referring to a red blood cell because researchers were unsure of the cell of origin. It became more easily identifiable in the 1970s. There are approximately 600 new cases diagnosed every year in the United States, making up about 2% of the adult cases of leukemia each year.

HCL is found in cells located in the blood. There are three types of cells found in the blood: the red blood cells that carry oxygen to all the parts of the body; the white blood cells that are responsible for fighting **infection** and protecting the body from diseases; and the platelets that help in the clotting of blood. Hairy cell leukemia affects a type of white blood cell called the lymphocyte. Lymphocytes are made in the bone marrow, spleen, lymph nodes, and other organs. It specifically affects B-lymphocytes, which mature in the bone marrow. However, extremely rare variants of HCL have been discovered developing from T-lymphocytes, which mature in the thymus.

When hairy cell leukemia develops, the white blood cells become abnormal both in the way they appear (by acquiring hairy projections) and in the way they act (by proliferating without the normal control mechanisms). Further, the cells tend to accumulate in the spleen, causing it to become enlarged. The cells may also collect in the bone marrow and prevent it from producing normal blood cells. As a result, there may not be enough normal white blood cells in the blood to fight infection.

Demographics

The median age at which people develop HCL is 52 years. Though it occurs in all ages, HCL more commonly develops in the older population. Men are four times more likely to develop HCL than women. There have been reports of familial aggregation of disease, with higher occurrences in Ashkenazi Jewish men. A potential genetic link is undergoing further investigation.

Causes and symptoms

The cause of hairy cell leukemia is not specifically known. However, exposure to radiation is a known cause of leukemia in general. Familial involvement is another theory, suggesting that there is a genetic component associated with this disease.

HCL is a chronic (slowly progressing) disease, and the patients may not show any symptoms for many years. As the disease advances, the patients may suffer from one or more of the following symptoms:

- weakness
- fatigue
- recurrent infections
- fever
- anemia
- bruising
- pain or discomfort in the abdominal area

A magnified image of white blood cells with "hairy" projections. *(Photograph by M. Abbey, Photo Researchers, Inc. Reproduced by permission.)*

- weight loss (uncommon)
- night sweats (uncommon)

Pain and discomfort are caused by an enlarged spleen, which results from the accumulation of the abnormal hairy cells in the spleen. Blood tests may show abnormal counts of all the different types of cells. This happens because the cancerous cells invade the bone marrow as well and prevent it from producing normal blood cells. Because of the low white cell count in the blood, the patient may have frequent infections. **Fever** often accompanies the infections. The patient is most susceptible to bacterial infections, but infections of any kind are the major cause of death. The low red cell count may cause **anemia**, **fatigue**, and weakness, and the low platelet count may cause the person to bruise and bleed easily.

Diagnosis

When a patient suffers from the above symptoms, the doctor will palpate (examine with fingers) the abdomen and may order scans to see if the spleen is enlarged (splenomegaly). An enlarged spleen is present in 80% of patients. An enlarged liver is less common, but can occur.

If the spleen is enlarged, the doctor may order several blood tests. In these tests, the total numbers of each of the different types of blood cells (CBC) are reported. Sixty to eighty percent of patients suffer from pancytopenia, which is a dramatic reduction in the number of red blood cells, white blood cells, and platelets circulating in the blood.

If the blood tests are abnormal, the doctor may order a **bone marrow aspiration and biopsy**. In order to establish a diagnosis, hairy cells must be present in the bone marrow.

Treatment team

If the patient is seeing a primary care provider, the provider may perform the initial diagnostic tests. However, in order to diagnose and treat HCL comprehensively, the primary care provider will refer the patient to an oncologist (cancer specialist). Radiologists and pathologists will also be involved to read scans and examine tissue samples. Other specialists involved with the treatment of hairy cell leukemia will be nurses and dieticians who are available to explain side effects of treatment and offer suggestions on eating healthy meals that may help fight the side effects.

Clinical staging, treatments, and prognosis

When physicians perform blood tests, they will determine the level of hemoglobin (the oxygen-transporting molecule of red blood cells). Serum hemoglobin levels and the size of the spleen, which can be measured on exam and by using an x ray, are proposed criteria for determining the stage of HCL. The following are the three proposed stages and their criteria:

- Stage I: Hemoglobin greater than 12 g/dL (1 g = approximately 0.02 pint and 1 dL = approximately 0.33 ounce) and spleen less than or equal to 10 cm (3.9 inches).

- Stage II: Hemoglobin between 8.5 and 12 g/dL and spleen greater than 10 cm (3.9 inches).

- Stage III: Hemoglobin less than 8.5 g/dL and spleen greater than 10 cm (3.9 inches).

Since there is generally no accepted staging system, another method for evaluating the progression of HCL is to group patients into two categories: untreated HCL and progressive HCL, in which hairy cells are present after therapy has been administered.

Some people with hairy cell leukemia have very few or no symptoms at all, and it is reasonable to expect that 10% of patients may not need any treatment. However, if the patient is symptomatic and needs intervention, HCL is especially responsive to treatment.

There are three main courses of treatment: **chemotherapy**, **splenectomy** (surgical removal of the spleen), and immunotherapy. Once a patient meets treatment criteria, purine analogues, particularly the drugs, **pentostatin** and **cladribine**, are the first-line therapy. Pentostatin is administered at 5mg/m^2 for two days every other week until total remission is achieved. Patients may experience side effects such as

fever, **nausea and vomiting**, photosensitivity, and keratoconjuctivitis. However, follow-up studies estimate a relapse-free survival rate at 76%. Cladribine (2-CdA) taken at 0.1mg/kg/day for seven days also has an impressive response. Eighty-six percent of patients experience complete remission after treatment, while 16% experience partial remission. Fever is the principal side effect of 2-CdA.

Biological therapy (also called immunologic therapy or immunotherapy), where the body's own immune cells are used to fight cancer, is also being investigated in **clinical trials** for hairy cell leukemia. A substance called interferon that is produced by the white blood cells of the body was the first systemic treatment that showed consistent results in fighting HCL. The FDA approved interferon-alpha (INF-alpha) to fight HCL. The mechanism by which INF-alpha works is not clearly understood. However, it is known that interferon stimulates the body's natural killer cells that are suppressed during HCL. The standard dosage is 2 MU/m^2 three times a week for 12 months. Side effects include fever, myalgia, malaise, rashes, and gastrointestinal complaints.

If the spleen is enlarged, it may be removed in a surgical procedure known as splenectomy. This usually causes a remission of the disease. However, 50% of patients who undergo splenectomy require some type of systemic treatment such as chemotherapy or immunotherapy. Splenectomy is not the most widely used course of treatment as it was many years ago. Although the spleen is not an indispensable organ, it is responsible for helping the body fight infection. Therefore, other therapies are preferred in order to salvage the spleen and its functions.

Most patients have excellent prognosis and can expect to live 10 years or longer. The disease may remain silent for years with treatment. Continual follow-up is necessary to monitor the patient for relapse and determine true cure rates.

Alternative and complementary therapies

Many individuals choose to supplement traditional therapy with complementary methods. Often, these methods improve the tolerance of side effects and symptoms as well as enrich the quality of life. The American Cancer Society recommends that patients talk to their doctors to ensure that the methods they are using are safely supplementing traditional therapy. Some complementary treatments include the following:

- yoga
- meditation
- religious practices and prayer

- music therapy
- art therapy
- massage therapy
- aromatherapy

Coping with cancer treatment

The treatment and the disease interfere with the patient's ability to produce red blood cells, white blood cells, and platelets, causing the patient to be vulnerable to anemia and life-threatening infection and bleeding. Transfusions can be given to patients in order to increase the number of red blood cells and platelets in the blood. In addition, colony-stimulating factors are being studied. These increase the number of the patient's own white blood cells.

Nausea and **vomiting** can result from chemotherapy and are often controlled by prescription drugs called **antiemetics**. Patients can also curb nausea and vomiting by eating slowly and avoiding large meals. Drinking water an hour before meals and staying away from foods that are sweet or fried is also helpful. Many times, chemotherapy is handled better if the patient is eating well. Nurses and dieticians can aid patients in choosing healthful foods to incorporate into their diet.

Patients can fight anemia and fatigue by getting plenty of rest and minimizing strenuous activities. A well-balanced diet can also counter anemia and fatigue.

Although physicians will do everything possible to keep a patient's blood count high, there are precautions that can be taken by patients in order to reduce their risk of infection. Patients should regularly wash their hands, especially before and after eating meals and after using the restroom. Patients should avoid individuals who are contagious with colds, the flu, or the chicken pox. It is also helpful if patients do not cut themselves or do anything to expose deeper layers of the skin where bacteria can contaminate and cause infection. Finally, patients should avoid large crowds.

Clinical trials

Clinical trials are being performed to improve the effectiveness of treatment and to minimize the side effects. Patients may choose to volunteer for a clinical trial if they do not respond to standard therapy or if they want to reduce side effects. Clinical trials for the treatment of HCL involving purine analogues were being researched in 2005. Clinical trials are being performed all over the United States, and patients should discuss options with their doctors or contact the Cancer Information Service at (800) 4-CANCER (800-422-6237).

In many cases, insurance companies will not cover procedures that are part of clinical trials. Patients should talk with their doctor and insurance company to determine which procedures are covered.

Prevention

Since the cause for the disease is unknown and there are no specific risk factors, there is no known prevention.

Special concerns

Cancer treatments and their side effects can take a physical and psychological toll on cancer patients and their families. To deal with the psychological impact, there are many different support groups and psychotherapists that can help. Psychiatrists can prescribe medication to help with **depression**. Support groups can encourage and strengthen the psyche by relating to one another through shared experiences and success stories. Relying on faith practices is also beneficial for cancer patients to deal with their condition. Patients should discuss all options with their physician to determine what is available to them.

See also Tumor staging.

Resources

BOOKS

Bast, Robert C. *Cancer Medicine*. Lewiston, NY: B.C. Decker Inc., 2000.

Haskell, Charles M. *Cancer Treatment*. 5th ed. Philadephia: W.B. Saunders Company, 2001.

OTHER

"Coping With Side Effects." *National Cancer Institute*. [cited July 2, 2005]. <http://cancernet.nci.nih.gov/chemo therapy/chemoside.html>.

NCI/PDQ Patient Statement, "Hairy cell leukemia." National Cancer Institute, 2001.

ORGANIZATIONS

American Cancer Society (National Headquarters). 1599 Clifton Road, N.E. Atlanta, Georgia 30329. (800) 227-2345. http://www.cancer.org.

Cancer Research Institute (National Headquarters). 681 Fifth Avenue, New York, N.Y. 10022. (800) 992-2623. http://www.cancerresearch.org.

Hairy Cell Leukemia Research Foundation. 2345 County Farm Lane, Schaumburg, IL 60194. (800) 693-6173.

Leukemia Society of America, Inc. National Office, 600 Third Avenue, 4th Floor, New York, NY 10016. (800) 955-4LSA.

National Cancer Institute. 9000 Rockville Pike, Building 31, Room 10A16, Bethesda, Maryland, 20892. (800) 422-6237. http://wwwicic.nci.nih.gov.
Oncolink. University of Pennsylvania Cancer Center. http://cancer.med.upenn.edu.

Lata Cherath, Ph.D.
Sally C. McFarlane-Parrott

Haloperidol *see* **Antiemetics**

Hand-foot syndrome

Definition

Hand-foot syndrome (HFS), also called palmar-plantar erythrodysesthesia syndrome (PPES) or chemotherapy-induced acral erythema, is a relatively common side effect associated with high-dosage **chemotherapy** treatments involving **fluorouracil** (5-FU) and drugs belonging to the chemical class called anthracyclines. It was first reported in 1974.

Demographics

There are no reliable statistics about the frequency of hand-foot syndrome as a complication of **cancer** chemotherapy.

Description

Anthracyclines have been widely used since the 1960s as dose-limited chemotherapy drugs for a variety of cancers, particularly leukemia, metastatic **breast cancer**, **ovarian cancer**, and colorectal cancer. The most familiar anthracyclines are **capecitabine** (Xeloda), **daunorubicin** (Cerubidine), **doxorubicin** (Adriamycin), **idarubicin** (Idamycin), and **vinorelbine** (Navelbine). Each of these drugs is broken down into 5-FU by chemicals inside the cancer cells.

A dose-limited drug is a drug for which the maximum dose is determined by the reactions of an individual patient. Symptoms of HFS usually indicate that a patient is receiving too much 5-FU or a particular anthracycline. In such a case, the dosage of the drug that is causing HFS is usually decreased until these symptoms either disappear completely or become tolerable to the patient.

Risk factors

The primary risk factor for HFS is cancer therapy involving anthracycline medications. There are no indications as of 2009 that sex, race, or age affects a person's risk of developing HFS.

Causes and symptoms

Causes

The symptoms of HFS are believed to be caused by some of the chemicals that 5-FU is broken down into by the natural biochemical processes of the body. Since all anthracycline drugs chemically breakdown into 5-FU, these drugs will all eventually be broken down into the chemicals that can cause the symptoms of HFS. For reasons that are not clear, some patients seem more prone to developing symptoms of HFS than other patients.

The direct cause of HFS is leakage of the chemotherapy drug from tiny blood vessels called capillaries into the skin on the palms of the hands and soles of the feet. The amount of drug leakage from the capillaries is increased by friction or heat. The leakage results in redness, tenderness, and possibly peeling of the skin on the palms and soles. The rash often looks like sunburn.

Symptoms

The symptoms of HFS may begin anywhere from days to weeks after the beginning of chemotherapy. The primary symptom of HFS is a tingling sensation and/or numbness of the skin, particularly on the palms of the hands or the soles of the feet. Swelling and redness (erythema) often accompany this symptom. In severe cases, the skin may peel, develop ulcerations or blisters, and cause severe pain. In the most extreme cases, symptoms of HFS may make it difficult, or impossible for the patient to grasp small objects, walk, or conduct other normal daily activities.

In a few cases, patients develop HFS on the knees and elbows as well as on the hands and feet.

Diagnosis

The diagnosis of HFS is based on a combination of the patient's history of chemotherapy and the appearance of the characteristic reddening and peeling of the skin on the extremities. It is important for cancer patients to consult their doctor as soon as they notice redness or tenderness on their palms or soles, before the skin starts to peel.

Treatment

Traditional

The symptoms of HFS are usually alleviated by lowering the dosage of the drug that the patient is receiving. In severe cases of HFS, it may be necessary to discontinue the use of the drug that is causing these symptoms. In some, but not all, patients the symptoms of HFS are reduced by treatment with such steroid-containing skin creams as hydrocortisone.

Other measures that help some patients are the application of cold in an ice pack or even a package of frozen food for 15–20 minutes at a time; or gently applying moisturizers like Lubriderm or Bag Balm to the palms and soles. It is important not to use pressure in applying moisturizers, however, as friction can worsen HFS.

Drugs

Some doctors recommend taking acetaminophen (Tylenol), an over-the-counter pain reliever, to ease the discomfort of HFS.

Alternative

Treatment of the hands and feet with an aloe vera-containing skin cream may help to alleviate some of the symptoms of HFS. Topical treatment of the skin with dimethyl sulfoxide (DMSO) has also been suggested as an alternative treatment.

Another alternative treatment that is sometimes recommended is vitamin therapy, specifically taking vitamin B_6.

Prognosis

HFS clears up in most cases when the medication dose is adjusted or the drug discontinued.

Prevention

Taking steps to reduce heat or friction on the hands and feet can help to prevent HFS:

- Avoid exposing the skin to hot water for long periods of time. Take short showers and baths, or bathe in lukewarm rather than hot water.
- Do not use rubber gloves when washing dishes as they trap heat against the skin.
- Avoid direct contact with detergents, bleach, ammonia, and other harsh household chemicals.
- Avoid jogging, power walking, jumping, tennis, softball, baseball, or aerobics as forms of exercise.
- Limit sun exposure.
- Make sure that shoes fit properly and do not put too much pressure on the feet.
- Wear loose, well-ventilated clothing.
- Avoid using garden and household tools that force the hand against a hard surface, such as chopping knives, screwdrivers, and some power tools.

These preventive measures should be taken within a week of starting intravenous anthracycline drugs and should be followed all the time when taking oral anthracyclines.

Resources

BOOKS

Airley, Rachel. Cancer Chemotherapy. Hoboken, NJ: Wiley-Blackwell, 2009.

McKay, Judith, and Tamera Schacher. The Chemotherapy Survival Guide: Everything You Need to Know to Get through Treatment, 3rd ed. Oakland, CA: New Harbinger Publications, 2009.

Spencer, Peter, and Walter Holt, eds. Anticancer Drugs: Design, Delivery and Pharmacology. Hauppauge, NY: Nova Science Publishers, 2009.

PERIODICALS

Cicek, D., et al. "Localized Palmar-Plantar Hyperplasia Associated with Use of Sorafenib." Clinical Drug Investigation 28 (December 2008): 803–07.

Eng, C. "Toxic Effects and Their Management: Daily Clinical Challenges in the Treatment of Colorectal Cancer." Nature Reviews: Clinical Oncology 6 (April 2009): 207–18.

Goutos, I., et al. "'Hand-foot Syndrome'—An Unusual Case of Plantar Pathology Presenting to a Burns Unit." Journal of Burn Care and Research 30 (May-June 2009): 529–32.

Sivaramamoorthy, C., et al. "Hand-foot Syndrome after Treatment with Docetaxel." Medical Journal of Australia 191 (July 6, 2009): 40.

OTHER

American Society of Clinical Oncology (ASCO). Hand-Foot Syndrome or Palmar-Plantar Erythrodysesthesia. http://www.cancer.net/patient/Diagnosis + and + Treatment/Treating + Cancer/Managing + Side + Effects/Hand-Foot + Syndrome + or + Palmar-Plantar + Erythrodysesthesia.

Cleveland Clinic Foundation. Hand-Foot Syndrome. http://www.chemocare.com/managing/handfoot_syndrome.asp.

National Cancer Institute (NCI). Managing Chemotherapy Side Effects: Skin and Nail Changes. http://www.cancer.gov/cancertopics/chemo-side-effects/skin-and-nail.

ORGANIZATIONS

American Cancer Society, 250 Williams Street NW, Atlanta, GA, 30303, 800-ACS-2345 (227-2345), www.cancer.org.

American Society of Clinical Oncology (ASCO), 2318 Mill Road, Suite 800, Alexandria, VA, 22314, 571-483-1300, 888-282-2552, membermail@asco.org, http://www.asco.org/ASCOv2?edition=default.

National Cancer Institute, 6116 Executive Blvd., Room 3036A, Bethesda, MD, 20892-8322, 800-422-6237, cancergovstaff@mail.nih.gov, www.cancer.gov.

Paul A. Johnson, Ed.M.
Rebecca J. Frey, PhD

False color scintigram (gamma camera scan) showing metastatic (secondary) cancer affecting the cervical (neck) vertebrae (white area). *(Copyright CNRI, Science Source/Photo Researchers, Inc. Reproduced by permission.)*

Head and neck cancers

Definition

The term head and neck cancers refers to a group of cancers found in the head and neck region, excluding tumors of the eyes, the thyroid gland and tumors which originate in the brain.

Tumors classified as head and neck tumors are found in:

- The oral cavity (mouth). The lips, the tongue, the teeth, the gums, the lining inside the lips and cheeks, the floor of the mouth (under the tongue), the roof of the mouth and the small area behind the wisdom teeth are all included in the oral cavity.

Cancers of the head and neck

Cancer types	Cancer occurs in
Hypopharyngeal cancer	Lowest section of the pharynx (region behind mouth)
Laryngeal cancer	Larynx (front of neck, near Adam's apple)
Nasopharyngeal cancer	Behind nose
	Pharynx
Oral cancer	Lips
	Lining of lips and cheeks
	Front two-thirds of tongue
	Teeth
	Gums
	Under tongue
Oropharyngeal cancer	Back one-third of tongue
	Upper section of pharynx
	Area around tonsils
Parathyroid cancer	Parathyroid glands (found behind the thyroid gland)
Thyroid cancer	Thyroid gland (found at front of neck, below the Adam's apple)

(Table by GGS Creative Resources. Cengage Learning, Gale.)

- The oropharynx, which includes the back one-third of the tongue, the back of the throat and the tonsils.
- Nasopharynx, which includes the area behind the nose).
- Hypopharynx, the lower part of the throat.
- The larynx (voice box, located in front of the neck, in the region of the Adam's apple). In the larynx, the cancer can occur in any of the three regions: the glottis (where the vocal cords are); the supraglottis (the area above the glottis); and the subglottis (the area that connects the glottis to the windpipe).
- The paranasal sinuses, which include the ethmoid and maxillary sinuses.
- The salivary glands.

The most frequently occurring cancers of the head and neck area are **oral cancers** and laryngeal cancers. Almost half of all the head and neck cancers occur in the oral cavity, and a third of the cancers are found in the larynx. By definition, the term "head and neck cancers" usually excludes tumors that occur in the brain.

Demographics

Roughly 3% of all cancers in the United States develop in the oral cavity, pharyngeal area or in the larynx. The most common cancers of the head and neck area are oral cancers, and **laryngeal cancer**. Half of all head and neck cancers occur in the oral cavity and pharynx and almost 20% originate in the larynx. The American Cancer Society estimates that in 2009 approximately 12,290 new cases of laryngeal

cancer will be diagnosed and that 3,660 people will die of this disease. Oral and oropharyngeal cancers are more prevalent with an estimated 35,720 new cases diagnosed in 2009. Approximately 7600 individuals are expected to die from these types of cancer in 2009. Numbers of new cases and deaths from laryngeal and oral cancers have been steadily decreasing in the last three decades. This decrease is attributed to the decrease in smoking.

Description

The tumors associated with head and neck cancers are found in several regions, including the lips, tongue, mouth, nasal passages, pharynx, larynx (voice box), and salivary gland. Many head and neck cancers interfere with the functions of eating and breathing. Laryngeal cancer affects speech. Loss of any of these functions is significant. Therefore, early detection and appropriate treatment is of utmost importance.

Risk factors

Tobacco is regarded as the single greatest risk factor contributing to the occurrence of oral and laryngeal cancer: 75–80% of these patients are smokers. Heavy alcohol use has also been included as a risk factor. A combination of tobacco and alcohol use increases the risk for oral cancer by 6 to 15 times more than for users of either substance alone. Exposure to asbestos appears to increase the risk of developing laryngeal cancer. **Infection** with the human papillomavirus (HPV) is a risk factor for some squamous cell cancers of the oropharynx.

The risk for both oral cancer and laryngeal cancer seems to increase with age. Most of the cases occur in individuals over 40 years of age, and the average age at diagnosis is 60. While oral cancer is diagnosed in men twice as often as it does women, laryngeal cancer is four times more common in men than in women. Both diseases are more common in African Americans than among whites.

Causes and symptoms

Use of tobacco products and alcohol, and in particular, the combination of the two play a major role in the development of cancers of the head and neck. Infection with HPV is linked to the development of **oropharyngeal cancer**.

There are many types of head and neck cancers. Signs and symptoms of the various types of cancer are often specific to the original location of the cancer.

- Oral cancers occur in the mouth, or oral cavity, which includes the lips, the lining inside the lips and cheeks, the front two-thirds of the tongue, the teeth, the gums, the floor of the mouth (under the tongue), the roof of the mouth, and the small area behind the wisdom teeth. Symptoms and signs include a mouth sore that does not heal within two weeks, unusual bleeding from the teeth or gums, or a lump in the gums, mouth, or tongue.

- Lip cancers occur on the inside or outside surface of the lips. Signs of this cancer include a lump on the inside of the lip or a sore on the outside, which is usually a form of skin cancer.

- Oropharyngeal cancer is found on the back one-third of the tongue, the upper section of the pharynx, and the area around the tonsils. Symptoms include a lump in the back of the mouth or throat, ear pain, or difficulty swallowing.

- Nasopharyngeal cancer is found in the area behind the nose and the upper section of the pharynx, the area just behind the mouth. Symptoms include difficulty breathing or speaking, pain or ringing in ears, frequent headaches, or trouble hearing.

- Hypopharyngeal cancer is found only in the bottom section of the pharynx. Symptoms include a sore throat that does not subside, difficulty swallowing, a lump in the neck, or ear pain.

- Laryngeal cancer starts in the larynx, which is located in front of the neck, in the region of the Adam's apple. Symptoms include pain when swallowing, a sore throat that does not subside, a change in voice, or ear pain.

- Paranasal sinus cancer and nasal cancer develop in the small, hollow spaces in the nose called the sinuses and in the nasal cavity, which is the passageway for air moving to the throat during breathing. Symptoms include frequent sinus infections, nosebleeds, a sore inside the nose that does not heal, or pain in the sinus area.

- Salivary gland tumors form in the salivary glands, which produce saliva to help prevent the mouth from drying out and aids with digestion. They are located under the jaw, in front of the ears, underneath the tongue, and in other regions of the digestive tract. Symptoms include swelling under the chin or around the jawbone, facial numbness, muscles in the face that will not move, or persistent pain in the face, chin, or neck.

Diagnosis

Specific diagnostic tests used to detect cancers of the head and neck depend on the location of the cancer. The standard tests are:

Physical examination

The first step in diagnosis is a complete and thorough examination of the oral and nasal cavity, using mirrors and other visual aids. The tongue and the back of the throat are examined as well. Any suspicious looking lumps or lesions are examined with fingers (palpation). In order to look inside the larynx, the doctor may sometimes perform a procedure known as **laryngoscopy**. In indirect laryngoscopy, the doctor looks down the throat with a small, long handled mirror. Sometimes the doctor inserts a lighted tube (laryngoscope or a fiber-optic scope) through the patient's nose or mouth. As the tube goes down the throat, the doctor can observe areas that cannot be seen by a simple mirror. This procedure is called a direct laryngoscopy. Sometimes patients may be given a mild sedative to help them relax, and a local anesthetic to ease any discomfort. An endoscopic examination under anesthesia may also be required as part of the work-up for head and neck cancer.

Blood tests

The doctor may order blood or other immunological tests. In cases where oropharyngeal cancer is suspected, HPV testing is recommended.

Imaging tests

X rays of the mouth, the sinuses, the skull, and the chest region may be required. **Computed tomography** scans (CT scan), a procedure in which a computer takes a series of x-ray pictures of areas inside the body, and/or **magnetic resonance imaging** (MRI) and **positron emission tomography** (PET scans) may be ordered. Patients with cancers of the nasopharynx may also undergo imaging tests with PET scans and/or CT scans to determine presence of distant metastatic lesions.

Dental, speech, and swallowing evaluations may also be conducted.

Biopsy

When a sore does not heal or a suspicious patch or lump is seen in the mouth, larynx, nasopharynx, or throat, a **biopsy** may be performed to rule out the possibility of cancer. The biopsy is the most definitive diagnostic tool for detecting the cancer. If cancerous cells are detected in the biopsied sample, the doctor may perform more extensive tests in order to find whether, and to where, the cancer may have spread.

Treatment

Most head and neck cancers are treated initially with surgery and/or **radiation therapy. Chemotherapy** may be administered as primary systemic therapy or concurrently with radiation therapy. Chemotherapy drugs currently used in the treatment of head and neck cancers are **cisplatin, fluorouracil** (5-FU), **carboplatin, docetaxel,** paclitaxel, docetaxel, **methotrexate, ifosfamide, bleomycin,** and **gemcitabine.** The monoclonal antibody, **cetuximab,** may also be used to treat head and neck cancers.

A newer form of radiotherapy that has proved beneficial to patients with head and neck cancer is intensity-modulated radiation therapy, or IMRT. IMRT allows the radiologist to deliver controlled doses of radiation to cancerous tissues while leaving nearby normal tissues and organs unaffected. IMRT has proven especially useful in the treatment of oropharyngeal, paranasal sinus, and nasopharyngeal cancers by reducing radiation doses to adjacent non-cancerous tissues and structures. The use of IMRT to treat other head and neck cancers is evolving. 3D and 2D conformal radiation therapy techniques may also be utilized. Another radiation technique which may be used is the Simultaneous Integrated Boost (SIB) technique which integrates IMRT, target volume dosing, and fractionation of radiation therapy.

One of the most difficult aspects of treating head and neck cancer for many years has been the necessity of **reconstructive surgery** and rehabilitation therapy following removal of the patient's lips, tongue, voice box, or other structures. Recent advances in reconstructive surgery, however, have provided patients with better functioning as well as appearance, thus improving their quality of life as well as length of survival.

Prognosis

The survival rates for head and neck cancers vary from good to poor, depending on the specific cancer, stage of the cancer at diagnosis, and the overall physical condition of the patient. Five year relative survival rates for laryngeal cancer range from 41–83% for patients diagnosed in Stage I to 20–43% for patients diagnosed in Stage IV. The average survival for patients diagnosed with laryngeal cancer has not improved significantly since the early 1970s. Five year relative survival rates for patients diagnosed with oral/oropharyngeal cancers range from 57–83% diagnosed in Stage I to 27–47% diagnosed in Stage IV.

Prevention

Refraining from the use of all tobacco products (**cigarettes**, cigars, pipe tobacco, chewing tobacco), consuming alcohol in moderation, and practicing good oral hygiene are some of the measures that one

QUESTIONS TO ASK YOUR DOCTOR

- What specific type of head and neck cancer do I have?
- What are the current treatment recommendations for this type of cancer?
- Will I require surgery? If so, how extensive will my surgery be?
- What types of treatment can I expect after surgery?
- How long will these treatments last?
- Will the surgery or any of my other treatments affect my ability to speak and/or swallow?

can take to prevent head and neck cancers. Since there is an association between excessive exposure to the sun and lip cancer, people who spend a lot of time outdoors in the sun should protect themselves from the sun's harmful rays. Regular physical examinations, or mouth examination by the patient himself, or by the patient's doctor or dentist, can help detect oral cancer in its very early stages.

Since working with asbestos has been shown to increase one's risk of getting cancer of the larynx, asbestos workers should follow safety rules to avoid inhaling asbestos fibers. Also, malnutrition and vitamin deficiencies have been shown to have some association with an increased incidence of head and neck cancers. The American Cancer Society, therefore, recommends eating a healthy diet, consisting of at least five servings of fruits and vegetables every day, and six servings of food from other plant sources such as cereals, breads, grain products, rice, pasta and beans. Reducing one's intake of high-fat food from animal sources is advised.

See also Alcohol consumption; Cigarettes; Laryngeal nerve palsy; Squamous cell carcinoma of the skin.

Resources

PERIODICALS

Bonner, J.A., Harari, P.M., Giralt, J, et al."Radiotherapy Plus Cetuximab for Squamous Cell Carcinoma of the Head and Neck."*N Engl J Med*354(2006):567–78.

Lee, N.Y., O'Meara, W., Chan,K., et al."Concurrent Chemotherapy and Intensity-Modulated Radiotherapy for Locoregionally Advanced Laryngeal and Hypopharyngeal Cancers."*Int J Radiat Oncol Biol Phys* 69(2007):459–68.

Ozyigit, G., T. Yang, and K. S. Chao. "Intensity-Modulated Radiation Therapy for Head and Neck Cancer." *Current Treatment Options in Oncology* 5 (February 2004): 3–9.

Porceddu, S., G. Hope, J. Wills, et al. "Intensity-Modulated Radiotherapy: Examples of Its Utility in Head and Neck Cancer." *Australasian Radiology* 48 (March 2004): 51–57.

Vermorken, J.B., Mesia, R., Revera, F., et al, "Platinum-based Chemotherapy Plus Cetuximab in Head and Neck Cancer."*N Engl J Med* 359(2008):1116–27.

Vural, E. "Surgical Reconstruction in Patients with Cancer of the Head and Neck." *Current Oncology Reports* 6 (March 2004): 133–140.

ORGANIZATIONS

American Academy of Facial Plastic and Reconstructive Surgery (AAFPRS). 310 South Henry Street, Alexandria, VA 22314. (703) 299-9291. www.facemd.org.

American Society of Plastic Surgeons (ASPS). 444 East Algonquin Road, Arlington Heights, IL 60005. (847) 228-9900. www.plasticsurgery.org.

Support for People with Oral and Head and Neck Cancer (SPOHNC). P.O. Box 53, Locust Valley, NY 11560-0053. (800) 377-0928. http://www.spohnc.org.

OTHER

American Cancer Society (ACS). "Laryngeal Cancer." http://www.cancer.org/docroot/CRI/content/CRI_2_ 4_1X_What_are_the_key_statistics_for-Laryngeal_ and hypolaryngeal_cancer_23.asp?rnav = cri. May 7, 2009 [cited September 23, 2009].

National Comprehensive Cancer Network. "NCCN Practice Guidelines in Oncology Head and Neck Cancer," vol. 1. 2009. http://www.nccn.org/professio nals/physician_gls/PDF/head-and-neck.pdf [cited September 23, 2009].

Lata Cherath, Ph.D.
Rebecca J. Frey, Ph.D.
Melinda Granger Oberleitner, R.N., D.N.S.,
A.P.R.N., C.N.S.

Health insurance

Definition

Health insurance is insurance that pays for all or part of a person's health care bills. The types of health insurance are group health plans, individual plans, workers' compensation, and government health plans such as Medicare and Medicaid.

Health insurance can be further classified into fee-for-service (traditional insurance) and managed care.

KEY TERMS

Clinical trial—A study to determine the efficacy and safety of a drug or medical procedure. This type of study is often called an experimental or investigational procedure.

Health care provider—A doctor, hospital, lab, or other professional person or facility offering health care services.

Health insurance claim—A bill for health care services that is turned in to the health insurance company for payment.

Both group and individual insurance plans can be either fee-for-service or managed care plans.

The following are types of managed care plans:

- Health Maintenance Organization (HMO)
- Preferred Provider Organization (PPO)

Purpose

The purpose of health insurance is to help people cover their health care costs. Health care costs include doctor visits, hospital stays, surgery, procedures, tests, home care, and other treatments and services.

Description

Health insurance is available to groups as well as individuals. Government plans, such as Medicare, are offered to people who meet certain criteria.

Group and individual plans can be further classified as either fee-for-service or managed care. **Cancer** patients may have specific concerns, such as the freedom to select specialists, that play a factor in choosing a health care plan. Fee-for-service plans traditionally

offer greater freedom when choosing a health care professional. Managed care often limits a patient to health care professionals listed by the managed care insurance company.

Group health plans

A group health plan offers health care coverage for employers, student organizations, professional associations, religious organizations, and other groups. Many employers offer group health plans to employees and their dependents as a benefit of working with that particular employer (medical benefits). The employer may pay for part or all of the insurance cost (premium).

When an employee leaves a job he or she may be eligible for continued health insurance as a result of the Consolidated Omnibus Budget Reconciliation Act of 1986 (COBRA). This federal law protects employees and their families in certain situations by allowing them to keep his or her health insurance for a specified amount of time. The individual must, however, pay a premium to keep their insurance plan in effect It is important to note that COBRA only applies under certain conditions, such as job loss, death, divorce, or other life events. The COBRA law usually applies to group health plans offered by companies with more than 20 employees. Some states have laws that require employers to offer continued health care coverage for people who do not qualify for COBRA. Each state's insurance board can provide additional information.

Individual plans

These type of health care plans are sold directly to individuals.

Fee-for-service

Fee-for-service is traditional health insurance in which the insurance company reimburses the doctor, hospital, or other health care provider for all or part of the fees charged. Fee-for-service plans may be offered to groups or individuals. This type of plan gives people the highest level of freedom to choose a doctor, hospital, or other health care provider. A person may be able to receive medical care anywhere in the United States and, often, in the world.

Under this type of insurance a premium is paid and there is usually a yearly deductible, which means benefits do not begin until this deductible is met. After the person has paid the deductible (an amount specified by the terms of the insurance policy) the insurance company pays a portion of covered medical services. For example, the deductible may be $250 so the patient pays the first $250 of yearly covered medical expenses. After that he or she may pay 20% of covered services while the insurance company pays 80%. The exact percentages and deductibles will vary with each policy. The person may have to fill out forms (claims) and send them to the insurance company to have their claims paid.

People who have cancer may be attracted to the freedom of choice that traditional fee-for-service plans offer. However, they will most likely have higher out-of-pocket costs than they would in a managed care plan.

Managed care

Managed care plans are also sold to both groups and individuals. In these plans a person's health care is managed by the insurance company. Approvals are needed for some services, including visits to specialist doctors, medical tests, or surgical procedures. In order for people to receive the highest level of coverage they must obtain services from the doctors, hospitals, labs, imaging centers, and other providers affiliated with their managed care plan.

People with cancer who are considering a managed care plan should check with the plan regarding coverage for services outside of the plan's list of participating providers. For example, if a person wants to travel to a cancer center for treatment, he or she should find out what coverage will be available. In these plans coverage is usually much less if a person receives treatment from doctors and hospitals not affiliated with the plan.

HEALTH MAINTENANCE ORGANIZATION (HMO). An HMO is a type of managed care called a prepaid plan. This type of coverage was designed initially to help keep people healthy by covering the cost of preventive care, such as medical checkups. The patient selects a primary care doctor, such as a family physician, from an HMO list. This doctor coordinates the patient's care and determines if referrals to specialist doctors are needed. People pay a premium, usually every month, and receive their health care services (doctor visits, hospital care, lab work, emergency services, etc.) when they pay a small fee called a copayment. The HMO has arrangements with caregivers and hospitals and the copayment only applies to those caregivers and facilities affiliated with the HMO. This type of coverage offers less freedom than fee-for-service, but out-of-pocket health care costs are generally lower and more predictable. A person's out-of-pocket costs will be much higher if he or she receives care outside of the HMO unless prior approval from the HMO is received.

PREFERRED PROVIDER ORGANIZATION (PPO). A PPO combines the benefits of fee-for-service with the features of an HMO. If patients use health care providers (doctors, hospitals, etc.) who are part of the PPO network, they will receive coverage for most of their bills after a deductible and, perhaps a copayment, is met. Some PPOs require people to choose a primary care physician who will coordinate care and arrange referrals to specialists when needed. Other PPOs allow patients to choose specialists on their own. A PPO may offer lower levels of coverage for care given by doctors and other professionals not affiliated with the PPO. In these cases the patient may have to fill out claim forms to receive coverage.

Government health plans

Medicare and Medicaid are two health plans offered by the U.S. government. They are available to individuals who meet certain age, income, or disability criteria. TRICARE Standard, formerly called CHAMPUS, is the health plan for U.S. military personnel.

MEDICARE. Medicare, created in 1965 under Title 18 of the Social Security Act, is available to people who meet certain age and disability criteria. Eligible people include:

- those who are age 65 years and older
- some younger individuals who have disabilities
- those who have end-stage renal disease (permanent kidney failure)

Medicare has two parts: Part A and Part B. Part A is hospital insurance and helps cover the costs of inpatient hospital stays, skilled nursing centers, **home health services**, and **hospice care**. Part B helps cover medical services such as doctors' bills, ambulances, outpatient therapy, and a host of other services, supplies, and equipment that Part A does not cover.

MEDICAID. Medicaid, created in 1965 under Title 19 of the Social Security Act, is designed for people receiving federal government aid such as Aid to Families with Dependent Children. This program covers hospitalization, doctors' visits, lab tests, and **x rays**. Some other services may be partially covered.

TRICARE. Eligible military families may enroll in TRICARE Prime, which is an HMO; TRICARE Extra, which offers an expanded choice of providers; or TRICARE Standard, which is the new name for CHAMPUS.

Supplemental insurance

Supplemental insurance covers expenses that are not paid for by a person's health insurance. Cancer insurance is a specific form of supplemental insurance that covers expenses that are not normally covered by health insurance but are specifically related to cancer treatments.

Workers' compensation

Workers' compensation covers health care costs for an injury or illness related to a person's job. Medical conditions that are unrelated to work are not covered under this plan. In some cases an evaluation is done to determine whether or not the medical condition is truly related to a person's employment.

Special concerns

There are a variety of special concerns that people with cancer have regarding health insurance.

Waiting period

Insurance may not take effect immediately upon signing up for a policy. Sometimes a waiting period exists, during which time premiums are not paid and benefits are not available. Health care services received during this period are not covered.

Preexisting condition

A preexisting condition, such as cancer, is a concern when choosing insurance. If a person received medical advice or treatment for a medical problem within six months of enrolling in new insurance, this condition is called preexisting, and it can be excluded from the new coverage. The six-month time lapse before a person enrolls in a new health insurance policy is called the look-back period. If a person received medical advice, recommendations, prescription drugs, diagnosis, or treatment for a health problem during the look-back period, he or she is considered to have a preexisting condition. People should check with their state insurance boards to determine preexisting condition rules.

Coverage renewal

Some people with diseases such as cancer worry about group health plans renewing their coverage. As long as the person meets the plan's eligibility requirements and the plan covers similar cases, the coverage must be offered. Coverage cannot be cancelled for health reasons.

Experimental/investigational treatments

Experimental/investigational treatments are often a concern for people with cancer. These treatments may or may not be covered by a person's health insurance. Some states mandate coverage for investigational treatments. People should check with their insurance plans

and state insurance boards to determine if coverage is available.

A clinical trial is a type of investigational treatment. Costs involved include patient care costs and research costs. Usual patient care costs that may be covered by insurance are visits to the doctor, stays in the hospital, tests, and other procedures that occur whether a person is part of an experiment or is receiving traditional care. Extra patient care costs that may or may not be covered by insurance are the special tests required as part of the research study.

Health insurance plans have policies regarding coverage for **clinical trials**. People should determine their level of health insurance coverage for clinical trials, and they should learn about the costs associated with a particular study.

In 2000, Medicare began covering certain clinical trials. The trials must meet specific criteria in order to be covered. In eligible trials treatments and services such as tests, procedures, and doctor visits that are normally covered by Medicare are covered. Some items may not be covered including investigational items like the experimental drug itself or items that are used only for data collection in the clinical trial. Patients should check to see if the clinical trial sponsor is providing the investigational drug at no charge.

Complementary therapies

Complementary cancer therapies are another coverage consideration. A cancer patient undergoing this type of therapy should check with his or her insurance policy regarding coverage.

Cancer screening coverage

Cancer screening coverage is an important consideration. Forty-four states mandate insurance coverage of screenings for at least one of these cancers: breast, cervical, prostate, and colorectal. **Breast cancer** screening coverage is most commonly mandated. Most mandates refer to screenings that follow the American Cancer Society guidelines. A Women's Health Initiative Observational Study investigated the use of cancer screenings by more than 55,000 women between September 1994 and February 1997. The study found that the type of insurance a woman had was linked with the number of cancer screenings she reported. Women age 65 years and older who had Medicare plus prepaid insurance were more likely to report that they had screenings than those who had Medicare alone.

Health care regulations

The Health Insurance Portability and Accountability Act (HIPAA), passed by the U.S. Congress in 1996, offers people rights and protections regarding their health care plans. Because of HIPAA, there are limits on preexisting condition exclusions, people cannot be discriminated because of health factors, there are special enrollment requirements for people who lose other group plans or have new dependents, small employers are guaranteed group health plan availability, and all group plans have guaranteed renewal if the employer wishes to renew. In summary these rights and protections include:

- Portability. This is the ability for a person to get new health insurance if a change is desired or needed.
- Availability. This refers to whether or not health insurance must be offered to a person and his or her dependents.
- Renewability. This refers to whether or not a person is able to renew his or her health plan.

The Women's Health and Cancer Rights Act of 1998 requires health insurance plans to cover **breast reconstruction** related to a **mastectomy** if the patient chooses to have reconstruction and if the health plan covered the mastectomy. The law became effective for different health plans on different dates, with the earliest date of effect being October 21, 1998.

Resources

PERIODICALS

Hsia, Judith, et al., "The Importance of Health Insurance as a Determinant of Cancer Screening: Evidence from the Women's Health Initiative." *Preventive Medicine* September 2000: 261-70.

Rathore, Saif S., et al., "Mandated Coverage for Cancer-Screening Services: Whose Guidelines Do States Follow?" *American Journal of Preventive Medicine* August 2000: 71-8.

OTHER

"Supplemental Insurance Policies May Be Offered Under a Flex Plan, IRS Says" In *Flex Plan Handbook: November 1999.* [cited May 9, 2001and July 5, 2005]. <http://207.226.10.52/tpg/pen_ben/flex/flexnov99.html>.

ORGANIZATIONS

Agency for Health Care Research and Quality, *Checkup on Health Insurance Choices* [cited 27 March 2005] http://www.ahcpr.gov/consumer/insuranc.htm.

Health Care Choices *Our Newsletter: Better Health Choices* (January 1999) [cited May 9, 2005]. http://www.healthcarechoices.org/newslet/news199brreconst.htm.

Health Care Financing Administration *HIPAA Online* [cited March 27, 2005]. http://www.hcfa.gov.

National Cancer Institute, *Cancer Trials and Insurance Coverage: A Resource Guide* [cited May 4, 2005]. <http://cancertrials.nci.nih.gov/understanding/indepth/insurance>.

TRICARE *The History of CHAMPUS and its Evolving Role* [cited May 9, 2005]. http://www.tricare.osd.mil/fact sheets/history.pdf.

Rhonda Cloos, R.N.

Hemolytic anemia

Definition

Hemolytic **anemia** is a form of red blood cell (RBC) deficiency in which the RBCs break down at a faster than normal rate either inside the blood vessels or elsewhere in the body. The term *hemolytic* comes from two Greek words that mean "blood" and "disintegration."

Red blood cells live on average about 120 days in the circulation and then die. They are replaced by new RBCs produced in the bone marrow. What happens in hemolytic anemia is that the bone marrow cannot produce enough RBCs quickly enough to keep pace with their early death. Premature destruction of the RBCs inside the blood vessels is called intravascular hemolytic anemia, while their destruction elsewhere in the body (usually in the spleen and liver) is called extravascular hemolytic anemia. Hemolytic anemia can also be classified according to whether it is inherited or whether it is acquired later in life as a complication of another disease or disorder.

Demographics

The overall incidence of hemolytic anemia is approximately 4 per 100,000 people in the United States and Canada. Hemolytic anemia accounts for about 5% of all cases of anemia.

Most types of hemolytic anemia are not sex-specific or specific to any race or ethnic group. The incidence of hemolytic anemia in other countries is thought to be close to the United States figures.

Description

Red blood cells (erythrocytes) transport oxygen and carbon dioxide in the bloodstream, maintain a normal acid-base balance, and determine how thick or thin the blood is. Hemolytic anemia refers to the premature increased destruction of erythrocytes. Hemolysis is the process in which these erythrocytes rupture with the release of hemoglobin into the plasma, and anemia is a reduced delivery of oxygen to the tissues. Some of the symptoms of hemolytic anemia include nosebleeds, bleeding gums, shortness of breath, **fatigue**, rapid heartbeat, pale skin color or yellow skin color (jaundice), chills, and dark-colored urine.

Risk factors

Risk factors for hemolytic anemia include:

- Race or ethnicity. A few types of inherited hemolytic anemia are more common in some racial or ethnic groups than in others. African Americans are at increased risk of sickle cell anemia, while the Amish are at increased risk of pyruvate kinase deficiency, and people of Southeast Asian or Mediterranean ancestry are at increased risk of thalassemia.
- Sex. Men are at increased risk of G6PD deficiency while women over 40 are at increased risk of hemolytic anemia related to lupus and other autoimmune disorders.
- Having certain types of cancer, particularly non-Hodgkin's lymphoma and chronic lymphocytic leukemia.
- Having certain viral infections, particularly Epstein-Barr virus (EBV), cytomegalovirus (CMV), and HIV infection.
- Having a form of bacterial pneumonia caused by *Mycoplasma pneumoniae*.
- Exposure to diseases caused by parasites, like malaria and babesiosis.
- Taking high doses of penicillin, methyldopa, ribavirin, or some other medications.
- Having artificial heart valves or extensive vascular surgery.
- Having liver disease.
- Working in an occupation that involves exposure to toxic chemicals or venomous snakes and insects.

Causes and symptoms

Causes

Erythrocyte (red blood cell) formation takes place in the red bone marrow in an adult and in the liver, spleen, and bone marrow of the fetus. Their formation requires an adequate supply of iron, cobalt, copper, amino acids, and certain **vitamins**. When the bone marrow loses its ability to compensate for the destruction of the erythrocytes by increasing their production, hemolytic anemia occurs. There are many types of hemolytic anemia, which are classified according to the location of this inability to produce red blood cells.

If the problem lies within the red blood cell itself, it is referred to as an intrinsic factor, and if the problem is outside the red blood cell, it is referred to as an extrinsic factor.

Rh factor incompatibility refers to genetically determined substances capable of producing an **immune response** (antigens). This can cause hemolytic anemia not only during pregnancy when the mother is Rh negative and the fetus is Rh positive, but in mismatched blood transfusions as well. There are a number of industrial poisons that produce hemolytic anemia. These include:

- antimalarial agents
- organic solvents (benzene)
- certain chemotherapies
- hypersensitivity to certain antibiotics
- metals (chromium, platinum salts, nickel, lead, copper)
- pyridium
- arsenic
- some herbs used in traditional Chinese medicines
- intravenous (IV) water (an IV that is not normal or half-normal saline)
- snake bites (if the venom contains hemolytic toxins) These are all factors external to the red blood cell and thus are extrinsic in nature.

One important extrinsic factor in the cause of hemolytic anemia is in the course of widespread **cancer**, leukemia, **Hodgkin's disease**, acute alcoholism and liver disease. Many of the **chemotherapy** agents (**cisplatin, carboplatin** and nonplatinum drugs) utilized in treating various cancers have side effects that cause a suppression of bone marrow activity, which results in severe hemolytic anemia. In essence, an individual is not only anemic as a result of cancer, but this anemia is worsened by the treatment. Since **nausea, vomiting**, and lack of appetite are also side effects of chemotherapy, it is extremely difficult for the patient to overcome this type of anemia with diet and supplements. Eventually, severe hemolytic anemia is the end result.

Intrinsic factors would include disorders in the immune response and such genetically inherited disorders as glucose-6-phosphate dehydrogenase (G6PD) deficiency, an essential enzyme. People with this disorder do not display any symptoms until exposed to certain medications or stress. Aspirin and **nonsteroidal anti-inflammatory drugs** (NSAIDs) can precipitate this reaction. This disorder is more common among African-American males, with approximately 10% to 14% of the population being affected. Other genetic disorders include sickle cell anemia, thalassemia, and spherocytosis. All of these produce structurally abnormal red blood cells to varying degrees.

Symptoms

The symptoms of hemolytic anemia depend on its severity and to some extent on its cause. People with only mild hemolytic anemia may not have any noticeable symptoms. The most common symptom of moderate to severe hemolytic anemia, however, is fatigue. It is a particularly troublesome symptom in cancer patients. Other symptoms of hemolytic anemia typically include shortness of breath; dizziness, especially when standing up; headache; cold, clammy hands or feet; pale skin, gums, and nail beds; and chest pain. Severe hemolytic anemia may produce jaundice or pain in the upper abdomen from an enlarged spleen. People with sickle cell anemia may also develop leg ulcers and severe pain in different parts of the body.

The low level of red blood cells in the patient's blood means that the heart must work harder to supply the body with oxygenated blood. This extra work load may lead to enlargement of the heart, heart murmurs, or abnormal heart rhythms.

Diagnosis

Hemolytic anemia is usually diagnosed by a combination of a careful patient history and the results of laboratory tests. The doctor will ask the patient about a family history of anemia as well as the patient's occupation, prescription and over-the-counter medications, and a history of liver disease, infections, or heart valve replacement or other procedures that can damage red blood cells. Hemolytic anemia can be diagnosed by family doctors, although in some cases the patient may be referred to a hematologist or infectious diseases specialist.

Examination

An office examination for hemolytic anemia will include listening to the patient's breathing and heartbeat for any irregularities; checking the skin and eyeballs for evidence of discoloration due to jaundice; feeling the patient's abdomen to see whether the spleen and liver are enlarged; and performing a rectal examination to check for occult (hidden) bleeding from the digestive tract.

Tests

There are several different types of blood tests that may be performed to diagnose the severity and cause of the patient's anemia:

- Complete blood count (CBC). This test measures the number of RBCs, white blood cells (WBCs), and platelets in the patient's blood. It also measures the hematocrit (proportion of blood volume occupied by red blood cells) and the amount of hemoglobin in the blood.
- Reticulocyte count. Reticulocytes are immature RBCs. Measuring the number of them in a blood sample tells whether the bone marrow is producing new RBCs at the correct rate.
- Peripheral smear. This test tells the doctor whether the red blood cells have normal or abnormal shapes.
- Coombs test. This test detects the presence of antibodies in the blood that may be destroying red blood cells. It can also be used to test blood prior to transfusions to prevent transfusion reactions.
- Tests for bilirubin (a breakdown product of hemoglobin) and liver function.

If blood tests do not help to diagnose the cause of the patient's hemolytic anemia, the doctor may order tests of the patient's bone marrow and kidney function, or have the patient tested for possible lead poisoning or vitamin deficiencies.

Treatment

Treatment of hemolytic anemia has three goals: stopping the premature destruction of red blood cells; raising the patient's RBC count to a healthy level; and treating the underlying condition. Inherited hemolytic anemias typically require lifelong treatment, while acquired hemolytic anemias often clear up once the cause is identified and treated.

Traditional

The treatment depends upon the cause and severity of the anemia. Medicines like **folic acid** and **corticosteroids** may be used to treat the anemia if it is not severe. Severe hemolytic anemia may be very quickly fatal and immediate hospitalization is required for transfusion of washed and packed red blood cells. Severe anemias can aggravate preexisting heart disease, lung disease and cerebrovascular disease.

Frequently with cancer treatments, a patient may undergo numerous blood transfusions to make up for the severe anemia suffered as a result of chemotherapy. Researchers investigating ways to enhance the quality of life for chemotherapy patients have primarily looked at controlling pain and loss of appetite (**anorexia**). Recent studies, however, have examined the use of **erythropoietin** (also called epoetin alfa; a protein hormone that stimulates red blood cell production) in improving fatigue symptoms and enhancing overall quality of life.

Once-weekly therapy with erythropoietin was found to increase hemoglobin levels, decrease transfusion requirements, and improve quality of life in patients with cancer and anemia undergoing chemotherapy. The downside of erythropoietin therapy is that it may stimulate some types of tumors and cause them to grow faster. The National Cancer Institute (NCI) recommends that cancer patients discuss the risks and benefits of this treatment with their doctor.

Alternative

Avoiding exposure to chemicals that precipitate the reaction, eating natural, whole grain foods, avoiding stress, and taking vitamin supplements can be helpful to patients with hemolytic anemia. With cancer patients, yoga and meditation provide a means of enhancing relaxation, reducing stress, and incorporating visualization for healing. Those patients who attend and participate in support groups have an increased quality of life with better outcomes from mainstream treatments.

Prognosis

The prognosis of hemolytic anemia depends on its cause. Some inherited anemias like sickle cell anemia lead to shortened life spans, while some acquired anemias have an excellent prognosis. Few patients die as a direct result of hemolytic anemia; however, elderly people and those with heart disease are at increased risk of health crises brought about by increased strain on the heart caused by the anemia.

Prevention

Inherited types of hemolytic anemia cannot be prevented as of 2009, with the exception of G6PD deficiency. People born with this deficiency can avoid fava beans, naphthalene (found in some brands of moth balls) and certain medications as advised by their doctor.

Acquired hemolytic anemia caused by a blood transfusion mismatch can be prevented by careful matching of blood donors and recipients. Hemolytic anemia caused by Rh-factor incompatibility can be prevented by prenatal care during pregnancy.

Resources

BOOKS

Bridges, Kenneth R., and Howard A. Pearson, eds. *Anemias and Other Red Cell Disorders*. New York: McGraw-Hill, 2007.

PERIODICALS

American Academy of Family Physicians. "Information from Your Family Doctor: Thalassemia." *American Family Physician* 80 (August 15, 2009): 371.

Elyassi, C. A., and M.H. Rowshan. "Perioperative Management of the Glucose-6-phosphate Dehydrogenase Deficient Patient: A Review of Literature." *Anesthesia Progress* 56 (Fall 2009): 86–91.

Khurana, V., et al. "Microangiopathic Hemolytic Anemia Following Disseminated Intravascular Coagulation in Aluminum Phosphide Poisoning." *Indian Journal of Medical Sciences* 63 (June 2009): 257–59.

Kotwal, R.S., et al. "Central Retinal Vein Occlusion in an Army Ranger with Glucose-6-phosphate Dehydrogenase Deficiency." *Journal of Special Operations Medicine* 9 (Summer 2009): 59–63.

Lai, J. I., and W. S. Wang. "Acute Hemolysis after Receiving Oxaliplatin Treatment: A Case Report and Literature Review."*Pharmacy World and Science* 31 (October 2009): 538–41.

Shen, Y. "Autoimmune Hemolytic Anemia Associated with a Formulation of Traditional Chinese Medicines." *American Journal of Health-System Pharmacy* 66 (October 1, 2009): 1701–03.

OTHER

Dhaliwal, Gurpreet, Patricia A. Cornett, and Lawrence M. Tierney, Jr. "Hemolytic Anemia." *American Family Physician* 69 (June 1, 2004): 2599–2606.http://www.aafp.org/afp/20040601/2599.html

National Cancer Institute (NCI). *Cancer Topics: Fatigue.* http://www.cancer.gov/cancertopics/pdq/supportive care/fatigue/patient/allpages

National Heart, Lung, and Blood Institute (NHLBI). *Hemolytic Anemia.* http://www.nhlbi.nih.gov/health/dci/Diseases/ha/ha_whatis.html

Schick, Paul. "Hemolytic Anemia." *eMedicine*, April 27, 2009. http://emedicine.medscape.com/article/201066-overview

ORGANIZATIONS

American Cancer Society, 250 Williams Street NW, Atlanta, GA, 30303, 800-ACS-2345 (227-2345), www.cancer.org.

American Society of Hematology (ASH), 1900 M Street, NW, Washington, DC, 20036, 202-776-0544, 202-776-0545, http://www.hematology.org/.

National Cancer Institute, 6116 Executive Blvd., Room 3036A, Bethesda, MD, 20892-8322, 800-422-6237, cancergovstaff@mail.nih.gov, www.cancer.gov.

National Heart, Lung, and Blood Institute (NHLBI), Health Information Center, P.O. Box 30105, Bethesda, MD, 20824-0105, 301-592-8573, 240-629-3246, nhlbiinfo@nhlbi.nih.gov, http://www.nhlbi.nih.gov/.

Linda K. Bennington, C.N.S., M.S.N.
Rebecca J. Frey, PhD

Hemoptysis

Definition

Hemoptysis is the coughing up of blood or bloody sputum from the respiratory tract. It is a symptom of a disease or disorder rather than a disease in its own right. The blood can come from the nose, mouth, throat, airway passages leading from the lungs, or the lungs themselves. Hemoptysis may be either self-limiting or recurrent. Massive hemoptysis is defined as 200–600 mL of blood coughed up within a period of 24 hours or less.

Description

Hemoptysis can range from small quantities of bloody sputum to life-threatening amounts of blood. The patient may or may not have chest pain. Massive hemoptysis is considered a medical emergency. Up to 75 percent of patients with massive hemoptysis die from asphyxiation (lack of oxygen) caused by too much blood in the airway.

Hemoptysis refers specifically to the spitting up of blood that comes from the respiratory tract. Often when persons spit up blood, they are not spitting up blood from the respiratory tract, but from somewhere else. When the blood comes from somewhere other than the respiratory tract, such as from a bloody nose or from the gastrointestinal tract, the symptom is called pseudohemoptysis. **Vomiting** blood from the gastrointestinal tract, which is called hematemesis, is one type of pseudohemoptysis. It is important to distinguish between true hemoptysis and pseudohemoptysis because they often involve very different parts of the body and the treatments are radically different. Hematemesis differs from hemoptysis in that the vomited blood is usually dark brown or black rather than pink or red; is usually mixed with food particles; and resembles coffee grounds rather than having a liquid or foamy appearance.

Risk factors

Risk factors for hemoptysis include:

- Smoking
- Occupational exposure to asbestos, nickel, or chromium
- Frequent travel to countries where parasitic and other infections are endemic
- HIV infection (This is a risk factor for **Kaposi's sarcoma** of the lung and for such opportunistic infections as aspergillosis.)
- History of bronchitis or other lung disorders

Causes and symptoms

Hemoptysis can be caused by a range of disorders:

- Infections. These include pneumonia; tuberculosis; aspergillosis; and parasitic diseases, including ascariasis, amebiasis, and paragonimiasis. Infection is the most common single cause of hemoptysis in adults, accounting for 60–70% of cases.
- Tumors that erode blood vessel walls. Cancers associated with hemoptysis include bronchial carcinoma, bronchial adenoma, respiratory tract hemangioma, and occasionally by metastatic cancer to the lungs. Primary lung cancers account for 23% of cases of hemoptysis in North America.
- Drug abuse. Cocaine can cause massive hemoptysis.
- Trauma. Chest injuries can cause bleeding into the lungs.
- Vascular disorders, including aneurysms, pulmonary embolism, and malformations of the blood vessels.
- Bronchitis. Its most common cause is long-term smoking.
- Foreign object(s) in the airway. This is a common cause of hemoptysis in children, second only to upper respiratory infections.
- Blood clotting disorders.
- Bleeding following such surgical procedures as bronchial biopsies and heart catheterization.
- Thoracic endometrial syndrome (TES). TES is a rare disorder marked by endometrial (uterine lining) tissue growing in the tissue covering the lungs or in the airway. A woman with TES will have catamenial hemoptysis, or hemoptysis related to her menstrual periods.

Diagnosis

The diagnosis of hemoptysis is complicated by the number of possible causes. For this reason, the doctor must take a thorough patient history, including the patient's occupation, recent travels, tobacco use, and a history of **cancer** or cancer treatment. It is important for the doctor to distinguish between blood from the lungs and blood coming from the nose, mouth, or digestive tract. Patients may aspirate, or breathe, blood from the nose or stomach into their lungs and cough it up. They may also swallow blood from the chest area and then vomit. The doctor will ask about stomach ulcers, repeated vomiting, liver disease, alcoholism, smoking, tuberculosis, mitral valve disease, or treatment with anticoagulant medications.

Examination

The doctor will examine the patient's nose, throat, mouth, and chest for bleeding from these areas and for signs of chest trauma. The most important consideration is to either identify or rule out bleeding from the upper airway. The doctor also listens to the patient's breathing and heartbeat for indications of heart abnormalities or lung disease. In some cases asking the patient whether they can identify the sensation of the bleeding may help the doctor pinpoint the location.

Tests

Laboratory tests for hemoptysis include blood tests to rule out clotting disorders, and to look for food particles or other evidence that the blood comes from the stomach. Sputum can be tested for fungi, bacteria, or parasites.

Procedures

Chest **x rays** and **bronchoscopy** are the most important studies for evaluating hemoptysis. They are used to evaluate the cause, location, and extent of the bleeding. The bronchoscope is a long, flexible tube used to identify tumors or remove foreign objects.

Computed tomography scans (CT scans) are used to detect aneurysms and to confirm x-ray results. Ventilation-perfusion scanning is used to rule out pulmonary embolism. The doctor may also order an angiogram to rule out pulmonary embolism, or to locate a source of bleeding that could not be seen with the bronchoscope.

In spite of the number of different diagnostic tests, the cause of hemoptysis cannot be determined in 30–40% of cases.

Treatment

Traditional

Massive hemoptysis is a life-threatening emergency that requires treatment in an intensive care unit. The patient will be intubated (the insertion of a tube to help breathing) to protect the airway, and to allow evaluation of the source of the bleeding. Patients with lung cancer, bleeding from an aneurysm (blood clot), or persistent traumatic bleeding require chest surgery.

The goal of treatment for patients with hemoptysis is to stop the bleeding as soon as possible while also treating the cancer or other underlying disorder that is causing the hemoptysis. When large amounts of blood have been lost, the patient may also require intravenous (IV) fluids and/or a blood transfusion.

Mild hemoptysis generally will stop spontaneously and no treatment is necessary, apart from reassurance of the patient that this condition will resolve on its own. Therefore, the general treatment for hemoptysis is to keep the patient calm and to ensure complete bed rest.

In the most severe cases of hemoptysis, surgery to remove the cancer that is causing the spitting up of blood may be necessary to relieve the symptoms of hemoptysis. Other treatment modalities include PDT (**photodynamic therapy**).

Foreign objects in the airway are removed with a bronchoscope.

If the cause of the bleeding cannot be determined, the patient is monitored for further developments.

Drugs

If the coughing that accompanies the hemoptysis is troublesome or aggravating the condition, cough suppressant medications may be recommended.

Patients with tuberculosis, aspergillosis, or bacterial **pneumonia** are given **antibiotics**.

Patients with pain associated with hemoptysis should not be given sedatives or opioid pain relievers (morphine, fentanyl, oxycodone, etc.) because these medications slow down respiration.

Alternative

Inhalation of the fumes of a tea made from the bark of the wild cherry (*Prunus virginiana*) tree has been an herbal remedy for many respiratory tract ailments, including tuberculosis and hemoptysis among the Native Americans for centuries.

Hydrazine sulfate, a naturally occurring mono-amine oxidase inhibitor (MAOI), has also been suggested as a treatment for hemoptysis.

Prognosis

The prognosis depends on the underlying cause. Patients with mild hemoptysis usually recover completely within 6 months of evaluation. In cases of massive hemoptysis, the mortality rate is about 15%. The rate of bleeding, however, is not a useful predictor of the patient's chances for recovery.

Prevention

Hemoptysis is a condition that is difficult to prevent because it has so many different possible causes. Avoiding or quitting smoking, however, is a preventive measure that can reduce a person's susceptibility to upper respiratory infections and lung cancer—two common causes of hemoptysis.

Resources

BOOKS

Fiebach, Nicholas H., et al, eds. *Principles of Ambulatory Medicine*. Philadelphia: Lippincott Williams and Wilkins, 2007.

Goroll, Allan H., and Albert G. Mulley Jr., eds. *Primary Care Medicine: Office Evaluation and Management of the Adult Patient*, 6th ed. Philadelphia : Wolters Kluwer Health/Lippincott Williams and Wilkins, 2009.

Porter, Robert S., ed. *The Merck Manual of Patient Symptoms: A Concise, Practical Guide to Etiology, Evaluation, and Treatment*. Whitehouse Station, NJ: Merck Research Laboratories, 2008.

PERIODICALS

Gross, A.M., et al. "Management of Life-threatening Haemoptysis in an Area of High Tuberculosis Incidence." *International Journal of Tuberculosis and Lung Disease* 13 (July 2009): 875–80.

Izumi, N., et al. "Primary Pulmonary Meningioma Presenting with Hemoptysis on Exertion." *Annals of Thoracic Surgery* 88 (August 2009): 647–48.

Lane, M. A., et al. "Human Paragonimiasis in North America Following Ingestion of Raw Crayfish." *Clinical Infectious Diseases* 49 (September 15, 2009): 55–61.

Lau, E.M., et al. "Recombinant Activated Factor VII for Massive Hemoptysis in Patients with Cystic Fibrosis." *Chest* 136 (July 2009): 277–81.

Parker, C.M., et al. "Catamenial Hemoptysis and Pneumothorax in a Patient with Cystic Fibrosis." *Canadian Respiratory Journal* 14 (July-August 2007): 295–97.

Prasad, R., et al. "Lessons from Patients with Hemoptysis Attending a Chest Clinic in India." *Annals of Thoracic Medicine* 4 (January 2009): 10–12.

OTHER

Bidwell, Jacob L., and Robert W. Pachner. "Hemoptysis: Diagnosis and Management." *American Family Physician* 72 (October 1, 2005): 1253–60. http://www.aafp.org/afp/20051001/1253.html

Merck Manual of Diagnosis and Therapy. *Hemoptysis.* http://www.merck.com/mmpe/sec05/ch045/ch045e.html

ORGANIZATIONS

American Cancer Society, 250 Williams Street NW, Atlanta, GA, 30303, 800-ACS-2345 (227-2345), www.cancer.org.

American College of Emergency Physicians (ACEP), 1125 Executive Circle, Irving, TX, 75038-2522, 972-550-0911, 800-798-1822, 972-580-2816, http://www.acep.org/.

American Lung Association (ALA), 1301 Pennsylvania Avenue NW, Suite 800, Washington, DC, 20004, 212-315-8700, 800-548-8252 (helpline), http://www.lungusa.org/.

Centers for Disease Control and Prevention (CDC), 1600 Clifton Road, Atlanta, GA, 30333, 800-232-4636, cdcinfo@cdc.gov, http://www.cdc.gov.

National Cancer Institute, 6116 Executive Blvd., Room 3036A, Bethesda, MD, 20892-8322, 800-422-6237, cancergovstaff@mail.nih.gov, www.cancer.gov.

National Heart, Lung, and Blood Institute (NHLBI), Health Information Center, P.O. Box 30105, Bethesda, MD, 20824-0105, 301-592-8573, 240-629-3246, nhlbiinfo@nhlbi.nih.gov, http://www.nhlbi.nih.gov/.

Paul A. Johnson, Ed.M.
Rebecca J. Frey, PhD

Heparin

Definition

Heparin is a drug that helps prevent blood clots from forming and belongs to the family of drugs called anticoagulants (blood thinners), although it does not actually thin the blood. It is sold in the United States under the brand names of Calciparine, Liquaemin, Calciparine, Hepalean, and Heparin Leo, and Calcilean in Canada.

Purpose

Heparin is used to decrease the clotting ability of the blood and to help prevent harmful clots from forming in the blood vessels. Heparin will not dissolve blood clots that have already formed, but it may prevent the clots from becoming larger and causing more serious problems. Heparin possesses several antithrombotic mechanisms. It is often used as a treatment for certain blood vessel, heart, and lung conditions and is also used to prevent blood clotting during open-heart surgery, bypass surgery, and dialysis. Heparin is used in low doses to prevent the formation of blood clots in certain patients, especially those who must have certain types of surgery or who must remain in bed for a long time. It is also used for the long-term treatment of thromboembolic disease, a common side effect of **cancer**.

One of the most common hematological complications is disordered coagulation. Approximately 15% of all cancer patients are affected by thromboembolic disease, which is the second leading cause of death for cancer patients. However, thromboembolic disease may represent only one of many complications in end-stage patients. Thromboembolic disease includes superficial and deep venous thrombosis, pulmonary emboli, thrombosis of venous access devices, arterial thrombosis, and embolism. The cancer itself or cancer treatments may induce coagulation. For example, **chemotherapy** can increase the risk of thromboembolic disease. An increased risk for arterial thrombosis has been observed with chemotherapy treatment.

Cancer and its treatment can affect all three causes of thromboembolic disease, including the alteration of blood flow, damage to endothelial cells (the cells in blood vessels), and enhancing procoagulants (causing the blood to clot). Cancer can affect blood flow by mechanically affecting blood vessels close to a tumor. In addition, tumors cause angiogenesis, which may create complexes of blood vessels that have a disordered appearance and flow (varying in magnitude and direction). Chemotherapy or tumors may directly damage endothelial cells. Procoagulants may be secreted into the blood stream by cancer cells or can be increased on the surface of cancer cells.

Antithrombotic treatment, in the form of the low-molecular-weight heparin reviparin, has been shown for the first time to safely improve the outcomes of patients

KEY TERMS

Angiogenesis—The formation of new blood vessels that occurs naturally under certain circumstances, for example, in the healing of a cut.

Anticoagulant—Anticoagulants are nonhabit-forming medications that prevent the formation of new blood clots and keep existing blood clots from growing larger.

Blood clot—A clump of blood that forms in or around a vessel as a result of coagulation. The formation of blood clots when the body has been cut is essential because without blood clots to cease the bleeding, a person would bleed to death from a relatively small wound.

Coagulation—The blood's natural tendency to clump and stick.

Embolism—An embolism occurs when a clump of material such as a broken-off piece of plaque, a blood clot, or air travels through the bloodstream and becomes lodged in a blood vessel.

Endothelial cells—The cells lining the inside of blood vessels.

Parenteral—Medications administered through intravenous, subcutaneous, or intramuscular injection.

Procoagulants—Inducing the blood to clot.

Thromboembolism—Another word for embolism (see embolism).

Thrombosis—The formation of a blood clot in an artery or vein that may be accompanied by inflammation. If untreated in arteries, thrombosis can lead to death of the nearby tissue.

with an acute myocardial infarction. The new findings show that reviparin "clearly improves the outcomes of patients who undergo thrombolysis with streptokinase or urokinase, and it also appears to be a useful adjunct for patients treated with primary percutaneous coronary intervention [PCI]," said Dr. Anderson, associate chief of the division of cardiology at LDS Hospital in Salt Lake City. The study has some limitations.

Description

Heparin is the most common anticoagulant used and the generic name product may be available in the United States and Canada.

Mechanisms of action:

Heparin increases the release of specific proteins, like tissue plasminogen activator and tissue factor pathway inhibitor (TFPI), into the blood in order to inhibit blood coagulation. It can also increase the activity of these proteins. Heparin augments the activity of anti-thrombin III, a natural compound that inhibits activated clotting factors from contributing to more coagulation. Furthermore, heparin has been found to inhibit substances that may contribute to angiogenesis, including vascular endothelial growth factor, tissue factor, and platelet-activating factor.

Whether anticoagulants like heparin may also improve cancer survival rates independent of their effect on thromboembolism has been investigated. In fact, experimental and clinical data have demonstrated that heparin is an effective compound in preventing metastases. Many investigators have shown that heparin inhibits tumor **metastasis** in experimental animals; a few **clinical trials** also suggest a positive effect in humans with cancer.

Recommended dosage

Heparin is available only with a doctor's prescription, in parenteral and injection (United States and Canada) dosage forms. A doctor will need to prescribe a specific dose for an individual's based on the type of heparin, as well as the patient's medical condition and body weight.

Dosing schedule

Heparin should be taken under the doctor's direction and at the same time every day. If a dose is missed, take it as soon as possible. However, if a dose is missed until the following day, patients should not double-dose, but just take the usual daily dose. Double-dosing may cause bleeding.

Precautions

Some medications should not be combined. Over-the-counter medicines, **vitamins**, and herbal products may cause interactions when combined with heparin, so the patient should check with the doctor monitoring the heparin medication before taking any new medication, even when prescribed by another doctor.

Patients who are pregnant, breastfeeding, have given birth recently, or using an IUD for birth control should consult their doctors. The doctor should also be notified if radiation treatments, surgery, or a fall or other injury has recently occurred.

The presence of other medical problems may affect the use of heparin. Patients should be sure to tell their doctors about any other medical problems, in particular:

- allergies or asthma (or history of)
- blood disease or bleeding problems
- colitis or stomach ulcer (or history of)
- diabetes mellitus
- high blood pressure (hypertension)
- kidney disease
- liver disease
- tuberculosis (active)

Side effects

The doctor should be contacted immediately if any of these side effects are present:

- wheezing or trouble breathing
- skin rash, itching, or hives
- red or "coffee ground" vomit
- unexplained nosebleeds
- swelling in the face, lips, or tongue
- blood in urine or stools
- black tarry stools

Interactions

Using any of the following medicines together with heparin may increase the risk of bleeding. Again, candidates for heparin should alert their physicians if they are taking any of these medications:

- aspirin
- persantine
- carbenicillin by injection (Geopen)
- cefamandole (Mandol)
- cefoperazone (Cefobid)
- cefotetan (Cefotan)
- dipyridamole (Persantine)
- divalproex (Depakote)
- medicine for inflammation or pain (Motrin, Aleve), except narcotics
- medicine for overactive thyroid
- pentoxifylline (Trental)
- plicamycin (Mithracin)
- probenecid (Benemid)
- sulfinpyrazone (Anturane)
- ticarcillin (Ticar)

• valproic acid (Depakene)
• medicines via intramuscular injection

See also Low molecular weight heparin; Warfarin.

Crystal Heather Kaczkowski, MSc.

Hepatic arterial infusion

Definition

Hepatic arterial infusion (HAI) therapy, delivers chemotherapeutic agents directly to the liver through a catheter placed in the hepatic artery. The hepatic artery is the main route of blood supply to liver tumors. HAI is also known as regional **chemotherapy**.

Purpose

Approximately 106,000 patients are diagnosed with **colon cancer** in the United States each year. The **cancer** spreads to the liver in about 70% of those patients. For patients with colorectal liver metastases, tumor progression within the liver is typically the primary cause of death.

Systemic chemotherapy using various agents hassome efficacy, but the side effects can have a profound negative impact on the patient's quality of life during treatment. HAI therapy may be an effective option because it delivers chemotherapy medication directly to the site of the tumor, making it appropriate as an alternative or adjuvant treatment to systemic chemotherapy. When metastases is limited to the liver, HAI with **floxuridine** (FUDR) or radioactive microspheres through an implantable pump under the skin or an external pump worn on the belt may be a better option than systemic chemotherapy.

HAI may extend life expectancy and reduce the chance that more liver tumors will develop.

Precautions

• Strict aseptic techniques should be used to prevent infection during all procedures.
• Pump flow rate will vary depending on factors such as body temperature, altitude, arterial pressure at the catheter tip, and solution viscosity.
• Patients should not attempt to resterilize the pump.

KEY TERMS

Adjuvant treatment—A treatment that is added to increase effectiveness of the first treatment.

Cancer—A term for diseases in which abnormal cells divide without control. Cancer cells can invade nearby tissues and can spread through the bloodstream and lymphatic system to other parts of the body.

Catheter—A flexible tube used to administer or withdraw fluids. During a course of chemotherapy, an indwelling catheter can be placed in a vein to administer intravenous fluids and chemotherapy. Catheters can stay in place for several weeks or months with proper care.

Chemotherapy—A cancer treatment using medicines.

Hepatic—Refers to the liver.

Implant—A device inserted into the body to either treat cancer or to replace or substitute for a lost part or ability.

Metastases—The spread of cancer to other body parts.

Tumor—An abnormal mass of tissue that serves no purpose. Tumors may be either benign (non-cancerous) or malignant (cancerous).

• The manufacturer's instructions should be followed regarding drug preparation, dosage, and administration.
• FUDR should be used with added caution in patients with impaired liver or kidney function.

Systemic therapy should be considered for patients with disease known to extend beyond the area capable of being infused.

Description

HAI enhances cancer therapy by increasing drug delivery directly to the site of the tumor (the liver) while minimizing systemic drug exposure and side effects. Development of fully implanted infusion systems have allowed for long-term delivery of hepatic regional chemotherapy.

Benefits of HAI therapy:
• yields higher tumor response rates and delays cancer progression
• trend toward increased survival rates
• enhances quality of life
• reduced systemic side effects

Preparation

Patient selection criteria

Successful results depend on careful patient selection. Candidates for HAI therapy should:

- have primary liver cancer or liver metastases from primary colorectal cancer
- show an absence of tumors outside the liver
- have demonstrated portal vein patency
- be a suitable surgical candidate
- show no evidence of infection
- be willing to participate in frequent pump refill appointments

Studies have demonstrated that patients with metastatic colorectal cancer who had liver disease only, had less than 70% of their liver involved with metastases, and had a good performance status responded best to HAI. When metastases are also located outside of the liver, HAI does not offer an advantage over systemic chemotherapy.

Aftercare

During the course of treatment, pump pocket infections occur rarely. At the first sign of **infection** at the pump pocket, systemic **antibiotics** need to be started. The pump needs to be moved to a new location in a newly created pocket if the infection does not resolve itself. The old pocket should be opened and drained.

Risks

The major problems with HAI are not surgical. They include gastritis, duodenitis, and biliary sclerosis.

Drug toxicity and medication side effects may occur. The most commonly reported side effects for FUDR are **nausea and vomiting**, **diarrhea**, and intestinal inflammation.

Other possible complications include:

- Arterial thromboses.
- Catheter dislodgement.
- The catheter may erode through the wall of the duodenum when the pump has been in place for more than a year.
- Overdose or underdose of medication if certain conditions affect the rate at which the pump delivers medication, i.e. pump damage due to strenuous activity, high heat, or a change in air pressure.
- Disruption in therapy if the pump is damaged by improper handling or filling.

Normal results

Morbidity or mortality occurring as a result of this procedure should be close to zero. Appropriate selection of patients and new combinations of chemotherapy should provide at least a 70% response rate from HAI for the treatment of hepatic metastases from colorectal primary tumors. This response rate is at least twice that of current systemic chemotherapies.

When used in conjunction with traditional chemotherapy, HAI therapy has been shown to extend life expectancy and reduce recurrence of liver tumors after two years for certain patients.

Abnormal results

Complications that can occur with surgery:

- infection
- fluid build up around the implant site
- skin erosion over the site of the implant
- incision breakdown
- drugs may be delivered to organs other than the liver

Resources

PERIODICALS

Henderson, C.W. "Combined Criteria Predict Response to Hepatic Arterial Infusion Chemotherapy." *Cancer Weekly* (August 1, 2000/).

Link, Karl H., Marko Kornmann, et al. " Thymidylate Synthase Quantitation and In Vitro Chemosensitivity Testing Predicts Responses and Survival of Patients with Isolated Nonresectable Liver Tumors Receiving Hepatic Arterial Infusion Chemotherapy." *Cancer* 89, no 12 (July 15, 2000): 288–9.

Venook, Alan, Betsy Althaus, et al. " Hepatic Arterial Infusion of Chemotherapy for Metastatic Colorectal Cancer." *New England Journal of Medicine* 342, no. 20 (May 18, 2000): 1524.

Crystal Heather Kaczkowski, M.S.

Hepatocellular carcinoma *see* **Liver cancer, primary**

Herceptin

Definition

Herceptin is a medicine that is used to slow or stop the growth of a cancerous tumor.

Purpose

Herceptin is used to treat **breast cancer** that has spread to other parts of the body in women whose tumor cells produce an overabundance of a protein known as the human epidermal growth factor receptor 2 (HER2).

Description

Also known by its generic name, **trastuzumab**, Herceptin is an antineoplastic drug manufactured by Genentech, Inc. A monoclonal antibody, Herceptin works differently than **chemotherapy** or hormonal **anticancer drugs**. It targets **cancer** cells that make too much of the HER2 protein, which is found on the surface of the cancer cells and thought to fuel cancer growth. Used only to treat cancers that make an overabundance of HER2 protein, Heceptin works by binding to the protein's particles and blocking its effect, thereby slowing down or stopping the cancer cell growth. The HER2 proteins with Herception are removed from the surface the cell. When this happens, they cannot tell the cell to grow and divide.

In addition, Genentech, Inc. explains that there may be two other factors that account for Herceptin's effectiveness; Herceptin signals the immune system and works with chemotherapy. After Herceptin binds to the HER2 protein, the natural killer cells of the immune system are attracted to Herceptin. Herceptin, in turn, binds to the natural killer cells and determines which cells are abnormal and helps to kill them. When this occurs, chemotherapy may be ehanced. Although Herceptin and chemotherapy work differently, Genentech points out that when used together, "the two drugs can be synergistic. Treatment with Herceptin prevents DNA repair following the impact of DNA-damaging chemotherapy that stops the tumor cells from growing."

According to the National Cancer Institute, approximately 25-30% of breast cancers make too much HER2 protein. These kinds of tumors tend to grow faster and are more likely to recur. The amount of HER2 that is present in a tumor is determined by a lab test and a score from 0, which is a negative score, to 3+, which is a highly positive score, is assigned. Only patients with high scores are expected to benefit from Herceptin treatment.

Clinical Trial Results and FDA Approval

Two groundbreaking **clinical trials** were conducted to test the safety and efficacy of Herceptin. One of them, conducted by Slamon and colleagues, produced data that led to Herceptin's approval by the U.S. Food and Drug Administration (FDA) in 1998. In 2001, The *New England Journal of Medicine* published the study results by Slamon and colleagues, which involved 234 randomly assigned patients who received chemotherapy alone and 235 patients who received chemotherapy plus Herceptin. All the patients in the study were diagnosed with metastasic breast cancer that overproduced HER2. Ultimately, Slamon and colleagues concluded that the addition of Herceptin to chemotherapy was associated with "a longer time to disease progression, a higher rate of response [to the treatment], longer survival, and a 20% reduction in the risk of death," as compared to treatment with chemotherapy alone. Specifically, for example, Herceptin combined with paclitaxel proved to be especially valuable; the overall response rate rose from 15% in women treated with paclitaxel to 38% in women treated with Herceptin and paclitaxel. All factors considered Herceptin seems to increase the clinical benefits of first-line chemotherapy.

In another clinical trial, as explained by the National Cancer Institute, "Women were given only Herception. In 14% of these women, the tumor got smaller or disappeared." Therefore, in September 1998, the FDA announced its approval of Herceptin for the treatment of metastatic breast cancer. Herceptin was specifically approved in combination with paclitaxel as therapy for HER2 breast cancer. It is also used alone as a therapy after other therapies have failed." Used by itself or with chemotherapy, Herceptin is the first FDA-approved therapy that targets a particular genetic defect known to play a role in cancer development.

Other Possible Uses for Herceptin

Herceptin is also being studied as an adjuvant therapy for the treatment of nonmetastatic breast cancer that has spread to the lymph nodes, but not anywhere else.

Herceptin may also be useful in fighting cancers of the lung, colon, prostate, and bladder in patients whose tumors have an overabundance of HER2. Several studies are underway to test the effectiveness of Herceptin with and without other anticancer drugs.

Recommended dosage

Herceptin is administered intravenously on a weekly basis in a hospital or clinic setting. Based on the patient's body weight, the typical dosage is 0.9 to 3.6 mg per pound.

Precautions

It is important to have periodic blood tests while taking Heceptin, because it can cause **anemia** and a low white blood cell count in many patients. Guarding the cardiac health of patients taking Herceptin is imperative, because using it can lead to congestive heart failure. Therefore, some patients may not be able to take Herceptin.

It isn't known whether Herceptin is safe to take while a patient is pregnant. Nonetheless, patients should avoid becoming pregnant while they are taking Herceptin. Pregnant patients should talk with their physicians regarding any possible risks to the fetus. Mothers should not breastfeed their babies while they are being treated with Herceptin, because it does pass to the breast milk. In fact, mothers should not breastfeed for at least 6 months after being treated with Herceptin.

Side effects

The two most serious side effects associated with the use of Herceptin are cardiac amd lung related. Damage to the heart muscle, which can cause heart failure, and lung complications, which can cause serious breathing problems can occur. In both cases, immediate medical attention is required. Whether during or after treatment, patients experiencing difficulty breathing or any of the signs associated with heart failure, such as shortness of breath, a fast heartbeat, or swelling in the feet or legs, should contact their physicians without delay. Cardiac side effects are more frequently experienced by elderly patients. Also, in clinical trials, it was found that patients receiving Herceptin with anthracycline chemotherapy were more likely to experience cardiac dysfunction than those who did not receive anthracyclines. Patients treated with Herceptin must be monitored carefully and screened prior to their treatment for any lung or heart problems. It is sometimes necessary to discontinue treatment with Herceptin.

The National Cancer Institute cautions patients that Herceptin can cause severe allergic reactions, such as low blood pressure, shortness of breath, rashes, and wheezing. These reactions are usually more common in patients who already suffer from lung disease.

Fever and chills are common during the first infusion and occur less frequently thereafter. Throughout Herceptin treatment it is not uncommon for patients to experience **nausea**, **vomiting**, **diarrhea**, dizziness, sleeplessness, appetite loss, cough, abdominal and back pain, headache, and sore throat. **Depression**, tingling in the hands or feet, fluid retention, sinus irritation, and flu-like symptoms are less commonly reported. Uncommon side effects are acne, cold sores, and urinary **infection**, as well as pain in the joints, bones, or nerves. As reminded by the National Cancer Institute, it is important to note that patients being treated with Herceptin alone in comparison to patients being treated with Herceptin and chemotherapy may have different side effects. For example, when Herceptin is used in combination with chemotherapy, patients are more likely to experience anemia leukopenia, diarrhea, and infection. Therefore, blood tests may be required more frequently for patients being treated with both Herceptin and chemotherapy. Rare side effects can develop in any part of the body, however, regardless of whether a patient is being treated with Herceptin only or in combination with chemotherapy. Patients should inform their physicians when they experience any side effects, regardless of whether the side effects are mild or severe. Some side effects, such as pain, can be managed medically.

Whether in the early or advanced stages, cancer itself can cause pain. In fact, numerous studies, such as the one by Reuben and colleagues published in 1998 in the Archives of Internal Medicine, have validated that patients with advanced cancer are likely to have a number of symptoms in addition to pain, such as insomnia, depression, and **fatigue**. Therefore, it is valuable, if possible, to determine the source of the pain whether is the drug therapy or the cancer itself causing the pain it. Once the source of the pain is determined, it is easier to decide what the next course of action should be. Patients should be their own health care advocates and work as closely as possible with their physicians regarding treatment strategies for adverse side effects and cancer-related pain. Patients should talk with their physicians about a variety of treatment modalities that range from conventional options to alternative therapies, such as acupuncture, for example.

Pain intensity should also be considered when developing a treatment plan to cope with unpleasant side effects. Certain pain measurement tools, such as the Visual Analogue Pain Scale (VAPS) and the McGill Pain Questionnaire, are commonly used by physicians to assess pain intensity. Patients having difficulty coping with the pain associated with cancer and cancer drugs might find it helpful to be referred to a physician who specializes in **pain management** or a pain clinic. Physicians specializing in the treatment of pain come from a variety of medical backgrounds, such as anesthesiology, obstetrics and gynecology, neurology, and surgery. Because of the complicated nature of cancer and cancer-related pain, ideally a pain management team should be formed that works with the patient's primary care physician, oncologist, and radiologist to provide comprehensive care to the patient.

Advances in cancer treatment lengthen survival among cancer patients. It is important for cancer patients to understand that they are not alone. Support groups exist to help patients cope not only with the physical aspects of having cancer, but with the psychological ones as well. In addition, the positive support (both emotional and otherwise) provided by caregivers can help to improve a patient's quality of life.

Interactions

There are no known food interactions. However, as mentioned earlier, cardiac dysfunction was especially high in patients who received Herceptin in combination with anthracycline chemotherapy. Patients should discuss any medications (over-the counter, herbal, and prescription) that they are taking with their physician so that an assessment can be made regarding the risk of interactions.

There are, in fact, a multitude of precautions and interactions related to chemotherapy treatment. The best thing for patients to do that are undergoing chemotherapy is to discuss all the precautions and interactions with their physicians. Usually a patient's doctor will provide patient education pamphlets regarding chemotherapy treatment. Pamphlets are also available from local cancer centers and the American Cancer Society.

Resources

BOOKS

Lema, Mark J., Day, Miles, Myers, David P., et al. Cancer Pain. In *Pain Medicine: A Comprehensive Review, edited by P. Prithvi Raj and Lee Ann Paradise.* St. Louis, MO: Mosby, 2003, pp.110–118.
Silverman, Harold M., editor. *The Pill Book.* 10th ed. New York, NY: Bantam Books, 2002.

PERIODICALS

Reuben, D. B., Mor, V., Hiris, J. "Clinical symptoms and length of survival in patients with terminal cancer." *Archives of Internal Medicine* 148 (1998): 1586.

Slamon, D. J., Leyland-Jones, B., Shak, S., et al. "Use of chemotherapy plus a monoclonal antibody against HER2 for metastic breast cancer that overexpresses HER2." *New England Journal of Medicine* 344 (2001): 782–792.

OTHER

"Herceptin Fact Sheet." *Genentech, Inc.* March 2005. 19 Mar. 2005 http://www.gene.com/gene/products/infor mation/oncology/herceptin/factsheet.jsp.
"Herceptin (Trastuzumab): Questions and Answers." *National Cancer Institute.* February 2002. 19 Mar. 2005 http://cis.nci.nih.gov/fact/7_45.htm.

Lee Ann Paradise

Herpes simplex

Definition

Herpes simplex is a virus that causes blister-like open sores, usually on the mouth or genitals of the infected person.

Demographics

There are two distinct types: herpes simplex virus type 1 (HSV-1) and herpes simplex virus type 2 (HSV-2). Both types of HSV are common worldwide. HSV-1 is transmitted from person to person by close contact, such as kissing. In the United States, by age 30, half of all individuals of high socioeconomic status are infected

Color digitized electron micrograph image of herpes simplex virus. Cancer patients, especially those who are undergoing chemotherapy or radiation treatments, are at greater risk of herpes infections. *(Custom Medical Stock Photo. Reproduced by permission.)*

with HSV-1, and 80% of all individuals of low socio-economic status carry the virus, although many of those infected do not show symptoms.

HSV-2 is transmitted through sexual contact, thus its distribution is related to the age at which sexual activity begins and the extent of sexual activity within a population. **Infection** is more common in women than men, and in the United States infection is more common among blacks than whites. As many as 90% of people infected with HSV-2 are unaware that they carry the virus because they have either no symptoms or very mild symptoms. The number of people infected with HSV-2 has been increasing worldwide since the mid-1990s.

Description

HSV-1 usually is associated with infections of the lips, mouth, and face. HSV-1 sores are referred to as oral herpes, cold sores, or **fever** blisters. HSV-2, or genital herpes, is a sexually transmitted disease (STD) and usually is associated with genital ulcers or sores. The first symptoms often occur within 2–20 days after contact with an infected person, although individuals may be infected with HSV-1 and/or HSV-2 and not develop any symptoms or the development of symptoms may be delayed.

Risk factors

Risk factors for HSV-2 infection include having many sexual partners and having unprotected sex. HSV-2 can also be transmitted by oral sex and cause sores on the lips. **Cancer** patients, especially those who are undergoing **chemotherapy** or radiation treatments, are at greater risk of primary (first) and secondary (recurrent) herpes infections, as are individuals with HIV/AIDS or other conditions in which the immune system is weakened.

Causes and symptoms

HSV virus causes sores on mucous membranes, most often in the mouth and in the genital region. Once HSV enters the body it spreads to nearby mucosal areas through nerve cells. Typically, 50–80% of people with oral herpes experience a prodrome (symptoms of oncoming disease) of pain, burning, **itching**, or tingling at the site where blisters will form. This prodrome stage may last anywhere from a few hours to one to two days. The herpes infection prodrome occurs in both the primary infection and recurrent infections.

Symptoms of the primary infection usually are more severe than those of recurrent infections. The primary infection can cause symptoms similar to

those experienced in other viral infections, including lack of energy, headache, fever, and swollen lymph nodes in the neck. The first sign of infection is formation of fluid-filled blisters that may last up to two weeks. However, the pain in the area may last much longer.

Once an individual becomes infected with HSV, the virus remains in the body for the life of that individual. During periods of latency there are no symptoms. At times the infected person may shed the virus, even in the absence of visible symptoms, and infect others. Individuals infected with the virus can have recurrent infections or flare-ups; however, recurrent infections usually have milder and shorter symptoms. Nevertheless, cancer patients and others with compromised immune systems can have severe recurrences and serious complications.

Women who develop their first (primary) HSV-2 infection during pregnancy are at greater risk of delivering babies with birth defects. An active genital herpes sore at the time of birth can cause extremely serious results, including blindness, birth defects, and even death. Cesarean section may be advisable for mothers with active herpes sores at the time of delivery.

Diagnosis

Often, herpes infection is diagnosed from symptoms and by visually examining the sores.

Tests

Testing for neonatal herpes infections may include special smears and/or viral cultures, blood antibody levels, and polymerase chain reaction (PCR) testing of spinal fluid. Cultures are usually obtained from skin vesicles, eyes, mouth, rectum, urine, stool, and blood. For older children and adults, if there is a question as to the cause of a sore, a tissue sample or culture can be taken to determine what type of virus or other microorganism is responsible. For herpes, it is preferable to have this test done within the first 48 hours after symptoms first show up for a more accurate result.

Treatment

Drugs

There is no cure for HSV infection, although antiviral drugs have some effect in lessening the symptoms, decreasing the length of herpes outbreaks, and preventing complications in immunocompromised individuals. There is evidence that some of these drugs also may prevent future outbreaks. For the best results drug treatment should begin during the prodrome stage before blisters are visible. Depending upon the length of the outbreak, drug treatment could continue up to 10 days.

Acyclovir (Zovirax) is often the drug of choice for herpes infection and can be given intravenously or taken by mouth. It can be applied directly to sores as an ointment but is not very useful in this form. A liquid form for children is also available. Acyclovir is effective in treating both the primary infection and recurrent outbreaks. When taken by mouth to prevent an outbreak, acyclovir reduces the frequency of herpes outbreaks. Other antiviral drugs used to treat HSV infection include penciclovir (Denavir), valacyclovir (Valtrex), and famciclovir (Famvir).

Alternative and complementary therapies

A number of steps may relieve the symptoms of herpes infections. It is important to keep the blisters or sores clean and dry with an agent such as cornstarch. One should avoid touching the sores, and wash hands frequently. Local application of ice may relieve the pain. Over-the-counter medication for fever, pain, and inflammation, such as aspirin, acetaminophen, or ibuprofen, may help. Children should never be given aspirin because of the possible development of Reye's syndrome.

Sexual intercourse should be avoided during both the active stage and the prodrome stages. During an outbreak of cold sores salty foods, citrus foods (oranges etc.), and other foods that irritate the sores should be avoided. Over-the-counter lip products that contain the chemical "phenol" (such as Blistex Medicated Lip Ointment) and numbing ointments (such as Anbesol) help to relieve the pain of cold sores. A bandage may be placed over the sores to protect them and prevent spreading the virus to other sites on the lips or face.

A diet rich in the amino acid lysine may help prevent recurrences of cold sores. Foods that contain high levels of lysine include most vegetables, legumes, fish, turkey, and chicken. Oral lysine supplements in the amount of 1000 mg per day may help sores heal faster. There is a belief that foods with high lysine-to-arginine ratio will help prevent outbreaks of herpes simplex. That has not been proven, and it is important to include foods that have a low lysine-to-arginine ratio also, such as nuts, onion, garlic, and green vegetables. It is also suggested that the amount of arginine in the diet be limited as there is a belief that arginine is needed for herpes virus growth. This amino acid is found in peanuts, beer, chocolate, gelatin, and raisins.

QUESTIONS TO ASK YOUR DOCTOR

- How do I know which type of HSV I have?
- How will HSV infection affect my sex life?
- What can I do to help prevent spreading HSV-1 to family members?
- What are the possible serious complications of this infection, and when should I call the doctor?

Prognosis

Infection is permanent. Although symptom-free periods are common, during these times individuals may still shed the virus into their saliva and genital secretions and infect others. Life-threatening neurological complications may occur in individuals who are immunocompromised, and HSV-2 infection during pregnancy and delivery can cause birth defects or serious harm to the infant.

Prevention

It is almost impossible to prevent HSV-1 infection. Limiting the number of sexual partners reduces the likelihood of becoming with HSV-2. Using a condom may help discourage infection, but does not fully protect against spread of the virus.

Resources

BOOKS

Ebel, Charles and Anna Wald. *Managing Herpes: Living and Loving With HSV*. Research Triangle Park, NC: American Social Health Association, 2007.

Warren, Terri. *The Good News About the Bad News: Herpes, Everything You Need to Know*. Oakland, CA: New Harbinger Publications, 2009.

OTHER

"Genital Herpes." United States Center for Disease Control and Prevention. February 26, 2009 [August 29, 2009]. http://www.cdc.gov/std/Herpes.

"Herpes simplex." MedlinePlus. August 14, 2009 [August 29, 2009]. http://www.nlm.nih.gov/medlineplus/herpessimplex.html.

ORGANIZATIONS

American Social Health Association, PO Box 13827, Research Triangle Park, NC, 27709, (919) 361-8400, (800) 227-8922, (919) 361-8425, http://www.ashastd.org.

National Institute of Allergy and Infectious Diseases Office of Communications and Government Relations, 6610

Rockledge Drive, MSC 6612, Bethesda, MD, 20892-6612, (301) 496-5717, (866) 284-4107 or TDD: (800)877-8339 (for hearing impaired), (301) 402-3573, http://www3.niaid.nih.gov.

Belinda M. Rowland, Ph.D.
Tish Davidson, A.M.

Herpes zoster

Description

Herpes zoster, also called shingles, and referred to as "zosteer," gets its name from both the Latin and French words for belt or girdle and refers to belt-like skin eruptions that may occur on the trunk of the body. The virus that causes chickenpox, the varicella zoster virus (VSV), can become dormant in nerve cells after an episode of chickenpox and later re-emerge as

Shingles, or herpes zoster, on patient's buttocks and thigh.
(Custom Medical Stock Photo. Reproduced by permission.)

shingles. Any individual who has had chickenpox can develop shingles. People of all ages, even children, can be affected, but the incidence increases with age. There are many other conditions which can predispose people to developing shingles, including newborn infants, bone marrow and other transplant recipients, and individuals with immune systems weakened by diseases like HIV or **cancer**, or drugs, such as those used in **chemotherapy**.

Shingles erupts along the course of the affected nerve, producing lesions anywhere on the body and may cause severe nerve pain. The most common areas to be affected are the face and trunk, which correspond to the areas where the chickenpox rash is most concentrated. The disease is caused by a reactivation of the chickenpox virus that has been dormant in certain nerves following an episode of chickenpox. Exactly how or why this reactivation occurs is not clear; however, it is believed that the reactivation is triggered when the immune system becomes weakened as in the examples described above. Early signs of shingles are often vague and can easily be mistaken for other illnesses. The condition may begin with **fever** and malaise (a vague feeling of weakness or discomfort). Within two to four days, severe pain, **itching**, and numbness/tingling (paresthesia) or extreme sensitivity to touch (hyperesthesia) can develop, usually on the trunk and occasionally on the arms and legs. Pain may be continuous or intermittent, usually lasting from one to four weeks. It may occur at the time of the eruption, but can precede the eruption by days, occasionally making the diagnosis difficult. Signs and symptoms may include the following:

- itching, tingling, or severe burning pain
- red patches that develop into blisters
- grouped, dense, deep, small blisters that ooze and crust
- swollen lymph nodes

Immunocompromised patients usually have a more severe course that is frequently prolonged for weeks to months. They develop shingles frequently and the **infection** can spread to the skin, lungs, liver, gastrointestinal tract, brain, or other vital organs.

Potentially serious complications can result from herpes zoster. Many individuals continue to experience persistent pain long after the blisters heal. This pain, called post-herpatic neuralgia, can be severe and debilitating. Post-herpetic neuralgia can persist for months or years after the lesions have disappeared.

Other complications include a secondary bacterial infection, and rarely, potentially fatal inflammation of the brain (encephalitis) and the spread of an infection throughout the body. These rare, but extremely serious, complications are more likely to occur in those individuals who have weakened immune systems (immunocompromised).

Causes

Herpes zoster has been reported in patients with many different types of cancer. However, the cancers that affect an individual's immune system, such as leukemia or **lymphoma**, are the types that place people at particular risk. Herpes zoster is also a particular problem after the various forms of cancer therapy. A study performed in 1998 looked at 766 episodes of herpes zoster infection at a large cancer center from 1972 to 1980. The highest risk of infection was present among patients with lymphoma and leukemia. In those who received radiation treatment and then developed herpes zoster, half of them developed this within seven months. They developed zoster on the area of their body where the radiation was given. This study showed that a period of months can pass before developing zoster as a consequence of radiation. In those who developed zoster after being treated with chemotherapy, half of them developed zoster within a month.

A study in 1999 looked at 215 consecutive patients who had received high-dose chemotherapy and autologous stem cell rescue to help determine what the incidence and severity of herpes zoster infection was. Herpes zoster was developed in 40 people. Over 80% of these infections occurred within six months of receiving the autologous stem cell rescue. Similar rates of herpes zoster have been seen in patients who received bone marrow transplants. A 1996 study looked at 107 children who had received bone marrow transplants for various malignancies. Thirty-three percent of these children developed herpes zoster. Approximately 90% of the cases developed within one year from the time of bone marrow transplant.

Treatments

Shingles almost always resolves spontaneously and may not require any treatment except for the relief of symptoms. In most people, the condition clears on its own in one or two weeks and seldom recurs. The antiviral drugs acyclovir, valacyclovir, and famciclovir can be used to treat shingles. These drugs may shorten the course of the illness. Their use results in more rapid healing of the blisters when drug therapy is started within 72 hours of the onset of the rash. In fact, the earlier the drugs are administered, the better, because early cases can sometimes be stopped. If taken later, these drugs are less effective but may still lessen the pain. Antiviral drug treatment does not seem to reduce the incidence of post-herpetic neuralgia, but recent studies suggest famciclovir may cut the duration of post-herpetic neuralgia in half. Side effects of typical oral doses of these antiviral drugs are minor with headache and **nausea** reported by 8-20% of patients. Severely immunocompromised individuals, such as those with cancer, may require intravenous administration of antiviral drugs. Preventive administration of acyclovir to seropositive patients (people who have evidence in their blood of past infection with varicella) who undergo leukemia induction or bone marrow transplant not only effectively prevents herpes zoster recurrence but also reduces the severity of chemotherapy-induced **mucositis**. Therefore, acyclovir prophylaxis should be considered in seropositive patients, especially if they have had a recurrence during previous chemotherapy cycles.

Alternative and complementary therapies

Cool, wet compresses may help reduce pain. If there are blisters or crusting, applying compresses made with diluted vinegar will make the patient more comfortable. The patient can mix one-quarter cup of white vinegar in two quarts of lukewarm water, and use the compress twice each day for 10 minutes. The patient should stop using the compresses when the blisters have dried up.

Soothing baths and lotions such as colloidal oatmeal baths, starch baths or lotions, and calamine lotion may help to relieve itching and discomfort. The skin should be kept clean, contaminated items should not be re-used. While the lesions continue to ooze, the person should be isolated to prevent infecting other susceptible individuals.

Later, when the crusts and scabs are separating, the skin may become dry, tight, and cracked. If that happens, the patient can rub on a small amount of plain petroleum jelly three or four times a day.

There are non-medical methods of prevention and treatment that may speed recovery. For example, getting lots of rest, eating a healthy diet, exercising regularly, and minimizing stress are always helpful in preventing disease. Supplementation with vitamin B_{12} during the first one to two days and continued supplementation with vitamin B complex, high levels of vitamin C with bioflavonoids, and calcium, are recommended to boost the immune system. Herbal antivirals such as echinacea can be effective in fighting infection and boosting the immune system. Patients should consult physician before taking supplements.

Although no single alternative approach, technique, or remedy has yet been proven to reduce the pain, there are a few options which may be helpful. For example, topical applications of lemon balm (*Melissa officinalis*) or licorice (*Glycyrrhiza glabra*) and peppermint (*Mentha piperita*) may reduce pain and blistering. Homeopathic remedies include *Rhus toxicodendron* for blisters, *Mezereum* and *Arsenicum album* for pain, and *Ranunculus* for itching. Practitioners of Eastern medicine recommend self-hypnosis, acupressure, and acupuncture to alleviate pain. All of these or similar alternative therapies should be discussed with the treating physician before using.

See also Antiviral therapy.

Resources

BOOKS

Berger, Joseph. *Cecil Textbook of Medicine.* 21st ed. Philadelphia: W.B. Saunders Company, 2000.

PERIODICALS

Bilgrami, S., et al. "Varicella zoster virus infection associated with high-dose chemotherapy and autologous stem-cell rescue."*Bone Marrow Transplant* 23 (March 1999): 469–74.

David Greenberg, M.D.

Hickmann lines *see* **Vascular access**

Histamine 2 antagonists

Definition

Histamine 2 antagonists are drugs that block the production of acid in the stomach.

Purpose

Histamine 2 antagonists are used to treat the pre-cancerous condition of **Barrett's esophagus**. They are also used to treat **Zollinger-Ellison syndrome** and multiple endocrine neoplasia, rare cancerous conditions in which the stomach makes too much acid and to prevent the development of gastric (stomach) and duodenal (upper part of the small intestine) ulcers.

Description

Histamine 2 blockers are familiar to most people as the over-the counter heartburn medications Tagamet (cimetidine), Pepcid, (famotidine), and Zantac (ranitidine). Axid (nizatidine) is less well known. These drugs also come in prescription strengths. Histamine 2

blockers work by reducing the amount of acid the stomach produces.

The esophagus is a tube 10–13 inches long and about 1 inch wide that carries food from the mouth to the stomach. Normally, the esophagus is lined with cells that are similar to skin cells and look smooth and pinkish-white.

The stomach makes acid to help digest food. A different type of cell that is resistant to acid lines the stomach. These cells look red and velvety. At the place where the esophagus meets the stomach, there is a ring of muscle called a sphincter that normally keeps acid stomach juices from backflowing into the esophagus. When this sphincter is not working correctly, stomach acid enters the bottom portion of the esophagus. This backflow is called reflux or heartburn. When reflux occurs frequently over an extended period of time, it is called gastroesophageal reflux disease (GERD).

Barrett's esophagus is a pre-cancerous condition in which normal cells lining the esophagus are repeatedly exposed to stomach acid and are replaced with abnormal cells that, in some people, develop into a type of **cancer** of the esophagus called **adenocarcinoma**. Histamine 2 blockers are given to reduce acid in the stomach and eliminate exposure of the esophageal cells to acid.

Histamine 2 blockers are also used to treat two rare cancerous conditions: multiple endocrine neoplasia (MEN) and Zollinger-Ellison syndrome, both of which can cause the stomach to produce too much acid. In MEN, an inherited form of cancer, tumors form in more than one gland. Depending on which glands are affected, the stomach may be stimulated to produce excess acid. In Zollinger-Ellison syndrome, a tumor in the digestive tract secretes a hormone called gastrin that stimulates the production of stomach acid. These tumors are malignant (cancerous) in 50–65% of people with Zollinger-Ellison syndrome.

Histamine 2 blockers are sometimes given in advance of **chemotherapy** to help reduce the gastrointestinal side effects of chemotherapy drugs. Cimetidine was the first histamine 2 blocker approved by the United States Food and Drug Administration (FDA) in 1976.

Recommended dosage

Recommended dose varies depending on how much stomach acid is produced. Histamine 2 blockers are available in low doses without a prescription and in higher doses with a prescription. They are available in tablet, chewable tablet, liquid, and injectable liquid form. In 2004, the FDA also approved a 25 mg effervescent tablet form of ranitidine (Zantac 25 Efferdose). If histamine 2 inhibitors are unsuccessful in controlling acid reflux, proton pump inhibitors (Prevacid, Prilosec) are usually given as an alternative.

Precautions

People who have trouble with heartburn should stay away from acidic foods such as orange, grapefruit, and tomato juice, coffee, and carbonated drinks (sodas) because these all increase stomach acid. Waiting at least two hours after eating before lying down, avoiding smoking, limiting drinking of alcohol, losing excess weight, and avoiding wearing tight-fitting clothes are other ways to prevent heartburn. Although animal studies show that histamine 2 blockers appear to be safe during pregnancy, these drugs pass into breast milk and should not be taken by nursing mothers.

Side effects

Histamine 2 blockers have few side effects. These drugs are excreted by the kidney, and may slow the excretion of other drugs excreted by the kidney. People with reduced kidney function may need a reduced dose of histamine 2 blockers.

Rare cases of irregular heart rhythms and high blood pressure have been reported when histamine 2 blockers are given intravenously (IV, injected directly into a vein). Mild **diarrhea** has been reported by some people taking these drugs.

Interactions

Histamine 2 blockers are reported to have few interactions with other drugs. However, because they reduce the level of acid in the stomach, they may inhibit the uptake of drugs such as ketoconazole that depend on an acid environment in the stomach to work. These drugs should be administered at least two hours before histamine 2 blockers are taken. Prior to starting any over-the-counter medications, herbal medications, or new medications, patients should notify their physician and check with their pharmacists for any potential drug interactions.

Resources

PERIODICALS

"Does Eating Slowly Prevent Heartburn? Determining Which Lifestyle Measures Stave Off Acid Reflux." *Tufts University Health & Nutrition Newsletter* (April 2000): 1.
"FDA Approved Ranitidine 25 mg Effervescent Tablets." *Formulary* (May 2004): 240.

Tish Davidson, A.M.

Histiocytosis X

Definition

Histiocytosis X is a generic term that refers to an increase in the number of histiocytes, a type of white blood cell, that act as scavengers to remove foreign material from the blood and tissues. Since recent research demonstrated Langerhans cell involvement as well as histiocytes, this led to a proposal that the term Langerhans Cell Histiocytosis (LCH) be used in place of histiocytosis X. Either term refers to three separate illnesses (listed in order of increasing severity): eosinophilic granuloma; Hand-Schuller-Christian disease; and Letterer-Siwe disease.

Description

Epidermal (skin) Langerhans cells (a form of dendritic cell) accumulate with other immune cells in various parts of the body and cause damage by the release of chemicals. Normally, Langerhans cells recognize foreign material, including bacteria, and stimulate the immune system to react to them. Langerhans cells are usually found in skin, lymph nodes, lungs, and the gastrointestinal tract. Under abnormal conditions these cells affect skin, bone, and the pituitary gland as well as the lungs, intestines, liver, spleen, bone marrow, and brain. Therefore, the disease is not confined to areas where Langerhans cells are normally found. The disease is more common in children than adults and tends to be most severe in very young children.

Histiocytosis X or LCH is a family of related conditions characterized by a distinct inflammatory and proliferative process but differs from each other in which parts of the body are involved. The least severe of the histiocytosis X/LCH family is eosinophilic granuloma. Approximately 60–80% of all diagnosed cases are in this classification, which usually occurs in children aged 5–10 years. The bones are involved 50–75% of the time, which includes the skull or mandible, and the long bones. If the bone marrow is involved, **anemia** can result. With skull involvement, growths can occur behind the eyes, bulging them forward. One recent case study involved swelling of the eyes caused by histiocytosis in a three-year-old girl. The lungs are involved less than 10% of the time, and this involvement signals the worst prognosis.

Next in severity is Hand-Schuller-Christian disease, a chronic, scattered form of histiocytosis. It occurs most commonly from the age of one to three years and is a slowly progressive disease that affects the softened areas of the skull, other flat bones, the eyes, and skin. Letterer-Siwe disease is the acute form of this series of diseases. It is generally found from the time of birth to one year of age. It causes an enlarged liver, bruising and skin lesions, anemia, enlarged lymph glands, other organ involvement, and extensive skull lesions.

Causes and symptoms

This is a rare disorder affecting approximately 1 in 200,000 children or adults each year. The International Histiocyte Society formed a registry in 2000 that has registered a total of 274 adults from 13 countries as of 2003. Because histiocytic disorders are so rare, little research has been done to determine their cause. Over time, histiocytosis may lessen in its assault on the body but there are still problems from damage to the tissues. There are no apparent inheritance patterns in these diseases with the exception of a form involving the lymphatic system; of the 274 adults in the international registry, only one came from a family with a history of the disease.

The symptoms of histiocytosis are caused by substances called cytokines and prostaglandins, which are normally produced by histiocytes and act as messengers between cells. When these chemicals are produced in excess amounts and in the wrong places, they cause tissue swelling and abnormal growth. Thus, symptoms may include painful lumps in the skull and limbs as well as rashes on the skin. General symptoms may include: poor appetite, failure to gain weight, recurrent **fever**, and irritability. Symptoms from other possible sites of involvement include:

- Gums: swelling, usually without significant discomfort.
- Ear: chronic discharge.
- Liver or spleen: abdominal discomfort or swelling.
- Pituitary: This gland at the base of the brain is affected at some stage in approximately 20%–30% of children causing a disturbance in water balance to produce thirst and frequent urination.
- Eyes: Due to the bony disease, behind-the-eye bulging may occur (exophthalmos).
- Lungs: Breathing problems.

Diagnosis

The diagnosis can be made only by performing a **biopsy**, that is, taking a tissue sample under anesthesia from a site in the patient thought to be involved. Blood and urine tests, chest and other **x rays**, **magnetic resonance imaging** (MRI) and **computed tomography** scans (CAT scans) (to check the extent of involvement), and possibly bone marrow or breathing tests may be required to confirm the diagnosis.

Treatments and prognosis

Although this disease is not **cancer**, most patients diagnosed with it are treated in cancer clinics. There are two reasons for this:

- Historically, cancer specialists treated it before the cause was known.

- The treatment requires the use of drugs typically required to treat cancer.

Any cancer drugs utilized are usually given in smaller doses, which diminishes the severity of their side effects. **Radiation therapy** is rarely used, and special drugs may be prescribed for skin symptoms. If there is only one organ affected, steroids may be injected locally, or a drug called indomethacin may be used. Indomethacin is an anti-inflammatory medication that may achieve a similar response with less severe side effects.

The disease fluctuates markedly. If only one system is involved, the disease often resolves by itself. Multisystem disease usually needs treatment although it may disappear spontaneously. The disease is not normally fatal unless organs vital to life are damaged. In general, the younger the child at diagnosis and the more organs involved, the poorer the outlook. If the condition resolves, there could still be long-term complications because of the damage done while the disease was active.

Resources

BOOKS

Beers, Mark H., MD, and Robert Berkow, MD, editors. "Histiocytic Syndromes." In *The Merck Manual of Diagnosis and Therapy*. Whitehouse Station, NJ: Merck Research Laboratories, 2007.

Behrman, Richard E., Robert Kliegman, and Hal B. Jenson, editors. *Nelson Textbook of Pediatrics*. Philadelphia: W. B. Saunders, 2000.

PERIODICALS

Arico, M., M. Girschikofsky, T. Genereau, et al. "Langerhans Cell Histiocytosis in Adults. Report from the International Registry of the Histiocyte Society." *European Journal of Cancer* 39 (November 2003): 2341–2348.

Eckhardt, A., and A. Schulze. "Maxillofacial Manifestations of Langerhans Cell Histiocytosis: A Clinical and Therapeutic Analysis of 10 Patients." *Oral Oncology* 39 (October 2003): 687–694.

Kobyahsi, M., O. Yamamoto, Y. Suenaga, and M. Asahi. "Electron Microscopic Study of Langerhans Cell Histiocytosis." *Journal of Dermatology* July 27, 2000: 453–7.

Levy, J., T. Monos, J.Kapelushnik, et al. "Langerhans Cell Histiocytosis with Periorbital Cellulitis." *American Journal of Ophthalmology* 136 (November 2003): 939–942.

OTHER

"Immunity Disorders." *Nurse Minerva*. [cited June 26, 2001]. <http://nurseminerva.co.uk/immunity.htm>.

ORGANIZATIONS

Histiocytosis Association of America. 302 North Broadway, Pitman, NJ 08071. 800–548–2758 (USA and Canada). http://www.histio.org.

Linda K. Bennington, C.N.S., M.S.N.
Rebecca J. Frey, Ph.D.

Hodgkin's disease

Definition

Hodgkin's disease is a rare **lymphoma**, a **cancer** of the lymphatic system.

Description

Hodgkin's disease, or Hodgkin's lymphoma, was first described in 1832 by Thomas Hodgkin, a British physician. Hodgkin clearly differentiated between this disease and the much more common non-Hodgkin's

A scanning electron micrograph (SEM) image of dividing Hodgkin's cells from the pleural effusions (abnormal accumulations of fluid in the lungs) of a 55-year-old male patient. *(Photograph by Dr. Andrejs Liepins, National Audubon Society Collection/Photo Researchers, Inc. Reproduced by permission.)*

Swollen lymph nodes of a Hodgkin's disease patient. *(Custom Medical Stock Photo. Reproduced by permission.)*

KEY TERMS

Antibody—An immune system protein that recognizes a specific foreign molecule.

Biopsy—The removal of a small sample of tissue for examination under a microscope; used for the diagnosis of cancer and to check for infection.

Bone marrow—Tissue inside the bones that produce red and white blood cells.

Chemotherapy—Treatment with various combinations of chemicals or drugs, particularly for the treatment of cancer.

Epstein-Barr virus (EBV)—Very common virus that infects immune cells and can cause mononucleosis.

Interferon—A potent immune-defense protein produced by viral-infected cells; used as an anti-cancer and anti-viral drug.

Interleukins—A family of potent immune-defense molecules; used in various medical therapies.

Laparotomy—A surgical incision of the abdomen.

Leukapheresis—A technique that uses a machine to remove stem cells from the blood; the cells are frozen and then returned to the patient following treatment that has destroyed the bone marrow.

Lymph nodes—Small round glands, located throughout the body and containing lymphocytes that remove foreign organisms and debris from the lymphatic fluid.

Lymphatic system—The vessels, lymph nodes, and organs, including the bone marrow, spleen, and thymus, that produce and carry white blood cells to fight disease.

Lymphocyte—White blood cells that produce antibodies and other agents for fighting disease.

PBSCT—Peripheral blood stem cell transplant; a method for replacing blood-forming cells that are destroyed by cancer treatment.

Radiotherapy—Disease treatment involving exposure to x rays or other types of radiation.

Reed-Sternberg cells—An abnormal lymphocyte that is characteristic of Hodgkin's disease.

Spleen—An organ of the lymphatic system, on the left side of the abdomen near the stomach; it produces and stores lymphocytes, filters the blood, and destroys old blood cells.

Splenectomy—Surgical removal of the spleen.

Staging—The use of various diagnostic methods to accurately determine the extent of disease; used to select the appropriate type and amount of treatment and to predict the outcome of treatment.

Stem cells—The cells from which all blood cells are derived.

Thymus—An organ of the lymphatic system, located behind the breast bone, that produces the T lymphocytes of the immune system.

Thyroid—A gland in the throat that produces hormones that regulate growth and metabolism.

lymphomas. Prior to 1970, few individuals survived Hodgkin's disease. Now, however, the majority of individuals with this cancer can be cured.

The lymphatic system

The lymphatic system is part of the body's immune system, for fighting disease, and a part of the blood-producing system. It includes the lymph vessels and nodes, and the spleen, bone marrow, and thymus. The narrow lymphatic vessels carry lymphatic fluid from throughout the body. The lymph nodes are small organs that filter the lymphatic fluid and trap foreign substances, including viruses, bacteria, and cancer cells. The spleen, in the upper left abdomen, removes old cells and debris from the blood. The bone marrow, the tissue inside the bones, produces new red and white blood cells.

Lymphocytes are white blood cells that recognize and destroy disease-causing organisms. Lymphocytes are produced in the lymph nodes, spleen, and bone marrow. They circulate throughout the body in the blood and lymphatic fluid. Clusters of immune cells also exist in major organs.

Hodgkin's lymphoma

Hodgkin's disease is a type of lymphoma in which antibody-producing cells of the lymphatic system begin to grow abnormally. It usually begins in a lymph node and progresses slowly, in a fairly predictable way, spreading via the lymphatic vessels from one group of lymph nodes to the next. Sometimes it invades organs that are adjacent to the lymph nodes. If the cancer cells spread to the blood, the disease can reach almost any site in the body. Advanced cases of Hodgkin's disease may involve the spleen, liver, bone marrow, and lungs.

QUESTIONS TO ASK THE DOCTOR

- What type of Hodgkin's disease do I have?
- What is the stage of my disease?
- What are the choices for treatment and what do you recommend?
- Should I obtain a second opinion?
- What are the short-term side effects of the treatment and what can be done about them?
- What are the possible long-term side effects of the treatment?
- Are there other risks from the treatment?
- How should I prepare for the treatment?
- How long will the treatment continue?
- What is the recovery time following the treatment?
- What are the chances of success?
- Are there clinical trials which may be appropriate for me?
- Are there complementary or alternative therapies that may be helpful?
- What is the likelihood that the cancer will return? How will a recurrence be diagnosed?
- Is a recurrence more likely with one treatment than with another?

There are different subtypes of Hodgkin's disease:

- nodular sclerosis (30–60% of cases)
- mixed cellularity (20–40% of cases)
- lymphocyte predominant (5–10% of cases)
- lymphocyte depleted (less than 5% of cases)
- unclassified

Demographics

The American Cancer Society estimates that there will be 8,510 new cases of Hodgkin's disease in the United States in 2009—3,870 in females and 4,640 in males. It is estimated that 800 men and 490 women in the United States will die of the disease in 2009.

Hodgkin's disease can occur at any age. However, the majority of cases develop in early adulthood (ages 15–40) and late adulthood (after age 55). Approximately 10–15% of cases are in children under age 17. It is more common in boys than in girls under the age of 10. The disease is very rare in children under five.

Causes and symptoms

The cause of Hodgkin's disease is not known. It is suspected that some interaction between an individual's genetic makeup, environmental exposures, and infectious agents may be responsible. Immune system deficiencies also may be involved.

Early symptoms of Hodgkin's disease may be similar to those of the flu:

- fevers, night sweats, chills
- fatigue
- loss of appetite (anorexia)
- weight loss
- itching
- pain after drinking alcoholic beverages
- swelling of one or more lymph nodes

Sudden or emergency symptoms of Hodgkin's disease include:

- sudden high fever
- loss of bladder and/or bowel control
- numbness in the arms and legs and a loss of strength

As lymph nodes swell, they may push on other structures, causing a variety of symptoms:

- pain due to pressure on nerve roots
- loss of function in muscle groups served by compressed nerves
- coughing or shortness of breath due to compression of the windpipe and/or airways, by swollen lymph nodes in the chest
- kidney failure from compression of the ureters, the tubes that carry urine from the kidneys to the bladder
- swelling in the face, neck, or legs, due to pressure on veins
- paralysis in the legs due to pressure on the spinal cord

As Hodgkin's disease progresses, the immune system becomes less effective at fighting **infection**. Thus, patients with Hodgkin's lymphoma become more susceptible to both common infections caused by bacteria and unusual (opportunistic) infections. Later symptoms of Hodgkin's disease include the formation of tumors.

Significantly, as many as 75% of individuals with Hodgkin's disease do not have any typical symptoms.

Diagnosis

As with many forms of cancer, diagnosis of Hodgkin's disease has two major components.

- identification of Hodgkin's lymphoma as the cause of the patient's disease

- staging of the disease to determine how far the cancer has spread

The initial diagnosis of Hodgkin's disease often results from abnormalities in a chest x ray that was performed because of nonspecific symptoms. The physician then takes a medical history to check for the presence of symptoms and conducts a complete physical examination.

Lymph node biopsy

The size, tenderness, firmness, and location of swollen lymph nodes are determined and correlated with any signs of infection. In particular, lymph nodes that do not shrink after treatment with **antibiotics** may be a cause for concern. The lymph nodes that are most often affected by Hodgkin's disease include those of the neck, above the collarbone, under the arms, and in the chest above the diaphragm.

Diagnosis of Hodgkin's disease requires either the removal of an entire enlarged lymph node (an excisional **biopsy**) or an incisional biopsy, in which only a small part of a large tumor is removed. If the node is near the skin, the biopsy is performed with a local anesthetic. However, if it is inside the chest or abdomen, general anesthesia is required.

The sample of biopsied tissue is examined under a microscope. Giant cells called Reed-Sternberg cells must be present to confirm a diagnosis of Hodgkin's disease. These cells, which usually contain two or more nuclei, are named for the two pathologists who discovered them. Normal cells have only one nucleus (the organelle within the cell that contains the genetic material). Affected lymph nodes may contain only a few Reed-Sternberg cells and they may be difficult to recognize. Characteristics of other types of cells in the biopsied tissue help to diagnose the subtype of Hodgkin's disease.

A fine needle aspiration (FNA) biopsy, in which a thin needle and syringe are used to remove a small amount of fluid and bits of tissue from a tumor, has the advantage of not requiring surgery. An FNA may be performed prior to an excisional or incisional biopsy, to check for infection or for the spread of cancer from another organ. However an FNA biopsy does not provide enough tissue to diagnose Hodgkin's disease.

Occasionally, additional biopsies are required to diagnose Hodgkin's disease. In rare instances, other tests, that detect certain substances on the surfaces of cancer cells or changes in the DNA of cells, are used to distinguish Hodgkin's disease from **non-Hodgkin's lymphoma**.

Clinical staging

Staging is very important in Hodgkin's disease. This is because the cancer usually spreads in a predictable pattern, without skipping sets of lymph nodes until late in the progression of the disease.

IMAGING. Imaging of the abdomen, chest, and pelvis is used to identify areas of enlarged lymph nodes and abnormalities in the spleen or other organs. **Computed tomography** (CT or CAT) scans use a rotating x-ray beam to obtain pictures. **Magnetic resonance imaging** (MRI) uses magnetic fields and radio waves to produce images of the body. Chest **x rays** also may be taken. These images will reveal rounded lumps called nodules in the affected lymph nodes and other organs.

Another imaging technique for Hodgkin's disease is a **gallium scan**, in which the radioactive element gallium is injected into a vein. The cancer cells take up the gallium and a special camera that detects the gallium is used to determine the location and size of tumors. Gallium scans are used when Hodgkin's disease is in the chest and may be hard to detect by other methods. Gallium scans also are used to monitor progress during treatment.

A lymphangiogram, a radiograph of the lymphatic vessels, involves injecting a dye into a lymphatic vessel in the foot. Tracking of the dye locates the disease in the abdomen and pelvis. This method is used less frequently and is usually not used with children.

Positron emission tomography (PET) scans are an extremely accurate method for staging Hodgkin's disease. A very low dose of radioactive glucose, a sugar, is injected into the body. The glucose travels to metabolically active sites, including cancerous regions that require large amounts of glucose. The PET scan detects the radioactivity and produces images of the entire body that distinguish between cancerous and non-cancerous tissues.

BONE MARROW. Anemia (a low red-blood-cell count), fevers, or **night sweats** are indications that Hodgkin's disease may be in the bone marrow. In these cases, a **bone marrow aspiration and biopsy** may be ordered. In biopsy, a large needle is used to remove a narrow, cylindrical piece of bone. Alternatively, an aspiration, in which a needle is used to remove small bits of bone marrow, may be used. The marrow usually is removed from the back of the hip or other large bone. This procedure may help to determine cancer spread.

Pathological staging

Sometimes further staging, called pathological staging or a staging laparotomy, is used for Hodgkin's disease. In this operation, a surgeon checks the abdominal lymph nodes and other organs for cancer and removes small pieces of tissue. A pathologist examines the tissue samples for Hodgkin's disease cells. Usually the spleen is removed (a **splenectomy**) during the laparotomy. The splenectomy helps with staging Hodgkin's disease, as well as removing a disease site.

Treatment team

The cancer care team for Hodgkin's disease includes a medical oncologist (a physician specializing in cancer), oncology nurses, technicians, and social workers. A surgeon performs the biopsies, as well as the laparotomy and splenectomy if required. Pathologists examine the biopsy specimens for the presence of Reed-Sternberg and other abnormal cells.

In the United States, most children with Hodgkin's disease are treated at children's cancer centers. Here, the treatment team includes psychologists, child life specialists, nutritionists, and educators, as well as a pediatric oncologist.

Clinical staging, treatments, and prognosis

The stages

All of the available treatments for Hodgkin's disease have serious side effects, both short and long-term. However, with accurate staging, physicians and patients often can choose the minimum treatment that will cure the disease. The staging system for Hodgkin's disease is the Ann Arbor Staging Classification, also called the Cotswold System or the Revised Ann Arbor System.

Hodgkin's disease is divided into four stages, with additional substages:

- Stage I: The disease is confined to one lymph node area
- Stage IE: The disease extends from the one lymph node area to adjacent regions
- Stage II: The disease is in two or more lymph node areas on one side of the diaphragm (the muscle below the lungs)
- Stage IIE: The disease extends to adjacent regions of at least one of these nodes
- Stage III: The disease is in lymph node areas on both sides of the diaphragm
- Stage IIIE/IIISE: The disease extends into adjacent areas or organs (IIIE) and/or the spleen (IIISE)
- Stage IV: The disease has spread from the lymphatic system to one or more other organs, such as the bone marrow or liver

Treatment for Hodgkin's disease depends both on the stage of the disease and whether or not symptoms are present. Stages are labeled with an A if no symptoms are present. If symptoms are present, the stage is labeled with a B. These symptoms include:

- loss of more than 10% of body weight over the previous six months
- fevers above 100° F (37.8° C)
- drenching night sweats

Treatments

RADIATION THERAPY. **Radiation therapy** and/or **chemotherapy** (drug therapy) are the standard treatments for Hodgkin's disease. If the disease is confined to one area of the body, radiotherapy is usually used. This treatment, with x rays or other high-energy rays, also is used when the disease is in bulky areas such as the chest, where chemotherapeutic drugs cannot reach all of the cancer. External-beam radiation, a focused beam from an external machine, is used to irradiate only the affected lymph nodes. This procedure is called involved field radiation.

More advanced stages of Hodgkin's disease may be treated with mantle field radiation, in which the lymph nodes of the neck, chest, and underarms are irradiated. Inverted Y field radiation is used to irradiate the spleen and the lymph nodes in the upper abdomen and pelvis. Total nodal irradiation includes both mantle field and inverted Y field radiation.

Since external-beam radiation damages healthy tissue near the cancer cells, the temporary side effects of radiotherapy can include sunburn-like skin damage, **fatigue**, **nausea**, and **diarrhea**. Other temporary side effects may include a sore throat and difficulty swallowing. Long-term side effects depend on the dose and the location of the radiation and the age of the patient. Since radiation of the ovaries causes permanent sterility (the inability to have offspring), the ovaries of girls and young women are protected during radiotherapy. Sometimes the ovaries are surgically moved from the region to be irradiated.

CHEMOTHERAPY. If the Hodgkin's disease has progressed to additional lymph nodes or other organs, or if there is a recurrence of the disease within two years of radiation treatment, chemotherapy is used.

Chemotherapy utilizes a combination of drugs, each of which kills cancer cells in a different way. The most common chemotherapy regimens for Hodgkin's disease are MOPP (either **mechlorethamine** or **methotrexate** with Oncovin, **procarbazine**, prednisone) and ABVD (Adriamycin or **doxorubicin**, **bleomycin**, **vincristine**, dacarbazine). Each of these consists of four different drugs. ABVD is used more frequently than MOPP because it has fewer severe side effects. However MOPP is used for individuals who are at risk for heart failure. The chemotherapeutic drugs may be injected into a vein or muscle, or taken orally, as a pill or liquid.

Children who are sexually mature when they develop Hodgkin's disease, and whose muscle and bone mass are almost completely developed, usually receive the same treatment as adults. Younger children usually are treated with chemotherapy, since radiation will adversely affect bone and muscle growth. However, radiation may be used in low dosages, in combination with chemotherapy. The chemotherapy for children with Hodgkin's disease usually includes more drugs than ABVD and MOPP.

The side effects of chemotherapy for Hodgkin's disease depend on the dose of drugs and the length of time they are taken. Since these drugs target rapidly dividing cancer cells, they also affect normal cells that grow rapidly. These include the cells of the bone marrow, the linings of the mouth and intestines, and hair follicles. Damage to bone marrow leads to lower white blood cell counts and lower resistance to infection. It also leads to lower red blood cell counts that can result in fatigue and easy bleeding and bruising. Damage to intestinal cells leads to a loss of appetite (**anorexia**), and **nausea and vomiting**. Mouth sores and hair loss (**alopecia**) also are common side effects of chemotherapy. These side effects disappear when the chemotherapy is discontinued. Some drugs can reduce or prevent the nausea and **vomiting**.

Chemotherapy for Hodgkin's disease may lead to long-term complications. The drugs may damage the heart, lungs, kidneys, and liver. In children, growth may be impeded. Some chemotherapy can cause sterility, so men may choose to have their sperm frozen prior to treatment. Women may stop ovulating and menstruating during chemotherapy. This may or may not be permanent.

Treatment for higher-stage Hodgkin's disease often involves a combination of radiotherapy and chemotherapy. Following three or four chemotherapy regimens, involved field radiation may be directed at the most affected areas of the body. The long-term side effects often are more severe when radiation and chemotherapy are used in combination.

The development of a second type of cancer is the most serious risk from radiation and chemotherapy treatment for Hodgkin's disease. In particular, there is a risk of developing leukemia, **breast cancer**, bone cancer, or **thyroid cancer**. Chemotherapy, particularly MOPP, or chemotherapy in conjunction with radiotherapy, significantly increases the risk for leukemia.

RESISTANT, PROGRESSIVE, AND RECURRENT HODGKIN'S DISEASE. Following treatment, the original diagnostic tests for Hodgkin's disease are repeated, to determine whether all traces of the cancer have been eliminated and to check for long-term side effects of treatment. In resistant Hodgkin's disease, some cancer cells remain following treatment. If the cancer continues to spread during treatment, it is called progressive Hodgkin's disease. If the disease returns after treatment, it is known as recurrent Hodgkin's disease. It may recur in the area where it first started or elsewhere in the body. It may recur immediately after treatment or many years later.

Additional treatment is necessary with these types of Hodgkin's disease. If the initial treatment was radiation therapy alone, chemotherapy may be used, or vice versa. Chemotherapy with different drugs, or higher doses, may be used to treat recurrent Hodgkin's. However, radiation to the same area is never repeated.

BONE MARROW AND PERIPHERAL BLOOD STEM CELL TRANSPLANTATIONS. An autologous bone marrow and/or a peripheral blood stem cell transplantation (PBSCT) often is recommended for treating resistant or recurrent Hodgkin's disease, particularly if the disease recurs within a few months of a chemotherapy-induced remission. These transplants are autologous because they utilize the individual's own cells. The patient's bone marrow cells or peripheral blood stem cells (immature bone marrow cells found in the blood) are collected and frozen prior to high-dosage chemotherapy, which destroys bone marrow cells. A procedure called leukapheresis is used to collect the stem cells. Following the high-dosage chemotherapy, and possibly radiation, the bone marrow cells or stem cells are reinjected into the individual.

Alternative and complementary therapies

Most complementary therapies for Hodgkin's disease are designed to stimulate the immune system to destroy cancer cells and repair normal cells that have been damaged by treatment. These therapies are used in conjunction with standard treatment.

Immunologic therapies, also known as immunotherapies, biological therapies, or biological response modifier therapies, utilize substances that are produced by the immune system. These include interferon (an immune system protein), **monoclonal antibodies** (specially engineered antibodies), colony-stimulating (growth) factors (such as **filgrastim**), and **vaccines**. Many immunotherapies for Hodgkin's disease are experimental and available only through **clinical trials**. These biological agents may have side effects.

Coenzyme Q10 (CoQ10) and polysaccharide K (PSK) are being evaluated for their ability to stimulate the immune system and protect healthy tissue, as well as possible anti-cancer activities. Camphor, also known as 714-X, green tea, and hoxsey (which is a mixture of a number of substances), have been promoted as immune system enhancers. However there is no evidence that they are effective against Hodgkin's disease. Hoxsey, in particular, can produce serious side effects.

Prognosis

Hodgkin's disease, particularly in children, is one of the most curable forms of cancer. Approximately 90% of individuals are cured of the disease with chemotherapy and/or radiation.

The one-year relative survival rate following treatment for Hodgkin's disease is 93%. Relative survival rates do not include individuals who die of causes other than Hodgkin's disease. The percentage of individuals who have not died of Hodgkin's disease within five years of diagnosis is 90–95% for those with stage I or stage II disease. The figure is 85–90% for those diagnosed with stage III Hodgkin's and approximately 80% for those diagnosed with stage IV disease. The 15-year relative survival rate is 63%. Approximately 75% of children are alive and cancer free 20 years after the original diagnosis of Hodgkin's.

Acute myelocytic leukemia, a very serious cancer, may develop in as many as 2–6% of individuals receiving certain types of treatment for Hodgkin's disease. Women under the age of 30 who are treated with radiation to the chest have a much higher risk for developing breast cancer. Both men and women are at higher risk for developing lung or thyroid cancers as a result of chest irradiation.

Individuals with the type of Hodgkin's disease known as nodular lymphocytic predominance have a 2% chance of developing non-Hodgkin's lymphoma. Apparently, this is a result of the Hodgkin's disease itself and not the treatment.

Coping with cancer treatment

Sufficient rest and good nutrition are important for relieving the side effects of treatment for Hodgkin's disease. As strength returns, a weekly exercise routine should be initiated. Support groups can be beneficial for helping with emotional problems that may arise during treatment.

Clinical trials

At least 115 clinical trials for the treatment of Hodgkin's disease were recruiting or planning to recruit participants. A number of these studies are directed at treating resistant (refractory) or recurrent (relapsed) Hodgkin's disease in both children and adults. Some are aimed at specific stages or subtypes of Hodgkin's disease. Some trials are for previously treated individuals and others are for those who have not yet received treatment.

Clinical trials of new treatments for Hodgkin's disease include:

- new drugs
- new chemotherapies
- monoclonal antibody therapy
- interferon, interleukin-2, and interleukin-12
- a vaccine made from cancer cells that contain the Epstein-Barr virus
- bone marrow and umbilical cord blood transplantations
- PBSCT
- various combinations of treatments.

There also are ongoing genetic studies of children and adults with Hodgkin's disease and quality-of-life studies of children who are undergoing treatment.

Prevention

There are very few known risk factors for Hodgkin's disease. A family history of the disease and the presence of the **Epstein-Barr virus** are associated with an increased risk. Individuals with acquired immunodeficiency syndrome (AIDS) are particularly susceptible to Hodgkin's disease.

Special concerns

Follow-up examinations continue for many years following treatment for Hodgkin's disease. Women who have had chest irradiation must have frequent mammograms and clinical and breast self examinations for early detection of breast cancer. Frequent physical exams and chest x rays may help to detect lung or thyroid cancer. Treatment with mantle field radiation causes hyperthyroidism, which requires thyroid medication and annual thyroid function tests.

Individuals with Hodgkin's disease do not have normal immune system function, a problem that can be intensified by chemotherapy, radiation, and removal of the spleen. Therefore, vaccinations and prompt treatment of infections are very important.

See also Amenorrhea; Bone marrow transplantation; Childhood cancers; Fertility and cancer; Imaging studies; Immune response.

Resources

BOOKS

Mauch, Peter M., et al., editors. *Hodgkin's Disease*. Philadelphia: Lippincott Williams & Wilkins, 1999.

OTHER

FS-8 - Complementary and Alternative Therapies for Leukemia, Lymphoma, Hodgkin's Disease, and Myeloma. The Leukemia and Lymphoma Society. [cited Mar.27, 2005]. http://www.leukemia-lymphoma.org.

"Hodgkin's Disease." *CancerNet*. National Cancer Institute. NIH Publication No. 99-1555. [cited Mar. 27, 2005]. >http://cancernet.nci.nih.gov/wyntk_pubs/hodgkins.htm>.

"Hodgkin's Disease." *Cancer Resource Center*. 10 Dec. 1999. American Cancer Society. [cited Mar. 27, 2005]. <http://www3.cancer.org>.

"Hodgkin's Lymphoma." *Diseases & Conditions*. MayoClinic.com. [cited Mar. 27, 2005]. http://www.mayohealth.org.

National Cancer Society. "NCI/PDQ Patient Statement: Adult Hodgkin's Disease." *Oncolink*. Nov. 2000. University of Pennsylvania Cancer Center. [cited Mar. 27, 2005]. http://www.oncolink.upenn.edu/pdq_html/2/engl/200003.html.

National Cancer Society. "NCI/PDQ Patient Statement: Childhood Hodgkin's Disease." *Oncolink*. Feb. 2001. University of Pennsylvania Cancer Center. [cited Mar. 27, 2005]. http://www.oncolink.upenn.edu/pdq_html/2/engl/203043.html.

"PET Scans Help Doctors Treat Hodgkin's Disease." *ACS News Today*. American Cancer Society. [cited Mar. 27, 2005]. <http://www2.cancer.org>.

ORGANIZATIONS

American Cancer Society. (800) ACS-2345. http://www.cancer.org. Provides information, funds for cancer research, prevention programs, and patient services, including education and support programs for patients and families, temporary accommodations for patients, and camps for children with cancer.

ClinicalTrials.gov. U. S. National Library of Medicine. National Institutes of Health. 8600 Rockville Pike, Bethesda, MD 20894. <http://clinicaltrials.gov/ct/gui/c/a1b/screen/BrowseAny/action/GetStudy?JServSessionIdcs_current=mgdpq4z7pm>. Information about clinical trials involving Hodgkin's disease.

Cure for Lymphoma Foundation. 215 Lexington Avenue, New York, NY 10016. (212) 213-9595. (800)-CFL-6848. infocfl@cfl.org. http://www.cfl.org/home.html. An advocacy organization that provides education and support programs, research grants, and information on clinical trials for Hodgkin's and non-Hodgkin's lymphomas.

The Leukemia and Lymphoma Society. 600 Third Avenue, New York, NY 10016. (800) 955-4572. (914) 949-5213. http://www.leukemia-lymphoma.org Provides information, support, and guidance to patients and health care professionals.

The Lymphoma Research Foundation of America, Inc. 8800 Venice Boulevard, Suite 207, Los Angeles, CA 90034. (310) 204-7040). http://www.lymphoma.org. Supports research into treatments for lymphoma and provides educational and emotional support programs for patients and families.

National Cancer Institute. Public Inquiries Office, Building 31, Room 10A31, 31 Center Drive, MSC 2580, Bethesda, MD 20892-2580. (800)-4-CANCER. http://www.nci.nih.gov/. <http://cancernet.nci.nih.gov>. Provides information on cancer and on clinical trials; conducts cancer research.

Rosalyn S. Carson-DeWitt, M.D.
Margaret Alic, Ph.D.

Home health services

Definition

Home health services refers to those health care services provided to the patient in his or her own home.

Description

Home health services can vary depending on the insurance coverage, but usually include nursing, physical therapy, occupational therapy, speech therapy, home health aides, social work, nutritional education, infusion therapy, blood drawing, and other laboratory services. Such services may also include bringing medical

A home healthcare nurses tends to a patient. *(Photograph by Carl Glassman. The Image Works Reproduced by permission.)*

KEY TERMS

Home parenteral nutrition (HPN)—HPN provides liquid nutrition via infusion for patients who are malnourished, or who have had surgery altering the usual process of chewing, swallowing, or digesting food.

Meditation—Meditation is a technique in which the individual focuses on a word or phrase to the exclusion of other thoughts. It has been shown to lower blood pressure and reduce stress.

Respite care—A form of temporary home health care that allows family members some time away from patient care. Respite care is usually short-term, ranging from a few hours to a weekend.

T'ai chi—An Asian practice of breathing and slow physical movements that develops strength and reduces stress.

Telehealth—The use of the telephone, Internet, and other forms of telecommunication to support long-distance health care, education of health care professionals, and public health concerns.

QUESTIONS TO ASK THE DOCTOR

- What kind of home care will I need?
- For how long will I need the different services?
- What happens if my condition worsens?
- Will my insurance cover the services you are prescribing?
- What kind of care is available to help my family care for me?
- Are there alternative therapies that would help my condition?
- Are any of these therapies covered by my insurance?
- Are there any side effects to these therapies?
- Who is in charge of making sure my pain is well controlled?

equipment into the home for patient use. Home health services do not provide around-the-clock care, but rely on the patient having other caregivers, such as family members, friends, or other community resources.

Home care services can be provided by many different organizations, such as the Visiting Nurses Association (VNA), home health agencies (which vary in the range of services provided), hospice organizations, providers of home medical equipment, and pharmacies with delivery services. Patients requiring a range of specialized services may find more continuity of care if one agency is able to provide all, or almost all, of the services they need. **Hospice care** is care provided to patients who are terminally ill. Most hospices care for their clients within the home. The goal of hospice is to help the client and their family deal with the physical, emotional, and spiritual issues associated with dying. Excellent **pain management** is a priority.

Nursing care

Skilled nursing care provides the backbone for home care. Visits may include wound and ostomy care; infusion therapy such as home **chemotherapy**, **antibiotics**, or home parenteral nutrition (HPN); patient and caregiver teaching; ongoing assessment of the client's physical and emotional condition and progress; pain control; psychological support; and

supervision of home health aides. The nurse may function as a case manager and coordinate the various other services the client is receiving. The nurse assesses the home environment for safety and for appropriateness of continued home care.

Physical therapy

Physical therapists develop a plan for the client to restore (as much as possible) the physical condition lost following surgery or as a result of a decline due to the disease process. They also teach patients how to prevent further injury or deterioration and how to maintain gains made.

Occupational therapy

Occupational therapists assist patients in restoring or enhancing their ability to perform their tasks of daily living. Patients may need to learn how to use adaptive equipment such as a prosthesis. The goal is to achieve the highest level of functioning possible.

Speech therapy

Speech therapists work with clients who have difficulty swallowing or clearly communicating.

Home health aides

Home health aides function under the supervision of a registered nurse. They provide care with personal hygiene, such as bathing and dressing, feeding, and ambulating. They may assist a nurse in providing patient care. They may provide homemaking services and companionship, or those tasks may be covered by a homemaker or attendant.

Social work

Social workers may assist clients in accessing the services that are available to them based on their insurance, and in learning what community resources exist. They may also facilitate the referral process, and provide counseling and patient advocacy.

Nutritional education

Nutritionists and registered dieticians may educate clients on their nutritional needs, and on how to go about attaining them. They may also be involved if HPN is required.

Infusion therapy

Some patients may receive their chemotherapy or antibiotics at home, or may require infusion of liquid nutrition (HPN). While these services may be provided by a nurse, a separate agency or company may provide the equipment and products.

Laboratory work

Blood drawing and other laboratory services may be provided by a nurse, a phlebotomist, or a laboratory technician.

Home medical equipment

Following surgery or treatment in a hospital, patients may need the delivery and servicing of items such as special beds, wheelchairs, walkers, catheters, and wound care and ostomy supplies.

Volunteers

Volunteers may provide a range of assistance such as respite care for the primary caregiver(s), caring for the home, cooking, cleaning, emotional support, companionship, running errands, making telephone calls, child care, elder care, and providing transportation. They may come from the patient's circle of friends or religious organization, or from such agencies as Meals on Wheels.

Causes

Many individuals with conditions that do not necessitate care in a hospital setting often require short-term or long-term home care. They may need care to assist them in regaining their health similar to that prior to their illness, or may need ongoing care as their condition deteriorates due to metastatic disease. One trend that is gathering speed in the early 2000s is an increase in home health care services as opposed to nursing home care.

Special concerns

Insurance coverage plays a major role in funding home health care. In organizing home care the patient must fully understand which services will be fully covered, covered but with a co-payment, or not covered at all. Insurance coverage may vary depending on whether the service provider is within a specified approved network. It must also be clear how often and for how long the services will be needed, and whether the insurance benefits cover the entire time period of anticipated care. The patient's safety must always remain a priority. The patient and the caregiver(s) may suffer from isolation and **depression**. Primary caregivers may become overwhelmed with caring for the patient, and there may come a point at which the level of care needed may no longer be able to be provided in the home setting. The health of the primary caregiver must periodically be assessed.

Treatments

Treatments provided in the home include wound and ostomy care, intravenous (IV) chemotherapy or antibiotics, HPN, and physical, occupational, and speech therapy.

Newer trends and future concerns

One trend in home health care is greater use of the telephone and Internet for contact between home health care workers and medical professionals, and for information gathering. The U. S. Department of Health and Human Services has sponsored a new web site intended to help consumers as well as professionals make informed choices about home health care agencies. In addition, the growth of so-called telehealth systems has already had an impact on nursing education and practice in the home health care field. The field of telehealth is expected to expand dramatically in the early 2000s, as experts estimate that home health care is 10–15 years behind other fields in its use of computers.

Another trend is the growing emphasis on culturally sensitive home health care. In many cases, patients from minority ethnic groups and cultures are more comfortable being cared for in their homes by caregivers who share their background or have been trained to understand it than to be sent to large urban nursing homes where they are isolated from familiar customs and language. Studies of the feasibility of home health care for Native Americans in remote locations are presently being conducted in Canada.

One worrisome concern for the future is the increasing difficulty of recruiting and retaining high-quality home health care workers in the United States and Canada. The aging of the general North American population coupled with the high turnover in the field of home health care poses a serious problem for policy makers.

Alternative and complementary therapies

Clients may contract to have home acupuncture or massage therapy. On their own they may engage in yoga, t'ai chi, meditation, guided imagery, visualization, or other stress-reducing techniques that help them better cope with their situation. They may also choose to investigate herbal supplements and medications; all supplemental medications should be approved by a physician before use.

Resources

BOOKS

Levin, Bernard. *American Cancer Society: Colorectal Cancer.* New York: Villard Books, 1999.

Runowicz, Carolyn D., Jeanne A. Petrek, and Ted S. Gansler. *American Cancer Society: Women and Cancer.* New York: Villard Books/Random House, 1999.

Teeley, Peter, and Philip Bashe. *The Complete Cancer Survival Guide.* New York: Doubleday, 2000.

PERIODICALS

Applebaum, R. A., S. A. Mehdizadeh, and J. K. Straker. "The Changing World of Long-Term Care: A State Perspective." *Journal of Aging and Social Policy* 16 (January 2004): 1–19.

Fermazin, M., M. O. Canady, P. R. Milmine, et al. "Home Health Compare: Web Site Offers Critical Information to Consumers, Professionals." *Lippincott's Case Management* 9 (March-April 2004): 89–95.

Hotson, K. E., S. M. Macdonald, and B. D. Martin. "Understanding Death and Dying in Select First Nations Communities in Northern Manitoba: Issues of Culture and Remote Service Delivery in Palliative Care." *International Journal of Circumpolar Health* 63 (March 2004): 25–38.

Lee, H., and M. Cameron. "Respite Care for People with Dementia and Their Carers." *Cochrane Database Systems Review* February 2004: CD004396.

Stone, R. I. "The Direct Care Worker: The Third Rail of Home Care Policy." *Annual Review of Public Health* 25 (2004): 521–537.

Williams, K. "Preparing Nurses for Telehealth: A Home Health Care Example." *Medinfo* 2004(CD): 1908.

ORGANIZATIONS

The American Cancer Society. 800–ACS–2345. http://www.cancer.org.

National Association for Home Care. 228 7th Street, S.E. Washington, D.C. 20003. 202–547–7424. http://www.nahc.org.

National Cancer Institute. Building 31, Room 10A31, 31 Center Drive, MSC 2580, Bethesda, MD 20892–2580. 301–435–3848. http://www.nci.nih.gov.

National Center for Complementary and Alternative Medicine. NCCAM Clearinghouse, P.O. Box 8218, Silver Spring, MD 20907–8218. 888–644–6226. <http://nccam.nih.gov>.

Office for the Advancement of Telehealth. 5600 Fishers Lane, Room 7C-22, Rockville, MD 20857. (301) 443-0447. Fax: (301) 443-1330. <http://telehealth.hrsa.gov>.

Visiting Nurse Association of America. 11 Beacon Street, Suite 910; Boston, MA 02108. 617–523–4042. Fax: 617-227–4843. http://www.vnaa.org.

Esther Csapo Rastegari, R.N., B.S.N., Ed.M.
Rebecca J. Frey, Ph.D.

Horner's syndrome

Description

William Edmonds Horner (1793–1853) first described a small muscle at the angle of the eyelid (tensor tarsi) as well as a description of an ingenious operation to correct problems with the lower lid in 1824 in the *American Journal of the Medical Sciences.* Since that time, his name has been associated with the syndrome of a small, regular pupil, drooping of the eyelid on the same side and occasional loss of sweat formation on the forehead of the affected eye. In appearance, it occurs on one side of the face with a sinking in of the eyeball (enophthalmos), drooping upper eyelid (ptosis), slight elevation of the lower lid, excessive contraction of the pupil of the eye (miosis), narrowing of the eyelid, and an absence of facial sweat on the affected side (anhidrosis). Other symptoms may include a variation in eye color of the iris and changes in the consistency of tears.

Causes

Horner's syndrome is caused by damage or interruption of the sympathetic nerve to the eye. There are two major divisions of the nervous system: the voluntary (conscious control) and involuntary (without conscious control). The involuntary (autonomic nervous system) has two divisions: sympathetic and parasympathetic nervous systems. Under normal conditions, there is a fine balance between sympathetic and parasympathetic stimulation. If an individual is threatened by a situation, the pupils dilate, blood is shifted to the muscles and the heart beats faster as the person prepares to fight or flee. This is sympathetic stimulation. The eye has both sympathetic (responds to challenges) and parasympathetic (slows the body down) innervation. The nerve that carries the sympathetic innervation travels down the spinal cord from the brain (hypothalamus), emerges in the chest cavity, and then finds it way up the neck along with the carotid artery and jugular vein through the middle ear and into the eye. If these sympathetic impulses were blocked, the eye would have an overbalance of parasympathetic supply, which would result in a constriction of the pupil, relaxation of all the muscles around the eye and a sinking of the eye into the orbit—Horner's syndrome. Thus, damage that occurs anywhere along the course of this nerve's route from the brain to the eye can evoke this syndrome.

If the syndrome exists from birth (congenital), it is typically noted around the age of two years with the presence of a variation in the color of the iris and the lack of a crease in the drooping eye. Since eye color is completed by the age of two, a variation in color is an uncommon finding in Horner's syndrome acquired later in life.

The common causes of acquired Horner's syndrome include aortic dissection (a tear in the wall of the aorta to create a false channel where blood becomes trapped), carotid dissection, tuberculosis, Pancoast tumor (a tumor in the upper end of the lung), **brain tumors**, spinal cord injury in the neck, trauma to the cervical or thoracic portions of the spinal cord, cluster migraine headache, vertebrae destruction or collapse, compression of the spinal cord by enlarged lymph nodes, and neck or thyroid surgery.

The diagnosis and localization of this disorder is made with the use of pharmacological testing by an ophthalmologist. The physician places drops of a 10% liquid cocaine into the eyes, blocking the parasympathetic nerves so the sympathetic nervous system can be evaluated. After thirty minutes, the dilation of the pupils is noted and a Horner's pupil dilates poorly. A positive cocaine test does not, however, localize the area of the damage. After waiting for 48 hours, other medications are used to determine where the nerve interruption occurs. This solution routinely has been hydroxyamphetamine bromide. However, it has not been routinely available and in 2004, a study reported that a phenylephrine solution works as well. An individual's urine can test positive for cocaine up to two days following the initial test.

Treatments

Treatment for congenital cases

Children who are diagnosed with Horner's syndrome of a congenital origin may undergo surgical correction to strengthen the muscle of the eyelid and give it an appearance similar to the unaffected eye. The surgery improves the appearance of the child but does not alleviate the syndrome. For these cases a plastic surgeon may be preferred. Occasionally Horner's syndrome may be seen in a newborn with a **neuroblastoma** (tumor originating from nerve cells). This is almost always a sign of a localized tumor and is associated with a relatively good prognosis. In these cases, a neurologist may be consulted for treatment since their specialty is the nervous system.

Treatment for acquired cases

The treatment for acquired Horner's syndrome depends upon the cause and is focused toward eliminating the disease that produces the syndrome. Frequently, there is no treatment that improves or reverses the condition, but recognition of the signs and symptoms is extremely important for early diagnosis and treatment. Early detection of the syndrome may facilitate treatment related to those caused by tumors as they can be removed before extensive damage is done. Causes related to an interruption in nerve transmission once the nerve leaves the spinal cord are usually related to blood circulation and are easier to treat. Any numbness or paralysis on one side of the body means the problem is within the spinal cord or brain and is more difficult to treat. Some acquired Horner's may be corrected slightly by plastic surgery for appearance changes.

Alternative and complementary therapies

Acupuncture may be utilized to enhance disruptions in nerve transmissions and herbs or supplements that improve circulation may benefit some cases of acquired syndrome. These herbs and supplements would include Gingko biloba and vitamin E. As with any complementary treatment, patients should notify their physician of any herbal or over-the-counter medications they are taking.

Resources

BOOKS

Jarvis, Carolyn. *Physical Examination and Health Assessment*. Philadelphia: W.B. Saunders Company, 2000.

PERIODICALS

Danesh-Meyer, H.V., P. Savino, and R. Sergott. "The Correlation of Phenylephrine 1% With Hydroxyamphetamine

1% in Horner's Syndrome." *British Journal of Ophthalmology* April 2004: 592–594.

OTHER

Handbook of Ocular Disease Management. [cited July 6, 2005]. http://www.revoptom.com.

Linda K. Bennington, C.N.S., M.S.N.
Teresa G. Odle

Hospice care

Definition

Hospice care is palliative care given to individuals who are terminally ill with an expected survival of six months or less. The focus of hospice care is on meeting the physical, emotional, and spiritual needs of the dying individual, while fostering the highest quality of life possible.

Description

Hospice services provide palliative care to individuals with a life expectancy of six months or less. Most hospice care is provided in the home, but may take place in a hospice home or a hospice/palliative care area within a medical facility. Requesting hospice care may be the first time that individuals, or their families, acknowledge that their condition is not treatable. It may be the first time that they have to deal with their death as a reality taking place within a few months. The emotional journey to be able to deal with these issues may take a while, and therefore may delay the time when the person begins to receive hospice care.

The focus of hospice is not on treatment, but on pain and symptom management, comfort measures, acknowledging that the individual will die, supporting the family, and trying to provide the best quality of life for the time remaining. Hospice functions under the philosophy that although some terminally ill patients may no longer receive treatment, they still require and deserve care.

Hospice care is interdisciplinary in nature, providing the services of physicians, nurses, social workers, physical, speech, or occupational therapists, clergy or other spiritual guides, health care aides, and volunteers. Home hospice care relies on the family and friends of the patient to provide most of the daily care. Nursing and other services are provided daily or weekly, but with 24 hours, 7 days a week on-call access. Addressing the

KEY TERMS

Meditation—Meditation is a technique in which the individual focuses on a word or phrase to the exclusion of other thoughts. It has been shown to reduce stress and anxiety.

Palliative care—Care focused on providing comfort, not cure.

Respite care—A form of temporary home health care that allows family members some time away from patient care. Respite care is usually short-term, ranging from a few hours to a weekend.

T'ai chi—An Asian practice of breathing and slow physical movements that develops strength and reduces stress.

Telehealth—The use of the telephone, Internet, and other forms of telecommunication to support long-distance health care, education of health care professionals, and public health concerns.

spiritual needs of the hospice client is a fundamental aspect of hospice care.

Some studies about hospice care have gleaned the following:

- When asked their preference, about two-thirds of cancer patients said they preferred to die in their own home.
- The majority of patients still die in the hospital.
- When surveyed, about 95% of families who received hospice care said that it had been helpful.
- Although satisfied with hospice care, caregivers report the job of caregiving as having a negative impact on their own quality of life, and felt the job was burdensome.
- When compared to a control group of noncaregivers, caregivers had higher levels of depression, anxiety, anger, and health problems. Caregivers had a higher rate of deteriorating health, social, and occupational functioning.
- Quality of life was influenced by the individual's spiritual well-being.
- Hospice patients expressed feelings of conflict between a hope for living, and "living in hope," being able to reconcile with others and coming to terms with death.
- Although hospice is focused on helping people in the last six months of their life, most hospice patients only receive about one month of hospice care prior to their death.

QUESTIONS TO ASK THE DOCTOR

- What do you think is my prognosis?
- What choices are there to manage my pain and other symptoms?
- What level of symptom management can I expect to receive?
- What types of care, conventional or alternative, would improve the quality of the time I have left?
- Will my insurance cover the care you suggest?
- If I choose hospice care, how will that affect my relationship with my doctors and treatment team?
- What kind of support is there for my family, both until I die and afterwards?

- Only 20% of physicians' prognoses about a patient's survival was accurate. Sixty-three percent were overly optimistic, and 17% were overly pessimistic. The more experience the physicians had, the better their accuracy of prognosis.

Causes

Hospice care was first established in the United States in 1974 in Branford, Connecticut. The Branford hospice was patterned on St. Christopher's Hospice in London, which was established by Dame Cicely Saunders in 1967. In 1969, the book *On Death and Dying*, by Dr. Elizabeth Kugler-Ross identified five stages that a terminally ill person goes through. In the book, Dr. Kubler-Ross addressed the importance of patients having a role in the decisions affecting the quality of their life and death. In 1972 she testified at the first U.S. Senate national hearing on dying with dignity.

Deciding on hospice care is a choice made by the terminally ill individual. To be eligible, one's physician needs to document that the individual's survival is expected to be six months or less. Should the patient recover, and the prognosis change, the relationship with hospice is terminated, but can be reestablished when needed at a later date. Not all patients will choose hospice. If only home hospice care is available, individuals who would be eligible may decide that hospice is not a good choice for them. Reasons for not choosing home hospice include:

- The patient lives alone, with little or no family support available.
- The patient has a need for 24-hour nursing care.

- The patient has family, but they are unable to provide the supportive care required.
- The patient is concerned about being a burden to the caregiver.
- The patient feels more secure in a hospital environment.

Special concerns

A study looking at the communication between physicians and their dying patients found these issues to be very important:

- Being honest and straightforward with patients.
- A willingness to talk about dying.
- Being sensitive when conveying bad news.
- Listening to patients.
- Encouraging patients to ask questions.
- Finding a balance between being honest without discouraging hope.

A *Journal of the American Medical Association* article found that patients at the end of their life expressed these issues as important:

- being mentally aware
- not being a burden
- having their funeral arrangements planned
- helping others
- coming to peace with God
- freedom from pain
- talking about the meaning of death
- Among nine issues, dying at home was rated the least important.

Because time is limited for patients in hospice, patients and their caregivers need to act swiftly on areas of dissatisfaction, such as quality of care being provided or insufficient symptom management.

Treatments

Curative treatments are not a part of hospice care. However, hospice places great importance on minimizing or alleviating pain and symptoms such as appetite loss (**anorexia**), **fatigue**, weakness, constipation, difficulty breathing, confusion, **nausea**, **vomiting**, cough, and dry or sore mouth. For many with advanced **cancer**, fatigue may be their worst symptom. Research has shown that a tailored exercise program can increase activity tolerance without increasing fatigue. In addition, patients reported an increase in quality of life and decreased anxiety. Patients who expressed the most fatigue showed the most decrease in fatigue with the exercise program. Many hospice patients have breakthrough pain in addition to their chronic pain. Research using an indwelling subcutaneous needle for pain control showed 88% pain control with this method when pain was not well controlled with oral medications. Chronic pain requires ongoing pain relief, such as might be handled with a pump or patch. Good pain control may mean waking the patient up at night for oral medication to prevent the pain from mounting during sleep.

Alternative and complementary therapies

Dealing with the issues of death may be addressed through talking with others, writing in a journal, creative expression such as painting, writing a poem, or composing music. Meditation may be beneficial to some patients. Gentle body movements such as with t'ai chi or yoga may be helpful, depending on the patient's activity tolerance.

Recent trends

A recent development in facilitating hospice care in the patient's home is night respite service. In general, respite care refers to home health care offered by volunteers or home health caregivers that allows the patient's family a few hours or a weekend away from direct patient care. Night respite care in a hospice setting involves trained aides who care for the patient in his or her home overnight, thus allowing other family members to catch up on necessary sleep. Studies indicate that many patients as well as family members feel that night respite care is a good option that allows patients to remain at home rather than being transferred to an inpatient hospice.

One trend in hospice care that has attracted considerable interest in the early 2000s is ethnically and culturally sensitive hospice care. As of 2004, hospice services in the United States and Canada are utilized disproportionately by Caucasians. One innovative Native American hospice program that is working well is a palliative care program at the Pueblo of Zuni in New Mexico. The Zuni program combines tribal-based home health care with inpatient care at an Indian Health Service (IHS) hospital.

Another significant trend in hospice care is the greater use of webcams, video phones, and other devices that have been introduced along with the computerization of hospital and hospice facilities. The rapid growth of "telehealth" since the mid-1990s indicates that technological innovations in telecommunications will affect hospice care as they have home health care and other outpatient settings.

Resources

BOOKS

Teeley, Peter and Philip Bashe. *The Complete Cancer Survival Guide.* New York: Doubleday, 2000.

PERIODICALS

Finke, B., T. Bowannie, and J. Kitzes. " Palliative Care in the Pueblo of Zuni." *Journal of Palliative Medicine* 7 (February 2004): 135–143.

Kristjanson, L. J., K. Cousins, K. White, et al. "Evaluation of a Night Respite Community Palliative Care Service." *International Journal of Palliative Nursing* 10 (February 2004): 84–90.

Lyke, J., and M. Colon. "Practical Recommendations for Ethnically and Racially Sensitive Hospice Services." *American Journal of Hospice and Palliative Care* 21 (March-April 2004): 131–133.

Oliver, D. R., and G. Demiris. "An Assessment of the Readiness of Hospice Organizations to Accept Technological Innovation." *Journal of Telemedicine and Telecare* 10 (March 2004): 170–174.

Steinhauser, K. E., et al. "Factors Considered Important at the End of Life by Patients, Family, Physicians, and Other Care Providers." *Journal of the American Medical Association* November 15, 2000: 2476–482.

OTHER

Cancer Resources. 457 West 22nd Street, Suite B, New York, NY 10011. 800-401-2233. Fax: 212-243-1063. e-mail: info@cancerresources.com. http://www.cancerresouces.com.

ORGANIZATIONS

American Cancer Society. 800-ACS-2345. http://www.cancer.org.

American Pain Society. 4700 W. Lake Ave., Glenview, IL 60025. 847-375-4715. <http://ampainsoc.org>.

Hospice Association of America. 228 Seventh Street, SE; Washington, DC 20003. 202-546-4759. Fax: 202-547-9559. www.hospice-america.org.

National Association for Home Care. 228 7th Street, S.E. Washington, D.C. 20003. 202-547-7424. http://www.nahc.org.

National Cancer Institute. Building 31, Room 10A31, 31 Center Drive, MSC 2580, Bethesda, MD 20892-2580. 301-435-3848. http://www.nci.nih.gov.

National Center for Complementary and Alternative Medicine. NCCAM Clearinghouse, P.O. Box 8218, Silver Spring, MD 20907-8218. 888-644-6226. <http://nccam.nih.gov>.

Office for the Advancement of Telehealth. 5600 Fishers Lane, Room 7C-22, Rockville, MD 20857. (301) 443-0447. Fax: (301) 443-1330. <http://telehealth.hrsa.gov>.

Esther Csapo Rastegari, R.N., B.S.N., Ed.M.
Rebecca J. Frey, Ph.D.

HPV *see* Human papilloma virus

Human growth factors

Definition

Human growth factors are compounds made by the body that function to regulate cell division and cell survival. Some growth factors are also produced in the laboratory by genetic engineering and are used in biological therapy.

Description

Human tumors express large amounts of growth factors and their receptors. A tumor will not grow beyond the size of a pinhead without new blood vessels to supply oxygen and nutrients. Growth factors are significant because they can induce angiogenesis, the formation of blood vessels around a tumor. These growth factors also encourage cell proliferation, differentiation, and migration on the surfaces of the endothelial cells—cells found inside the lining of blood vessels. Of the approximately 20 proteins that activate endothelial cell growth, two growth factors in particular, vascular endothelial growth factor (VEGF) and basic fibroblast growth factor (bFGF), are expressed by many tumors and appear important in contributing to tumor growth and promoting tumor spread throughout the body. Several compounds that block VEGF or its receptor are now in **clinical trials**.

See also Angiogenesis inhibitors.

Crystal Heather Kaczkowski, MSc.

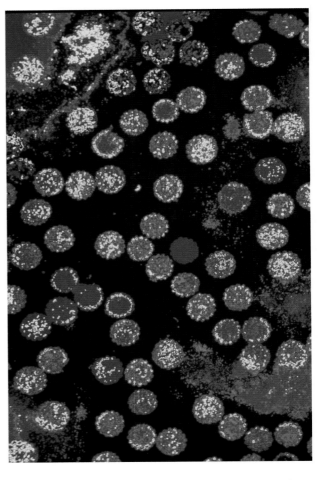

Transmission electron micrograph of human papilloma virus, magnified 40,000 times. HPV is the cause of warts, including genital warts, and has been implicated in cervical cancer. *(Custom Medical Stock Photo. Reproduced by permission.)*

Human papilloma virus

Definition

HPV **infection** is a sexually transmitted disease (STD) caused by 30–40 of the 130 or so known strains of human papillomavirus, the name of a group of viruses that infect the skin and mucous membranes of humans and some animals. In humans these sexually transmitted strains can cause genital warts, precancerous changes in the tissues of the female vagina, or **cervical cancer**. Other strains of HPV are responsible for warts on the soles of the feet (plantar warts), common warts on the hands, and flat warts on the face or legs.

Large brown genital wart of a female. *(Custom Medical Stock Photo. Reproduced by permission.)*

Demographics

In recent years HPV infection has become the most common STD in the United States. Approximately 20 million Americans are infected with HPV as of 2009, and another 6.2 million people become newly infected each year. According to one study, 27 percent of women between the ages of 14 and 59 are infected with one or more types of HPV, and 35% of homosexual men. The Centers for Disease Control and Prevention (CDC) estimates that more than 80 percent of American women will contract at least one strain of genital HPV by age 50. About 75–80 percent of sexually active Americans of either sex will be infected with HPV at some point in their lifetime.

As far as is known, men and women are at equal risk of being infected with HPV, as are members of all races and ethnic groups.

In terms of specific illnesses associated with HPV, 11,000 women are diagnosed with cervical **cancer** each year in the United States and 3,900 women die of the disease. Another 5,800 women are diagnosed with cancers of the vagina and the external female genitals, while 3,300 men are diagnosed with cancer of the penis or the anal area. The risk of **anal cancer** is 17 to 31 times higher among gay and bisexual men than among heterosexual men.

Description

The family of human papilloma viruses includes a large number of genetically related viruses. Many of these cause warts, including the warts commonly found on the skin. Another group of HPV preferentially infect the mucosal surfaces of the genitals, including the penis, vagina, vulva, and cervix. These are spread among adults by sexual contact. One group of HPV that infect the genitals causes soft warts, often designated condylomata acuminata. These genital warts are quite common and rarely if ever become cancerous. The most common of these low-risk HPV types are designated HPV 6 and 11.

The second group of viruses, termed high-risk HPV types, is associated with the development of cervical cancer. Individuals infected with these viruses are at higher risk for the development of precancerous lesions. Typically, infection with these viruses is common in adolescents and women in their twenties, and usually do not result in cancerous growth. The most common high-risk HPV is type 16. The appearance of abnormal cells containing high-risk HPV types is seen most frequently in women over the age of 30 who have abnormal Pap smears.

It is possible that other viruses work together with human papilloma viruses to produce precancerous changes in tissue. Cases of tongue cancer have been reported in which HPV was found together with **Epstein-Barr virus**, or EBV. Smoking, the use of oral contraceptives for birth control for longer than 5 years, and suppression of the immune system are also thought to be factors that combine with HPV infection to lead to precancerous lesions in tissue.

Risk factors

Some people are at greater risk of sexually transmitted HPV than others:

- Gay and bisexual men.
- People with HIV or other diseases that weaken the immune system.
- Males or females below age 25. Younger people appear to be more biologically vulnerable to the HPV virus.
- People who have large numbers of sexual partners.
- People in relationships with partners who have sex with many other people.
- People who must take drugs that suppress the immune system.

Causes and symptoms

Causes

The cause of sexually transmitted HPV infection is one or more strains of the human papillomavirus. The virus enters the body through small breaks in the skin surface or in the mucous membranes lining the genitals. In most cases the body fights off the virus within a few weeks. In some people, however, HPV remains dormant for a period ranging from a few weeks to three years in one of the lower layers of skin cells. The virus then begins to replicate (copy itself) when these cells mature and move upward to the surface of the skin. The virus affects the shape of the cells, leading to the formation of noticeable warts, precancerous changes in skin cells, or cervical cancer. About 1 percent of sexually active adults in the United States have genital warts at any one time; about 10 percent of women with high-risk HPV in the tissues of their cervix will develop long-lasting HPV infections that put them at risk for cervical cancer.

The percentages of cancers caused by high-risk types of HPV are as follows:

- cervical cancer: 100%
- anal cancer: 90%
- cancer of the vulva: 40%

- vaginal cancer: 40%
- oropharyngeal cancer: 12%
- oral cancer: 3%

Symptoms in adults

Symptoms of sexually transmitted HPV infection may include:

- Genital warts. These appear as bumps or clusters of fleshy outgrowths around the anus or on the genitals. Some may grow into large cauliflower-shaped masses. Genital warts usually appear within weeks or months after sexual contact with an infected person. If left untreated, genital warts may go away, remain unchanged, or increase in size or number but will not turn into cancers. It is possible, however, for a person to be infected with a high-risk strain of HPV as well as one of the strains that cause genital warts; therefore the appearance of genital warts does not necessarily mean that the person is not at risk of cancer.
- Precancerous changes in the tissues of the female cervix. These are flat growths on the cervix that cannot be seen or felt by the infected woman.
- Cancer. High-risk strains of HPV can cause cancers of the mouth and throat as well as cancers of the anal area and the male and female genitals. These typically take years to develop after infection. In men, symptoms of anal cancer may include bleeding, pain, or a discharge from the anus, or changes in bowel habits. Early signs of cancer of the penis may include thickening of the skin, tissue growths, or sores.

It is not fully understood as of 2009 why most infections with high-risk HPV are of short duration, while a small percentage persist and eventually transform cervical cells to a state of cancerous growth.

Symptoms in children

In addition to producing precancerous lesions in some patients, HPV infections in women are a health concern because they can be transmitted to the respiratory tract of a baby during childbirth. This type of HPV infection may lead to a rare disorder known as juvenile-onset recurrent respiratory papillomatosis (JO-RRP) or laryngeal papillomatosis, in which papillomas or warts form in the child's airway, producing hoarseness or partial blockage of the windpipe. Although laryngeal papillomatosis can occur in HPV-infected adults, 60–80% of cases occur in children, most of them younger than three years.

Laryngeal papillomatosis is usually diagnosed by **laryngoscopy**. Surgery, whether traditional or laser surgery, is the usual treatment for JO-RRP, but the warts often recur and require additional surgery to remove them. In extreme cases, the patient may be given a tracheotomy, a procedure in which a hole is cut through the throat into the windpipe and a tube is inserted to keep the breathing hole open. A newer treatment for the disorder is **photodynamic therapy** or PDT. In PDT, a special light-sensitive dye is injected into the patient's blood. The dye collects in the tumors rather than in healthy tissue. When bright light of a specific wavelength is shined on the throat, it destroys the tumors containing the dye.

Cidofovir and interferon are often given as adjuvant treatments for this disease as of the early 2000s. JO-RRP is a serious illness, leading to death in a significant number of affected children. In a very few cases, respiratory papillomatosis can lead to cancer as well as breathing difficulties.

Diagnosis

There is no general blood, urine, or imaging test for HPV infection. The diagnosis of genital warts is obvious based on their location and appearance. The doctor may, however, use a vinegar solution to identify HPV-infected areas on the skin of the genitals. The vinegar solution will turn white if HPV is present. Since genital warts are caused by low-risk strains of HPV, the doctor does not need to identify the specific strain of the virus that is present.

Sexually active women should be screened periodically for the presence of changes in the tissues of the cervix. The most common test is the Papanikolaou test or Pap smear, invented by a Greek physician in the 1940s. To perform a Pap smear, the doctor takes a small spatula to obtain cells from the outer surface of the cervix and smears the collected cells on a slide that is then examined in a laboratory for signs of any abnormal cells. If abnormal or questionable cells are found, the doctor may order an HPV DNA test, which can identify the DNA of 13 high-risk types of HPV in cells taken from the cervix.

There are no HPV screening tests for men as of 2009; however, some doctors are suggesting that anal Pap smears for men who have sex with men would be useful in early detection of anal cancer..

Tests

The relationship among HPV, precancerous cellular changes, and cervical cancer have led to the suggestion that testing for the presence of HPV can be a useful addition to Pap tests. Pap tests involve microscopic analysis of cells removed from the cervix. The results of these tests are generally reported as either normal or consistent with the presence of cancer or a precancerous condition. Patients receiving the latter diagnosis usually are treated either by excisional or ablative therapy surgery or some other means in order to remove the tumor or precancerous lesion.

In some cases the cytologist or pathologist examining a Pap test reports a "borderline" result when abnormal cells are observed, but it is not possible to distinguish whether the changes seen are due to early precancerous changes or to inflammation caused by some infectious agent or irritant. In these cases, some physicians and scientists believe that testing for the presence of HPV can help to identify those women who should be closely followed for the development of early cancerous lesions, or who should undergo colposcopy, a procedure to examine the cervix for precancerous lesions. These cancer precursors, termed cervical intraepithelial neoplasia (CIN) when identified early, before they have become invasive, can almost always be completely removed by minor surgery, essentially curing the patient before the cancer has had a chance to develop. The cervical tissue removed, which includes the precancerous tissue, is examined as part of a **biopsy** to confirm the diagnosis, and if requested by a doctor, can be tested for the presence of high-risk HPV types.

Treatment

Patients with genital warts should *never* use over-the-counter-preparations designed to remove common or flat warts from the hands or face. Doctors can treat genital warts with various medical or surgical techniques:

- Cryotherapy. Cryotherapy uses liquid nitrogen to freeze the warts. The dead tissue in the wart falls away from the skin beneath in about a week.
- Imiquimod. Imiquimod (Aldara) is a topical cream that gets rid of genital warts by stimulating the body's immune system to fight the virus that causes the warts.
- Podofilox. Podofilox (Condylox) is a topical medication available in liquid or gel form that destroys the wart tissue.
- Surgery. The doctor can remove the wart by drying it out with an electric needle and then scraping the tissue with a sharp instrument called a curette. Lasers can also be used to remove genital warts.

Low-grade precancerous changes in the tissue of the female cervix are not usually treated directly because most of them will eventually go away on their own without developing into cancer. The patient should, however, see the doctor for follow-up Pap smears to make sure that the tissues are returning to normal. High-risk

QUESTIONS TO ASK YOUR DOCTOR

- Do you think I should have an HPV test if my Pap smear results are abnormal?
- Based upon my Pap smear result and HPV testing, when should I have my next Pap smear?
- What can I do to decrease my risk of becoming (re)infected with HPV?
- What is your opinion of HPV vaccination for men?

precancerous lesions are removed, usually by surgery, **cryotherapy**, electrocauterization, or laser surgery.

Since the incidence of latent and recurrent infections is high, the eradication of HPV is not always 100% effective. It is essential to be aware that HPV is a sexually transmitted disease and women must engage in safe sex practices to decrease the risk of spreading the virus or becoming reinfected. A vaccine effective against four of the HPV types most likely to cause genital warts or cervical cancer was approved for use in 2006; it is described more fully under Prevention below. As of 2009, researchers are working on developing **vaccines** that protect against additional types of the HPV virus.

Prognosis

The prognosis of sexually transmitted HPV infections depends on the patient's age, number of sexual partners, gender, and the condition of their immune system. Women are significantly more likely than men to develop cancers following HPV infection. However, most people of either sex with normally functioning immune systems who are infected with HPV will clear the infection from their bodies within two years.

Prevention

Preventive measures that people can take to lower their risk of HPV infection include:

- Abstaining from sex, or having sex only with an uninfected partner who is faithful.
- Reducing the number of sexual partners.
- Using condoms regularly during sexual intercourse.
- For women, using a new vaccine called Gardasil. Approved by the Food and Drug Administration (FDA) in 2006, Gardasil is a vaccine that protects against the four types of HPV that cause most cervical cancers and genital warts. The vaccine is recommended for 11- and 12-year-old girls. It is also

recommended for girls and women age 13 through 26 who have not yet been vaccinated or completed the vaccine series. Gardasil works best in girls who have not yet been sexually active. It is given as a series of three shots over a six-month period.

A second human papillomavirus vaccine, Cervarix, was approved in Europe, Australia, and the Philippines in 2007. It is awaiting FDA approval for use in the United States as of September 2009.

In addition to giving the available preventive vaccines to women, some doctors think it might be a useful preventive measure to vaccinate men as well to protect their female partners against infection. As of 2009, however, male vaccination for HPV is still under discussion rather than being put into clinical practice.

Resources

BOOKS

Gonzales, Lissette. *Frequently Asked Questions about Human Papillomavirus.* New York: Rosen, 2009.

Krueger, Hans, et al. *HPV and Other Infectious Agents in Cancer: Opportunities for Prevention and Public Health.* New York: Oxford University Press, 2010.

Marr, Lisa. *Sexually Transmitted Diseases: A Physician Tells You What You Need to Know,* 2nd ed. Baltimore, MD: Johns Hopkins University Press, 2007.

Nardo, Don. *Human Papillomavirus (HPV).* Detroit, MI: Lucent Books, 2007.

Rosenblatt, Alberto. *Human Papillomavirus.* New York: Springer, 2009.

PERIODICALS

Burki, T. "Should Males Be Vaccinated against HPV?" *Lancet Oncology* 10 (September 2009): 845.

Haug, C. "The Risks and Benefits of HPV Vaccination." *Journal of the American Medical Association* 302 (August 19, 2009): 795–95.

Hershey, J.H., and L.F. Velez. "Public Health Issues Related to HPV Vaccination." *Journal of Public Health Management and Practice* 15 (September-October 2009): 384–92.

Lindsey, K., et al. "Anal Pap Smears: Should We Be Doing Them?" *Journal of the American Academy of Nurse Practitioners* 21 (August 2009): 437–43.

O'Connor, M. B., and C. O'Connor. "The HPV Vaccine for Men." *International Journal of STD and AIDS* 20 (April 2009): 290–91.

Printz, C. "HPV Status Predicts Survival of Oropharyngeal Cancer Patients." *Cancer* 115 (September 15, 2009): 4045.

Samara, R. N., and S. N. Khleif. "HPV as a Model for the Development of Prophylactic and Therapeutic Cancer Vaccines." *Current Molecular Medicine* 9 (August 2009): 766–73.

Wang, Z., et al. " Detection of Human Papilloma Virus Subtypes 16 and P16(ink4a) in Invasive Squamous Cell Carcinoma of the Fallopian Tube and Concomitant Squamous Cell Carcinoma in Situ of the Cervix." *Journal of Obstetrics and Gynaecology Research* 35 (April 2009): 385–89.

OTHER

Centers for Disease Control and Prevention (CDC). *Human Papillomavirus (HPV) Infection.* http://www.cdc.gov/std/hpv/default.htm.

Centers for Disease Control and Prevention (CDC) Fact Sheet. *HPV and Men.* http://www.cdc.gov/std/hpv/STDFact-HPV-and-men.htm.

Gearhart, Peter A., and Thomas C. Randall. "Human Papillomavirus." *eMedicine,* August 4, 2009. http://emedicine.medscape.com/article/219110-overview.

Mayo Clinic. *HPV Infection.* http://www.mayoclinic.com/health/hpv-infection/DS00906

National Cancer Institute (NCI). http://www.cancer.gov/cancertopics/factsheet/Risk/HPV.

National Institute of Allergy and Infectious Diseases (NIAID). *Human Papillomavirus and Genital Warts.* http://www3.niaid.nih.gov/topics/genitalWarts.

National Institute on Deafness and Other Communication Disorders (NIDCD). *Laryngeal Papillomatosis.* http://www.nidcd.nih.gov/health/voice/laryngeal.htm.

ORGANIZATIONS

American College of Obstetricians and Gynecologists (ACOG), 409 12th St., S.W., P.O. Box 96920, Washington, DC, 20090-6920, (202) 638-5577, resources@acog.org, http://www.acog.org/.

American Social Health Association (ASHA), P.O. Box 13827, Research Triangle Park, NC, 27709, (919) 361-8400, (800)227-8922, (919)361-8425, http://www.ashastd.org/index.cfm.

Centers for Disease Control and Prevention (CDC), 1600 Clifton Road, Atlanta, GA, 30333, (800)232-4636, cdcinfo@cdc.gov, http://www.cdc.gov.

National Cancer Institute, 6116 Executive Blvd., Room 3036A, Bethesda, MD, 20892-8322, (800) 422-6237, cancergovstaff@mail.nih.gov, www.cancer.gov.

National Institute of Allergy and Infectious Diseases (NIAID), 6610 Rockledge Drive, MSC 6612, Bethesda, MD, 20892-6612, (301) 496-5717, (866) 284-4107, (301) 402-3573, http://www3.niaid.nih.gov.

National Institute on Deafness and Other Communication Disorders (NIDCD), 31 Center Drive, MSC 2320, Bethesda, MD, 20892-2320, (800) 241-1044, (301) 770-8977, nidcdinfo@nidcd.nih.gov, http://www.nidcd.nih.gov/index.asp.

Warren Maltzman, PhD
Rebecca J. Frey, PhD

Hydrocodone *see* **Opioids**

Hydrocortisone *see* **Corticosteroids**

Hydromorphone *see* **Opioids**

Hydroxyurea

Definition

Hydroxyurea, also known by its trade name Hydrea, is an antineoplastic agent, meaning it is used to treat **cancer**. It is taken orally.

Purpose

Hydroxyurea is used to treat the following conditions:

- Melanoma
- Chronic myelocytic leukemia that is resistant to other therapies
- Ovarian cancer that is recurrent, metastatic or inoperable.
- Squamous cell carcinoma of the head and neck, excluding the lip. (In this case, hydroxyurea is given with radiation therapy.)
- Sickle cell anemia
- Other: Hydroxyurea has shown promise in the management of thrombocytosis, a condition in which platelet levels are abnormally high

Description

Hydroxyurea belongs to antimetabolites, a group of compounds that interfere with the production of nucleic acids. Hydroxyurea exerts its anticancer activity by inhibiting ribonucleotide reductase, an enzyme required for DNA synthesis. When used in conjunction with **radiation therapy**, the effectiveness of hydroxyurea increases because it also inhibits the ability of cells damaged by radiation to repair themselves.

Recommended dosage

Hydroxyurea dosages are calculated based on a person's weight as milligrams per kilogram (mg/kg). Doctors will usually use whichever value is lowest—the patient's actual weight or the patient's ideal weight—to calculate dosages. The drug is not given if white blood cell levels drop below 2500 mm^3, or if red blood cell levels drop below 100,000 mm^3. Usually, bone marrow recovery is rapid, and few doses are missed. Hydroxyurea is usually given for six weeks before its effectiveness can be adequately evaluated.

Hydroxyurea is administered in a capsule form, each containing 500 mg of the drug. If a patient is unable to swallow the capsule, its contents can be dissolved in a glass of water and swallowed immediately. The drug will not completely dissolve in water.

KEY TERMS

Mucositis—A painful inflammation of the mucous membranes.

Mutagen—An agent capable of causing DNA changes.

Myelosuppression—Diminished bone marrow activity resulting in decreased red blood cells, white blood cells, and platelets.

Plateletpheresis—A procedure in which platelets are removed from whole blood.

Dosages have not been established for children in part because the cancers for which hydroxyurea is useful do not normally occur in that age group.

In the treatment of solid tumors, such as ovarian cancers, patients are usually given 80 mg/kg once every three days. Alternatively, a dose of 20–30 mg/kg may be given every day.

In **head and neck cancers** also treated with radiation, 80 mg/kg of hydroxyurea is given once every three days. The drug should be started a week before radiation therapy begins, and should continue for some time after radiation therapy.

When it is used to treat resistant **chronic myelocytic leukemia**, hydroxyurea is given in the dosage of 20–30 mg/kg once a day.

In thrombocytosis, doses of 15–30 mg/kg taken once a day are usually effective. Platelet levels return to a normal level within two to six weeks of therapy. In more severe cases, doses of 1.5–3.0 grams per day have been given with plateletpheresis, a procedure that removes platelets from the blood.

Precautions

This drug should not be administered to a person who has had a previous allergic reaction to it. Liver and kidney function should be evaluated prior to, and during, treatment. The drug may interfere with certain lab tests. For example, creatinine levels may be elevated. Patients taking hydroxyurea should stay well-hydrated, drinking up to 12 glasses per day of water or other fluids.

Hydroxyurea is potentially mutagenic, meaning that it causes mutations in DNA. Patients taking the drug should discuss the potential effects on their future conception plans. Hydroxyurea should not be administered to pregnant women, and women taking the drug should use birth control methods to prevent pregnancy.

Hydroxyurea is excreted in breast milk; therefore, women taking the drug should not breast-feed.

Side effects

Hydroxyurea and radiation therapy each cause adverse side effects. When they are used together, the incidence and severity of side effects may increase.

Bone marrow suppression is the major side effect of hyroxyurea therapy, and may develop within two days of the first dose. Blood tests are performed routinely to monitor for changes. Usually, leukopenia (decreased white blood cells) develops first. Reduced red blood cells and platelets can also occur, but generally not as frequently. If **anemia** develops, it should be corrected with whole blood transfusions. Hydroxyurea causes red blood cell abnormalities that are not severe and that do not reduce the red blood cell survival time.

Gastrointestinal symptoms are not as common as **myelosuppression** and are usually mild. These symptoms may include **nausea, vomiting, diarrhea,** and constipation. Usually, medications can control **nausea and vomiting. Mucositis,** a painful swelling of the mucous membranes, may also develop, especially if the patient is undergoing radiation treatment to the head and neck. Mucositis can be managed with medicated mouthwashes, good oral hygiene, and hydration to keep the mouth moist.

Headache and dizziness may occur. With long-term use, skin changes, such as hyperpigmentation of the skin and nails, have also been reported.

Hydroxyurea has also been linked to leg ulcers. Studies suggest that leg ulcers have been reported mainly in older patients who might be at an increased risk. There have also been reports of hydroxyurea causing leg ulceration when it is used in psoriasis for a prolonged period.

Interactions

Patients at risk for bone marrow suppression should inform their doctor about all medications they are taking, both prescription and non-prescription. Many over-the-counter medications contain aspirin, which acts as a blood-thinner, increasing the potential for bleeding. Patients with reduced platelets should not take aspirin.

Tamara Brown, R.N.

Hypercalcemia

Description

Hypercalcemia is an abnormally high level of calcium in the blood, usually more than 10.5 milligrams per deciliter of blood. It is the most common life-threatening metabolic disorder associated with **cancer.**

Calcium plays an important role in the development and maintenance of bones in the body. It is also needed in tooth formation and is important in other body functions. As much as 99% of the body's calcium is stored in bone tissue. A healthy person experiences a constant turnover of calcium as bone tissue is built and reshaped. The remaining 1% of the body's calcium circulates in the blood and other body fluids. Calcium in the blood plays an important role in the control of many body functions, including blood clotting, transmission of nerve impulses, muscle contraction, and other metabolic activities.

Cancer-caused hypercalcemia produces a disruption in the body's ability to maintain a normal level of calcium. This abnormally high level of calcium in the blood develops because of increased bone breakdown and release of calcium from the bone. The disorder occurs in approximately 10-20% of all cancer cases. The most common cancers associated with hypercalcemia are breast, prostate, and lung cancer, as well as **multiple myeloma** or other tumors with extensive **metastasis** to the bone. It may also occur in patients with head and neck cancer, **cancer of unknown primary, lymphoma,** leukemia, **kidney cancer,** and gastrointestinal cancer. Hypercalcemia most commonly develops as a late complication of cancer, and its appearance constitutes an emergency.

Several clinical symptoms are associated with cancer-related hypercalcemia. Symptoms may appear gradually and often look like signs of other cancers and diseases. The symptoms of hypercalcemia are not only related to the elevated level of calcium in the blood, but—more importantly—to how rapidly the hypercalcemia develops. The severity of the symptoms is often dependent upon factors such as previous cancer treatment, reactions to medications, or other illnesses a patient may have. Most patients do not experience all of the symptoms of hypercalcemia, and some may not have any signs at all. Rapid diagnosis of hypercalcemia may be complicated because the symptoms are often nonspecific and are easily ascribed to other factors. These symptoms include:

- decreased muscle tone and muscle weakness
- delirium, disorientation, incoherent speech, and psychotic symptoms such as hallucinations and delusion

- constipation
- fatigue
- poor appetite, nausea and/or vomiting
- frequency of urination and increased thirst
- pain

Causes

The fundamental cause of cancer-related hypercalcemia is increased movement of calcium out of the bones and into the bloodstream, and secondarily, an inadequate ability of the kidneys to get rid of higher calcium levels. Normally, healthy kidneys are able to filter out large amounts of calcium from the blood, getting rid of the excess that is unneeded by the body and keeping the amount of the calcium the body does need. However, the high levels of calcium in the body caused by cancer-related hypercalcemia may cause the kidneys to become overworked, thus making them unable to excrete the excess. Another problem is that some tumors produce a substance that may cause the kidneys to get rid of too little calcium.

Two types of cancer-caused hypercalcemia have been identified: osteolytic and humoral. Osteolytic occurs because of direct bone destruction by a primary or metastatic tumor. Humoral is caused by certain factors secreted by malignant cells, which ultimately cause calcium loss from the bones. Certain types of hormonal therapy may precipitate hypercalcemia and the use of some diuretics may contribute to the disorder.

Because immobility causes an increase in the loss of calcium from bone, cancer patients who are weak and spend most of their time in bed are more prone to hypercalcemia. Cancer patients are often dehydrated because they take in inadequate amounts of food and fluids and often suffer from **nausea and vomiting**. Dehydration reduces the ability of the kidneys to remove excess calcium from the body, and therefore is another contributing factor in the development of hypercalcemia in cancer patients.

Treatments

Individuals at risk for developing hypercalcemia may be the first to recognize symptoms, such as **fatigue**. The patient and family should be aware of the signs and symptoms so that a health care professional can be notified as early as possible should they occur. Patients can take several preventative measures like ensuring adequate fluid intake, controlling **nausea** and **vomiting**, maintaining the highest possible mobility, and avoiding drugs that affect the functioning of the kidneys. This includes avoiding those medications containing calcium, vitamin D, or vitamin A. Since absorption of calcium is usually decreased in individuals with hypercalcemia, dietary calcium restriction is unnecessary.

The mortality rate for untreated hypercalcemia is quite high. Early diagnosis and prompt treatment are essential. The magnitude of hypercalcemia and the severity of symptoms is usually the basis for determining what type of treatment is indicated.

For those patients who have mild hypercalcemia, are experiencing no symptoms, and have cancer that is responsive to treatment, giving intravenous fluids and observing the patient may be all that is necessary to treat the condition. If the patient is experiencing symptoms or has a cancer that is expected to respond poorly to treatment, then medication to treat the hypercalcemia should be initiated. Additional treatment focuses on controlling nausea and vomiting, encouraging activity, and avoiding any medication that causes drowsiness.

In treating moderate or severe hypercalcemia, replacing fluids is the first treatment intervention. Though providing fluid replacement will not restore normal calcium levels in all patients, it is still the most important initial step. Improvement in mental status and nausea and vomiting is usually apparent within 24 hours for most patients. However, rehydration is only a temporary measure. If the cancer is not treated, then drugs that will help to control the hypercalcemia are necessary. Many drugs are used to treat hypercalcemia, including **calcitonin**, **plicamycin** (formerly mithramycin), **gallium nitrate**, and **bisphosphonates**. Bisphosphonates are some of the most effective drugs for controlling hypercalcemia. Loop diuretics like furosemide are often given because they help to increase the excretion of excess serum calcium. For severe hypercalcemia that is complicated by kidney failure, dialysis is an option. Because of the large amounts of intravenous fluids given to treat hypercalcemia, the health care team will carefully observe for any signs of overhydration or other electrolyte imbalances.

The severity of hypercalcemia determines the amount of treatment necessary. Severe hypercalcemia should be treated immediately and aggressively. Less severe hypercalcemia should be treated according to the symptoms. A positive response to the treatment is exhibited by the disappearance of the symptoms and a decreased level of calcium in the blood. Mild hypercalcemia does not usually need to be treated aggressively. After calcium levels return to normal, urine and blood should continue to be checked often to make certain the treatment is still working.

GALE ENCYCLOPEDIA OF CANCER 3

711

Alternative and complementary therapies

There are no known proven alternative treatments for cancer-related hypercalcemia. Some of the medications used are more effective than others, and the patient and family should discuss which ones are the most appropriate for the patient's needs.

Hypercalcemia usually develops as a late complication of cancer, and its appearance is very serious. The outlook is often quite grim. However, it is not clear if death occurs because of the hypercalcemia crisis or because of the advanced cancer. Because hypercalcemia is often a complication that occurs in the final stages of cancer, the decision to treat it depends upon the overall goals of treatment determined by the patient, family, and physician. The natural course of untreated hypercalcemia will progress to loss of consciousness and coma. Some patients may prefer this at the end of life rather than have unrelieved suffering and/or untreatable symptoms. It is therefore important for the patient and caregivers to discuss what supportive care measures are wanted.

Resources

BOOKS

Prucha, Edward J., editor. *Cancer Sourcebook*. Detroit: Omnigraphics, 2000.

OTHER

National Cancer Institute. Building 31, Room 10A31, 31 Center Drive, MSC 2580, Bethesda, MD 20892-2580. (800) 4-CANCER. [cited July 5, 2005]. http://www.nci.nih.gov.

Deanna Swartout-Corbeil, R.N.

Hypercoagulable states, Trousseau's syndrome, Blood clots *see* **Hypercoagulation disorders**

Hypercoagulation disorders

Description

Hypercoagulation disorders (or hypercoagulable states or disorders) cause an increased tendency for clotting of the blood. In normal hemostasis (the stoppage of bleeding) clots form at the site of the blood vessel's injury. However, in hypercoagulation disorders the clots can develop in circulating blood. This may put a patient at risk for obstruction of veins and arteries (phlebitis, thrombosis, or thrombophlebitis). The hypercoagulable state and thrombophlebitis is

common cases of **cancer** involving solid tumors such as pancreatic, breast, ovarian, and **prostate cancer**.

Hypercoagulation disorders can cause clots throughout the body's blood vessels, a condition known as thromboembolic disease. Thromboembolic disease can lead to infarction (death of tissue as a result of blocked blood supply to the tissue). Other serious results of hypercoagulation make this a dangerous condition. Clotting (thrombosis) in the veins and arteries leading to the lungs can prevent blood flow, causing sudden and severe loss of breath and chest pain. These clots, called pulmonary embolisms, are potentially fatal. Clots in the blood vessels of the brain can result in a stroke, and clots in the heart's blood vessels can result in a heart attack.

Symptoms of hypercoagulation disorders include swelling or discoloration of the limbs, pain or tenderness of the skin, visible obstructions in the surface veins, and ulcers of the lower parts of the legs.

The diagnosis of hypercoagulation disorders is completed with a combination of physical examination, **imaging studies**, and blood tests. The presence of deep clots can be determined using Doppler ultrasound examination—special x-ray techniques called venography or arteriography (in which a solution is injected into the blood vessel to aid in imaging), or a specific type of blood pressure test called plethysmography. There are a number of blood tests that can determine the presence or absence of proteins, clotting factors, and platelet counts in the blood. Among the tests used to detect hypercoagulation is the Antithrombin III assay. Protein C and Protein S concentrations can be diagnosed with immunoassay or plasma antigen level tests.

Causes

Hypercoagulation disorders are associated with cancer of the pancreas. About half of patients with **pancreatic cancer** experience incidence of thrombosis. Approximately 10% of patients with pancreatic cancer develop a specific type of hypercoagulation disorder known as migratory thrombophlebitis, or Trousseau's syndrome. In Trousseau's syndrome the blood vessels become inflamed and clots in the blood vessels spontaneously appear and disappear. Other types of cancer may also result in hypercoagulation disorders.

In order for blood coagulation to occur, platelets (small, round fragments in the blood) help contract blood vessels to lessen blood loss and also to help plug damaged blood vessels. The conversion of platelets into actual clots is a complicated process involving proteins that are identified clotting factors. The factors are carried in the plasma, or liquid portion, of the blood. Proteins C and S are two of the clotting factors that are present in the plasma to help regulate or activate parts of the clotting process. It is believed that pancreatic tumors produce chemicals that promote clotting, or coagulation, of the blood (procoagulants), or that they activate platelet function. It is also possible that tumors interfere with the functions of proteins C and S.

Treatments

The treatment for patients with hypercoagulation disorders varies depending upon the severity of the clotting and the other conditions it may have caused. Medications may include blood thinners (anticoagulants) such as **heparin** and **warfarin**, which prevent the formation of new blood clots; antiplatelet drugs such as aspirin; or thrombolytic drugs to dissolve existing clots. Pain medications and nonsteroidal anti-inflammatory medications may be given to reduce pain and swelling. **Antibiotics** will be prescribed if **infection** has occurred.

Resources

BOOKS

Deloughery, Thomas G. *Hemostasis and Thrombosis.* Georgetown, TX: Landes Bioscience, 1999.
Goodnight, Scott H., and William E. Goodnight. *Disorders of Hemostasis and Thrombosis.* 2nd ed. New York: McGraw-Hill, 2000.

OTHER

American Academy of Family Physicians. *Hypercoagulation: Excessive Blood Clotting.* (15 April 2001). [cited July 5, 2005]. http://familydoctor.org/handouts/244.html.

ORGANIZATIONS

National Heart, Lung and Blood Institute. Building 31, Room 4A21, Bethesda, MD 20892. (301) 496-4236. http://www.nhlbi.nih.gov.
National Hemophilia Foundation. 116 West 32nd St., 11th Floor, New York, NY 10001. 800-42-HANDI. http://www.hemophilia.org.

Paul A. Johnson, Ed.M.

Hyperthermia

Definition

Hyperthermia refers to the use of heat to treat various cancers on and inside the body. It is also called hyperthermia therapy or thermotherapy.

Hyperthermia therapy for **cancer** should not be confused with heat therapy, which is a treatment that involves the application of mild heat from heating pads or warm compresses to localized areas of the body to relieve muscle and joint pain or stiffness. Hyperthermia therapy is specifically intended to kill or weaken tumors rather than to temporarily relieve discomfort caused by arthritis, sprains and strains, or similar conditions. It can be applied to a very small area (local hyperthermia), an entire limb or organ (regional hyperthermia), or the patient's entire body (whole-body hyperthermia).

Purpose

The purpose of hyperthermia is to shrink and hopefully destroy cancerous tissues without harming noncancerous cells. It can be used to treat cancer in many areas of the body, including the brain, thyroid, lung, breast, and prostate. It is thought that high temperatures, up to 106 degrees Fahrenheit, can help shrink cancerous tumors. Hyperthermia is starting to be more widely used because it does not usually have severe side effects like such other forms of cancer treatment as radiation or **chemotherapy**. In most instances, hyperthermia is used at the same time with other forms of cancer therapy.

Demographics

Although hyperthermia treatment was considered an experimental form of cancer therapy in the 1980s, its proponents believe that the treatment has been accepted by many physicians, and that use of hyperthermia will increase as more cancer centers install the high-tech equipment necessary for regional and whole-body hyperthermia. As of 2009, cancer care centers offering whole-body treatment are limited in number; however, there are several in larger cities across the United States that offer local hyperthermia. In general, hyperthermia is used more often in Europe as an adjuvant treatment for cancer than in North America.

The American Cancer Society has acknowledged that hyperthermia can make the cancer cells of some cancers more responsive to treatment, but still considers the treatment experimental, especially in whole-body form. The Cancer Treatment Centers of America (CTCA), however, lists local hyperthermia as a conventional treatment under the larger heading of **radiation therapy**. The National Cancer Institute (NCI) is sponsoring ongoing **clinical trials** of hyperthermia in cancer treatment; there are 71 such trials underway as of late 2009. The types of cancer being studied in these trials include breast, prostate, bladder, cervical, uterine, head and neck, ovarian, thyroid, and liver cancers. Several studies are concerned with late-stage metastatic and soft-tissue cancers. All age groups are represented in these clinical trials, including children.

Precautions

Patients who have extensive **metastasis** (spreading of the cancer throughout their body) are not considered the best candidates for hyperthermia, although they can receive whole-body treatment. Patients must be free of major infections and able to tolerate the high temperatures of the treatment. Caution must be used when areas of the body are heated with such external heat sources as heating pads to avoid potentially dangerous burns.

Other types of patients who should be treated cautiously with hyperthermia include:

- Pregnant women.
- People who are anemic.
- People known to be sensitive to high temperatures.
- Diabetics.
- People with tuberculosis.
- People with seizure disorders.

Description

Hyperthermia can be used on the body from very small areas of the body to the entire body itself. Local hyperthermia refers to heating just one area of body, usually where the tumor is located. The heat is applied for about an hour. Heat can be applied from outside the body using microwaves or high-frequency radio waves. Heat can be applied from inside the body or even inside the tumor itself by the use of thin heated wires, small tubes filled with hot water, implanted microwave antennae, or radiofrequency electrodes. Some cancer centers use ultrasound to produce heat within the tumor. Ultrasound is more easily focused than other energy modalities, and can be applied to tumors located on the skin surface or up to 3 inches (8 cm) inside the body.

If heat is used to treat an entire organ or limb, it is referred to as regional hyperthermia. High-energy magnets or other devices that produce high energy, and thus heat, are placed over the larger areas to be heated. Magnetic fluid hyperthermia involves the injection of a fluid containing magnetic nanoparticles directly into the malignant tumor. When the nanoparticles are placed in an alternating magnetic field with frequencies similar to FM radio signals, they generate heat and destroy the tumors.

Another method of regional hyperthermia is the use of perfusion. Hyperthermia perfusion is a technique that uses the patient's own blood; the blood is removed, heated outside the body, then pumped back into the area that contains the cancer. A warmed solution containing **anticancer drugs** may also be used as part of perfusion hyperthermia. One form of perfusion hyperthermia that is used to treat abdominal cancers is called continuous hyperthermic peritoneal perfusion or CHPP. Performed during open surgery, this procedure involves the circulation of heated anticancer drugs through the abdominal cavity to raise the temperature of the internal organs to 106–108°F (41–42°C).

For treatment of cancers that have spread throughout the body, whole-body hyperthermia can be considered. Various methods are used to heat up a patient's entire body, including warm-water or electric blankets, hot wax, or thermal chambers which are very much like incubators used to warm newborn babies, except much larger.

Origins

Hyperthermia has a long history; the earliest report of heat treatment to cure systemic disease is found in the writings of Hippocrates (c. 400 B.C.). A century before Hippocrates, another Greek philosopher/physician named Parmenides (520–450B.C.) thought that an artificially induced **fever** could cure any disease. In ancient India, practitioners of Ayurveda used regional and whole-body hyperthermia to treat various disorders. In North America in more recent times, many Native American tribes used sweat lodges for healing rituals or to purify warriors wounded in battle.

The use of heat as a cancer treatment in scientific medicine dates from the nineteenth century. A German physician reported in 1866 that a patient with a neck **sarcoma** was cured of the tumor after surviving a high fever. In 1893, a Swedish gynecologist named Westermark experimented with fevers induced by bacterial toxins and the use of a coil filled with hot water to treat uterine tumors. No controlled studies were conducted at the time, however, and reports of successful cancer treatment using heat were considered anecdotal.

Interest in heat as a possible treatment for cancer declined in the early twentieth century but rose again in the 1960s when some researchers working with cancer cells in mice thought that the malignant cells might be more sensitive to heat than normal cells. Unfortunately, later studies demonstrated that cancer cells are not necessarily more sensitive to heat by itself than normal cells. Doctors presently think that hyperthermia is effective only in combination with radiotherapy or chemotherapy.

Preparation

Patients should be prepared for hyperthermia by an explanation of the specific technique that is to be used and what to expect during and after the procedure. In most cases the patient will be given a local anesthetic when temperature probes are inserted to monitor the heat levels in the part of the body being treated. **Radiofrequency ablation** or perfusion of the peritoneal cavity usually requires general anesthesia.

Aftercare

Patients will usually need to rest afterward. Those who have had general anesthesia will need to be monitored during recovery. Patients who have had whole-body hyperthermia may need aftercare for **nausea and vomiting**. Patients who have had perfusion hyperthermia may need aftercare for tissue swelling or bleeding.

Risks

The major risks of hyperthermia use are pain and external burns. Heat applied directly to the skin can cause minor discomfort to significant pain, especially when high temperatures are used. Blistering and actual burning of the skin can also occur at higher temperatures, although with careful application of the instrument or device, these side effects are very rare. As of 2009, many cancer centers use **magnetic resonance imaging** (MRI) not only to locate the tumor, but to guide the application of hyperthermia to the cancerous cells.

Risks associated with perfusion hyperthermia include swollen tissues, blood clots, and bleeding; these side effects are usually temporary, however. Risks associated with whole-body hyperthermia include **nausea**, **vomiting**, and **diarrhea**. Rare side effects with whole-body hyperthermia include heart and vascular disorders.

Results

Normal results

The goal of hyperthermia is to control the growth and shrink hyperthermia-sensitive tumors. As stated earlier, hyperthermia can also be used to help sensitize tumors to such other cancer treatment modalities as radiation and chemotherapy. While hyperthermia is considered effective in shrinking tumors or making them more sensitive to other therapies, there is little evidence as of 2009 that it extends patients' survival time. It does, however, improve their quality of life, as several European studies have reported.

QUESTIONS TO ASK YOUR DOCTOR

- Should I consider hyperthermia as an adjuvant therapy?
- What is your opinion of hyperthermia?
- What type of hyperthermia would you recommend?
- Can you recommend a cancer center with the necessary equipment and experience in this form of treatment?
- Should I consider participation in a clinical trial of hyperthermia as an adjunctive treatment for my type of cancer?
- What are the risks of hyperthermia?

Abnormal results

Hyperthermia has fewer severe side effects than radiation therapy or chemotherapy. As noted above, tissue swelling and bleeding may be temporary side effects in some patients, while some experience nausea and other gastrointestinal disturbances following whole-body hyperthermia. Such side effects as pain and burning from external heat sources can be minimized with careful application of the heat.

Health care team roles

Hyperthermia usually requires at least two doctors to administer, an oncologist and a radiologist. An anesthesiologist will be needed if the specific procedure requires the patient to be under general anesthesia. Nursing staff are required to monitor patients for vital signs and possible side effects during the recovery period.

Alternatives

As of 2009, radiofrequency ablation (RFA) is used more frequently than perfusion or whole-body hyperthermia to deliver heat to malignant tumors. RFA makes use of a special probe inserted directly into a tumor that uses radiofrequency waves to heat the tumor above 122°F (50°C), a temperature that is high enough to kill the tumor cells. This is a higher temperature level than can be used with hyperthermia. In addition to its ability to actually kill malignant cells, RFA has the additional advantage of targeting malignant tumors precisely with minimal risk to nearby healthy tissue.

Research and general acceptance

While radiofrequency ablation is a proven mainstream alternative to regional or whole-body hyperthermia, one type of hyperthermia therapy that is not only unproven but potentially dangerous is intra-cellular hyperthermia, also called 2-4-dinitrophenol or DNP therapy. DNP is an organic substance injected directly into the body to cause an artificial fever. There is no evidence that dinitrophenol is effective in treating cancer; moreover, some patients have died as a result of DNP injections.

Caregiver concerns

Hyperthermia is administered in a clinic or hospital rather than at home. Caregivers should, however, monitor patients who have received whole-body hyperthermia after they return home for possible side effects.

Resources

BOOKS

Abeloff, Martin D., et al., eds. *Abeloff's Clinical Oncology*, 4th ed. Philadelphia: Churchill Livingstone/Elsevier, 2008.

Ades, Terri, et al., editors. *American Cancer Society Complete Guide to Complementary and Alternative Cancer Therapies*, 2nd ed. Atlanta, GA: American Cancer Society, 2009.

Baronzio, Gian Franco, and E. Dieter Hager, eds. *Hyperthermia in Cancer Treatment: A Primer*. New York: Springer Science + Business Media, 2006.

PERIODICALS

Bakshandeh-Bath, A., et al. "Preclinical and Clinical Aspects of Carboplatin and Gemcitabine Combined with Whole-body Hyperthermia for Pancreatic Adenocarcinoma." *Anticancer Research* 29 (August 2009): 3069–3077.

Chua, T.C., et al. "Intraoperative Hyperthermic Intraperitoneal Chemotherapy after Cytoreductive Surgery in Ovarian Cancer Peritoneal Carcinomatosis: Systematic Review of Current Results." *Journal of Cancer Research and Clinical Oncology* 135 (December 2009): 1637–45.

Corchero, J.L., and A. Villaverde. "Biomedical Applications of Distally Controlled Magnetic Nanoparticles." *Trends in Biotechnology* 27 (August 2009): 468–76.

Helm, C.W. "The Role of Hyperthermic Intraperitoneal Chemotherapy (HIPEC) in Ovarian Cancer." *Oncologist* 14 (July 2009): 683–94.

Piso, P., et al. "Quality of Life after Cytoreductive Surgery and Hyperthermic Intraperitoneal Chemotherapy for Peritoneal Surface Malignancies." *Journal of Surgical Oncology* 100 (September 15, 2009): 317–20.

Riley, W. "Belmont Hyperthermia Pump in the Conduct of Intra-operative Heated Chemotherapy." *Perfusion* 24 (March 2009): 115–118.

Salloum, M., et al. "Enhancement in Treatment Planning for Magnetic Nanoparticle Hyperthermia: Optimization of the Heat Absorption Pattern." *International Journal of Hyperthermia* 25 (June 2009): 309–21.

Schildkopf, P., et al. "Hyperthermia in Combination with X-irradiation Induces Inflammatory Forms of Cell Death." *Autoimmunity* 42 (May 2009): 311–313.

OTHER

American Cancer Society (ACS). *Heat Therapy*. http://www.cancer.org/docroot/ETO/content/ETO_5_3X_Heat_Therapy.asp.

Cancer Treatment Centers of America (CTCA). *Local Hyperthermia*. [Includes 2-minute video] http://www.cancercenter.com/conventional-cancer-treatment/local-hyperthermia.cfm.

National Cancer Institute (NCI) Fact Sheet. *Hyperthermia in Cancer Treatment: Questions and Answers*. http://www.cancer.gov/cancertopics/factsheet/Therapy/hyperthermia.

ORGANIZATIONS

American Cancer Society, 250 Williams Street NW, Atlanta, GA, 30303, 800-ACS-2345 (227-2345), www.cancer.org.

Cancer Treatment Centers of America (CTCA), 800-931-0599, http://www.cancercenter.com/.

National Cancer Institute, 6116 Executive Blvd., Room 3036A, Bethesda, MD, 20892-8322, 800-422-6237, cancergovstaff@mail.nih.gov, www.cancer.gov.

National Center for Complementary and Alternative Medicine (NCCAM), 9000 Rockville Pike, Bethesda, MD, 20892, 888-644-6226, info@nccam.nih.gov, http://nccam.nih.gov/.

International Clinical Hyperthermia Society (ICHS), U.S. contact: Dr. James Haim I. Bicher, 12099 W. Washington Blvd., #304, Los AngelesCA, United States, 90066, 310-398-0013, inforequest@hyperthermia-ichs.org, http://www.hyperthermia-ichs.org/.

Edward R. Rosick, D.O., M.P.H.
Rebecca J. Frey, PhD

Hypocalcemia

Definition

Hypocalcemia is a type of electrolyte disturbance in which the level of calcium in the blood is too low. It occurs when the concentration of free calcium ions in the blood falls below 4.0 mg/dL (dL = a deciliter or one-tenth of a liter, about 3.4 fluid ounces). The normal concentration of free calcium ions in the blood serum is 4.0–6.0 mg/dL. Hypocalcemia can be caused by a range of conditions or disorders that either decrease the entry of calcium into the blood or increase the loss of calcium from the blood.

Demographics

It is difficult to estimate the frequency of hypocalcemia in the general population because many people, particularly those with mild forms of the disorder, have no noticeable symptoms. Studies of hospitalized patients admitted to intensive care units have indicated that 15–50% have hypocalcemia.

Hypocalcemia can affect persons of any age, depending on the disorder or condition causing the imbalance. As far as is known, both sexes and all races are equally likely to develop hypocalcemia.

Description

Calcium is an important mineral for maintaining human health. It is not only a component of bones and teeth, but is also essential for normal blood clotting and necessary for normal muscle and nerve functioning. In the human body, 99% of the total calcium is in the bones and teeth, and 1% is in the blood plasma.

The calcium ion (Ca^{2+}) has two positive charges. In bone, calcium ions occur as a complex with phosphate to form crystals of calcium phosphate. In the bloodstream, calcium ions also occur in complexes, and here calcium is found combined with proteins and various nutrients. However, in the bloodstream, calcium also occurs in a free form. Normally, about 47% of the calcium in the blood plasma is free, while 53% occurs in a complexed form.

Although all of the calcium in the bloodstream serves a useful purpose, only the concentration of free calcium ions has a direct influence on the functioning of our nerves and muscles. For this reason, the measurement of the concentration of free calcium is more important in the diagnosis of disease than measuring the level of total calcium or of complexed calcium. The level of total calcium in the blood serum is normally 8.5–10.5 mg/dL, while the level of free calcium is normally 4–5 mg/dl.

Risk factors

Risk factors for hypocalcemia include:

- history of kidney disorders
- history of thyroid disorders
- poor nutrition, especially vitamin D deficiency
- eating disorders
- alcoholism
- diagnosis of breast or prostate cancer
- being treated with chemotherapy for cancer
- heavy use of laxatives or other medications containing magnesium
- pancreatitis

- treatment for heavy metal poisoning
- diGeorge syndrome and other congenital disorders characterized by failure of the parathyroid gland to develop normally

Causes and symptoms

Causes

Hypocalcemia has several different possible causes. It can be caused by hypoparathyroidism, by failure to produce 1,25-dihydroxyvitamin D, by low levels of plasma magnesium, or by failure to get adequate amounts of calcium or vitamin D in the diet. Hypoparathyroidism involves the failure of the parathyroid gland to make parathyroid hormone. In some cases hypoparathyroidism results from surgical removal of the parathyroid gland or from genetic disorders that affect the normal development of the parathyroid gland.

Parathyroid hormone controls and maintains plasma calcium levels. The hormone exerts its effect on the kidneys, where it triggers the synthesis of 1,25-dihydroxyvitamin D. Thus, hypocalcemia can be independently caused by damage to the parathyroid gland or to the kidneys. 1,25-Dihydroxyvitamin D stimulates the uptake of calcium from the diet and the mobilization of calcium from the bone. Bone mobilization refers to the natural process by which the body dissolves part of the bone in the skeleton in order to maintain or raise the levels of plasma calcium ions.

Low plasma magnesium levels (hypomagnesemia) can result in hypocalcemia. Hypomagnesemia can occur with alcoholism or with diseases characterized by an inability to properly absorb fat. Magnesium is required for parathyroid hormone to play its part in maintaining plasma calcium levels. For this reason, any disease that results in lowered plasma magnesium levels may also cause hypocalcemia.

Hypocalcemia may also result from the consumption of toxic levels of phosphate. Phosphate is a constituent of certain enema formulas. An enema is a solution that is used to cleanse the intestines via a catheter or tube inserted into the rectum. Cases of hypocalcemia have been documented in which people swallowed enema formulas or an enema had been administered to an infant.

Other causes of hypocalcemia include:

- Cancers that metastasize (spread) from other organs to the bone and destroy the bone. The most likely cancers of this type are breast cancer and prostate cancer.
- Certain cancer chemotherapy drugs, particularly cisplatin, leucovorin, and 5-fluorouracil.

- Severe pancreatitis (inflammation of the pancreas).
- Chelation therapy. Chelation therapy involves the use of such chemicals as EDTA to treat heavy metal poisoning. The chelating agent binds to the mercury, lead, or other heavy metal and enables the body to excrete the toxic substance safely. Hypocalcemia is a side effect of chelation therapy, however.
- Hungry bone syndrome. Hungry bone syndrome is a disorder that develops in some patients after surgical removal of the parathyroid gland.
- Sepsis (whole-body inflammatory response to severe infection).
- Toxic shock syndrome.

Symptoms

Symptoms of severe hypocalcemia include numbness or tingling around the mouth or in the feet and hands, as well as in muscle spasms in the face, feet, and hands. These involuntary muscle spasms are called tetany. Hypocalcemia can also result in **depression**, memory loss, or hallucinations. Severe hypocalcemia occurs when serum free calcium is under 3 mg/dL. Chronic and moderate hypocalcemia can result in cataracts (damage to the eyes). In this case, the term "chronic" means lasting one year or longer.

Diagnosis

Hypocalcemia is frequently asymptomatic. When suspected, it is diagnosed by taking a careful patient history, a physical examination, and taking a sample of blood serum. The blood is tested for the concentraton of free calcium using a calcium-sensitive electrode. Hypocalcemia has several causes; hence a full diagnosis requires assessment of the parathyroid gland, kidneys, and plasma magnesium concentration.

The patient should be asked about a history of eating disorders, vitamin deficiencies, treatment for alcoholism, kidney or liver problems, disorders of the pancreas or digestive tract, thyroid or parathyroid disorders, recent neck or bowel surgery, or epilepsy.

Examination

Physical examination of a patient with suspected hypocalcemia includes an examination of the patient's skin, mouth, and hair. Patients with hypocalcemia often have dry skin, brittle hair and nails, teeth in bad condition, skin rashes or **itching** skin, and cataracts in the eye. If the patient has a disorder of the parathyroid gland, they may also be shorter than average, have a round "moon" face, and possibly mentally retarded.

The doctor may hear wheezing or rattling noises when listening to the patient's breathing. An electrocardiogram (EKG) may indicate some irregularities in heart rhythm.

The patient may complain of muscle cramps or spasms, intestinal cramping, difficulty swallowing, coughing spells, facial twitching, general aching sensations in the muscles, numbness in fingers or toes, or tingling sensations.

In severe hypocalcemia, the patient may have such neurological symptoms as seizures, hallucinations, and confusion.

Tests

The doctor will usually order blood tests to evaluate the level of calcium and other electrolytes (particularly magnesium and phosphate levels) in the blood as well as tests of liver and kidney function. The level of parathyroid hormone will be checked by means of an antibody-mediated radioimmunoassay. The doctor will also order an EKG if one was not performed in the office in order to evaluate abnormal heart rhythms.

Two diagnostic tests that may be performed are the Chvostek and Trousseau tests. In the Chvostek test, the doctor taps over the facial nerve along the jawline about an inch in front of the ear. A patient with hypocalcemia will develop twitching at the corner of the mouth, the nose, the eye, and the other facial muscles. In the Trousseau test, a blood pressure cuff is placed on the patient's arm and inflated above the level of the systolic pressure for 3 minutes. A patient with hypocalcemia will develop spasms in the hand and forearm and the wrist will flex upward.

Treatment

Traditional

The method chosen for treatment depends on the exact cause and on the severity of the hypocalcemia. Mild hypocalcemia may require nothing more than a thorough office examination and laboratory testing. Severe hypocalcemia requires admission to the hospital for supportive care and immediate injection of calcium ions, usually in the form of calcium gluconate. In severe cases, emergency room physicians will need to consult one or more specialists, including surgeons, neurologists, oncologists, dietitians, internists, endocrinologists, and toxicologists.

Drugs

Oral calcium supplements are prescribed for long-term treatment (non-emergency) of hypocalcemia. The oral supplements may take the form of calcium carbonate, calcium chloride, calcium lactate, or calcium gluconate. Where hypocalcemia results from kidney failure, treatment includes injections of 1,25-dihydroxyvitamin D. Oral vitamin D supplements can increase gastrointestinal absorption of calcium. Where hypocalcemia results from hypoparathyroidism, treatment may include oral calcium, 1,25-dihydroxyvitamin D, or other drugs. Where low serum magnesium levels occur, concurrently with hypocalcemia, the magnesium deficiency must be corrected to effectively treat the hypocalcemia.

Prognosis

The prognosis for hypocalcemia from simple dietary deficiencies is excellent. In most cases, however, the prognosis depends on the disorder or condition causing the hypocalcemia. Patients with alcoholism or eating disorders may need psychiatric intervention as well as medical treatment in order to recover fully. Severe symptomatic hypocalcemia can result in seizures, low blood pressure that does not respond to fluid, and irregular heart rhythms. In a few cases, cardiovascular collapse brought on by hypocalcemia has resulted in death.

Prevention

The first and most obvious way to help prevent hypocalcemia is to ensure that adequate amounts of calcium and vitamin D are consumed each day, either in the diet or as supplements. Hypocalcemia that may occur with damage to the parathyroid gland or to the kidneys cannot be prevented. Hypocalcemia resulting from overuse of enemas can be prevented by reducing enema usage. Hypocalcemia resulting from magnesium deficiency tends to occur in chronic alcoholics, and this type of hypocalcemia can be prevented by reducing **alcohol consumption** and increasing the intake of healthful food.

Resources

BOOKS

Fiebach, Nicholas H., et al, eds. *Principles of Ambulatory Medicine*. Philadelphia: Lippincott Williams and Wilkins, 2007.

Jameson, J. Larry, ed. *Harrison's Nephrology and Acid-base Disorders*. New York: McGraw-Hill Medical, 2010.

Kleerekoper, Michael, Ethel S. Siris, and Michael McClung, eds. *The Bone and Mineral Manual: A Practical Guide*, 2nd ed. Burlington, MA: Elsevier Academic Press, 2005.

PERIODICALS

Athappan, G., and V. K. Ariyamuthu. "Images in Clinical Medicine. Chvostek's Sign and Carpopedal Spasm." *New England Journal of Medicine* 360 (April 30, 2009): e24.

Ferron, M., and G. Karsenty. "The Gutsy Side of Bone." *Cell Metabolism* 10 (July 2009): 7–8.

Jordan, R., et al. "An Alcoholic Presenting Fits." *Clinical Medicine* 9 (June 2009): 291–92.

Oztas, E., et al. "Oral Fleet Phospho-Soda Laxative Induced Symptomatic Hypocalcemia in an Adult Patient with Celiac Disease." *American Journal of Gastroenterology* 104 (June 2009): 1607–08.

Zhou, P., and M. Markowitz. "Hypocalcemia in Infants and Children." *Pediatrics in Review* 30 (May 2009): 190–92.

OTHER

Beach, Christopher B. "Hypocalcemia." *eMedicine*, March 9, 2009. http://emedicine.medscape.com/article/767260-overview.

Lewis, James L., III. "Disorders of Calcium Concentration: Hypocalcemia." *Merck Manual of Diagnosis and Treatment*. http://www.merck.com/mmpe/sec12/ch156/ch156g.html#sec12-ch156-ch156g-837.

Skugor, Mario. "Hypocalcemia." *Cleveland Clinic Disease Management Project*. http://www.clevelandclinicmeded.com/medicalpubs/diseasemanagement/endocrinology/hypocalcemia/.

ORGANIZATIONS

American Association of Clinical Endocrinologists (AACE), 245 Riverside Ave., Suite 200, Jacksonville, FL, 32202, 904-353-7878, http://www.aace.com/.

American College of Emergency Physicians (ACEP), 1125 Executive Circle, Irving, TX, 75038-2522, 972-550-0911, 800-798-1822, 972-580-2816, http://www.acep.org/.

American Society for Nutrition (ASN), 9650 Rockville Pike, Bethesda, MD, 20814, 301-634-7050, 301-634-7892, info@nutrition.org, http://www.nutrition.org/.

Food and Drug Administration (FDA), 10903 New Hampshire Ave., Silver Spring, MD, 20993, 888-463-6332, http://www.fda.gov/.

National Toxicology Program (NTP), P.O. Box 12233, MD K2-03, Research Triangle Park, NC, 27709, 919-541-0530, http://ntp.niehs.nih.gov/.

Tom Brody, PhD
Rebecca J. Frey, PhD

Ibritumomab

Definition

Ibritumomab is a radioimmunotherapy used to treat **non-Hodgkin's lymphoma** (NHL).

Purpose

Ibritumomab is used to treat individuals with low grade follicular NHL that has failed to respond or that has stopped responding to the drug **rituximab** (Rituxan).

NHL is a **cancer** that arises in the organs of the lymph system. It is the most common type of **lymphoma** in the United States. The lymph system is important in creating and transporting blood cells called lymphocytes that fight **infection** throughout the body. The major organs of the lymph system are the spleen, thymus, tonsils, and bone marrow. These organs produce several different kinds of cells that fight infection. The major ones are called T-cells and B-cells. Ibritumomab specifically targets both mature and immature B-cells.

In NHL, abnormal (cancerous) lymphocytes grow out of control. So many of these abnormal lymphocytes develop that they prevent other immune system cells and blood vessel from forming. There are several types of NHL. One form is called follicular lymphoma. In this form, the cancerous cells clump together. They may grow quickly, in which case the disease is called a high-grade lymphoma, or they may grow slowly, in which case the cancer is called low-grade lymphoma.

Standard treatments for NHL include **chemotherapy, radiation therapy**, stem cell therapy, and a newer form of therapy called biologic therapy. Biologic therapy uses the biopharmaceutical rituximab. Ibritumomab is used in patients with low-grade B-cell NHL who have failed to respond or who have relapsed after standard treatment.

Description

Ibritumomab, which is also called ibritumomab tiuxetan, is manufactured in the United States and sold under the brand name Zevalin by IDEC Pharmaceuticals. It was approved for use in February 2002 and was the first radioimmunotherapy approved by the United States Food and Drug Administration (FDA). Generic substitutes are not available, and currently there is only one American manufacturer.

Radioimmunotherapy is a form of biologic therapy that combines a protein that attaches to the target cell with a small dose of radioactive material that disrupts and kills the cell. Unique proteins called antigens exist on the surface of every cell. The body monitors these proteins, and when it recognizes a cell as foreign or defective, it creates other antigen-specific proteins called antibodies to attach to the unwanted cells and disable them. With NHL, this system of protection fails and defective cancerous cells are allowed to continue growing.

Ibritumomab is an antibody made of mouse (murine) protein that comes from Chinese hamster ovary cells. It binds with the a protein called CD20 that is found on the surface of both normal and malignant B-cells. Ibritumomab alone does not kill B-cells, so it is bound to a radioactive material, either Indium-111 (In-111) or Yttrium-90 (Y-90). The role of ibritumomab is to deliver the radioactive material to specific target cells and bind it there. The radioactive rays given off by IN-111 or Y-90 disrupt the cell's functions, resulting in cell death. This therapy kills both healthy and cancerous B-cells.

Recommended dosage

Ibritumomab is given only in a two-step cycle in conjunction with another non-radioactive antibody called rituximab. Rituximab attacks the same B-cells as ibritumomab but does not deliver a dose of radioactive material to the cell. The two-step cycle of administration of ibritumomab is intended to occur only once.

The material needed for the therapeutic administration of ibritumomab is sold under the name Zevalin. The ibritumomab carrier antibody is mixed with the radioactive material by the physician shortly before use.

Step 1 includes a single dose of rituximab. The dose is determined by the patient's body size. Rituximab is infused slowly into a vein while the physician watches for hypersensitivity reactions. Within four hours following administration of rituximab, a single dose of 5.0 milliCuries (mCi) ibritumomab tiuxetan that contains the radioactive material In-111 is injected intravenously (IV) over a period of 10 minutes.

Step 2 follows seven to nine days after Step 1. The patient is given another IV dose of rituximab, again based on body size. Within four hours following the rituximab, the patient is injected with a dose of radioactive ibritumomab Y-90. This dose is also based on body size up to a total maximum allowable dose of 32.0 mCi. This completes the active part of the therapy, but patients must continue to have their blood count monitored for several months, as the therapy continues to kills cells for weeks.

Precautions

People who are allergic to any type of mouse (murine) protein, rituximab, yttrium chloride or indium chloride should not use this therapy. Ibritumomab can cause harm to the developing fetus and should not be used by pregnant women. Women should use birth control for 12 months after receiving this therapy. It has not been established whether this therapy is safe to use in breastfeeding women. A pediatric dose has not been established.

Zevalin is radioactive when it is being administered, and care should be taken to minimize exposure of patients and health care providers.

Side effects

Side effects are many and varied. Serious but rare side effects include:

- potentially fatal infusion hypersensitivity reactions, usually to the first dose of rituximab, that can cause low blood pressure, difficulty breathing, heart attack, and anaphylactic shock
- severe drop in platelet count (thrombocytopenia) or neutrophil count (neutropenia); uncontrolled bleeding
- development of secondary malignancies that arise from the therapy

More common but less serious side effects include:

- susceptibility to infections; fever or chills
- nausea, vomiting, diarrhea, black, tarry stools
- loss of appetite
- anemia
- joint pain
- dizziness
- increased cough or hoarseness
- rash, swelling, or puffiness around the face and neck

Interactions

It is important to tell the physician about all prescription medications, over-the counter medications, and herbal or alternative remedies that are being taken before treatment with Zevalin is begun. No formal drug interaction studies have been completed, however, Zevalin therapy does interfere with blood clotting and should not be used while individuals are taking blood thinners such as **warfarin** (Coumadin) or clopidogrel bisulfate (Plavix). Individuals who have a very low platelet count may not be able to use this therapy.

Individuals should not be vaccinated with a live virus vaccine prior to or soon after receiving this therapy. The interaction of live virus **vaccines** and this therapy has not been investigated, but it is recommended that individuals receiving ibritumomab avoid people who have recently been vaccinated with live virus oral polio vaccine.

Tish Davidson, A. M.

Idarubicin

Definition

Idarubicin is a medication that kills **cancer** cells.

Purpose

Idarubicin is approved to treat only one single cancer, acute myelocytic leukemia (AML) in adults. Recent research suggests that using idarubicin rather than the more traditional **daunorubicin** in treating AML results in higher rates of complete remission (CR) and longer survival for patients. CR is the total elimination of all diseased cells detectable following therapy. The Food and Drug Administration (FDA) has not approved idarubicin as treatment for **acute lymphocytic leukemia** (ALL).

Much research involving idarubicin is now being conducted. Some of this has involved acute lymphocytic leukemia (ALL) as well as AML. For example, a recent study was conducted in patients with either AML or ALL who had received **bone marrow transplantation** and then relapsed. Patients received a combination of **cytarabine**, idarubicin, and **etoposide**, as well as a medicine called G-CSF (**filgrastim**). This treatment achieved a high CR rate in these patients.

Another recent study looked at the use of idarubicin in children with AML. All of the children received cytarabine and etoposide. In addition, some of the children received idarubicin, while some received daunorubicin. Overall, patients in both groups fared equally well in terms of survival length. However, patients who had larger numbers of cells known as blasts (immature cells) tended to do better if they received idarubicin rather than daunorubicin. In addition, high-risk patients tended to do better with idarubicin than with daunorubicin. No subgroup of patients achieved better outcomes with daunorubicin than with idarubicin.

For older patients with acute nonlymphocytic leukemia, treatment with Idarubicin is effective and has acceptable side effects. According to recent research from Italy, "There is growing interest in autologous stem cell transplantation (ASCT) for elderly patients with acute myeloid leukemia (AML). While mortality and toxicity from ASCT have been reduced, relapse rate is still high."

Description

Idarubicin is an antibiotic, although doctors do not use this drug to attack infections. Its only use is to

KEY TERMS

Bilirubin—A pigment produced when the liver processes waste products. A high bilirubin level causes yellowing of the skin.

Blasts—Immature cells

Complete remission (CR)—Complete remission is the total elimination of all diseased cells detectable following therapy.

Necrosis—The sum of the morphological changes indicative of cell death. It may affect groups of cells or part of a structure or an organ.

kill cancer cells. It does so by affecting how the DNA of cancer cells work.

Recommended dosage

In the treatment of AML, 12 mg of idarubicin per square meter may be given over a period of two to three days every three weeks in combination with other medications. Patients with liver problems may be given lower doses than other patients receive. Idarubicin is not typically given by mouth, as an insufficient amount of the medication would be transported through the stomach wall if this were done. Rather, this medication is usually administered through an intravenous (IV) procedure. During this time, it circulates widely throughout the body.

A new formulation of idarubicin has been developed. This permits idarubicin to be taken orally. However, this formulation is currently available only in France and only for older patients who are not good candidates for intensive intravenous treatment. There is little information currently available on the effectiveness of this oral formulation. The studies that have been performed suggest that it is less effective than other formulations of idarubicin.

Precautions

Idarubicin may be associated with excessive toxicity in patients with congestive heart failure, liver function characterized by a high bilirubin level, or prior chest radiation to the heart.

Side effects

Like daunorubicin and **doxorubicin**, idarubicin may adversely affect the patient's heart. However, doctors are not certain how much of the drug it takes to cause such harm and, therefore, how to limit dosage so that such harm is not caused. However, idarubicin appears to be less likely to cause heart damage than similar drugs such as daunorubicin and doxorubicin. Another serious side effect that limits how much of the drug is given to patients is its potential adverse effect upon the bone marrow, where blood cells are produced.

Idarubicin may cause **nausea and vomiting**, baldness (**alopecia**), and stomach problems. In addition, idarubicin may cause blistering if extravasation occurs. Extravasation is when **chemotherapy** gets outside of the vein during infusion. If this occurs, the drug may cause severe local pain, swelling, or tissue necrosis that may require plastic surgery.

Patients receiving idarubicin in conjunction with certain other **anticancer drugs** may develop a type of leukemia. However, this is extremely rare.

In the few studies that have been conducted on the oral formulation of idarubicin, the most prominent side effects seen are low blood cell counts, **nausea**, **vomiting**, **diarrhea**, and alopecia.

Bob Kirsch

Ifosfamide

Definition

Ifosfamide is an anticancer (antineoplastic) agent. It also acts as a suppressor of the immune system. It is available under the brand name IFEX.

Purpose

Ifosfamide is approved by the Food and Drug Administration (FDA) to treat germ cell **testicular cancer**. It is generally prescribed in combination with another medicine (**mesna**), which is used to prevent the bladder problems that may be caused by ifosfamide alone.

Ifosfamide also has activity against other cancers and is prescribed in practice for these **cancer** types:

- **pancreatic cancer**
- **stomach cancer**
- **soft-tissue sarcoma**
- **Ewing's sarcoma**
- acute and **chronic lymphocytic leukemia**
- **bladder cancer**

- bone cancer
- **breast cancer**
- **cervical cancer**
- **head and neck cancers**
- lung cancer
- **lymphomas**
- neuroblastomas
- **ovarian cancer**
- **Wilms' tumor**

Description

Ifosfamide chemically interferes with the synthesis of the genetic material (DNA and RNA) of cancer cells by cross-linking of DNA strands, which prevents these cells from being able to reproduce and continue the growth of the cancer.

Recommended dosage

Ifosfamide may only be taken as an injection into the vein. The dosage prescribed varies widely depending on the patient, the cancer being treated, and whether or not other medications are also being taken. Examples of common doses for adults are: 50 mg per kg per day, or 700–2,000 mg per square meter of body surface area for five days every three to four weeks. Another alternative regimen is 2,400 mg per square meter of body surface area for three days or 5000 mg per square meter of body surface area as a single dose every three to four weeks. Examples of common dosing regimens for children are: 1,200 to 1,800 mg per square meter of body surface area per day for three to five days every 21 to 28 days; 5,000 mg per square meter of body surface area once every 21 to 28 days; or 3,000 mg per square meter of body surface area for two days every 21 to 28 days.

Precautions

Ifosfamide can cause an allergic reaction in some people. Patients with a prior allergic reaction to ifosfamide should not take this drug.

Ifosfamide should always be taken with plenty of fluids.

Ifosfamide can cause serious birth defects if either the man or the woman is taking this drug at the time of conception or if the woman is taking this drug during pregnancy. Contraceptive measures should be taken by both men and women while on this drug. Because ifosfamide is easily passed from mother to child through breast milk, breast feeding is not recommended during treatment.

Ifosfamide suppresses the immune system, and its excretion from the body is dependent on a normal functioning kidney and liver. For these reasons, it is important that the prescribing physician is aware of any of the following pre-existing medical conditions:

- a current case of, or recent exposure to, chickenpox
- **herpes zoster** (shingles)
- all current infections
- kidney disease
- liver disease

Also, because ifosfamide is such a potent immuno-suppressant, patients taking this drug must exercise extreme caution to avoid contracting any new infections.

Side effects

Inflammation and irritation of the bladder, causing blood in the urine, is the most common and severe side effect of ifosfamide. However, this side effect can be prevented and controlled with the administration of the bladder protectant drug mesna and vigorous hydration with intravenous fluids before, during, and after **chemotherapy**. Patients should also urinate frequently (at least every 2 hours) to enhance removal of the drug from the body, and drink 2 to 3 liters of fluids a day for 2 to 3 days after discontinuation of the chemotherapy.

Other common side effects of ifosfamide are:

- confusion
- hallucinations
- drowsiness
- dizziness
- temporary hair loss (**alopecia**)
- increased susceptibility to infection
- increased risk of bleeding (due to a decrease of the platelets involved in the clotting process)
- **nausea and vomiting** (can be prevented with prescribed **antiemetics**)

Less common side effects include:

- increased coloration (pigmentation) of the skin and fingernails
- loss of appetite (**anorexia**)
- diarrhea
- nasal stuffiness
- skin rash, itching, or hives

A doctor should be consulted immediately if the patient experiences any of these side effects:

- painful or difficult urination
- increase in frequency or feeling of urgency to urinate
- blood in the urine
- blood in the stool
- severe diarrhea
- mental status changes such as confusion, drowsiness, or hallucinations
- signs of infection such as cough, sore throat, fever and chills
- shortness of breath
- chest or abdominal pain
- pain in the lower back or sides
- unusual bleeding or bruising
- tiny red dots on the skin

Interactions

Ifosfamide should not be taken in combination with any prescription drug, over-the-counter drug, or herbal remedy without prior consultation with a physician.

Paul A. Johnson, Ed.M.

Imaging studies

Definition

Imaging studies are tests performed with a variety of techniques that produce pictures of the inside of a patient's body. They have become indispensable tools in **cancer** screening and detection.

Description

Imaging tests are performed using sound waves, radioactive particles, magnetic fields, or **x rays** that are detected and converted into images after passing through body tissues. Dyes are sometimes used as contrasting agents with x-ray tests so that organs or tissues not seen with conventional x rays can be enhanced. The operating principle of the various techniques is based on the fact that rays and particles interact differently with various types of tissues, especially when cancerous growths are present. In this way, the interior of the body can be visualized and pictures are provided of normal structure and function as well as of abnormalities.

Imaging tests differ from endoscopic tests, which are carried out with a flexible, lighted piece of tubing connected to a viewing lens or camera.

Imaging studies are used to detect cancer in its early stages in a procedure called screening. Screening is performed in patients who have no obvious cancer symptoms. Imaging studies are also used to locate tumors in patients who have symptoms which the physician may wish to investigate further so as to distinguish between benign growths or cancerous tumors. They are also used to determine the extent of a cancer and indicate how a given treatment is unfolding. As such, they represent crucial tools for cancer diagnosis and management.

Major imaging techniques

Computed tomography scan (CT scan)

Computed tomography scans show a cross-section of a part of the body. In this technique, a thin beam is used to produce a series of exposures detected at different angles. The exposures are fed into a computer which overlaps them so as to yield a single image analogous to a slice of the organ or body part being scanned. A dye is often injected into the patient so as

to improve contrast and obtain images that are clearer than images obtained with x rays.

Magnetic resonance imaging (MRI)

Magnetic resonance imaging also produces cross-sectional images of the body using powerful magnetic fields instead of radiation. MRI is especially useful to detect and locate cancers of the liver and the central nervous system, which occur in the brain or the spinal cord. It uses a cylinder housing a magnet which will induce the required magnetic field. The patient lies on a platform inside the scanner. The magnetic field aligns the hydrogen atoms present in the tissue being scanned in a given direction. Following a burst of radio-frequency radiation, the atoms flip back to their original orientation while emitting signals which a fed into a computer for conversion into a two- or three-dimensional image. Dyes can also be injected into patients to produce clearer images.

Mammography

Mammography is an x-ray examination of the breast. It is often used as a screening tool to detect breast abnormalities and cancers before they can be felt. Mammograms (the image produced) are acquired using an x-ray machine working at lower radiation levels than conventional x ray. The breast is compressed between two plates so as to allow the low-level x-ray radiation to produce a film.

Nuclear scan

Nuclear scans, also called radionuclide imaging or scintigraphy, use substances called tracers or radionuclides that release low levels of radioactivity. The test is based on the principle that the tracers will be absorbed to a different degree by different tissues, thus allowing to distinguish between normal and cancerous tissues. Common **nuclear medicine scans** for cancer patients to receive are bone scans; liver, spleen, and thyroid scans are also frequently performed.

Position emission tomography (PET)

Positron emission tomography uses a form of sugar that contains a radioactive atom which emits particles called positrons. The positrons are absorbed to a different extent by cells varying in their metabolic rate. PET scans are especially useful for brain imaging studies and are widely applied to the assessment of the spread of cancers in the lungs. PET scans are also being used experimentally in the assessment of breast, colon, rectum, and ovarian cancers.

X rays

X rays produce shallow images of certain specific organs or tissues. X rays are a form of high-energy radiation and tissues of the body can absorb it to varying degrees. For example, bones absorb less x rays than soft tissue. After passing through the body, the x rays are directed on a film, where the dense tissue appears as a white shadow, thus providing contrast with the soft tissue, which produces a darker impression on the film. X rays produce a single image.

Chest x rays are used to detect lung and bronchial cancers, and also to evaluate a patient's symptoms, such as shortness of breath. Other types of x rays, such as abdominal x rays, may also be ordered to assess a patient's symptoms, but are not used as cancer screening tools as chest x rays may be used.

X rays with dye studies

Dye studies are usually performed by injecting the contrasting agent in the patient's circulatory system or in the target organ. These studies are used to produce angiograms, cystograms, myelograms, lymphangiograms and fistulograms.

ANGIOGRAM. An angiogram is an examination of the blood vessels using x rays. It is usually performed with intravenous injection of fluorescein dye followed by multiframe photography. The doctor inserts a small tube (catheter) into the blood vessel and then injects the dye that makes the vessels visible when the x-ray pictures are acquired.

CYSTOGRAM. A cystogram is a scan of the bladder and ureters. The ureters are passages that lead from the kidneys to the bladder. A catheter is inserted into the bladder or a radioactive material, called a radio-isotope, is introduced into the bladder. An oral cholecystogram (OCG) is an x-ray examination of the gallbladder, the organ that helps release bile into the small intestine for the digestion of fats. The gallbladder is not seen well on conventional x-ray pictures and special tablets are ingested by mouth to enhance contrast.

MYELOGRAM. A myelogram is an x ray of the spine and spinal cord. The spinal cord is the nerve tissue enclosed in the vertebral column that goes from the bottom of the brain to halfway down the back. During a myelogram, x-ray dye is injected into the spinal fluid and mixes with it, flowing around the spinal cord which can then be seen and recorded on x-ray film.

LYMPHANGIOGRAM. A lymphangiogram is an x ray of the lymphatic system, also carried out with dye injection for contrasting purposes. It is used to screen for lymph node involvement in cancer.

FISTULOGRAM. A fistula is an abnormal passage within body tissue. For example, a fistula may connect two organs inside the body that are not normally connected. A fistula may also lead from an internal organ inside the body to the surface outside. Examples are: between the skin and the bowel (enterocutaneous fistula), between the stomach and the colon (gastrocolic fistula). A fistulogram is an x-ray examination of this abnormal passage. The contrasting agent is injected directly into the fistula so that it will show up on x-ray pictures.

Fluoroscopy

Fluoroscopy is one of the oldest areas of diagnostic radiology. It is similar to x ray in that a small dose of x rays is directed through a body part but the image obtained is displayed on a monitor rather than on the conventional x-ray film. The fluoroscope provides images of internal body parts as they move, similar to a movie. A continuous x-ray beam is passed through the body part being examined, and is transmitted to an image-intensifying tube, which is a TV-like monitor so that the body part and its motion can be seen in detail.

During fluoroscopy, the patient is placed between the x-ray source and the monitor. The live images generated by the x-ray source strike the image-intensifying tube and allow doctors to see the size, shape, and structure of a patient's internal structures. Because the radiation is blocked more effectively by dense tissue, such as that of a tumor, the result is a dark shadow of the tumor on the screen, against a light background. Most fluoroscopy devices include television or video cameras attached to the image-intensifier tube. The camera output can be digitized and sent through a computer for image enhancement.

In fluoroscopic studies, the radiologist can either insert an intravenous (IV) catheter (hollow tube inserted into blood vessels or into an organ) to **biopsy** a tumor or he can use a contrast agent to visualize the organ or area of interest. The contrast agent allows the image to be viewed more clearly. Contrast agents may be introduced into the patient's body by injection, swallowing, or an enema. Fluoroscopic exams include the following types of tests: barium swallow, **barium enema**, and intravenous pyelography (also called **intravenous urography**).

BARIUM SWALLOW. Used for GI series. The patient drinks a chalky, milkshake-like concoction containing barium, which coats the esophagus and stomach. The barium absorbs the x rays so that the lining of the upper digestive tract can be clearly seen. In barium x rays, fluoroscopy allows the physician to see the movement of the intestines as the barium moves through them.

BARIUM ENEMA. In a lower GI series, the patient receives a barium enema, which coats the intestines and rectum. A gap in the image in the stomach or small intestine could indicate an ulcer and bubbles in the normally smooth large intestinal lining may be abnormal growths.

INTRAVENOUS PYELOGRAPHY (IVP). Pyelography, also called urography, consists of several x rays of all the urinary system, meaning kidneys, ureter, bladder and urethra. A contrast agent is injected through a vein, to make the organs visible for the x rays.

See also Screening test; Ultrasonography.

Resources

BOOKS

Seeram, E. *Computed Tomography: Physical Principles, Clinical Applications and Quality Control.* Philadelphia: W. B. Saunders & Co., 2001.

von Schulthess, G. K., editor. *Clinical Positron Emission Tomography.* Philadelphia: Lippincott, Williams & Wilkins, 1999.

Westbrook, C. *Handbook of MRI Techniques.* Malden, MA: Blackwell Science, 1999.

PERIODICALS

Frassica, F. J., J. A. Khanna, and E. F. McCarthy. "The role of MR imaging in soft tissue tumor evaluation:perspective of the orthopedic oncologist and musculoskeletal pathologist." *Magnetic Resonance Imaging, Clin. N. Am.* 8 (November 2000): 915-27.

Hopper, K. D., K. Singapuri, and A. Finkel. "Body CT and oncologic imaging." *Radiology* 215 (April 2000): 27-40.

Jain, P., and A. C. Arroliga. "Spiral CT for lung cancer screening: is it ready for prime time?" *Cleveland Clinical Journal of Medicine* 68 (January 2001): 74-81.

Pomper, M. G., and J. D. Port. "New techniques in MR imaging of brain tumors." *Magnetic Resonance Imaging, Clin. N. Am.* 8 (November 2000): 691-713.

Roelcke, U., and K. L. Leenders. "PET in neuro-oncology." *Journal of Cancer Research and Clinical Oncology* 127 (January 2001): 2-8.

OTHER

"Imaging Information." *American Cancer Society.* 15 October 1999. [cited July 11, 2005]. <http://www3.cancer.org/cancerinfo/load_cont.asp?ct=1&doc=66>.

ORGANIZATIONS

National Cancer Information Center. 1-800-ACS-2345.

National Cancer Institute. Public Inquiries Office, Building 31, Room 10A31, 31 Center Drive, MSC 2580, Bethesda, MD 20892-2580. (301)435-2848. Imaging Information and data sheets. http://search.nci.nih. gov/search97cgi/s97_cgi.

Monique Laberge, Ph.D.

Imatinib mesylate

Definition

Imatinib mesylate is an enzyme inhibitor used for **cancer** therapy. Imatinib mesylate is also known as STI571 and is sold under the brand name, Gleevec. It was given the name STI571 during early development. STI stands for signal transduction inhibitor.

Purpose

Imatinib mesylate is approved by the U. S. Food and Drug Administration to treat a rare cancer called chronic myeloid leukemia (CML). (CML is also called chronic myelogenous leukemia or **chronic myelocytic leukemia**, as well.)

Description

Imatinib mesylate is the first drug of its kind developed. It fights cancer by turning off an enzyme called tyrosine kinase that causes CML cells to lose their ability to die so they can multiply at an abnormal rate. Its function is different from other cancer drugs because it specifically targets an enzyme that allows the growth of CML cells. This drug has been shown to significantly reduce the number of cancer cells in the blood and bone marrow of treated patients.

Patients who are diagnosed with CML in the three phases of disease can be treated with imatinib mesylate. Chronic myeloid leukemia appears to respond within one to three months following administration of this drug.

Recommended dosage

A doctor experienced in the treatment of patients with CML should initiate therapy.

To minimize the risk of gastrointestinal irritation, imatinib mesylate should be taken with food and a large glass of water. The recommended dosage varies according to clinical circumstances and phase of disease, but generally ranges between 300 and 600 mg per day. As long as the patient continues to benefit, treatment should be continued.

Precautions

Studies have not been performed with imatinib mesylate to determine if it is a carcinogen (cancer causing); therefore it is not known whether this drug may cause mutations or may have cancer-causing effects. In addition, imatinib mesylate's safety and

KEY TERMS

CYP3A4—An enzyme that is predominately responsible for the metabolism of imatinib mesylate.

Enzyme—Any protein that acts as a catalyst, increasing the rate of a chemical reaction.

Kinase—An enzyme.

Leukemia—A type of cancer in which the bone marrow produces an excessive number of abnormal (leukemic) white blood cells. White blood cells protect the body against infection but the abnormal cells suppress the production of normal white blood cells.

Tumor—An abnormal mass of tissue that serves no purpose. Tumors may be either benign (non-cancerous) or malignant (cancerous).

Tyrosine—A non-essential amino acid. Amino acids are the building blocks of protein. They are the raw materials used by the body to make protein. Tyrosine is labeled "nonessential" because, when the amino acids are lacking in the diet, they can be manufactured in the body.

effectiveness has not been established in pediatric patients.

- Fluid retention and edema. If patients experience swelling or weight gain from water retention, they should inform their doctor and should be closely monitored. Signs and symptoms of fluid retention should be closely monitored and patients should be weighed regularly. Appropriate treatment must be provided if an unexpected rapid weight gain occurs. The likelihood of edema is increased with higher doses and in those over age 65 years.

- gastrointestinal irritation

- hematologic toxicity (toxicity of the blood)

- hepatotoxicity (toxicity of the liver)

- toxicities from long-term use

Side effects

Commonly reported side effects include **nausea and vomiting**, muscle cramps, edema (water retention), skin rash, **diarrhea**, heartburn, and headache. Serious side effects occur less frequently, but if they occur may include severe edema liver toxicity, and the potential for bleeding especially in the elderly.

Interactions

Imatinib mesylate interacts with many other drugs. In some cases, side effects may be increased because imatinib mesylate might increase blood levels of certain drugs. Alternatively, imatinib mesylate may decrease blood levels of the drugs, thus reducing their effectiveness. In addition, the blood levels of imatinib mesylate may rise or fall because of other drugs. Therefore, side effects of imatinib mesylate may be increased or effectiveness may be reduced. The patient must discuss all of their medications with their doctor due to many potential drug-drug interactions.

CYP3A4 is an enzyme that is predominately responsible for the metabolism of imatinib mesylate.

The following drugs or families of drugs may interact with imatinib mesylate:

- Inhibitors of the CYP3A4 family, such as ketoconazole, itraconazole, erythromycin.

- Co-medications that induce CYP3A4, such as dexamethasone, phenytoin, carbamazepine, rifampicin, phenobarbital or St. John's wort). No formal studies have been conducted on these medications and imatinib mesylate together.

- CYP3A4 substrates, such as cyclosporine or pimozide.

- CYP3A4 metabolized drugs, such as certain HMG-CoA reductase inhibitors, triazolo-benzodiazepines, and dihydropyridine calcium channel blockers.

- Warfarin. Patients needing anticoagulant therapy while taking imatinib mesylate should be prescribed low-molecular weight or standard heparin.

This list is not all-inclusive of all possible interactions. Patients must inform their doctors of any drugs they are taking in order to avoid drug interactions.

Investigators also evaluated the effect of St. John's wort, an herb used to treat mild to moderate **depression**, on the pharmacokinetics of imatinib. Studies showed that the administration of St. John's wort along with imatinib mesylate reduced absorption and increased elimination of imatinib, reducing drug exposure by as much as 42%. Since clinical efficacy of imatinib is dependent on drug dose and concentration, the interaction with St. John's wort could result in a loss of therapeutic effect. Therefore, the concurrent use of St. John's wort and imatinib should be avoided.

See also Low molecular weight heparins.

Crystal Heather Kaczkowski, MSc.

Immune globulin

Definition

Immune globulin is a concentrated solution of antibodies, pooled from donated blood, which is sometimes given to **cancer** patients whose own immune systems are either not working or are suppressed as a side effect of treatment. Immune globulin can also be called gamma globulin; in the United States some of the brand names are Gamimune, Gammagard, Gammar-P, Iveegam, Polygam, Sandoglobulin, and Venoglobulin.

Purpose

A healthy human body produces proteins called antibodies that act to destroy microorganisms (bacteria and viruses) that invade the body. Some cancer patients, due to the illness itself or side effects of treatment, become depleted of these proteins and therefore susceptible to serious infections. Immune globulin is given to these patients to restore their body's immunity. The use of immune globulin in this way is also called passive immunization. For example, immune globulin is given to bone marrow transplant recipients to prevent the development of severe bacterial infections while their own immune systems are not functioning, and **chronic lymphocytic leukemia** patients (of the type whose antibody-producing cells are the malignant cells) are given immune globulin to prevent the recurrent infections these patients sometimes suffer. Use in this disorder also allows the use of aggressive **chemotherapy** that will destroy the patient's own cancerous antibody-producing cells.

Immune globulin is also used to treat other diseases such as **Lambert-Eaton myasthenic syndrome,** a rare neurological disorder that sometimes occurs in association with **small cell lung cancer**. Also called Eaton-Lambert syndrome, it is an autoimmune disease in which a patient's own antibodies attack nerve cells. The use of immune globulin appears to cause the body to reduce its own production of antibody, thereby improving the neurological disorder.

Description

Immune globulin primarily consists of antibody proteins of the type called IgG or gamma, although the solution may contain small amounts of other antibody types as well as sugars, proteins, and salt.

It is produced by pooling donated blood from at least 1,000 people who have been tested to be free of blood-borne diseases like HIV or hepatitis. The

---

---

antibody proteins are then separated out of the whole blood, and the pH of the immune globulin solution is adjusted to match the normal pH of blood. The preparation is also treated to remove any contaminants, including infectious bacteria or viruses.

Recommended dosage

The dose of immune globulin used varies with the specific problem that it is being used for. When immune gobulin is used in patients with Eaton-Lambert Syndrome, the effective dose is usually about 1 g/kg of body weight/day. (One gram equals 0.035274 ounce; one kilogram equals 2.2046 pounds.) When used to counteract immunodeficiency, the dose is designed to produce an antibody level that stays at an effective threshold over a period of time.

When immune globulin is given to bone marrow transplant recipients, it is usually begun at the time of the transplant and continued for 100 days thereafter, with the objective of maintaining the level of IgG in the patient's blood above 400 mg per deciliter. (A deciliter equals 3.38 fluid ounces.) In patients with chronic lymphocytic leukemia (B-cell type) the target threshold for antibodies in the patient's blood is usually about 600 mg/dL. Although the amount required to maintain these levels varies from patient to patient (because different patients metabolize the drug at different rates) a dose between 10 and 200 mg/kg of body weight, given every 3-4 weeks, is usually sufficient.

Immune globulin is usually given intravenously, although intramuscular shots are available.

Precautions

Some people may have experienced severe reactions, including allergy-type reactions, to other antibody preparations. Generally, these people should not be given intravenous immune globulin. Patients with deficiency of antibody IgA, specifically, should also avoid the use of immune globulin. People with a tendency to form blood clots, or those with kidney problems should also avoid the use of this product, especially if elderly. While many pregnant women have been treated with immune globulin for different problems that have occurred during their pregnancy, since the method of action and specific effects on the fetus are not completely understood, pregnant women should avoid the use of immune globlulin unless it is clearly necessary. Any patient who is given immune globulin should be watched carefully, and epinephrine should be kept available in case a severe allergic reaction is experienced. Immune globulin which was made to be given through intramuscular injection should never be administered intravenously.

Side effects

Administration of intramuscular immune globulin may result in tenderness, swelling, and possibly hives at the site of the injection.

Intravenous immune globulin may cause more severe reactions related to rapid introduction into the blood system. Possible side effects include headache, backache, aching muscles, **fever**, low blood pressure, and chest pain. More commonly, fever accompanied by chills or **nausea and vomiting** may be experienced. If these side effects occur, they are usually related to the immune globulin being administered too rapidly. If the rate of infusion is reduced, or if the infusion is stopped temporarily, negative effects will generally disappear. Rare, but potentially serious, side effects observed have been kidney failure and aseptic meningitis.

Interactions

Use of immune globulin may reduce the effectiveness of vaccinations (for example, measles, mumps, and rubella) for a few months following the use of the immune globulin preparation. Patients who have been given immune globulin should notify their doctors before any vaccinations are given. In addition, in some situations patients may need to have antibody levels measured to determine whether or not they have had previous **infection** with a specific microorganism. Use of immune globulin can create the false

impression of prior exposure to the organism due to the donated antibodies in their blood.

See also Immunologic therapies.

Wendy Wippel, M.S.

Immune response

Definition

The ability of any given cell in the body to distinguish self from nonself is called the immune response.

All cells in the body are recognized as self. Any microorganism (for example, a foreign body or tumor) that invades or attacks the cells is recognized as nonself—or foreign—requiring the immune system to mount a combat against the nonself.

Immune system

The immune system is comprised of a network of immune cells that are generated in the bone marrow stem cell (a cell whose daughter cells may develop into other types of cells). From stem cells different types of immune cells originate that can handle specific immune functions. Phagocytes (cell eaters), serve as the first line of defense, engulfing dead cells, debris, virus, and bacteria. Macrophages are an important type of phagocyte, often presenting the antigen—which is usually a foreign protein—to other immune cells and thus are also called "antigen-presenting cells" (APC). T and B lymphocytes, important immune-system cells, are also capable of recognizing the antigen and become activated. T lymphocytes are classified into two subtypes: killer T cells (also called cytotoxic T cells) and helper T cells. Killer T cells recognize and kill the infected or **cancer** cells that contain the antigen or the foreign protein. Helper T cells release cytokines (chemical messengers) upon activation that either directly destroy the tumor or stimulate other cells to kill the target (tumor). B lymphocytes produce antibodies after recognizing the antigens. The antibodies, which help protect the body from the antigen, are normally specific to that particular antigen. In cases of tumor the specific antibodies attach to tumor cells and, through various mechanisms, impair the functions of the tumor, ultimately leading to the death of the cancer cell.

In addition to these lymphocytes are natural killer (NK) cells that particularly perform the task of eliminating foreign cells. Natural killer cells differ from killer T cells in that they target tumor cells and do not have to recognize an antigen before activation. These cells have been shown to be of potential use in treating cancer.

Immune system and cancer

The immune system serves as one of the primary defenses against cancer. When normal tissue becomes a tumor or cancerous tissue, new antigens develop on their surface. These antigens send a signal to immune cells such as the cytotoxic T lymphocytes, NK cells, and macrophages, which in turn directly kill the tumor cells or release substances like cytokines that may bring about tumor cell death. Thus, under normal circumstances, the immune system provides continued surveillance and eliminates cells that become cancers. However, tumors may survive by hiding or disguising their tumor antigens, or by producing substances that allow suppressor T cells (cells that block cytotoxic, or killer T cells that would normally attack the tumor) to proliferate (multiply).

Biological response modifiers in cancer therapy

Researchers have been working on stimulating the immune cells during cancer with substances broadly classified as **biological response modifiers**. Cytokines are one such substance. These are proteins that are predominantly released by immune cells upon activation or stimulation. During the 1990s the number of cytokines identified increased enormously and the functions associated with them are of immense potential in diagnostics and immune therapy. Some of the key cytokines that have proven therapeutic value in cancer are interleukin-2 (IL-2), Interferon gamma, and interleukin-12 (IL-12). Cytokines are normally injected directly to cancer patients; however, there are other cases where a cancer patient's own lymphocytes are modified under laboratory conditions and injected back into the patient. Examples of these are lymphokine-activated killer (LAK) cells and tumor-infiltrating lymphocytes (TILs). These modified cells are capable of devouring cancer cells.

Immunoprevention of cancer

Immunotherapy is emerging as one of the management strategies for cancer. However, established tumors or large masses of tumor do not respond well to immunotherapy. There is clinical evidence, however, that suggests that patients with minimal residual cancer cells (a few cells left after other forms of cancer treatment) are potential candidates for effective immunotherapy. In these cases immunotherapy often results in a prolonged tumor-free survival. Thus, immune responses can be manipulated to prevent recurrence, even though it does not destroy large tumors. Based on results of immunotherapy trials, most immune therapies are geared towards designing immunoprotective strategies such as cancer **vaccines**.

Cancer vaccines

Cancer vaccines can be made either with whole, inactivated tumor cells, or with fragments or cell surface substances (called cell-surface antigens) present in the tumors. In addition to the whole cell or antigen vaccines, biological modifiers, like cytokines, serve as substances that boost immune response in cancer patients.

Since cancer vaccines are still under clinical evaluation, caution should be exercised while choosing them as the mode of therapy. The cancer care team will provide further insight on whether or not cancer vaccine or cytokine therapy will be beneficial after they assess the patient's stage and the various modes of treatments available.

Resources

PERIODICALS

"Genetic Vaccines." *Scientific American* July 1999.
"Immunoprevention of Cancer: Is the Time Ripe?" *Cancer Research* 60 (May 15, 2000): 2571-2575

OTHER

"Treating Cancer with Vaccine Therapy." *National Cancer Institute*. 2000. [cited July 5, 2005]. <http://cancertrials.nci.nih.gov/news/features/vaccine/html/page05.html>.

Kausalya Santhanam, Ph.D.

Immunoelectrophoresis

Definition

Immunoelectrophoresis, also called gamma globulin electrophoresis, or immunoglobulin electrophoresis, is a method of determining the blood levels of three major immunoglobulins: immunoglobulin M (IgM), immunoglobulin G (IgG), and immunoglobulin A (IgA).

Purpose

Immunoelectrophoresis is a powerful analytical technique with high resolving power as it combines

KEY TERMS

Antibody—A protein manufactured by the white blood cells to neutralize an antigen in the body. In some cases, excessive formation of antibodies leads to illness, allergy, or autoimmune disorders.

Antigen—A substance that can cause an immune response, resulting in production of an antibody, as part of the body's defense against infection and disease. Many antigens are foreign proteins not found naturally in the body, and include germs, toxins, and tissues from another person used in organ transplantation.

Autoimmune disorder—A condition in which antibodies are formed against the body's own tissues, for example, in some forms of arthritis.

separation of antigens by electrophoresis with immunodiffusion against an antiserum. The increased resolution is of benefit in the immunological examination of serum proteins. Immunoelectrophoresis aids in the diagnosis and evaluation of the therapeutic response in many disease states affecting the immune system. It is usually requested when a different type of electrophoresis, called a serum **protein electrophoresis**, has indicated a rise at the immunoglobulin level. Immunoelectrophoresis is also used frequently to diagnose **multiple myeloma**, a disease affecting the bone marrow.

Precautions

Drugs that may cause increased immunoglobulin levels include therapeutic gamma globulin, hydralazine, isoniazid, **phenytoin** (Dilantin), procainamide, oral contraceptives, methadone, steroids, and tetanus toxoid and antitoxin. The laboratory should be notified if the patient has received any vaccinations or immunizations in the six months before the test. This is mainly because prior immunizations lead to the increased immunoglobulin levels resulting in false positive results.

It should be noted that, because immunoelectrophoresis is not quantitative, it is being replaced by a procedure called immunofixation, which is more sensitive and easier to interpret.

Description

Serum proteins separate in agar gels under the influence of an electric field into albumin, alpha 1,

alpha 2, and beta and gamma globulins. Immunoelectrophoresis is performed by placing serum on a slide containing a gel designed specifically for the test. An electric current is then passed through the gel, and immunoglobulins, which contain an electric charge, migrate through the gel according to the difference in their individual electric charges. Antiserum is placed alongside the slide to identify the specific type of immunoglobulin present. The results are used to identify different disease entities, and to aid in monitoring the course of the disease and the therapeutic response of the patient with such conditions as immune deficiencies, autoimmune disease, chronic infections, chronic viral infections, intrauterine fetal infections, multiple **myeloma**, and monoclonal gammopathy of undetermined significance.

There are five classes of antibodies: IgM, IgG, IgA, IgE, and IgD.

IgM is produced upon initial exposure to an antigen. For example, when a person receives the first tetanus vaccination, antitetanus antibodies of the IgM class are produced 10 to 14 days later. IgM is abundant in the blood but is not normally present in organs or tissues. IgM is primarily responsible for ABO blood grouping and rheumatoid factor, yet is involved in the immunologic reaction to other infections, such as hepatitis. Since IgM does not cross the placenta, an elevation of this immunoglobulin in the newborn indicates intrauterine **infection** such as rubella, cytomegalovirus (CMV) or a sexually transmitted disease (STD).

IgG is the most prevalent type of antibody, comprising approximately 75% of the serum immunoglobulins. IgG is produced upon subsequent exposure to an antigen. As an example, after receiving a second tetanus shot, or booster, a person produces IgG antibodies in five to seven days. IgG is present in both the blood and tissues, and is the only antibody to cross the placenta from the mother to the fetus. Maternal IgG protects the newborn for the first months of life, until the infant's immune system produces its own antibodies.

IgA constitutes approximately 15% of the immunoglobulins within the body. Although it is found to some degree in the blood, it is present primarily in the secretions of the respiratory and gastrointestinal tract, in saliva, colostrum (the yellowish fluid produced by the breasts during late pregnancy and the first few days after childbirth), and in tears. IgA plays an important role in defending the body against invasion of germs through the mucous membrane-lined organs.

IgE is the antibody that causes acute allergic reactions; it is measured to detect allergic conditions. IgD, which constitutes the smallest portion of the immuno-globulins, is rarely evaluated or detected, and its function is not well understood.

Preparation

This test requires a blood sample.

Aftercare

Because this test is ordered when either very low or very high levels of immunoglobulins are suspected, the patient should be alert for any signs of infection after the test, including **fever**, chills, rash, or skin ulcers. Any **bone pain** or tenderness should also be immediately reported to the physician.

Risks

Risks for this test are minimal, but may include slight bleeding from the blood-drawing site, fainting or feeling lightheaded after venipuncture, or bruising.

Normal results

Reference ranges vary from laboratory to laboratory and depend upon the method used. For adults, normal values are usually found within the following ranges (1 mg = approximately .000035 oz. and 1 dL = approximately 0.33 fluid oz.):

- IgM: 60–290 mg/dL
- IgG: 700–1,800 mg/dL
- IgA: 70–440 mg/dL

Abnormal results

Increased IgM levels can indicate Waldenström's macroglobulinemia, a malignancy caused by secretion of IgM at high levels by malignant lymphoplasma cells. Increased IgM levels can also indicate chronic infections, such as hepatitis or mononucleosis and autoimmune diseases, like rheumatoid arthritis.

Decreased IgM levels can be indicative of AIDS, immunosuppression caused by certain drugs like steroids or dextran, or leukemia.

Increased levels of IgG can indicate chronic liver disease, autoimmune diseases, hyperimmunization reactions, or certain chronic infections, such as tuberculosis or sarcoidosis.

Decreased levels of IgG can indicate Wiskott-Aldrich syndrome, a genetic deficiency caused by inadequate synthesis of IgG and other immunoglobulins. Decreased IgG can also be seen with AIDS and leukemia.

Increased levels of IgA can indicate chronic liver disease, chronic infections, or inflammatory bowel disease.

Decreased levels of IgA can be found in ataxia, a condition affecting balance and gait, limb or eye movements, speech, and telangiectasia, an increase in the size and number of the small blood vessels in an area of skin, causing redness. Decreased IgA levels are also seen in conditions of low blood protein (hypoproteinemia), and drug immunosuppression.

Resources

BOOKS

Fischbach, Frances T. *A Manual of Laboratory Diagnostic Tests.* Philadelphia: Lippincott Williams & Wilkins, 1999.
Pagana, Kathleen D., and Timothy J. Pagana. *Mosby's Manual of Diagnostic and Laboratory Tests.* St. Louis: Mosby, Inc., 1999.

Janis O. Flores

Immunohistochemistry

Definition

Immunohistochemistry is a method of analyzing and identifying cell types based on the binding of antibodies to specific components of the cell. It is sometimes referred to as immunocytochemistry.

Purpose

Immunohistochemistry (IHC) is used to diagnose the type of **cancer** and to help determine the patient's prognosis. In cases such as metastases or **carcinoma of unknown primary** origin, where it may be difficult to determine the type of cell from which the tumor originated, immunohistochemistry can identify cells by the characteristic markers on the cell surface. IHC can also help distinguish between benign and malignant tumors.

Description

Immunohistochemistry requires a sample of tissue from a **biopsy**; usually the tissue sample is examined fresh, but frozen or chemically preserved material can be used. A blood sample or bone marrow may also be examined. The tissue sample is sliced extremely thinly, so that it is approximately one cell thick, then the sample is fixed onto a glass slide. The tumor cells in the sample have characteristic markers, or antigens, on their cell surfaces which can be used to help identify the specific type of tumor cell. Antibodies against these characteristic antigens are added to the sample on the slide, and the antibodies bind wherever the antigens are present. Excess antibody is then washed away. The antibodies that remain bound to the cell have labels on them that either fluoresce (glow) or undergo a chemical reaction that makes them visible by microscope. The pathologist is able to see the specially labeled tumor antigens as they appear in the patient's tissue.

The pathologist will try to assess the level of maturity of the tumor cells, which will help him to determine their origin. He will be checking for cell types that are found in an inappropriate part of the body, for example prostate cells in a lymph node. He will also look for cell characteristics that will indicate if the tumor is benign or malignant. Proteins involved in the replication of genetic material and cell growth may be present in greater amounts; for example, antibodies against the antigen Ki-67 are used to evaluate malignant melanomas, breast carcinomas, and non-Hodgkin's lymphomas. Hormone receptors may also be examined. The presence of receptors to estrogen and progesterone indicate a good prognosis for **breast cancer** patients. Pathologists may also look for an increase in tumor suppressor proteins. A wide variety of antibodies are available to help determine the origin of the tumor, whether it is growing rapidly, and whether it is a type of tumor that responds well to particular treatments.

Preparation

The physician will choose the type of sample to be taken based on the type of tumor. If the patient has a solid tumor, a tissue sample may be biopsied; if the entire tumor is being removed a biopsy may be taken during surgery. In this case the patient should prepare for the surgery or the biopsy as the physician suggests. A routine blood sample may also be required; in most cases, no additional preparation is required.

Aftercare

The only aftercare that might be required is from the sample collection process.

Risks

The risks associated with IHC are the risks associated with the sample collection, either the biopsy of the tumor or the drawing of blood. The only other concern is the possibility that the test could yield unclear results.

Normal results

Normal results will simply look like normal cells. The cells will have a high level of maturity and be located only in sites appropriate to their cell type. For example, analysis of lymph nodes will show only the cells that belong there, not cells that would normally be present in the breast. No specific tumor antigens will be present in increased numbers.

Abnormal results

An abnormal result would consist of cells which appear immature or poorly differentiated, or that are found in an inappropriate tissue for their cell type. The pathologist may test for the presence of a particular antigen, such as Ki-67, carcinoembryonic antigen (CEA), or prostate specific antigen (PSA). In this case, there may be a numerical standard value to compare normal to abnormal results and help the physician in determining prognosis.

See also Receptor analysis; Tumor markers.

Resources

BOOKS

Javois, Lorette C. *Immunocytochemical Methods and Protocols.* Totowa, NJ:Humana Press Inc., 1999.

PERIODICALS

Bendayan, Moise. "Worth Its Weight in Gold." *Science* 291 (February 16, 2001): 1363–1365.

Cote, R. J., et al. "Role of Immunohistochemical Detection of Lymph-Node Metastases in Management of Breast Cancer." *The Lancet* 354 (September 11, 1999): 896–900.

Gastl, Gunther, et al. "Ep-CAM Overexpression in Breast Cancer as a Predictor of Survival." In *The Lancet* 356 (9 December 2000): 1981–1982.

Racquel Baert, M.S.

Immunologic therapies

Definition

Immunologic therapy is the treatment of disease using medicines that boost the body's natural **immune response**. Some forms of immunologic therapy are intended to bypass the body's weakened immune system while others are intended to repair or direct it.

Purpose

Immunologic therapy is used to improve the immune system's natural ability to fight diseases such as **cancer**, hepatitis and AIDS. These drugs may also be used to help the body recover from immunosuppression resulting from treatments such as **chemotherapy** or **radiation therapy**.

Description

Most drugs in this category are synthetic versions of substances produced naturally in the body. In their natural forms, these substances help defend the body against disease. For example, **aldesleukin** (Proleukin) is an artificially made form of interleukin-2, which helps white blood cells work. Aldesleukin is administered to patients with kidney cancers and skin cancers that have spread to other parts of the body. **Filgrastim** (Neupogen) and **sargramostim** (Leukine) are versions of natural substances called colony stimulating factors, which drive the bone marrow to make new white blood cells. Another type of drug, epoetin (Epogen, Procrit), is a synthetic version of human **erythropoietin** that stimulates the bone marrow to make new red blood cells. **Thrombopoietin** stimulates the production of platelets, disk-shaped bodies in the blood that are important in clotting. **Interferons** are substances the body produces naturally using immune cells to fight infections and tumors. The synthetic interferons carry brand names such as Alferon, Roferon or Intron A. Some of the interferons that are currently in use as drugs are Recombinant Interferon Alfa-2a, Recombinant Interferon Alfa-2b, Interferon Alfa-n1, and Interferon Alfa-n3. Alfa interferons are used to treat **hairy cell leukemia**, malignant **melanoma**, and AIDs-related **Kaposi's sarcoma**. In addition, interferons are also used for other conditions such as laryngeal papillomatosis, genital warts, and certain types of hepatitis.

Recommended dosage

The recommended dosage depends on the type of immunologic therapy. For some medicines, the physician will decide the dosage for each patient, taking into account a patient's weight and whether he/she is taking other medicines. Some drugs used in immunologic therapy are given only in a hospital, under a physician's supervision. For those that patients may give themselves, check with the physician who prescribed the medicine or the pharmacist who filled the prescription for the correct dosage.

Most of these drugs come in injectable form. These drugs are generally administered by the cancer care provider.

Precautions

Aldesleukin

This medicine may temporarily increase the chance of getting infections. It may also lower the number of platelets in the blood, and thus possibly interfering with the blood's ability to clot. Taking these precautions may reduce the chance of such problems:

- Avoid people with infections, if possible.

- Be alert to signs of infection, such as fever, chills, sore throat, pain in the lower back or side, cough, hoarseness, or painful or difficulty with urination. If any of these symptoms occur, get in touch with a physician immediately.

- Be alert to signs of bleeding problems, such as black, tarry stools, inky red spots on the skin, blood in the urine or stools, or any other unusual bleeding or bruising.

- Take care to avoid cuts or other injuries. Be especially careful when using knives, razors, nail clippers, and other sharp objects. Check with a dentist for the best ways to clean the teeth and mouth without injuring the gums. Do not have dental work done without checking with a physician.

KEY TERMS

AIDS—Acquired immunodeficiency syndrome. A disease caused by infection with the human immunodeficiency virus (HIV). In people with this disease, the immune system breaks down, increasing vulnerability to other infections and some types of cancer.

Bone marrow—Soft tissue that fills the hollow centers of bones. Blood cells and platelets (disk-shaped bodies in the blood that are important in clotting) are produced in the bone marrow.

Chemotherapy—Treatment of an illness with chemical agents. The term is usually used to describe the treatment of cancer with drugs.

Clot—A hard mass that forms when blood gels.

Dendritic cells—Immune system cells derived from a type of white blood cell called monocytes. Dendritic cells help to activate the B cells, helper T cells, and killer T cells in the immune system.

Hepatitis—Inflammation of the liver caused by a virus, chemical, or drug.

Immune response—The body's natural, protective reaction to disease and infection.

Immune system—The system that protects the body against disease and infection through immune responses.

Inflammation—Pain, redness, swelling, and heat that usually develop in response to injury or illness.

Psoriasis—A skin disease that manifests itself with itchy, scaly, red patches on the skin.

Seizure—A sudden attack, spasm, or convulsion.

Shingles—A disease caused by an infection with the Herpes zoster virus—the same virus that causes chickenpox. Symptoms of shingles include pain and blisters along one nerve, usually on the face, chest, stomach, or back.

Sickle cell anemia—An inherited disorder in which red blood cells contain an abnormal form of hemoglobin, a protein that carries oxygen. The abnormal form of hemoglobin causes the red cells to become sickle-shaped. The misshapen cells may clog blood vessels, preventing oxygen from reaching tissues and leading to pain, blood clots and other problems. Sickle cell anemia is most common in people of African descent and in people from Italy, Greece, India, and the Middle East.

• Wash hands frequently, and avoid touching the eyes or inside of the nose unless the hands have just been washed.

Aldesleukin may make some medical conditions worse, such as chickenpox, shingles (**herpes zoster**), liver disease, lung disease, heart disease, underactive thyroid, psoriasis, immune system problems, and mental problems. The medicine may increase the chance of seizures (convulsions) in people who are prone to having them. Also, the drug's effects may be greater in people with kidney disease, because their kidneys are slow to clear the medicine from their bodies.

Colony stimulating factors

Certain drugs used in treating cancer reduce the body's ability to fight infections. Although colony stimulating factors help restore the body's natural defenses, the process takes time. Getting prompt treatment for infections is important, even while taking this medicine. Call the physician at the first sign of illness or **infection**, such as a sore throat, **fever**, or chills.

People with certain medical conditions could have problems if they take colony stimulating factors.

People who have kidney disease, liver disease, or conditions caused by inflammation or immune system problems can worsen these problems with colony stimulating factors. Those who have heart disease may be more likely to experience side effects such as water retention and heart rhythm problems while taking these drugs. Finally, patients who have lung disease might increase their chances of suffering from shortness of breath. Those who have any of these medical conditions should check with their personal physicians before using colony stimulating factors.

Epoetin

Epoetin is a medicine that may cause seizures (convulsions), especially in people who are prone to having them. No one who takes these drugs should drive, use machines, or do anything considered dangerous in case of a seizure.

Epoetin helps the body make new red blood cells, but it is not effective unless there is adequate iron in the body. The physician may recommend taking iron supplements or certain **vitamins** that help supply the body with iron. It is necessary to follow the physician's advice in this instance—recommendations for iron in this case, as with any supplements should only come from a physician.

In studies of laboratory animals, epoetin taken during pregnancy caused birth defects, including damage to the bones and spine. However, the drug has not been reported to cause problems in human babies whose mothers take it. Women who are pregnant or who may become pregnant should check with their physicians for the most up-to-date information on the safety of taking this medicine during pregnancy.

People with certain medical conditions may have problems if they take this medicine. For example, the chance of side effects may be greater in people with high blood pressure, heart or blood vessel disease, or a history of blood clots. Epoetin may not work properly in people who have bone problems or sickle cell **anemia**.

Interferons

Interferons can add to the effects of alcohol and other drugs that slow down the central nervous system, such as antihistamines, cold medicine, allergy medicine, sleep aids, medicine for seizures, tranquilizers, some pain relievers, and muscle relaxants. They may also add to the effects of anesthetics, including those used for dental procedures. Those taking interferons should check with their physicians before taking any of the above.

Some people experience dizziness, unusual **fatigue**, or become less alert than usual while being treated with these drugs. Because of these possible problems, anyone who takes these drugs should not drive, use machines, or do anything else considered dangerous until they have determined how the drugs affect them.

Interferons often cause flu-like symptoms, including fever and chills. The physician who prescribes this medicine may recommend taking acetaminophen (Tylenol) before—and sometimes after—each dose to keep the fever from getting too high. If the physician recommends this, follow instructions carefully.

Like aldesleukin, interferons may temporarily increase the chance of getting infections and lower the number of platelets in the blood, leading to clotting problems. To help prevent these problems, follow the precautions for reducing the risk of infection and bleeding listed for aldesleukin.

People who have certain medical conditions may have problems if they take interferons. For example, the drugs may worsen some medical conditions, including heart disease, kidney disease, liver disease, lung disease, diabetes, bleeding problems, and mental problems. In people who have overactive immune systems, these drugs can even increase the activity of the immune system. People who have shingles or chickenpox, or who have recently been exposed to chickenpox may increase their risk of developing severe problems in other parts of the body if they take interferons. People with a history of seizures or mental problems could at risk if taking interferon.

In teenage women, interferons may cause changes in the menstrual cycle. Young women should discuss this possibility with their physicians. Older people may be more sensitive to the effects of interferons. This may increase the chance of side effects.

These drugs are not known to cause fetal death, birth defects, or other problems in humans when taken during pregnancy. Women who are pregnant or who may become pregnant should ask their physicians for the latest information on the safety of taking these drugs during pregnancy.

Women who are breastfeeding their babies may need to stop while taking this medicine. Whether interferons pass into breast milk is not known. Because of the chance of serious side effects to the baby, breastfeeding while taking interferon is discouraged. Check with a physician for advice.

General precautions for all types of immunologic therapy

Regular physician visits are necessary during immunologic therapy treatment. This gives the physician a chance to make sure the medicine is working and to check for unwanted side effects.

Anyone who has had unusual reactions to drugs used in immunologic therapy should let the physician know before resuming the drugs. Any allergies to foods, dyes, preservatives, or other substances should also be reported.

Side effects

Aldesleukin

In addition to its helpful effects, this medicine may cause serious side effects. Generally, it is given only in a hospital, where medical professionals can watch for early signs of problems. Medical tests might be performed to check for unwanted effects.

Anyone who has breathing problems, fever, or chills while being given aldesleukin should check with a physician immediately.

Other side effects should be brought to a physician's attention as soon as possible:

- dizziness
- drowsiness
- confusion
- agitation
- depression
- nausea and vomiting
- diarrhea
- sores in the mouth and on the lips
- tingling of hands or feet
- decrease in urination
- unexplained weight gain of five or more pounds

Some side effects are usually temporary and do not need medical attention unless they are bothersome. These include dry skin; itchy or burning skin rash or redness followed by peeling; loss of appetite; and a general feeling of illness or discomfort.

Colony stimulating factors

As this medicine starts to work, the patient might experience mild pain in the lower back or hips. This is nothing to cause undue concern, and will usually go away within a few days. If the pain is intense or causes discomfort, the physician may prescribe a painkiller.

Other possible side effects include headache, joint or muscle pain and skin rash or **itching**. These side effects tend to disappear as the body adjusts to the medicine, and do not need medical treatment. If they continue, or they interfere with normal activities, check with a physician.

Epoetin

This medicine may cause flu-like symptoms, such as muscle aches, **bone pain**, fever, chills, shivering, and sweating, within a few hours after it is taken. These symptoms usually go away within 12 hours. If they do not, or if they are troubling, check with a physician. Other possible side effects that do not need medical attention are **diarrhea**, **nausea** or **vomiting** and fatigue or weakness.

Certain side effects should be brought to a physician's attention as soon as possible. These include headache, vision problems, increased blood pressure, fast heartbeat, weight gain and swelling of the face, fingers, lower legs, ankles or feet.

Anyone who has chest pain or seizures after taking epoetin should seek professional emergency medical attention immediately.

Interferons

This medicine may cause temporary hair loss (**alopecia**). While upsetting, it is not a sign that something is seriously wrong. The hair should grow back normally after treatment ends.

As the body adjusts to the medicine many other side effects usually go away during treatment. These include flu-like symptoms, **taste alteration**, loss of appetite (**anorexia**), **nausea and vomiting**, skin rash, and unusual fatigue. If these problems persist, or if they interfere with normal life, check with a physician.

A few more serious side effects should be brought to a physician's attention as soon as possible:

- confusion
- difficulty thinking or concentrating
- nervousness
- depression
- sleep problems
- numbness or tingling in the fingers, toes and face

General caution regarding side effects for all types of immunologic therapy

Other side effects are possible with any type of immunologic therapy. Anyone who has unusual symptoms during or after treatment with these drugs should should contact the physician immediately.

Interactions

Anyone who has immunologic therapy should let the physician know all other medicines being taken. Some combinations of drugs may interact, that can increase or decrease the effects of one or both drugs or can increase the likelihood of side effects. Consultation with a physician is highly recommended to get the insight on whether the possible interactions can interfere with drug therapy or cause harmful effects.

Immunoprevention

Considering that most of the biological modifiers such as cytokines elicit immune response that inhibit incipient tumors before they are clinically evident, immunoprevention has been proposed as a recent strategy for combating cancer. Treatment involving immune molecules (such as cytokines) prepared synthetically or that are not produced by the patients themselves is called as passive immunotherapy. Conversely, a vaccine is a form of active immune therapy because it elicits an immune response in patients. A cancer vaccine may be made of whole tumor cell or of substances or fragments contained in the tumor called antigens.

Newer types of immunologic therapy that are still considered investigational as of 2003 include cell-based therapies. Instead of using synthetic chemicals that resemble substances produced by the body, cell-based therapies use modified stem cells or dendritic cells as **vaccines** against cancer. Stem cells are undifferentiated cells whose daughter cells can develop into various types of specialized cells, while dendritic cells are cells that are able to initiate and modify the immune system's responses to cancer by activating B cells and T cells. Dendritic cells appear to offer a promising new form of immunotherapy for cancer.

Another investigational form of treatment is the development of cell-free tumor-specific peptide vaccines. Peptides are subunits of protein molecules that contain two or more amino acids. Peptide vaccines are intended to induce responses in the patient's T cells that inhibit tumor growth. As of late 2003, however, peptide-based tumor vaccines have been shown to shrink cancerous tumors only in patients with limited disease.

Adoptive immunotherapy

Adoptive immunotherapy involves stimulating T lymphocytes by exposing them to tumor antigens. These modified cells are grown in the laboratory and then injected into patients. Since the cells taken from a different individual for this purpose often results in rejection, patients serve both as donor and recipient of their own T cells. Adoptive immunotherapy is particularly effective in patients who have received massive doses of radiation and chemotherapy. In such patients, therapy results in immunosuppression (weakened immune systems), making them vulnerable to viral infections. For example, CMV-specific T cells can reduce the risk of cytomegalovirus (CMV) infection in transplant patients.

Resources

BOOKS

Reiger, Paula T. *Biotherapy: A Comprehensive Overview.* Sudbury: Jones and Bartlett, Inc. 2000.

Stern, Peter L., P. C. Beverley, and M. Carroll. *Cancer Vaccines and Immunotherapy.* New York: Cambridge University Press, 2000.

PERIODICALS

Fishman, M. N., and S. J. Antonia. "Cell-Based Immune Therapy for Metastatic Renal Cancer." *Expert Review of Anticancer Therapy* 3 (December 2003): 837–849.

"Immunoprevention of Cancer: Is the time Ripe?" *Cancer Research* 60 (May 15, 2000): 2571–2575.

National Cancer Institute. *Treating Cancer with Vaccine therapy* 2000. [cited June 29, 2005]. <http://cancertrials.nci.nih.gov/news/features/vaccine/html/page05.htm>.

Nieda, M., M. Tomiyama, and K. Egawa. "Ex vivo Enhancement of Antigen-Presenting Function of Dendritic Cells and Its Application for DC-Based Immunotherapy." *Human Cell* 16 (December 2003): 199–204.

Paczesny, S., H. Ueno, J. Fay, et al. "Dendritic Cells as Vectors for Immunotherapy of Cancer." *Seminars in Cancer Biology* 13 (December 2003): 439–447.

Rosenberg, S. A. "Progress in Human Tumor Immunology and Immunotherapy." *Nature* 411, no. 6835 (2001): 380–385.

Scheibenbogen, C., A. Letsch, A. Schmittel, et al. "Rational Peptide-Based Tumour Vaccine Development and T Cell Monitoring." *Seminars in Cancer Biology* 13 (December 2003): 423–429.

Rebecca J. Frey, Ph.D.

Immunotherapy *see* **Immunologic therapies**

Implantable subcutaneous ports *see* **Vascular access**

Incontinence, cancer-related

Definition

Cancer-related **incontinence** is the inability to control bladder or bowel function (or both) as a result of the direct effects of **cancer** on the body or the effects of various forms of cancer therapy. In some patients, cancer-related incontinence can be easily treated and controlled, but requires specialized consultation and treatment in others.

Demographics

The demographics of urinary and fecal incontinence vary widely according to the type of cancer and the treatments for it. One study reported that about 35% of women treated for cancers of the female reproductive system developed urinary incontinence, while another found that 80% of women treated for cancer of the uterus with **radiation therapy** developed urinary incontinence. Between 50 and 80% of patients receiving **irinotecan** (Camptosar), a drug given to treat **colon cancer**, develop severe **diarrhea** and fecal incontinence. About 99% of patients given opioid drugs to relieve pain develop constipation, which can lead to fecal incontinence if untreated.

Description

Incontinence is the loss of normal control of the bowel or bladder. Incontinence can involve the involuntary voiding of urine (urinary incontinence) or of stool and gas (fecal or bowel incontinence). There are several types of urinary incontinence. Those most frequently seen as side effects of cancer include overflow incontinence, urge incontinence, and stress incontinence. In rare cases incontinence occurs as the result of cancer, but more commonly it is a side effect of treatment.

Because the subjects of bowel and bladder control are perceived as socially unacceptable, those affected with incontinence often feel ashamed or embarrassed by the problem. Instead of seeking medical attention, these individuals try to hide the problem or manage it themselves. For this reason, incontinence is sometimes referred to as "the silent affliction." The psychological effects of incontinence include low self-esteem, social withdrawal and isolation, and **depression**. In most cases incontinence can be successfully treated, so affected individuals should discuss the problem with a doctor.

Risk factors

Risk factors for cancer-related incontinence include:

- Previous history of irritable bowel syndrome, Crohn's disease, diabetes, or multiple sclerosis.
- Being diagnosed with Alzheimer's or Parkinson's disease in addition to the cancer.
- In women, previous history of childbirth by vaginal delivery.
- In men, diagnosis of and treatment for prostate cancer.
- Any cancer treatment that involves surgical removal of part of the digestive tract.
- Radiation therapy to the stomach or abdomen as part of cancer treatment.
- Cancers that arise in or spread to the brain and spinal cord.
- Anticancer drugs that affect the nervous system.
- Pain relievers that contain opium or opium derivatives. These drugs include fentanyl, morphine, codeine, oxycodone, tramadol, and dextropropoxyphene. Opioids can cause constipation that can lead in turn to fecal incontinence.

Causes and symptoms

Incontinence can result from damage to the muscle, nerves, or the structure of the body parts involved in the control of voiding. Complex systems of hollow organs (such as the bladder) and tube-shaped structures (such as the rectum and urethra) work together to store and release waste. Special muscles, including sphincters, are especially important in maintaining the tight seals that hold in waste. When physical damage to muscle or organ structure occurs, the system can no longer maintain these tight seals, and waste can leak out.

Nerves carry messages between the brain and the bowel and bladder systems. Injury to these nerves, or the related part of the brain, interferes with the delivery of these messages, which can prevent the body from recognizing the signals telling it when to void. Without these signals and messages, an individual cannot coordinate the brain with the bowel and bladder systems, and incontinence results.

Several types of cancer and its treatments are associated with incontinence. Usually, it is the treatment of cancer that causes incontinence, rather than the cancer itself. Fecal incontinence frequently results from **anticancer drugs** that cause either diarrhea or constipation. Anticancer drugs that can cause constipation include the vinca alkaloids, oxaliplatins, taxanes, and **thalidomide**. Drugs that can cause diarrhea include the fluoropyrimidines, adriamycin, **cisplatin**, and irinotecan; in one study, 80% of cancer patients receiving these drugs developed severe diarrhea.

Prostate cancer

The treatment of **prostate cancer** is one of the most common causes of cancer-related urinary incontinence, largely because the prostate is located so closely to the nerves, muscles, and structures involved in urine control. Surgical removal of the prostate, or **prostatectomy**, carries the highest risk of urinary incontinence as a side effect; the risk from radiation therapy is somewhat lower. The incontinence (typically stress or urge incontinence) is often temporary, but in a small percentage of men it may be long lasting.

Prostate cancer itself seldom causes incontinence. However, this depends on the location and size of the cancer; a large cancerous prostate can interfere with the flow of urine and result in overflow incontinence.

Bladder cancer

Incontinence is only occasionally the direct result of **bladder cancer**, but it is a common side effect of some treatments. For early-stage cancer where treatment does not require the bladder to be removed, incontinence almost never occurs. But removal of the bladder and surrounding structures is often necessary to treat more advanced cancer. This requires creation of an artificial system for storing and releasing urine and carries a risk of long-term incontinence.

Colon cancer and rectal cancer

Muscles in the anal and rectal region largely control bowel evacuation, with the colon storing stool and gas. When these regions are removed or damaged during cancer treatment, or if injury to the related nerves occurs, fecal incontinence can result. Fecal incontinence is most commonly a side effect of surgery. Weakening of bowel muscles or damaging of nerves by radiation therapy can also cause incontinence, but this type is more likely to be mild and temporary, and will often improve as these areas heal. However, in some patients, radiation causes permanent and severe fecal incontinence; this condition is known as radiation **enteritis**.

Other causes

Loss of voluntary bowel and bladder control is less commonly associated with other cancers of the genital and urinary systems, mainly as a side effect of treatment. Incontinence can also result from cancer or treatment damage in the brain and spinal cord. Other cancers indirectly cause incontinence; for example, constant coughing from lung cancer can lead to stress incontinence. Incontinence can be a side effect of certain other medications.

Diagnosis

The diagnosis of incontinence is usually obvious on the basis of the patient's treatment history and reported symptoms.

Treatment

Traditional

The method of treatment depends on the cause and type of incontinence. Surgical treatment is usually reserved for severe or long-lasting incontinence. An artificial pouch for storing urine or stool can be placed inside the body as a substitute for a removed bladder, colon, or rectum. Placement of an artificial sphincter successfully treats other cases. For mild or temporary incontinence, treatment may include medications, dietary changes, muscle-strengthening exercises, or behavioral training, such as establishing a time pattern for voiding. A small group of patients, however, requires a permanent **colostomy** or **urostomy**.

Electrical stimulation therapy, which targets involved muscles with low-current electricity, can be used to treat either urinary or fecal incontinence.

Biofeedback uses electronic or mechanical devices to improve bladder or bowel control by teaching an individual how to recognize and respond to certain body signals.

Embarrassment may lead some people to manage the symptoms of incontinence themselves by wearing absorbent pads to prevent the soiling of their clothes. However, many treatments exist to successfully restore or improve control of bowel and bladder function, so individuals experiencing incontinence should speak to a doctor or nurse.

Cancer patients who have difficulty with frequent or occasional incontinence may find the following tips helpful:

- Always use the bathroom before leaving home.
- Always carry a backpack or tote containing cleansing towelettes and a change of underwear.
- Locate public restrooms before the need to use them is urgent.
- If the problem is specifically fecal incontinence, try taking an oral fecal deodorant. Over-the-counter products approved by the Food and Drug Administration (FDA) include Devrom and Nullo. These products work by reducing the number of odor-causing bacteria in stool.
- Wear disposable undergarments or sanitary pads if an episode of incontinence seems likely.

Drugs

Constipation caused by cancer therapy can be treated by one or more stimulant **laxatives**, stool softeners, lubricant laxatives, or agents that increase the bulk of the stools. Patients whose constipation is caused by opioid pain relievers can be given a drug called methylnaltrexone (Relistor), which will relieve the constipation without affecting the patient's pain control.

Diarrhea caused by cancer treatment can be treated by giving the patient loperamide, a drug that slows down intestinal motility. Other medications include absorbent materials like pectin or methylcellulose; these absorb excess liquid in the digestive tract. As of 2009, the most promising drug to treat diarrhea associated with cancer **chemotherapy** is octreotide (Sandostatin).

Alternative

Good results for cancer-related fecal incontinence have been reported for biofeedback training, although the subject is still being researched. In successful cases, patients regain complete control over defecation, or at

QUESTIONS TO ASK YOUR DOCTOR

- Is my incontinence caused by the cancer or by cancer therapy?
- Is it possible to change the dosage of my chemotherapy drug or try a different drug?
- Is it safe to take over-the-counter preparations for constipation or diarrhea caused by cancer treatment?
- What is the prognosis of my incontinence?
- Where can I go for advice about my specific difficulties with incontinence?

least improve their control, by learning to contract the external part of the anal sphincter whenever stools enter the rectum.

Home remedies

In some cases, patients with fecal incontinence related to cancer treatment may be helped by eating small, frequent meals and avoiding certain foods. The most frequent offenders include milk and dairy products, spicy foods, alcohol, caffeine-containing foods and beverages (including coffee, tea, and cola), certain fruit juices, gas-forming foods and beverages, high-fiber foods, and high-fat foods.

Prognosis

Success in treating cancer-related incontinence depends on the location of the cancer and the methods used to treat it. In most cases the patient can obtain at least partial relief. When incontinence remains a problem despite medical treatment, disposable underwear and other commercial incontinence products are available to make life easier. Doctors and nurses can offer advice on coping with incontinence, and people should never be embarrassed about seeking their assistance. Counseling and information are also available from support groups.

Prevention

Incontinence related to cancer or cancer treatment is difficult to prevent, in part because researchers do not understand as of 2009 why some patients become incontinent with cancer or cancer therapy and others do not.

Resources

BOOKS

Airley, Rachel. *Cancer Chemotherapy*. Hoboken, NJ: Wiley-Blackwell, 2009.

DeAngelis, Lisa M., and Jerome B. Posner. *Neurologic Complications of Cancer*, 2nd ed. New York: Oxford University Press, 2009.

Leupold, Nancy E., and James J. Scubba, eds. *Meeting the Challenges of Oral and Head and Neck Cancer: A Survivor's Guide*. San Diego, CA: Plural Publishing, 2008.

McKay, Judith, and Tamera Schacher. *The Chemotherapy Survival Guide: Everything You Need to Know to Get through Treatment*, 3rd ed. Oakland, CA: New Harbinger Publications, 2009.

Perry, Michael P., ed. *The Chemotherapy Source Book*. Philadelphia: Wolters Kluwer Health/Lippincott Williams and Wilkins, 2008.

Pettit, Paul, editor in chief. *Mayo Clinic on Managing Incontinence*. Rochester, MN: Mayo Clinic, 2005.

PERIODICALS

Bartlett, L., et al. "Impact of Fecal Incontinence on Quality of Life." *World Journal of Gastroenterology* 15 (July 14, 2009): 3276–82.

Chamlou, R., et al. " Long-term Results of Intersphincteric Resection for Low Rectal Cancer." *Annals of Surgery* 246 (December 2007): 916–921.

Govaert, B., et al. "Neuromodulation for Functional Bowel Disorders." *Best Practice and Research: Clinical Gastroenterology* 23 (April 2009): 545–53.

Keating, N. L. "Physical and Mental Health Status of Older Long-term Cancer Survivors." *Journal of the American Geriatrics Society* 53 (December 2005): 2145–52.

Lange, M.M., and C. J. van de Velde. "Faecal and Urinary Incontinence after Multimodality Treatment of Rectal Cancer." *PLoS Medicine* 5 (October 7, 2008): 202.

Muehlbauer, P. M., et al. " Putting Evidence into Practice: Evidence-based Interventions to Prevent, Manage, and Treat Chemotherapy- and Radiotherapy-induced Diarrhea." *Clinical Journal of Oncology Nursing* 13 (June 2009): 336–41.

Parsons, B. A., et al. "Prostate Cancer and Urinary Incontinence." *Maturitas* 63 (August 20, 2009): 323–28.

OTHER

American Cancer Society (ACS). *Managing Incontinence after Prostate Cancer Treatment*. http://www.cancer.org/docroot/NWS/content/NWS_2_1x_Managing_Incontinence.asp.

American Cancer Society (ACS). *Managing Side Effects of Chemotherapy*. http://www.cancer.org/docroot/MBC/content/MBC_2_1x_Managing_Side_Effects_of_Chemotherapy.asp?sitearea=MBC.

American Cancer Society (ACS). *Radiation Therapy to the Stomach and Abdomen*. http://www.cancer.org/docroot/MBC/content/MBC_2_3X_What_Side_Effects_Occur_With_Radiation_Therapy_to_the_Stomach_and_Abdomen_Area.asp?sitearea=MBC.

American Society of Clinical Oncology (ASCO). *Managing Side Effects of Cancer Treatment: Diarrhea.* http://www.cancer.net/patient/Diagnosis + and + Treatment/Treating + Cancer/Managing + Side + Effects/Diarrhea + - + ASCO + curriculum.

American Society of Clinical Oncology (ASCO). *Managing Side Effects of Cancer Treatment: Nervous System Side Effects.* http://www.cancer.net/patient/Diagnosis + and + Treatment/Treating + Cancer/Managing + Side + Effects/Nervous + System + Side + Effects.

International Foundation for Functional Gastrointestinal Disorders (IFFGD). *About Incontinence.* http://www.aboutincontinence.org/.

Mayo Clinic. *Fecal Incontinence.* http://www.mayoclinic.com/health/fecal-incontinence/DS00477.

National Association for Continence (NAFC). *Incontinence Overview.* http://www.nafc.org/bladder-bowel-health/what-is-incontinence/.

National Cancer Institute (NCI). *Coping with Cancer: Gastrointestinal Complications.* http://www.cancer.gov/cancertopics/pdq/supportivecare/gastrointestinalcomplications/healthprofessional/allpages.

National Cancer Institute (NCI). *Managing Chemotherapy Side Effects: Urination Changes.* http://www.cancer.gov/cancertopics/chemo-side-effects/urination.

National Institute of Diabetes and Digestive and Kidney Diseases (NIDDK). *Fecal Incontinence.* http://digestive.niddk.nih.gov/ddiseases/pubs/fecalincontinence/index.htm

ORGANIZATIONS

American Cancer Society, 250 Williams Street NW, Atlanta, GA, 30303, 800-ACS-2345 (227-2345), www.cancer.org.

American College of Gastroenterology, P.O. Box 342260, Bethesda, MD, 20827-2260, 301-263-9000, http://www.acg.gi.org/.

American Society of Clinical Oncology (ASCO), 2318 Mill Road, Suite 800, Alexandria, VA, 22314, 571-483-1300, 888-282-2552, membermail@asco.org, http://www.asco.org/ASCOv2?edition = default.

National Association for Continence (NAFC), P.O. Box 1019, Charleston, SC, 29402, 843-377-0900, 800-BLADDER, 843-377-0905, memberservices@nafc.org, http://www.nafc.org/.

National Cancer Institute, 6116 Executive Blvd., Room 3036A, Bethesda, MD, 20892-8322, 800-422-6237, cancergovstaff@mail.nih.gov, www.cancer.gov.

National Institute of Diabetes and Digestive and Kidney Diseases (NIDDK), Building 31. Rm 9A06, 31 Center Drive, MSC 2560, Bethesda, MD, 20892-2560, 301-496-3583, http://www2.niddk.nih.gov/Footer/Contact NIDDK.htm, http://www2.niddk.nih.gov/.

International Foundation for Functional Gastrointestinal Disorders (IFFGD), P.O. Box 170864, MilwaukeeWI, United States, 53217-8076, 414-964-1799, 414-964-7176, iffgd@iffgd.org, http://www.iffgd.org/.

Stefanie B.N. Dugan, M.S.
Rebecca J. Frey, PhD

Infection and sepsis

Definition

In its most general sense, an infection represents the harmful colonization of a host by organisms of another species. The infecting organism seeks to exploit the host's resources to multiply, usually at the expense of the host. Sepsis is a serious medical condition characterized by an inflammatory response of the entire body and the presence of a suspected or known infection.

Because the term *sepsis* was used somewhat loosely before the 1990s, the American College of Chest Physicians and the Society of Critical Care Medicine drew up a set of definitions in 1992 to clarify the definitions of sepsis syndromes in order of severity:

- Sepsis: the presence of a systemic inflammatory response syndrome (SIRS) in the setting of an infection.
- Severe sepsis: infection with evidence of end-organ dysfunction as a result of hypoperfusion (inadequate blood supply to tissues and organs).
- Septic shock: severe sepsis with persistent low blood pressure despite fluid resuscitation and resulting tissue hypoperfusion.

Demographics

According to the U.S. National Center for Health Statistics, the incidence of sepsis increased threefold between 1979 and 2000, from 83 cases to 240 cases per year per 100,000 population. Severe sepsis accounts for more than 500,000 visits to hospital emergency departments each year in Canada and the United States. There are several reasons for this increase: the growing proportion of elderly in the general population; more efficient diagnosis of severe disease; a sharp rise in the number of invasive procedures and organ transplantation; increased use of immunosuppressive agents and **chemotherapy** in **cancer** patients; increased use of indwelling lines and devices in hospitalized patients; and a rise in such chronic diseases as end-stage renal disease and HIV infection.

As of 2009, African Americans—particularly males—have twice the risk of sepsis as members of other races, but this disparity is thought to reflect differences in access to treatment as well as differences in the severity of underlying conditions. Men of all races are at greater risk of severe sepsis and septic shock than women, but it is not known as of 2009 whether these data reflect more severe underlying conditions in men, a higher incidence of lung disease in men, or whether women have some inherent protection against the inflammation present in severe sepsis.

The incidence rate of sepsis in cancer patients in North America is estimated at 45%. Mortality rates from sepsis in cancer patients exceed 30%.

Description

Infection is characterized by an inflammatory response to the presence of microorganisms in the body. This response may include **fever**, chills, redness, swelling, pus formation, and other responses. The most common cause of illness and death in patients with cancer is infection. Patients with cancer who are treated with chemotherapy, **radiation therapy**, and/or surgery are at increased risk of developing an infection. Mortality from infection in cancer patients decreased during the late 1900s due to the development of new types of **antibiotics**, the use of hematopoietic growth factors (HGFs) which activate proliferation (multiplication) and maturation of blood cell lines, and due to the prophylactic (preventive) use of antifungal and antiviral agents. Blood cell lines, markedly decreased due to chemotherapy, are required to fight infections. Most infections in cancer patients are due to bacteria; however, fungal infections are usually the cause of fatal infections.

If left untreated, or if inadequately treated, infection can progress to sepsis. Several conditions indicate sepsis, including a temperature of greater than 38 degrees Celsius (100.4° Fahrenheit) or less than 36°C (96.8°F), heart rate greater than 90 beats per minutes, and respiratory rate greater than 20 breaths per minute.

Risk factors

Risk factors for infection and sepsis include:

- Weakened immune system.
- Hospitalization. Many infections are acquired during a hospital stay.
- Surgery, dental work, catheter or pacemaker insertion, placement of a prosthesis or artificial joint, or other procedures that involve cutting into or injuring tissue.
- Concurrent HIV infection.
- Treatment for cancer.
- Homelessness.
- Poor personal hygiene.
- Being treated for severe burns. Like cancer patients, burn patients are highly susceptible to infections.
- Age below 1 year or over 35 years.

- Pregnancy.
- History of lung disease.
- Using injected drugs of abuse.
- Abnormalities of the heart valves.

Causes and symptoms

Causes

There are many possible causes of infection in patients with cancer. For example, certain cancers interfere with the body's immune system response, which results in increased risk of infection to the patient. These cancer types include acute leukemia, **chronic lymphocytic leukemia**, **multiple myeloma**, **Hodgkin's disease**, and **non-Hodgkin's lymphoma**. Certain therapies used to treat cancer, such as chemotherapy (which interrupts bone marrow production of white blood cells, red blood cells, and platelets), radiation therapy, **bone marrow transplantation**, and treatments using **corticosteroids**, can lead to infection in the patient with cancer.

The protein-calorie malnutrition that some cancer patients experience can result in suppression of the immune system, which results in increased risk for infection. Many cancer patients develop infections from procedures which break the integrity of the skin, which then leads to the introduction of microorganisms into the body. These procedures include such common interventions in the care of cancer patients as venipunctures, biopsies, insertion of urinary catheters, and use of long-term central venous catheters. Infection rates associated with long-term central venous catheter use in cancer patients are estimated to be as high as 60%. If the cancer patient's immune system is severely compromised, infection can occur from food sources, plants, and/or air the patient comes in contact with.

Myelosuppression is the term used to describe the decrease in numbers of circulating white blood cells (WBC), red blood cells (RBC), and platelets. Myelosuppression is often a side effect of treatment with chemotherapy and/or radiation therapy. Blood counts usually begin to fall one to three weeks after treatment with chemotherapy, depending upon the type of chemotherapy and the lifespan of the blood cell. The counts generally begin to recover to normal levels within two to three weeks. The neutrophil, which is a component of the white blood cells, is the body's first line of defense against infection caused by bacteria. A state of **neutropenia** exists when the number of neutrophils is decreased. Neutropenia is the single greatest predictor of infection in patients with cancer. Three key factors are important in predicting the potential of a patient to experience an infectious episode when myelosuppressed. These factors include: 1) the degree of neutropenia, i.e., the lower the neutrophil count the more likely the patient will become infected; 2) the duration of the neutropenia, i.e., the longer a patient is neutropenic, the greater the likelihood of infection; and 3) the rate at which neutropenia develops—the more rapidly it develops, the greater the risk of infection.

Bacterial infections in cancer patients develop quickly, especially in the neutropenic patient, and account for 85–90% of the microorganisms associated with neutropenia accompanied by fever. The most serious episodes occur from infections attributed to such gram-negative organisms as *Enterobacteriaceae* or *Pseudomonas aeruginosa*. However, infections from such gram-positive organisms as *Staphylococcus, Streptococcus, Corynebacteria*, and *Clostridia* have increased in the 1990s, probably due to the increased use of implanted central venous catheters and prophylactic antibiotics (to which these organisms develop an immunity). Listeriosis, a severe bacterial infection caused by *Listeria monocytogenes*, is another infection on the increase in cancer patients. Listeriosis has become a common complication of bone marrow transplantation in the early 2000s as well as a frequent cause of patient death.

Other organisms that cause infections in the immunocompromised cancer patient include such herpesviruses as **herpes simplex** virus 1 and 2 (HSV-1, HSV-2), varicella zoster virus (VZV), cytomegalovirus (CMV), and **Epstein-Barr virus** (EBV). Sources of secondary infections include the fungus *Candida albicans*. Common causes of secondary infection in severely immunosuppressed patients include CMV and the filamentous fungus *Aspergillus*. Aspergillosis is an increasingly common and often fatal infection in patients with hematologic (blood-related) cancers.

The incidence of sepsis and septic shock increases when the patient remains neutropenic for longer than seven days. Other factors that put the cancer patient at high risk for the development of sepsis include infection with a gram-negative organism, presence of a central venous catheter, history of prior infection, malnutrition, history of frequent hospitalization, increased age of patient, and concurrent (at the same time) presence of such other diseases as diabetes, cardiovascular, gastrointestinal, hepatic, pulmonary, and/or renal disease. Sites of infection that most often lead to sepsis include infection of the lungs, invasive lines, and urinary tract.

Symptoms

Sepsis manifests (develops) with both local and systemic symptoms that involve the neurologic,

endocrine, immunologic, and cardiovascular systems. Signs of sepsis and septic shock include changes in blood pressure, heart rate and respiratory rate, among others. If left untreated, the patient can progress to septic shock which may result in death even if the shock episode is treated. Factors that appear to increase the patient's chances of survival include rapid admission to an intensive care unit and aggressive treatment with antibiotics.

Diagnosis

The diagnosis of sepsis is based on the following criteria:

- Temperature above 101°F or below 96°F.
- Heart rate above 90 beats per minute (bpm).
- Respiration more than 20 breaths per minute.
- WBC higher than $12,000/mm^3$ or lower than $4,000/mm^3$.
- Low blood pressure: lower than 90 mmHg or a reduction of 40 mmHg or more from the patient's baseline blood pressure.
- Abnormalities in platelet count.
- Altered mental status: delirium, confusion, anxiety, and/or agitation.
- Reduced output of urine (oliguria).

A patient does not have to meet all these criteria to be diagnosed with severe sepsis or septic shock.

Examination

In addition to abnormalities in the patient's vital signs, the doctor may also observe changes in mental status or the condition of the patient's skin. In the early stages of septic shock, the patient's skin is often warm to the touch; in later stages, the skin may become clammy and cool to the touch. It may also develop a pale, grayish, or mottled color. The doctor will listen to the patient's breathing for evidence of fluid accumulation in the lungs. If the infection appears to be localized, the doctor will evaluate that portion of the patient's body for redness, swelling, pain, or a discharge.

Tests

Standard laboratory tests for infection and suspected sepsis include a complete blood cell count (CBC) and a blood chemistry panel; measurement of hemoglobin levels; a blood culture to identify the organism causing the infection; liver function tests; urine tests; and a test of the patient's sputum when **pneumonia** is suspected.

Imaging tests are ordered as appropriate for the location of the infection. They may include chest x rays, abdominal ultrasounds, CT or MRI imaging, or x-ray studies of the extremities when soft tissue infections are suspected. The patient will also usually be given an EKG to check for abnormal heart rhythms.

Procedures

Patients with severe sepsis or septic shock are usually intubated to keep the airway open. Other procedures that may be performed include a **lumbar puncture** (spinal tap) if meningitis is suspected; placement of a urinary catheter to monitor the patient's urine output; and surgical drainage of any abscesses.

Treatment

Traditional

Sepsis is a medical emergency and is usually treated in an intensive care unit (ICU). It includes maintenance of ventilation, oxygenation, fluid volume, and cardiac output as well as antibiotic treatment and **nutritional support**. Patients may be placed on a mechanical ventilator to assist with breathing or given supplemental oxygen if needed. Speed of treatment is essential; several studies have shown that for every hour of delay in the administration of appropriate antibiotic therapy, there is an associated 7% rise in mortality.

Drugs

Empiric antibiotic therapy is the mainstay of treatment for infection in the cancer patient. Empiric therapy refers to initiation of antibiotic therapy prior to the identification of the infecting organism. Broad-spectrum antibiotics, antibiotics effective against both gram-negative and gram-positive organisms, are administered. Commonly used agents include aminoglycosides, fluoroquinolones, glycopeptides, and beta-lactams such as penicillins, cephalosporins, carbapenems, and monobactams.

Empiric **antifungal therapy** is initiated 5–7 days after empiric antibiotic therapy has been started if the patient remains febrile (with a fever). Antiviral agents may be administered if there is evidence of a viral infection. The Infectious Diseases Society of America (IDSA) recommends a minimum of five to seven days further treatment with parenteral (introduced in other ways than intestinal absorption) antibiotic therapy after the fever resolves (returns to normal). Continued monitoring of bacterial and fungal culture results is

essential. This allows the use of more tailored antibiotics for the specific infectious agents.

The neutropenic patient with fever can progress quickly to sepsis and septic shock if left untreated. The patient may also progress to septic shock if empiric antibiotic coverage is inadequate. The most common cause of septic shock in cancer patients is infection with gram-negative bacteria.

In addition to antibiotics, patients with sepsis may also be given corticosteroids to bring down inflammation.

Patients with severe sepsis or septic shock can be treated with drotrecogin alfa (Xigris; also known as activated protein C), which is an artificially produced human protein that prevents inflammation and blood clotting. It is thought to reduce the risk of death from severe sepsis and septic shock. Xigris was approved for the treatment of severe sepsis by the Food and Drug Administration (FDA) in 2001; it can be administered only in an ICU by a doctor qualified in critical care medicine, however.

Prognosis

The mortality rate for severe sepsis and septic shock is frequently quoted as anywhere from 20% to 50%. The most detailed recent study gives a death rate of 30%. Other studies report that between 20% and 35% of patients with severe sepsis and 40–60% of patients with septic shock die within 30 days of hospital admission. Risk factors for mortality with infection and sepsis include delayed antibiotic treatment; male sex; older age (especially age over 50); the presence of two or more other illnesses; altered mental status; and acquiring the infection in a hospital.

Prevention

Strategies that can be used to prevent or minimize infection in the neutropenic patient include:

- Identification of patients at highest risk for infection.

- Avoiding practices by health care team members that increase colonization of microorganisms.

- Implementation of fewer invasive procedures when possible.

Cancer patients at risk for neutropenia may also benefit from treatment with two new hematopoietic growth factors, pegfilgrastim (Neulasta) and darbepoietin alfa (Aranesp). These drugs appear to be effective in reducing the risk of opportunistic infections in cancer patients as well as improving their overall quality of life.

Specific interventions in the hospital setting that can be used to prevent or minimize infection include:

- scrupulous handwashing by patient, staff, and visitors.

- good personal hygiene, including an oral care protocol by the patient.

- ambulation (movement).

- aggressive efforts to promote lung expansion.

- elimination of uncooked fruits and vegetables from the diet.

- removal of plants and other sources of stagnant water from the patient's room.

- screening and minimizing outside visitors to avoid those with infection

In addition, the hospitalized patient should be assessed by the staff at least every four hours and laboratory results collected and analyzed to determine risk for and presence of neutropenia.

A newer method to prevent infection in the cancer patient works by decreasing the duration of neutropenia. This method decreases the period of maximum risk for infection by using hematopoietic growth factors (HGFs). These growth factors are administered daily beginning 24 hours after chemotherapy, and shorten the duration and severity of neutropenia. Therefore, the period of risk for infection is shortened. HGFs work by activating the production and maturation of RBCs, WBCs, and platelet cell lines. Specific HGFs stimulate the production and maturation of aggressive neutrophils and macrophages, which are effective in destroying pathogens (bacteria or viruses that cause infection or disease).

Sepsis can be avoided by preventing infection in immunocompromised patients and by recognizing risk factors and altering those factors whenever possible.

Resources

BOOKS

Daniels, Ron, and Tim Nutbeam, eds. *ABC of Sepsis.* Hoboken, NJ: BMJ Wiley-Blackwell, 2010.

Perrin, Kathleen Ouimet. *Understanding the Essentials of Critical Care Nursing.* Upper Saddle River, NJ: Pearson Prentice Hall, 2009.

Rello, Jordi, and Marcos I. Restrepo, eds. *Sepsis: New Strategies for Management.* Berlin: Springer, 2008.

PERIODICALS

Annane, D., et al. "Corticosteroids in the Treatment of Severe Sepsis and Septic Shock in Adults: A Systematic Review." *Journal of the American Medical Association* 301 (June 10, 2009): 2362–75.

Cohen, J. "Sepsis and Septic Shock: Inching Forward." *Clinical Medicine* 9 (June 2009): 256–57.

Cull, L.F., and M.B. Nolan. "Treating Neutropenic Fever in the Emergency Department: Delays May Be Deadly!" *Journal of Emergency Nursing* 35 (January 2009): 36–39.

Hirasawa, H., et al. "Blood Glucose Control in Patients with Severe Sepsis and Septic Shock." *World Journal of Gastroenterology* 15 (September 7, 2009): 4132–36.

Mann, H.J., et al. "Protein C in Critical Illness." *American Journal of Health-System Pharmacy* 66 (June 15, 2009): 1089–96.

Marraro, G. A. "Treatment of Septic Shock and Use of Drotrecogin Alfa (Activated) in Children." *Expert Review of Anti-infective Therapy* 7 (September 2009): 769–72.

Panwar, R., et al. "Plasma Protein C Levels in Immunocompromised Septic Patients Are Significantly Lower Than Immunocompetent Septic Patients: A Prospective Cohort Study." *Journal of Hematology and Oncology* 2 (October 19, 2009): 43.

Park, H.Y., et al. "Outcome and Prognostic Factors of Patients with Acute Leukemia Admitted to the Intensive Care Unit for Septic Shock." *Leukemia and Lymphoma* 49 (October 2008): 1929–34.

da Silva, E.D., et al. "Risk Factors for Death in Children and Adolescents with Cancer and Sepsis/Septic Shock." *Journal of Pediatric Hematology/Oncology* 30 (July 2008): 513–18.

OTHER

Filbin, Michael R. "Shock, Septic." *eMedicine*, August 12, 2009. http://emedicine.medscape.com/article/786058-overview.

JAMA Patient Page. "Sepsis." *Journal of the American Medical Association* 301 (June 17, 2009): 2516. http://jama.ama-assn.org/cgi/reprint/301/23/2516.pdf.

Mayo Clinic. "Blood Poisoning: What Does It Mean?" http://www.mayoclinic.com/health/blood-poisoning/AN00716.

Young, Lowell S. "Sepsis and Septic Shock." *Merck Manual of Medical Information*, 2nd home edition. http://www.merck.com/mmhe/print/sec17/ch191/ch191c.html.

ORGANIZATIONS

American College of Emergency Physicians (ACEP), 1125 Executive Circle, Irving, TX, 75038-2522, 972-550-0911, 800-798-1822, 972-580-2816, http://www.acep.org/.

Centers for Disease Control and Prevention (CDC), 1600 Clifton Road, Atlanta, GA, 30333, 800-232-4636, cdcinfo@cdc.gov, http://www.cdc.gov.

Infectious Diseases Society of America (IDSA), 1300 Wilson Boulevard, Suite 300, Arlington, VA, 22209, 703-299-0200, 703-299-0204, info@idsociety.org, http://www.idsociety.org/.

National Institute of Allergy and Infectious Diseases (NIAID), 6610 Rockledge Drive, MSC 6612, Bethesda, MD, 20892-6612, 301-496-5717, 866-284-4107, 301-402-3573, http://www3.niaid.nih.gov.

International Sepsis Forum (ISF), US mailing address: 7024 Palmetto Pines Lane, Land O'LakesFL, United States, 34637, 813-235-9813 (US only), 813-235-9014 (US only), elaine@sepsisforum.org, http://www.sepsis forum.org/.

World Health Organization (WHO), Avenue Appia 20, 1211 Geneva 27, Switzerland, + 41 22 791 21 11, + 41 22 791 31 11, info@who.int, http://www.who.int/en/.

Melinda Granger Oberleitner, R.N., D.N.S.
Rebecca J. Frey, Ph.D.

Infertility *see* Fertility issues

Intensity modulated radiation therapy

Definition

Intensity modulated **radiation therapy** uses a computer to deliver precise, three-dimensional doses of **x rays** to a tumor to treat **cancer**.

Purpose

As a new and special form of radiation therapy, intensity modulated radiation therapy (IMRT) offers special treatment options for cancer patients. When a patient has cancer, he or she may have radiation therapy to destroy the tumor or cancerous cells. The radiation therapy may be the only treatment given or a treatment prescribed along with surgery and/or **chemotherapy**.

The radiation aimed at the cancerous cells also can destroy nearby healthy cells. IMRT is an advanced treatment method that allows physicians to target the cancer so effectively that healthy tissue receives little to no radiation, even when the tumor is wrapped around a vital organ. This makes IMRT a good choice for many cancer patients, particularly those with small tumors, brain and spinal cord tumors, **prostate cancer**, cancer of the head and neck, many children, infants with certain muscle tumors, and some patients who have previously received radiation treatments. Research continues on expanding use of IMRT for a number of cancers; **clinical trials** are underway around the world.

Precautions

Any time a patient is considered for radiation therapy, physicians weigh the risks and benefits of the procedure. IMRT, like any external radiation therapy procedure, introduces x rays (ionizing radiation) to the patient's skin, tissues, and organs near the treatment area. Some patients will not be candidates for treatment. IMRT will require frequent trips to the radiation oncology facility for the prescribed treatment plan and careful following of instructions to deal with radiation side effects. On the positive side, the accuracy of IMRT means some patients who may not have been candidates for radiation therapy under older, less precise methods now can have radiation treatment. IMRT can deliver radiation to the intended target more precisely and do a better job of sparing surrounding organs and tissues. The oncology treatment team should discuss all risks and benefits of IMRT with the patient.

Description

Physicians have used radiation to treat cancer for more than 100 years. The damaging effects of x rays can destroy cancerous cells in the body and help rid the patient of the pain or related spread and complications of some cancers. For some patients, radiation therapy is the first treatment physicians choose; for others the treatment is used after surgery or chemotherapy or at the same time as chemotherapy. Radiation therapy also sometimes is called "radiotherapy."

The goal of radiation therapy is to destroy as many cancer cells as possible, while limiting damage to nearby healthy tissue. To accomplish this, complicated dose measurements are made based on information gathered by studying the tumor before radiation treatment begins. Today, physicians can use procedures such as **computed tomography** (CT) to produce three-dimensional models that can better pinpoint the tumor. Planning radiation treatments in three dimensions allows physicians to target the radiation beams at the tumor's height, width, and depth. This newer technique is called "3-D conformal radiation therapy."

IMRT is a new type of 3-D conformal radiation therapy that uses beams of varying intensities. By doing so, the beams, which can strike the tumor from three dimensions, also can deliver different doses to small areas of tissue at once. This offers more individualized targeting of the tumor than in the past, so that the radiation oncologist (a physician who specializes in using radiation to treat cancer) can plan higher doses to the tumor and lower doses to the nearby tissue. Insurance companies have found IMRT a valuable treatment for many cancers in recent years because of its effectiveness.

Tomotherapy is a form of IMRT that delivers the radiation dose by rotating the beams over a small slice of tissue.

Most IMRT procedures are performed at a cancer center, radiation oncology physician office or outpatient facility, or in a hospital. The radiation oncologist oversees the patient's plan, working closely with a team of professionals. A medical physicist has special training in radiation physics and the operation and repair of radiology and radiation therapy equipment. The physicist also may help develop the patient's treatment plan. A medical dosimetrist works under the direction of the radiation oncologist and medical physicist to calculate radiation dose. IMRT treatments normally are performed by a radiation therapist, a specially trained technologist who positions the patient and runs the equipment. A radiation oncology nurse also may help with managing care, side effects, and explaining the treatments.

As the treatment begins, the patient is positioned on a treatment table in a precise location that has been set in treatment planning or simulation sessions. A special molding or other device may be applied to help keep the patient from moving during the procedure. The radiation therapist can observe the patient throughout the entire procedure through a window or closed circuit television. The therapist may reposition the patient during the procedure. A treatment session usually lasts about 15 to 30 minutes. The procedure should be painless, but if the patient is uncomfortable, the therapist can stop the machine. The number of treatments a patient must return for will depend on the type and stage of cancer. Some patients may receive treatments every day for a period of a several weeks.

Preparation

Before beginning IMRT treatment, the radiation oncologist and treatment team will need to know the precise location of the tumor in the body (anatomical position). This means the patient may have to go for several **imaging studies** in addition to those already completed to diagnose the cancer. Computed tomography (CT), **positron emission tomography** (PET) scans, and **magnetic resonance imaging** (MRI) may be used to provide three-dimensional information for the IMRT system. These imaging visits and the resulting work of the treatment team often are called treatment simulation. The patient also may have to go to the radiation therapy facility prior to treatment for a planning session. At this session, a special device may be molded to help the patient maintain an exact treatment position. The patient also may receive a mark or tattoo with colored ink to help align and target the equipment once treatment begins.

Aftercare

The radiation oncologist, radiation therapist, or radiation oncology nurse will provide instructions on IMRT aftercare. Since some effects of radiation therapy do not begin to show up until after several treatments, these instructions may vary throughout the course of treatment. Some side effects of radiation therapy occur soon after treatment begins, but others occur later. The most common side effects of external radiation therapy are **fatigue** and skin changes.

People undergoing radiation therapy who become fatigued may need to reduce their routines somewhat and not try to do too much. It is best to keep in touch with the treatment team for advice on feelings of fatigue and care for its effects. If skin becomes irritated, it also is important to follow the team's instructions concerning washing, sun exposure, and use of skin care products.

Risks

Radiation therapy carries the risk of radiation reaching and damaging normal tissues or organs near the area being targeted. However, IMRT treatment is more precise than other external radiation therapy procedures. There also is a small risk of dose being calculated incorrectly and a patient receiving too much radiation, but equipment should be run by FDA-approved software. Facilities have many quality processes in place to ensure the correct dose is given to the precise location on the correct patient. Radiation therapy also can cause low levels of white blood cells and platelets. White blood cells help fight **infection** and platelets help blood clot. Radiation therapy causes other side effects and risks, depending on the area being treated, though many only last a short time. For example, radiation treatment to the head can cause hair loss (**alopecia**), but the hair eventually will grow back.

Normal results

After completion of IMRT treatments, cancer cells should stop dividing and growing, which should slow tumor growth. Often, cancer cells completely die and a tumor shrinks or disappears. With IMRT, there should be little radiation damage to the normal, healthy tissues around the tumor and fewer resulting side effects.

Abnormal results

The treatment may not always completely eliminate cancer cells. A cancer may still partially remain or recur at a later date. Physicians usually follow up with imaging studies to see how the treatment is progressing and set up a future schedule check for cancer recurrence.

Resources

PERIODICALS

"Beyond Conventional Radiation" *RN* (June 1998):34–38.
"IMRT and Image-guided Tumor Localization Improve Radiotherapy in Prostate Cancer." *Health & Medicine Week* (April 5, 2004):691.
"IMRT Reduces Radiation Dose to Healthy Breast Tissue." *Cancer Weekly* (Oct. 26, 2004):30.
Leaver, Dennis. "IMRT Part I." *Radiation Therapist* (Fall 2002):106–124.
"Study Finds IMRT Is Cost-effective Compared to Previous Conformal Technique." *Medical Devices & Surgical Technology Week* (October 31, 2004):291.

OTHER

*External Radiation Therapy.*Web page. American Cancer Society, 2004. http://www.cancer.org.

*Intensity-modulated Radiation Therapy (IMRT).*Web page. Radiological Society of North America, 2005. http://www.radiologyinfo.org.

ORGANIZATIONS

American Society for Therapeutic Radiology and Oncology. 12500 Fair Lakes Circle, Suite 375, Fairfax, VA 22033-3882. 800-962-7862. http://www.astro.org.

Teresa G. Odle

Interferons

Definition

Interferons are in a class of naturally occurring small proteins or glycoproteins called cytokines. They are produced by white blood cells called leucocytes and T lymphocytes (T cells) and by fibroblasts, as part of an **immune response** to **infection** or other biological stimuli. Interferons are synthesized or produced through genetic engineering for use as immunotherapy medications in the treatment of viral infections, **cancer**, and multiple sclerosis (MS).

Purpose

The first interferon was discovered in 1957 as an immune-system agent that was produced in response to viral infection and interfered with the production of new viral particles—hence the name "interferon." Recombinant DNA technology has since been adapted to produce interferons for research and drug treatments. Interferons attach to specific receptors on the surfaces of cell membranes, where they have a variety of effects on the immune system including the stimulation and inhibition of enzymes, inhibition of cell proliferation, and enhancement of macrophage and T-lymphocyte activities.

There are several different classes of interferons, including alfa, beta, gamma, tau, and omega. These classes are further broken into subclasses designated with Arabic numerals and letters. Alfa and beta interferons are type I interferons that are produced by white blood cells and fibroblasts (a type of connective-tissue cell). Gamma interferon is a type II interferon produced by T cells when they are activated by infection or another stimulus.

Alfa interferons are used to treat viral infections and cancer:

- Interferon alfacon-1 is a synthetic interferon used to treat chronic hepatitis C infection. It binds to the same receptor that binds the hepatitis C virus, thereby preventing the virus from entering and infecting host cells.
- Interferons alfa-2a and alfa-2b are used to treat both cancer and viral infections.
- Peginterferon is interferon alfa combined with polyethylene glycol, which keeps the interferon active longer. Peginterferon alfa-2a and alfa-2b are used to prevent further liver damage in patients with chronic hepatitis C infections, often in combination with the antiviral drug ribavirin. Peginterferon alfa-2a is also used to treat chronic hepatitis B infections.
- Interferon alfa-n3 is used to treat recurring or refractory genital or venereal warts.

In cancer immunotherapy alfa interferons activate tumor-specific cytotoxic T lymphocytes that destroy tumor cells, although the molecular details of this activity remain unclear. Interferons may cause antigens on the exposed tumor surface to more readily stimulate the immune system's T-cell response. Tumor growth may also be slowed by interferon-mediated damage to the blood cells that nourish the tumor. Alfa interferons are used to treat **hairy cell leukemia**, malignant **melanoma**, and Kaposi's **sarcoma**, an AIDS-related cancer. Alfa interferons are used off-label to treat many other cancers including kidney and bladder cancers, **chronic myelocytic leukemia**, carcinoid tumors, non-Hodgkin's **lymphoma**, **ovarian cancer**, and skin cancers. Alfa interferons may be combined with other chemotherapeutic drugs such as **doxorubicin**.

Interferons beta-1a and beta-1b are used to decrease the number of symptomatic episodes or flare-ups of MS and to slow the progression of the disease in patients with relapsing-remitting MS. Interferon does not help patients with chronic progressive MS in which symptoms are always present. MS is an autoimmune disease in which the body's own immune system demyelinates the myelin sheaths enclosing nerve cells. Demyelination causes malfunctions in the transmission of impulses from nerve to nerve and from nerve to muscle. Interferon beta-1a is in a class of medications called immunomodulators, but it is not known exactly how it decreases MS flare-ups.

Interferon beta-1b is a synthetic version of a human protein that is in a class of medications known as biologic response modifiers. It enhances T-cell activity while simultaneously reducing the production of inflammatory cytokines. Interferon beta-1b also retards the exposure of antigens on the surfaces of cells, thereby reducing the immune response to the antigen and slowing the appearance of lymphocytes in the central nervous system. This dampening of the immune response can reduce both symptomatic episodes of MS and damage to neurons in the brain. In 2006 the U.S. Food and Drug Administration (FDA) extended approval of interferon beta 1-b for use in patients who are at high risk of developing MS.

Interferon gamma-1b is a synthetic version of a naturally occurring interferon. It is used to treat chronic granulomatous disease, an inherited immune-system disorder.

Description

There are no generic forms of interferon. Interferons are always administered by injection, usually by the patient or caregiver. They cannot be taken by mouth because they are destroyed by stomach acids. The injections can be either intramuscular (IM; into a muscle) or subcutaneous (SC). SC injections are made under the skin, between the fat layer and the muscle, often in the abdomen, thigh, buttocks, or upper arm—anywhere that there is a fat layer between the skin and muscle, except around the waist or near the navel. Each injection is at a different site than the previous one, because side effects at the injection site are common. Injections are always on the same day(s) of the week at approximately the same time of day, usually late afternoon or evening before bedtime, so that the worst of the side effects occur during sleep.

U.S. brand names

- Infergen (interferon alfacon-1, SC injection) supplied as a 30-microgram (mcg) per milliliter (ml) solution of 0.3 or 0.5 ml
- Roferon-A (interferon alfa-2a, recombinant)
- Intron A (interferon alfa-2b, recombinant)

- Pegasys (peginterferon alfa-2a), for SC injection, supplied in a 1.2-ml-solution vial of 180 mcg per ml or a pre-filled syringe with 180 mcg in 0.5 ml
- PEG-Intron (peginterferon alfa-2b), for SC injection, supplied as powder in a vial to which solution is added or as a single-dose injection pen
- Alferon N (interferon alfa-n3) supplied as a 1-ml 5-million-unit solution.
- Avonex (interferon beta-1a, IM injection) supplied as a liquid in a pre-filled syringe or as a powder in a single-use vial that is mixed into a solution
- Rebif (interferon beta-1a, SC injection) supplied in 22-mcg pre-filled syringes
- Betaseron (interferon beta-1b, SC injection) supplied with pre-filled syringes to which the medication is added; also available in an autoinjector
- Actimmune (interferon gamma-1b)

Canadian brand names

- Infergen (alfacon-1)
- Alferon N (alfa-n3)
- Pegasys (peginterferon alfa-2a)
- PEG-Intron (peginterferon alfa-2b)
- Avonex (beta-1a)
- Betaseron (beta-1b)

International brand names

- Infergen, Inferax (alfacon-1)
- Pegintron, ViraferonPeg (peginterferon alfa-2b)

Recommended dosage

- Interferon alfacon-1 is injected three times per week at 9 mcg per dose for 24 weeks. For patients who do not respond or have relapsed, the dosage may be increased to 15 mcg for six months.
- Dosages of interferons alfa-2a and -2b depend on various factors including the condition being treated, the patient's weight, and other medications that are being administered. They are generally injected daily for 10–24 weeks during what is called the induction period. During the following maintenance period, the drug is injected once every three weeks. Treatment usually continues for at least six months.
- The usual adult dosage of peginterferon alfa-2a is 180 mcg (less if side effects are severe) once per week for 24 or 48 weeks, injected into the abdomen or thigh.
- Peginterferon alfa-2b is injected once per week at a dosage that depends on body weight. Treatment usually continues for one year.

- Interferon alfa-n3 (0.05 ml; 250,000 units) is injected into each wart twice weekly for a maximum of eight weeks. The treatment is not repeated for at least three months.
- The usual dosage of interferon beta-1a is 30–44 mcg. Avonex is injected once per week. Rebif is injected three times per week, with at least 48 hours between injections. The initial dosage of Rebif is usually 8.8 mcg, gradually increased to 44 mcg over a four-week period.
- Interferon beta-1b is usually injected every other day at an initial dose of 62.5 mcg, gradually increased over six weeks to 250 mcg.
- Interferon gamma-1b is SC injected three times per week.

Precautions

Interferons can reduce the number of white blood cells in the body, causing increased susceptibility to infection. Patients on interferon should avoid contact with people who have infections and should consult their physicians immediately if they believe they are developing an infection. Patients should take care not to cut themselves, should not touch their eyes or inside of their nose with unwashed hands, and should take care when brushing their teeth so as not to cause bleeding. Patients are often advised to drink extra water to avoid low blood pressure. Patients on interferon beta should have periodic liver function tests.

Pediatric

Most interferon treatments have not been studied for safety in children under age 18. However beta interferon is approved for treating MS in children.

Geriatric

Although interferon treatment has not been studied in elderly patients, they may require lower dosages.

Pregnant or breastfeeding

Alpha interferons have not been shown to cause problems in fetuses. The fetal effects of beta interferons are unknown and they are not approved for use during pregnancy. Women of childbearing potential should use reliable birth control while on beta interferon. The FDA has required interferon manufacturers to develop pregnancy registers to monitor the outcomes in women who have become unintentionally pregnant while receiving beta interferon. Because it is not known whether interferons cross into breast milk, women should not breastfeed while undergoing interferon treatment.

Other conditions and allergies

The following conditions may be exacerbated by interferons:

- bleeding problems
- depression or other mental problems
- convulsions
- diabetes mellitus
- heart disease
- heart attack
- liver disease
- kidney disease
- lung disease
- an overactive immune system

Patients who have had or are at risk for seizures, as well as those with heart disorders such as angina, congestive heart failure, or an irregular heartbeat, should be closely monitored following interferon injection. Before receiving an interferon injection patients should notify their doctors if they are allergic to immunoglobulins or egg whites.

Side effects

The side effects of interferon treatment vary from the uncomfortable to the severe. The most common side effects of interferons are general flu-like symptoms including:

- headache
- loss of appetite
- nausea and vomiting
- fatigue
- fever
- chills
- sweating
- muscle aches
- an unusual metallic taste in the mouth
- irritability

These symptoms tend to diminish with time. Physicians may suggest taking acetaminophen (e.g., Tylenol) or ibuprofen (e.g., Advil) before each dosage.

Interferons sometimes cause serious side effects from their actions on the central nervous system. Since most side effects are dose-dependent, severe side effects may require dosage modification. Symptoms of central nervous system side effects include:

- difficulty concentrating
- confusion

- mental depression
- nervousness
- numbness or tingling of fingers, toes, and face Although uncommon, patients who are already clinically depressed may develop suicidal feelings during interferon treatment.

Other side effects may include:

- infection, swelling, inflammation, bruising, or necrosis (cell death) at the site of injection
- menstrual cycle changes in women
- liver and thyroid malfunction
- decreases in platelets and red and white blood cells
- a variety of other—sometimes very serious—side effects, depending on the specific interferon

Other conditions and allergies

Interferon induces an allergic reaction in some people. However the massive and sometimes fatal allergic reaction termed anaphylaxis is rare with interferons.

Interactions

Interferons can interact with a variety of other medications, in some cases increasing their effects. Interferons should not be combined with any other medications except under a physician's supervision.

Most medications that interact with alfa interferons are those that affect the central nervous system including:

- antihistamines
- sedatives
- tranquilizers
- sleeping medications
- prescription pain medicines

- seizure medications
- muscle relaxants
- narcotics
- barbiturates

Other drugs that may interact with interferons include:

- Warfarin
- Clozapine, an antipsychotic
- Theophylline
- Prednisone

Alfa interferons can increase the effects of alcohol. Alcohol can worsen the side effects of beta interferons. During interferon treatment alcohol should be consumed only with the physician's consent. Alcohol should never be consumed by patients with hepatitis.

Resources

BOOKS

Pitha, Paula M. *Interferon: The 50th Anniversary*. New York: Springer, 2007.

Plotnikoff, Nicholas P. *Cytokines: Stress and Immunity*, 2nd ed. Boca Raton, FL: CRC/Taylor & Francis, 2007.

Stephensen, Frank Harold. *DNA: How the Biotech Revolution Is Changing the Way We Fight Disease*. Amherst, NY: Prometheus Books, 2007.

PERIODICALS

Coghlan, Andy. "Cheap Drug Dodges Big Pharma Patents." *New Scientist* 193, no. 2585 (January 6–12, 2007): 14.

Cooper, Chet. "MS in Children." *Ability Magazine* 2007, no. 5 (2007): 56–61.

Criscuolo, Domenico. "A Place for Proteins." *Applied Clinical Trials* (May 2009): 6–8.

OTHER

"Avonex (Interferon Beta 1a)." *National Multiple Sclerosis Society*. http://www.nationalmssociety.org/about-multiple-sclerosis/treatments/medications/interferon-beta-1a-avonex/index.aspx.

"Betaseron (Interferon Beta 1b)." *National Multiple Sclerosis Society*. http://www.nationalmssociety.org/about-multiple-sclerosis/treatments/medications/interferon-beta-1b/index.aspx.

"Biological Therapies for Cancer: Questions and Answers." *National Cancer Institute*. http://www.cancer.gov/cancer topics/factsheet/Therapy/biological.

"Interferons-alfa." *American Cancer Society*. http://www.cancer.org/docroot/CDG/content/CDG_interferons_alfa.asp.

National Digestive Diseases Information Clearinghouse. "Chronic Hepatitis C: Current Disease Management." *NIH Publication No. 07-4230*. http://digestive.niddk.nih.gov/ddiseases/pubs/chronichepc/.

"Rebif (Interferon Beta 1a)." *National Multiple Sclerosis Society*. http://www.nationalmssociety.org/about-multiple- sclerosis/treatments/medications/interferon-beta-1a-rebif/index.aspx.

ORGANIZATIONS

American Cancer Society, 1599 Clifton Road NE, Atlanta, GA, 30329-4251, (800) ACS-2345, http://www.cancer.org.

National Cancer Institute, NCI Public Inquiries Office, 6116 Executive Boulevard, Room 3036A, Bethesda, MD, 20892-8322, (800) 4-CANCER, http://www.cancer.gov.

National Digestive Diseases Information Clearinghouse, 2 Information Way, Bethesda, MD, 20892-3570, (800) 891-5389, (703) 738-4929 , nddic@info.niddk.nih.gov, http://www.digestive.niddk.nih.gov.

National Multiple Sclerosis Society, 733 Third Avenue, New York, NY, 10017, (800) 344-4867, http://www.nationalmssociety.org.

U.S. Food and Drug Administration, 10903 New Hampshire Ave., Silver Spring, MD, 20993-0002, (888) INFO-FDA, http://www.fda.gov.

Sally C. McFarlane-Parrott
Brian Douglas Hoyle, PhD
Margaret Alic, PhD

Interleukin 2

Definition

Interleukin-2 (IL-2) is a protein produced naturally in the body in very small amounts. It is produced by a type of white blood cell called a T-lymphocyte and acts as part of the immune system by helping white blood cells work. **Aldesleukin** is a biological response modifier, a synthetic form of interleukin-2.

Purpose

Interleukin-2 (IL-2) is a naturally occurring chemical, called a cytokine, produced by certain cells of the immune system. It is also manufactured and administered as a drug to augment immune responses. While it is approved by the U.S. Food and Drug Administration (FDA) only for the treatment of **kidney cancer**, it is also used in the treatment of HIV and AIDS. Inhaled interleukin-2 may halt disease progression in patients with kidney **cancer** that has spread to the lungs. Aldesleukin, a synthetic version of interleukin-2, is used to treat cancer of the kidney and **skin cancer** that has spread to other parts of the body.

Aldesleukin is approved by the United States Food and Drug Administration (FDA) for treatment of metastatic malignant **melanoma** (skin cancer that has spread to other parts of the body) and metastatic renal cell **carcinoma** (kidney cancer that has spread to other parts of the body). It has also been used in combination with other drugs in treatment of AIDS and **cutaneous t-cell lymphoma**.

Description

The kidneys are a pair of bean-shaped organs, located on the sides of the spine. The kidneys filter the blood and eliminate waste in the urine through a complex system of filtration tubules. All of the blood in the body passes through the kidneys approximately twenty times an hour. Renal cell cancer (RCC) is an uncommon form of cancer that is most often characterized by the presence of cancer cells in the lining of the filtration tubules of the kidney. Advanced (metastatic) RCC refers to cancer that has spread outside the kidneys to other locations in the body. The only agent approved for metastatic RCC is high-dose Proleukin (interleukin-2). One site of cancer spread in metastatic RCC is the lungs, referred to as pulmonary **metastasis**.

Recommended dosage

IL-2 is usually administered by injection into a vein but can also be injected under the skin (subcutaneous injection). It can be given in a hospital or clinic setting by a healthcare professional and is sometimes given at home. The dosage depends on the height and weight of the patient. It is given as an infusion for 15 minutes every eight hours for up to five days followed by nine days without the drug and then another five-day cycle of infusion. Up to four subsequent maintenance cycles of IL-2 can be given with four-week intervals without the drug to patients who have

responded favorably to the treatment. About 15% of patients respond to treatment. It is difficult to estimate the cost of IL-2 treatment since the dose and number of treatment cycles given varies according to patients' individual responses; however, the cost is quite high, perhaps as much as $2,000 for one cycle. A six-cycle regimen of IL-2 may cost about $14,100. Because of the high cost and low effectiveness of interleukin-2, it is often not covered by insurance plans, especially HMOs. It is covered by Medicare if given in a hospital.

Precautions

IL-2 is highly toxic and usually makes patients feel generally unwell. Any side effects should be reported to a physician, but the course of medicine should continue even though the patient feels ill, unless the physician or healthcare professional tells the patient to stop. While using aldesleukin, IL-2 patients will be more susceptible to **infection**. They should avoid people with colds, flu, and bronchitis. They should not have any vaccinations without their IL-2 prescriber's approval, and they should avoid anyone who has recently had an oral polio vaccine. Patients should drink several glasses of water a day to help reduce possible kidney problems.

Aldesleukin should not be used by lactating mothers. It should also be avoided in patients with the following conditions:

- acute s-t elevation myocardial infarction
- angina pectoris
- atrial fibrillation
- bacterial infection
- bradycardia
- capillary leak syndrome
- coma
- epilepsy
- fungal infections
- impaired cognition
- intestinal perforation
- ischemic bowel disease
- neoplasm metastatic to the central nervous system
- organ transplantation
- pericardial tamponade
- protozoal infection
- pulmonary disease
- renal failure
- supraventricular tachycardia
- toxic psychosis

- ventricular tachycardia
- viral infection

According to <medscape.com>, the drug should be avoided or used with extreme care in patients with the following:

- arthritis
- bone marrow depression
- bullous pemphigoid
- cerebral arteritis
- cholecystitis
- Crohn's disease
- diabetes mellitus
- disease of liver
- glomerulonephritis
- myasthenia gravis
- psychotic disorder
- renal disease
- scleroderma thyroiditis
- untreated hypothyroidism

According to <MedlinePlus.com>, the drug should be avoided by people who have the following conditions:

- chicken pox (including recent exposure)
- herpes zoster (shingles)
- heart disease
- immune system problems
- liver disease
- lung disease
- psoriasis
- underactive thyroid
- infection
- kidney disease
- mental problems
- history of seizures

Side effects

When IL-2 is given by intravenous infusion, the most common side effect is called capillary leak syndrome. This condition causes weight gain, swelling, low blood pressure, and other problems. At lower doses, people taking IL-2 get flu-like symptoms, including **fever** and muscle aches. Because IL-2 stimulates the immune system, it can make some immune disorders get worse, including arthritis, psoriasis, and diabetes. It can also reduce the number of neutrophils, a particular type of infection-fighting cell, and can cause low levels of thyroid.

When IL-2 is given by subcutaneous injection, the side effects are usually milder than with intravenous infusions. There is the added side effect of irritation at the site of the injection. Side effects show up from two to six hours after injection of IL-2 and disappear quickly after the end of each cycle. IL-2 can cause mood changes, including irritability, insomnia, confusion, or **depression**. These can continue for several days after IL-2 is stopped.

Interleukin-2 has a number of other side effects. More common ones are fever or chills, shortness of breath, agitation, confusion, **diarrhea**, dizziness, drowsiness, mental depression, **nausea and vomiting**, sores in the mouth and on the lips, tingling of hands or feet, unusual decrease in urination, unusual tiredness, a weight gain of five to ten pounds or more, **anemia**, heart problems, kidney problems, liver problems, low blood pressure, low platelet counts in blood, low white blood cell counts, other blood problems, under active thyroid, dry skin, loss of appetite, skin rash or redness with burning or **itching** followed by peeling, and an unusual feeling of general discomfort or illness.

Less common problems include black and tarry stools, skin blisters, blood in the urine, bloody vomit, chest pain, cough or hoarseness, lower back or side pain, painful or difficult urination, pinpoint red spots on the skin, severe stomach pain, unusual bleeding or bruising, bloating and mild stomach pain, blurred or double vision, faintness, fast or irregular heartbeat, loss of taste, rapid breathing, redness, swelling, and soreness of the tongue, trouble in speaking, yellow eyes and skin, constipation, headache, joint pain, and muscle pain.

Rare problems include changes in menstrual periods, clumsiness, coldness, convulsions, listlessness, muscle aches, pain or redness at site of injection, sudden inability to move, swelling in the front of the neck, swelling of the feet or lower legs, and weakness.

Interactions

Interleukin-2 can adversely interact with the anti-cancer drug **dacarbazine** and hormones such as prednisone or cortisone.

Ken R. Wells

Intimacy *see* **Sexuality**

Intraocular melanoma *see* **Melanoma**

Intrathecal chemotherapy

Definition

Intrathecal **chemotherapy** is a method of administration in which the chemotherapy drugs and other drugs are introduced directly into the cerebrospinal fluid.

Purpose

Intrathecal chemotherapy is used primarily to treat leukemas and lymphomas. The chemotherapy drugs are injected directly into the cerebrospinal fluid (CSF), which is the fluid that surrounds the brain and the spinal cord. Intrathecal chemotherapy is used to kill **cancer** cells that have entered the CSF, but it is not used as a therapy if tumors have begun to grow on the spinal cord or brain. Intrathecal chemotherapy frequently is used in the treatment of leukemias.

Precautions

Intrathecal chemotherapy is not appropriate for everyone. Chemotherapy drugs can cause serious side effects. Women who are pregnant or breastfeeding should discuss risks and alternatives with their doctors.

Description

Intrathecal chemotherapy introduces chemotherapy drugs directly in the cerebrospinal fluid to kill cancer cells that exist there. To introduce the chemotherapy drugs into the CSF, two methods are commonly used. The first, called **lumbar puncture** (sometimes called a spinal tap) injects the chemotherapy drugs into the spinal column. The second

A spinal tap is one method of administering intrathecal chemotherapy. *(Alix/Photo Researchers, Inc. Reproduced by permission).*

introduces the drugs directly into the fluid around the brain using a device called a **Ommaya reservoir**.

Regular chemotherapy procedures, such as giving chemotherapy by mouth or intravenously, usually are not effective for killing cancer cells that exist in the CSF. This is because most chemotherapy drugs cannot move past the blood-brain barrier. The blood brain barrier is made up of special, very tightly packed cells that allow some small molecules, such as oxygen, through but do not allow larger molecules to pass into the CSF. This helps to protect the brain from bacteria, viruses, and other cells and molecules that may be harmful to it. Unfortunately, the blood brain barrier also restricts the passage of most chemotherapy drugs. Therefore, to get chemotherapy drugs into the CSF they must be injected directly.

Lumbar Puncture

The lumbar puncture procedure introduces chemotherapy drugs directly into the fluid surrounding the spinal cord. To begin the procedure, the patient usually lays face down on a table, and a small area of back above the spine is treated with local anesthetic. A small device (called a stopcock) is then inserted into the spinal column. The stopcock allows for the injection of chemotherapy drugs and the removal of CSF without repeated punctures. A small needle is inserted through the stopcock into the spinal column. Some of the CSF may be withdrawn for diagnostic tests or for use in flushing the stopcock after the injection of the chemotherapy drugs. The chemotherapy drugs are then injected through the stopcock, and the stopcock is flushed and removed. After removal of the stopcock the area around the puncture site is cleaned and bandaged.

Ommaya Reservoir

The Ommaya reservoir is used to introduce chemotherapy drugs directly into the fluid surrounding the brain. An Ommaya reservoir is a small plastic dome-shaped device that has a catheter (thin tube) attached to it. The placement of the Ommaya reservoir requires a surgical procedure. An area of hair is shaved, and then a small hole is made in the skull into which the reservoir is placed. The reservoir is very small, and it remains in place throughout the duration of chemotherapy treatment. It allows the doctor to remove fluid samples for testing or introduce chemotherapy drugs without requiring a new surgical incision in the skull each time. To perform intrathecal chemotherapy, a very small needle is inserted into the Ommaya reservoir, and the chemotherapy drugs are injected into the fluid surrounding the brain.

Preparation

Each patient is given individual instructions on how to prepare for the intrathecal chemotherapy by his or her cancer care team. Patients may be advised not to eat any solid foods for three or more hours before the procedure. Patients may also be advised to drink plenty of clear liquids. In some cases, CSF is removed during the procedure, and good hydration can help the body replace the fluid more quickly.

Some patients may be given anti-nausea drugs before the procedure. **Nausea and vomiting** are common side-effects of chemotherapy, and taking anti-nausea drugs before the procedure can help reduce the severity of these problems and in some cases prevent them altogether.

Some patients may be asked to stop taking specific medications a day or more before the procedure. Anti-coagulants such as **warfarin** (Coumadin) and aspirin may increase the risk of bleeding during and after the procedure, so patients may be instructed to stop taking the medications several days before the procedure. The cancer care team should provide an individualized set of instructions about which medications should be stopped and when they can be started again. Patients should never stop taking medication without consulting their physician.

Aftercare

After the procedure the patient may be instructed to lie flat on his or her stomach for up to eight hours. This helps to reduce the side effects of the lumbar puncture, and can help the chemotherapy drugs to distribute evenly throughout the CSF. Activities may need to be limited for 24 hours after the procedure.

Risks

Women who are pregnant should talk to their doctors carefully about the risks and benefits of intrathecal chemotherapy, as the chemotherapy drugs can pose a significant risk to the fetus. Women who are breastfeeding should talk to their doctors about alternatives to breastfeeding as chemotherapy drugs may pass to the nursing infant through the breast milk.

The risks of intrathecal chemotherapy differ depending on the type and amount of chemotherapy drug being used. Risks include bleeding, soreness, and **infection** at the injection site, dizziness, **nausea** or **vomiting**, and **fatigue**. Headaches are a relatively common side effect of lumbar punctures. In some cases the headaches can be severe, although they usually resolve within hours after the procedure. Lying prone (flat and face-down) and drinking plenty of fluids can

help reduce this risk. If the headache is very severe or does not resolve in a few hours patients should alert their doctors.

Chemotherapy commonly causes hair-loss, dryness of the mouth and throat, and sores in the mouth. It also frequently causes intestinal problems that can cause **diarrhea** and upset stomach. Decreased interest in sex, hormone changes, and kidney and bladder irritation are also common side effects. Individuals undergoing chemotherapy are also at increased risk of infection because chemotherapy drugs kill many good immune system cells that are needed to combat infection as well as killing cancer cells.

Results

Results of intrathecal chemotherapy vary. Each person's body reacts to chemotherapy differently, and each type of cancer is different. Results can depend on the stage of the cancer, the type of chemotherapy drug used, any health problems the patient has in addition to cancer, and a variety of other factors. Patients should ask their physician and cancer care team about the expected results for their specific situation.

Health care team roles

Intrathecal chemotherapy is administered by a hematologist (doctor who specializes in treating diseases of the blood) or an oncologist (doctor who specializes in treating cancer). The doctor may be assisted by another doctor during the procedure. One or more nurses may assist by helping to prepare the patient, administering local anesthetic, and providing other assistance. The chemotherapy drugs are mixed by a pharmacist with specialized knowledge of chemotherapy drugs.

Caregiver concerns

Intrathecal chemotherapy affects different people in different ways. Some individuals may have few or no side-effects from the treatment, but many individuals will feel tired, sore, and/or nauseated after the procedure.

If the intrathecal chemotherapy is being given on an out-patient basis, the patient will need someone to help him or her get home after treatment. If the car ride home is very long, the patient may need to lie as flat as possible in the car to help reduce side effects from the lumbar puncture and to help the chemotherapy drugs spread correctly. The patient may vomit on the way home; caregivers should be prepared for this.

During a course of chemotherapy treatment patients often feel nauseated and foods that were once enjoyed may seem unappealing. Caregivers may want to organize friends and loved ones to help provide nutritious, high-calorie meals and snacks.

Helping with housework, childcare, errands, and chores can be a great way to help an individual undergoing intrathecal chemotherapy. Individuals undergoing chemotherapy are often very tired, and juggling chemotherapy with other responsibilities can be overwhelming.

Resources

BOOKS

Aryan, Henry E. *Spinal Tumors: A Treatment Guide for Patients and Family*. Sudbury, MA: Jones and Bartlett Publishers, 2010.

McKay, Judith, and Tamera Schacher. *The Chemotherapy Survival Guide: Everything You Need to Know to Get Through Treatment*, 3rd ed. Oakland, CA: New Harbinger Publications, 2009.

Perry, Michael C., ed. *The Chemotherapy Source Book*, 4th ed. Philadelphia: Wolters Kluwer Health/Lippincott Williams and Wilkins, 2008.

Polovich, M., White, J.M., Olsen, M. (Eds.)(2009) *Chemotherapy and Biotherapy Guidelines and Recommendations for Practice*, 3rd edition. Pittsburgh, PA: Oncology Nursing Society.

ORGANIZATIONS

American Cancer Society, 1599 Clifton Rd., NE, Atlanta, GA, 30329, (404) 320-3333, (800) ACS-2345, http://www.cancer.org.

National Cancer Institute Public Inquires Office., 6116 Executive Boulevard, Room 3036A, Bethesda, MD, 20892-8322, (800) 4-CANCER. TTY (800) 332-8615, http://www.cancer.gov.

Tish Davidson, A.M.

Intravenous urography

Definition

Intravenous urography is a test that **x rays** the urinary system using intravenous dye for diagnostic purposes.

The kidneys excrete the dye into the urine. X rays can then create pictures of every structure (kidney, renal pelvis, ureter, bladder, urethra) through which the urine passes.

The procedure has several variations and many names:

- Intravenous pyelography (IVP)
- Urography
- Excretory urography
- Pyelography

Intravenous urography showing contrast in distal ureter. Ureter is the narrow tube shown at the lower right of the image, and the dye has traveled from the kidney (above) and is traveling to the bladder. *(Custom Medical Stock Photo. Reproduced by permission.)*

- Antegrade pyelography differentiates this procedure from "retrograde pyelography," which injects dye into the lower end of the system, therefore flowing backward or "retrograde." Retrograde pyelography is better able to define problems in the lower parts of the system and is the only way to get x rays if the kidneys are not working well.

- Nephrotomography is somewhat different in that the x rays are taken by a moving x ray source onto a film moving in the opposite direction. By accurately coordinating the movement, all but a single plane of tissue is blurred, and that plane is seen without overlying shadows.

Every method available gives good pictures of this system, and the question becomes one of choosing among many excellent alternatives. Each condition has special requirements, while each technique has distinctive benefits and drawbacks.

- Nuclear medicine scans rely on the radiation given off by certain atoms. Chemicals containing such atoms are injected into the bloodstream. They reach the kidneys, where images are constructed by measuring the radiation emitted. The radiation is no more dangerous than standard x rays. The images require considerable training to interpret, but unique information (e.g. blood flow, kidney function, etc.) is often available using this technology. Different chemicals can concentrate the radiation in different types of tissue. This technique may require several days for the chemical to concentrate at its destination. It also requires a special detector to create the image.

- Ultrasound is a quick, safe, simple, and inexpensive way to obtain views of internal organs. Although less detailed than other methods, it may be sufficient, especially to detect obstructions.

- Retrograde pyelography is better able to define problems in the lower parts of the system and is the only way to get x rays if the kidneys are not working well. Dye is usually injected through an instrument (cystoscope) passed into the bladder through the urethra.

- A computed tomography scan (CT or CAT scanning) uses the same kind of radiation used in x rays, but it collects information by computer in such a way that three dimensional images can be constructed, eliminating interference from nearby structures. CT scanning requires a special apparatus, but often gives better information on masses within the kidney.

- Magnetic resonance imaging (MRI) uses magnetic fields and radio frequency signals, instead of ionizing radiation, to create computerized images. This form of energy is entirely safe as long as the patient does not have any implanted metal such as artificial joints,

aneurysm clips, etc. The technique is far more versatile than CT scanning as it can not only demonstrate masses, but also look at the blood vessels. However, MRI requires special apparatus and, because of the powerful magnets needed, even a special, separate building. It is quite expensive and only occasionally is this degree of detail required.

Purpose

IVP will provide information concerning most diseases of the kidneys, ureters, and bladder. The procedure is comprised of two phases. First, it requires a functioning kidney to filter the dye out of the blood into the urine. The time required for the dye to appear on x rays correlates accurately with kidney function. The second phase gives detailed anatomical images of the urinary tract. Within the first few minutes the dye "lights up" the kidneys, a phase called the nephrogram. Subsequent pictures follow the dye down the ureters and into the bladder. A final film taken after urinating reveals how well the bladder empties.

IVPs are most often done to assess structural abnormalities or obstruction to urine flow. If kidney function is at issue, more films are taken sooner to catch the earliest phase of the process.

- Stones, tumors and congenital malformations account for many of the findings.

- Kidney cysts and cancers can be seen.

- Displacement of a kidney or ureter suggests a space-occupying lesion (like a cancer of the colon, rectum, or gynecological organs) pushing it out of the way.

- Bad valves where the ureters enter the bladder will often show up.

- Bladder cancers and other abnormalities are often outlined by the dye in the bladder.

- An enlarged prostate gland will show up as incomplete bladder emptying and a bump at the bottom of the bladder.

Precautions

The only serious complication of an IVP is allergy to the iodine-containing dye that is used. Such an allergy is rare, but it can be dramatic and even lethal. Emergency measures taken immediately are usually effective.

Description

IVPs are usually done in the morning. In the x ray suite, the patient undresses and lies down. There are two methods of injecting the dye. An intravenous line can be established, through which the dye is consistently fed through the body during the procedure. The other method is to give the dye all at once through a needle that is immediately withdrawn. X rays are taken until the dye has reached the bladder, an interval of half an hour or less. The patient is asked to empty the bladder before one last x ray. A compression device (a wide belt containing 2 balloons that can be inflated) may be used to keep the contrast material in the kidneys. The patient needs to urinate after the compression device is removed. Another picture is taken after the bladder is emptied to see how empty the bladder is.

In the past, of the many ways to obtain images of the urinary system, the intravenous injection of a contrast agent has been considered the best. Recent studies are showing, however, that while intravenous urography is a useful technique, there may be other imaging techniques, such as B mode ultrasound, Doppler ultrasound, renal scintigraphy with angiotensin-converting enzyme inhibitors, intra-venous and intra-arterial catheter **angiography**, computed tomographic angiography, and magnetic resonance angiography, that are better or less costly.

Preparation

Emptying the bowel with **laxatives** or enemas prevents bowel shadows from obscuring the details of the urinary system. An empty stomach prevents the complication of **vomiting**, a rare effect of the contrast

agent. Therefore, the night before the IVP the patient is asked to evacuate the bowels and to drink sparingly.

Preparation for infants and children depends on the age of the infant or child.

Aftercare

Feeling weak, nauseous, and/or lightheaded for a short time after the procedure is a possibility.

Risks

Allergy to the contrast agent is the only risk. Anyone with a possible iodine allergy, a previous reaction to x ray dye, or an allergy to shellfish must be particularly careful to inform the x ray personnel.

Exposure to x ray radiation should be noted. Most experts agree that the risk of exposure to low radiation is low compared to the benefits. Pregnant women and children are more sensitive to the risks of x rays.

Normal results

X-ray images of the kidney and bladder structures appear normal.

Abnormal results

An abnormal intravenous urography result may indicate kidney disease, birth defect, tumor, kidney stone, and/or inflammation caused by infections.

Resources

BOOKS

Ballinger, Philip W., and Eugene D. Frank. *Merrill's Atlas of Radiographic Positions and Radiologic Procedures.* 9th ed. St. Louis: Year Book Medical Publishers, 1999.

PERIODICALS

Aitchson, F., and A. Page. "Diagnostic Imaging of Renal Artery Stenosis" *Journal of Human Hypertension* September 1999: 595–603.

Dalla–Palma, L. "What is Left of I.V. Urography?" *European Radiology* March 2001: 931–939.

Hession, P., et al. "Intravenous Urography in Urinary Tract Surveillance in Carcinoma of the Bladder." *Clinical Radiology* July 1999: 465–467.

Little, M. A., et al. "The Diagnostic Yield of Intravenous Urography." *Nephrology Dialysis Transplantation* February 2000: 200–204.

ORGANIZATIONS

American Cancer Society (National Headquarters). 1599 Clifton Road, N.E., Atlanta, GA 30329. (800) 227-2345. http://www.cancer.org.

Cancer Research Institute (National Headquarters). 681 Fifth Avenue, New York, NY 10022. (800) 992-2623. http://www.cancerresearch.org.

Kidney Cancer Association. 1234 Sherman Avenue, Suite 203, Evanston, IL 60202-1375. (800) 850-9132. http://www.kidneycancerassociation.org.

National Cancer Institute. 9000 Rockville Pike, Building 31, Room 10A16, Bethesda, MD 20892. (800) 422-6237. http://www.nci.nih.gov.

National Kidney Cancer Association. 1234 Sherman Avenue, Suite 203, Evanston, IL 60202-1375. (800) 850-9132.

National Kidney Foundation. 30 East 33rd Street, New York, NY 10016. (800) 622-9010. http://www.kidney.org.

J. Ricker Polsdorfer, M.D.
Laura Ruth, Ph.D.

Investigational drugs

Definition

"Investigational drugs" refers to drugs that have received FDA approval for human testing, including those drugs still undergoing **clinical trials**, but are not approved for marketing to the general public.

Description

Investigational drugs represent interesting and novel new agents in the fight against **cancer**. These agents include **chemotherapy** designed to treat specific cancers, to provide palliative therapy for pain and symptoms, and to reduce invasive cancers in high-risk patients. The challenge faced by private and commercial investigators is to reduce the lag time in bringing an investigational drug to market without compromising drug quality or patient safety. The guidelines that insure the correct procedures are being followed in the process of drug development and approval fall under the direction of the Food and Drug Administration (FDA).

At present, the cycle of investigational drug research and development, to clinical trials, to FDA approval can easily cover a period of 10-12 years. Under exceptional circumstances, provisions can be made for patient use of investigational drugs under the guidance of specially trained and registered oncologists. These specific investigational drugs are classified as "Group C" drugs, and have demonstrated a high level of reproducible activity in pre-clinical testing. There is also the route of "Accelerated FDA Approval" for some investigational drugs.

Accelerated approval relies on specific indicators that suggest that a particular investigational drug is likely to have beneficial effects before the benefits have been clinically verified. All investigational drugs that have been granted accelerated approval must undergo follow-up testing in order to receive final FDA approval. Some researchers are presently working on a format to combine traditional clinical testing of investigational drugs with a global database of drug information. This integrated system would give FDA monitoring agencies and healthcare providers access to the most comprehensive source of archived data available on investigational drugs. This combined approach is another attempt to reduce approval time for investigational drugs and make these agents available to the cancer patient for treatment.

Resources

PERIODICALS

Johnson, Dale E., and Grushenka H.I. Wolfgang. "Predicting human safety: screening and computational approaches." *Drug Discovery Today* 5, no.10 (October 2000): 445-454.

OTHER

Preclinical Development of Investigational Agents: The Developmental Therapeutics Program *CTEP* Info CTEP. [cited May 8, 2009]. http://www.CTEP.info.nih.gov.

Understanding the Approval Process for New Cancer Drugs. *Understanding Trials*. NCI Cancer Trials. [cited May 18, 2009]. http://www.cancertrials.nci.nih.gov.

Jane Taylor-Jones, Research Associate, M.S.

Irinotecan

Definition

Irinotecan is a drug used to treat certain types of **cancer**. Irinotecan, also known as CPT-11, is available under the trade name Camptosar, and may also be referred to as irinotecan hydrochloride or camptothecin-11.

Purpose

Irinotecan is an antineoplastic agent used to treat cancer. A primary use of the drug is treatment of colon or rectal cancers that have recurred or progressed while the patient was on 5-FU (**fluorouracil**) therapy. Irinotecan also can be given as first line therapy with 5-FU and **leucovorin** for patients with metastatic colon or **rectal cancer**. Other uses for irinotecan include treatment of **small cell lung cancer**, nonsmall cell lung cancer, **ovarian cancer**, **stomach cancer**, **breast cancer**, **pancreatic cancer**, leukemia, **lymphoma**, and **cervical cancer**.

Several studies showed some potential uses for irinotecan. One reported that a combination of irinotecan and **docetaxel** can help patients with **esophageal cancer** who have been extensively pretreated with **cisplatin**. Weekly use of irinotecan has shown preliminary results in treating patients with nonsmall cell lung cancer with minimal side effects. Another study reported that when used in combination with cancer drugs cisplatin and **epirubicin**, irinotecan might have promising broad antitumor activity. In the future, irinotecan might be used in combination therapies to treat many types of tumors.

Description

Irinotecan is a synthetic derivative of the naturally occurring compound camptothecin. Camptothecin belongs to a group of chemicals called alkaloids and is extracted from plants such as *camptotheca acuminata*. Captothecin was initially investigated as a chemotherapeutic agent due to its anti-cancer activity in laboratory studies. The chemical structure and biological action of irinotecan is similar to that of camptothecin and **topotecan**.

Irinotecan inhibits the normal functioning of the enzyme topoisomerase I. The normal role of topoisomerase I is to aid in the replication, recombination, and repair of deoxyribonucleic acid (DNA). Higher levels of topoisomerase I have been found in certain cancer tumors compared to healthy tissue. Inhibiting topoisomerase I causes DNA damage. This damage leads to apoptosis, or programmed cell death.

Recommended dosage

Patients should be carefully monitored during irinotecan treatment for toxicity. Irinotecan is given at a dose of 125 mg per square meter of body surface area per week for four weeks, followed by a two week rest period. Other dosing schedules include 100 mg per square meter of body surface area per day for three days every three weeks, or 100–115 mg per square meter of body surface area per week, or 200–350 mg per square meter of body surface area every three weeks. The drug is administered through the vein over a 90-minute period. The initial dose of irinotecan may be adjusted downward depending on patient tolerance to the toxic side effects of irinotecan.

Treatment may be continued as long as intolerable side effects do not develop and patients continue to benefit from the treatment.

Precautions

Irinotecan should only be used under the supervision of a physician experienced in the use of cancer chemotherapeutic agents. Special caution, especially in those 65 years and older, should be taken to monitor the toxic effects of irinotecan, particularly **diarrhea**, **nausea**, and **vomiting**. Because irinotecan is administered intravenously, the site of infusion should be monitored for signs of inflammation. Should inflammation occur, flushing the site with sterile water and applying ice are recommended. Irinotecan may cause **nausea and vomiting**, and premedication with antiemetic agents is recommended.

Neither the effects of irinotecan in patients with significant liver dysfunction nor the safety of irinotecan in children have been established. Irinotecan should not be administered to pregnant women. Women of child-bearing age are advised not to become pregnant during treatment with this drug.

Side effects

Early- or late-onset diarrhea are common side effects of irinotecan. Late-onset diarrhea, occurring more than 24 hours after irinotecan administration, can be life-threatening and should be treated promptly. Patients should immediately report diarrhea to their physician. Patients can also take the antidiarrheal drug loperamide as prescribed by their physician at the first sign of diarrhea. Suppression of bone marrow function is another serious side effect commonly observed in this treatment. Additional side effects, including nausea, vomiting, **anorexia** (loss of appetite), pain, **fatigue**, and hair loss (**alopecia**) may occur.

Interactions

Irradiation treatment during the course of irinotecan treatment is not recommended. Patients who have received prior pelvic or abdominal irradiation treatment should notify their physician. Since irinotecan may cause diarrhea, the use of **laxatives** should be avoided. The use of diuretics should be closely monitored. The adverse side effects caused by irinotecan may be increased by other **antineoplastic agents** having similar adverse effects and should generally be avoided.

Resources

PERIODICALS

"Cisplatin, Irinotecan, and Epirubicin Have Promising Broad Antitumor Activity." *Cancer Weekly* October 14, 2003:12.

"Irinotecan and Docetaxel Shows Some Activity in Extensively Pretreated Patients." *Clinical Trials Week* October 13, 2003: 25.

"Weekly IrinotecanShowed Antitumoral Activity and Minimum Toxicity in NSCCLC." *Clinical Trials Week* October 13, 2003: 25.

Marc Scanio
Teresa G. Odle

Islet cell carcinoma *see* **Pancreatic cancer, endocrine**

Itching

Description

Itching, also called pruritus, is an unpleasant sensation of the skin that causes a person to scratch or rub the area to find relief. Itching can be confined to one spot (localized) or over the whole body (generalized). Severe scratching can injure the skin causing redness, bumps, and scratches. Injured skin is prone to **infection**.

Itching can profoundly affect quality of life. It can torment the patient and cause discomfort, stress, loss of sleep, concentration difficulty, and constant concern.

Causes

The biology underlying itching is not fully understood. It is believed that itching results from the interactions of several different chemical messengers. Although itching and pain sensations were at one time thought to be sent along the same nerve pathways, researchers reported the discovery in 2003 of itch-specific nerve pathways. Nerve endings that are specifically sensitive to itching have been named pruriceptors.

Research into itching has been helped by the recent invention of a mechanical device called the Matcher, which electrically stimulates the patient's left hand. When the intensity of the stimulation equals the intensity of itching that the patient is experiencing elsewhere in the body, the patient stops the stimulation and the device automatically records the measurement. The Matcher was found to be sensitive to immediate changes in the patient's perception of itching as well as reliable in its measurements.

Itching is associated with a variety of factors including skin diseases, blood diseases, emotions, and drug reactions as well as by **cancer** and cancer treatments. Itching can be a symptom of cancer including **Hodgkin's disease**, **non-Hodgkin's lymphoma**, leukemia, **Bowen's disease**, **multiple myeloma**, central nervous system (brain and spinal cord) tumors, **germ cell tumors**, and invasive squamous cell **carcinoma**. The buildup of toxins in the blood, caused by kidney, gallbladder, and liver disease, can cause itching. Cancer treatments that are associated with itching are: **radiation therapy**, **chemotherapy**, and **biological response modifiers** (drugs that improve the patient's immune system). Skin reactions are more severe when both chemotherapy and radiation therapy are used. Patients treated with **bone marrow transplantation** may develop itching resulting from **graft-vs.-host disease**. Itching can be caused by infection.

General medications that may be used by cancer patients can cause itching. Itching can be caused by drug reactions from **antibiotics**, **corticosteroids**, hormones, and pain relievers (analgesics).

Itching can be a sign that the patient is very sensitive to a particular chemotherapy drug.

Chemotherapy drugs and biological response modifiers that cause itching include:

- allopurinol
- aminoglutethimide
- bleomycin
- carmustine
- chlorambucil
- cyclophosphamide
- cytarabine
- daunorubicin
- doxorubicin
- hydroxyurea
- idarubicin
- interleukin (aldesleukin)
- mechlorethamine
- megestrol acetate
- mitomycin-C
- tamoxifen
- topiramate

Itching commonly occurs during radiation therapy. Parts of the body that are particularly sensitive to radiation are the underarms, groin, abdomen, breasts, buttocks, and skin around the genitals (perineum) and anus (perianal). Itching is usually caused by skin dryness when the oil (sebaceous) glands are damaged by the radiation. Radiation also causes skin darkening, redness, and skin shedding, which can all cause itching.

Itching caused by cancer usually disappears once the cancer is in remission or cured. Chemotherapy-induced itching usually disappears within 30 to 90 minutes after the drug has been administered. Itching caused by radiation therapy will resolve once the injured skin has healed.

Treatments

There are three aspects in the treatment of itching: managing the underlying cancer, maintaining skin health, and relief of itching.

Patients should avoid the particular things that cause or worsen their itching. Also, patients can take measures to maintain skin health. Suggestions include:

- taking short baths in warm water
- using mild soaps and rinsing well
- applying bath oil or moisturizing cream after bathing
- avoiding use of cosmetics, perfumes, deodorants, and starch-based powders
- avoiding wool and other harsh fabrics

- using mild laundry detergents and rinsing thoroughly
- avoiding use of dryer anti-static sheets
- wearing loose-fitting cotton clothing
- avoiding high-friction garments such as belts, pantyhose, and bras
- maintaining a cool environment with a 30% to 40% humidity level
- using cotton sheets
- avoiding vigorous exercise (if sweating causes itching)
- avoiding skin products that are scented or contain alcohol or menthol

To reduce skin injury caused by scratching the patient should keep fingernails short, wear soft cotton mittens and socks at night, and keep the hands clean. Gently rubbing the skin around the itch or applying pressure or vibration to the itchy spot may reduce itching. Using a soft infant toothbrush to gently stroke the itchy area may relieve itching. Itching may be relieved by applying a cool washcloth or ice to the itchy area.

The most effective way to relieve itching is to treat the underlying disease. Sometimes, itching disappears as soon as a tumor is treated or removed.

Itching may be relieved by applying any of a variety of different products to the skin. The patient may need to try several before the most effective one is found. The patient's physician should be consulted before any anti-itch products are used. Topical treatments include:

- Corticosteroids, such as hydrocortisone, reduce inflammation and itching.
- Calamine lotions can cool and soothe itchy skin. These products can be drying, which may be helpful for weeping or oozing rashes.
- Antihistamine creams stop itching that is associated with the chemical messenger histamine.
- Moisturizers treat dry skin which helps to relieve itching. Moisturizers that are recommended to cancer patients include brand names Alpha Keri, Aquaphor, Eucerin, Lubriderm, Nivea, Prax, and Sarna. Moisturizers should be applied after bathing and at least two or three times daily.
- Gels that contain a numbing agent (e.g. lidocaine) can be used on some parts of the body.

Itching may be treated with whole-body medications. Some of these systemic treatments include:

- antihistamines
- tricyclic antidepressants
- sedatives or tranquilizers

- such selective serotonin reputake inhibitors as paroxetine (Paxil) and sertraline (Zoloft)
- binding agents (such as cholestyramine which relieves itching associated with kidney or liver disease).
- aspirin
- cimetidine

Alternative and complementary therapies

A well-balanced diet that includes carbohydrates, fats, minerals, proteins, **vitamins**, and liquids will help to maintain skin health. Capsules that contain eicosapentaenoic acid, which is obtained from herring, mackerel, or salmon, may help to reduce itching. Vitamin A plays an important role in skin health. Vitamin E (capsules or ointment) may reduce itching. Patients should check with their treating physician before using supplements.

Homeopathy has been reported to be effective in treating systemic itching associated with hemodialysis.

Baths containing oil with milk or oatmeal are effective at relieving localized itching. Evening primrose oil may soothe itching and may be as effective as corticosteroids. Calendula cream may relieve short-term itching. Other herbal treatments that have been recently reported to relieve itching include sangre de drago, a preparation made with sap from a South American tree; and a mixture of honey, olive oil, and beeswax.

Distraction, music therapy, relaxation techniques, and visualization may be useful in relieving itching. Ultraviolet light therapy may relieve itching associated with conditions of the skin, kidneys, blood, and gallbladder. There are some reports of the use of acupuncture and transcutaneous electrical nerve stimulators (TENS) to relieve itching.

Resources

BOOKS
Beers, Mark H., MD, and Robert Berkow, MD, editors. "Pruritus." In *The Merck Manual of Diagnosis and Therapy*. Whitehouse Station, NJ: Merck Research Laboratories, 2007.

PERIODICALS
Al-Waili, N. S. "Topical Application of Natural Honey, Beeswax and Olive Oil Mixture for Atopic Dermatitis or Psoriasis: Partially Controlled, Single-Blinded Study." *Complementary Therapies in Medicine* 11 (December 2003): 226–234.
Browning, J., B. Combes, and M. J. Mayo. "Long-Term Efficacy of Sertraline as a Treatment for Cholestatic Pruritus in Patients with Primary Biliary Cirrhosis." *American Journal of Gastroenterology* 98 (December 2003): 2736–2741.
Cavalcanti, A. M., L. M. Rocha, R. Carillo, Jr., et al. "Effects of Homeopathic Treatment on Pruritus of Haemodialysis Patients: A Randomised Placebo-Controlled Double-Blind Trial." *Homeopathy* 92 (October 2003): 177–181.
Ikoma, A., R. Rukwied, S. Stander, et al. "Neurophysiology of Pruritus: Interaction of Itch and Pain." *Archives of Dermatology* 139 (November 2003): 1475–1478.
Jones. K. "Review of Sangre de Drago (*Croton lechleri*)—A South American Tree Sap in the Treatment of Diarrhea, Inflammation, Insect Bites, Viral Infections, and Wounds: Traditional Uses to Clinical Research." *Journal of Alternative and Complementary Medicine* 9 (December 2003): 877–896.
Ochoa, J. G. "Pruritus, a Rare but Troublesome Adverse Reaction of Topiramate." *Seizure* 12 (October 2003): 516–518.
Stener-Victorin, E., T. Lundeberg, J. Kowalski, et al. "Perceptual Matching for Assessment of itch; Reliability and Responsiveness Analyzed by a Rank-Invariant Statistical Method." *Journal of Investigative Dermatology* 121 (December 2003): 1301–1305.
Zylicz, Z., M. Krajnik, A. A. Sorge, and M. Costantini. "Paroxetine in the Treatment of Severe Non-Dermatological Pruritus: A Randomized, Controlled Trial." *Journal of Pain and Symptom Management* 26 (December 2003): 1105–1112.

Belinda Rowland, Ph.D.
Rebecca J. Frey, Ph.D.

Itraconazole *see* **Antifungal therapy**
IVP, Excretory urography, Intravenous pyelography *see* **Intravenous urography**

K

Kaposi's sarcoma

Definition

Kaposi's **sarcoma** (KS) is a **cancer** of the skin, mucous membranes, and blood vessels; it is the most common form of cancer in AIDS patients. It was named for Dr. Moritz Kaposi (1837–1902), a Hungarian dermatologist who first described it in 1872. As of 2009, researchers disagree as to whether KS is a true cancer or a disorder of the skin that develops as a reaction to **infection** by a herpes virus.

Description

The formal medical term for Kaposi's sarcoma is multiple idiopathic hemorrhagic sarcoma. This term means that KS develops in many different sites on the patient's skin or internal organs; that its cause is unknown; and that it is characterized by bleeding. The lesions (areas of diseased or damaged skin), which are usually round or elliptical in shape and a quarter of an inch to an inch in size, derive their characteristic purple or brownish color from blood leaking out of capillaries (small blood vessels) in the skin. In KS, the capillaries begin to grow too rapidly and irregularly, which causes them to become leaky and eventually break. The lesions themselves may become enlarged and bleed, or cause the mucous membranes of the patient's internal organs to bleed.

There are three types of KS lesions, defined by their appearance:

- Nodular. These are reddish-purple, but are sometimes surrounded by a border of yellowish or brown pigment. Nodular lesions may appear to be dark brown rather than purple in patients with dark skin.

- Infiltrating. Infiltrating lesions may be large or have a raised surface. They typically grow downward under the skin.

- Lymphatic. These lesions are found in the lymph nodes and may be confused with other causes of swollen lymph nodes.

KS is classified into five types:

- Classic KS. This form of KS is sometimes called indolent KS because it is slow to develop. Classical KS is most commonly found in males between 50 and 70 years of age, of Italian or Eastern European Jewish descent.

- African KS. This form of the disease appears in both an indolent and an aggressive form in native populations in equatorial Africa. It accounts for almost 10% of all cancers in central Africa.

- Immunosuppressive treatment-related KS. The third form of KS occurs in kidney transplant patients who have been given drugs to suppress their immune systems-usually prednisone and azathioprine. This form of KS is sometimes called iatrogenic KS, which means that it is caused unintentionally by medical treatment.

- Epidemic KS. Epidemic KS was first reported in 1981 as part of the AIDS epidemic. Most cases of epidemic KS in the United States have been diagnosed in homosexual or bisexual men.

- Non-epidemic gay-related KS. This form of KS occurs in homosexual men who do not develop HIV infection. Non-epidemic gay-related KS is an indolent form of the disease that primarily affects the patient's skin.

Demographics

The demographic distribution of KS varies considerably across its five types:

- Classic KS. Classic KS is considered a rare disease, with a male/female ratio of 10:1 or 15:1. In North America and Europe, most patients are between 50 and 70 years old. Classic KS is more common in men from Mediterranean countries and in Ashkenazic Jews.

Purple-colored (violaceous) plaques of Kaposi's sarcoma on the heel and side of foot. *(Centers for Disease Control.)*

This HIV-positive patient is afflicted with Kaposi's sarcoma inside the mouth. The tumor is toward the back of the mouth, to the right. *(Custom Medical Stock Photo. Reproduced by permission.)*

- African KS. African KS has the same male/female ratio as classic KS, although most patients with African KS are younger. A form of African KS that attacks the lymphatic system primarily affects children, with a male/female ratio of 3:1.

- Immunosuppresive treatment-related KS. This form of KS occurs mostly in kidney-transplant patients, at a rate of 150 to 200 times as often as in the general population. It represents 3% of all tumors that occur in kidney-transplant patients. The male/female ratio is 2:1.

- Epidemic KS. Epidemic KS is overwhelmingly a disease of adult homosexual or bisexual males. It is 20,000 times more common in people with AIDS than in those without HIV infection. According to the National Institutes of Health (NIH), 95% of all

the cases of epidemic KS in the United States have been diagnosed in homosexual or bisexual males. Epidemic KS is far more prevalent among homosexual or bisexual males with AIDS than among hemophiliacs or intravenous drug users with AIDS. Prior to 1995, about 26% of all homosexual males with AIDS had KS as their first symptom or eventually developed KS, as compared with fewer than 3% of heterosexual intravenous drug users with AIDS. This clustering of KS cases among a subpopulation of AIDS patients led to the hypothesis that a blood factor transmitted by sexual contact is a partial cause of KS. The number of new cases of AIDS-related KS has declined in recent years, for reasons that are not yet clear. Some researchers think that the introduction of highly active antiretroviral therapy, or HAART, is related to the decline in the number of cases of epidemic KS. Only about 12% of AIDS patients develop KS.

- Non-epidemic, gay-related KS. This small group of KS patients is entirely male.

Causes and symptoms

Causes

GENETIC FACTORS. The role of genetic factors in KS varies across its five types. Classic KS is the only form associated with specific ethnic groups. In addition, patients with classic KS and immunosuppressive treatment-related KS have a higher incidence of a genetically determined immune factor called HLA-DR.

MALE HORMONES. The fact that all forms of KS affect men more often than women may indicate that androgens (male sex hormones) may be a factor in the development of KS.

IMMUNOSUPPRESSION. In addition to organ transplant patients receiving immunosuppressive drugs, patients who are taking high-dose **corticosteroids** are also at increased risk of developing KS.

INFECTIOUS AGENTS. Some researchers think that cytomegalovirus (CMV) and **human papilloma virus** (HPV) may be involved in the development of KS because fragments of these two types of virus have been found in KS tumor samples. The most likely candidate for an infectious agent, however, is human herpesvirus 8 (HHV-8), which is sometimes called KS-associated herpesvirus (KSHV). Fragments of the HHV-8 genome were first detected in 1994 by using a technique based on polymerase chain reaction (PCR) analysis. HHV-8 belongs to a group of herpesviruses called rhadinoviruses, and is the first herpesvirus of this subtype to be found in humans. HHV-8 is, however, closely related to the human herpesvirus called **Epstein-Barr virus** (EBV). EBV is known to cause infectious mononucleosis as well as tumors of the lymphatic system, and may be involved in other malignancies, including the African form of **Burkitt's lymphoma**, **Hodgkin's disease**, and **nasopharyngeal cancer**. HHV-8 has been found in tissue samples from patients with African KS, classic KS, and immunosuppression treatment-related KS as well as epidemic KS. HHV-8 is also associated with a rare non-cancerous disease called Castleman's disease, which affects the lymph nodes. Some KS patients have been found to have KS and Castleman's disease occurring together in the same lymph node.

OTHER CAUSES. Some practitioners of alternative medicine regard environmental toxins, psychological distress, and constitutional weaknesses as probable or partial causes of KS. These theories are discussed in more detail under the heading of alternative treatments.

Symptoms

CLASSIC KS. The symptoms of classic KS include one or more reddish or purplish patches or nodules on one or both legs, often on the ankles or soles of the feet. The lesions slowly enlarge over a period of 10-15 years, with additional lesions sometimes developing. It is rare for classic KS to involve the patient's internal organs, although bleeding from the digestive tract sometimes occurs. About 34% of patients with classic KS eventually develop **non-Hodgkin's lymphoma** or another primary cancer.

AFRICAN KS. The symptoms of the indolent form of African KS resemble those of classic KS. The aggressive form, however, produces tumors that may penetrate the tissue underneath the patient's skin, and even the underlying bone.

EPIDEMIC KS. Epidemic KS has more varied presentations than the four other types of KS. Its onset is usually, though not always, marked by the appearance of widespread lesions at many different points on the patient's skin and in the mouth. Most HIV-infected patients who develop KS skin and mouth lesions feel healthy and have no systemic symptoms. On the other hand, KS may affect the patient's lymph nodes or gastrointestinal tract prior to causing skin lesions.

Patients with epidemic KS almost always develop disseminated (widely spread) disease. The illness progesses from a few localized lesions to lymph node involvement and further spread to other organs. Disseminated KS is defined by the appearance of one or more of the following: a count of 25 or more external lesions; the appearance of 10 or more new lesions per month; and the appearance of visible lesions in the patient's lungs or stomach lining.

In some cases, disseminated KS causes painful swelling (edema) of the patient's feet and lower legs. The lesions may also cause the surrounding skin to ulcerate or develop secondary infections. The spread of KS to the lungs, called pleuropulmonary KS, usually occurs at a late stage of the disease. KS involvement of the lungs causes bleeding, coughing, shortness of breath, and eventual respiratory failure. Most patients who die directly of KS die from its pleuropulmonary form.

Diagnosis

Physical examination and patient history

The diagnosis of any form of KS requires a careful examination of all areas of the patient's skin. Even though the characteristic lesions of classic KS appear most frequently on the legs, all forms of KS can produce lesions on any area of the skin. An experienced doctor, who may be a dermatologist, an internist, or a primary care physician, can make a tentative diagnosis of KS on the basis of the external appearance of the skin lesions (size, shape, color, and location on the face or body), particularly when they are accompanied by evidence of lymph node involvement, internal bleeding, and other symptoms associated with disseminated KS. The doctor may touch or press on the lesions to find out whether they turn pale (blanch) ; KS plaques and nodules do not blanch under fingertip pressure. In addition, KS lesions are not painful when they first appear.

Other signs of KS may appear on the soft palate or the membrane covering the eye (conjunctiva). In addition, the doctor will press on the patient's abdomen in order to detect any masses in the liver or spleen.

A thorough history is necessary in order to determine whether the patient's ethnic background, lifestyle, or medical history places him or her in a high-risk category for KS.

Biopsy

A definitive diagnosis of KS requires a skin **biopsy** in order to rule out bacillary angiomatosis, a bacterial infection resembling cat-scratch disease. It is caused by a bacillus, *Bartonella henselae*. Collecting a tissue sample for a biopsy is not difficult if the patient has skin lesions, but can be complicated if the nodules are primarily internal. An endoscopy of the upper end of the digestive tract may be performed in order to obtain a tissue sample from an internal KS lesion.

Under the microscope, an AIDS-related KS lesion will show an unusually large number of spindle-shaped cells mixed together with small capillaries. The origin of the spindle-shaped cells is still unknown. The tumor cells in a KS lesion resemble smooth muscle cells or fibroblasts, which are cells that help to form the fibers in normal connective tissue.

If the patient's lymph nodes are enlarged, a biopsy may be done in order to rule out other causes of swollen lymph nodes.

Other tests

Other diagnostic tests may be performed if the patient appears to have disseminated KS. These tests include:

- Chest x ray. A radiograph of the patient's lungs will show patchy areas of involved tissue.

- Gallium scan. The results will be negative in KS.
- Bronchoscopy. This procedure allows the doctor to examine the patient's bronchial pathways for visible KS lesions. It is not, however, useful for obtaining tissue samples for biopsy.
- Endoscopy. Examination of the patient's stomach allows the doctor to examine the mucous lining for KS lesions as well as to obtain a tissue sample.

Treatment team

KS patients may receive treatment for skin lesions from a dermatologist or radiologist as well as treatment for lung or lymphatic involvement from internists or primary care practitioners. A surgeon may be called in to remove lesions in the digestive tract if they are bleeding or blocking the passage of food. Children with KS may be treated by pediatricians or by primary care physicians who specialize in treating AIDS patients.

Clinical staging, treatments, and prognosis

Staging

The NIH recommends individualized staging of patients with classic KS, due to the age of most patients, the localized nature of the lesions, the slow progression of the disease, and the low risk of spread to the internal organs.

The criteria for staging epidemic KS have evolved over the past decade in response to changes in the treatment of HIV infection and to the recognition that KS does not fit well into standard categories of tumor assessment. Several different systems have been used to stage epidemic KS, but none is completely satisfactory.

NYU STAGING SYSTEM. One staging system that originated at New York University divides KS patients into four groups according to the following symptom clusters:

- Skin lesions that are indolent (slow-growing) and limited to relatively small areas of the body.
- Skin lesions limited to specific regions of the body but aggressive in growth. There may or may not be involvement of lymph nodes.
- General involvement of the skin and mucous membranes, with or without lymph node involvement.
- Involvement of the internal organs.

AIDS CLINICAL TRIALS GROUP (ACTG) STAGING SYSTEM. The ACTG Oncology Committee published a staging system for epidemic KS in 1989. This system was reevaluated in 1995 and is undergoing continued assessment. It is based on three criteria: extent of tumor; condition of the patient's immune system; and presence of systemic illness:

- Tumor (T): Good risk (0) is a tumor limited to the skin and/or lymph nodes and/or minimal oral disease (limited to the palate). Poor risk (1) is any of the following: edema associated with the tumor; widespread KS in the mouth; KS in the digestive tract; KS in other viscera.

- Immune system (I): Good risk (0) is a CD4 cell count greater than 200 per cubic millmeter. Poor risk (1) is a CD4 cell count lower than 200 per cubic millimeter.

- Systemic illness (S): Good risk (0) is no history of opportunistic infections (OI) or thrush; no "B" symptoms (unexplained fever, night sweats, diarrhea lasting more than 2 weeks, weight loss greater than 10%); performance status above 70 on the Karnofsky scale. Poor risk (1) is any of the following: history of OI or thrush; presence of "B" symptoms; Karnofsky score lower than 70; and other HIV-related illnesses.

Treatment

Treatment of KS depends on the form of the disease.

CLASSIC KS. Radiation therapy is usually quite effective if the patient has small lesions or lesions limited to a small area of skin. Low-voltage photon radiation or electron beam therapy give good results. Surgical removal of small lesions is sometimes done, but the lesions are likely to recur. The best results are obtained from surgical treatment when many small lesions are removed over a period of years.

For widespread skin disease, radiation treatment with electron beam therapy is recommended. Classic KS has not often been treated with **chemotherapy** in the United States, but some researchers report that treatment with **vinblastine** or **vincristine** has been effective. Disease that has spread to the lymph nodes or digestive tract is treated with a combination of chemotherapy and radiation treatment.

IMMUNOSUPPRESSIVE TREATMENT-RELATED KS. The standard pattern of therapy for this form of KS begins with discontinuing the immunosuppressive medications if they are not essential to the patient's care. Treatment of the KS itself may include radiation therapy if the disease is limited to the skin, or single- or multiple-drug chemotherapy.

EPIDEMIC KS. As of 2001, there is no cure for epidemic KS. Treatment is aimed at reducing the size of skin lesions and alleviating the discomfort of open ulcers or swollen tissue in the legs. There are no data

that indicate that treatment prolongs the survival of patients with epidemic KS. In addition to treatment of the KS itself, these patients also need ongoing retroviral therapy and treatment of any opportunistic infections that may develop. An additional complication in treating epidemic KS is that highly active antiretroviral therapy, or HAART, is not the "magic bullet" that some had hoped when it was introduced in 1998. HAART uses three- or four-drug combinations to treat HIV infection. Problems with HAART include severe psychiatric as well as physical side effects, in addition to the patient's risk of developing a drug-resistant form of HIV if even one dose of medication is missed. The complex dosing schedules as well as the medication side effects make it difficult to assess the effectiveness of treatments aimed at the KS by itself.

Small KS lesions respond very well to radiation treatment. They can also be removed surgically or treated with **cryotherapy**, a technique that uses liquid nitrogen to freeze the lesion. Lesions inside the mouth (on the palate) can be treated with injections of vinblastine. In addition, the patient may be given topical alitretinoin (Panretin gel), which is applied directly to the lesions. Alitretinoin received FDA approval for treating KS in 1999.

Systemic treatments for epidemic KS consist of various combinations of anti-cancer drugs, including vincristine (Oncovin), vinblastine (Velban), **bleomycin** (Blenoxane), **doxorubicin** (Adriamycin), **daunorubicin** (DaunoXome), interferon-alpha (Intron A, Roferon-A), **etoposide** (VePesid), or paclitaxel (Taxol). The effectiveness of systemic treatments ranges from 50% for high-dose therapy with interferon-alpha to 80% for combinations of vincristine, vinblastine, bleomycin, doxorubicin, and etoposide. The drawbacks of systemic treatment include the toxicity of these drugs and their many side effects. Interferon-alpha can be given only to adult patients with relatively intact immune systems and no signs of lymphatic involvement. The side effects of systemic chemotherapy include hair loss (**alopecia**), **nausea and vomiting**, **fatigue**, **diarrhea**, headaches, loss of appetite (**anorexia**), allergic reactions, back pain, abdominal pain, and increased sweating.

As of 2005, the standard for first-line treatment of epidemic KS is one of the FDA-approved anthracyclines such as liposomal doxorubicin (Doxil) or liposomal daunorubicin (DaunoXome), rather than a combination drug regimen. Liposomes are small sacs consisting of an outer layer of fatty substances used to coat an inner core of another medication. In addition to concentrating the drug's effects on the tumor, liposomes moderate the side effects.

In 1997, the FDA approved paclitaxel (Taxol) for epidemic KS resistant to treatment. Paclitaxel is a drug derived from the bark of the Pacific yew tree that prevents the growth of cancer cells by preventing the breakdown of normal cell structures called microtubules. After paclitaxel treatment, cancer cells become so clogged with microtubules that they cannot grow and divide. The drug has serious side effects, most notably suppression of the patient's bone marrow.

Experimental treatments for AIDS-related KS include retinoic acid, which is derived from vitamin A; and other drugs that inhibit the formation of new blood vessels (angiogenesis) in tumors. The reason for inhibiting angiogenesis is that new blood vessels keep a cancer supplied with oxygen and nutrients, which help the cancer grow and spread to other parts of the body. Antiangiogenic agents that have been proposed for treating KS include Fumagillin, SP-PG, and Platelet 4 factor. As of 2005, the effectiveness of these substances in humans is not yet known. Approval by the Food and Drug Administration will require several years after the test results are known.

Prognosis

The prognosis of KS varies depending on its form. Patients with classic KS often survive for many years after diagnosis; death is often caused by another cancer, such as non-Hodgkin's **lymphoma**, rather than the KS itself. The aggressive form of African KS has the poorest prognosis, with a fatality rate of 100% within three years of diagnosis. Patients with immunosuppressive treatment-related KS have variable prognoses; in many cases, however, the KS goes into remission once the immune-suppressing drug is discontinued. The prognosis of patients with epidemic KS also varies, depending on the patient's general level of health. As a rule, patients whose KS has spread to the lungs have the poorest prognosis.

Alternative and complementary therapies

SHARK CARTILAGE. The only alternative treatment for epidemic KS that has been evaluated by the NIH is shark cartilage. Shark cartilage products are widely available in the United States as over-the-counter (OTC) preparations that do not require FDA approval. A 1995 review of alternative therapies found more than 40 brand names of shark cartilage products for sale in the United States to treat arthritis and psoriasis as well as KS. The cartilage can be taken by mouth or by injection.

The use of shark cartilage to treat KS derives from a popular belief that sharks and other cartilaginous fish (skates and rays) do not get cancer. This belief is countered by findings from samples of captured sharks that they do in fact develop various kinds of tumors. There are three explanations of the role of shark cartilage in preventing KS. Some researchers have proposed that it kills cancer cells directly. A second explanation is that cartilage stimulates the human immune system. The third theory, which has more evidence in its favor than the first two, is that the cartilage slows down or prevents angiogenesis. Two complex proteins in shark cartilage, identified as U-995 and SCF2, have been shown to inhibit angiogenesis in laboratory studies. As of December 2000, only three studies using human subjects had been published; the results were inconclusive. The complete results of three other studies using shark cartilage in human subjects have not yet been published in complete form. Preliminary reports of NIH-sponsored **clinical trials** are also not yet available; however, all three studies being currently conducted have received the lowest rating (3iii) for the statistical strength of the study's design.

The side effects of treatment with shark cartilage include mild to moderate **nausea**, **vomiting**, abdominal cramps, constipation, low blood pressure, abnormally high levels of blood calcium (**hypercalcemia**), and general feelings of weakness.

OTHER ALTERNATIVE THERAPIES. Other alternative treatments for KS are aimed almost completely at epidemic KS. Most are based on assumptions that AIDS victims have had their immune systems weakened by such environmental toxins as lead and radioactive materials, or by psychological stress generated by societal disapproval of homosexuality. Naturopaths would add such life-style stresses as the use of tobacco and alcohol, as well as poor sleep patterns and nutritional deficiencies. Homeopaths believe that AIDS is the product of hereditary predispositions to disease called miasms, specifically two miasms related to syphilis and gonorrhea respectively.

Alternative topical treatments for the skin lesions of AIDS-related KS include homeopathic preparations made from periwinkle, **mistletoe**, or phytolacca (poke root). Other alternative skin preparations include a selenium solution made from aloe gels, selenium, and tincture of silica; a mixture of aloe vera and dried kelp (seaweed); and a mixture of aloe vera, tea tree oil, and tincture of St. John's wort. Alternative treatments for KS lesions on the internal organs include a mixture of warm wine and Yunnan Paiyao powder, a Chinese patent medicine made from ginseng; castor oil packs; or a three-to seven-day grape fast repeated every 120 days.

Alternative systemic treatments for AIDS-related KS include:

- Naturopathic remedies: High doses of vitamin C, zinc, echinacea, or goldenseal to improve immune function; or preparations of astragalis, osha root, or licorice to suppress the HIV virus.
- Homeopathic remedies: These include a homeopathic preparation of cyclosporine and another made from a dilution of killed typhoid virus.
- Ozone therapy: There are isolated reports from Europe and the United States of AIDS-related KS going into several months of remission after treatment with ozone given via rectal insufflation.

Alternative treatments aimed at improving the quality of life for KS patients include Reiki, reflexology, meditation, and chromatherapy.

Coping with cancer treatment

Studies of treatment side effects in patients with epidemic KS are complicated by the difficulty of distinguishing between side effects caused by treatment aimed at the HIV retrovirus itself and those caused by treatment for KS. Common problems related to KS treatment include damage to the bone marrow, hair loss, and nerve damage from medications.

Other treatment-related problems include **weight loss** due to poor appetite, and swelling of body tissues due to fluid retention. Patients may be given nutritional counseling, medications to stimulate the appetite, and radiation treatment or diuretics to reduce the level of fluid in the tissues.

Clinical trials

By 2009, there are 21 open and active clinical trials being conducted for treatments for KS, twelve for epidemic KS and one for unspecified KS. Some of these are comparing the relative effectiveness of doxorubicin, daunorubicin, and paclitaxel. Others are studies of other agents, including interleukin-11, interleukin-12, cidofovir, and **filgrastim**. One is a study of the effects of HAART on AIDS-related KS. The National Cancer Institute (NCI) reported that clinical trials of **thalidomide** indicated that the drug has some activity against epidemic KS. Updated information about the content of and patient participation in clinical trials can be obtained at the web site of the National Cancer Institute: http://cancertrials.nci.nih.gov.

Prevention

The only known preventive strategy for reducing one's risk for epidemic KS is abstinence from intercourse or modification of sexual habits. Homosexual or bisexual males can reduce their risk of developing KS by avoiding passive anal intercourse. Women can reduce their risk by avoiding vaginal or anal intercourse with bisexual males.

Kidney transplant patients who are at increased risk of developing KS as a result of taking prednisone or other immunosuppressive drugs should consult their primary physician about possible changes in dosage.

Special concerns

The two special concerns most likely to arise with epidemic KS are social isolation due to the disfigurement caused by KS lesions on the patient's face, and spiritual or psychological concerns related to the tumor's connection to AIDS and homosexuality. There are many local and regional support groups for cancer patients that can help patients deal with concerns about appearance. With regard to religious/spiritual issues, most major Christian and Jewish bodies in the United States and Canada have task forces or working groups dealing with AIDS-related concerns. The National Catholic AIDS Network (NCAN) maintains an information database and web site (http://www.ncan.org) and accepts call-in referrals at (707) 874-3031.

Resources

BOOKS

Beers, Mark H., MD, and Robert Berkow, MD, editors. "Hematology and Oncology." Section 11 In *The Merck Manual of Diagnosis and Therapy*. Whitehouse Station, NJ: Merck Research Laboratories, 2004.

Kubota, Marshall K., MD. "Human Immunodeficiency Virus Infection and Its Complications," In *Conn's Current Therapy*, edited by Robert E. Rakel, MD. Philadelphia: W. B. Saunders Company, 2000.

PERIODICALS

Correspondence: Kaposi's Sarcoma. *New England Journal of Medicine* 343, no. 8 (August 24, 2000).

San Francisco AIDS Foundation. *Bulletin of Experimental Treatments for AIDS*.

ORGANIZATIONS

AIDS Clinical Trials Group (ACTG). c/o William Duncan, PhD, National Institutes of Health. 6003 Executive Boulevard, Room 2A07, Bethesda, MD 20892.

American Cancer Society (ACS). 1599 Clifton Road, NE, Atlanta, GA 30329. (404) 320-3333 or (800) ACS-2345. Fax: (404) 329-7530. Web site: http://www.cancer.org.

National Cancer Institute, Office of Cancer Communications. 31 Center Drive, MSC 2580, Bethesda, MD 20892-2580. (800) 4-CANCER (1-800-422-6237). TTY: (800) 332-8615. Web site: http://www.nci.nih.gov.

NIH National Center for Complementary and Alternative Medicine (NCCAM) Clearinghouse. P. O. Box 8218,

Silver Spring, MD 20907-8218. TTY/TDY: (888) 644-6226. Fax: (301) 495-4957.
San Francisco AIDS Foundation (SFAF). 995 Market Street, #200, San Francisco, CA 94103. (415) 487-3000 or (800) 367-AIDS. Fax: (415) 487-3009. Web site: http://www.sfaf.org.

Rebecca J. Frey, Ph.D.

Ketoconazole *see* **Antifungal therapy**

Ki67

Definition

Ki67 is a molecule that can be easily detected in growing cells in order to gain an understanding of the rate at which the cells within a tumor are growing.

Purpose

Detection of Ki67 is carried out on biopsies, samples of tumor tissue. The goal of this assay is to evaluate an important characteristic of the cells within the tumor, the percentage of tumor cells that are actively dividing and giving rise to more **cancer** cells. The number obtained through this examination is termed the S-phase, growth, or proliferative fraction. This information can play an important part in deciding the best treatment for a cancer patient.

Precautions

This test is performed on tissue or cells that have been removed during the initial surgery or diagnostic procedure used to determine the precise nature of the cancer. It usually does not require any new surgery or blood draw on the patient and, so, does not entail any additional precautions for the patient.

Description

Cancer is a group of diseases characterized by abnormal, or neoplastic, cellular growth in particular tissues. In many instances this growth is abnormal because cells are growing more rapidly than is normal. This unregulated growth is how a tumor is formed. A tumor is more or less a collection of cells that grow more rapidly than the surrounding normal tissue. Most importantly, this difference in growth rate is central to how many cancer drugs, termed cytotoxic agents, work. The ability of these drugs to eliminate cancer cells depends on their ability to kill cells that are actively proliferating, but do less damage to cells that

KEY TERMS

Immunocytochemistry—Method for staining cells or tissues using antibodies so that the location of a target molecule can be determined

Nucleus—The part of the cell containing chromosomes

S phase—The part of the cell division cycle during which the genetic material, DNA, is duplicated

are not actively dividing. This makes it useful to know how actively the cells in tumor are growing compared to the surrounding tissue. The measurement of Ki67 is one of the most common ways to measure the growth fraction of tumor cells. This molecule can be detected in the nucleus of only actively growing cells.

Analysis of Ki67 in tumors is accomplished by a pathologist who examines a piece of the tumor tissue using special techniques. The technique used is termed immunocytochemistry. This involves the preparation of a histologic section, a very thin piece of tumor tissue placed on a glass microscope slide. These kinds of tissue sections are used in the diagnosis of cancer. In the case of Ki67 assays, the section is incubated with antibodies that can react with the Ki67 molecule, and then treated with special reagents that cause a color to appear where antibody has bound. In this way, when the pathologist looks at the section using a microscope the fraction of growing cells, whose nuclei are stained for Ki67, can be determined for the tumor cells and compared with the normal tissue. In some instances, depending on the particular type of cancer, the pathologist might feel it more appropriate to use a different technique to assess the growth fraction for a specific tumor or leukemia.

Preparation, Aftercare, and Risks

Because this test is performed on tissue or cells that had been removed during an initial **biopsy** or other diagnostic procedure, and because no new surgery or sample is required, no additional recommendations regarding preparation, aftercare, or risks are necessary.

Results

The proliferative or growth fraction as determined by Ki67 analysis is interpreted in view of what is normal for the tissue in which the tumor has been found or from which it originated. In the case of certain types of tissue—for example, brain—there is little cellular growth in normal tissue. In other cases,

An extracted cancerous kidney. *(Photo by Robert Riedlinger. Custom Medical Stock Photo. Reproduced by permission.)*

such as breast or the cells that line the colon, cellular growth is a normal part of the function of that tissue. The significance of an increased proliferative fraction is interpreted in light of the experience of the oncologist as well as the knowledge and experience of other clinicians as reported in the medical literature. The Ki67 result, often termed the "Ki67 labeling index," can be used in some cases as a prognostic indicator for some cancers. For example, for **brain tumors**, such as astrocytomas and glioblastomas, a high Ki67 labeling index is one factor that predicts a poor prognosis. For breast tumors, the clinician will consider the proliferative fraction in conjunction with other factors such as patient age, results of receptor assays, and whether or not there is evidence of spread of the disease to lymph nodes or other sites within the body. The value of Ki67 is not as firmly established for other cancers such as bladder or **pituitary tumors**.

Resources

PERIODICALS

Chassevent, A., et al. "S-Phase Fraction and DNA Ploidy in 633 T1T2 Breast Cancers: A Standardized Flow Cytometric Study." *Clinical Cancer Research* 7 (2001): 909-17.

Warren Maltzman, Ph.D.

Kidney cancer

Definition

Kidney **cancer** is a disease in which the cells in certain tissues of the kidney start to grow uncontrollably and form tumors. Renal cell **carcinoma**, sometimes referred to as hypernephroma, occurs in the cells lining the kidneys (epithelial cells). It is the most common type

Background of illustration and to left: a pair of kidneys. One kidney is normal, while the other is cancerous. The foreground of the illustration and in color: a cutaway of the cancerous kidney. *(Custom Medical Stock Photo. Reproduced by permission.)*

of kidney cancer. Eighty-five percent of all kidney tumors are renal cell carcinomas. **Wilms' tumor** is a rapidly developing cancer of the kidney most often found in children under four years of age.

Description

The kidneys are a pair of organs shaped like kidney beans that lie on either side of the spine just above the waist. Inside each kidney are tiny tubes (tubules) that filter and clean the blood, taking out the waste products and making urine. The urine that is made by the kidney passes through a tube called the ureter into the bladder. Urine is held in the bladder until it is discharged from the body. Renal cell carcinoma (RCC) generally develops in the lining of the tubules

KEY TERMS

Biopsy—The surgical removal and microscopic examination of living tissue for diagnostic purposes.

Bone scan—An x-ray study in which patients are given an intravenous injection of a small amount of a radioactive material that travels in the blood. When it reaches the bones, it can be detected by x ray to make a picture of their internal structure.

Chemotherapy—Treatment with anticancer drugs.

Computed tomography (CT) scan—A medical procedure in which a series of x-ray images are made and put together by a computer to form detailed pictures of areas inside the body.

Cryoablation—A technique for removing tissue by destroying it with extreme cold.

Hematuria—Blood in the urine.

Immunotherapy—Treatment of cancer by stimulating the body's immune defense system.

Intravenous pyelogram (IVP)—A procedure in which a dye is injected into a vein in the arm. The dye travels through the body and concentrates in the urine to be discharged. It outlines the kidneys, ureters, and the urinary bladder. An x-ray image is then made and any abnormalities of the urinary tract are revealed.

Magnetic resonance imaging (MRI)—A medical procedure used for diagnostic purposes in which pictures of areas inside the body can be created using a magnet linked to a computer.

Nephrectomy—A medical procedure in which the kidney is surgically removed.

Primary tumor—A cancer's origin or initial growth.

Radiation therapy—Treatment with high-energy radiation from x-ray machines, cobalt, radium, or other sources.

Renal ultrasound—A painless and non-invasive procedure in which sound waves are bounced off the kidneys. These sound waves produce a pattern of echoes that are then used by the computer to create pictures of areas inside the kidney (sonograms).

---

that filter and clean the blood. Cancer that develops in the central portion of the kidney (where the urine is collected and drained into the ureters) is known as **transitional cell carcinoma** of the renal pelvis. Transitional cell cancer is similar to **bladder cancer**. Wilms' tumor is the most common type of childhood kidney cancer and is distinct from kidney cancer in adults.

Background of illustration and to left: a pair of kidneys. One kidney is normal, while the other is cancerous. The foreground of the illustration and in color: a cutaway of the cancerous kidney.

Demographics

Kidney cancer accounts for approximately 2–3% of all cancers. In the United States, kidney cancer is the tenth most common cancer and the incidence has increased by 43% since 1973; the death rate has increased by 16%. According to the American Cancer Society, 57,760 Americans will be diagnosed with kidney cancer in 2009, and 12,980 died from the disease. RCC accounts for 90–95% of malignant neoplasms that originate from the kidney.

Kidney cancer occurs most often in men over the age of 40. The median age of diagnosis is 65. The male:female ratio is about 3:2.

Causes and symptoms

The causes of kidney cancer are unknown, but there are many risk factors associated with kidney cancer. The risk factors listed from greatest to smallest include:

- von Hippel-Lindau disease (>100)
- chronic dialysis (32)
- obesity (3.6)
- tobacco use (2.3)
- first-degree relative with kidney cancer (1.6)
- hypertension (1.4)
- occupational exposure to dry cleaning solvents (1.4)
- diuretics(non-hypertension use) (1.3)
- trichloroethylene exposure (1.0)
- heavy phenacetin use (1.1–6.0)
- polycystic kidney disease (0.8–2.0)
- cadmium exposure (1.0–3.9)
- arsenic exposure (1.6)
- asbestos (1.1–1.8)

The most common symptom of kidney cancer is blood in the urine (hematuria). Other symptoms include painful urination, pain in the lower back or on the sides, abdominal pain, a lump or hard mass that can be felt in the kidney area, unexplained **weight loss**, **fever**, weakness, **fatigue**, and high blood pressure.

Diagnosis

A diagnostic examination for kidney cancer includes taking a thorough medical history and making a complete physical examination in which the doctor will probe (palpate) the abdomen for lumps. Blood tests will be ordered to check for changes in blood chemistry caused by substances released by the tumor. Laboratory tests may show abnormal levels of iron in the blood. Either a low red blood cell count (**anemia**) or a high red blood cell count (erythrocytosis) may accompany kidney cancer. Occasionally, patients will have high calcium levels.

If the doctor suspects kidney cancer, an intravenous pyelogram (also called an IVP or **intravenous urography**) may be ordered. An IVP is an x-ray test in which a dye is injected into a vein in the arm. The dye travels through the body, and when it is concentrated in the urine to be discharged, it outlines the kidneys, ureters, and the urinary bladder. On an x-ray image, the dye will reveal any abnormalities of the urinary tract. The IVP may miss small kidney cancers.

Renal ultrasound is a diagnostic test in which sound waves are used to form an image of the kidneys. Ultrasound is a painless and non-invasive procedure that can be used to detect even very small kidney

tumors. Imaging tests such as **computed tomography** (CT) scans and **magnetic resonance imaging** (MRI) can be used to evaluate the kidneys and the surrounding organs. These tests are used to check whether the tumor has spread outside the kidney to other organs in the abdomen. If the patient complains of **bone pain**, a special x ray called a bone scan may be ordered to rule out spread to the bones. A chest x ray may be taken to rule out spread to the lungs.

A kidney **biopsy** is used to positively confirm the diagnosis of kidney cancer. During this procedure, a small piece of tissue is removed from the tumor and examined under a microscope. The biopsy will give information about the type of tumor, the cells that are involved, and the aggressiveness of the tumor (tumor stage).

Staging, treatment, and prognosis

Staging

Staging guidelines for kidney cancer are as follows (2.5 cm equals approximately 1 in):

- Stage I: Primary tumor is 5 cm or less in greatest dimension and is limited to the kidney, with no lymph node involvement.
- Stage II: Primary tumor is larger than 5 cm in greatest dimension and is limited to the kidney, with no lymph node involvement.
- Stage III: Primary tumor may extend into major veins or invade adrenal glands or perinephric tissues, but not beyond Gerota's fascia. There may be metastasis in a single lymph node.
- Stage IV: Primary tumor invades beyond Gerota's fascia. Metastasis in more than one lymph node. Possible metastasis to distant structures in the body.

Treatment

Each person's treatment is different and depends on several factors. The location, size, and extent of the tumor have to be considered in addition to the patient's age, general health, and medical history. In addation, much has changed in the treatment and management of kidney cancer since the 1980s, including new surgical techniques, new **anticancer drugs**, and the development of effective treatments for advanced disease.

The primary treatment for kidney cancer that has not spread to other parts of the body, which is a Stage I, II, or III tumor, is surgical removal of the diseased kidney (**nephrectomy**). Because most cancers affect only one kidney, the patient can function well with the remaining one. Two types of surgical procedure are used. Radical nephrectomy removes the entire kidney and the surrounding tissue. Sometimes, the lymph nodes surrounding the kidney are also removed. Partial nephrectomy removes only part of the kidney along with the tumor. This procedure is used either when the tumor is very small or when it is not practical to remove the entire kidney. It is not practical to remove a kidney when the patient has only one kidney or when both kidneys have tumors. There is a small (5%) chance of missing some of the cancer. Nephrectomy can also be useful for Stage IV cancers, but alternative surgical procedures such as transarterial angioinfarction may be used.

The rapid development and widespread use of laparoscopic techniques has made it possible for surgeons to remove small tumors while sparing the rest of the kidney. Most tumors removed by **laparoscopy** are 4 cm (1.6 in) in size or smaller. Laparoscopy also allows the surgeon to remove small tumors with **cryoablation** (destroying the tumor by freezing it) rather than cutting.

Radiation therapy, which consists of exposing the cancer cells to high-energy gamma rays from an external source, generally destroys cancer cells with minimal damage to the normal tissue. Side effects are **nausea**, fatigue, and stomach upsets. These symptoms disappear when the treatment is over. In kidney cancer, radiation therapy has been shown to alleviate pain and bleeding, especially when the cancer is inoperable. However, it has not proven to be of much use in destroying the kidney cancer cells. Therefore radiation therapy is not used very often as a treatment for cancer or as a routine adjuvant to nephrectomy. Radiotherapy, however, is used to manage metastatic kidney cancer.

Treatment of kidney cancer with anticancer drugs (**chemotherapy**) has not produced good results. However, new drugs and new combinations of drugs continue to be tested in **clinical trials**. One new drug, semaxanib (SU5416), is reported to have good results in treating patients with kidney cancer. As of 2004, however, semaxanib is still undergoing clinical trials in the United States.

Immunologic therapy (or immunotherapy), a form of treatment in which the body's immune system is harnessed to help fight the cancer, is a new mode of therapy that is being tested for kidney cancer. Clinical trials with substances produced by the immune cells (**aldesleukin** and interferon) have shown some promise in destroying kidney cancer cells. These substances have been approved for use but they can be very toxic and produce severe side effects. The benefits derived from the treatment have to be weighed very carefully against the side effects in each case. Immunotherapy is the most promising systemic therapy for metastatic kidney cancer.

Prognosis

Because kidney cancer is often caught early and sometimes progresses slowly, the chances of a surgical cure are good. It is also one of the few cancers for which there are well-documented cases of spontaneous remission without therapy.

Alternative and complementary therapies

There are several healing philosophies, approaches, and therapies that may be used as supplemental or instead of traditional treatments. All of the items listed may have varying effectiveness in boosting the immune system and/or treating a tumor. The efficacy of each treatment also varies from person to person. None of the treatments, however, have demonstrated safety or effectiveness on a consistent basis. Patients should research such treatments for any potential dangers (laetrile, for example, has caused death due to cyanide poisoning) and notify their physician before taking them.

- 714-X
- antineoplastons
- Cancell
- cartilage (bovine and shark)
- coenzyme Q10
- Gerson Therapy
- Gonzalez Protocol
- Hydrazine sulfate
- immuno-augementative therapy
- Laetrile
- mistletoe

Coping with cancer treatment

Side effects of treatment, as well as nutrition, emotional well-being, and other complications, are all parts of coping with cancer. There are many possible side effects for a cancer treatment that include:

- constipation
- delirium
- fatigue
- fever, chills, sweats
- nausea and vomiting
- mouth sores, dry mouth, bleeding gums
- pruritus (itching)
- sexuality
- sleep disorders

Anxiety, **depression**, loss, post-traumatic stress disorder, **sexuality**, and **substance abuse** are all possible emotional side-effects. Nutrition and eating before, during, and after a treatment can also be of concern. Other complications of coping with cancer include fever and pain.

Clinical trials

As of 2009, the National Cancer Institute (NCI) listed many clinical trials in place across the United States studying new types of radiation therapy and chemotherapy, new drugs and drug combinations, biological therapies, ways of combining various types of treatment for kidney cancer, side effect reduction, and improving quality of life. Immunostimulatory agents and gene-therapy techniques that modify tumor cells, antiangiogenesis compounds, cyclin-dependent kinase inhibitors, and differentiating agents are all being investigated as possible therapies. One may consult http:// clinicaltrials.gov and a doctor for a list of kidney cancer clinical trials.

Prevention

The exact cause of kidney cancer is not known, so it is not possible to prevent all cases. However, because a strong association between kidney cancer and tobacco has been shown, avoiding tobacco is the best way to lower one's risk of developing this cancer. Using care when working with cancer-causing agents such as asbestos and cadmium and eating a well-balanced diet may also help prevent kidney cancer.

See also Renal pelvis tumors; von Hippel-Lindau syndrome.

Resources

BOOKS

Beers, Mark H., MD, and Robert Berkow, MD, editors. "Renal Cell Carcinoma (Hypernephroma; Adenocarcinoma of the Kidney)." In *The Merck Manual of Diagnosis and Therapy*. Whitehouse Station, NJ: Merck Research Laboratories, 2007.

PERIODICALS

Brauch, H., G. Weirich, B. Klein, et al. "VHL Mutations in Renal Cell Cancer: Does Occupational Exposure to Trichloroethylene Make a Difference?" *Toxicology Letters* 151 (June 15, 2004): 301–310.

Dutcher, J.P. "Immunotherapy: Are We Making a Difference?" *Current Opinion in Urology* September 2000: 435–9.

Godley, P.A., and K.I. Ataga. "Renal Cell Carcinoma." *Current Opinion in Oncology* May 2000: 260–4.

Griffiths, T. R., and J. K. Mellon. "Evolving Immunotherapeutic Strategies in Bladder and Renal Cancer." *Postgraduate Medical Journal* 80 (June 2004): 320–327.

Jennens, R. R., M. A. Rosenthal, G. J. Lindeman, and M. Michael. "Complete Radiological and Metabolic Response of Metastatic Renal Cell Carcinoma to SU5416 (Semaxanib) in a Patient with Probable von Hippel-Lindau Syndrome." *Urologic Oncology* 22 (May-June 2004): 193–196.

Lam, J. S., O. Svarts, and A. J. Pantuck. "Changing Concepts in the Surgical Management of Renal Cell Carcinoma." *European Urology* 45 (June 2004): 692–705.

Lotan, Y., D. A. Duchene, J. A. Cadeddu, et al. "Changing Management of Organ-Confined Renal Masses." *Journal of Endourology* 18 (April 2004): 263–268.

Moon, T. D., F. T. Lee, Jr., S. P. Hedican, et al. "Laparoscopic Cryoablation under Sonographic Guidance for the Treatment of Small Renal Tumors." *Journal of Endourology* 18 (June 2004): 436–440.

OTHER

American Cancer Society (ACS). *Cancer Facts & Figures 2004*.http://www.cancer.org/downloads/STT/ CAFF_finalPWSecured.pdf.

ORGANIZATIONS

American Cancer Society (National Headquarters). 1599 Clifton Rd. NE, Atlanta, GA 30329. (800) 227-2345. http://www.cancer.org.

American Foundation for Urologic Disease. E-mail: admin@afud.org.

American Urological Association. 1120 N. Charles St., Baltimore, MD 21201. (410) 727-1100. http://www.auanet. org/patient_info/find_urologist/index.cfm.

Cancer Research Institute (National Headquarters). 681 Fifth Ave., New York, NY 10022. (800) 992-2623. http://www.cancerresearch.org.

Kidney Cancer Association. 1234 Sherman Ave., Suite 203, Evanston, IL 60202-1375. (800) 850-9132. http:// www.kidneycancerassociation.org.

National Cancer Institute (NCI). 9000 Rockville Pike, Building 31, Room 10A16, Bethesda, MD 20892. (800) 422-6237. http://www.nci.nih.gov.

National Kidney Cancer Association. 1234 Sherman Ave., Suite 203, Evanston, IL 60202-1375. (800) 850-9132.

National Kidney Foundation. 30 East 33rd St., New York, NY 10016. (800) 622-9010. http://www.kidney.org.

Lata Cherath, Ph.D.
Laura Ruth, Ph.D.
Rebecca Frey, Ph.D.